Health Promotion

Throughout the Life Span

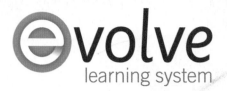

evolve
learning system

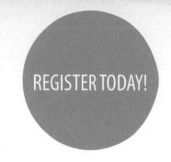

REGISTER TODAY!

To access your Student Resources, visit the web address below:

http://evolve.elsevier.com/Edelman/

Evolve Student Resources for Edelman/Mandle: *Health Promotion Throughout the Life Span,* 7th Edition, offer the following features:

- ### WebLinks

  An exciting resource that lets you link to numerous websites carefully chosen to supplement the content of the textbook

- ### Website Resources

  Resources such as forms, assessment tools, illustrations, and tables that supplement the chapter discussions

- ### Study Questions

  Multiple choice questions to help your review and assess your knowledge of chapter content

- ### Glossary

  Comprehensive list of all Key Terms and their definitions. Search capability allows searching by term, definition, or chapter

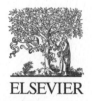

ELSEVIER

Health Promotion

Throughout the Life Span

Carole Lium Edelman, APRN, BC, CMC
Director of Geriatric Care Management
Waveny Care Network
New Canaan, Connecticut

Carol Lynn Mandle, PhD, AP, RN, CNS, FNP
Associate Professor
Connell School of Nursing
Boston College
Chestnut Hill, Massachusetts;
Massachusetts General Hospital
Boston, Massachusetts

Seventh Edition

3251 Riverport Lane
St. Louis, Missouri 63043

HEALTH PROMOTION THROUGHOUT THE LIFE SPAN   ISBN: 978-0-323-05662-5

Notice

Knowledge and best practice in this field are constantly changing. As new research and experience broaden our knowledge, changes in practice, treatment and drug therapy may become necessary or appropriate. Readers are advised to check the most current information provided (i) on procedures featured or (ii) by the manufacturer of each product to be administered, to verify the recommended dose or formula, the method and duration of administration, and contraindications. It is the responsibility of the practitioner, relying on their own experience and knowledge of the patient, to make diagnoses, to determine dosages and the best treatment for each individual patient, and to take all appropriate safety precautions. To the fullest extent of the law, neither the Publisher nor the Authors assumes any liability for any injury and/or damage to persons or property arising out of or related to any use of the material contained in this book.

The Publisher

Previous editions copyrighted 2006, 2002, 1998, 1994, 1990, 1986

Library of Congress Cataloging-in-Publication Data

Health promotion throughout the life span / [edited by] Carole Lium Edelman, Carol Lynn Mandle. -- 7th ed.
   p. ; cm.
   Includes bibliographical references and index.
   ISBN 978-0-323-05662-5 (pbk. : alk. paper) 1. Health promotion. 2. Nursing. 3. Medicine, Preventive.
I. Edelman, Carole. II. Mandle, Carol Lynn.
   [DNLM: 1. Nursing Care. 2. Health Promotion. WY 100 H4343 2010]
RT90.3.H435 2010
613--dc22
                                                                    2009009174

Acquisitions Editor: Nancy O'Brien
Developmental Editor: Carlie Irwin
Publishing Services Manager: Deborah Vogel
Project Manager: Brandilyn Tidwell
Designer: Margaret Reid

Printed in Canada

Last digit is the print number: 9 8 7 6 5 4 3 2 1

Working together to grow
libraries in developing countries

www.elsevier.com | www.bookaid.org | www.sabre.org

ELSEVIER   BOOK AID International   Sabre Foundation

Contributors

Gary P. Austin, PT, PhD
Associate Professor
Director, Orthopaedic Physical Therapy Residency
    Program
Department of Physical Therapy and Human Movement
    Science
Sacred Heart University
Fairfield, Connecticut
Chapter 12, Exercise

Lenny Chiang-Hanisko, RN, PhD
Assistant Professor
College of Nursing
Kent State University
Kent, Ohio
Chapter 11, Nutrition Counseling for Health Promotion

Kevin K. Chui, PT, PhD, GCS
Assistant Professor
Department of Physical Therapy and Human Movement
    Science
Graduate Program in Geriatric Health and Wellness
College of Education and Health Professions
Sacred Heart University
Fairfield, Connecticut
Chapter 12, Exercise

Helene Dixon, CNM, MSN
Instructor, ADN Program
University of Texas at Brownsville and Texas Southmost
    College
Brownsville, Texas
Chapter 23, Middle-Age Adult

Martha Driessnack, PhD, APRN
Assistant Professor
College of Nursing
The University of Iowa
Iowa City, Iowa
*Chapter 15, Overview of Growth and Development
    Framework*
Chapter 18, Toddler
Chapter 21, Adolescent

Carole Lium Edelman, APRN, BC, CMC
Director of Outpatient Programs
Waveny Care Center
New Canaan, Connecticut
*Chapter 1, Health Defined: Objectives for Promotion and
    Prevention*

Pamela J. Grace, APRN, PhD
Associate Professor of Nursing and Ethics
William F. Connell School of Nursing
Boston College
Chestnut Hill, Massachusetts
Chapter 5, Ethical Issues Relevant to Health Promotion

Philip A. Greiner, DNSc, RN
Associate Dean for Public Health & Entrepreneurial
    Initiatives
School of Nursing
Fairfield University
Fairfield, Connecticut
*Chapter 1, Health Defined: Objectives for Promotion and
    Prevention*

Suzy Harrington, DNP, MS, RN, CHES
Executive Director
HIP on Health
Prosper, Texas
Chapter 9, Screening

Susan A. Heady, PhD, RN
Professor and Chair
Nursing Department
Webster University
St. Louis, Missouri
Chapter 10, Health Education

June Andrews Horowitz, PhD, RN, CNS-BC, FAAN
Professor
William F. Connell School of Nursing
Boston College
Chestnut Hill, Massachusetts
Chapter 4, The Therapeutic Relationship
Chapter 13, Stress Management

Debora Elizabeth Kirsch, RN, MS, CNS, PhDc
Clinical Assistant Professor
Director of Undergraduate Studies
College of Nursing
SUNY Upstate Medical University
Syracuse, New York
Chapter 3, Health Policy and the Delivery System

Elizabeth C. Kudzma, DNSc, MPH, RNC
Professor
Division of Nursing
Curry College
Milton, Massachusetts
Chapter 22, Young Adult

Gina C. Lowry, PhD, RN
Lecturer
College of Nursing
University of Kentucky
Lexington, Kentucky
Chapter 14, Holistic Health Strategies

Carol Lynn Mandle, PhD, AP, RN, CNS, FNP
Associate Professor
Connell School of Nursing
Boston College
Chestnut Hill, Massachusetts;
Massachusetts General Hospital
Boston, Massachusetts
Chapter 5, Ethical Issues Relevant to Health Promotion

Anne Rath Rentfro, MSN, RN
Associate Professor
School of Health Sciences
The University of Texas at Brownsville and Texas
  Southmost College
Brownsville, Texas
Chapter 6, Health Promotion and the Individual
Chapter 7, Health Promotion and the Family
Chapter 8, Health Promotion and the Community
Chapter 19, Preschool Child

Susan Scott Ricci, ARNP, MSN, MEd
Nursing Faculty
College of Nursing
University of Central Florida
Orlando, Florida
Chapter 16, The Prenatal Period
Chapter 17, Infant

Ratchneewan Ross, PhD, RN
Assistant Professor
College of Nursing
Kent State University
Kent, Ohio
*Chapter 25, Health Promotion for the Twenty-First
  Century*

Leslie Kennard Scott, PhD, PN-BC, CDE
College of Nursing/Pediatric Endocrinology
University of Kentucky
Lexington, Kentucky
Chapter 20, School-Age Child

Geraldine Valencia-Go, PhD, MA, RN, CS
Associate Professor
School of Nursing
College of New Rochelle
New Rochelle, New York
Chapter 2, Emerging Populations and Health

Meredith Wallace, PhD, APRN
Associate Professor
School of Nursing
Yale University
New Haven, Connecticut
Chapter 24, Older Adult

Ancillary Contributors
Darlene Nebel Cantu, MSN, RNC
Faculty, Department of Nursing Education
San Antonio College;
Director, Baptist Health System
San Antonio, Texas
Study Questions

Bernadette Madara, PhD, BC, APRN
Professor of Nursing
Southern Connecticut State University
New Haven, Connecticut
Test Bank

Kathleen Sparbel, PhD, APRN, BC
Postdoctoral Fellow in Clinical Genetics
College of Nursing
University of Iowa
Iowa City, Iowa
PowerPoint Slides

Concettina Tolomeo, DNP, RN, APRN, FNP-BC, AE-C
Director, Program Development
Yale University School of Medicine
New Haven, Connecticut
Test Bank

Reviewers
Dolores S. Aguilar, APRN, MS
Clinical Instructor
School of Nursing
University of Texas at Arlington
Arlington, Texas

Linda F. Garner, PhD, RN
Professor
Louise Herrington School of Nursing
Baylor University
Dallas, Texas

Judy Hightower, MS, MEd, RN
Clinical Assistant Professor
College of Nursing and Healthcare Innovation
Arizona State University
Phoenix, Arizona

Mariatu Kargbo, MSN, RN, cFNP
Founder and Executive Director
Global Health Nurse Training Services
Alexandria, Virginia

Kathryn Lever, MSN, WHNP-C
Associate Professor
Department of Nursing and Health Sciences
University of Evansville
Evansville, Indiana

Joanne Turka, RN, MSN, CCRN
Critical Care Nurse Educator
Department of Nursing Education and Research
University of Pittsburgh Medical Center
Shadyside Hospital
Pittsburgh, Pennsylvania

Jody K. Williams, MA, EdM, EdD, RN
Assistant Professor of Nursing
Ramapo College of New Jersey
Mahwah, New Jersey

Mary E. Abrums, RN, MN
Marinda Allender, RN, MSN, CPN
Douglas Bloomquist, PhD
Philip Boyle, PhD
Carolyn Spence Cagle, PhD, RNC
Jacqueline Clinton, PhD, RN, FAAN
Joni Cohen, RN, MN
Rebecca Cohen, RN, EdD
Katherine Smith Detherage, PhD, RN, CNAA
Lea Edwards, BSN, MEd
James A. Fain, PhD, RN, RAAN
Gail Park Fast, MN
Marilyn Frank-Stromberg, EdD, NP
Carol Scheel Gavan, EdD, RN
Heather O'Brien Gillespie, MSPT
Qalvy Grainzvolt, BS
Sheila Grossman, PhD, APRN-BC
Krishan Gupta, MD
Lois Hancock, MSN, ARNP
Carolyn Hayes, PhD, RN
Janice Hooper, PhD, RN, CS
James S. Huddleston, MS, PT

Kathleen Huttlinger, PhD, FNP
Dennis T. Jaffe, PhD
Sally Stark Johnson, RN, MSN
Jeanette Lancaster, RN, PhD, FAAN
Margaret K. Macali, MS, RN, CS
William Martimucci, MD
Ann Marie McCarthy, RN
Nancy Curro McCarthy, RN, EdD
Nancy Milio, PhD, FAAN, FAPHA
Katherine E. Murphy, MN, FNP
Lisa Newton, PhD
Jean M. O'Connor, MS, MPH, RNC, FNP
Reverend James O'Donahue, SJ, PhD
Ellen F. Olshansky, DNSc, RNC
Johanne Quinn, PhD, RN
Gurpal K. Sandhu, PhD
Jan Schurman, MN, FNP
Linda Snetselaar, PhD, RD
Arlene Spark, EdD, RD
Marie Truglio-Londrigan, PhD, RN, GNPC
Carol L. Wells-Federman, MS, MEd, RN, CS

Preface

PURPOSE OF THE BOOK

The case for promoting and protecting health, and preventing disease and injury has been established by many accomplishments as we begin the twenty-first century. Americans are taking better care of themselves, and public concern about physical fitness, good nutrition, and avoidance of health hazards such as smoking has gone beyond a fad, and has become ingrained in the American lifestyle.

Encouraging positive health changes has been a major effort of individuals, the government, health professionals, and society in general. In the United States, public and private attempts to improve the health status of individuals and groups traditionally have focused on reducing communicable diseases and health hazards. Now growing concerns exist to improve access to and reduce costs of health services and to improve the overall quality of life for all people. Americans increasingly recognize that the health of each individual is influenced by health-environments of all individuals worldwide.

Indirect health information and informed decision or direct health education and resulting health-promotion, health-protection, and disease- and injury-prevention practices can all lead to the adoption of healthy lifestyles.

Health-promotion advances require a better understanding of health risks, behaviors, and intervention measures. Ten examples of categories are identified as important determinants of health status:

1. Smoking
2. Nutrition
3. Alcohol use
4. Habituating drug use
5. Driving
6. Exercise
7. Sexual practices and contraceptive use
8. Family relationships
9. Risk management
10. Coping and adaptation

Outcome measures designed to assist individual efforts to change and improve behavior in these areas can lead to decreases in morbidity and mortality.

Professionals who undertake health-promotion strategies also need to understand the basics of health protection and disease and injury prevention. Health protection is directed at population groups of all ages and involves adherence to standards, infectious disease control, and governmental regulation and enforcement. The focus of these activities is on reducing exposure to various sources of hazards, including those related to air, water, foods, drugs, motor vehicles, and other physical agents.

Health care providers present individuals, families, and communities with disease- and injury-prevention services, which include immunizations, screenings, health education, and counseling. To implement prevention strategies effectively, it is essential to develop activities targeted to and tailored for all age groups in various settings, including schools, industries, the home, the health care delivery system, and the community.

Throughout the history of the United States, the public health community has assessed the health of Americans. In 1789, the Reverend Edward Wigglesworth developed the first American mortality tables through his study in New England. The *Report of a General Plan for the Promotion of Public and Personal Health* was completed by Lemuel Shattuck in 1880. *Healthy People, The Surgeon General's Report on Health Promotion and Disease Prevention* was first published in 1979, and was followed by *Healthy People 2000: National Health Promotion and Disease Prevention Objectives*, which listed three goals to be achieved by the year 2000:

1. Increase the span of healthy life for Americans.
2. Reduce health disparities among Americans.
3. Achieve access to preventive services for all Americans.

Healthy People 2010 addresses these health problems by establishing goals and objectives for the first decade of the new millennium. The vision for *Healthy People 2010* is "Healthy People in Healthy Communities" because, as nursing has long recognized, the health of each individual is inseparable from the health of families, communities, the nation, and the world. Health is significantly affected by the environments in which each individual lives, works, travels, and plays. Dimensions of the environment are not only physical but also psychosocial and spiritual, including the behaviors, attitudes, and beliefs of each individual. Specific objectives in 28 focus areas support two major goals:

1. Increase quality and years of healthy life.
2. Eliminate health disparities.

The 28 focus areas of *Healthy People 2010* were developed by the lead federal agencies with the most relevant scientific expertise. The development process was informed by a Healthy People Consortium and Alliance of more than 350 national membership organizations and 250 health and environmental agencies. In addition, through a series of regional and national meetings and an interactive website, more than 11,000 public comments on the draft objectives were received.

Healthy People 2020 will reflect these assessments of major risks to health, changing public health priorities, and emerging issues related to our nation's health preparedness and prevention.

Public participation across the country is shaping the development of *Healthy People 2020*, which will be released in two phases. In 2010, *Healthy People 2020* objectives will be released along with guidance for achieving the new ten-year targets (subscribe to the Healthy People listserv for the latest information and to receive email notices of related news, events, and publications at *http://healthypeople.gov/ hp2020*).

These databases continue to provide assessments of health status and risk for evaluations and future planning, not only for health policy makers and health care providers, but for individuals, families, and communities (local, regional, national, and global).

The information in this edition of *Health Promotion Throughout the Life Span* includes these and other data and recommendations for health promotion, health protection, preventive services, and surveillance data systems, including those of the U.S. Preventive Services Task Force (*www. ahrq.gov/clinic/cps*) and the Guide to Community Preventive Services (*www.thecommunityguide.org*).

APPROACH AND ORGANIZATION

This edition presents health data and related theories and skills that are needed to understand and practice when providing care. This book focuses on primary prevention intervention, based on the Leavell and Clark model; its three main components are (1) health promotion, (2) specific health protection, and (3) prevention of specific diseases. Health promotion is the intervention designed to improve health, such as providing adequate nutrition, a healthy environment, and ongoing health education. Specific protection and prevention, such as massive immunizations, periodic examinations, and safety features in the workplace, are the interventions used to protect against illness.

In addition to primary prevention, this book discusses secondary prevention intervention, focusing specifically on screening. Such programs include blood pressure, glaucoma, and diabetes screening and referral (the acute component of secondary prevention is not addressed in this book).

This text is presented in five parts, each forming the basis for the next.

Unit One, *Foundations for Health Promotion*, describes the foundational concepts of promoting and protecting health, and preventing diseases and injuries, including diagnostic, therapeutic, and ethical decision-making based on the nursing emphasis of health patterns as described by Margaret Newman.

Unit Two, *Assessment for Health Promotion*, focuses on individuals, families, and communities and the factors affecting their health. The functional health pattern assessments developed by Gordon serve as the organizing framework for assessing the health of individuals, families, and communities.

Unit Three, *Interventions for Health Promotion*, discusses theories, methodologies, and case studies of nursing interventions, including screening, health education counseling, stress management, and crisis intervention.

Unit Four, *Application of Health Promotion*, also uses Gordon's functional health patterns, emphasizing developmental, cultural, ethnic, and environmental variables in assessing the developing person. The intent is to address the health concerns of all Americans regardless of gender, race, age, or sexual orientation. Although the human development theories discussed are primarily based on the research of male subjects, emerging theories based on female subjects have been included. The hope is to describe human development that more accurately reflects the complexity of human experiences throughout the life span.

Unit Five, *Challenges in the Twenty-First Century*, presents a single chapter that discusses changing population groups and their health needs, and related implications for research and practice in the twenty-first century. Throughout the text, research abstracts have been added to highlight the science of nursing practice and to demonstrate to the reader the relationship among research, practice, and outcomes.

Throughout these units, the evolving health care professions and the changing health care systems, including future challenges and initiatives for health promotion, are described. Emphasis is placed on the current concerns of reducing health care costs while increasing life expectancy and improving the quality of life for all Americans. This promotes the reader's immediate interest in and thoughts about the content of the chapters.

Key Features

- A **full-color design**, including color photos, has been implemented throughout for better accessibility of content and visual enhancement.
- Each chapter starts with a list of **objectives** to help focus the reader and emphasize the content the reader should acquire through reading the book. **Key Terms** are listed at the front to acquaint readers with the important terminology of the chapter.
- Each chapter's narrative begins with **Think About It**, the presentation of a clinical issue or scenario that relates to the topic of the chapter, followed by critical thinking questions. This promotes the reader's immediate interest in and thought about the chapter.
- **Research Highlights** boxes provide brief synopses on current health promotion research studies that demonstrate the links between research, theory, and practice.
- **Multicultural Awareness** boxes offer cultural perspectives on various aspects of health promotion.
- **Hot Topics** explores current issues, controversies, and ethical dilemmas with respect to health promotion, providing an opportunity for critical analysis of care issues.

- **Health Teaching** boxes present special tips and guidelines to use when educating people about health-promotion activities.
- The **Case Study** highlights a real-life clinical situation relevant to the chapter topic.
- The **Care Plan** relates to the Case Study with the standardized sections of *Defining Characteristics, Related Factors, Expected Outcomes,* and *Interventions,* and details nursing diagnoses relevant to health-promotion activities and the related interventions.
- **Innovative Practice** boxes highlight inventive and resourceful projects, programs, and research studies that draw upon new ways of implementing health promotion.
- *Healthy People 2010* boxes present a list of selected objectives that are relevant to the chapter's topic. *Healthy People 2020* objectives were available in 2010.
- **Website Resources** include expanded chapter resources, such as assessment tools, developmental charts, and immunization schedules.
- **Study Questions** are located on the book's website to offer additional review and self-study practice.

New Features

- **Updated photos and figures** throughout the book
- **Midcourse Review objectives** of *Healthy People 2010* (*http://healthypeople.gov*) and a link to new listings of the developing data and goals for 2020 on the book's Evolve website
- Specific emphasis on growth and development throughout the life span
- **Expanded content in Chapter 3** on financing health care, global health, historical perspectives, concierge medical practices, and the hospitalist movement
- A new **Case Study and Care Plan on Genetic Screening Programs** in Chapter 5
- Updated information on the **Dietary Guidelines for Americans and MyPyramid** in Chapter 11
- **Completely revised Chapter 25, Health Promotion in the Twenty-First Century** now includes up-to-date information on malnutrition in developing and underdeveloped nations, emerging infections, global violence, and bioterrorism

evolve ONLINE TEACHING/LEARNING PACKAGE

The expanded website for this book provides materials for both students and faculty, and is accessible at **http://evolve.elsevier.com/Edelman/**.

For Students

Website Resources: Resources that supplement the chapter discussion
WebLinks: Organized by chapter, these are direct links to numerous websites related to the chapter content
Study Questions: Multiple choice and in NCLEX-format
Glossary: Comprehensive list of all Key Terms and their definitions. Search capability allows searching by term, definition, or chapter

For Instructors

Chapter Outlines
Learning Objectives
Research Evaluation and Critique article
Image Collection, with all images from the book
Lecture Slides, in PowerPoint
Test Bank, 700 questions in NCLEX format, including the new innovative item format

The current trend to emphasize the developing health of people mandates that health care professionals understand the many issues that surround individuals, families, and communities in social, work, and family settings, including the biological, inherited, cognitive, psychological, environmental, and sociocultural factors that can put their health at risk. Most important is that they develop interventions to promote health by understanding the diverse roles these factors play in the person's beliefs and health practices, particularly in the areas of disease and injury prevention, protection, and health promotion. Achieving such effectiveness requires collaboration with other health care providers and the integration of practice and policy while developing interventions and considering the ethical issues within individual, family, and community responsibilities for health.

Carole Lium Edelman
Carol Lynn Mandle

Acknowledgments

We had the good fortune of receiving much assistance and support from many friends, relatives, and associates. Our colleagues read chapters, gave valuable advice and criticism, helped clarify concepts, and provided case examples.

We also acknowledge the contributions of all the authors. In developing this text, they gave the project their total commitment and support. Their professional competence aided greatly in the development of the final draft of the manuscript. Special thanks goes to Josheko Coleman for assistance with typing the manuscript.

The editors worked and learned from each other during the planning and development of this book; throughout the entire process, close contact prevailed. They seemed to become the book and, in turn, the book now reflects them.

Both family and friends helped in the work and fulfilled the many responsibilities requested of them.

I am fortunate to have faith in the Lord, who gives courage and strength to face life's difficulties in a positive manner. My children, John and Megan Gillespie, Tom and Heather Gillespie, and Deirdre O'Brien, and my grandchildren, Ryan, Caroline, Meredith, and Colleen bring joy to me as an author and editor. Their patience and love are truly appreciated. Rachel Pennacchia provides much encouragement and support. Fredric Edelman gives continued joy and happiness in our marriage.

Carole Lium Edelman

In the continued development of health, I acknowledge our faith in God and the joy of friends; the love of marriage and family with Robert, Elizabeth, Jonathan, Stephanie, and David; the commitments of nurses to social justice in the care of all people; and the knowledge we are continually becoming . . .

Carol Lynn Mandle

*To our wonderful families, friends, students, and colleagues—
that they promote health in themselves and others.*

Contents

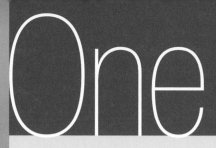

One

Unit

Foundations for Health Promotion

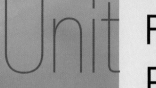

Chapter 1

Philip A. Greiner
Carole Lium Edelman

Health Defined: Objectives for Promotion and Prevention

objectives

After completing this chapter, the reader will be able to:

- Analyze concepts and models of *health* as it has been used historically and as they are used in this textbook.
- Evaluate the consistency of *Healthy People 2010* goals with various concepts of health.
- Analyze the progress made in this nation from the original *Healthy People* document to the foci in *Healthy People 2010* and the developing *Healthy People 2020*.
- Differentiate between health, illness, disease, disability, and premature death.
- Compare the three levels of prevention (primary, secondary, and tertiary) with the levels of service provision available across the lifespan.
- Critique the role of research and the nurse's role in the research process for the promotion of health for individuals and populations.

key terms

Adaptive model of health	Eudaimonistic	Qualitative studies
Applied research	Eudaimonistic model of health	Quality of life
Asset planning	Evidence-based practice	Quantitative studies
Clinical model of health	Functional health	Racism
Community-based care	Health	Role performance model of health
Cultural competence	Health disparities	
Disease	Health promotion	Well-being
Ecological model of health	*Healthy People 2010*	Wellness
Empathy	High-level wellness	Wellness-illness continuum
Epidemiology	Illness	
Ethnocentrism	Levels of prevention	

website materials

evolve These materials are located on the book's website at *http://evolve.elsevier.com/Edelman/*.
- WebLinks
- Study Questions
- Glossary
- Website Resources
  1A: Twenty-One Competencies for the Twenty-First Century

THINK About It

Use of Complementary and Alternative Therapies

One of the biggest challenges to health care providers is the blending of Western medicine and health practices with the health practices from other cultures and ethnic groups. The federal government formed the National Center for Complementary and Alternative Medicine (NCCAM) [http://nccam.nih.gov/] to conduct and support basic and applied research and training and to disseminate information on complementary and alternative medicine to practitioners and the public. As demographics of the United States shift, more people use a combination of therapies in self-care and for the treatment of specific illnesses.

1. What questions should the student ask to obtain information from people about their use of nontraditional therapies?

2. What information should the student know about the benefits or drawbacks of using complementary therapies, such as acupuncture, spiritual healing, herbal remedies, or chiropractic?

3. What resources should the student trust for information on the efficacy and use of herbal remedies relative to prescription medications?

4. Which ideas of health would be most compatible with the use of alternative therapies?

5. How can alternative therapies be integrated into *Healthy People 2020* objectives, given that the emphasis of these objectives is the use of available community resources and the development of partnerships?

Health is a core concept in society. This concept is modified with qualifiers such as *excellent, good, fair,* or *poor,* based on a variety of factors. These factors may include age, gender, race or ethnic heritage, comparison group, current health or physical condition, past conditions, social or economic situation, or the demands of various roles in society. In addition, there is growing recognition that larger societal and environmental concerns determine health outcomes. This chapter will discuss health as a concept and related concepts such as wellness, illness, disease, disability, and functioning. These concepts are frequently embedded in theories, such as theories of health behavior (Pender et al., 2006) or health planning (Issel, 2004). Some motivating factors behind the move to disease prevention and health promotion in society will be examined with an introduction to *Healthy People 2010,* the federal government's health objectives for the nation. The implementation of these concepts as nursing actions will also be addressed from ideal and pragmatic standpoints. Research supporting these concepts and recommendations for further research will be presented.

Nurses understand the pivotal role they play in promoting health and preventing disease, the important role of research in the knowledge of what is "healthy", and the central role of **epidemiology** (the study of health and disease in society) and public health theories in the everyday practice of nursing.

EXPLORING CONCEPTS OF HEALTH

Newman (2003) states that definitions of health in the nursing literature can be classified broadly within two major paradigms. The first paradigm is the **wellness-illness continuum**, a dichotomized portrayal of health and illness ranging from high-level wellness at the positive end to depletion of health at the negative end. **High-level wellness** is further conceptualized as a sense of **well-being**, life satisfaction, and **quality of life**. Movement toward the negative end of the continuum includes adaptation to disease and disability through various levels of functional ability.

The wellness-illness conceptualization was the focus of early research and is consistent with some of the categories Smith (1983) identified in her philosophical analysis of health. Research based on this paradigm conforms primarily to scientific methods that seek to control contextual effects, provide the basis for causal explanations, and predict future outcomes.

The second paradigm characterizes health as a perspective developmental phenomenon of unitary patterning of the person-environment. The developmental perspective of health has been present in the nursing literature since 1970, but it was not identified clearly with health until the late 1970s and early 1980s. It has been conceptualized as expanding consciousness, pattern or meaning recognition, personal transformation, and, tentatively, self-actualization. This shift toward a developmental perspective has had clear implications for the way in which health is conceptualized (Newman, 2003). Although not endorsing the developmental perspective to the extent of Rogers (1970) and Reed (1983), Pender et al. (2006), Allen & Warner (2002), and Grzywacz & Fuqua (2000) state that health is an outcome of ongoing patterns of person and environment interaction throughout the lifespan. Research within this paradigm seeks to address the dynamic whole of the health experience through behavioral and social mechanisms over time. Health can be better understood if each person is seen as a part of a complex, interconnected, biological, and social system. A more recent and comprehensive developmental approach is the **ecological model of health** (IOM, 2003), which is useful for promoting health at individual, family, community, and societal levels. In this way, the ecological model of health is more compatible with Smith's descriptions of health as adaptation and eudemonia (self-actualization). Each of these ideas will be examined in more detail throughout this chapter.

People involved in health promotion should consider the meaning of health for themselves and for others. Recognizing differences in the meaning of health can clarify outcomes and expectations in health promotion and enhance the quality of health care. Because health is used to describe a number of entities, including a philosophy of care (health promotion and health maintenance), a system (health care delivery system), practices (evidence-based health practices), behaviors (personal health behaviors), costs (health care costs), and insurance (uninsured health care), the reason that confusion continues regarding the use of the term "health" becomes clear. People's use of the term "health", and its incorporation into these various entities, has also changed over time.

Americans born before 1940 have experienced the greatest changes in how health is defined. Because infectious diseases claimed the lives of many children and young adults at that time, health was viewed as the absence of disease. The physician in independent practice was the primary provider of health care services, with services provided in the private office. The federal government was just establishing its role in working with states to address public health and welfare issues (Barr et al., 2003).

As the national economy expanded during and after World War II in the 1940s and 1950s, the idea of role performance became a focus in industrial research and entered the health care lexicon. Health became linked to a person's ability to fulfill a role in society. Increasingly, the physician was asked to complete physical examination forms for school, work, military, and insurance purposes as physician practice became linked more directly to hospital-based services. The federal government expanded its role through funding for hospital expansion and establishment of a new Department of Health, Education, and Welfare (DHEW), currently the Department of Health and Human Services (DHHS) (Barr et al., 2003). It was recognized that a person might recover from a disease yet be unable able to fulfill family or work roles because of residual changes from the illness episode. The work or school environment was viewed as a possible contributor to health or illness.

From the 1960s to the present, there have been incredible changes in the health care delivery system as federal and state governments have attempted to control spending and health care costs have escalated (Barr et al., 2003). Primary care providers, including nurse practitioners and other advanced practice nurses, now attempt to involve individuals and their families in the delivery of care, and teaching individuals about individual responsibilities and lifestyle choices has become an important part of their job. Health care has become an interdisciplinary endeavor even as managed care companies limit the health promotion options available under insurance plans. During this time, the idea of adaptation had an important influence on the way Americans view health. Increasingly health became linked to individuals' reactions to the environment rather than being viewed as a fixed state. Adaptation fit well with the self-help movement during the 1970s and with the progressive growth in knowledge from research about disease prevention and health promotion at the individual level.

More recently, emphasis is being placed on the quality of a person's life as a component of health (USDHHS, 2000). Research on self-rated health (Cano et al., 2003; Idler & Benyamini, 1997) and self-rated function (Greiner et al., 1999) indicates that there are multiple factors contributing to a person's perception of his or her health, sometimes referred to as **functional health** or *health-related quality of life* (Andresen et al., 2003; Gordon, 2006).

Models of Health

Throughout history, society has entertained a variety of concepts of health (David, 2000). Smith (1983) describes four distinct models of health in her classic work:

Clinical Model

In the clinical model health is defined by the absence, and illness by the conspicuous presence, of signs and symptoms of disease. People who use this model may not seek preventive health services or they may wait until they are very ill to seek care. The clinical model is the conventional model of the discipline of medicine.

Role Performance Model

The **role performance model of health** defines health in terms of individuals' ability to perform social roles. Role performance includes work, family, and social roles, with performance based on societal expectations. Illness would be the failure to perform roles at the level of others in society. This model is the basis for occupational health evaluations, school physical examinations, and physician-excused absences. The idea of the "sick role," which excuses people from performing their social functions, is a vital component of the role performance model. It is argued that the sick role is still relevant in health care today (Shilling, 2002).

Adaptive Model

In the **adaptive model of health,** people's ability to adjust positively to social, mental, and physiological change is the measure of their health. Illness occurs when the person fails to adapt or becomes maladaptive to these changes. As the concept of adaptation has entered other aspects of American culture, this model of health has become more accepted. For example, spirituality can be useful in adapting to a decreased level of functioning in older adults (Haley et al., 2001).

Eudaimonistic Model

In the eudaimonistic model exuberant well-being indicates optimal health. This model emphasizes the interactions between physical, social, psychological, and spiritual aspects of life and the environment that contribute to goal attainment and create meaning. Illness is reflected by a denervation or languishing, a lack of involvement with life. Although these ideas may appear to be new when compared with the **clinical model of health**, aspects of the eudaimonistic model predate the clinical model of health. This model is also more congruent with integrative modes of therapy (NIH/NCCAM, 2007), which are used increasingly by people of all ages in the United States and the world. In this eudaimonistic model, a person dying of cancer may still be healthy if she is finding meaning in her life at this stage of development.

These ideas of health provide a basis for how people view health and disease and how they view the role of nurses, physicians, and other health care providers. For example, in the clinical model of health, a person may expect to see a health care provider only when there are obvious signs of illness. Personal responsibility for health may not be a motivating factor for this individual because the provider is responsible for dealing with the health problem and returning the person to health. Therefore attempts to teach health-promoting activities may not be effective with this person. On the other hand, those who adopt a **eudaimonistic model of health** may find that practitioners working under a clinical model do not address their more comprehensive health needs. They may instead seek out a practitioner of alternative medicine or the council of a priest, rabbi, or minister to complement the services of the more traditional health provider.

Wellness-Illness Continuum

The wellness-illness continuum, as stated earlier, is a dichotomous depiction of the relationship between the concepts of health and illness. In this paradigm, **wellness** is a positive state in which incremental increases in health can be made beyond the midpoint (Figure 1-1). These increases involve improved physical and mental health states. The opposite end of the continuum is illness, with the possibility of incremental decreases in health beyond the midpoint. This depiction of the relationship of wellness and illness fits well with the clinical model of health.

High-Level Wellness

From a dichotomous representation of health and illness as opposites, Dunn (1961) developed a health-illness continuum that assessed a person not only in terms of his or her relative health compared with that of others but also in terms of the favorability of the person's environment for health and wellness (see Figure 1-1). Adding this second dimension to the health-illness continuum created a matrix in which a favorable environment allows high-level wellness to occur and an unfavorable environment allows low-level wellness to exist.

With this addition, it became possible to combine the clinical model of health with models based on social and environmental parameters. The concept demonstrates that a person can have a terminal disease and be emotionally prepared for death, while acting as a support for other people and achieving high-level wellness. High-level wellness involves progression toward a higher level of functioning, an open-ended and ever-expanding future with its challenge of fuller potential and the integration of the whole

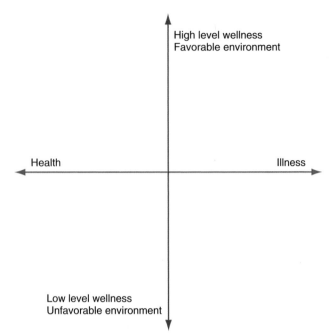

Figure 1-1   Wellness-illness continuum with high-level wellness added. Moving from the center to the right demonstrates movement toward illness. Moving from the center to the left demonstrates movement toward health. Moving above the line demonstrates movement toward increasing wellness. Moving below the line demonstrates movement toward decreasing wellness. (Adapted from U.S. Department of Health and Human Services, Public Health Service, 1982.)

being (Ardell, 2007). This definition of high-level wellness contains ideas similar to those in the eudaimonistic model of health. Additionally, high-level wellness emphasizes the interrelationship between the environment and the ability to achieve health on both a personal and a societal level.

Health Ecology

An evolving view of health recognizes the interconnection between people and their physical and social environments. Newman (2003) expressed this interconnection within a developmental framework, and the work of Gordon (2006) applies this interconnection to functional health patterns as presented in subsequent chapters. Health from an ecological perspective is multidimensional, extending from the individual into the surrounding community, and including the context within which the person functions. It incorporates a systems approach within which the actions of one portion of the system affect the functioning of the system as a whole (IOM, 2003). This view of health expands on high-level wellness by recognizing that there are social and environmental factors that can enhance or limit health and healthy behaviors. For example, most people can benefit from physical activity such as walking, and people are more likely to walk in areas where there are sidewalks or walking paths and where they feel safe. Nurses can encourage people to walk, but may also need to advocate for safe areas for people to walk and work with others to plan for people-friendly community development.

Functioning

One of the defining characteristics of life is the ability to function. Functional health can be characterized as being present or absent, high level or low level, and influenced by neighborhood and society. Functioning is integral to health. There are physical, mental, and social levels of function, and these are reflected in terms of performance and social expectations. Function can also be viewed from an ecological perspective, as in the example of walking used previously. Loss of function may be a sign or symptom of a disease. For example, sudden loss of the ability to move an arm or leg may indicate a stroke. The inability to leave the house may indicate overwhelming fear. In both cases, the loss of function is a sign of disease, a state of ill health. Loss of function is a good indicator that the person may need nursing intervention. Research in older adults indicates that decline in physical function may predict future loss of physical function and death (Greiner et al., 1996).

HEALTH

Health, as defined in this text, is a state of physical, mental, spiritual, and social functioning that realizes a person's potential and is experienced within a developmental context. While health is, in part, an individual's responsibility, health also requires collective action to ensure a society and an environment in which people can act responsibly to support health. The culture and beliefs of people can also influence health action. This definition is consistent with the World Health Organization (WHO) definition of health as the state of complete physical, mental, and social well-being and not merely the absence of disease and infirmity (2004), but moves beyond this definition to encompass spiritual, developmental, and environmental aspects over time. This broader definition is applicable across the lifespan, as well as in situations where illness may be a chronic state. For example, in this broader definition of health, a person with diabetes may be considered healthy if she is able to adapt to her illness and live a meaningful, spiritually satisfying life.

ILLNESS, DISEASE, AND HEALTH

It is easy to think of health or wellness as the lack of disease and to consider illness and disease as interchangeable terms. However, health and disease are not simply antonyms and disease and illness are not synonyms. Disease literally means "without ease." **Disease** may be defined as the failure of a person's adaptive mechanisms to counteract stimuli and stresses adequately, resulting in functional or structural disturbances. This definition is an ecological concept of disease, which uses multiple factors to determine the cause of disease rather than describing a single cause. This multifactorial approach increases the chances of discovering multiple points of intervention to improve health.

Illness is made up of the subjective experience of the individual and the physical manifestation of disease (Hollingsworth & Didelot, 2005). Both are social constructs in which people are in an imbalanced, unsustainable relationship with their environment and are failing in their ability to survive and create a higher quality of life. Illness can be described as a response characterized by a mismatch between a person's needs and the resources available to meet those needs. Additionally, illness signals to individuals and populations that the present balance is not working. Within this definition, illness has social, psychological, spiritual, and social components. A person can have a disease without feeling ill (e.g., asymptomatic hypertension). A person can also feel ill without having a diagnosable disease (stress). Our understanding of disease and illness within society, overlaid with our understanding of the natural history of each disease, creates a basis for promoting health.

PLANNING FOR HEALTH

Public health has always had the prevention of disease in society as its focus. However, over the past 30 years, the promotion of health has moved to the forefront within public health and has become a driving force in health care.

A key milestone in promoting health was the advent of *Healthy People* (U.S. Department of Health, Education, and Welfare [USDHEW], Public Health Service, 1979), the first Surgeon General's report on health promotion and disease prevention issued in the later years of President Carter's administration. This document identified five national health goals addressing the reduction of death in adults and children and the reduction of sick days in older adults.

1. To continue to improve infant health, and, by 1990, to reduce infant mortality by at least 35 percent, to fewer than 9 deaths per 1000 live births
2. To improve child health, foster optimal childhood development, and, by 1990, reduce deaths among children ages 1 to 14 years by at least 20 percent, to fewer than 34 per 100,000
3. To improve the health and health habits of adolescents and young adults, and, by 1990, to reduce deaths among people ages 15 to 24 by at least 20 percent, to fewer than 93 per 100,000
4. To improve the health of adults, and, by 1990, to reduce deaths among people ages 25 to 64 by at least 25 percent, to fewer than 400 per 100,000
5. To improve the health and quality of life for older adults, and, by 1990, to reduce the average annual number of days of restricted activity due to acute and chronic conditions by 20 percent, to fewer than 30 days per year for people 65 and older

Further, the document identified three causes of the major health issues in the United States as careless habits, pollution of the environment, and permitting harmful social conditions (e.g., hunger, poverty, and ignorance) to persist that destroy health, especially for infants and children.

Healthy People was a call to action and an attempt to set health goals for the United States for the next 10 years by issuing 226 health objectives. Unfortunately, a change in political leadership, a lack of political and social willpower, and the spiraling costs of hospital-based health care caused this document to be placed on the back burner for seven years. The need to report on progress toward the national objectives led a larger, renewed effort in the form of *The 1990 Health Objectives for the Nation: A Midcourse Review* (USDHHS, Public Health Service, 1986). This midcourse review noted that, although many goals were achievable, the unachieved goals were hindered by current health status, limited progress on risk reduction, difficulties in data collection, and a lack of public awareness.

Healthy People 2000 (USDHHS, Public Health Service, 1990) and its *Midcourse Review and 1995 Revisions* (USDHHS, Public Health Service, 1996) were landmark documents in that a consortium of people representing national organizations worked with U.S. Public Health Service officials to create a more global approach to health. Additionally, a management-by-objectives approach was used to address each problem area. These two documents became the blueprints for each state as funding for federal programs became linked to meeting these national health objectives. As the objectives became more widely implemented, methods for collecting data became formalized and the data flowed back into the system to form the revisions set in 1995. The core of these health objectives remained: that is, prevention of illness and disease was the foundation for health. *Healthy People 2000* set out three broad goals:

1. Increase the span of healthy life.
2. Reduce **health disparities**.
3. Create access to preventive services for all.

Additionally, the work included 22 specific areas for achievement, with objectives in each area based on age, health disparities, and health needs. By 1995, progress was made on 70% of these objectives. However, on 30% of the objectives, movement on goals was either in the wrong direction, had experienced no change, or could not be determined because the data were insufficient.

HEALTHY PEOPLE 2010

Healthy People 2010 (USDHHS, Public Health Service, 2000), the latest of the *Healthy People* documents, sets out 2 overarching goals, with 28 specific areas for health improvement and 467 objectives.

Healthy People 2010 Goals

The two main goals of *Healthy People 2010* are to:

1. Increase quality and years of healthy life.
2. Eliminate health disparities.

Each goal is important. The first goal addresses the issues of longevity and quality of life. Increasing the years of healthy life addresses the concern that people are living longer, but frequently with numerous chronic health problems that interfere with the quality of their lives. However, quality of life is also an issue for people who are unable to achieve a long life. Combining these two ideas places an emphasis on both longevity and quality of life as areas that need

---

Healthy People 2010

Selected National Health Promotion and Disease Prevention Objectives for Nutrition and Overweight

- 19-1. Increase the proportion of adults who are at a healthy weight.
- 19-2. Reduce the proportion of adults who are obese.
- 19-3. Reduce the proportion of children and adolescents who are overweight or obese.
- 19-5. Increase the proportion of persons aged 2 years and older who consume at least two daily servings of fruit.
- 19-6. Increase the proportion of persons aged 2 years and older who consume at least three daily servings of vegetables, with at least one third being dark green or deep yellow vegetables.
- 19-7. Increase the proportion of persons aged 2 years and older who consume at least six daily servings of grain products, with at least three being whole grains.
- 19-8. Increase the proportion of persons aged 2 years and older who consume less than 10 percent of calories from saturated fat.
- 19-9. Increase the proportion of persons aged 2 years and older who consume no more than 30 percent of calories from fat.
- 19-10. Increase the proportion of persons aged 2 years and older who consume 2400 mg or less of sodium daily.

From U.S. Department of Health and Human Services, Public Health Service. (2000). *Healthy people 2010* (conference edition, in two volumes). U.S. Department of Health and Human Services. Washington, DC: U.S. Government Printing Office.

improvement. The second goal, eliminating health disparities, addresses the continuing problems of access to care; differences in treatment based on race, gender, ability to pay; and related issues such as urban versus rural health, insurance coverage, Medicare and Medicaid reimbursement for care, and satisfaction with service delivery.

Together, these two goals set out the territory in which health promotion and disease prevention efforts take place. Research in a variety of areas has clearly indicated that health disparities are directly and indirectly linked to longevity and quality of life issues. For example, it is known that Black men and women live fewer years than do White men and women. Recent research from the Agency for Health Care Research and Quality demonstrates that Black men and women are also provided with less invasive and less expensive interventions for cardiac disease than are White men and women (Canto et al., 2000). By choosing not to offer reperfusion therapy to one racial group when it is warranted and to offer the same therapy to another group contributes to the racial disparity in health and health care in this country and to the increased mortality of Blacks as compared with Whites (see Multicultural Awareness box).

MULTICULTURAL AWARENESS

Influence of Personal Cultural Values on Health Care Delivery

Culture influences every aspect of human life, including beliefs, values, and customs regarding health care. As health care providers, nurses need to be aware of their beliefs, values, and customs and how these ideas translate into behavior. It is easy to assume that an individual's own perspective is correct and shared by others. This is especially true when working with other health care providers who share the same culture. This concept is referred to as **ethnocentrism** and can lead to a devaluing of the beliefs, values, and customs of others, known as **racism**. Although it is impossible for any person to ignore the cultural influences on their lives, nurses and other health care providers have a special obligation to be aware of their own cultural biases and to focus more on the cultural influences in the lives of their clients through the development of **cultural competence**. This ability to view other persons' situations from their perspective is known as **empathy**. Multicultural health issues will continue to challenge providers to lifelong learning about the persons for whom they provide care as the racial and ethnic mix in society changes.

Box 1-1   The 28 Focus Areas in *Healthy People 2010*

- Access to quality health services
- Arthritis, osteoporosis, and chronic back conditions
- Cancer
- Chronic kidney disease
- Diabetes
- Disability and secondary conditions
- Educational and community-based programs
- Environmental health
- Family planning
- Food safety
- Health communication
- Heart disease and stroke
- Human immunodeficiency virus
- Immunization and infectious diseases
- Injury and violence prevention
- Maternal, infant, and child health
- Medical product safety
- Mental health and mental disorders
- Nutrition and overweight
- Occupational safety and health
- Oral health
- Physical activity and fitness
- Public health infrastructure
- Respiratory diseases
- Sexually transmitted diseases
- Substance abuse
- Tobacco use
- Vision and hearing

From U.S. Department of Health and Human Services, Public Health Service. (2000). *Healthy people 2010* (conference edition, in two volumes). U.S. Department of Health and Human Services. Washington, DC: U.S. Government Printing Office. *www.healthypeople.gov*.

The 2006 Midcourse Review provides updated information on each of these topic areas, including changes in subobjective wording and outcome measures for the 2010 evaluation. Go to *www.healthypeople.gov/Data/midcourse/* for further information.

The *Healthy People 2010* focus areas and objectives are the road map for this territory and a guide for health care research, practice, education, policy, and communications. They should allow the health care community to measure progress on the broader goals.

The detailed objectives can be found on the Internet at *www.healthypeople.gov*. The 28 specific focus areas are listed alphabetically in Box 1-1. A quick look through these focus areas indicates of the scope of the *Healthy People 2010* areas compared with earlier *Healthy People* documents. These focus areas span age categories from conception to death and incorporate prevention, access, treatment, and follow-up at the individual, family, provider, work site, and community levels. *Healthy People 2010* is centered on 10 leading health indicators that "reflect the major public health concerns in the United States and were chosen based on their ability to motivate action, the availability of data to measure their progress, and their relevance as broad public health issues" (USDHHS, Public Health Service, 2000, p. 11) (Box 1-2). One example is used here for illustration of the scope of this project.

Objective 22-2. Increase the proportion of adults who engage regularly, preferably daily, in moderate physical activity for at least 30 minutes per day. This objective directly addresses the first two leading health indicators: physical activity and weight (obesity). Arguably, other indicators such as tobacco and substance abuse and mental health are indirectly related to this objective. A person who smokes or uses drugs regularly is limited in the ability to meet this objective. Nevertheless, physical activity can contribute to positive mental health through stress reduction and physical

fitness. Access to health care to obtain a complete physical examination before starting to exercise and the quality of the work or neighborhood environment available for exercise can contribute to success or failure of this objective. This objective is related to other objectives such as nutrition and control of high blood pressure.

Additionally, current knowledge about physical activity and specific populations was considered when creating the *Healthy People 2010* objectives. Women, low-income populations, Black and Hispanic peoples, people with disabilities, and those over the age of 75 exercise less than do White men with moderate-to-high incomes. These health disparities can influence the number of people in these groups who develop high cholesterol or high blood pressure, which further increases their risk of heart disease and stroke. Although this objective addresses adults, other objectives address the need for beginning exercise activities at an early age and encouraging young adults to be actively engaged in exercise. How might this objective be adjusted to the needs of an older adult population?

| Box **1-2** | The 10 Leading Health Indicators in *Healthy People 2010* (and the Specific Objectives and Subobjectives Used to Track Their Progress) |

PHYSICAL ACTIVITY:
Objective 22-2
Increase the proportion of adults who engage in moderate physical activity for at least 30 minutes per day 5 or more days per week or vigorous physical activity for at least 20 minutes per day 3 or more days per week.

Objective 22-7
Increase the proportion of adolescents who engage in vigorous physical activity that promotes cardiorespiratory fitness 3 or more days per week for 20 or more minutes per occasion.

OVERWEIGHT AND OBESITY:
Objective 19-2
Reduce the proportion of adults who are obese.

Objective 19-3c
Reduce the proportion of children and adolescents aged 6 to 19 who are overweight or obese.

TOBACCO USE:
Objective 27-1a
Reduce tobacco use by adults—cigarette smoking.

Objective 27-2b
Reduce tobacco use by adolescents—cigarettes.

SUBSTANCE ABUSE:
Objective 26-10a
Increase the proportion of adolescents not using alcohol or any illicit drugs during the past 30 days.

Objective 26-10c
Reduce the proportion of adults using any illicit drug during the past 30 days.

Objective 26-11c
Reduce the proportion of persons aged 18 years and older engaging in binge drinking of alcoholic beverages.

RESPONSIBLE SEXUAL BEHAVIOR:
Objective 13-6
Increase the proportion of sexually active persons who use condoms.

Objective 25-11
Increase the proportion of adolescents who abstain from sexual intercourse or use condoms if currently sexually active.

MENTAL HEALTH:
Objective 18-9b
Increase the proportion of adults aged 18 years and older with recognized depression who receive treatment.

INJURY AND VIOLENCE:
Objective 15-5
Reduce deaths caused by motor vehicle crashes.

Objective 15-32
Reduce homicides.

ENVIRONMENTAL QUALITY:
Objective 8-1a
Reduce the proportion of persons exposed to air that does not meet the U.S. Environmental Protection Agency's health-based standards for harmful air pollutants—ozone.

Objective 27-10
Reduce the proportion of nonsmokers exposed to environmental tobacco smoke.

IMMUNIZATION:
Objective 14-24
Increase the proportion of young children and adolescents who receive all vaccines that have been recommended for universal administration for at least 5 years.

Objective 14-29a
Increase the proportion of noninstitutionalized adults who are vaccinated annually against influenza.

Objective 14-29b
Increase the proportion of noninstitutionalized adults who are ever vaccinated against pneumococcal disease.

ACCESS TO HEALTH CARE:
Objective 1-1
Increase the proportion of persons with health insurance.

Objective 1-4a
Increase the proportion of persons of all ages who have a specific source of ongoing care.

Objective 16-6a
Increase the proportion of pregnant women who receive early and adequate prenatal care beginning in the first trimester of pregnancy.

Data from: U.S. Department of Health and Human Services, Public Health Service. (2000). *Healthy people 2010* (conference edition, in two volumes). U.S. Department of Health and Human Services. Washington, DC: U.S. Government Printing Office and from U.S. Department of Health and Human Services, Public Health Service. (2006). *Healthy People 2010 Midcourse Review*. Accessed on February 2, 2008, at *www.healthypeople.gov/Data/midcourse/*.

Another important feature of *Healthy People 2010* is its emphasis on responsibility. Individuals need to accept responsibility for their lifestyle choices and behaviors. This emphasis on personal responsibility gives each individual a role in the quality of his or her life and the length of healthy life each may have.

Health care providers need to be responsible for offering health promotion, preventive health services, and monitoring behaviors. Unfortunately, many of the financial incentives for providers are to do tasks and procedures rather than to counsel and help individuals choose between various behaviors. Providers need to take the time to discuss behaviors that may improve the quality of life and extend years of life. For example, the addictive nature of tobacco and its effect on the development and course of a variety of chronic health conditions is now well recognized. Providers should be asking every person if they use tobacco and should be providing them with ways to quit smoking, including economic and social incentives.

Providers also need to look for partnership in the community through which they can better serve the needs of individuals. *Healthy People 2010* emphasizes the efforts of partnerships and partnership building as essential to health promotion. One approach to partnerships is the development and use of community nursing centers (*http://nncc.us/*). The Health Promotion Center (HPC) operated by Fairfield University School of Nursing in Fairfield, Connecticut, is one example. The nurses and nursing students who provide health education, screening, and referral services at the HPC work with existing community organizations to better meet the health care needs of underserved people. The HPC works with senior housing and senior centers to provide comprehensive cardiovascular screenings and medication review. As an extension of this work, funding was secured for a program called *Step Up to Health*, a project to increase physical activity in this population through interactive planning and consumer ownership of the activities. The project was part of the National Blueprint Project supported by the Robert Wood Johnson Foundation (*www.agingblueprint. org*). The project engaged older adults in walking programs, line dancing, gardening, and low impact exercise programs, including the People with Arthritis Can Exercise (PACE) program from the National Arthritis Foundation (*www. arthritis.org/events/getinvolved/ProgramsServices/PACE.asp*). Another approach to partnerships is to have providers serve as active participants on community boards and advisory committees, which enables providers to become more aware of the service needs in the community and the resources available to help meet those needs.

Work sites and communities need to become partners in providing opportunities for people to lead healthy lives through flexible work schedules, work site wellness programs, safe parks, and the availability of exercise facilities. Converting empty lots into community gardens provides beautification of the area, an opportunity for exercise in caring for the garden, and a source of fresh vegetables.

Churches, temples, and mosques can be a vital partners in meeting *Healthy People 2010* objectives. Faith communities can cut across economic, social, racial, and gender barriers, making them an excellent source for sharing information on health promotion and disease prevention. Parish nurses are becoming increasingly prevalent and they incorporate *Healthy People 2010* objectives into their activities (Berry, 2004).

Public health officials at all levels are necessary partners in meeting *Healthy People 2010* objectives. As part of the core public health functions of assessment, policy development, and assurance, the U.S. Public Health Service and all state, county, and local health departments need to collect data, make information available to the public, create policies that support *Healthy People 2010* objectives, and ensure that needed services are available from a competent workforce.

Healthy People 2010 can form the basis for planning, service delivery, evaluation, and research in every aspect of the health care system. The nurse needs to be familiar with this document and its intent. Nurses should compare their practices with the objectives in *Healthy People 2010*. Additionally, the nurse needs to be aware of the research and practice changes that occur as a result of the work toward these objectives.

Healthy People 2010 Update

The Mid-Course Review of *Healthy People 2010* came out in 2006. It is available at *www.healthypeople.gov/data/ midcourse/pdf/ExecutiveSummary.pdf*. The mid-course review uses data available in 2005 as the basis for decision making about progress on each of the 467 objectives and subobjectives. Only 6% (29) of the objectives were met during the mid-course review period. Another 30% (138) demonstrated some movement toward meeting the objectives. A total of 31% (114) of the objectives had no change from baseline, mixed changes (some positive and some negative), or negative movement from the baseline. Approximately 158 objectives could not be assessed, of which 28 objectives were dropped from the list. This leaves 439 objectives and subobjectives with continuing measurement for 2010. Only 36% of the objectives demonstrated consistent and positive movement in the past 5 years measured. While this accounts for only 5 of the 10 years in the assessment period, it does reflect the limited amount of funding that supports health promotion activities and the focus of our health care system on illness care.

The comments about progress on *Healthy People 2010* objectives are organized around the two primary goals: Increase Quality and Years of Healthy Life and Eliminate Health Disparities.

With regard to the first goal, Increase Quality and Years of Healthy Life, life expectancy continues to improve, with women living longer than men and Whites living longer than Blacks. Total life expectancy is now 77.2 years, with life expectancies of 79.8 years for women, 74.5 years for men, 77.7 years for Whites, and 72.2 years for Blacks. While these figures show overall improvement, they also demonstrate health disparities related to life expectancies by gender and race. In addition, the three measures selected for measuring health, activity limitations, and chronic disease demonstrate similar trends, with women doing better than men and Whites doing better than Blacks. All groups, however, decreased in the measure of "Expected years free of selected chronic diseases," indicating an increasing concern about developing chronic diseases.

For the second goal of Eliminating Health Disparities, the results at mid-course were decidedly mixed. Trend data indicated that, overall, disparities have not changed significantly. Specifically, the disparities between men and women improved for 25 objectives, but got worse for 15 objectives. There was no change on 83% of the objectives. Some may look at these data and see a positive trend in that health disparities are not getting worse. However, the goals were set for realistic improvement, so the expectation was for movement away from the baseline, not maintenance of that baseline. For example, the overall percentage of people with health insurance did not change significantly from the 1997 benchmark data. This result may be due to the stable nature of employment from 2000 to 2005, since having health insurance is linked directly to employment. Viewed through the first perspective, the stable nature of the percentage of people with health insurance may indicate a reversal of the trend of fewer people without health insurance. However, the objective was to increase the number of people with health insurance, not to maintain the status quo. Therefore, the lack of progress in insuring people against health problems is problematic. There were similar changes in disparities across racial and ethnic groups. Most striking is that disparities among education groups showed the most negative change. The group with the highest level of education did better than those groups with lower levels of education. These disparities have yet to be reflected in income and geographic variables, although people with higher incomes continued to do better than those with lower incomes in this area. Data suggest that disparities by education groups will eventually be demonstrated in income and racial/ethnic categories, thus maintaining the disparities seen at the beginning of data collection in 2000.

Even though some progress is demonstrated on about 70% of the objectives and subobjectives and the life expectancy in the United States continues to improve, our life expectancy continues to be less than the life expectancy in other developed countries. In addition, there is little evidence to indicate reductions in health disparities in the United States. These data from the Mid-Course Review (USDHHS, 2006) and the data being analyzed for *Healthy People 2020* (both at *www.healthypeople.gov*) support the need for increased effort and more targeted funding for health promotion and disease prevention, particularly among men, racial/ethnic groups, and those with high school or less education.

CASE STUDY

Refer to the Case Study that appears at the end of this chapter along with the Care Plan. Read carefully, because some of the concepts covered in those boxes are applied in the following sections.

Problem Identification

How many problems does Frank's situation present? The answer depends on who is asked the question and his or her position in relation to Frank. Each point of view focuses on different aspects of Frank's life. His physician, using a clinical model of health, might say that Frank has coronary heart disease with an acute myocardial infarction, hypertension, hyperlipidemia, chronic bronchitis, and obesity. But

Frank's problems also represent a failure to meet several of the *Healthy People 2010* objectives on a personal level. His nurse can add that he has paid little attention to his lifestyle, even after changes were recommended. He continues to overeat, drink too much, smoke, not exercise, and live a stressful life. Frank's employer sees a man who has potential, but who is now too disabled to take on new responsibilities and perhaps unable to continue performing his previous duties. Frank's children might feel that he can no longer take them on jaunts or play with them. His wife, Sada, knows that their plans for educating their children, and for travel and enjoyment, might suffer. The human resource personnel who manage Frank's health insurance and pension programs would say that he has an expensive disease, and the state health planner would point out that Frank's problem is only one of a growing number of disabling illnesses that result from preventable causes. A reviewer planning for *Healthy People 2020* might see Frank as part of the aggregated data on heart disease, indicating a continuing increase in heart disease among Black non-Hispanic men.

To Frank, his health problems are multidimensional. His initial fear of dying, pain, dependence, and frustration decreased as he began to feel better, but his realization that he might never be able to achieve his dreams for himself and his family haunt him. Although theoretically in his prime, Frank suddenly sees himself as far older than his years, both in body and in social achievement. He believes he has reached his limit and that he will never again have the freedom to choose his future. He and his family needed to evaluate their situation and make alternative plans based on asset planning. A care plan has been developed based on the situation of Frank and his family. (See Care Plan at the end of this chapter.)

Planning Interventions

Rather than emphasizing the chronic health issues and related problems, the nurse can begin with asset planning within the family. **Asset planning** is a planning approach that, given the realities of the present, helps focus the family and their providers on the building blocks for their future. It focuses on the assets or strengths of the individual, the family, and the community, applying those assets to improve or maintain the current level of functioning.

Frank's physician and nurse can begin with the fact that Frank survived his first myocardial infarction. The coronary damage resulting from this event becomes the baseline for determining future change in the lives of Frank and his family. Earlier, Frank's physician had taken a broader time perspective when he advised Frank to cut down on smoking, which was contributing to both his bronchitis and his hypertension, and to change his high-fat diet and sedentary habits, which contributed to his weight problem and aggravated his high blood pressure. These lifestyle changes now become tools for Frank's recovery and for change within his family. His cardiac event also becomes a risk factor for heart disease in the lives of his children.

Looking at the immediate future, Frank's employer saw the effect of the event on Frank's position within the company. Frank would have a long recovery that could be successful if he adhered to his cardiac rehabilitation program. Asset planning at this level means examining how to move Frank back into his work role without further jeopardizing his health. Frank and Sada also need to examine if he could continue in this position, given its potential effect on his health.

Frank and his family used a broader perspective than the medical personnel or the corporation. They knew that to achieve the family's economic and educational goals and still spend time together, they had to make decisions that would ultimately affect Frank's health. Similar to many Americans, they had been willing to live with Frank's job pressures and stressful lifestyle. The family members were aware of their impoverished roots and had no wish to go back to them. However, they also recognized that the strength of their family, their ability to work together to achieve goals, and their faith were assets that were missing in some families.

Frank's social network of friends, relatives, and church members became an additional asset. They helped the family through the difficult initial weeks at home by providing meals, taking care of the yard work and laundry, and providing companionship so Sada could shop and have time alone. As Frank recovered, they would provide support for the social and lifestyle changes that Frank and his family needed to make.

The nurse-led cardiovascular rehabilitation group played a vital role in Frank's recovery. As the physician continued to monitor Frank's cardiac status, the nurse began the long process of working with Frank to change his habits. He had stopped smoking while in the hospital, but with more free time than usual, he was craving to smoke again. Using an asset planning approach and Gordon's functional health patterns (2006), the nurse identified the changes that Frank needed to make to decrease the risk of a second heart attack. A plan was developed to help Frank begin to take control of his life through behavior changes. These changes included relaxation techniques, diet modification, smoking cessation, and mild chair exercises. The support of the family was enlisted to reinforce the changes Frank was willing to make, since social support and environmental changes are shown to enhance personal decision making. His employer was contacted and agreed to a plan enabling Frank to work from home using a computer while the workplace became smoke free. Frank became an asset to the workplace, serving as a spokesperson for the benefits of lifestyle change. He was enlisted to talk with other employees about stress management, exercise, weight reduction, and smoking cessation based on his personal experiences.

Health planners and public health officials used the broadest perspective in asset planning by viewing Frank as an example of a person whose potential shifted as a result of a preventable, disabling illness. The planners looked to public and private community patterns and policies that increase healthful habits and living conditions. Work schedules and work load; stress and safety in work environments; affirmative action programs for jobs and wages; availability of public transportation systems, recreational facilities, and economically accessible housing; farm price subsidies for food and tobacco crops that affect buying patterns; excise taxes and regulation of health-damaging drugs such as alcohol and nicotine were all taken into consideration (Grzywacz & Fuqua, 2000). The asset planning approach emphasized the positive actions that could be made at the personal, employment, community, and societal levels to minimize the effects of Frank's illness and related diseases, thereby addressing all levels of the ecological model of health.

What was the Actual Cause of Frank's Problem?

It is not possible to separate one cause from another because heart disease is a multifactoral disease. In Frank's case, the sources of illness were found in the many interrelationships in his life. Attempting to treat or change each factor as a separate entity can have but a limited effect on the improvement of overall health. Frank's health problems were numerous. In addition to a poor diet, weight gain, lack of exercise, and smoking, his hyperlipidemia, an adaptive biological response to the pressures in his life, further debilitated him. It eventually clogged his coronary vessels and they became maladaptive. His hypertension, resulting from his diet and time-constrained lifestyle and complicated by the buildup of plaque secondary to hyperlipidemia, was also a biological attempt to adjust to a situation that contributed to an imbalance between his personal resources and the demands of his family and the economic world. Frank's smoking was a psychosocial means to help him relieve some of the emotional pressures. It may have served this short-term purpose, but only at a silently rising cost to his health. Cigarette use by persons who have hypertension or high serum cholesterol levels multiplies their risk of coronary heart disease (Izzo & Black, 2003).

Evaluation of the Situation

The health status of an individual or population depends on a sustainable balance of the complex responses between physiological, psychological, and social and environmental factors. Health was initially conceived as a biological state, with genetic endowment as the starting point. However, health involves psychological and social aspects and is interpreted within the context of the immediate environment.

The interconnections between biophysical, psychological, and environmental causes and consequences did not end with Frank's heart attack. His heart attack was only the most dramatic sign that health-damaging responses outweighed health-promoting ones. The "tip of the iceberg" analogy is frequently used to illustrate the importance of identifying individuals with subclinical symptoms. High blood lipid levels, high blood pressure, obesity, smoking, and persistent worrying were no less important than the infarction in shaping the status of Frank's health. To repair the damage to Frank's heart without changing his lifestyle, habits, and work environment would only buy a brief amount of time before further damage would occur.

The infarction and resulting disability also permanently reshaped Frank's environment. After a few months of working full time, Frank realized that he needed to find a less stressful job. He recognized that his sales administration skills were an asset and began interviewing in the nonprofit sector. Ultimately, he landed a job at half his previous salary, but with excellent benefits and a flexible work environment. His reduced income meant that his children's educational opportunities were more limited than they were before his heart attack, but his family responded by writing for tuition support from community organizations. Frank found that his contacts in both the corporate and the nonprofit sectors increased his value to his new employer. Frank's entire life, internal and external, had changed. He had learned to adapt to his health problems and had developed a more **eudaimonistic** approach to health and life.

Frank's situation illustrates how causes and effects in life and health tend to merge into constant, inseparable interconnections between individuals and their worlds. A person's health status is a reflection of a web of relationships that characterize that person's life. Health is not an achievement or a prize, but a high-quality interaction between a person's inner and outer worlds that provides the capacity to respond to the demands of the biological, psychological, and environmental systems of these worlds.

After reviewing the list of *Healthy People 2010* Focus Areas listed in Box 1-1, which of the focus areas apply to the promotion of Frank's health? Clearly, the area of heart disease and stroke is most applicable. The *Healthy People 2010* website (*www.healthypeople.gov*) has a number of objectives that relate directly to the prevention of heart disease, hypertension, and hyperlipidemia, including objectives that relate to treatment options and training the public to recognize and respond to heart attacks and stroke. Based on the information about Frank and his experience, determine what his children should be taught based on the *Healthy People 2010* objectives in this focus area.

LEVELS OF PREVENTION

Prevention, in a narrow sense, means averting the development of disease in the future. In a broad sense, prevention consists of all measures, including definitive therapies, that limit disease progression. Leavell and Clark (1965) defined three **levels of prevention**: primary, secondary, and tertiary (Figure 1-2). While the levels of prevention are related to the natural history of disease, they can be used to prevent disease and provide nurses with starting points in making effective, positive changes in the health status of their clients. Within the three levels of prevention, there are five steps. These steps include health promotion and specific protection (primary prevention); early diagnosis, prompt treatment, and disability limitation (secondary prevention); and restoration and rehabilitation (tertiary prevention).

Some confusion exists in the interpretation of these concepts; therefore, a consistent understanding of primary, secondary, and tertiary prevention is essential. The levels of prevention operate on a continuum, but may overlap in practice. The nurse must clearly understand the goals of each level to intervene effectively in keeping people healthy.

Primary Prevention

Primary prevention precedes disease or dysfunction. However, primary prevention is therapeutic in that it includes health as beneficial to well-being, it uses therapeutic treatments, and, as a process or behavior towards enhancing health, it involves symptom identification when teaching stress reduction techniques. Primary prevention intervention includes health promotion, such as health education about risk factors for heart disease, and specific protection, such as immunization against hepatitis B. Its purpose is to decrease the vulnerability of the individual or population to disease or dysfunction. Interventions at this level encourage individuals and groups to become more aware of the means of improving health and the things they can do at the primary preventive health level and the optimal health level. People are also taught to use appropriate primary preventive measures. However, primary prevention can also include advocating for policies that promote the health of the community and electing public officials who will enact legislation that protects the health of the public.

Health Promotion

The **health promotion** definitions vary. O'Donnell (1987, p. 4) has defined health promotion as "the science and art of helping people change their lifestyle to move toward a state of optimal health." Kreuter and Devore (1980) propose a more complex definition in a paper commissioned by the U.S. Public Health Service. They state that health promotion is "the process of advocating health in order to enhance the probability that personal (individual, family, and community), private (professional and business), and public (federal, state, and local government) support of positive health practices will become a societal norm" (Kreuter & Devore, 1980, p. 26).

The Theoretical Basis of Health Promotion The theoretical underpinnings for health promotion have evolved since the early 1980s. Most of these theories are behaviorally based, derived from the social sciences, and extensively researched. These theories include the theory of reasoned action by Ajzen & Fishbein (1980), theories of behavior by Bandura (1976, 1999, 2004), the health belief model by Rosenstock (Janz et al., 2002), Pender's Health Promotion Model (Pender et al., 2006), and stages of change theories by Prochaska (Prochaska et al., 2004). Internet searches on each of these theories will provide numerous sites where more detailed information is available.

The Social Nature of Health Promotion Health promotion goes beyond providing information. It is also proactive

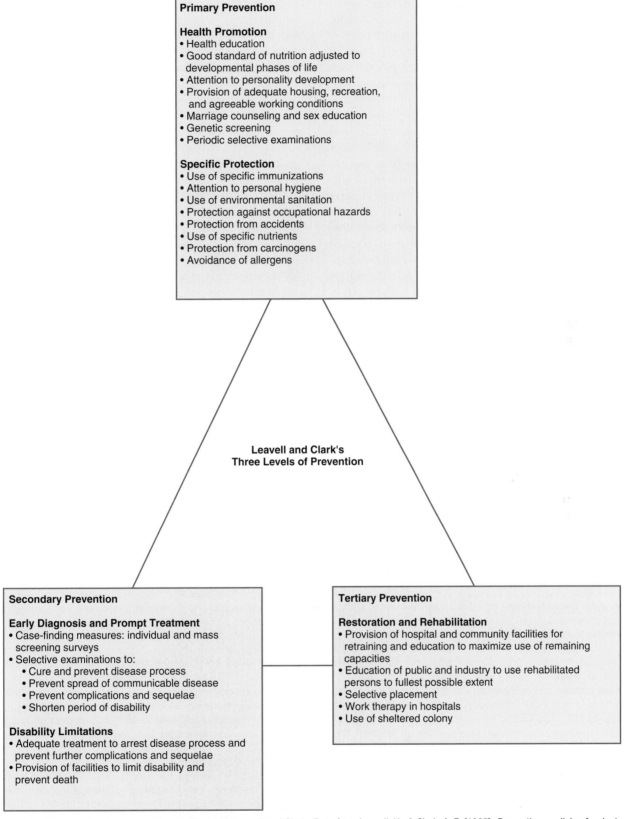

Primary Prevention

Health Promotion
- Health education
- Good standard of nutrition adjusted to developmental phases of life
- Attention to personality development
- Provision of adequate housing, recreation, and agreeable working conditions
- Marriage counseling and sex education
- Genetic screening
- Periodic selective examinations

Specific Protection
- Use of specific immunizations
- Attention to personal hygiene
- Use of environmental sanitation
- Protection against occupational hazards
- Protection from accidents
- Use of specific nutrients
- Protection from carcinogens
- Avoidance of allergens

**Leavell and Clark's
Three Levels of Prevention**

Secondary Prevention

Early Diagnosis and Prompt Treatment
- Case-finding measures: individual and mass screening surveys
- Selective examinations to:
  - Cure and prevent disease process
  - Prevent spread of communicable disease
  - Prevent complications and sequelae
  - Shorten period of disability

Disability Limitations
- Adequate treatment to arrest disease process and prevent further complications and sequelae
- Provision of facilities to limit disability and prevent death

Tertiary Prevention

Restoration and Rehabilitation
- Provision of hospital and community facilities for retraining and education to maximize use of remaining capacities
- Education of public and industry to use rehabilitated persons to fullest possible extent
- Selective placement
- Work therapy in hospitals
- Use of sheltered colony

Figure 1-2   The three levels of prevention developed by Leavell and Clark. (Data from Leavell, H., & Clark, A. E. [1965]. *Preventive medicine for doctors in the community.* New York: McGraw-Hill.)

decision-making at all levels of society as reflected in the *Healthy People* (*www.healthypeople.gov*) objectives. Health promotion holds the best promise for lower-cost methods of limiting the constant increase in health care costs and for empowering people to be responsible for the aspects of their lives that can enhance well-being. Based on the need for health promotion activities within the health care system, efforts must be made to identify the multiple determinants of health, identify relevant health promotion strategies, and delineate issues relevant to social justice and access to care. Individuals, families, and communities must be active participants in this process so that the actions taken are socially relevant, economically feasible, and supportive of changes at the individual level.

The Active and Passive Nature of Health Promotion
Health promotion efforts, unlike those efforts directed at specific protection from certain diseases, focus on maintaining or improving the general health of individuals, families, and communities (see Health Teaching box). These activities are carried out at the public level (government programs promoting adequate housing), at the community level (Habitat for Humanity), and at the personal level (voting for improved low-income housing). Nursing interventions are actions directed toward developing people's resources to maintain or enhance their well-being—a form of assets-based planning.

Two strategies of health promotion involve the individual and may be either passive or active. Passive strategies involve the individual as an inactive participant or recipient. Examples of passive strategies are public health efforts to maintain clean water and sanitary sewage systems to decrease infectious diseases and improve health, and efforts to introduce vitamin D in all milk to ensure that children will not be at high risk for rickets when there is little sunlight. These passive strategies must be used to promote the health of the public when individual participation might be low.

Active strategies depend on the individual becoming personally involved in adopting a proposed program of health promotion. Two examples of lifestyle change are daily exercise as part of a physical fitness plan and a stress-management program as part of daily living. A combination of active and passive strategies is best for making an individual healthier. Reexamine the Case Study to determine when Frank could have incorporated some of these strategies to decrease his risk of heart disease.

This text is concerned almost entirely with active strategies and the nurse's role in these strategies. Some passive strategies are presented, but they are presented with the implicit belief that each individual must take responsibility for improving health. It is undeniable that passive strategies also have a valuable role, but they must be used within a context of encouraging and teaching individuals to assume more responsibility for their health.

An Application of Theory to the Practice of Health Promotion The Transtheoretical Model (TTM) is an excellent example and can be applied to this case study. TTM incorporates Stages of Change (readiness to take action), Decisional Balance (benefits to and detractors from changing a behavior), Self-Efficacy (personal confidence in making a change), and Processes of Change (cognitive, affective, and behavioral activities facilitating

---

HEALTH TEACHING   Process for Assessing, Evaluating, and Treating Overweight and Obesity in Adults

Overweight and obesity are major concerns in public health because they contribute to other health problems such as high cholesterol, high blood pressure, Diabetes Mellitus, heart disease, functional limitations, and disability. As part of the National Heart, Lung, and Blood Institute's (NHLBI) Obesity Education Initiative, titled Aim for a Healthy Weight, nurses have an important role to play in health education related to obesity prevention and control. Complete information can be retrieved from: *www.nhlbi.nih.gov/health/public/heart/obesity/lose_wt/index.htm*.

Make the Most of the Client Visit and Set an Effective Tone for Communication: Nurses need to be able to ask individuals about their weight history, weight-related health risks, and desire to lose weight. The approaches used need to be respectful of a person's lifestyle, habits, and cultural influences. Discussions need to be nonjudgmental and goal directed.

Assess Client's Motivation/Readiness to Lose Weight: Nurses need to be able to explain body mass index and why it is the preferred method of determining overweight and obesity in adults. They need to understand the methods of data collection and measurement of height and weight, as well as waist circumference, risk factors, and comorbidities. Nurses need to develop skill in determining readiness and motivation to lose weight in their clients.

Build a Partnership with an Individual: Nurses should work with individuals to determine what each person is willing to do to achieve a lower weight. This approach includes knowing the best practices in weight management and weight loss. Fad diets, dietary supplements, and weight loss pills may be inappropriate for most people, and formal weight loss programs may be too expensive for low- and moderate-income families. Use recommended diets that restrict caloric intake, set activity goals with your clients, encourage the person to keep a Weekly Food and Activity Diary, and provide information on diet and activity. Be sure to record individual goals and the treatment plan, including a health education plan. Nurses are knowledgeable about current treatment options and their success. Holistic approaches are needed, since food behaviors are influenced by many factors. Listen to the individual stories about food and its role in their lives. Therapies should fit the individual's goals and lead to lifestyle change.

change). The bases of TTM are the stages of change—six stages that people spiral through on a path toward making and sustaining a behavioral change to promote health. These stages are:

Precontemplative	Not considering change
Contemplative	Aware of but not considering change soon
Preparation	Planning to act soon
Action	Has begun to make behavioral change (recent)
Maintenance	Continued commitment to behavior (long-term)
Relapse	Reverted to old behavior

Each stage provides opportunities for the nurse to provide information and support behavioral change. Encouraging people and suggesting changes to their environment that support behavioral change can increase their self-efficacy and their chances of maintaining a change. This model also recognizes that people need multiple opportunities to make behavioral change before achieving success and that relapse should be expected (Prochaska et al., 2004).

Although health promotion would seem to be a practical and effective mode of health care, the major portion of health care delivery is geared toward responding to acute and chronic disease. Preventing or delaying the onset of chronic disease and adding new dimensions to the quality of life are not as easy to implement because they take time to implement and evaluate and require personal action. These actions are more closely associated with everyday living and the lifestyles adopted by individuals, families, communities, and nations. Habits such as eating, resting, exercising, and handling anxieties appear to be transmitted from parent to child and from social group to social group as part of a cultural, not a genetic, heritage. These activities may be taught in subtle ways, but they influence behavior and have as much of an influence on health as does genetic inheritance. Although the public may not appreciate the causal relationships between behavior and health, it should be apparent to health professionals. Arguably, the concept of risk is the most basic of all health concepts, since health promotion and disease protection are based on this concept.

Health promotion strategies have the potential of enhancing the quality of life from birth to death. For example, good nutrition is adjusted to various developmental phases in life to account for rapid growth and development in infancy and early childhood, physiological changes associated with adolescence, extra demands during pregnancy, and the many changes occurring in older adults. Good nutrition is known to enhance the immune system, enabling individuals to fight off infections that could lead to disabling illnesses. Other individual activities are adapted to the person's needs for optimal personality development at all ages. As seen in Unit Four, much

can be done on a personal or group basis, through counseling and properly directed parent education, to provide the environmental requirements for the proper personality development of children. Community participation is also an important factor in promoting individual, family, and group health (see Chapters 6, 7, and 8).

Personal health promotion is usually provided through health education (see Chapter 10). An important function of nurses, physicians, and allied health professionals, health education is principally concerned with eliciting useful changes in human behavior based on current research. The goal is to inculcate a sense of responsibility in individuals for their own health and a shared sense of responsibility for avoiding injury to the health of others. For example, encouraging child-rearing practices that foster normal growth and development (personal, social, and physical) addresses both the individual parent and the needs of society. Health education nurtures health-promoting habits, values, and attitudes that must be learned through practice. These must be reinforced through systematic instruction in hygiene, bodily function, physical fitness, and use of leisure time. Another goal is to understand the appropriate use of health services. For example, a semiannual visit to a dentist may teach a child better oral health habits and to visit the dentist regularly, although this is not the primary purpose of the visit. Parents, teachers, and caregivers play a vital role in health education. In addition to teaching individuals, nurses need to develop skills in group teaching and in providing education within community organizations.

Available research clearly shows an increase in longevity, a decrease in mortality and morbidity, and an improvement in the quality of life for individuals who have been involved in health promotion activities such as physical activity and avoidance of smoking. It must be emphasized that health promotion requires lifestyle change. Once a lifestyle change has been adopted, vigilance is needed to ensure that the lifestyle change is maintained and modified to fit developmental and environmental changes.

Empirical data linking risk factors, health promotion activities, and outcomes are sufficient to drive the development of the *Healthy People 2010* objectives and to be incorporated into quality improvement measures in managed care. One of the challenges posed in *Healthy People 2010* is the development of measurable outcome objectives that are based on more realistic economic models.

Health promotion is an important concept for nursing because it embodies many other concepts that nursing is concerned with today. As stated earlier, much of the nursing role is involved with health teaching. Standard 5B of the *Nursing: Scope and Standards of Practice* document (ANA, 2004, p. 28) requires nurses "to promote health and a safe environment" through health teaching and evaluation of teaching effectiveness in clinical practice (Hot Topics box). Health education is clearly a nursing role.

HOT topics

HEALTH PROMOTION PROGRAM INCENTIVES

The concept of health promotion program incentives is multi-dimensional. Incentives are best defined relative to their purpose, type, and form for either groups or individuals.

An incentive is a reward designed to influence an individual to make a desired change where he/she might otherwise not make the behavioral change solely on the intrinsic benefit of the changed behavior. For example, a person may not choose to stop smoking because of the cost of the smoking cessation materials. If the person is given the smoking cessation materials for free and provided with a $10 incentive each week for using the materials, then that person might decide to make the change. The benefits of not smoking were not enough of an incentive to stop smoking, but the incentives helped to make the behavioral change possible.

One example of an integrated incentive program in an employee wellness program is the HEALTH Plus program at Vanderbilt University (2008) (*www.vanderbilt.edu/HRS/wellness/healthplus.htm*). Full-time employees and faculty can participate in an incentive program that rewards them for participation and achievement of specific health and wellness goals. Participants receive monetary incentives for completing a Health Risk Assessment on line. They can then select a level of behavior change based on increasing levels of commitment (bronze, silver, or gold). For each level, participants choose wellness categories and actions they are willing to take within each category. They then work on those actions over the next year and complete another Health Risk Assessment at the end of the year to note specific achievement. Information is available on each category and action, and wellness staff can assist participants in reaching desired goals. The incentive for the participants is an additional $10 to $15 in each paycheck, participation in groups working on specific actions, and recognition of achievement of each level. The university benefits from healthier employees, which increases productivity, limits health care costs, and improves quality of life.

Specific Protection

This aspect of primary prevention focuses on protecting people from injury and disease, for example, by providing immunizations and reducing exposure to occupational hazards, carcinogens, and other environmental health risks. These hazards and risks include work-related injuries ranging from back injuries for nurses to dismemberment for machinists, exposure to chemicals in boat repair to inhaled sawdust by carpenters, and exposure of children to diesel emissions to damage to a fetus due to radiation.

Primary prevention interventions are considered health protection when they emphasize shielding or defending the body (or the public) from specific causes of injury or disease. Implementing nursing interventions that prevent a specific health problem may seem easier than promoting well-being among individuals, groups, or communities because: (1) the variables are delineated more clearly in prevention than in promotion and (2) the potential influences are less diverse.

Examples Two examples may help demonstrate these differences. Immunization for influenza is quite popular and has become a regular activity for people at risk each autumn. Nurses can participate in this specific protection role by giving the influenza injections in clinics and offices. Another example is creating nut-free schools to protect hypersensitive children from life-threatening allergic reactions to peanut products. Such initiatives have largely been the result of grassroots parent organizations working with formal community organizations to adopt policies that protect the health of these children. Nurses may be involved in the parent organizations or the school or public health boards that review the proposed policies. Additionally, nurses must be able to address the need to protect portions of the population at risk.

Secondary Prevention

Although primary prevention measures have decreased the hazards of chronic diseases such as cardiovascular disease, conditions that preclude a healthy quality of life are still prevalent. Secondary prevention ranges from providing screening activities and treating early stages of disease to limiting disability by averting or delaying the consequences of advanced disease.

Screening is secondary prevention because the principle goal is to identify individuals in an early, detectable stage of the disease process. However, screening provides an excellent opportunity to offer health teaching as a primary preventive measure. Screening activities now play an important role in the control of diseases such as heart disease, stroke, and colorectal cancer. Additionally, screening activities provide early diagnosis and treatment of nutritional, behavioral, and other related problems. Nurses play an important role in screening activities because they provide clinical expertise and educationally sound health information during the screening process.

Delayed recognition of disease results in the need to limit future disability in late secondary prevention. Limiting disability is a vital role for nursing since preventive measures are primarily therapeutic and are aimed at arresting the disease and preventing further complications. The paradox here is that health education and disease prevention activities are similar to those used in primary prevention, but applied to a person or population with an existing disease. Modifications to the teaching plan must be made based on the individual's current health status and ability to modify behavior. In the case study, Frank needed secondary prevention after his heart attack. The lifestyle changes needed to prevent a second heart attack were similar to the steps he could have taken to prevent his initial heart attack, but with a recognition that his coronary status was now compromised. As a result, exercise had to be increased gradually as part of a cardiac rehabilitation program and diet modifications had to be made with support from a registered dietitian to ensure adequate nutrition and weight loss.

Tertiary Prevention

Tertiary prevention occurs when a defect or disability is permanent and irreversible. The process involves minimizing the effects of disease and disability by surveillance and maintenance activities aimed at preventing complications and deterioration. Tertiary prevention focuses on rehabilitation to help people attain and retain an optimal level of functioning regardless of their disabling condition. The objective is to return the affected individual to a useful place in society, maximize remaining capacities, or both. The responsibility of the nurse is to ensure that persons with disabilities receive services that enable them to live and work according to the resources that are still available to them. When a person has a stroke, rehabilitating this individual to the highest level of functioning and teaching lifestyle change to prevent future strokes are examples of tertiary prevention.

THE NURSE'S ROLE

Evolving demands are placed on the nurse and the nursing profession as a result of changes in society. Emphasis is shifting from acute, hospital-based care to preventive, **community-based care**, which is provided in nontraditional health care settings in the community. This demand for community-based services, with the home as a major community setting for care, is closely related to the changing demographics of the U.S. As the home and community become the existing sites for care, nurses must assume more blended roles, with a knowledge base that prepares them to practice across settings using **evidence-based practice**. Within these roles, nurses assume a more active involvement in the prevention of disease and the promotion of health. Nurses can be more independent in their practice, place a greater emphasis on promoting and maximizing health, and more than ever, are accountable morally and legally for their professional behavior.

Nursing Roles in Health Promotion and Protection

Although nurses often work with persons on a one-to-one basis, they seldom work in isolation. Within today's health care system, nurses collaborate with other nurses, physicians, social workers, nutritionists, psychologists, therapists, individuals, and community groups. In this collaborative capacity, nurses play a variety of roles.

Advocate

As advocates nurses help individuals obtain what they are entitled to receive from the health care system, try to make the system more responsive to individual and community needs, and help persons develop the skills to advocate for themselves. In the role of advocate, the nurse strives to ensure that all persons receive high-quality, appropriate, and cost-effective care. The nurse may spend a great deal of time identifying and coordinating resources for complex cases. Other examples of advocacy will be seen in subsequent chapters.

Care Manager

The nurse acts as a care manager to prevent duplication of services and to reduce costs. Information gathered from reliable data sources enables the care manager to help individuals avoid care that is unproven, ineffective, or unsafe. Reliable sources of information on best practices, evidence-based practices, and standard protocols are available from Internet sites sponsored by the federal government (e.g., *www.nih.gov*, *www.cdc.gov*), specialty organizations (e.g., *www.arthritis.org*, *www.nursingworld.org*, *www.caremanager. org*), and private foundations (e.g., *www.rwjf.org*, *www.jhartfound.org*). Successful care management depends on a collaborative relationship among the care manager, other nurses and physicians, the individual and his or her family, the payer, and other care providers who work with the person. The wishes of the individual and family need to be clear to the care manager. Facilitating communication among parties is one of the care manager's most important functions.

Consultant

Nurses may provide knowledge about health promotion and disease prevention to individuals and groups as a consultant. Some nurses have specialized areas of expertise or advanced practice standing, such as in gerontology, women's health, or community/public health, and they are equipped to provide information as consultants in these areas of specialization (ANA, 2004). For example, a gerontological nurse specialist might be on a community planning board offering advice about what types of health promotion activities should be considered in planning a new senior housing development. In contrast to independent consultation, all nurses need to develop consultation skills that can be integrated into practice and allow the individual nurse to take advantage of opportunities to provide support on an individual level or for future development at the organizational level (Norwood, 2003).

Deliverer of Services

The core role of the nurse is the delivery of direct services such as health education, flu shots, and counseling in health promotion. Visible, direct delivery of nursing care is the foundation for the public image of nursing. The public demands that nurses be knowledgeable and competent in their delivery of services. This role is clearly expressed in the Nursing's Social Policy Statement (ANA, 2003) and in the ANA Code of Ethics (ANA, 2008).

Educator

Health practices in the United States are derived from the theory that health components such as good nutrition, industrial and highway safety, immunization, and specific drug therapy should be within the grasp of the total population. Even with its rich resources, society falls far short of attaining the goal of maximal health for all. The problem is not a lack of knowledge, but rather the lack of application; therefore it is incumbent on nurses to be excellent health educators. To teach effectively, the nurse must know essential facts abut how people learn and the teaching-learning process (see Chapter 10).

In addition to their storehouse of scientific knowledge, nurses who are committed to their teaching role know that individuals are unique in their response to efforts to change their behavior. Teaching may range from a chance remark by the nurse, based on a perception of desirable individual behavior, to structurally planned teaching according to individual needs. Selection of the methods most likely to succeed involves the establishment of teacher-learner goals. Health promotion and protection rely heavily on the individual's ability to use appropriate knowledge. Health education is one of the primary prevention techniques available to avoid the major causes of disability and death today and is a critical role for nurses.

Healer

The role of healer requires the nurse to help individuals integrate and balance the various parts of their lives (McKivergin, 2004). Healing resides in the ability to glimpse or intuit the "interior" of an individual, to sense and identify what is important to that other person, and to incorporate the specific insight into a care plan that helps that person develop his or her own capacity to heal. It requires a mindful blending of science and subjectivity (Siegel, 2007). Nurses have a special ability to help people heal. The art of nursing is the extraordinary ability to manage a broad array of information to create something meaningful, sensible, and whole (see Chapter 14).

Researcher

In today's health care environment, nurses are constantly striving to understand and interpret research findings that will enhance the quality and value of individual care. To provide optimal health care, nurses need to use research findings as their foundation for clinical decision-making. When nurses or other clinicians use research findings and the best evidence possible to make decisions, the outcome is termed evidence-based practice. Evidence-based practice is defined as the conscientious, explicit, and judicious use of current best evidence in making decisions about the care of individuals. The practice of evidence-based medicine means integrating individual clinical expertise with the best available external clinical evidence from systematic research (ANA, 2004).

The National Institute of Nursing Research (NINR) serves as the focal point in developing research themes for the future of the profession. NINR supports research to establish a scientific base for the care of individuals throughout the lifespan, from management of individuals during illness and recovery to the reduction of risks for disease and disability. The four themes NINR has identified are: (1) promoting health and preventing disease, (2) improving quality of life, (3) eliminating health disparities, and (4) setting directions for end-of-life research (NINR Strategic Plan, 2006). Notice that health promotion is the basis for all of these themes.

Evidence-based practice involves tracking down the best evidence with which to answer clinical research questions. Research evidence can be gathered from **quantitative studies** that describe situations, correlate different variables related to care, or test causal relationships between variables related to care. Such studies become incorporated into screening and treatment standards such as those from the U.S. Preventive Services Task Force (2007). Research evidence can also be gathered from **qualitative studies** that describe phenomena or define the historical

---

research highlights

Update on Health Literacy

People change their behavior when presented with information on the benefits of change and/or the harm done if changes are not made. Key to this process is the ability of people to obtain, process, and understand basic health information to make appropriate health decisions, known as health literacy. The most comprehensive research on this topic comes from the U.S. Department of Education, National Center for Educational Statistics, National Assessment of Adult Literacy, *The Health Literacy of America's Adults: Results from the 2003 National Assessment of Adult Literacy* (Kutner et al., 2006). Why is health literacy important? Research into this issue demonstrates the following:

- 36% of all adults have health literacy at or below the basic level.
- 66% of Hispanic adults have health literacy at or below the basic level.
- 58% of Black adults have health literacy at or below the basic level.

- Those adults who have less than a high school education score, on average, below the basic level of health literacy.
- 63% to 69% of those adults who rate their health as fair to poor have health literacy at or below the basic level.
- 55% to 60% of those adults who have Medicare, Medicaid, or no insurance have health literacy at or below the basic level.

In all situations where the nurse is attempting to educate about health behavior, assessment of health literacy is important. Cloonan (2004) found that few schools of nursing include health literacy in their curricula. More recently, Riley et al. (2006) examined the scope of the health literacy problem and its impact in the critical care environment. Given the importance placed by the federal government on health promotion and health literacy, nurses need to incorporate health literacy into health promotion protocols as research is expanded in this area.

From Kutner, M., Greenberg, E., Jin, Y., and Paulsen C. (2006). *The Health Literacy of America's adults: Results from the 2003 National Assessment of Adult Literacy* (NCES 2006-483). U.S. Department of Education. Washington, DC: National Center for Education Statistics.

nature, cultural relevance, or philosophical basis of aspects of nursing care. **Applied research** is done to directly affect clinical practice (Burns & Grove, 2003). Sackett and colleagues (1996) stressed the use of the best evidence available to answer clinical questions and explore the next best evidence when appropriate. The next best evidence may include the individual clinical judgment that nurses acquire through clinical experience and clinical practice and other qualitative approaches to research.

Nurses need to recognize research is important as a basis of evidence for their practice and that they often participate in the research process. For example, both home health nurses and nurses in long-term care facilities are required to collect extensive data on the cognitive and physical functioning of their clients through the OASIS and MDS assessment tools. These data are used as part of the quality improvement process to indicate areas for improvement in care, thereby contributing to nursing protocols.

Chapters 16 to 24 contain specific health promotion research studies. Time should be taken to review these studies and explore the relationship between behavior and disease, to identify which populations groups are at risk, and to discover what types of health promotion programs work and why they work. Through knowledge of research, nurses can strengthen their confidence in making daily decisions about quality care.

IMPROVING PROSPECTS FOR HEALTH
Population Effects

Cultural and socioeconomic changes within the population unequivocally influence lay concepts of health and health promotion. Currently there are areas of the United States where the Hispanic population is larger than any other population group. By the year 2050, it is predicted that the majority of people in the United States will not be of White European descent. Taken together as a portent for future health promotion strategies, these predictions about the population indicate that current knowledge about and approaches to health promotion may not meet the needs of the future U.S. population (see Chapter 2).

In addition to changes in the ethnic and racial distribution within the population, the projected changes in age distribution will affect health promotion practice. Considerable growth is expected in the proportion of the population that is 25 years of age and older. For example, the post–World War II baby boom will increase the number of persons in the 65-and-older age group between the years 2010 and 2030. While there was a drop in births after 1960, this decrease has been offset by an increase in immigration, both legal and illegal. More restrictive immigration rules related to Homeland Security have limited legal immigration since 2002 (U.S. Department of Homeland Security, 2003). Analysis of these population trends and projections helps health professionals determine changing needs. Additionally, analysis of the social environment is necessary for social policy concerning health.

SHIFTING PROBLEMS

The provision of personal health services must be informed by environmental health. Environmental pollution is a complex and increasingly hazardous problem. Diseases related to industry and technology, including asthma and trauma, have also become important threats to health.

The physical and psychological stresses of a rapidly changing and fast-paced society present daily problems, such as psychosocial and spiritual poor health habits. Obesity, for example, partly attributed to a lack of exercise and increasing food portion size, is a growing health issue. The ingestion of potentially toxic, non-nutritious, high-fat foods is another contributing factor (see Chapter 11). The abuse of tobacco, drugs, and alcohol also negatively affects health.

The emphasis on treating disease through the application of complex technology is not only costly, but it also contributes minimally to the improvement of health. An orientation toward illness clearly focuses on the effects rather than the causes of disease.

A substantial change in wellness patterns is occurring. Infectious and acute diseases were the major causes of death in the early part of the twentieth century, whereas chronic conditions, heart disease, cerebrovascular accident (stroke), and cancer are the major causes today. An emphasis on the diagnosis and treatment of disease, which were highly successful in the past, are not the answers for today's needs, which are closely related to and affected by the individual's biochemical functioning, genetics, environment, and personal choices.

MOVING TOWARD SOLUTIONS

Solutions are neither simple nor easy, but they can be focused in two major directions: individual involvement and government involvement. The first direction concentrates on actions of the individual, especially actions related to lifestyle choices across the lifespan. The learning and the inherent changes that are involved require the adoption of a new set of skills by people who will need the assistance of nurses to make those changes. Approximately one fifth of the population in the United States is faced with the problem of getting the basic necessities of food and shelter. The other four fifths, whose basic needs are met, must overcome problems resulting from affluence (U.S. Department of Health and Human Services, 2006).

Motivational factors play a large role in influencing attitudinal change. As discussed in Chapter 10, programs for health promotion and health education are only part of the answer. Financial incentives for prevention may be another motivating factor, and health advocacy by professionals in the health field is critical. Additionally, private and public action at all levels is needed to reduce social and environmental health hazards. Toxic agents in the environment such as particles from diesel emissions and social conditions such as school overcrowding can present health hazards that may not be detected for years; therefore, it is necessary for individuals and government to play a role.

Legislation and financing that relate to primary prevention are discussed in Chapter 3. Government activity, in the form of legislation, is currently increasing in this area. For example, bicycle safety, seat belts, and a graduated tax on cigarettes are specific areas for governmental intervention. Health ecology and planning are important areas for government involvement in the future. The redirection of the existing health care delivery system, putting more emphasis on primary prevention, is probably the most difficult and the most far-reaching goal; however, an emphasis on a wellness system is necessary to improve the health of the U.S. population.

SUMMARY

The ways individuals define health and health problems are important because definitions influence attempts to improve health and care delivery. In the case study, Frank Thompson's health was affected by obvious, immediate, and personal factors, such as his diet and employment pressures. Nevertheless, his problems had their roots in the social and economic conditions of his parents; in his own early history of illness, education, and work; and in his and his family's hopes and aspirations. His physician defined Frank's prob-

---

CASE STUDY

Health Assessment: Frank Thompson and Family

Frank Thompson's large brick home is located off a sparsely traveled country road. A few yards away stands the uninhabited shack where Frank was born during World War II.

Frank was raised knowing the odds that he faced as a poor tenant farmer. He helped his father, Ben, with their small tobacco and corn crops. They were unaware that the hazardous chemicals in the pesticides they used would later affect Ben's life. As his father often reminded him, Frank had to do better than others in school so he would not be doomed to the tenant farmer's life. However, Frank's school attendance was erratic because it was interrupted by the frequent demand of tending field crops. Thin and often tired, he had recurrent infections. The school nurse helped the Thompson family obtain the necessary medication for Frank's initial infection, but the family was never able to afford the penicillin that was necessary to prevent recurrent infections.

Inspired by the early work of Martin Luther King, Jr., Frank was intent on helping at home and building something better for his future. Frank managed to more than make up for his lost time at school. He passed his college entrance examinations and was awarded one of the new equal opportunity grants, which offered him a choice of attending any of the Ivy League schools in the Northeast. Instead, he chose the prestigious Southern University and eventually earned a Masters of Business Administration (MBA) degree. He married Sada, his longtime girlfriend, and the two planned their future.

With a good job in a large local sales firm, Frank built his house and started a family. He moved from a salesman to a division head and often traveled to regional meetings, sometimes accompanied by Sada and their three children. Frank's dream of sharing his success with his family included using part of his earnings to help his brothers and sisters with their education.

This new way of life meant little time for relaxation and frequent attendance at business luncheons and career-promoting social occasions. He kept late hours and worked long weekends. Good food, drinks, and cigarettes helped him relax before and after important business and social encounters; these softened the edges of hard bargaining and were status symbols.

Not surprisingly, Frank gained weight. He had a persistent cough, which was probably a result of the smoking habit that developed dur-

ing the early years of his career. Frank's physician, with whom Frank visited regularly at the corporation's health maintenance organization (HMO), said Frank's blood pressure and serum lipid levels were both higher than normal and that he had chronic bronchitis. The physician urged Frank to do what Frank already knew: cut down on smoking, drinking, saturated fats, and calories; get more exercise; and find ways to relax. However, Frank's life was too busy for exercise. He had to work harder as he moved up in his company, but he also had to appear relaxed, which was an essential characteristic for a prospective vice president. To meet these goals, he tended to drink and smoke more. He also refused to take medication for problems he could not see. Without the outward signs of disease, Frank believed he was out of shape, but generally healthy. Then Sada pointed out that his chance for promotion might actually improve if he lost some weight; therefore, he registered for a physical fitness program for executives that he could attend on Sunday mornings and before work during the week. At his first workout, the classic sharp pain gripped his chest and Frank had a massive heart attack.

Weeks later, Frank was convalescing at home after being released from the university's coronary care facility. He was lucky to survive the heart attack, and he was also lucky to have most of the services covered by his medical insurance plan and 80% of his earnings were protected by the company's disability pension. (Most people in the United States do not have this protection.)

However, Frank's dreams of promotion were shattered. For many months he could go to the office only two or three times a week at most, simply to deal with routine matters. He could not travel, for business or otherwise, for a long time. He was also skeptical about his cardiac rehabilitation program because his heart attack happened during exercise.

Reflective Questions:
1. As a nurse, how would you explain to Frank that his heart attack was not caused by his exercise?
2. How might a family approach to diet and exercise work with this family, given its structure and background?
3. Are there negative behaviors in your life that you see as status symbols?

lem in immediate biomedical terms. Public health planners, who saw Frank's problem on a longer-term population basis, sought policy solutions to the problem of preventing cardiovascular disease.

The view taken in this text is that a broad and longer-term perspective of health is the best guide to promoting health more effectively, even as nurses deal with individual problems on a day-to-day basis. Health is a sustainable balance between internal and external forces. Health allows people to move through life free from the constraints of illness and allows healing to take place.

Illness represents an imbalance that human choices (intertwined social, political, spiritual, professional, and personal choices) create. In the United States, communities may yet have time to slow the onslaught of chronic disability and shift the direction, slow the pace, and humanize the scope of economic and social life.

To shift directions in today's health care patterns may be possible only when nurses and other health profession-

als do what is expected of them as leaders in the care of health: to work with others through open processes; to provide leadership in finding the vision and the path; and to inform, educate, and reeducate themselves, their colleagues, the media, and the general public using research findings and evidence-based practice methods. **Website Resource 1A** presents 21 competencies for health professionals in the twenty-first century developed by the Pew Health Professions Commission.

The responsibility of nurses as health professionals today is to see the health problem in new ways and help others to do the same. Responsibility means developing new roles and looking at the problem through others' eyes, including the eyes of individuals, the public, other professionals, and other nations. Responsibility also means evaluating the social and individual consequences, the long-term and short-term effects, and the public and private interests that are involved when deciding on the set of tools to use in the care of health.

CARE PLAN

Health Assessment: Frank Thompson and Family

Nursing Diagnosis: Risk for Ineffective Coping Due to Change in Role Performance and Self-Esteem

DEFINING CHARACTERISTICS

- Inability to complete tasks
- Lack of focus on needs
- Feelings of inadequacy
- Inability to make decisions
- Sense of being overwhelmed
- Rest and sleep disturbance
- Frequent stress-related headaches
- Emotional fragility
- Assessment of situations does not match assessments of others

RELATED FACTORS

- Unexpected life changes
- Diagnosis of chronic disease
- Stressful life events
- Unsure of family supports
- Unrealistic expectations of self
- Unpredictable future
- Need to reassess abilities
- Insecure job status

EXPECTED OUTCOMES

- The person will develop realistic expectations of capabilities based on rehabilitation potential.

- The nurse and person will set mutually agreeable milestones for resuming functions.
- The person will develop a revitalized sense of self.
- The person and family will use available resources to examine social and role shifts that affect the family.
- The person and spouse will express to each other their hopes and fears about the future.

INTERVENTIONS

- Listen to the concerns of the person and spouse regarding job, social, family, and medical concerns.
- Counsel the individual and spouse about realistic goals and expectations of cardiac rehabilitation.
- Assist the individual in setting realistic and reachable short-term goals.
- Assist the individual in developing more effective problem-solving skills.
- Provide support and positive feedback as short-term goals are met.
- Explore available community services that match the goals of the family.
- Facilitate family access to needed services through advocacy and supportive guidance.
- Supervise and teach about the use of prescribed and other medications.
- Coordinate communications between providers, employers, and other organizations to meet coping needs of the individual and his or her family.

REFERENCES

Ajzen, A., & Fishbein, M. (1980). *Understanding attitudes and predicting social behavior.* NJ: Prentice-Hall.

Allen, F. M., & Warner, M. (2002). A developmental model of health and nursing. *Journal of Family Nursing, 8*(2), 96–135.

American Nurses Association. (2003). *Nursing's social policy statement.* Washington, DC: ANA Publications.

American Nurses Association. (2004). *Nursing: Scope and standards of practice.* Washington, DC: ANA Publications.

American Nurses Association. (2008). *Code of ethics for nurses with interpretive statements.* Washington, DC: ANA Publications.

Andresen, E. M., Catlin, T., Wyrwich, K. W., & Jackson-Thompson, J. (2003). Retest reliability of surveillance questions on health related quality of life. *Journal of Epidemiology and Community Health, 57*(5), 339–343.

Ardell, D. B. (2007). *What is wellness.* Retrieved January 18, 2007, from *www.seekwellness.com/wellness/articles/what_is_wellness.htm.*

Bandura, A. (1976). *Social learning theory.* NJ: Prentice-Hall.

Bandura, A. (1999). *Self-efficacy: The exercise of control.* NY: W. H. Freeman Company.

Bandura, A. (2004). Health promotion by social cognitive means. *Health education Behavior, 31*(2), 143–164.

Barr, D., Lee, P., & Benjamin, A. (2003). Health care and health policy in a changing world. In H. Wallace (Ed.), *Health and welfare for families in the 21st century* (2nd ed.). Boston: Jones & Bartlett.

Berry, R. (2004). Community-oriented nurse as parish nurse. In M. Stanhope & J. Lancaster (Eds.), *Community & public health nursing* (pp. 1092–1113). St. Louis: Mosby.

Burns, N., & Grove, S. K. (2003). *Understanding nursing research* (3rd ed.). Philadelphia: Saunders.

Cano, A., Scaturo, D., Sprafkin, R., Lantinga, L., Fiese, B., & Brand, F. (2003). Family support, self-rated health, and psychological distress. *Primary Care Companion Journal of Clinical Psychiatry, 5,* 111–117.

Canto, J. G., Allison, J. J., Kiefe, C. I., Fincher, C., Farmer, R., Sekar, P., et al. (2000). Relation of race and sex to the use of reperfusion therapy in Medicare beneficiaries with acute myocardial infarction. *New England Journal of Medicine, 342*(15), 1094–1100.

Cloonan, P. (2004). *Health literacy in public health nursing education.* Abstract retrieved August 30, 2004, from *http://apha.confex.com/apha/132am/techprogram/paper_85683.htm.*

David, R. (2000). *Keynote address: Leadership for innovation in health care.* In *Ford Foundation, John F. Kennedy School of Government, Summary of Proceedings, Local Innovations in Health Care Conference,* Cambridge, MA. June 28–30, 2000.

Dunn, H. (1961). *High-level wellness.* Arlington, VA: R.W. Beatty Co.

Gordon, M. (2006). *Manual of nursing diagnosis* (11th ed.). Sudbury, MA: Jones & Bartlett Publishers.

Greiner, P., Snowdon, D., & Greiner, L. (1996). The relationship of self-rated function and self-rated health to concurrent functional ability, functional decline, and mortality: Findings from the Nun Study. *The Journal of Gerontology. Series B, Psychological Sciences and Social Sciences, S, 51B*(5), S234–S241.

Greiner, P., Snowdon, D., & Greiner, L. (1999). Self-rated function, self-rated health, and postmortem evidence of brain infarcts: Findings from the Nun Study. *The Journal of Gerontology. Series B, Psychological Sciences and Social Sciences, 54*(4), S219–S222.

Grzywacz, J., & Fuqua, J. (2000). The social ecology of health: Leverage points and linkages. *Behavioral Medicine, 26*(3), 101–115.

Haley, K., Koenig, H., & Bruchett, B. (2001). Relationship between private religious activity and physical functioning in older adults. *Journal of Religion and Health, 40*(2), 302–312.

Hollingsworth, L., & Didelot, M. (2005). *Illness: The redefinition of self and relationships.* Paper presented at the 4th Global Conference—Making Sense of: Health, Illness, and Disease, Mansfield College, Oxford, Great Britain.

Idler, E., & Benyamini, Y. (1997). Self-rated health and mortality: A review of twenty-seven community studies. *Journal of Health and Social Behavior, 38*(1), 21–37.

Institute of Medicine. (2003). *The future of the public's health in the 21st century.* Washington, DC: National Academies Press.

Institute of Medicine. (2004). *Health literacy: A prescription to end confusion.* Washington, DC: National Academies Press.

Issel, L. M. (2004). *Health program planning and evaluation: A practical, systematic approach for community health.* Sudbury, MA: Jones & Bartlett.

Izzo, J., & Black, H. (Eds.). (2003). *Hypertension primer* (3rd ed.). Philadelphia, PA: Lippincott, Williams, and Wilkins.

Janz, N., Champion, V., & Strecher, V. (2002). The health belief model. In K. Glanz, B. Rimer, & F. Lewis (Eds.), *Health behavior and health education: Theory, research and practice* (3rd ed.). San Francisco: Jossey-Bass.

Johnson, R., & Wolinsky, F. (1993). The structure of health status among older adults: Disease, disability, functional limitation, and perceived health. *Journal of Health and Social Behavior, 34,* 105–121.

Kreuter, M., & Devore, R. (1980). Update: Reinforcing the case for health promotion. *Family & Community Health, 10,* 106.

Leavell, H., & Clark, A. E. (1965). *Preventive medicine for the doctor in his community.* New York: McGraw-Hill.

McKivergin, M. (2004). The nurse as an instrument of healing. In B. Dossey, L. Keegan, & C. Guzzetta (Eds.), *Holistic nursing: A handbook for practice* (pp. 233–254). Sudbury, MA: Jones and Bartlett.

National Heart, Lung, and Blood Institute. (2000). *The practical guide: Identification, evaluation, and treatment of overweight and obesity in adults.* NIH Publication No. 00-4084. Bethesda, MD: U.S. Government Printing Office.

National Institutes of Health, National Center for Complementary and Alternative Medicine. (2007). *What is CAM?* Retrieved December 20, 2007, from *http://nccam.nih.gov/health/whatiscam/.*

National Institute of Nursing Research (NINR). (2006). *NINR strategic plan.* U.S. Department of Health and Human Services, National Institutes of Health, Pub. No. 06-4832.

Newman, M. (2003). A world of no boundaries. *Advances in Nursing Science, 26*(4), 240–245.

Norwood, S. (2003). *Nursing consultation: A framework for working with communities* (2nd ed.). Upper Saddle River, NJ: Prentice Hall.

O'Donnell, M. (1987). Definition of health promotion. *American Journal of Health Promotion, 1*(1), 4–5.

Pender, N. J., Murdaugh, C. L., & Parsons, M. A. (2006). *Health promotion in nursing practice* (5th ed.). Upper Saddle River, NJ: Prentice Hall.

Prochaska, J., Gill, P., & Hall, S. (2004). Treatment of tobacco use in an inpatient psychiatric setting. *Psychiatric Services, 55,* 1265–1270.

Reed, P. G. (1983). Implications of the life-span developmental framework for well-being in adulthood and aging. *Advances in Nursing Science, 6*(1), 18–25.

Riley, J., Cloonan, P., & Norton, C. (2006). Low health literacy: A challenge to critical care. *Critical Care Nursing Quarterly, 29*(2), 174–178.

Rogers, M. (1970). *An introduction to the theoretical basis of nursing.* Philadelphia: F.A. Davis.

Sackett, D., Rosenberg, W., Gray, J., Haynes, R., & Richardson, W. (1996). Evidence based medicine: What it is and what it isn't. *British Medical Journal, 312,* 71–72.

Shilling, C. (2002). Culture, the "sick role" and the consumption of health. *The British Journal of Sociology, 53*(4), 621–638.

Siegel, D. (2007). *The mindful brain: Reflection and attunement in the cultivation of well-being.* New York: W.W. Norton & Co.

Smith, J. A. (1983). *The idea of health: Implications for the nursing profession.* New York: Columbia University Teachers College Press.

U.S. Department of Health, Education, and Welfare, Public Health Service. (1979). *Healthy people*. U.S. Department of Health and Human Services. Washington, DC: U.S. Government Printing Office.

U.S. Department of Health and Human Services, National Institutes of Health, National Heart, Lung, and Blood Institute, Obesity Education Initiative. Retrieved February 2, 2008, from *www.nhlbi.nih. gov/health/public/heart/obesity/lose_wt/index. htm*.

U.S. Department of Health and Human Services, Office of Disease Prevention and Health Promotion. (2003). *Communicating health: Priorities and strategies for progress*. U.S. Department of Health and Human Services. Washington, DC: U.S. Government Printing Office.

U.S. Department of Health and Human Services, Public Health Service. (1986).

The 1990 health objectives for the nation: A midcourse review. U.S. Department of Health and Human Services. Washington, DC: U.S. Government Printing Office.

U.S. Department of Health and Human Services, Public Health Service. (1990). *Healthy people 2000: The Surgeon General's report on health promotion and disease prevention*. U.S. Department of Health and Human Services (Publication No. 7955071). Washington, DC: U.S. Government Printing Office.

U.S. Department of Health and Human Services, Public Health Service. (1996). *Healthy people 2000 mid-course review and 1995 revisions*. Boston: Jones & Bartlett.

U.S. Department of Health and Human Services, Public Health Service. (2000). *Healthy people 2010 (conference edition, in two volumes)*. U.S. Department of Health and Human Services. Washington, DC: U.S. Government Printing Office.

U.S. Department of Health and Human Services, Public Health Service. (2006). *Healthy people 2010 midcourse review*. Retrieved February 2, 2008, from *www. healthypeople.gov/Data/midcourse/*.

U.S. Department of Homeland Security. (2003). *Yearbook of immigration statistics, 2002*. Washington, DC: U.S. Government Printing Office.

U.S. Preventive Services Task Force. (2007). *Guide to clinical preventive services, 2007*. Retrieved February 2, 2008, from *www. ahrq.gov/clinic/pocketgd.htm*.

Vanderbilt University. (2008). *HEALTH plus program*. Retrieved February 2, 2008, from *www.vanderbilt.edu/HRS/wellness/health-plus.htm*.

World Health Organization. (2004). *About the World Health Organization*. Retrieved July 18, 2004, from *www.who.int/about/en/*.

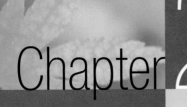

Chapter 2

Geraldine Valencia-Go

Emerging Populations and Health

After completing this chapter, the reader will be able to:

- Distinguish voluntary large scale migration from involuntary migration.
- Differentiate among ethnicity, ethnic group, race, and minority group.
- Describe demographic data relative to emerging populations:
  - Arab Americans
  - Asian Americans/Pacific Islanders
  - Black/African Americans
  - Latino/Hispanic Americans
  - Native Americans
  - Homeless Persons
  - HIV-AIDS–Afflicted Persons
- Discuss selected cultural factors that may have an impact on the health and well-being of emerging populations.
- Describe health concerns and issues of emerging populations.
- Contrast the folk healing system from the professional care system.
- Explain strategies of the nursing profession to meet the needs of emerging populations.
- Describe initiatives to address the health care concerns of emerging populations.

key terms

Acculturation
Bipolarity
Chi
Collectivism
Complementary and alternative medicine
Culture
Emerging populations
Ethnic group
Ethnicity
Ethnocentric perspective
Folk healing system
Genital mutilation
Gentrification

Health disparities
Homelessness
Hot and cold concept of disease
Imagery
Individualism
Involuntary migration
Jing
Massage
Meditation
Minority group
Post-westernization
Professional care systems
Race

Refugees
Relaxation
Shaman
Skid row
Sojourners
Taoism
Therapeutic touch
Transcultural nursing
Value orientations
Values
Voluntary large-scale migration
Yang
Yin

website materials

THINK About It

A New Brand of Outreach for Chemically Dependent Homeless People Living with HIV-AIDS

Access to health care services is often a major barrier for people who are considered underserved by the health care system. Community outreach programs have had some success in reaching persons with different types of health problems. However, outreach programs for certain marginalized populations have not always been successful in their efforts to reach the "hard-to-reach".

A new approach in outreach programs for chemically dependent homeless people living with HIV-AIDS is harm reduction. This approach "acknowledges the reality that drug use is a part of life. Rather than condemn or condone, harm reduction practitioners seek to work collaboratively with the client" (Shepard, 2007, p. 26).

Harm reduction as a part of outreach programs:

1. Aims to build on the ability of individuals to make decisions about their own lives
2. Views drug use along a spectrum, ranging from heavy use to abstinence
3. Honors self-determination and individual dignity
4. Functions as an alternative model of treatment that reinforces a hierarchical doctor-client relationship
5. Emphasizes incremental change in manageable steps for the client

Practitioners who view harm reduction as an essential component of outreach:

1. See the clients as experts of their lives and their addiction

2. Consider the structural factors that influence adoption of healthy lifestyles
3. Facilitate an egalitarian relationship between the client and the provider
4. Consider all the multiple pressures affecting client functioning in all spheres of life

With the above premises and beliefs, an outreach program explored the service utilization of chemically dependent persons living with HIV-AIDS. The study's purpose was to investigate whether hard-to-reach participants, lodged through a harm reduction program at single-room occupancy hotels, access health services at the same level as those who report at the agency's drop-in center (Shepard, 2007). Data indicate that low-threshold harm reduction outreach did increase access to health services by reducing barriers to services.

The researcher concluded that this component of outreach is a "valuable intervention for increasing utilization among this highly marginalized group" (p. 26). Will this philosophy of outreach be effective in helping persons with chronic illnesses such as diabetes, hypertension, obesity just to name a few? Something to think about!

From Shepard, B. (2007). Harm reduction outreach services and engagement of chemically-dependent homeless people living with HIV/AIDS: An analysis of service utilization data to evaluate program theory. *The Einstein Journal of Biology and Medicine, 23,* 26-32.

At the close of the twentieth century, there was a sense of optimism relative to the health of the U.S. population because of the progress in achieving of the goals of *Healthy People 2000*. A follow-up federally-supported initiative, *Healthy People 2010*, has 28 identified focus areas, and its goals are to increase quality of life and eliminate health disparities (U.S. Department of Health and Human Services, 2000). Predicted positive outcomes include "significant decreases in infant mortality, declines of death rates for coronary heart disease and stroke and advances in cancer management. The complex and dynamic interplay of economic, political, social, and technological factors will require active participation in advocating for health, home, community, business, state, and nation" (Valencia-Go, 2006, p. 42).

Health disparities have become a major focus of the work of health care professionals. They have been described as "chasms in health status between the advantaged and the disadvantaged" (Martino Maze, 2005, p. 546). One reason proposed to explain health disparities is that the populations who receive the latest and best health care are active participants in health research while those who receive less optimal care are less likely to be involved in such research. Participation of minorities in health research is characterized by low recruitment and retention (The Office of Minority Health, 2007a). Many reasons have been proposed for this. One reason, lack of cultural understanding on the part of White researchers and recruiters, could be effectively overcome through education for culturally competent care. The intent of this chapter is to provide an overview of the current status, culture, cultural aspects relative to health, and health issues of the major ethnic minority populations. Those groups considered to be disenfranchised—e.g., homeless persons and persons who are human immunodeficiency virus (HIV) positive and have acquired immune deficiency syndrome (AIDS)—are discussed as well. Information about these groups will hopefully facilitate the work of health care professionals, who in turn might take action to address health disparities.

EMERGING POPULATIONS IN THE UNITED STATES

Currently, **emerging populations** include ethnic minorities, persons who are homeless, and those persons afflicted with HIV-AIDS. Ethnic minority populations include Asian Americans–Pacific Islanders, Blacks/African Americans, Latinos/Hispanic Americans, Native Americans, and Arab Americans. It is important to note that people who reported only one race are identified under single-race population. For instance, "respondents who reported their race as one or more detailed Asian groups, but no non-Asian race, would be included in the single-race Asian population" (Reeves & Bennett, 2004, p. 2).

The presence in the U.S. of the major ethnic groups that are the foci of this chapter could be attributed to a number of factors. One major factor is **voluntary large-scale**

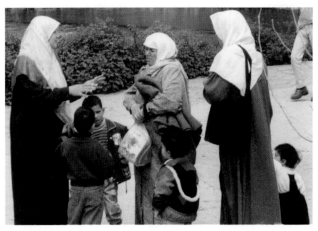

Arab American mothers with their children dressed in Western-style clothing.

migration, generally motivated by the quest of the individual or group for one or more goals including (a) educational opportunities, (b) economic benefits, (c) social improvements, and (d) political or religious freedom (Fox et al., 2001). Those who come to the U.S. for a more positive experience are identified as immigrants and those who "leave their homeland under threat of injury or loss of life due to political or religious persecution" (p. 778) as **refugees**. Orozco (2001) classifies immigrants on the basis of permanence in the new country. There are the immigrants whose move is permanent and "**sojourners**" (p. 7212) who stay for a specified length of time and then return to their homelands. Contract workers such as farm workers fall into this category as do those who travel back and forth from the adopted country and their homeland to see remaining family members, check on business enterprises, or temporarily escape the winter months.

Another type of migration is **involuntary migration**. Meilaender (2001) identified fleeing a hostile army, civil war, and political anarchy as reasons that cause involuntary movement of people to other lands. Natural disasters such as fires, floods, famines, earthquakes, and volcanic eruptions cause people to search for safer, more secure places to live. A more severe situation occurs when people are literally forced out of their countries as in the slave trade of Africans, who were considered to be an abundant source of cheap labor (Bookman, 2002). More recently, there is "indentured servitude" (p. 140), which is the plight of persons who have been lured by the promise of attractive job opportunities in another country only to find themselves trapped in low-paying menial jobs or prostitution.

Involuntary and voluntary migratory movements result in ethnic diversity that presents both problems and advantages. "Advantages might include a wide array of cultural activities such as festivals and restaurants. Problems include widespread uneven political representation, inequities in housing and employment, language instruction difficulties in schools, and interethnic tensions" (Vigil & Roseman, 2001, p. 410). As a nation of diverse peoples faces the challenges of the twenty-first century, will there be a unified quest to address the basic needs of every individual? Increasing awareness and understanding are key elements to achieving this goal.

ETHNICITY, ETHNIC GROUP, MINORITY GROUP, AND RACE

The U.S. Bureau of the Census, in its official reports, uses a system of classification that groups people into ethnic, racial, or minority groups (Holmes, 2003; Williams, 2000). However, the U.S. Office of Management and Budget issued a policy directive that established four races and two ethnicity categories. "The racial categories include White, Black, American Indian/Alaska Native, and Asian Pacific Islander. The ethnicity categories, Hispanic origin and not of Hispanic origin" (Holmes, 2003, p. 1) are used by the U.S. Bureau of the Census in presenting data about persons and families. There are, however, differences in these terms as proposed in numerous anthropological and sociological resources. It is reassuring to note that the U.S. Bureau of Census is continuing its work in refining the categories. This work is difficult and challenging given that many persons in the U.S. are "multiracial and multiethnic in ancestry" (Williams, 2001, p. 1436).

Race emphasizes "physical properties and biological heredity" (Bookman, 2002, p. 4). Early in the eighteenth century, race was used as a designation for "the descendants of a common ancestor, emphasizing kinship rather than skin color or other physical characteristics (Feagin, 2001, p. 12711). Later in the century, race evolved as a categorical system to designate persons with distinctive physical characteristics such as skin color, physique, hair texture, and facial features. Leading intellectuals of the late eighteenth and early nineteenth centuries "increasingly proclaimed the virtues and privileges of whiteness" (p. 12712). The crystallization of the distinction between "white race" and "inferior race" became widespread as "Europeans expanded their colonial adventures overseas. Colonizers developed racist rationalizations for their destruction of indigenous societies, enslavement of Africans, and other colonial pursuits" (Feagin, 2001, p. 12712).

The use of race to categorize persons is losing ground with research data indicating that "there is more variation within races than between them and although there are patterns to the distribution of genetic characteristics, our racial categories do not capture biological distinctiveness. Racial taxonomies are arbitrary, and race is more of a social category than a biological one" (Williams, 2001). In American society, race is socially constructed (Yancey, 2003). "Americans attach social meanings to the perceived biological differences associated with racial differences. This definition leads to the construction of a racial identity that has profound sociological implications" (pp. 10-11). Further, "race is only a rough proxy for socioeconomic status, culture, genes, but it precisely captures the social classification of people in a race-conscious society such as the United States" (Jones, 2000, p. 1212).

Ethnicity is a reference to a collective identity, a sense of uniqueness within the larger society, and a distinction from nonmembers. Ethnicity denotes a sharing of customs, food, dress, music, religion, and of symbols, such as language, among those who see themselves as fellow members of the group (Ben-Rafael, 2001; Gabaccia, 2002; Greene, 2000; Henslin, 2001). An **ethnic group** may have "common geographic origins, family patterns, language, religion, values, traditions, and symbols, music, dietary preferences, and employment patterns" (Williams, 2000, p. 210). The ethnic group includes those members with the sense of belonging to the collective identity. An "ethnic group is a group that is set apart by insiders or outsiders primarily on the basis of cultural or national origin characteristics subjectively selected" (Feagin, 2001, p. 12712). Although ethnic groups can share a range of phenotypic characteristics due to shared ancestry, the term *ethnicity* is typically used to highlight cultural and social characteristics instead of biological ones (Bookman, 2002; Williams, 2001). "Ethnic groups are socially organized groups with salient differences with respect to other groups in society" (Winkelman, 2001, p. 283). Ethnic groups provide some common identification with members. They are reference groups from which a member "acquires personal characteristics, social and psychological attachments, definitions of self, and a sense of common membership or group belonging" (p. 286).

Values and perceptions about health and illness evolve from the socialization process within a person's ethnic group. A sense of ethnicity also inspires the person to form a network of individual and group relationships that are maintained and nurtured by frequent interactions. The importance that individuals place on their families and other relatives as sources of formal and informal support during illness and crisis is a significant aspect of ethnic culture. Ethnicity plays an important role in relationships between people (Winkelman, 2001). Specific roles and expectations regarding different life situations facilitate optimal functioning of individuals. For example, "children learn basic facts of their family history and origins and the cultural content and practices associated with their ethnicity in their households" (Waters, 2001). Finally, ethnicity provides a basis for assessing the value systems of other groups (Winkleman, 2001).

The misuse of racial and ethnic group identity created another group category, the **minority group**. "Racial categories reflected a hierarchy of racial preferences: Whites at the top, Blacks at the bottom, and other groups in the middle." Therefore, "racial categories capture some of the inequalities that emerged as attitudes and beliefs about racial groups that became policies and societal arrangements to limit the opportunities and life chances of stigmatized groups" (Williams, 2000, p. 210). A minority group may be perceived as consisting of people who receive less

FEMALE GENITAL MUTILATION: TABOO OR TRADITION?

HOTtopics

Are the practices of people or groups to be condemned when these are deeply rooted in beliefs that such practices are essential aspects of life? Are practices considered to be taboo by some who do not share the same beliefs and that such practices are harmful? This is the case of female **genital mutilation** (FGM). What is the likelihood of health care providers having an encounter with circumcised women? Probably high because "although the incidence of FGM in women is worldwide, rough estimates range from 114-130 million women" (Little, 2003, p. 30). Migration of circumcised women to the U.S. and that "female circumcision has been practiced in U.S. since the 19th century" (Webber & Schonfeld, 2003, p. 65) increase the probability of these women's presence in health care settings. In countries that legally prohibit FGM, parents often feign a holiday or vacation to the native country and there have the young daughter circumcised.

Female circumcision and female genital mutilation have unknown origins. However, it is believed that the practice can be traced "in Africa as far back as the 5th century B.C. and has taken place in ancient Egypt, ancient Rome, Arabia, and Tsarist Russia" (Little, 2003, p. 30). There are four types of FGM:

1. Type 1, also known as clitoridectomy, is the excision of the clitoral prepuce and may also involve the excision of all or part of the clitoris.
2. Type 2 is the excision of the clitoris and may also involve the excision of all or part of the labia minora.
3. Type 3, also known as infibulation, involves excision of part or all of the external genitalia and the stitching or narrowing of the vaginal opening.
4. Type 4 refers to all other genital procedures (Momoh, 2004, p. 631).

It is a myth that FGM is advocated by specific individuals in cultures or societies that advocate and support this practice. Leval et al. (2004) analyzed the ways Swedish midwives discussed sexuality in circumcised African women. Their encounters with spouses in maternity wards dispelled the myth that men are the power holders. They were described as "always tender, caring, power shares, or even subordinates in the relationship" (p. 753). Support for this myth buster is seen in societies where adult women advocate and support the practice as an affirmation of their roles and high regard for their bodies (Little, 2003). Parents of young girls support the practice as an assurance of economic security for daughters (Gruenbaum, 2005). In some societies, powerful women leaders who are feared and respected promote this practice (Little, 2003).

There are many explanations for female circumcision. Gruenbaum (2005) offers a comprehensive discussion of these. Her analysis to approaches for proposed changes in the practice or its elimination through the passage of laws is extremely enlightening and provides a deep understanding of the complexities of FGM. There are cultural reasons, including health benefits, the preservation of virginity before marriage, a rite of passage, economic security for women as well as for the persons performing such acts, health (Gruenbaum, 2005; Little, 2003), and beliefs about sexuality and responses (Leval et al., 2004).

FGM has many complications. The immediate ones include hemorrhage, infections, abscesses, and urinary difficulties such as retention and straining. Long-term complications include difficulty voiding, urinary and reproductive tract infections, and incontinence. Other complications seen are infertility, painful intercourse, keloids, introital and vaginal stenosis, dermoid cysts, and pain. For the circumcised woman during labor, there is obstructed labor, fetal distress, perineal tears, perineal wound infection, and postpartum hemorrhage and sepsis (Little, 2004). Obermeyer (2005) contends that complications or consequences of FGM are poorly documented because of many methodological issues, including the quality of data collected. "Good quality research on the health consequences of female genital cutting has to overcome a number of difficulties, some of which are common to all epidemiological research—questions of variable definitions, sampling data collection—while others are specific to the problem of circumcision" (p. 445). Valid research on female circumcision is a fertile ground. Obermeyer's (2005) review of studies on FGM is an excellent resource for interested researchers.

What are the care implications for nurses? Midwives and nurses whose area of practice is women's health are more likely to have experiences with circumcised women. "It is essential that midwives recognize the cultural complexities of FGM and show sensitivity when caring and supporting women with FGM during pregnancy, labour, and the postnatal period" (Momoh, 2004, p. 634). Identification can start by asking, "Have you been closed? Did you have the cut or operation as a child?" (p. 634). Referrals to a specialist would facilitate discussion of legal issues and possible reversal of the procedure (infibulation). Procedures to reverse infibulation during labor might be performed. Other invasive procedures need to be avoided to eliminate possible sources of pain and stress. "Adequate pain relief is essential to prevent flashbacks and memories" (p. 634).

Following delivery, before reinfibulation or restitching is done, the health care provider needs to consider the laws governing this. Mother and baby, if female, are cared for with a view towards the future of the baby.

The information presented is but a very small representation of the continuing interests and work of people from diverse backgrounds. One powerful statement made by these scientists and caregivers is that whatever is done to eliminate FGM, "the cultural integrity of the people" (Little, 2003) must be preserved. Readers are strongly urged to read the cited references for a fuller understanding of FGM.

From Gruenbaum, E. (2005). Socio-cultural dynamics of female genital cutting: Research, findings, gaps, and directions. *Culture, Health & Sexuality, 7*(5), 420-441; Leval, A., Widmar, C., Tishelman, C., & Ahlberg, B. M. (2004). The encounters that rupture the myth: Contradictions in midwives' descriptions and explanations of circumcised women's sexuality. *Health Care for Women International, 25*, 743-760; Little, C. M. (2003). Female genital circumcision: Medical and cultural considerations. *Journal of Cultural Diversity, 10*(1), 30-34; Momoh, C. (2004). Attitudes to female genital mutilation. *British Journal of Midwifery 12*(10), 631-638; Obermeyer, C. M. (2005). The consequences of female circumcision for health and sexuality: An update on the evidence. *Culture, Health & Sexuality, 7*(5), 443-461; Webber, S. & Schonfeld, T. (2003). Cutting history, cutting culture: Female circumcision in the United States. *American Journal of Bioethics, 3*(2), 65-66.

than their share of wealth, power, or social status (Greene, 2000). "Minority status reflects the convergence of ethnic origin and socioeconomic disadvantage" (Williams, 2000, p. 211). In addition, minority group members "are subjected to unequal treatment through prejudice and discrimination by a dominant group" (p. 211).

CULTURE, VALUES, AND VALUE ORIENTATION

Ethnicity is evidenced in customs that reflect the socialization and cultural patterns of the group. **Culture**, as an element of ethnicity, consists of shared patterns of values and behaviors that characterize a particular group (Winkelman, 2001). It is "shaped by values, beliefs, norms, and practices that are shared by members of the same cultural group" (Giger & Davidhizar, 2008, p. 2).

Values are beliefs about the worth of something and serve as standards that influence behavior and thinking. "The value that an individual holds reflects cultural and social influences, relationships, and personal needs" (Ecker, 2003, p. 406). Cultural values "are unique, individual expressions of a particular culture that have been accepted as appropriate over time. They guide actions and decision-making that facilitate self-worth and self-esteem" (Giger & Davidhizar, 2008, p. 2). Relative to health, cultural values "shape human behaviors and determine what individuals will do to maintain their health status, how they will care for themselves, and others who become ill, and where and from whom they will seek health care" (Boyle, 2008, p. 266).

Value orientations, learned and shared through the socialization process, reflect the personality type of a particular society. The dominant value orientations are shared by the majority of the group. Kluckhohn's model (1953) of value orientations incorporates themes regarding basic human nature, the relationship of human beings to nature, human beings' time orientation, valued personality type, and relationships between human beings. **Website Resource 2A** shows various solutions to the questions proposed by Kluckhohn.

Health as a Value

Fifty years ago, Madeleine Leininger founded **transcultural nursing** "as a formal area of legitimate study and practice" (Leininger, 2000, p. 69), seeking to transform health care and help people of diverse cultures. Underlying her initiative was the belief that optimal health for all is an essential cultural value. Society generally believes that all people have a right to health care. "Educational programs, research projects, and clinical practices in transcultural nursing continue to be established and implemented to provide culturally sensitive, safe, competent, and meaningful care to people of diverse and similar cultures" (p. 69). An analysis of Leininger's vision for the work of transcultural nursing indicates that there are many barriers and issues in health care, particularly for persons from diverse cultures. For instance, health care for poor Americans and ethnic minorities is less than optimal because they are unable to pay for services because of lack

of insurance (Holmes, 2003). Health care insurance is not affordable for many poor Americans, whose priorities are the basic needs of health including food, clothing, and shelter rather than health care. Availability of health care facilities and resources does not mean accessibility because of multiple difficulties traveling to a facility, long waiting periods in clinics, the unattractive and impersonal surroundings of health care facilities, and lack of understanding of the process of obtaining care by health care consumers. Fragmentation of care and ethnocentric and impersonal attitudes of some health care providers place individuals in uncomfortable situations when intimate personal information is sought from them. For ethnic groups, health as a value may have different definitions and their behavior may reflect this.

Incongruent beliefs and attitudes about health and health care services among ethnic groups versus the rest of the population, particularly health care providers, are major barriers in improving the health status of ethnic group members. Leininger (2001) believes that "our rapidly growing multicultural world makes it imperative that nurses understand different cultures to work and function effectively with people having different values, beliefs, and ideas about nursing, health, caring, wellness, illness, death, and disabilities" (pp. 6-7). Health care providers need to become responsive to the cultural values of different peoples and how these could augment effective and humanistic care delivery.

FOLK HEALING AND PROFESSIONAL CARE SYSTEMS

A group has within its cultural and/or ethnic customs and traditions a healing system that incorporates the beliefs and practices deemed essential in maintaining and restoring health. Andrews (2008) identified three components of the healing systems of people including self-care, **professional care systems**, and folk healing systems. "Professional care is characterized by specialized education and knowledge, responsibility for care, and expectation of remuneration of services rendered" (p. 71). A **folk healing system** embodies the beliefs, values, and treatment approaches of a particular cultural group that are products of cultural development. Folk health practices are seen in a variety of settings, including community groups, kinship groups, private homes, and healers' shrines. Folk healers range from priests and medicine men and women to fortunetellers, astrologers, and geomancers. Unlicensed practitioners such as lay midwives, bone setters, and herbalists are part of the folk sector, as are religious practitioners such as spiritualists, Christian Scientists, and scientologists. Other areas of differences between folk and professional care systems are summarized in **Website Resource 2B**.

The choice of a health care system varies among ethnic groups and among individuals within the same group. Ethnic individuals' preference for their folk healing systems is motivated by their familiarity with the folk healer, who usually speaks the same language and is knowledgeable about the beliefs, customs, and traditions of the ethnic group. Easy access and the individual's ability to pay for the healer's services are real advantages when compared with the difficulty of getting appointments, the long waits, and the unfamiliar institutional settings in the professional care system. When folk healing practices are not effective, the individual may turn to the professional care system. Through a culturally sensitive assessment process, nurses can determine what specific folk remedies individuals are using and whether their continued use would interfere with the prescribed medical regimen. Andrews and Boyle (2008) and Giger and Davidhizar (2008) have developed transcultural assessment guides that nurses and other health care providers can use when working with ethnically diverse individuals. Selected cultural models by transcultural nurses can be found in **Website Resource 2C**. Health care professionals must avoid an ethnocentric perspective when working with ethnic groups. An **ethnocentric perspective**, which views other ways as inferior, unnatural, or even barbaric, can serve as a major obstacle in establishing and maintaining good working relationships with consumers of health care services.

Ethnic groups will continue to use folk remedies and healing. Therefore, health care professionals need to take a look at the many positive aspects of folk systems. A caring, holistic approach that incorporates family and support systems and considers the individual's viewpoint is one of the more positive aspects of folk systems. This approach is getting recognition by the professional care system. A blend of both systems would optimize health care for ethnic Americans.

ARAB AMERICANS

Arab Americans come from several countries; Lebanon is the home of most. Other countries include Syria, Palestine, Iraq, Egypt, Yemen, and Jordan. The term Arab is a "cultural, linguistic, and to some extent, political designation" (Abraham, 1995, p. 84). Politically, the Arab world is usually said to include 18 countries. In the linguistic sense, the term Arab "refers to those areas where most people speak Arabic as their native language" (Donner, 2002, p. 584). Arab Americans came to the U.S. in three immigration waves. The first wave of immigrants who came between the late 1800s and World War I were mostly from Greater Syria. The second wave came after the close of World War II and included many Muslims and refugees displaced by the 1948 Palestine War. The last wave occurred in the 1960s and consisted of many professionals, entrepreneurs, skilled and semiskilled laborers (Abraham, 1995; Stussy, 2000).

The U.S. Census of 2000 was a milestone survey because it recognized Arab Americans for the first time as a separate ethnic group. There are 1.2 million or 0.42% persons who reported an Arab ancestry. The three largest groups are the Lebanese, Syrians, and Egyptians. About 48% of the Arab population lives in California, Florida, Michigan, New York, and New Jersey. While the largest numbers reside in New York City, their proportion of the population is highest in Michigan (Brittingham & de la Cruz, 2005). Three major religions are represented among Arab Americans including Christianity, Judaism, and Islam (Chelala, 2002). Other statistical data on Arab Americans can be found in **Website Resource 2D**.

Health Care Issues of Arab Americans

There is a scarcity of health-related information (Kulwicki et al., 2000) and a paucity of scholarship about Arab Americans (Sayed, 2003). Available resources indicate that the most prevalent health problem is adult-onset diabetes, and coronary artery disease is on the rise (Hatahet et al., 2002). One of the largest groups of Arab Americans lives in Dearborn, Michigan (Jaber et al., 2003b). A study of the prevalence of diabetes among 542 participants revealed a 15.5% prevalence rate in women and 20.1% in men. Further, the prevalence for undiagnosed diabetes was 10%.

Several factors put Arab Americans at high-risk for diabetes including obesity, age, gender, low employment rates for both males and females, and lack of a high school education in women. The last two factors were examined in relation to the process of **acculturation**. Jaber et al. (2003a) suggested that acculturation issues play an important role in the development of diabetes. The phenomenon called **post-westernization** has been suggested to "explain the lower rates of diabetes associated with acculturation." "Acculturation is associated with the adoption of healthy western habits (such as isocaloric low fat diets and regular physical activity) rather than detrimental Western habits (such as hypercaloric high-fat diets and sedentary lifestyles)" (Jaber et al., 2003b, p. 2013).

Another health concern, where work has just begun, is mental health. Sayed (2003) looked at the concept of mental illness and mental health in Arab Americans. Analyses of several case studies indicate that therapists need to be fully aware of cultural meanings and significance of therapeutic approaches, such as psychotherapy, in order to bring about a comfortable therapist-client relationship. Similarly, Nassar-McMillan and Hakim-Larson (2003) looked at counseling considerations among Arab Americans. They suggested integrating Arab Americans' receptivity to counseling, cultural and religious backgrounds, and self-perceptions in counseling approaches. The last one is important as it relates to how an Arab American individual perceives the U.S. and thus how receptive that person would be to a non-Arab therapist.

Many barriers exist that prevent Arab Americans from using professional care services. These include religious beliefs and practices, cultural norms relating to modesty, family values of upholding the family's reputation, gender issues such as preference for same sex health provider, use of folk remedies, and stresses of assimilation and acculturation such as lack of English skills. There are also barriers related to the health providers including lack of culturally competent services and attitudes such as stereotyping and discrimination (Kulwicki et al., 2000; Nassar-McMillan & Hakim-Larson, 2003).

A health issue on the rise among Arab American adolescents is smoking, considered to be a major risk factor for many health problems affecting the respiratory and cardiovascular systems. Islam and Johnson (2003) looked at smoking behavior among 480 seventh to twelfth graders and found peer smoking to "exert a stronger influence on adolescents' susceptibility and experimentation than any other risk factor" (p. 331). Peer pressure was also found to be an important determinant of tobacco use in another study of Arab American adolescents by Kulwicki and Rice (2003). Islam and Johnson's (2003) data indicate that smoking rates were higher for males compared to females since males are more likely to spend time with other males. The researchers attributed the higher rates of smoking of Muslim Arab adolescents to their belief that smoking enhanced their masculinity. For females their lower rates of smoking reflect their concern for femininity, image, and reputation. Religion was also seen to exert a protective influence over experimentation for both genders. The researchers recommended that "including a religious perspective on smoking in preventive programs aimed at Muslim adolescents may be beneficial to protect them from progressing to habitual smoking" (p. 332).

Selected Health-Related Cultural Aspects

Arabs value the family and the ties it maintains. Therefore, the extended family, a clan, and tribe are common kinship groups. Customs center on hospitality around food, family, and friends (Abraham, 1995; Andrews, 2008; Donner, 2002). Religion plays an important part in Arab culture and there are dietary rules and prescribed rituals for praying and washing (Kavanaugh, 2008; Nassar-McMillan & Hakim-Larson, 2003). The male role is more dominant and women are expected to play a submissive role (Adib & Mikkey, 2003; Mikkey, 2003; Nagaty, 2003). The emphasis on preservation of female chastity and fidelity prohibits adult males from being alone with women, except for spouses. Some women do not shake hands with men and touching is done only within the marital relationship (Kavanaugh, 2008). Arab Americans are present oriented and view the future as uncertain (Kavanaugh, 2008).

ASIAN AMERICANS–PACIFIC ISLANDERS (AAPIs)

The AAPI population grew tremendously with two streams of immigration (Kim, 2001). Chinese, Koreans, and Filipinos, currently the three largest groups, came during the first stream and their numbers, 46.2% of all immigrants, added to the already large numbers in the U.S. In 2005, AAPIs numbered over 13 million (The 2007 Statistical Abstract, 2007). They were mostly highly educated and many came to join families and seek employment (Holmes, 2003). Current data can be found in **Website Resource 2E.** Native Hawaiians or Pacific Islanders include people from

Hawaii, Guam, Samoa, and other Pacific Islands (Reeves & Bennett, 2004). Asians include Asian Indians, Chinese, Filipinos, Japanese, Koreans, Vietnamese, and other Asians such as Cambodians, Laotians, Thais, Hmongs, and Malaysians (Qui & Ni, 2003). AAPIs are most likely to live in California, Washington, New York, Texas, and Utah (Reeves & Bennett, 2004).

AAPIs represent peoples from many different countries, so their origins, cultures, lifestyles, and religions are diverse. A look at the status of AAPIs, as a group, reveals that they are doing relatively well in the U.S. For instance, the median family income is $14,700, higher than the national median income for all households. Compared to other ethnic groups their poverty level is lower at 11% (Reeves & Bennett, 2004). In addition, AAPIs have surpassed all ethnic groups in educational achievement. Among first-time kindergartners, Asians surpassed all groups in persistence at tasks, eagerness to learn, and paying attention. Dropout rates for Asians ages 16 to 24 were the lowest among all ethnic groups and Whites (Holmes, 2003). A greater percentage earned bachelor's, master's, and doctoral degrees. Lastly, compared to 34% of the total population, about 44% are employed in management, professional, and related professions (Reeves & Bennett, 2004).

Health Care Issues of Asian American–Pacific Islanders

Variations in the health status of AAPIs are a result primarily of subcultures within the larger group. Additionally, little is known about the health issues of AAPIs because of the diversity among the different subgroups (Ozawa et al., 2006). Studies on the morbidity and mortality rates among the different subgroups of AAPIs are needed to fully understand their health issues. For instance a study of death rates during hospitalization for breast cancer indicates AAPI women come to treatment with more advanced stages of the disease. The study's researchers contend that "socioeconomic variables, combined with cultural beliefs and attitudes" (Polek et al., 2004, p. 72) might explain the hesitancy of AAPI women with breast cancer to seek early diagnosis and treatment. An integrative review on breast screening practice among Chinese, Korean, Filipino, and Asian Indian women found that "screening rates are far lower than the objectives targeted by *Healthy People 2010*" (Wu et al., 2005, p. 240). These researchers express their concern over the challenges faced by health care providers and policymakers in informing Asian women about "the benefits of breast health practices and the specific skills needed to perform screening practices at recommended intervals" (p. 243).

AAPIs have health problems similar to those of the U.S. population as a whole. Heart disease, cancers, and cerebrovascular problems are the leading causes of death. AAPI women are less likely to die from breast cancer, and mortality rates are lower compared to the other ethnic groups. However, AAPIs have the highest rates of tuberculosis, 36.6

cases per 100,000 persons. The infant death mortality rate of 5.5 deaths per 1000 live births is lower than that of any other race. Only 16.9% of AAPI women did not receive prenatal care, lower than all ethnic groups (Holmes, 2003). In 2003, AAPI men were 40% less likely to have prostate cancer compared to non-Hispanic Whites and less likely than White adults to die from heart disease. They have lower rates of HIV-AIDS. In general, AAPIs have lower rates of being overweight, lower rates of hypertension, and are less likely to be current cigarette users compared with White adults. In 2003, AAPI women were 30% less likely to have breast cancer compared to White women. However, they are 1.2 times likely to have cervical cancer compared to non-Hispanic Whites (The Office of Minority Health, 2007b).

Health care issues of AAPIs are relative to their status as immigrants and an ethnic group. Some Asian American immigrants have brought diseases from the home countries, and they may now experience new diseases because of their new lifestyle and living conditions. Others develop mental health issues such as depression relative to their inability to cope adequately in a new culture (Fox et al., 2001). Others exhibit a level of cultural rigidity that hinders their adjustment and thus access to the health care system that is wrought with multiple barriers. Important social problems that serve as barriers to health include (a) living in poverty, (b) socioeconomic conditions that stress intergenerational relationships when adult children cannot support and provide for older parents, (c) cultural norms that prevent people from seeking help outside the family, (d) incongruence between role expectations and fulfillment that strain spousal relationships, (e) change in child-rearing practices that challenge family harmony, and (f) loss of important social networks that could lead to depression and anxiety (Dhooper, 2003). These factors combined with poor access and underutilization of health services increase risks and produce more negative health outcomes in this group.

Mental health problems among Asian Americans can be attributed to the stresses of adjustment to a new culture including "pressure to succeed, immigration and acculturation stressors, shame and denial, discrimination and racism" (Kuramoto & Nakashima, 2000, p. 58). Leong and Lau (2001) looked at cognitive, affective, value orientation, and physical barriers to providing effective mental health services to Asian Americans. They found that cognitive barriers include thoughts that "encompass traditional Asian notions of the nature, causes, and cures of mental illness and of well-being" (p. 203). Thus, Asian Americans may not readily seek help for mental illness unless the behaviors are "upsetting to the social group" (p. 203). Further, most would first rely on folk healers. Affective barriers include "culturally-based affective responses" (p. 303) such as shame and stigma that are avoided at all costs to protect the reputation of the family. Closely related to the cognitive barriers are those that relate to value orientation. Asian Americans put emphasis on the family as a group rather than the individual. Hence, when "many traditional psychotherapy orientations place

high value on open communication, exploration of intra-psychic conflicts, and a focus on the individual" (p. 204), Asian Americans perceive these to be in conflict with their value of **collectivism** versus **individualism**. Physical barriers, not necessarily unique to Asian Americans, include "lack of awareness of available services due to economic and geographic realities" (Leong & Lau, 2001, p. 204).

Selected Health-Related Cultural Aspects

AAPIs share many traditional values. A comprehensive description of traditional values in several Asian groups indicates commonalities and differences (Andrews & Boyle, 2008; D'Avanzo & Geissler, 2003). A list of some of the most important values is summarized in **Website Resource 2F**.

The family is the most important social institution for AAPIs (Dhooper, 2003; Kavanagh, 2008). Although family dynamics and structure vary in the different AAPI subgroups, one can see that the family is often the source of functional and psychological support (Doutrich & Colclough, 2008; Earp, 2008; Miller & Lass, 2008; Stauffer, 2008; Vance, 2008; Xu & Chang, 2008). Traditional familial values such as respect for elders are part of everyday life. For instance among Filipinos, calling older persons by their first names is a sign of disrespect. Male friends of one's parents or grandparents are addressed as "Tito" (uncle) followed by the first name. For female friends it is "Tita" (aunt). These terms, denoting respect, have been substituted for Filipino terms that do not have English translations.

Many people find the task of parenthood in a new country difficult because some of their cultural values conflict with the mainstream cultural values—for example, passivity to avoid conflict versus assertiveness. Exposure of children

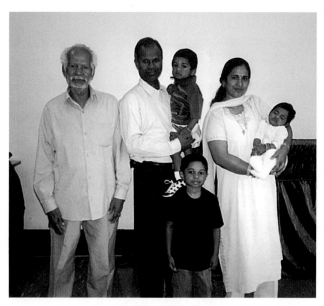

A three-generation Asian American/Pacific Islander family of Indian origin. The mother wears a sari, traditional Indian women's clothing.

to different cultures in schools and in their neighborhood facilitates their adoption of other cultural beliefs and attitudes in their socialization (Vance, 2008). Additionally, the employment of immigrant women outside the home has exposed their children to other caretakers. Grandparents are often the caretakers of young grandchildren. Filipino-American grandparents view their roles as part of their family responsibility (Kataoka-Yahiro et al., 2004).

Asian folk medicine and philosophies have a strong Chinese influence as a result of early Chinese migration throughout Asia. Therefore, the folk medicines of Filipinos, Japanese, Koreans, and Southeast Asians are all imbued with Chinese principles. **Taoism** was the philosophical and theoretical foundation of Chinese medicine. According to Tao doctrine, humans are microcosms within the universe. Achieving harmony between the two is essential because the energies of both intertwine. Two forces, **Yin** and **Yang**, keep innate energy, called **Chi**, and sexual energy, called **Jing**, in balance. Yin is feminine, negative, dark, and cold;

Yang is masculine, positive, light, and warm. An imbalance in energy can be caused, for instance, by yielding to strong emotions or eating an improper diet. In their interactions, humans and the universe are both susceptible to the elements of earth, fire, water, metal, and wood (Andrews, 2008; Kavanaugh, 2008; Yue et al., 2003).

Asian folk medicine uses a wide variety of herbs for healing purposes, including roots, leaves, seeds, tree bark, and parts of flowers. Some aspects of Asian folk medicine have gained popularity within the professional care system. In general the use or nonuse of healing traditions seems to be consistent with how closely Asians identify with their heritage (Tashiro, 2006). Of these, the best known is acupuncture (Andrews, 2008). Similar alternative treatment modalities that are slowly gaining wide acceptance are **meditation, therapeutic touch, massage, imagery, relaxation, and bipolarity**. The Research Highlights box discusses the rise of **complementary and alternative medicine (CAM)** among ethnic minority populations.

---

research highlights

Use of Complementary and Alternative Medicine (CAM) on the Rise Among Ethnic Minority Populations

Western medicine, supported by improved knowledge and advances in technology, has been successful in dealing with numerous illnesses. However, there remains a cadre of chronic illnesses and conditions that do not respond well to allopathic treatment. Persons who do not experience relief from chronic conditions often resort to complementary alternative medicine.

Complementary therapies are "those therapies used in addition to conventional treatment recommended by the person's health care provider" (Potter & Perry, 2006, p. 912). Acupuncture, biofeedback, relaxation, music therapy, massage, art, music, and dance therapy are some examples. Alternative therapies, on the other hand, include those approaches that become the person's choice of treatment as opposed to the conventional ones.

CAM use among ethnic minority populations has been the foci of several studies.

Kronenberg et al. (2006) looked at CAM use among non-Hispanic Whites, African Americans, Mexican Americans, and Chinese Americans. Data indicated that between one third and one half of persons from each group used at least one CAM modality. Furthermore, the use of CAM was an adjunct to traditional medicine rather than a substitute. There was also differential use among the groups. Since the Chinese Americans and Mexican Americans in the study were foreign-born, their use of different modalities, which were culturally based, was extensive as hypothesized by the researchers. Non-Hispanic White women, however, were found to be users of a wider

variety of approaches because of more social resources and greater access.

Looking at Asian Americans' use of CAM, Hsiao et al. (2006) conducted computer-assisted telephone interviews with 55,428 respondents. Data indicate that there are great variations in the use of CAM among the different subgroups. Chinese Americans used CAM more than the other subgroups and South Asians had the least usage. An important aspect of this study was the inclusion of spirituality as a predictor for CAM use. "Increased spirituality was associated with greater CAM use for all Asian-American subgroups" (p. 1009).

Finally, Owens and Dirksen (2004) reviewed and critiqued the literature of complementary and alternative therapy use among Hispanic/Latino women with breast cancer. The referent for this article can be attributed to the nondisclosure of CAM use by Hispanic/Latino women undergoing conventional therapies. Often adverse side effects, including death, have resulted when clients do not share CAM use with their health care providers. The researchers' review and critique of other studies provided an excellent start point for further studies that would focus on specific CAM modalities. They also provided a list of helpful questions that can be used as guidelines in assessing CAM use.

Overall, there is increasing concern over CAM use not only by ethnic minority populations but also by the other members of the U.S. population. The dynamic interplay of many factors that serve as barriers to accessing traditional health care and the person's own cultural beliefs warrant a close look at how CAM can greatly augment health care services.

Compiled from Hsiao, A., Wong, M.D., Goldstein, M.S., Becerra, L.S., Cheng, E.M. & Wenger, N.S. (2006). Complementary and alternative medicine use among Asian-American Subgroups: Prevalence, predictors, and lack of relationship to Acculturation and access top conventional health care. *The Journal of Alternative and Complementary Medicine, 12*(10), 1003-1010; Owens, B.O. & Dirksen, S.R. (2004). Review and critique of the literature of complementary and alternative therapy use among Hispanic/Latino women with breast cancer. *Clinical Journal of Oncology Nursing, 8*(2)151-156; Kronenberg, F, Wade, C.M. & Chao, M. T. (2006). Race/ethnicity and women's use of complementary and alternative medicine in the United States: Results of a national survey. Retrieved July 24, 2007, from *www.cinahl.cpm/cgi-bin/refsvc?jid=114&accno=2009227888*; Potter, P. A., & Perry, A. G. (2008). *Fundamentals of nursing* (7th ed.). St. Louis: Mosby.

LATINO/HISPANIC AMERICANS (LHAs)

In the last U.S. Census, the Latino/Hispanic population became the largest ethnic group. In 2005, there were 42,687,000 million Hispanics who accounted for 14.4% of the total U.S. population (The 2007 Statistical Abstract, 2007). "A high rate of immigration and high birth rate have combined to make Hispanic Americans one of the fastest-growing groups in the United States" (Garcia, 2001, p. 258). This ethnic group has relatively young members. The median age is 26 years compared with 35.4 years for the total population (Ramirez, 2004). For more statistical information see **Website Resource 2G**.

Hispanic Americans are also called *Latinos* because of their Latin American origins (Garcia, 2001). The Census Bureau revisited the term *Hispanic* and in 1996 redefined it and in 1997 "the Office of Management and Budget issued a standard by which the term Latino and Hispanic were to be used interchangeably" (Chong, 2002, p. 5). The largest Hispanic American subgroups are Mexicans, Puerto Ricans, and Cubans. Most Hispanics live in Texas, New York, Florida, and California (The Office of Minority Health, 2007c). Overall, LHAs tend to be urban dwellers (Benson, 2003; Garcia, 2001).

LHAs are making educational strides in spite of many barriers. "Discrimination continues to plague many Hispanic American students. Studies have shown that Hispanic students have often been assigned to classes for low achievers, forced to repeat grades, or classified as mentally handicapped because they do not speak English well or because of other cultural differences" (Garcia, 2001, p. 258). Among those 25 years of age and older, 52.4% completed high school. The percentage of those with some college and bachelor degrees is 40.7%. Finally, 3.8% have advanced degrees (Bauman & Graf, 2003).

Health Issues of Latino/Hispanic Americans

LHAs have many health issues complicated by multiple cultural, economic, political, and social factors. "Hispanics are the highest uninsured racial or ethnic group within the United States" (The Office of Minority Health, 2007c, p. 2). Lack of insurance can be attributed to employment of Hispanics in jobs that do not offer health insurance (Asamoa et al., 2004). In addition to lack of insurance, language and cultural barriers to preventive care have implications for their health (Sherrill et al., 2005). A study of LHA women found that excess risk of cervical cancer incidence and death are related to underutilization of preventive services. "Underutilization appeared to be strongly associated with possible indicators of low access to preventive services such as low income and uninsured status" (Asamoa et al., 2004, p. 658).

LHAs use and receive less preventive health care. They are at a "greater risk for reduced access to regular medical care, delays in getting necessary diagnosis and treatment, poorer health outcomes, increased suffering, and even death" (Lee & Estes, 2003). Most LHAs are employed in occupations that do not provide health insurance (Carter-Porkas & Zambrana, 2001; Holmes, 2003). Compared to other ethnic groups and the White population, only 49.9% of Hispanics have private insurance coverage. Several factors contribute to these barriers. LHAs might not have acquired citizenship; therefore, they have lower odds of being insured by employers. In addition, the lack of a high school education diminishes the opportunities to work in workplaces that offer health insurance. Many more Latinos are employed in agricultural, mining, service, domestic, and construction industries, which are not as likely to provide health coverage as other jobs (Carrillo et al., 2001).

Hispanic men and women have higher incidence and mortality rates for stomach cancer. Mexican American adults are two times more likely than non-Hispanic Whites to have diabetes and one and a half times as likely to die from this disease. Although cardiovascular disease and cancer are the first and second causes of morbidity and mortality among LHAs, their incidence in the general population is higher. Hispanic men were 20% less likely to die from stroke, and for women it is 30% compared to non-Hispanic Whites (The Office of Minority Health, 2007c)

Among adults 25 to 44 years of age in the Hispanic American population, HIV infection was ranked as the leading cause of death (Holmes, 2003). LHAs had the second-largest numbers of persons with HIV-AIDS at the close of 2005 (Centers for Disease Control and Prevention, 2005). "Even though Latinos are heavily impacted by HIV/AIDS, they may be reluctant to participate in HIV vaccine trials" (Brooks et al., 2007, p. 55). Mistrust and fear that the vaccine would jeopardize one's life, social repercussions of being HIV positive, and social stigma were found to be the barriers to participation. Among Hispanic American subgroups, socioeconomic status (SES) has been linked to health status. Cubans have a higher percentage (35%) of persons whose families earn $35,000 or more. Additionally, fewer families live below the poverty level. Overall, Puerto Ricans and Mexicans have the lowest incomes and have higher rates of living below the poverty level. Cubans report better health status compared with the other two subgroups. Health care contact and restricted activity days were lowest for Cubans (Hayat et al., 2000).

The difficulties experienced by LHAs in receiving appropriate health care services are identical to those of the poor and other ethnic minorities. Other barriers include the lack of racial and ethnic diversity in the leadership and workforce of the health care system. Lack of interpreter services for Spanish-speaking people and lack of or inadequate culturally appropriate health care resources serve as barriers in the delivery of care. Guendelman and Wagner's (2001) study of Hispanic experience within the health care system indicates the importance of emphasizing culturally appropriate personal interactions. These researchers propose that "culturally-appropriate personal interactions may serve as the basis for monitoring satisfaction with health care plans in the future" (p. 44). Poor access to health care providers and health care facilities also serve as a deterrent in obtaining care (Carrillo et al., 2001).

Many Hispanic Americans may not readily seek care because they have continued reliance on their folk system of healing. Their preference for this is logical given their lack of health insurance and perceived difficulties negotiating the health care system because of language and other sociocultural barriers.

One must note that underlying all the statistical data about the health status of LHAs is a major issue in the classification of ethnic groups in the U.S. "Racial and ethnic identification—and its public reporting—among Hispanics/Latinos in the United States is embedded in dynamic social factors. Ignoring these factors leads to significant problems in interpreting data and understanding the relationship of race, ethnicity, and health among Hispanics/Latinos" (Amaro & Zambrana, 2000, p. 1724). Furthermore, a careful study of the diversity of Latino and Hispanic cultures and more accurate reporting of demographic data based on a more effective system of surveying are essential in creating policies for the health and well-being of the largest ethnic group in the U.S.

Selected Health-Related Cultural Aspects

Each subgroup of the LHA population has distinct cultural beliefs and customs. However, a common heritage determines similar values and beliefs. For instance, the emphasis on family and religion are the two most important aspects of all Hispanic cultures. For older Hispanic Americans, the family is an important component of good health. The family is the most important source of support; therefore, the needs of the family as a whole supersede the needs of the individual. During times of illness and crisis, the family is there for the individual. Older family members and other relatives are accorded courtesy and respect and are often consulted on important matters (Andrews, 2008; Carbonell, 2003; Chong, 2002; Dumonteil & Gamboa-Leon, 2003).

LHAs' dependence on spiritual strength to aid them in illness and dying is evident in their use of prayer. They have "profound reverence for God and for other powerful forces they believe exist.… Furthermore, health and disease are believed to be consequences of God's approval or disapproval of a person's behavior" (Chong, 2002, pp. 26-27). LHAs attribute the origins of disease and illness to spiritual or natural punishments, hot and cold imbalances, magic, dislocation of internal organs, natural diseases, and emotional and mental issues. The **hot and cold concept of disease** was derived from the Hippocratic theory of pathology. Illness occurs when there is an imbalance. This concept of hot and cold guides Hispanics when they categorize illnesses and select appropriate treatments. For example, an elevated body temperature is managed by giving the person a cool drink to lower the fever. For a person who has a cold, drinking warm fluids would be considered therapeutic (Chong, 2002).

LHAs attribute illness and disease to many supernatural and psychological causes. The evil eye or the "mal de ojo" is an example. Fright or "susto" and hysteria or "ataque de nervios" are caused by strong emotions, crises, and traumatic experiences (Chong, 2002). LHAs still resort to many home remedies and consult folk healers including the curandero, spiritualist, *yerbero*, and the *sabador*. *Curanderos* use a variety of folk remedies, including prayers, rituals, herbs, and the laying on of hands. Spiritualists use medals, amulets, and prayers to affect a cure. The *yerbero* is knowledgeable in the use of herbs, while the *sabador* is an expert in massage and manipulation of bones and muscles (Andrews, 2008). Other Hispanic Americans, such as Cubans, practice *Santeria*. Persons who are ill may seek the advice of a "godfather" who is a member of the *Santeria*. Wearing White clothes for a year, performing rituals, and following dietary restrictions are involved in bringing forth a cure to an illness (Carbonell, 2003).

Folk remedies are used in combination with professional care approaches. The individual's belief in the folk remedy can have positive effects on the person's well-being. Therefore, professional care personnel need to find ways to blend the two systems to the optimal benefit of LHAs and their families.

BLACK/AFRICAN AMERICANS

There are currently 37 million BAAS (BAAs); they constitute 13% of the total U.S. population (The 2007 Statistical Abstract, 2007). More data on BAAs can be found in **Website Resource 2H**.

The immigration history of Blacks to America is significantly different from that of Europeans, Asians, and Hispanics. Most BAAs identify their ancestral heritage from

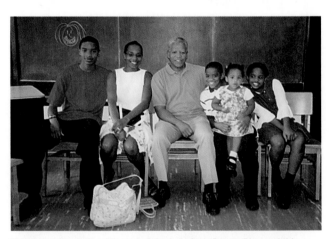

This father is a Latino/Hispanic American from Puerto Rico and this mother is a Black African American. Religion is important to both of these cultures. The family is photographed in a classroom at their church.

the western part of Africa that was controlled by three great and wealthy empires, Ghana, Mali, and Songhai. "Africans had practiced slavery during the ancient period. Slaves captured in warfare were sold to Arab traders of northern Africa" (Hornsby, 2001, pp. 136c-d). Portugal and Spain, as leaders in exploration and colonization, were involved in slave trade. Some believe that the first Blacks in America came with Christopher Columbus in 1492. Black slaves also traveled in other expeditions. The migration of BAAs can be identified as involuntary as this was forced, impelled, or imposed by explorers of the New World from Spain and Portugal. In the New World, many thriving industries had high demands for labor that the Native Americans could not fill; therefore, Africans were captured and sold as slaves (Black Americans, 2003)

The beginning of Black America is recorded as the time when "the first laborers were brought to Virginia from the Caribbean in 1619" (Gabaccia, 2002, p. 25). When these laborers completed their service, they were free to buy property. "But racial prejudice among White colonists forced most free Blacks to remain in the lowest level of colonial society" (Hornsby, 2001, p. 136d). Yancey (2003) contends that the "overarching feature of African American history is slavery, and the American slave system set the tone for future racism and alienation towards African Americans" (p. 44). Further, African Americans were not given the same treatment extended to other migrant groups who had the opportunity to assimilate into the dominant majority culture. "Slavery made it necessary for majority group members to maintain a caste system for African Americans that deprived them of any possible social acceptance, and despite the adoption by African slaves of many European American cultural aspects, such as Christianity, they were unable to engage in the process of assimilation that other racial and ethnic groups experienced" (Yancey, 2003, p. 45). As one of the largest ethnic groups in the U.S., Black/African Americans are considered a minority group, a label originating from their slavery roots. Therefore, they continue, in many ways, to experience extreme segregation and exclusion from mainstream society, and discrimination by the majority group.

BAAs have made substantial progress in many areas in the past century. However, there are still inequities in many areas such as business, education, political participation, and leadership. Educationally, BAAs have made substantial gains. In 2003, 72.3% completed high school; 42.5% attended college; 14.3% completed a bachelor's degree and 4.8% earned an advanced degree. Among the major ethnic groups discussed here, BAAs surpassed the Latinos/Hispanic and Native Americans. They still lag behind Whites in some levels of education (Bauman & Graf, 2003) as seen in **Website Resource 2I**. However, they have a higher percentage of registered nurses with masters and doctoral degrees, 14.2% compared with 13.2% among the White, non-Hispanic population (Health Resources and Services Administration, 2004).

Health Issues of Blacks/African Americans

A complex set of social, economic, and environmental factors can be identified as contributors to the current health status of Blacks/African Americans. However, poverty may be the most profound and pervasive determinant of health status. In the U.S., health care is a commodity that can be purchased according to an individual's ability to pay (Keith, 2000), and health care is expensive. Individuals and families who are below the poverty level or lack adequate resources are obviously the most affected. Poor people cannot afford health insurance. That limits their access to health care services such as prenatal and maternal care, childhood immunizations, dental checkups, well-child care, and a wide range of other health promotion preventive services. Decreased resources for preventive care may necessitate more expensive services, such as emergency room care and intensive care in times of severe illness (Mays et al., 2000). In 2003, only 51.5% of Black/African Americans had private insurance coverage compared to 65.6% of the total population. In 2005, 19.5% were uninsured (The Office of Minority Health, 2007d).

Two indices of the effects of poverty can be seen in the high rates of infant mortality and maternal mortality. Despite changes in living conditions, advances in infection control, and improved standards in neonatal care, BAAs still experience high infant and maternal mortality rates. In 2003, the infant mortality rate for BAAs was 2.4 times higher that of non-Hispanic Whites (The Office of Minority Health, 2007d). BAAs have the second-highest percentage of women who lack prenatal care in the first trimester of pregnancy (Holmes, 2003). Life expectancy for males is 68.3 years compared to 74.8 in White males. For BAA females, life expectancy is 75 years compared to 80 in White females (Holmes, 2003).

Black American children living below the poverty level experience numerous health problems, including malnutrition, anemia, and lead poisoning. These problems and the lack of immunizations combine to inhibit normal growth and development and affect school performance. Poverty-stricken families usually live in depressed socioeconomic areas where housing conditions are unsafe and unhygienic. Unsafe buildings and other environmental structures cause accidents and injuries among young children. Young children have fallen to their deaths from windows that were unprotected by metal railings. Older people have suffered falls and other injuries from poorly lit stairways and hallways. Other hazards include uncollected garbage and abandoned buildings that are used as dumpsites or as meeting places for a variety of illegal activities.

The incidence of cancer and mortality rates for BAAs is higher than that for White Americans. In 2003, BAAs were 1.4 times likely to have new cases of lung cancer and twice as likely to have stomach cancer. The five-year survival rate is lower for lung and pancreatic cancers. Men were 2.4 times more likely to die from prostate cancer than were to non-Hispanic White men. African American women are 36% more likely to die from breast cancer, and they are 2.2 times more likely to die from stomach cancer (The Office of Minority Health, 2007d). During 2005, among men, 41% living with HIV-AIDS were Black; among women, it was 64%. In 2005, 63% of the 166 children under the age of 14 diagnosed with HIV-AIDS were Black. In 2005 the total number of HIV-AIDS cases among BAAs was 18,121, (Centers for Disease Control and Prevention, 2005).

Severe high blood pressure is more common for Black Americans in both men and women. In 2003, there were 46.8 deaths per 100,000 BAAs compared with 12.8 deaths among Whites (Holmes, 2003). BAA adults are 30% more likely to have a stroke and males were 50% more likely to die from a stroke (The Office of Minority Health, 2007d).

Other health issues that are receiving more attention include obesity and its contributing factors (Adderly-Kelly & Williams-Stephens, 2003; James, 2004). Mental health concerns including depression and suicide are getting more attention. The work of Gary et al. (2003) on the epidemiology of suicide and Harley and Dillard's (2005) book on mental health issues are superlative resources for mental health professionals.

Selected Health-Related Cultural Aspects

Differences in cultural beliefs, attitudes, and practices exist between rural and urban Black Americans; however, they share some basic cultural beliefs. Black American culture is centered on the family and religion. The family, the strongest institution, provides strong extended kinship bonds with grandparents, aunts, uncles, and cousins. The family is considered the strongest source of support, especially in times of crisis and illness (Gary et al., 2003). Family members and relatives are consulted before BAAs seek care elsewhere. There is a "need to be involved in the family's caring, nurturing, and healing process" (Bailey, 2000).

Religion and religious behavior are an integral part of the BAA community. BAAs are said to be "the most religious group in the world" (McGadney-Douglass, 2000a, p. 202). The church, as the second most important institution for BAAs, has many purposes beyond worship and formation including (a) serving as a place to meet where members could pass news, take care of business, and find strength of purpose; (b) providing direct social welfare services; (c) acting as a stabilizing force in the community; (d) facilitating citizenship training and community social action; (e) serving as a transmitter of cultural history; and (f) providing the means for coping and surviving in a hostile world (McGadney-Douglass, 2000b).

The BAA church and spirituality also play an important role in health issues. For instance, prostate education for older men is received more favorably when done within the parish nursing approach (Lambert et al., 2002). An earlier study focused on African American churches as the sites where the perceived health needs of urban African American church congregants could best be considered. This study was an important milestone in establishing parish nursing where nurses, as members of the congregation, "may be uniquely positioned to work within the culture of the congregation and establish trusting, effective relationships" (Baldwin et al., 2001, p. 301). This is consistent with findings of earlier studies that indicated BAA beliefs that the disease is God's will (Kinney et al., 2002). Samaan (2000) looked at the influence of race, ethnicity, and poverty on the mental health of children. Although the views of Black children and White children regarding the importance of religion are not that different, Black children's attendance at religious services is "more pronounced" (p. 108). The researcher indicated that this factor could account for the lower rates of psychiatric illness attributed to the "communal buffering factor in attending church" (p. 108).

BAAS define *health* as a feeling of well-being and the ability to fulfill role expectations. Diseases can be caused by natural or spiritual forces (Bailey 2000; Kavanaugh, 2008). Therefore, BAAs' approach to health care is guided by these beliefs. Readers are referred to Bailey (2000) for an enlightening historical overview of African American alternative medicine. BAAs continue to use their own traditional health system, especially when they lack access to the professional care system (Fletcher, 2000). Family members, such as grandmothers and other community members, are often consulted for traditional home remedies. Traditionally, roots, herbs, potions, oils, powders, rituals, and ceremonies are still used in many Southern communities. The use of healers is also common, including the old lady, who is knowledgeable about folk remedies and child care; the spiritualist, who assists with financial, personal, spiritual or physical problems; and the voodoo priest or priestess, who is knowledgeable about herbs, signs, and omens (Andrews, 2008).

As noted with the folk health practices of Asian and Hispanic Americans, BAAs' folk healing beliefs and practices can augment the professional care system. Black Americans often find comfort in the support that their religious leader or traditional healer can give them. Health care providers must find an appropriate place for these nontraditional modalities when caring for BAAs.

NATIVE AMERICANS

Native Americans lived in America for thousands of years before the arrival of Europeans. Most scientists believe that Native American peoples came to Alaska via land bridges now known as the Bering Strait (Campbell, 2000; Fixico et al., 2001) although Native Americans themselves say they have always been here. Native Americans came to be known as Indians, a label given by Columbus when he encountered the native peoples in the West Indies that he mistook for the East Indies. This label was then extended to all the native peoples of North and South America, from the Arctic to Tierra del Fuego. Before 1492 there were an estimated 5 million Native Americans.

Columbus' discovery brought colonization and settlement by various European groups (Snipp, 2000). Thus, the ancestral lands of the Native Americans were usurped, and the people were forced to labor on farms and in mines. Thousands died from disease and hard labor or were killed in attempts to escape from slavery. Other events, such as the removal of the Southeastern tribes in 1830, the Navajos' Long March to Fort Sumner in 1864, and the massacre at Wounded Knee in 1890, caused the Native American population to dwindle to 250,000 by 1890 (Fixico et al., 2001).

The 1890 census, the first to obtain a complete count of Native Americans, reported an increase from 237,000 in 1900 to 357,000 in 1950. The period from 1950 to 1980 was a time of rapid growth. However, "conquest, subjugation, corruption, genocide, and ethnocide brought considerable transformations in the lives and governments of Native Americans from coast to coast" (Grinde, 2002, p. xiii). In 2005, Native Americans numbered 2,863,000 or about 1% of the total U.S. population (The 2007 Statistical Abstract, 2007). Other data can be found in **Website Resource 2J**. Native Americans are concentrated in Oklahoma, California, Arizona, New Mexico, Alaska, Washington, North Carolina, Texas, New York, and Michigan. Of the total Native American population of almost 2 million, 62.3% live off reservations and 37.7% live on Native American lands. There are 561 federally recognized tribes and more than 100 state-recognized tribes. The Cherokees make up the largest tribe (Ogunwole, 2006; Holmes, 2003).

Native Americans also experience minority group status. In important aspects of life, such as educational attainment and income levels, Native Americans lag behind Whites and other major ethnic groups. Native American percentages for higher education degrees are low in proportion to their total number. For example, in 2000 Native Americans ranked second lowest in members having some college education, bachelor's, and advanced degrees compared to other ethnic minority groups. The Latino/Hispanic group was ranked the lowest in these educational achievements. Among Native Americans, 70.9% are high school graduates compared to the 52.4% of the Latino/Hispanic group (Bauman & Graf, 2003). Native Americans have the lowest percentage, 0.3%, of the 311,177 registered nurses who reported ethnicity or race (Health Resources and Services Administration, 2004). Native Americans are making some progress in all levels of college education. However, low continuing educational attainment and income levels combined with higher rates of poverty are socioeconomic issues that affect health and the quality of life. Native Americans experience the many negative situations that confront poor people both on the reservations and in the larger society.

Health Care Issues of Native Americans

Many of the health problems of Native Americans can be linked directly to the social and economic conditions described here. These conditions predispose Native Americans to illnesses and health problems that afflict the poor. Some of these problems have been discussed in the section on BAAs. Although Native Americans have responded well to prevention and treatment of infectious diseases, other health problems are closely linked with poverty and harmful lifestyle practices (The Office of Minority Health, 2007e). For instance, Native Americans have the highest percentage of smoking compared with all groups of people in the United States. (Kegler et al., 2000).

Many Native American deaths can be attributed to unintentional injuries, cirrhosis, homicide, suicide, pneumonia, and complications of diabetes (U.S. Department of Health and Human Services, 2000). Among Native American men from 15 to 44 years of age, unintentional deaths from accidents and intentional deaths from suicide and homicide account for 80% of all deaths each year. Alcoholism-related deaths are 62.7% higher than for the overall U.S. population (Bohn, 2003). Alcohol use has been implicated as a major factor in the abuse of Native American women (Bohn, 2003; Lauderdale, 2003). "Living with abuse and becoming dependent on alcohol and other drugs are intertwined problems for many women, especially Native American women. The use and abuse of alcohol and/or drugs is one way of coping with an abusive relationship, but also places the woman and developing fetus at considerable health risk" (Lauderdale, 2003, p. 124). In a small sample of 30 Native American women, Bohn (2003) found that half of study participants reported a history of substance abuse, including alcohol.

Native American adults are 2.3 times more likely than White adults to have diabetes (The Office of Minority Health, 2007e). Harmful lifestyle practices, including poor nutrition and inadequate activity levels, are implicated in the development of diabetes, which kills twice as high a percentage of Native Americans compared to the White population. Hence, health researchers focus on lifestyle interventions to forestall the complications of diabetes (Gilliland et al., 2002). Boyle (2008) outlined the beliefs and practices related to diabetes. These beliefs include one's image and control of the body and illness as an unpleasant topic that needs to be avoided. A study by Wittig (2004) showed that "diabetes was cited most frequently by students as a disease that nurses should be knowledgeable about when caring for Native Americans because of the high incidence of this condition among the population" (p. 58).

Many mental health problems confront Native Americans. Difficult life situations and stresses of daily life contribute to an array of problems, including feelings of hopelessness, desperation, family dissolution, and substance abuse, specifically alcohol. In 1998, there were 13.4 suicides per 100,000 Native Americans, a higher incidence than for non-Hispanic Whites, non-Hispanic African Americans, and Hispanics (Holmes, 2003).

Native Americans are twice as likely to have hepatic cancer and more likely to be obese than White adults. They are more likely to have high blood pressure, and they are 60% more likely to have a stroke. Their AIDS rates are 40% higher compared to non-Hispanic Whites. "Socioeconomic characteristics of the population, such as poverty and unemployment, may indicate barriers to receiving HIV prevention messages and accessing or using intervention and treatment services" (McNaghten et al., 2005, p. 66). The infant mortality rate is 1.5 times that of non-Hispanic Whites (The Office of Minority Health, 2007e).

The health problems of Native Americans are complicated by difficult access to health care. Of all ethnic groups discussed here, Native Americans have the second highest percentage of persons who have not visited a dentist in the last 12 months. For instance, a survey of oral health care showed that nearly two thirds of Native Americans have unmet dental needs. Only 1% of Medicaid-eligible babies get a dental examination before 1 year of age (Benn, 2003). Persons who live on reservations and are served by the Indian Health Service may find that this federally funded agency does not provide the services they need. Persons who live in rural areas are underserved, with inadequate facilities and a lack of qualified personnel.

Selected Health-Related Cultural Aspects

Native Americans are generally present oriented: they emphasize events that are occurring now rather than events that will happen later. They take one day at a time and in times of illness, they cope by hoping for improvements the next day (Kavanaugh, 2008; Reid & Rhoades, 2000). Native Americans value cooperation rather than competition. Sharing of resources, even among the poor, is an important component of this cultural value. Native Americans place great importance on their families and relatives. Three or more generations form an extended kinship system, which is enlarged by the membership of nonrelatives who are included through various religious ceremonies (Boyle, 2008).

Despite the great diversity in Native American groups in their beliefs and practices concerning health, illness, and healing, they share a common philosophical base. Native Americans believe that a state of health exists when a person lives in total harmony with nature (Rhoades & Rhoades, 2001). The earth is seen as a living entity that should be treated with respect; failure to do so harms the body. Illness is viewed not as an alteration in a person's physiological state, but rather as an imbalance between the ill person and natural or supernatural forces (Boyle, 2008). Native Americans believe that a person's sickness can be traced directly to having committed a violation against natural and spiritual laws; an individual can also inherit such a violation. The violation causes the person to have an imbalance that causes illnesses mentally, physically, emotionally, and spiritually.

Traditional health practices are an important part of the Native American way of life (Buchwald et al., 2000).

Rituals and healing ceremonies that are believed to restore balance when illness occurs may be carried out by the medicine man or woman, who is believed to have hypnotic powers, the gift of mind-reading, and expertise in concocting drugs, medicine, and poisons. More recently, the terms *traditional*, **shaman**, or *medicine person* has to be considered imprecise. The term "traditional medicine is generally used to describe the healing and beliefs of the Indian population" (Rhoades & Rhoades, 2001, p. 401). The crystal gazer hand trembler identifies the cause of an illness, and the shaman is called to induce a cure. The shaman is usually a powerful individual in the tribe. Although the power and reverence given to shamans may vary among different tribes, they are treated with respect for their role in inculcating religious beliefs and promoting spirituality, good health, and good living for the people (Andrews, 2008; Boyle, 2008).

THE EMERGING RURAL AND URBAN POPULATIONS: HOMELESS PERSONS
Homelessness: A Continuing Saga

Homelessness is a complex social and economic problem that continues to persist and grow. It has been on the "American policy agenda for close to two decades" (Burt et al., 2001, p. 310). Many services and programs have been developed to address the issue, yet homelessness remains a significant problem.

A universal definition of homelessness has proven elusive; therefore, who is considered homeless is difficult to answer. Burt et al. (2001) proposed that there are three elements that characterize homelessness: "transience or instability of place, the instability or absence of connections to family, and the instability or absence of housing" (p. 2).

Transience or instability of place characterizes persons who have no fixed place to live, such as nomadic tribes, people who work in a circus, carnival workers and many migrant farm workers, peddlers, or itinerant menders of kettles and pans, who work or repair in an amateurish way. In the modern world, single people hired for construction or industries may have a place to stay, but not a fixed one. The instability or absence of connections can be seen in persons without a family such as the skid row population. **Skid row** is "a general term for an impoverished urban area where cheap housing, day labor, and marginal businesses can be found" (Hombs, 2001, p. 280). The Bowery in lower Manhattan, New York, is the most well-known domain for the skid row population. "The skid-row Bowery grew out of the Civil War which created homelessness on a vast-scale" (Isay & Abramson, 2000, p. xiv). The men in the Bowery had flophouses that offered the "shabbiest accommodations" (p. xiii). They had no connections with family. Some of the residents in these flophouses include recovering substance abusers, ex-prisoners, poor immigrants, persons discharged from mental institutions, just to name a few. Finally, persons who have unstable or no housing include those who have experienced fire, flood, or natural disasters. Loss of one's dwelling characterizes this third type of homeless persons. Additionally, a person whose family or community can no longer provide them housing or accommodation are considered homeless. This last type best fits the description of what "homeless" generally means in the U.S.

The Stewart B. McKinney Homeless Assistance Act (public law 100-77) defines *homelessness* as the lack of a fixed, regular, and adequate nighttime residence. A homeless person's nighttime residence may be a supervised or publicly-operated shelter designed as temporary living quarters, an institution serving as a temporary residence for persons who require institutionalization, and any public or private place not intended for regular sleeping accommodations (Hombs, 2001). This definition is extremely limited and presents multiple issues and problems in resolving the homeless situation.

Burt et al. (2001) maintain that inclusive definitions of homelessness become useless because then entire populations who are poor or poorly housed will be eligible for services and benefits. On the other hand, "if the definitions are too specific, they focus too exclusively on the homelessness of the moment" (p. 6). With these perspectives in mind, it is suggested that a look at the causes of homelessness would facilitate the formulation of a definition that would address all related issues.

Why Families and Persons Become Homeless

A look at homeless persons over the last two decades reveals that they are individuals who were affected by changing (a) housing markets for low-income families and single persons, (b) opportunities for persons with only a secondary education or less, and (c) institutional supports for persons with severe mental illness. In addition, persistent poverty and racial inequalities were identified as structural causes. There are also individual causes including (a) child and adult victimization, (b) mental illness, (c) substance abuse, (d) low levels of education, (e) poor or no work history, and (f) too early child-bearing (Burt et al., 2001; National Health Care for the Homeless Council [NHCHC], 2006). Both structural and personal factors alone or in combination lead to lack of resources to secure and/or maintain housing. Burt et al. (2001) propose that "housing affordability was and still is assumed to be the immediate cause of homelessness" (p. 8).

DePastino (2003) described the events in the 1980s, when many federal programs for social welfare and housing lost funding in the face of soaring poverty. There were also the changes in long-term economic and labor markets that had an impact on employment of men and women. The contraction of the government "safety net" resulted in many cuts of funding for programs such as the Aid to Families with Dependent Children. Women caring for dependent children were severely affected by this. There was also the move to **gentrification**, a process of "transformation of a neighborhood to a higher-income area, through the displacement

of lower-end tenants, renovation of buildings, and the opening of higher-priced business" (Hombs, 2001, p. 278). Further, the release of mentally ill persons into the community starting in the 1950s swelled the numbers of persons without affordable housing. Thus, the era of the new homeless came into being. "Old skid row refugees, displaced by urban renewal and gentrification, suddenly found themselves outnumbered by legions of newcomers: men, women, and even children pushed to the streets by the lack of affordable housing" (Depastino, 2003, p. 247). The new homeless consisted of "unprecedented proportions of women, children, and nonwhites living in shelters and on the street" (p. 256). "The homelessness of the late 20th century involved not only an economic crisis of shelter and housing, but also a cultural crisis of race, family, and gender" (p. 249).

A striking feature of the new homeless is the large numbers of adolescents—estimated to be between 1 and 2 million. "Each year more than 1.35 million children and youth experience life without a home, living in shelters or parks" (NHCNC, 2006, p. 3). "Adolescents who are homeless in the United States come from every socioeconomic stratum in urban, suburban, and rural areas. Homeless youth are both males and females of every racial/ethnic identity" (Rew, 2002, p. 423). In a descriptive study of homeless adolescents, Rew et al. (2001) found that nearly half of the sample reported a history of sexual abuse. "Over half (51%) were thrown out of their homes by their parents; 37% left home because their parents disapproved of their alcohol or drug use, and nearly one-third left home because parents sexually abused them" (p. 33). In another study, Rew et al. (2002) reported that 35% of a convenience sample of 425 homeless adolescents left home because of homosexual or bisexual orientation. Recognition of homeless youth as medically vulnerable warrants increased efforts to address their many issues relative to reasons for being homeless. A study on the perspective and experience of homeless youth found that the majority of them reported "positive experiences as research participants" (Ensign, 2006, p. 647). They valued the incentives provided and were interested in how their data were going to be used. This perspective by homeless youth is a refreshing piece of information given the known reluctance of other marginalized populations to be participants in research.

Other individuals who comprise the homeless population are U.S. veterans. Nyamathi and colleagues (2004) reviewed current literature and found (a) more than 250,000 may be homeless at any given night; (b) poverty, postmilitary mental illness, and social isolation are prevalent risk factors; (c) up to 70% have long-standing alcohol dependency; (d) they have high rates of posttraumatic stress disorder; and (e) they exhibit severe impairment in occupational and social functioning.

Selected characteristics from the profile of the homeless persons include more than 50% with less than a high school education, no health insurance, and reported substance abuse. History of victimization, incomes below poverty levels, many days without eating, and only a few days of temporary work add to the grim life of homeless persons (Hombs, 2001).

The multidimensionality of homelessness serves as a negative consideration: expansion of the definition would depend on availability of resources to alleviate the problem.

Estimates of Numbers of Homeless Persons

Given the multiple definitions of homelessness and the lack of a universal system for counting this population, estimates of the numbers of homeless vary from resource to resource. "Substantial problems of methodology exist in trying to count homeless people. Street counts have always been the Achilles heel of homeless studies" (Hombs, 2001, p. 8). Additionally, "the kinds of living arrangements defining one as [homeless] can vary considerably from one investigator to another, adding a further note of uncertainty and making historical or regional comparisons risky" (Hopper, 2003, pp. 60-61). There are estimates as low as 250,000 and as high as several million homeless persons. These cannot be taken as accurate without considering some basic issues of estimating or counting. Homeless persons "work very hard to obscure their homelessness by dress, appearance, and daily schedule. They try to make their homelessness invisible to those who might not otherwise recognize it" (p. 8). A segment of the homeless population is particularly hard to reach when outreach efforts are limited to shelters and soup kitchens (Tommasello et al., 2006, p. 911). Those who do not use shelters, where counts are done, sleep in abandoned buildings, in their cars, depots on the streets, or a tent in the woods. For example, a group of homeless persons were found in a shanty area "tucked among tall ferns, twisted tree branches, and a thicket of overgrown grass and weeds behind the Supreme Industrial Equipment Co." (Schienberg, 2004, p. A32).

The homeless situation is a problem not only of individuals, but also of families, communities, and societies. This problem needs to be addressed as a dynamic and not a static phenomenon. For as societies continue to change and evolve, there will always be those who are excluded and suffer consequences. These are the risks that must be actively anticipated so that strategic planning could forestall any devastating and long-lasting effects.

Health Issues of Homeless Persons and Families

The lives of homeless persons and families are constant battles for daily survival. Homeless persons experience exposure to extremes in temperatures, unsanitary living conditions, crowded shelters, poor nutrition, and unsafe situations, wherever they live. They experience the same situations relative to health care, i.e., poor access because of lack of health insurance and the resources to get to health facilities. A survey of health care access by homeless persons identified the predominant physical and psychological health problems. Homeless persons report respiratory ailments such as asthma and infections, ulcers, sexually transmitted diseases, dental caries, and vision difficulties. Psychological problems include alcohol and drug abuse, behavioral disorders, depression, and posttraumatic stress disorder. Pregnancy rates are higher than comparable cohorts in the general population (Hatton et al., 2001).

Homeless people lack preventive care and fail to return for follow-up care or comply with prescribed treatment (McCabe et al., 2001). Exceptions are veterans, who comprise almost 40% of the homeless population. Homeless veterans have better access to health care benefits but frequently do not utilize them (Nyamathi et al., 2004). Lack or nonuse of preventive care among the homeless population has often led to use of expensive emergency room care.

Han and Wells (2003) looked at whether the use of the Health Care for the Homeless Program services by homeless adults was associated with their reduced risk for inappropriate use of emergency care services. Data indicate that misuse was not from the lack of insurance but the inadequate access to primary care.

Homeless persons suffer from mental health problems, often the major cause of their homelessness. Homelessness also creates mental problems (Choucair, 2006). Multiple stresses of living in shelters and on the streets, physical problems, lack of resources, psychosocial issues such as shame and stigma, and feelings of hopelessness and despair often tax the homeless person's ability to cope.

Substance and drug abuse accompany their mental health problems (Fisk et al., 2006). Nyamathi et al. (2004) examined perception of health status by homeless U.S. veterans. The researchers used a nonveteran comparison group. Both groups reported alcohol dependency and use of crack cocaine. Perceptions of fair/poor health were associated with injection drug use and perceptions of worse health status were associated with symptoms of depression. Treatment for their mental illness is often wrought with difficulties because it is combined with their substance abuse, lack of insurance, and poverty, which serve as barriers to their receiving care from providers who may harbor negative attitudes toward them (Lafuente, 2003; Sochalski & Mark, 2001).

Currently, the large numbers of homeless youth and the problems and issues they face have caught the attention of nurse researchers such as Rew who has established a track record of research on this population. Homeless youth suffer the health problems of the general population of homeless persons. "Homeless adolescents must learn to survive in environments that are highly stressful and filled with greater health risks than those encountered by household youth. Although many have fled from homes that were chaotic, all of them find that having no permanent place for food, shelter, or social support creates a formidable challenge to healthy growth and development" (Rew, 2002, p. 425). Homeless youth have "higher incidence of trauma-related injuries, developmental delays, sinusitis, anemia, asthma, bowel dysfunction, eczema, visual, and neurological deficits, and poor academic performance" (Montauk, 2006, p. 1137). They have high risk for sexually transmitted diseases including HIV-AIDS (Rew et al., 2002). Substance abuse is also commonly seen; so are mental problems including depression, self-harm, and suicide (Rew, 2002).

A Mosaic of Strategies to Address Homelessness

Homelessness has long been recognized as a multidimensional problem of modern day society. A review of past strategies reveals that approaches must go beyond the shelter approach. In addition to shelters, other traditional approaches currently in use in varying degrees include (1) community-based residence programs, (2) residential services for the mentally ill, (3) foster family care, (4) halfway houses, (5) community lodges, and (6) satellite housing. Readers are encouraged to seek resources that these programs offer. A discussion of shelters as the predominant temporary residences for homeless persons was presented in the previous issues of this textbook.

Montauk (2006) and Hombs (2001) provide an extensive resource and services list on homelessness. Other professionals who have done extensive work on the topic of homelessness provide a variety of solutions and strategies to address the issue. One approach addresses mainstream social programs like "welfare, health care, mental health care, substance abuse treatment, veterans assistance and so on. These programs, however, are oversubscribed" (Hombs, 2001, p. 142). These social programs have been shifting their responsibility to the homeless assistance system that "ends homelessness for thousands of people everyday, but are quickly replaced by others" (p. 143). Chronically homeless persons and those who are chronically ill should be given housing that comes with supportive services. These two concurrent approaches, which "close the front door" and "open the back door," are believed to reduce the costs of "expensive public systems such as jails and hospitals" (p. 143).

Many initiatives to address the issues of homeless people are being implemented by the National Health Care for the Homeless Council, which provides advocacy, research, training, and clinical resources. Several major U.S. cities have developed their own programs to address the health care needs of the homeless. Boston, for example, provides care through the Boston Health Care for Homeless Persons program (O'Connell et al., 2004). The Access to Community Care and Effective Services and Supports (ACCESS), funded in New Haven in 1994, "was designed to test the impact of the integration of fragmented services in treating homeless persons with serious mental illness" (Fisk et al., 2006, p. 481).

Community health nurses, who are at the forefront of advocacy for the homeless, work to bring about changes and develop strategies to deal with their problems. An example is the work of Lashley (2007), who established a parish nurse practice in a small community. "This led to the establishment of a partnership with an inner-city, faith-based mission serving homeless addicts in a long-term residential recovery program" (p. 24). Other strategies include helping homeless persons to gain access to the health care system and benefits, working with the community to obtain services and resources, educating homeless persons about their health, and educating health care personnel about homeless persons. Nurses also advocate for adequate transportation, day care, "one-stop shopping" for services, elimination of stigma, and policies that promote a healthy community (Hatton et al., 2001).

The problem of homelessness centers on the person who is part of a family, a community, and society. How much data and information are needed to solve a problem? In the case of homelessness, there is a critical need to know more about these men and women. It is the author's belief that the solutions to alleviate this problem are at the basic level of the individual homeless person. A few selected works addressing this notion are worthy of mention. Rew's work on homeless youth, mentioned earlier, sheds light on how to address their health issues. One study on resilience showed that homeless youth who perceived themselves as resilient "reported feeling less lonely, less hopeless, and less engaged in life-threatening behaviors than those who perceived themselves as not being resilient" (Rew et al., 2001, p. 39). These researchers hypothesized that "in the banding together to form living arrangements, they interacted more with each other than they would have the mainstream world from which they may feel alienated" (p. 39). In another study, Rew (2002) looked at sexual health practices and recommended the use of "brief culturally-relevant interventions" (p. 144) for safe sex behaviors.

Communities also need to continue their in-kind work with homeless persons. Many schools and houses of religious worship have worked with local governments in extending support to the homeless. Food, clothing, night shelter, and short-term socializing have been provided. Parishioners may donate their time preparing meals, preparing the shelter, and serving as chaperones during the night. Much work is still needed to reduce homelessness. The needs of the recently identified rural homeless must be addressed. Every citizen should be educated so each person can serve as an advocate and neighborhood coalitions should be established to prevent the increase of homeless persons and to support the return of the homeless person as a dignified, contributing member of society. Health care providers must continue to seek effective ways to coordinate their efforts through the creation of comprehensive resource materials. Technology must be used at its maximal capability to facilitate assessment and monitoring. Preparation for nursing and health care for the homeless in both rural and urban settings should be strengthened as an essential part of the curriculums of the health care disciplines. Finally, more research regarding health care outcomes should be supported and data should be disseminated in a timely manner.

There is a greater degree of optimism today in dealing with the problems of homelessness. Individuals and communities are showing concern through increased involvement. Homelessness is everyone's problem, and people can ultimately affect the establishment of priorities to facilitate an improved quality of life. Increasing awareness and knowledge of the current status of homeless people will aid in understanding the problem and its ramifications. This understanding will serve as an excellent guide in providing input, taking necessary action, and making the final decision as to what will make a healthy nation.

People Living with HIV-AIDS

The HIV-AIDS epidemic is in its twenty-seventh year of known devastation to the lives of people, families, countries, and the world. In 2005 alone, there were 41,897 cases of AIDS. Through 2005, 984,155 persons had been reported as having AIDS in the U.S. and dependent areas. Persons aged 35 to 39 years had the highest incidence followed by the group of those aged 30 to 34 years. In 2005, the highest numbers of AIDS cases were from male-to-male sexual contact, followed by high-risk heterosexual contact, then through injection use, and finally from other causes (hemophilia, blood transfusion, perinatal, and risk not reported or identified). Through 2005 the cumulative estimates were highest in male-to-male sexual contact, followed by injection drug use, high-risk heterosexual contact, and other. Perinatal transmissions totaled 8460 cases. New York had the highest numbers in 2005 and also cumulatively through 2005. Florida had the second highest in 2005; but was third cumulatively through 2005. California was third highest in the number of cases in 2005, and was second in cumulative estimates through 2005 (Centers for Disease Control and Prevention, 2005). Selected data on HIV-AIDS can be found in **Website Resource 2K**.

Much has changed since the identification of HIV-AIDS more than 20 years ago. Once it was considered to be a disease of gay White persons. Currently, this disease has affected persons of all ages, both genders, and different populations in the U.S. Adults 50 years and over are the "fastest growing age-group with the disease. It's not just that more people who were diagnosed with the disease in their 30's and 40's are surviving. The number of new HIV infections in older adults is rising" (Stark, 2007, p. 30). Cumulatively through 2005 there were 118,370 AIDS cases among persons 50 years old and older. Of these 14,503 were 65 and older (Centers for Disease Control and Prevention, 2005). Older adults have low risk awareness and "have unprotected sex, use alcohol, or inject drugs" (Stark, 2007, p. 30). Lindau et al. (2006) looked at older women's attitudes, behavior, and communication about sex and HIV. Data indicate that many older women are active sexually, and a majority of them do not use condoms. In addition they believe that "physicians should address issues of sexuality and insufficient attention was paid to their sexual health" (p. 752). Age-related changes such as decline in immunity, cellular

deterioration, and decreased ability to fight infections put older adults at higher risk (Stark, 2007). Older adults with HIV-AIDS face difficult challenges as they live with this disease. They might find themselves "disconnected from family and again stigmatized by formal institutions" (Shippy & Karpiak, 2005, p. 252). Furthermore, data indicated that overall "the aging HIV/AIDS population will not be able to rely upon typical support networks (e.g., spouses, children, and other relatives) for needed emotional and instrumental support" (p. 252).

Among APIs there were 417 cases, or 1% of the total HIV-AIDS population in the U.S., at the close of 2005 (Centers for Disease Control and Prevention, 2005). Although the numbers of infected persons and those having the disease are low compared to the other groups, there is concern about this population because of rapid growth, high teen pregnancy, sexually transmitted disease rates, and increased mobility, immigration, and tourism (Centers for Disease Control and Prevention, 2001).

Like all the other ethnic groups, the Native American population has been witnessing increases in HIV-AIDS–afflicted members. At the close of 2005, a total of 195, or 1% of the total HIV-AIDS population, has been reported with the disease (Centers for Disease Control and Prevention, 2005). The small percentage of Native Americans with HIV-AIDS seems insignificant given the many health issues that pose as high risks for this disease. However, "socioeconomic characteristics of the population, such as poverty and unemployment, may indicate barriers to receiving HIV prevention messages and accessing or using intervention and treatment services" (McNaghten et al., 2005, p. 66).

LHAs accounted for 18% or 6782 cases of HIV-AIDS at the close of 2005. Hispanic males had over 3 times the AIDS rate compared to non-Hispanic males and were 2.7 times more likely to die from this disease. Hispanic females had over 5 times the AIDS rates compared to non-Hispanic females and are 4.5 times more likely to die from it. Among LHAs many barriers exist in accessing or receiving HIV-AIDS–related health care. They are underrepresented in HIV clinical trials. Brooks et al. (2007), using a focus group technique, explored "concerns, motivation, and intentions regarding participation in a preventive HIV-vaccine trial" (p. 53). Mistrust and fear of the government, concerns such physical side effects, vaccine-induced HIV, stigma, and false HIV-positive test results were cited as barriers by Spanish-speaking participants.

BAAs account for 13% of the U.S. population, but for about 49% of all persons who get HIV-AIDS. In 2005, 41% of men and 64% of women living with HIV-AIDS were Blacks. At the close of 2005, there were 18,121 cases, the highest among the ethnic groups discussed in this chapter. Cumulatively through 2005, there were 397,548 cases of HIV-AIDS, surpassing all the ethnic groups and the White, non-Hispanic U.S. population (Centers for Disease Control and Prevention, 2005). The most common way of getting HIV by males was having unprotected sex with another man who has HIV; for females it was having unprotected sex with a man who has HIV. In a study of HIV risk and prevention strategies, risk factors identified included unprotected sex, bisexuality, multiple partners, trust that the partner would not to sleep with others, "thinking people who were healthy looking did not have HIV and thinking people who had HIV were giving it away" (Brown & Hill, 2005, p. 363). Barriers to prevention and accessing care will be discussed in more detail in this next section. **Website Resource 2L** summarizes HIV-AIDS data on ethnic minorities.

Issues in HIV-AIDS Prevention and Management

Currently the most effective approaches to dealing with HIV-AIDS are prevention, rapid diagnosis, symptom management (Coyne et al., 2002) and highly active antiretroviral chemotherapy (HAART) (Comulada et al., 2003; Harris & Brown, 2001). Implementation of these approaches has been met with many insurmountable multidimensional barriers. There are the stigma, poverty, lifestyles, behaviors, culture, beliefs, and values of persons. Then there are the socioeconomic factors and political machinery of a nation. However, in the absence of a vaccine, there must be continued and sustained efforts to deal with the increase in numbers of infected persons and deaths from this disease. Since prevention is the most important goal to contain the HIV-AIDS epidemic, any strategy should have as its focal point individuals who are both the carriers and victims and their relationship with their families and communities. The discussion of prevention of HIV-AIDS is at best only cursory in this chapter because of space limitations. An advance apology is extended to those who work tirelessly in continuing the mission of prevention. The material presented here is not sufficient recognition of their commitment and dedication. Further, the material will emphasize the situation of BAAs who are most severely affected.

In the late 1990s, a sense of diminished priority for HIV-AIDS was considered to be the reason for the escalation of this problem among BAAs. Williams (2003) compiled an excellent HIV-AIDS profile of African Americans. Readers are encouraged to consult this resource for more comprehensive discussion of issues and suggested strategies. A look at the factors that contribute to the AIDS epidemic among BAAs indicates that these are applicable to the other ethnic groups discussed here. First, BAAs have low educational attainment (see **Website Resource 2I**). They are underrepresented in the health care professions. Of the 311,717 registered nurses who reported their ethnicity or race, only 4.2% are BAAs (Health Resources and Services Administration, 2004). The insufficient numbers of health care professionals have implications for culturally appropriate preventive care and management of HIV-AIDS in ethnic minority persons. Second, there are communication gaps between health care professionals and BAAs. "Cultural differences, lack of access to available services,

racism, and misconceptions are some of the barriers to effective HIV/AIDS education and health promotion services" (Williams, 2003, p. 297). Third, there are myths, misconceptions, apathy, and lack of awareness of the consequences of the disease and other related social problems. BAAs have many health issues as discussed previously. They also have high poverty levels that contribute to their lack of access to resources for understanding and dealing with the disease and its consequences. Further, they have a lingering mistrust of a health care system that exploited them without benefits for the population, as evidenced by The Tuskegee Syphilis Study. Compounding factors include "high levels of stress, street violence and crime, homelessness, as well as heavy alcohol and illicit drug use" (p. 298). Fourth, there is the evident sustained health disparity and the problem of drug abuse. "Sharing of hypodermic needles and trading sex for drugs are two ways that substance abuse can lead to HIV and other [sexually transmitted diseases] STD transmission" (p. 299).

Those who monitor the HIV-AIDS epidemic can attest to the important role that culture plays in prevention and management of the disease. In cultures where the value orientation relative to the human relationship to nature is fatalism (see **Website Resource 2A**), members perceive no control over their lives. African Americans (Plowden et al., 2000) and Asian Americans (Chng & Collins, 2000) have fatalistic orientations. Fatalism is defined as a "surrendering of power to external forces of life which destroy personality, potential, hope, and life" (Powe & Johnson, 1995, p. 123). Research studies indicate that "in communities where the fatalism was high, participation in primary and secondary screening programs was low" (Plowden et al., 2000, p. 89). Additionally, the importance of the family could serve as a deterrent in seeking early diagnosis. Fear of shame and stigmatization of family (Yoshioka & Schustack, 2001) prevent the individual from disclosing her/his diagnosis. On the other hand, loyalty and commitment to the family as a cultural norm could serve as strong motivators for providing assistance and support for HIV-AIDS–afflicted family members (Miner, 2000).

Since the early 1990s the Jemmotts and their colleagues have conducted intervention studies that emphasize preventive outcomes. Their research studies have incorporated what they know about preventive measures and approaches that are culturally appropriate and have sound theoretical bases. Further they study the most vulnerable groups that could exert the most significant impact on the prevention of the disease. A synthesis of these studies is found in an excellent resource, in which HIV-AIDS is discussed under lifestyle behaviors (Jemmott et al., 2001). These researchers' important contributions to the research on HIV-AIDS include not just the positive outcomes, but also the lessons that have been learned and the sharing of these lessons with the research community. "Racism, distrust of researchers, religious beliefs, homophobia, economic variables, and diversity within the community" (p. 329) must be addressed since these could serve as barriers. Additionally, substance abuse, women's issues, and adolescents' issues within the context of family and other relationships must also be considered in designing prevention strategies. The bases for interventions must be theoretical models that "suggest new ways of thinking about program elements and provide a framework for organizing program content" (p. 334). Knowledge taught should be complemented by skill-building content. "Several studies have suggested that interventions that address safer sex skills and perceived self-efficacy are more likely to be effective than information-only programs" (p. 335). Culturally sensitive approaches that consider social norms and values of the African American community should also be integrated in intervention programs. Culture plays an important role in HIV-AIDS because it "strongly affects values, beliefs about health, disease, pain and suffering, expectations regarding health care professionals, religious doctrine, and world views, in general" (Brown, 2001, p. 61). Relative to religious beliefs, faith communities remain strong cultural influences in the lives of African Americans. Therefore, "It is important that any work in the African American population takes into consideration the impact of religion and the faith community on behavior because faith communities serve as means of social support for many African Americans" (Plowden et al., 2000, p. 91). Finally, researchers should build a relationship with the community. Communities could provide "input in the design, planning, and implementation of risk-reduction studies" (Jemmott et al., 2001, p. 337).

There are two other aspects of prevention that must be addressed to limit the transmission of HIV. One aspect is early detection and the other is prevention of infection in women. "Unrecognized HIV infection is a major problem with important individual and public health implications" (Johnson et al., 2003, p. 277). "Failed early detection of HIV infection prevents any possible early educational interventions or behavior modification and precludes pre-AIDS treatment with highly active antiretroviral therapy (HARRT)" (p. 278). "Failed early detection is also failed secondary prevention. Persons with HIV infection who are unaware of their status may continue to engage in high-risk practices which promote transmission of the virus" (p. 280). "For some AIDS cases, delays have been long as several years. About 52% of AIDS cases were reported to CDC within 3 months of diagnosis and about 88% were reported within 1 year" (U.S. Department of Health and Human Services, 2002, p. 37). Weinstock et al. (2002) surveyed persons who attended sexually transmitted disease clinics. Of the 52,260 clients, 14,750, or 28%, of the clinic clients reported not having had an HIV test. Similarly, Johnson et al. (2003) conducted a survey of adults recently diagnosed with AIDS. The date of their first HIV positive test was one of the questions asked. Researchers found early HIV detection less likely for women and ethnic minorities. An important recommendation from this research is the expansion of "behavioral intervention programs to reduce HIV risk behaviors" (p. 281).

HIV prevention in women, particularly those of childbearing age, is a priority because of the potential devastation to future generations. Heterosexual contact among adult or adolescent females is the mode of transmission. In 2005, 12,388 women contacted HIV through heterosexual contact. Through 2005, HIV-AIDS affected a total of 65,881 women. Perinatal transmissions were up to 8460 in 2005 (Centers for Disease Control and Prevention, 2005).

There are many issues in HIV-AIDS prevention, particularly among women from ethnic minority populations. Amaro et al. (2001) describe the cultural, economic, educational, and social influences on HIV prevention among Latinas. Cultural factors include beliefs that there is nothing to do to prevent HIV. Hispanic culture is identified as having a fatalistic concept of the human being's relationship to nature (see **Website Resource 2A**, Cultural Value Orientations). Additionally, Latinas are identified with submissive roles in the marital relationship. Therefore, their negotiation skills with regard to condom use might be ineffective. Moreover, Latino men are more likely to view the use of a condom as interference with sexual pleasure. Many Latinas suffer from poverty, low educational attainment, and poor language skills that hinder opportunities for health education and knowledge crucial in prevention. Others are involved in abusive relationships that both hamper their abilities to control their lives and heighten their risks for HIV. Illegal status among many Latinas makes them vulnerable to victimization and exploitation. Given the complex set of factors that exert a strong influence in HIV prevention in Latinas, it is recommended that prevention efforts be concentrated on empowerment strategies that incorporate all the contextual factors and socioeconomic circumstances.

The need for HIV-AIDS prevention is beyond assessment. There is now a core body of knowledge that could guide the design and implementation of preventive programs and strategies. Continued and increased support from the government for research, collaboration of health care disciplines, involvement of individuals and families through community initiatives, political activism, and advocacy could bring a rapid halt to transmission with hopes for a vaccine in the near future.

Other HIV-AIDS Prevention Initiatives

Selected initiatives for prevention that consider the issues discussed in the previous section can be found in many communities in the U.S. The Alternative Co-Therapies project (ACTP) in New York City serves HIV-positive African American women and their families. Its services include child care, transportation support, comprehensive health care services, alternative cotherapies, increased accessibility of family members to health care services, and culturally competent clinicians (Miner, 2000). Another initiative is the Racial and Ethnic Approaches to Community Health

(REACH), "a two-phased five-year demonstration project to support community coalitions in the design and implementation of unique community-driven strategies to eliminate health disparities" (Ma'at et al., 2001, p. 94). One of the health problems addressed is HIV-AIDS. The U.S. Department of Health and Human Services in collaboration with the Congressional Black Caucus created Rapid Assessment, Response, and Evaluation (RARE), a community-based technical assistance strategy. "RARE methodologies can provide a means through which municipalities can augment the role played by public health research in curtailing the HIV-AIDS epidemic" (Needle et al., 2003, p. 978). Active work on HIV-AIDS prevention and management continues at the local, national, and global levels.

THE NATION'S RESPONSE TO THE HEALTH CHALLENGE

Healthy People 2010

Healthy People 2010 outlines a comprehensive, nationwide health promotion and disease-prevention agenda. This initiative is designed to serve as a roadmap for addressing and improving the health of all persons in the United States. *Healthy People 2010* is its foundation. With its 28 identified focus areas, the central goals are to increase quality of life and eliminate health disparities (U.S. Department of Health and Human Services, 2000). The anticipated success of *Healthy People 2010* would include significant decreases in infant mortality, declines of death rates for coronary heart disease and stroke, and advances in the management of cancer. The complex and dynamic interplay of economic, political, social, and technological factors will require active participation in advocating for health, home, community, business, state, and the nation. Selected objectives relevant to the foci of this chapter are found in the *Healthy People 2010* Box. In addition, the developing data and goals for 2020 can be accessed at *www.healthypeople.gov*.

Office of Minority Health

The U.S. Department of Health and Human Services has an Office of Minority Health. "On July 10, 2002, it convened the National Leadership Summit on Eliminating Racial and Ethnic Disparities in Health" (U.S. Department of Health and Human Services, 2002). To eliminate health disparities several strategies have been proposed, including "(a) broadening scientific research and data on racial and health disparities, (b) increasing awareness of the challenges facing minorities, (c) establishing partnerships to mobilize the larger community and stakeholders, (d) developing and enforcing policies, laws, and regulations to support the needs of racial and ethnic minorities and (e) ensuring access to critical health and human services" (p. 1).

Another initiative established by the Centers for Disease Control and Prevention is the Racial and Ethnic Approaches to Community Health (REACH) 2010. Its objective is to "eliminate disparities in health access and outcomes. These six health areas were selected for emphasis because they

Healthy People 2010

Selected National Health Promotion and Disease Prevention Objectives for Emerging Populations

1. Increase the number of persons with health insurance to 100%.
   (Baseline: 83% [lower in ethnic minorities] of persons under 65 years covered by health insurance in 1997)
2. Increase the proportion of persons who have a specific source of on-going care to 96%.
   (Baseline: 87% in 1998)
3. Reduce the overall cancer death rate.
   Target: 159.9 deaths per 100,000 of the population.
   (Baseline: 202.4 deaths per 100,000 of the population in 1998)
4. Prevent diabetes. Target: 2.5 new cases per 1000 per year.
   (Baseline: 3.5 new cases, 3-year average, 1994-1996)
5. Increase the proportion of persons with diabetes who receive formal diabetes education. Target: 60%.
   (Baseline: 45% of persons with diabetes received formal education in 1998)
6. Reduce coronary heart disease deaths.
   Target: 166 deaths per 100,000.
   (Baseline: 208 coronary artery disease deaths per 100,000 in 1998)
7. Reduce AIDS among adolescent and adults.
   Target: 1 new case per 100,000.
   (Baseline: 19.5 cases of AIDS, aged 13 and older in 1998)

From U.S. Department of Health and Human Services (2000). *Healthy people 2010, vol. 1.* Washington, DC: U.S. Government Printing Office. Also see developing data and goals for the *Healthy People 2020* at *www.healthypeople.gov*.

reflect areas of disparity that are known to affect multiple racial and ethnic minority groups at all life stages" (The Office of Minority Health and Health Disparities, 2007). These areas include (a) infant mortality, (b) deficits in breast and cervical cancer screening and management, (c) cardiovascular diseases, (d) diabetes, (e) HIV infections/AIDS, and (f) child and adult immunizations.

Other initiatives have been created to protect the health of minority communities. Initiatives address common health problems such as diabetes, substance abuse, and AIDS. Most recently the "Health Resources and Services Administration granted almost $150 million to nursing schools that offer programs focusing on underserved populations" (Carol, 2007, p. 47). Schools supported by this funding enroll students from any ethnic background. The anticipated success of these programs is almost a guarantee because in a similar project directed by the author, project participants are practicing in areas considered to be medically underserved. The project achieved its goal of preparing ethnic minority persons to return and serve their communities (Valencia-Go, 2005).

MULTICULTURAL AWARENESS

One of the core competencies of baccalaureate education entails the development of students' abilities to deliver culturally competent care (American Association of Colleges of Nursing, 2007). Transcultural concepts and/or a separate transcultural course are essential elements of a nursing curriculum that prepares graduates to meet this competency.

The author's academic institution prides itself on addressing this competency. First, the recognition of cultural diversity among the student body and the members of the college community is acknowledged and reflected in all college activities and publications. Second, in the baccalaureate nursing curriculum there is a separate course that formally prepares students to deliver culturally competent care. Third, faculty select learning resources that address cultural diversity. Fourth, the college community encourages and facilitates initiatives to showcase the work of students and faculty.

As an overall initiative to implement the goals of *Healthy People 2010*, the administration, faculty, and students plan and implement a campus-wide health program, Healthy Campus 2010. Senior nursing students are the overall coordinators, a role that also fulfills their course objectives. In order to fulfill the objectives of community-based care, seniors in the summer semester assess the health issues of the college community members. All students in the nursing program participate in the event. With the guidelines from *Healthy People 2010*, students address health issues identified as health disparities given the ethnic minority composition of the student body in the multiple campuses of the college.

Sophomore-level students address health promotion topics such as nutrition, physical safety, and medication education. In addition, there is an emphasis on cultural aspects.

For example, what are the cultural foods that a hypertensive Chinese or Jamaican person needs to avoid? What cultural folk healing practices support Western approaches? What are the different cultural physical activities that can enhance nutrition?

Junior-level students are able to address specific health problems since these are the foci of their classes. Awareness of health disparities determine their choice of topics and approaches. Students' wider and deeper knowledge facilitates their decisions regarding health care resources that they provide for participants in the event. For instance, students teach members of the college community how to read labels of ethnic foods and where participants could purchase appropriate foods at reasonable prices.

Senior nursing students, as event coordinators, act as a resource for all the other students and provide information on logistics, serve on the planning committee with the faculty, oversee all arrangements, and manage the evaluation of the event. The work of evaluation is ongoing, but an essential component is determining how the different student presentations have enhanced multicultural awareness and understanding by the participants, as well as by the presenters themselves.

The success of the event, held annually, has been astounding. Students progress in their curriculum with a stronger commitment to culturally competent care. Senior students exit the program with a high level of confidence in their abilities to address the health issues of multicultural populations. The college community gains a fuller appreciation of cultural diversity with its strengths and its areas of concern. The faculty continue to have a feeling of having done a "good job" and are inspired to think of creative ways to educate students about multiculturalism.

There are also minority health research initiatives sponsored by the National Institutes of Health, Centers for Disease Control and Prevention, and the Agency for Health care Research and Quality. Support for these initiatives and future ones must continue at all levels.

NURSING'S RESPONSE TO EMERGING POPULATIONS AND HEALTH

The American Nurses' Association's (ANA) Code of Ethics explicitly states the profession's commitment to provide service to people regardless of background or situation (American Nurses' Association, 1985). "Nurses need to understand the specific health needs and responses to illness of different populations," (Martino Maze, 2005, p. 551). The ANA's Council on Cultural Diversity supports the work of nurses in their development of culturally competent care. The organization and its leadership, through the Ethnic-Minority Fellowship Program, has had an essential role in supporting the work and efforts of AAPIs, BAAs, LHAs, and Native Americans with graduate and doctoral work. Nurses continue to make many positive moves toward understanding culturally diverse populations. See the Case Study and Care Plan about Mr. and Mrs. Arahan, an older adult immigrant couple, at the end of this chapter, which proposes nursing interventions to ensure their quality of life in their later years. Nurses' awareness and understanding of transcultural issues have been facilitated by the works of leaders such as Leininger, Giger, Davidhizar, Andrews, and Boyle, just to name a few. In addition, wide dissemination of research findings has been made possible through the *Journal of Transcultural Nursing* and through annual conferences and other sponsored workshops. Additionally, nurses with advanced preparation have committed their time and energy to developing approaches and models for transcultural nursing. These models can be found in **Website Resource 2C**.

Several nursing journals focus on cultural diversity, such as the *Journal of Cultural Diversity* and the *Journal of Multicultural Nursing and Health*. These journals and a variety of other publications are constantly increasing professionals' knowledge of health-related cultural issues. In addition, the *Minority Nurse Newsletter* provides excellent summaries of research studies, legislative updates affecting ethnic minorities, and relevant topics in education and practice. Ethnic nursing organizations are having an effect on greater cultural understanding through their dissemination of important works by clinicians, educators, and researchers.

HEALTH TEACHING   Student Health Promotion Project

When students are retaking a clinical nursing course, they have a unique opportunity to strengthen theoretical concepts introduced in their first attempt at the course. To avoid duplication of learning experiences, the faculty needs to be creative and resourceful in enhancing critical thinking and creating experiences that would support students' achievement of course objectives. In their first attempt at the course, students are often unsuccessful in course examinations that test higher levels of learning in the cognitive domain. Therefore, learning experiences must motivate students to overcome their anxiety about failing for the second time and also inspire them to do their best.

In the first attempt at the course a community-focused health promotion project is implemented at a senior citizen center. For the second attempt at the course students have dual roles, that of teacher and learner. First, students prepare for the experience by examining the health issues and concerns of young and middle adulthood, since these are the two age stages of the group members. The course textbook and multimedia resources in the learning center provide a review of developmental tasks, prevalent health problems, cultural aspects, and appropriate health care and nursing approaches. In a seminar format, students share their information with each other including their own experiences and perspectives as young or middle adults.

Second, students then survey the professional literature for appropriate resources, including assessment instruments on specific health issues and culturally appropriate approaches. Students agree that the prevalent issues of the group members are stress, unhealthy lifestyles, and time management.

Third, students agree on one tool to be used for the assessment, and data are collected as students interview one another. The data are comprehensive, and students are very much surprised at the commonalities among them. Results of their assessment indicate that all of the students have multiple roles, each with overwhelming demands on their time. In their pursuit of a nursing degree, students confront studying for many hours, reading voluminous numbers of pages, doing many written assignments, and reviewing for challenging examinations that they all agree tax their energy reserves. Sleep is often sacrificed, and most resort to unhealthy eating as a way to cope.

Fourth, the students develop a teaching plan using the concepts on client education taught to them during the first attempt of the course. The students formulate realistic and measurable objectives for themselves as learners. They have commented that selecting and writing these objectives seemed easier because they were the learners and realized the importance of achieving these. The healthy lifestyle strategies selected are those that they could implement with their busy schedule but would be effective nevertheless.

Fifth, the presentation of the project is held in a room that has multimedia capabilities. Using current technology, students present their material on stress and strategies to address unhealthy lifestyles through nutrition, exercise, and time management. An actual demonstration of exercises that can be done while studying or working in front of the computer are well received. Each student gets an opportunity to try out the exercises. Using a similar approach, the second group of students presents strategies on time management to cope with the multiple demands on each student's time. Student presenters discuss an awareness of one's body rhythms. They inform their peers of the value of matching the demand of the task on hand and one's corresponding energy and attention level. Culturally specific food recipes that can be prepared in a short period of time are shared with the group.

Sixth, the evaluation of the learning is done later in the semester as opposed to almost immediately after students taught at a senior center. Students see each other at least twice per week after the presentation. All the students believe that they have met the learning objectives and are continuing the strategies taught by their peers. They comment that the teaching "hit home" and that they have come to realize that as future health care professionals, health promotion activities should be for the self first before they can address the health issues of others. From the faculty's perspectives, students gain a better understanding of the concepts of client education and appreciation of a comprehensive assessment as well as use of culturally appropriate and creative approaches to teaching. The students' success in their second attempt at the course gives them a much stronger foundation for subsequent courses and a deeper appreciation of staying healthy as a priority goal of every future health care professional.

Major organizations such as the ANA, the National League for Nursing (NLN), and the American Association of Colleges of Nursing (AACN) publish culturally relevant materials to guide students, clinicians, and educators. Accrediting bodies for nursing education such as the NLN and the Commission on Collegiate Nursing Education (CCNE) support diversity with the inclusion of standards for dealing with diversity in the academic preparation of baccalaureate and masters students (American Association of Colleges of Nursing, 2007). Additionally, there is a cadre of nurses whose research on the cultural practices and beliefs of individuals and families gives professionals a sound base for improving practice and designing cost-effective and humanistic health care strategies. The quest to deliver culturally competent care has provided the impetus for nursing faculty to require transcultural courses in the nursing curriculum to facilitate awareness and understanding of cultural diversity. (See the Multicultural Awareness Box and Health Teaching Box.) Additionally, major textbooks focusing on specific clinical areas of practice devote material to health care issues of ethnic minorities. Other resources include a chapter or two on cultural diversity. In addition, discussion of specific health care problems and nursing care always includes cultural aspects. In the clinical setting, health care workers, through staff development and in-service programs, are provided opportunities to learn and develop culturally sensitive care approaches.

SUMMARY

This century will continue to be a time of great challenges as the population of the U.S. continues to be a nation of diverse peoples. The nation and its people have risen again and again through devastations by both nature and humankind itself. As citizens, emerging populations share similar concerns about life, including health, an acceptable standard of living, and quality of life. An array of cultural, economic, educational, social, and political barriers are being chipped away at the local, national, and global levels to ensure the health and well-being of the peoples of the U.S. The government, public and private industries, health care professions, and every individual are working together to reduce health disparities and ensure a healthy nation for future generations.

CASE STUDY

An Older Immigrant Couple: Mr. and Mrs. Arahan

Mr. and Mrs. Arahan, an older couple in their 70s, have been living with their oldest daughter, her husband of 15 years, and their two children, ages 12 and 14. They all live in a middle-income neighborhood in a suburb of a metropolitan city. Mr. and Mrs. Arahan are both college educated and worked full-time while they were in their native country. In addition, Mr. Arahan, the only offspring of wealthy parents, inherited a substantial amount of money and real estate. Their daughter came to the U.S. as a registered nurse and met her husband, a drug company representative. The couple came to the U.S. when their daughter became a U.S. citizen and petitioned them as immigrants. Since the couple was facing retirement, they welcomed the opportunity to come to the U.S.

The Arahans found life in the U.S. different from their home country, but their adjustment was not as difficult since both were healthy and spoke English fluently. Most of their time was spent taking care of their two grandchildren and the house. As the grandchildren grew older, the older couple found that they had more time on their hands. The daughter and her husband advanced in their careers and spent a great deal more time at their jobs. The family dinners during the week were seldom. On weekends, the daughter, her husband, and their children socialized with their own friends. The couple began to feel isolated and longed for a more active life.

Mr. and Mrs. Arahan began to think that perhaps they should return to the home country, where they still had relatives and friends. However, political and economic issues would have made it difficult for them to live there. Besides, they had gotten used to the way of life in the U.S. with all the modern conveniences and abundance of goods that are difficult to come by in their country. However, they also became concerned that they might not be able to tolerate the winter months and that minor health problems might get worse as they got older. They wondered who would take care of them if they became very frail and where they would live knowing that their daughter worked to save money for their grandchildren's college education. They expressed their sentiments to their daughter, who became very concerned about how her parents were feeling.

This older couple had been attending church on a regular basis, but had never been active in other church-related activities. The church bulletin announced the establishment of parish nursing with two retired registered nurses as volunteers. The couple attended the first opening of the parish clinic. Here, they met one of the registered nurses, who had a short discussion with them about the services offered. The registered nurse had spent a great deal of her working years as a community health nurse. She informed Mr. and Mrs. Arahan of her availability to help them resolve any health-related issues.

Reflective Questions:

1. What strategies could be suggested for this older adult couple to enhance their quality of life?
2. What community resources can they utilize?
3. What can the daughter and her family do to address the feelings of isolation of the older couple?
4. What health promotion activities can ensure a healthy lifestyle for them?

CARE PLAN

An Older Immigrant Couple: Mr. and Mrs. Arahan

Nursing Diagnosis: Risk for Continued Feelings of Isolation

DEFINING CHARACTERISTICS

- Couple no longer have a great deal of caretaking responsibilities
- Daughter and husband spend a great deal of time on their careers
- Family dinners during the week are seldom
- Daughter and her family socialize with their own friends
- Older adult couple are thinking of returning to native country
- Concern over life in the U.S. with harsh winters and their minor health problems
- Concern over advancing years and future living arrangements

EXPECTED OUTCOMES

The Arahans will:
- Join a senior citizen center for socialization and other activities
- Volunteer at a nearby hospital or school several mornings or afternoons per week
- Work with daughter and her family to plan at least one family get together per week
- Pursue some neglected hobbies
- Get involved in a church group or in a civic organization

- Begin a discussion on future alternate living arrangements
- Make periodic visits to the native country to see relatives and friends

SUGGESTED INTERVENTIONS

- Encourage the couple to have open discussions about their concerns with their daughter and her family
- Support them in their choice of meaningful activities such as joining the senior center and volunteering
- Provide information on resources on future living arrangements in the U.S.
- Develop a plan for health monitoring on a regular basis

- Provide a list of organizations that address issues and concerns of older adults such as the Association of Retired Persons (AARP)
- Utilize their experience and expertise (if any) in managing the parish nursing clinic
- Initiate an older support group in the parish with Arahans as the first members

The Arahans' situation is a very common one in most immigrant groups. The interventions outlined above would need to consider the cultural traditions, personal preferences, health status, motivation level, physical ability, and resources of the couple to ensure positive outcomes and goal achievement.

REFERENCES

Abraham, N. (1995). Arab Americans. In R. J. Vecoli, J. Galens, A., Sheets, R. V. Young (Eds.), Gale encyclopedia of multicultural America (Vol. 1, pp. 84–98). New York: Gale Research Inc.

Adderly-Kelly, B., & Williams-Stephens, E. (2003). The relationship between obesity and breast cancer. The ABNF Journal, 14(3), 61–65.

Adib, S. M., & Mikkey, I. F. (2003). Lebanon. In C. E. D'Avanzo & E. M. Geissler (Eds.), Cultural health assessment (3rd ed., pp. 443–449). St. Louis: Mosby.

Amaro, H., Vega, R. R., & Valencia, D. (2001). Gender, context, and HIV prevention among Latinos. In M. Aguirre-Molina, C. W. Molina, & R. E. Zambrana (Eds.), Health issues in the Latino community (pp. 301–324). San Francisco: Jossey-Bass.

Amaro, H., & Zambrana, R. E. (2000). Criollo, Mestizo, Mulato, LaitNegro, Indigena, White, or Black? The US Hispanic/Latino population and multiple responses in the 2000 Census. American Journal of Public Health, 90(11), 1724–1727.

American Association of Colleges of Nursing. (2007). Draft: Revision of the essentials of baccalaureate nursing education. Retrieved December 18, 2007, from www.aacn.nche.

American Nurses' Association. (1985). Code of ethics. Kansas City, MO: The Association.

Andrews, M. M. (2008). The influence of cultural health belief systems on health care practices. In M. M. Andrews & J. S. Boyle (Eds.), Transcultural concepts in nursing care (5th ed., pp. 66–81). Philadelphia: Wolters Kluwer Lippincott Williams & Wilkins.

Andrews, M. M., & Boyle, J. S. (2008). Andrews/Boyle transcultural nursing assessment guide for individuals and families. In M. M. Andrews & J. S. Boyle (Eds.), Transcultural concepts in nursing care (5th ed., pp. 453–457). Philadelphia: Wolters Kluwer Lippincott Williams & Wilkins.

Asamoa, K., Rodriguez, M., Gines, V., Varela, R., Dominguez, K., Mills, C. G., et al. (2004). Use of preventive health services by Hispanic/Latino women in two urban communities: Atlanta, Georgia and Miami, Florida, 2000 and 2001. Journal of Women's Health, 13(6), 654–661.

Bailey, E. (2000). African American alternative medicine: Using alternative medicine to prevent and control chronic diseases. Westport: Bergin & Garvey.

Baldwin, K. A., Humbles, P. L., Armmer, F. A., & Cramer, M. (2001). Perceived health needs of urban African American church congregants. Public Health Nursing, 18(5), 295–303.

Bauman, K. J., & Graf, N. L. (2003). Educational attainment: 2000, Census 2000 brief. US Department of Commerce Economics and Statistics Administration. Washington, DC: US Census Bureau.

Benn, D. K. (2003). Professional monopoly, social covenant, and access to oral health care in the United States. Journal of Dental Education, 67(10), 1080–1090.

Ben-Rafael, E. (2001). Sociology of ethnicity. In N. J. Smelser & P. B. Baltes (Eds.), International encyclopedia of the social & behavioral sciences (Vol. 7, pp. 4838–4842). United Kingdom: Cambridge University Press.

Benson, S. G. (Ed.). (2003). The Hispanic American almanac (3rd ed.). Detroit: Thomson/Gale.

Black Americans. (2007). A statistical sourcebook. Palo Alto, CA: Information Publications, Inc.

Bohn, D. K. (2003). Lifetime physical and sexual abuse, substance abuse, depression, and suicide attempts among Native American women. Issues in Mental Health Nursing, 24, 333–352.

Bookman, M. Z. (2002). Ethnic groups in motion: Economic competition and migration in multiethnic states. London: Frank Cass.

Boyle, J. S. (2008). Culture, family, and community. In M. M. Andrews & J. S. Boyle (Eds.), Transcultural concepts in nursing care (5th ed., pp. 261–296). Philadelphia: Wolters Kluwer Lippincott Williams & Wilkins.

Brittingham, A., & de la Cruz, G. P. (2005). We the people of Arab ancestry in the United States. US Department of Commerce Economics and Statistics Administration. Washington, DC: US Census Bureau.

Brooks, R. A., Newman, P. A., Duan, N., & Ortiz, D. J. (2007). HIV vaccine trial preparedness among Spanish-speaking Latinos in the US. AIDS Care, 19(1), 52–58.

Brown, E. J., & Hill, M. A. (2005). Perceptions of HIV risks and prevention strategies by rural and small city African Americans who use cocaine: Views from the inside. Issues in Mental Health Nursing, 26, 359–377.

Brown, G. (2001). The impact of HIV/AIDS on the African American woman and child: Epidemiology, cultural, and psychosocial issues and nursing management. The ABNF Journal, 12(3), 60–62.

Buchwald, D., Beals, J., & Manson, S. M. (2000). Use of traditional health practices among Native Americans in a primary care setting. Medical Care, 38(12), 1191–1199.

Burt, M., Aron, L. Y., Lee, E., & Valente, J. (2001). Helping America's homeless. Washington, DC: The Urban Institute Press.

Campbell, G. R. (2000). American Indian demographics. In C. J. Moose & R. Wildin (Eds.), Racial and ethnic relations in America (Vol. 1, pp. 63–66). Pasadena, California: Salem Press Inc.

Carbonell, A. A. (2002). Cuba. In C. E. D'Avanzo & E. M. Geissler (Eds.), Mosby's pocket guide to cultural health assessment (3rd ed., pp. 218–233). St. Louis: Mosby.

Carol, R. (2007). Majoring in minority health. Minority Nurse, Summer, 46–50.

Carrillo, J. E., Trevino, F. M., Betancourt, J. R., & Coustasse, A. (2001). Latino access to health care: The role of insurance, managed care, and institutional barriers. In M. Aguirre-Molina, C. W. Molina, & R. E. Zambrana (Eds.), Health issues in the Latino community (pp. 55–73). San Francisco: Jossey-Bass.

Carter-Porkas, O., & Zambrana, R. E. (2001). Latino health status. In M. Aguirre-Molina, C. W. Molina, & R. E. Zambrana (Eds.), Health issues in the Latino community (pp. 23–54). San Francisco: Jossey-Bass.

Centers for Disease Control and Prevention. (2001). *HIV/AIDS surveillance report, 13*(2), Atlanta, GA: Centers for Disease Control and Prevention.

Centers for Disease Control and Prevention. (2005). *Basic statistics: HIV/AIDS.* Retrieved September 24, 2007, from *www.cdc.gov/hiv/topics/surveillance/basic.htm.*

Chelala, C. (2002). A vibrant place: Arab Americans in New York. *Lancet, 360*(9330), 417–420.

Chng, C. L., & Collins, J. R. (2000). Providing culturally competent HIV prevention programs. *American Journal of Health Studies, 16*(1), 24–33.

Chong, N. (2002). *The Latino patient: A cultural guide for health care providers.* Maine: Intercultural Press.

Choucair, B. (2006). Health care for the homeless in America. *American Family Physician, 74*(7), 1099–1100.

Comulada, W. S., Swendeman, D. T., Rotheram-Borus, M. J., Mattes, K. M., & Weiss, R. E. (2003). Use of HAART among young people living with HIV. *American Journal of Health Behavior, 27*(4), 389–400.

Coyne, P. J., Lyne, M. E., & Watson, H. C. (2002). Symptom management in people with AIDS. *American Journal of Nursing, 102*(9), 48–56.

D'Avanzo, C. E., & Geissler, E. M. (Eds.). (2003). *Pocket guide to cultural health assessment* (3rd ed.). St. Louis, MO: Mosby.

DePastino, T. (2003). *Citizen Hobo: How a century of homelessness shaped America.* Chicago: The University of Chicago Press.

Dhooper, S. S. (2003). Health care needs of foreign-born Asian Americans: An overview. *Health and Social Work, 28*(1), 63–73.

Donner, F. M. (2002). Arabs. In *The world book encyclopedia* (Vol. 1, pp. 584–590). Chicago: World Book, Inc.

Doutrich, D. L., & Colclough, Y. (2008). Japanese Americans. In M. M. Andrews & J. S. Boyle (Eds.), *Transcultural concepts in nursing care* (5th ed., pp. 357–393). Philadelphia: Wolters Kluwer Lippincott Williams & Wilkins.

Dumonteil, E., & Gamboa-Leon, M. R. (2003). Mexico (United Mexican States). In C. E. D'Avanzo & E. M. Geissler (Eds.), *Pocket guide to cultural health assessment* (3rd ed., pp. 520–525). St. Louis: Mosby.

Earp, J. K. (2008). Korean Americans. In M. M. Andrews & J. S. Boyle (Eds.), *Transcultural concepts in nursing care* (5th ed.). Philadelphia: Wolters Kluwer Lippincott Williams & Wilkins.

Ecker, M. (2003). Ethnics and values. In P. A. Potter & A. G. Perry (Eds.), *Fundamentals of nursing* (5th ed., pp. 401–422). St. Louis: Mosby.

Ensign, B. J. (2006). Perspectives and experiences of homeless young people. *Issues and Innovations in Nursing Practice, 54*(6), 647–652.

Feagin, J. R. (2001). Racial relations. In *International encyclopedia of the social and behavioral sciences* (Vol. 19, pp. 12711–12116). St. Louis: Elsevier.

Fisk, D., Rakfeldt, J., & McCormack, E. (2006). Assertive outreach: An effective strategy for engaging homeless persons with substance abuse disorders into treatment. *The American Journal of Drug and Alcohol Abuse, 32*, 47–486.

Fixico, D., Kolata, A. L., & Neely, S. (2001). American Indian. In *The world book encyclopedia* (Vol. 10, pp. 136–185). Chicago: World Book.

Fletcher, A. B. (2000). African American folk medicine: A form of alternative therapy. *The ABNF Journal, 11*(1), 18–20.

Fox, P. G., Burns, K. R., Popovich, J. M. & Ilg, M. (2001). Depression among immigrant Mexican women and Southeast Asian refugee women in the U.S. *The International Journal of Psychiatric Nursing Research, 7*(1), 778–791.

Gabaccia, D. R. (2002). *Immigration and American diversity.* Massachusetts: Blackwell Publishers.

Garcia, H. D. (2001). *Hispanic Americans: The world book encyclopedia* (Vol. 9, pp. 244–259). Chicago: World Book.

Gary, F. A., Yarandi, H. N., & Scruggs, F. C. (2003). Suicide among African Americans: Reflections and a call to action. *Issues in Mental Health Nursing, 24*(3), 353–375.

Giger, J. N., & Davidhizar, R. E. (2008). Introduction. In J. Giger & R. Davidhizar (Eds.), *Transcultural nursing: Assessment and interventions* (5th ed., pp. 2–19). St. Louis: Mosby.

Gilliland, S. S., Azen, S. P., Perez, G. E., & Carter, J. S. (2002). Strong in body and spirit: Lifestyle intervention for Native American adults with diabetes in New Mexico. *Diabetes Care, 25*(1), 78–83.

Greene, R. (2000). *Social work with the aged and their families.* New York: Aldine de Guyter.

Grinde, D. A. (Ed.). (2002). *Native Americans.* Washington, DC: C Q Press.

Guendelman, S., & Wagner, T. (2001). Hispanics' experience within the health care system: Access, utilization, and satisfaction. In M. Aguirre-Molina, C. W. Molina, & R. E. Zambrana (Eds.), *Health issues in the Latino community* (pp. 15–46). San Francisco: Jossey-Bass.

Han, B., & Wells, B. L. (2003). Inappropriate emergency department visits and use of health care for the homeless program services by homeless adults in the northeastern United States. *Journal of Public Health Management Practice, 9*(6), 530–537.

Harley, D. A., & Dillard, J. M. (Eds.). (2005). *Contemporary mental health issues among African Americans.* Alexandria: American Counseling Association.

Hatahet, W., Khosla, P., & Fungwe, T. V. (2002). Prevalence of risk factors to coronary heart disease in an Arab-American population in southeast Michigan. *International Journal of Food Science and Nutrition, 53*, 325–335.

Hatton, D. C., Kleffel, D., Bennett, S., & Gaffrey, E. (2001). Homeless women and children's access to health care: A paradox. *Journal of Community Health Nursing, 18*(1), 25–34.

Hayat, A., Lucas, J. B., & Kington, R. (2000). *Health outcomes among Hispanic subgroups: Data from the National Interview Survey, 1992–1995. Advance Data.* Hyattsville, MD: U.S. Department of Health and Human Services.

Health Resources and Services Administration. (2004). *The registered nurse population: Findings from the 2004 national sample.* Retrieved November 13, 2007 from *http://bhpr.hrsa.gov/healthworkforce/msurvey04/3.htm.*

Henslin, J. M. (2001). *Race and ethnic relations: Measuring inequality.* In A. M. Garcia & R. A. Garcia (Eds.), *Race and ethnicity* (pp. 22–41). San Diego, CA: Greenhaven Press.

Holmes, T. (Ed.). (2003). *Minorities: A changing role in American society.* Detroit: Thomson-Gale.

Hombs, M. E. (2001). *American homelessness* (3rd ed.). Santa Barbara, CA: Contemporary World Issues.

Hopper, K. (2003). *Reckoning with homelessness.* Ithaca: Cornell University Press.

Hornsby, A. (2001). African Americans. In *The World Book Encyclopedia* (Vol. 1, pp. 136b–136h). Chicago: The World Book.

Isay, D., & Abramson, S. (2000). *Flophouse: Life on the Bowery.* New York: Random House.

Islam, S., & Johnson, C. A. (2003). Correlates of smoking behavior among Muslim Arab-American adolescents. *Ethnicity & Health, 8*(4), 319–337.

Jaber, L. A., Brown, M. B., Hammad, A., Nowak, S. N., Zhu, Q., Ghafoor, A., et al. (2003a). Epidemiology of diabetes among Arab Americans. *Diabetes care, 26*(2), 308–313.

Jaber, L. A., Brown, M. B., Hammad, A., Zhu, Q., & Herman, W. H. (2003b). Lack of acculturation is a risk for diabetes in Arab immigrants in the U.S. *Diabetes care, 26*(7), 2010–2014.

James, D. (2004). Factors influencing food choices, dietary intake, and nutrition-related attitudes among African Americans: Application of a culturally sensitive model. *Ethnicity and Health, 9*(4), 349–367.

Jemmott, L. S., Jemmott, J. B., III, & Hutchinson, K. M. (2001). HIV/AIDS. In R. L. Braithwaite & S. E. Taylor (Eds.), *Health issues in the Black community* (2nd ed., pp. 309–346). San Francisco: Jossey-Bass Publishers.

Johnson, D. F., Sorvillo, F. J., Wohl, A. R., Bunch, G., Harawa, N. T., Carruth, A., et al. (2003). Frequent failed HIV detection in a high prevalence area: Implications for prevention. *AIDS Patient Care and STDs, 17*(6), 277–282.

Jones, C. P. (2000). Levels of racism: A theoretic framework and a gardener's tale. *American Journal of Public Health, 90*(8), 1212–1215.

Kataoka-Yahiro, M., Ceria, C., & Yoder, M. (2004). Grandparent caregiving role in Filipino American families. *Journal of Cultural Diversity, 11*(3), 110–117.

Kavanaugh, R. R. (2008). Transcultural perspectiveness in mental health nursing. In M. M. Andrews & J. S. Boyle (Eds.), *Transcultural concepts in nursing care* (5th ed., pp. 226–259). Philadelphia: Wolter Kluwer Lippincott Williams & Wilkins.

Kegler, M. C., Cleaver, V. L., & Yazzie-Valencia, M. (2000). An exploration of the influence of family on cigarette smoking among American Indian adolescents. *Health Education Research, 15*(5), 547–557.

Keith, V. M. (2000). A profile of African Americans' health care. In C. J. Hogue, M. A. Hargraves, & K. S. Collins (Eds.), *Minority health in America* (pp. 47–76). Baltimore: The John Hopkins University Press.

Kim, H. (2001). Asian-Americans. In *The world book encyclopedia* (Vol. 1, pp. 812–814). Chicago: World Book.

Kinney, A. Y., Emery, G., Dudley, W. N., & Croyle, R. (2002). Screening behaviors among African American women at high risk for breast cancer: Do beliefs about God matter? *Oncology Nursing Forum, 29*(5), 835–843.

Kluckhohn, C. (1953). Dominant and variant value orientations. In C. Kluckhohn, H. A. Murray, & D. A. Schneider (Eds.), *Personality in nature, society, and culture* (2nd ed.). New York: Alfred A. Knopf.

Kulwicki, A. D., Miller, J., & Schim, S. M. (2000). Collaborative partnership for culture care: Enhancing health services for the Arab community. *Journal of Transcultural Nursing, 11*(1), 31–39.

Kulwicki, A. D., & Rice, V. H. (2003). Arab American adolescent perceptions and experiences with smoking. *Public Health Nursing, 20*(3), 177–183.

Kuramoto, F., & Nakashima, J. (2000). Developing an ATOD prevention campaign for Asian and Pacific Islanders: Some considerations. *Journal of Public Health Management Practice, 6*(3), 57–64.

Lafuente, C. (2003). Powerlessness and social disaffiliation in homeless men. *The Journal of Multicultural Nursing and Health, 9*(1), 46–54.

Lambert, S., Fearing, A., Bell, D., & Newton, M. (2002). A comparative study of prostate screening, health beliefs, and practices between African American men and Caucasian men. *The ABNF Journal, 13*(3), 61–63.

Lashley, M. (2007). Nurses on a mission: A professional service learning experience with the inner-city homeless. *Nursing education Perspectives, 28*(1), 24–26.

Lauderdale, J. (2003). Transcultural perspectives in childbearing. In M. M. Andrews & J. S. Boyle (Eds.), *Transcultural concepts in nursing care* (4th ed., pp. 95–131). Philadelphia: Lippincott Williams & Wilkins.

Lee, P. R., & Estes, C. L. (2003). *The nation's health.* (7th ed.). Sudbury, MA: Jones & Bartlett.

Leininger, M. (2000). Founder's focus: The third millennium and transcultural nursing. *Journal of Transcultural Nursing, 11*(1), 69.

Leininger, M. (2001). The theory of culture care diversity and universality. In M. M. Leininger (Ed.), *Culture care diversity and universality: A theory of nursing* (2nd ed., pp. 5–68). Boston: Jones and Bartlett Publishers.

Leong, F. T., & Lau, A. S. (2001). Barriers to providing effective mental health services to Asian Americans. *Mental Health Services Research, 3*(4), 201–214.

Lindau, S. T., Leitsch, S. A., Lundberg, K. L., & Jerome, J. (2006). Older women's attitudes, behavior, communication about sex and HIV: A community-based study. *Journal of Women's Health, 15*(6), 747–753.

Ma'at, I., Fouad, M., Grigg-Saito, D., Liang, S. L., McLaren, K., Pichett, J. W., et al. (2001). REACH 2010: A unique opportunity to create strategies to eliminate health disparities among women of color [Special Issue]. *American Journal of Health Studies, 17*(2), 93–101.

Martino Maze, C. D. (2005). Registered nurses' personal right vs. professional responsibility in caring for members of underserved and disenfranchised populations. *Journal of Clinical Nursing, 14*, 546–554.

Mays, V. M., Cochran, S. D., & Sullivan, J. G. (2000). Healthcare for African American and Hispanic women. In C. J. Hogue, M. A. Hargraves, & K. S. Collins (Eds.), *Minority health in America* (pp. 97–123). Baltimore: The John Hopkins University Press.

McCabe, S., Macnee, C. L., & Anderson, M. K. (2001). Homeless patients' experience of satisfaction with care. *Archives of Psychiatric Nursing, 15*(2), 78–85.

McGadney-Douglass, B. F. (2000a). The health care needs of the Black elderly: From well to frail. In S. L. Logan & E. M. Freeman (Eds.), *Health care in the Black community: Empowerment, knowledge, skills, and collectivism* (pp. 115–133). New York: The Haworth Press.

McGadney-Douglass, B. F. (2000b). The Black Church response to the mental health needs of the elderly. In S. L. Logan & E. M. Freeman (Eds.), *Health care in the Black community Empowerment, knowledge, skills, and collectivism* (pp. 199–214). New York: The Haworth Press.

McNaghten, A. D., Neal, J. J., Li, L., & Fleming, P. L. (2005). Epidemiologic profile of HIV and AIDS among American Indians/Alaska Natives in the USA through 2000. *Ethnicity and Health, 10*(1), 57–71.

Meilaender, P. C. (2001). *Toward a theory of immigration.* New York: Palgrave.

Mikhail, B. (2000). Prenatal care utilization among low-income African American women. *Journal of Community Health Nursing, 17*(4), 235–246.

Mikkey, I. F. (2003). Syria. In C. E. D'Avanzo & E. M. Geissler (Eds.), *Cultural health assessment* (3rd ed., pp. 748–754). St. Louis: Mosby.

Miller, S. W., & Lass, K. A. (2008). East Indian Hindu Americans. In M. M. Andrews & J. S. Boyle (Eds.), *Transcultural concepts in nursing care* (5th ed., pp. 537–561). Philadelphia: Wolters Kluwer Lippincott Williams & Wilkins.

Miner, J. (2000). Black women and HIV/AIDS: Culturally sensitive family health care. In S. L. Logan & E. M. Freeman (Eds.), *Healthcare in the Black community* (pp. 185–197). New York: Hawthorne Press.

Montauk, S. L. (2006). The homeless in America: Adapting your practice. *American Academy of Family Physicians, 24*(7), 1132–1139.

Nagaty, K. A. (2003). Egypt. In C. E. D'Avanzo & E. M. Geissler (Eds.), *Cultural health assessment* (3rd ed., pp. 748–754). St. Louis: Mosby.

Nassar-McMillan, S. C., & Hakim-Larson, J. (2003). Counseling considerations among Arab Americans. *Journal of Counseling and Developments, 81*, 150–159.

National Health Care for the Homeless Council. (2006). *The basics of homelessness.* Retrieved October 10, 2007, from *www.nhchc.org/Publications/basics_of_homelessness.html.*

Needle, R., Trotter II, R. T., Singer, M., Bates, C., Page, J. B., Metzger, D., et al. (2003). Rapid assessment of the HIV/AIDS crisis in racial and ethnic minority communities: An approach for timely community interventions. *American Journal of Public Health, 93*(6), 970–979.

Nyamathi, A., Sands, H., Pattatucci-Aragon, A., Berg, J., Leake, B., Hahn, J. E., et al. (2004). Perception of health status by homeless US veterans. *Family Community Health, 27*(1), 65–74.

O'Connell, J. J., et al. (2004). Old and sleeping rough: Elderly homeless persons on the streets of Boston. *Case Management Journals, 5*(2), 101–106.

Ogunwole, S. U. (2006). *We the people: American Indians and Alaska Natives in the United States.* US Department of Commerce Economics and Statistics Administration. Washington, DC: US Census Bureau.

Orozco, M. M. (2001). Immigration and migration: Cultural concerns. In M. J. Smelser & P. B. Baltes (Eds.), *International encyclopedia* of the social and behavioral sciences (Vol. 11, pp. 7211–7217). St. Louis: Elsevier.

Ozawa, C., Alpert, P. T., & Miller, S. K. (2006). Culturally sensitive treatment of metabolic syndrome in Asian Americans. Home Health Care Management & Practice, 18(5), 394–402.

Plowden, K. O., Miller, J. L., & James, T. (2000). HIV health crisis and African Americans: A cultural perspective. The ABNF Journal, 11(4), 88–93.

Powe, B. D., & Johnson, A. (1995). Fatalism as a barrier to cancer screening among African Americans: Philosophical perspectives. Journal of Religion and Health, 135(20), 119–124.

Polek, C., Klemm, P., Hardie, T., Wheeler, E., Birney, M., & Lynch, K. (2004). Asian/Pacific Islander American women: Age and death rates during hospitalization for breast cancer. Oncology Nursing Forum, 31(4), e69–e74.

Qiu, Y., & Ni, H. (2003). Utilization of dental care services by Asians and Native Hawaiian or other Pacific Islanders: United States, 1997–2000. Advance Data, #336. Hyattsville, Maryland: US Department of Health and Human Services.

Ramirez, R. R. (2004). We the people: Hispanics in the United States. US Department of Commerce Economics and Statistics Administration. Washington, DC: US Census Bureau.

Reeves, T. J., & Bennett, C. E. (2004). We the people: Asians in the United States. US Department of Commerce Economics and Statistics Administration. Washington, DC: US Census Bureau.

Reid, R. R., & Rhoades, E. R. (2000). Cultural considerations in providing care to American Indians. In E. R. Rhoades (Ed.), American Indian health (pp. 418–425). Baltimore: The John Hopkins University Press.

Rew, L. (2002). Characteristics and health care needs of homeless adolescents. Nursing Clinics of North America, 37, 423–431.

Rew, L., Fouladi, R. T., & Yockey, R. (2002). Sexual health practices of homeless youth. Journal of Nursing Scholarship, 34(2), 139–145.

Rew, L., Taylor-Seehafer, M., Thomas, N. Y., & Yockey, R. D. (2001). Correlates of resilience in homeless adolescents. Journal of Nursing Scholarship, 33(1), 33–40.

Rhoades, E. R., & Rhoades, D. A. (2001). Traditional Indian and modern western medicine. In E. R. Rhoades (Ed.), American Indian health (pp. 401–417). Baltimore: The John Hopkins University Press.

Samaan, R. A. (2000). The influences of race, ethnicity, and poverty on the mental health of children. Journal of Health Care of the Poor and Underserved, 11(1), 100–110.

Sayed, M. A. (2003). Psychotherapy of Arab patients in the West: Uniqueness, empathy, and "otherness." American Journal of Psychotherapy, 57(4), 445–459.

Schienberg, J. (2004). Day laborers on the outside. Newsday, April 14, A32.

Sherrill, W. W., Crew, L., Mayo, R. M., Mayo, W. F., Rogers, B. L., & Haynes, D. F. (2005). Educational and health services innovation to improve care for rural Hispanic communities in the US. Education for Health, 18(3), 356–367.

Shippy, R. A., & Karpiak, S. E. (2005). The aging HIV/AIDS population: Fragile social networks. Aging and Mental Health, 9(3), 246–254.

Snipp, C. M. (2000). Selected demographic characteristics of Indians. In E. R. Rhoades (Ed.), American Indian health (pp. 41–57). Baltimore: The John Hopkins University Press.

Soschalski, J., & Mark, H. D. (2001). Response to health service utilization patterns among homeless men in transition: Exploring the need for on-site shelter-based nursing care. Scholarly Inquiry for Nursing Practice: An International Journal, 15(4), 155–159.

Stark, S. W. (2007). The aging face of HIV/AIDS. American Nurse Today, 2(6), 30–34.

Stauffer, R. Y. (2008). Vietnamese Americans. In M. M. Andrews & J. S. Boyle (Eds.), Transcultural concepts in nursing care (5th ed., pp. 494–536). Philadelphia: Wolters Kluwer Lippincott Williams & Wilkins.

Stussy, S. A. (2000). Arab Americans. In C. J. Moose & R. Wilder (Eds.) Racial and ethnic relations in America (Vol. 1, pp. 102–107). Pasadena, CA: Salem Press.

Tashiro, C. J. (2006). Identity and health in the narratives of older mixed ancestry Asian Americans. Journal of Cultural Diversity, 13(1), 41–49.

The Office of Minority Health and Health Disparities. (2007). About minority health. Retrieved September 25, 2007, from www.cdc.gov/omhd/Amh/AMH.htm.

The Office of Minority Health. (2007a). The minority role in clinical trials. Retrieved October 10, 2007, from www.omhrc.gov/templates/content.aspx?ID=5147&1v1=2&1v11D+179.

The Office of Minority Health. (2007b). Asian American/Pacific Islander profile. Retrieved September 24, 2007, from www.omhrc.gov/templates/browse.aspx?1v1=1&1v11D=2.

The Office of Minority Health. (2007c). Hispanic/Latino profile. Retrieved September 24, 2007, from www.omhrc.gov/templates/browse.aspx?1v1+1&1v11D=2.

The Office of Minority Health. (2007d). African American profiles. Retrieved September 24, 2007, from www.omhrc.gov/templates/browse.aspx?1v1=1&1v11D=2.

The Office of Minority Health. (2007e). American Indian/Alaska Native profile. Retrieved September 24, 2007, from www.omhrc.gov/templates/browse.aspx?1v1=1&1v11D=2.

The 2007 Statistical Abstract. (2007). The national data book. Washington, DC: US Census Bureau. Retrieved November 11, 2007, from www.census.gov/compendia/statab/.

Tommasello, A. C., Gillis, L. M., Lawler, J. T., & Bujak, G. J. (2006). AIDS Care, 18(8), 911–917.

U.S. Department of Health and Human Services. (2000). Healthy People 2010. Understanding and improving health. Washington, DC: U.S. Government Printing Office.

U.S. Department of Health and Human Services. (2002). Cases of HIV infection and AIDS in the United States, 2002. HIV/AIDS surveillance report, 14. Atlanta, GA: Centers for Disease Control and Prevention.

Valencia-Go, G. N. (2005). Growth and access increase for nursing students: A retention and progression project. Journal of Cultural Diversity, 12(1), 18–25.

Valencia-Go, G. N. (2006). Emerging populations and health. In C. Edelman & C. Mandle (Eds.), Health promotion throughout the life span (6th ed., pp. 23–49). St Louis: Mosby.

Vance, A. R. (2008). Filipino Americans. In M. M. Andrews & J. S. Boyle (Eds.), Transcultural concepts in nursing care (5th ed., pp. 467–493). Philadelphia: Wolter Kluwer Lippincott Williams Wilkins.

Vigil, J. D., & Roseman, C. C. (2001). Teaching ethnicity and peace in the United States. In I. Susser & T. C. Patterson (Eds.), Cultural diversity in the United States (pp. 405–413). Massachusetts: Blackwell Publishers.

Waters, M. C. (2001). Personal identity and ethnicity. In A. M. Garcia & R. A. Garcia (Eds.), Race and ethnicity (pp. 66–71). San Diego, CA: Greenhaven Press.

Weinstock, H., Dale, M., Linley, L., & Gwinn, M. (2002). Unrecognized HIV infection among patients attending sexually transmitted disease clinics. American Journal of Public Health, 92(2), 280–283.

Williams, D. R. (2000). Race, stress, and mental health. In C. J. Hogue, M. A. Hargraves, & K. S. Collins (Eds.), Minority health in America (pp. 209–243). Baltimore: The John Hopkins University Press.

Williams, D. R. (2001). Ethnicity, race, and health. In The world book encyclopedia (Vol. 7, pp. 4831–4838). Chicago: World Book.

Williams, P. B. (2003). HIV/AIDS case profile of African Americans: Guidelines for ethnic-specific health promotion, education, and risk reduction activities for African Americans. Family Community Health, 26(4), 289–306.

Winkelman, M. (2001). Ethnicity and psycho cultural models. In I. Susser & T. C. Patterson (Eds.), Cultural diversity in the United States: A critical reader (pp. 281–301). Massachusetts: Blackwell Publishers.

Wittig, D. R. (2004). Knowledge, skills and attitudes of nursing students regarding culturally congruent care of Native Americans. Journal of Transcultural Nursing, 15(1), 54–61.

Wu, T. Y., Guthrie, B., & Bancroft, J. (2005). An integrative review of breast cancer screening practice and correlates among Chinese, Korean, Filipino, and Asian Indian American women. *Health Care for Women International, 26*(3), 225–246.

Xu, Y., & Chang, K. (2008). Chinese Americans. In M. M. Andrews & J. S. Boyle (Eds.), *Transcultural nursing concepts in nursing care* (5th ed., pp. 442–466). Philadelphia: Wolters Kluwer Lippincott Wilkins & Williams.

Yancey, G. (2003). *Who is White? Latinos, Asians, and the new Black/NonBlack divide*. Boulder, London: Lynne Rienner Publishers.

Yoshioka, M. R., & Schustack, A. (2001). Disclosure of HIV status: Cultural issues of Asian patients. *AIDS Patient Care and STDs, 15*(2), 77–82.

Yue, Z., Lee, W., & Wong, F. (2003). China. In C. E. D'Avanzo & E. M. Geissler (Eds.), *Pocket guide to cultural health assessment* (3rd ed., pp. 180–186). St. Louis: Mosby.

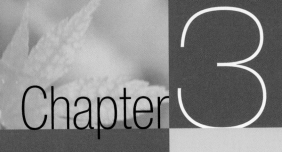

Chapter 3

Debora Elizabeth Kirsch

Health Policy and the Delivery System

objectives

After completing this chapter, the reader will be able to:

- Examine key developments in the history of health care that influenced the philosophical basis of American health care and separated preventive from curative measures.
- Differentiate between private and public sector functions and responsibilities in the delivery of health care.
- Describe the mechanisms by which health care in the United States is financed in both private and public sectors.
- Analyze the influence of health legislation on health care delivery.
- Differentiate between the purposes, benefits, and limitations of Medicare, Medicaid, and other government sponsored programs.
- Compare and contrast the health care delivery system of the United States with selected industrialized countries.
- Develop the nurse's role in influencing health policy with regard to cost, access, and quality.

key terms

Advanced practice nurses
Advocate
Capitation system
Concierge care
Fee-for-service
Gatekeeper
Health maintenance organizations
Health savings accounts
Hospitalist

Independent practice associations
Insurance
Lobbying
Lobbyist
Managed care
Medicaid
Medicare
Medicare Advantage
Nursing centers
Point-of-service

Policy decision-making
Politics
Preferred provider organizations
Primary care
Primary care provider
Self-insurance

website materials

evolve These materials are located on the book's website at *http://evolve.elsevier.com/Edelman/*.
- WebLinks
- Study Questions
- Glossary
- Website Resources
  3A: Medicare Insurance–Covered Services for 2004
  3B: Comparison of Medicare and Medicaid

THINK About It | Making Health Promotion a Reality

The inclusion of health promotion activities and preventive measures in primary health care is supported by evidence-based practice. Combining clinical preventive services with population-based health promotion activities—such as group smoking cessation programs, health education programs, and fitness programs in schools and on work sites—makes sense. These combined measures are not only cost-effective, but they are essential to improve and maintain the health of present and future citizens.

The nurse is a key player in planning for a new health program based on recommendations from a community assessment. The nurse proposes a community fitness program be established by building a new recreational center in combination with the current athletic facilities at the local public high school. This primary preventive intervention would benefit students while in school and family and community members outside of school hours, thus promoting the fitness of the community. Individuals and families would join the center paying a reasonable membership.

1. How can the nurse "sell" the idea of the fitness health-promotion center to school board and other community members?
2. Why is the fitness program cost-effective?

The health care delivery system in the United States is a complex, multilayered entity that has the capacity to provide the newest technological treatments and implement the most advanced scientific interventions in the world. Research findings have sparked the development of international gold standards for practicing evidence-based medical and nursing care. The market-driven American health care system is distinct from any other health care delivery system in the world, employing almost 9.7 million health care professionals. With 6200 hospitals, 16,700 nursing homes, 5400 inpatient mental health facilities, and 13,500 various types of health agencies (Shi & Singh, 2005), the American system is massive—but so is the cost. The rising cost of health care is consuming a growing percent of the nation's gross domestic product (GDP). Preliminary figures in 2006 indicate that 16% of the United States GDP ($2.1 trillion, or $7026 per person) is consumed by health care, the highest of all industrialized countries (NCHS, 2007). More than 25% of total federal government expenditures and 15.6% of state and local total expenditures went to health care in 2004 (NCHS, 2006).

Despite the vast resources devoted to financing the health care system, unequal access to care exists, especially among vulnerable populations. The rising cost of health **insurance** premiums is a growing burden to working American families, and the number of uninsured individuals and families is growing. Health care reform has consisted of incremental steps, but escalating health care costs and concern for improvement in the quality and safety of health care make it clear that more substantive effort is needed. Meeting the health needs of vulnerable populations will require a more comprehensive reform effort. Other industrialized countries have implemented various types of universal health care plans or national health insurance, but each system is plagued with problems. None has dealt effectively with the rising cost of health care, workforce shortages of health care professionals, or access and quality issues. Both the American free-market system and international universal health care systems share common problems, which include rising health care costs, issues of access and affordability, and workforce shortages of health care providers. Medical errors, quality of care concerns, and escalating medical malpractice costs are further complicating health care reform efforts in America.

THE HEALTH OF THE NATION

Health, United States is a published document prepared by the Department of Health and Human Resources reporting the health status of the nation by tracking a variety of specific, measurable health indicators. The annual report serves several key functions, but the main goal is to inform policymakers, the President, and Congress of the trends of the nation's health to guide the development of sound health policy and allocate resources to maintain and improve the health of the nation's citizens. The latest report, published in 2007, indicates the health of the nation has improved in many areas as a result of substantial funding of public health programs, research, provision of health care, and initiatives to support consumer education. Emerging trends indicate success in the reduction of morbidity and mortality of many diseases, control of widespread infectious diseases through widespread vaccination programs, improved motor vehicle safety, and reduction of cardiovascular-related deaths. Education regarding leading a healthy lifestyle, controlling hypertension, and using cholesterol-lowering medications has contributed to better health for Americans, but concern about sedentary lifestyle, rising obesity trends, and chronic disease is noted. Improvements in the nation's health have not been uniform as differences in health and health care and have been identified when considering an individual's income, race, gender, ethnicity, education level, and geographic location (NCHS, 2007).

Another indicator of the health of the nation is the status of the 28 focus areas identified in *Healthy People 2010*. The Healthy People Midcourse Review is conducted by the U.S. Department of Health and Human Services (USDHHS), federal agencies, and other experts who assess the data trends. At the completion of the review, objectives may be changed, deleted, or added depending on the availability of data, data trends, and emerging science.

Table 3-1 International Comparisons of Core Health Indicators for 2005

	Canada	France	Germany	Mexico	Sweden	United Kingdom	United States
Life expectancy at birth: males (years)	78.0	77.0	76.0	72.0	79.0	77.0	75.0
Life expectancy at birth: females (years)	83.0	84.0	82.0	77.0	83.0	81.0	80.0
Infant mortality rate (per 1000 live births)	5.0	4.0	4.0	22.0	3.0	5.0	7.0

Data from the World Health Organization: *Core health indicators.* Retrieved November 1, 2007, from: *www.who.int/whosis/database/core/core_select_process.cfm.*

Box 3-1 Vulnerable Populations

- Older adults
- Children
- Racial and ethnic minorities
- The poor
- The uninsured
- The chronically ill
- The physically disabled or handicapped
- The terminally ill
- The mentally ill
- Persons with AIDS
- Alcohol or substance abusers
- Homeless individuals
- Residents of rural areas
- Individuals who do not speak English
- Individuals with communication difficulties
- Low education levels or illiterate

From Shi, L. & Stevens, G. (2005). *Vulnerable populations in the United States.* San Francisco, CA: Jossey-Bass Publishers.

The December 2006 report, released in 2007, indicates that overall, the nation's health is improving with nearly 60 percent of the objectives that can be tracked either met or moved toward their targets. Twenty percent of the measurable objectives moved away from targets. Health disparities among vulnerable populations remain virtually unchanged (USDHHS, 2007a). Individuals once considered vulnerable may have been limited to populations such as older adults, children, those living in poverty, and the homeless, but vulnerable populations also include populations with low education levels, individuals who do not speak English, and residents of rural areas. A more complete list of vulnerable populations can be found in Box 3-1. Vulnerable populations are especially at risk for disparities in health care access and quality (Shi & Stevens, 2005). Also see data and goals for *Healthy People 2020* at *www.healthypeople.gov.*

Standard measures used to compare the health status of the population of one nation with another are actually death indicators. Although mortality-based indicators do not directly measure the health status of the living population, the data is more readily available through the World Health Organization (WHO). Table 3-1 compares the life expectancy by gender as well as infant mortality rates of selected countries. According to WHO statistics, life expectancy of a male in the United States in 2005 was 75 years compared to 79 years in Sweden and 78 years in Canada, while females in America were reported to have a life expectancy of 80 years compared to 84 years in France and Canada. Mexico was significantly lower for both males (72 years) and females (77 years). In 1950, life expectancy for combined genders in the United States was reported as 68.2 years (Turnock, 2004). Infant mortality rates, another indicator of health status, was reported in the United States as 7.0 deaths in the first year of life per 1000 live births in 2005, a dramatic improvement from 29.2 reported in 1950 but higher than in other industrialized nations (Turnock, 2004). Mexico has an infant mortality rate of 22.0, which is similar to other poorer nations. One reason the United States ranks lower in health indicators than other industrialized nations is attributed to the large disparities in health status by geographic areas, race, and ethnic groups as well as by social class (Schroeder, 2007). For example, *Health, United States 2007* reports that in 2004 the infant mortality rates for African Americans was more than twice that of Whites and Hispanics (Table 3-2). The infant mortality rates for Whites in the United States was 5.7, which is still higher than that of other industrial nations presented in Table 3-1. When examining infant mortality rates by women of similar socioeconomic rates as measured by years of education completed, large differences are readily apparent as shown in Table 3-3. Infant mortality rates of White mothers more than 20 years of age with college education is 4.2, well in line with those of other industrialized countries. African American women with less than a high school education have the highest infant mortality rates reported as 14.4. For most races and ethnicities the higher a women's education level is the lower infant mortality rate as shown in Table 3-3. To improve health indicators of a population, other variables such as education reform and raising health literacy need to be considered.

Healthy People 2010

The overarching goals of *Healthy People 2010* are to increase the quality and years of healthy life for all Americans as well as to eliminate health disparities. Achievement of the goals of *Healthy People 2010* requires a health care system that reaches all Americans integrating personal health care and population-based public health (USDHHS, 2007a). Public health nursing practice promotes and preserves the health of populations, looking at the community as a whole and its effect on the health of individuals, families, and groups. Community health nursing practice promotes, preserves, and maintains the health of populations through care provided to individuals, families, and groups and the effect of their health status on that of the community as a whole (Stanhope & Lancaster, 2008). Nies and McEwen (2007) define community as a group or collection of locality-based individuals interacting in social units and sharing common interests, characteristics, values, and/or goals. *Healthy People 2010* emphasizes the relationship between individual health and community health, which is the health of the community and the environment in which individuals live, work, and play. A community's health is affected by the collective behaviors, attitudes, and beliefs of all who live in it. The health of individuals is almost inseparable from that of the larger community, and the health of every community in every state determines that of the nation (NCHS, 2006).

Table 3-2	Infant Mortality Rate by Race/Ethnicity, 2004
Race/Ethnicity	**Infant Deaths per 1000 Births**
Asian and Native Hawaiian/ Pacific Islander	4.7
Hispanic	5.5
White, Non-Hispanic	5.7
American Indian/Alaska Native	8.4
African American, Non-Hispanic	13.2
All mothers	6.8

Note: Births are categorized according to race/ethnicity of mother.
From *Health, United States 2007*, Table 19. National Center for Health Statistics.

Nurses have a long tradition of involvement in health promotion, beginning with Florence Nightingale, the founder of modern nursing. While caring for wounded soldiers in the Crimean War, she fought for hospital reform by crusading for cleanliness and against overcrowding and lack of ventilation. Her careful recordings of care outcomes quantified needed reform in health promotion (Neuhauser, 2003). Later, Lillian Wald, appalled by the lack of medical care, ignorance, and living conditions of the poor in 1893, developed a settlement program in New York City that trained nurses, provided care to families, and developed education programs for the community. Wald, a leader in political activism, spearheaded organized public health in the direction of health promotion for families and communities (Holder, 2004). These pioneers and others set the stage for nurses' unique role in health promotion.

A SAFER SYSTEM

The health care delivery system in the United States is experiencing significant changes. The Institute of Medicine (IOM), a nonprofit organization, conducts research from a systems approach to improve the health care of the nation. A 1999 IOM research report, *To Err is Human: Building a Safer Health System*, focused on prevention of medical errors, which account for approximately 98,000 deaths in hospitals each year. The startling findings concluded that the health care system, not bad practitioners, is the basic cause of medical errors. In 2003 the IOM released another report, *Keeping Patients Safe: Transforming the Work Environment of Nurses*. This report shows that work environments in hospitals and nursing homes contribute to nurses' errors. Four main problem areas in nurses' work environments are identified: (1) organizational management, (2) workforce management, (3) work design, and (4) organizational culture. Increased client-to-nurse staffing ratios, fewer nurses, mandatory overtime, inadequate continuing education, and lack of nurse involvement in decisions about client care create an environment that contributes to error making. The data the IOM provided in this project support a direct link between nurse staffing and work environment and client outcomes (IOM, 2004; Kennedy, 2004). Other efforts by the IOM to improve the health of the nation include the 2006 report, *Preventing Medication Errors*, released in July of 2006. The report found

Table 3-3	Infant Mortality Rates for Mothers Age 20+ by Race/Ethnicity and Education, 2004					
	Black or African American	**American Indian/ Alaska Native**	**White**	**Asian and Native Hawaiian/Pacific Islander**	**Hispanic**	**All Mothers**
Less than 12 years	14.4	10.6	6.5	5.7	5.4	7.5
12 years of education	13.3	8.1	6.1	4.9	5.3	7.4
13 years or more of education	11.7	6.0	4.2	3.8	4.7	5.0

From *Health, United States, 2007*, Table 20. National Center for Health Statistics.

that medication errors were not only common but costly to the nation and recommended a comprehensive approach to decreasing the prevalence of medication errors by making changes in the health care system (IOM, 2006). To provide safe, evidence-based care nurses have a responsibility to understand the system in which they practice. Although health care often is equated with medical care, which focuses on the treatment of illness, this chapter presents the evolution and ongoing development of a broader concept of health based on the definition given in Chapter 1.

GLOBAL HEALTH

WHO's overriding objective is to influence health opportunities and outcomes for all people so that they can attain the highest possible level of health. WHO recognizes the importance of families and health promotion and has contributed to the family health policies of many nations by shaping global awareness for health promotion. The current agenda of WHO involves the following six goals: (1) promoting development; (2) fostering health security; (3) strengthening health systems; (4) harnessing research, information and evidence; (5) enhancing partnerships; and (6) improving performance (WHO, 2007). Internationally, shrinking health care budgets have resulted in a variable level of achievement of these goals. In developing nations, such as those in Latin America and Africa, huge inequities in health care persist.

Historical Perspectives

The complexities of the health care system necessitate an understanding of the system as a whole before focusing on the intermingled causative factors that have created a fragmented system. Many of today's problems have their roots in the decisions and directions of the past. It is not possible to identify and analyze current problems or to devise solutions without first exploring how the system developed. The relevance of the split between preventive and curative measures is apparent when the organization and financing of the delivery system is examined. The United States has established a system that uses two basic divisions of society to provide service: the public sector and the private sector. The merger of public health and welfare policies in the public sector is rooted in the Puritan ethic inherent in the historical development of the United States. The current focus on managed care as both an organizational strategy and a financing mechanism is highlighted in a discussion of how health care is delivered and financed. This discussion includes the role of the nurse as an advocate in the development of health policy.

HISTORY OF HEALTH CARE

Early Influences

Historical records of early civilizations (Egyptian, Indian, Chinese, Aztec, and Greek) show that ancient peoples were concerned with disease and practiced various methods of treatment. The earliest views of health can be seen as holistic in the sense that they sprang from an integrated worldview. Primitive peoples understood illness in mystical terms: sickness and cure theories were tied to the cosmic view of life, with natural and supernatural forces often inseparable. Most religions include a person's hygiene as part of their practice. For thousands of years, epidemics were viewed as divine judgments on human wickedness, with a gradual awareness that pestilence has natural causes such as climate and other aspects of the physical environment. During the Middle Ages, infectious diseases in epidemic proportions (leprosy, bubonic plague, smallpox, and tuberculosis [TB]) were the leading causes of death. Clearly, health was viewed in terms of survival and absence of disease.

Industrial Influences

The population of the Western world began to increase during the 1600s, when America was first being explored. The New World had many things to offer explorers. An adequate food supply made it possible for the population to live longer, and advances in transportation made distribution of food supplies and other goods and services possible. Manufacturing advances during the eighteenth century, through the invention of the flush toilet and cast iron pipe, made sanitary engineering possible, saving many lives by preventing diseases such as typhoid, paratyphoid, and gastroenteritis.

Socioeconomic Influences

Although the Elizabethan poor laws (1601) in England provided a system of relief for the poor, which included infants, sick and older people, and laborers in the workhouses, a new poor law was enacted in 1834 based on the harsher philosophy that regarded pauperism among able-bodied workers as a moral failing. If the worker did not earn a subsistence-level income, the attitude toward that worker was suspicious and punitive. These poor laws were the legal implementation of the Protestant work ethic that the Puritan forebears brought to the United States. According to this view, people are held directly accountable for their state in life, and health maintenance is the responsibility of the individual. The far-reaching implications of this ethic can be seen today in the organization, financing, and delivery of health services.

Public Health Influences

Edwin Chadwick (1800-1890) is known as the father of British and American public health. Chadwick established an English Board of Health, which emphasized environmental sanitation but excluded physicians outside times of crisis. Additionally, Chadwick was secretary of the Poor Law Commission, which strove to improve the health of the masses for economic reasons. Chadwick's rationale was that disease among the poor was a major factor in their inability to support themselves. Therefore governmental health and welfare policies have been joined in England since the nineteenth century.

Lemuel Shattuck, a leader of the public health, began the movement in the United States. He used the British system as the model, with public health services and welfare combined, despite the contradictory emphasis. Public health has focused on improving the health of the poor, whereas welfare has dictated subsistence at the minimal level. The influence of the Puritan ethic on the American health care system is apparent in the emphasis on the value of work and the attitude toward the poor. Today health and welfare departments continue their contradictory approach to the poor.

Scientific Influences

Until the twentieth century, epidemics of infectious disease (plague, cholera, typhoid, smallpox, and influenza) were the most critical health problems and major causes of death and disability for Americans. Scientific advances during the nineteenth century by Louis Pasteur (germ theory), Robert Koch (origin of bacterial infection), Joseph Lister (antisepsis), and Paul Ehrlich (chemotherapy) expanded public health from its earlier concentration on sanitation to control of communicable diseases through a broad biological base. Public health became an important force in decreasing death rates and increasing life expectancy through the application of bacteriology. International environmental conditions were improved by developing systems that safeguard water, milk, food supplies, promote sanitary sewage disposal, and monitor the quality of urban housing.

Between 1936 and 1954, the discovery and use of sulfonamides and other antibiotics to treat bacterial infections reduced the death rate to its lowest point in history, with deaths caused by primary infections reduced to 4%, as compared with 33% only 50 years earlier (in 1886). The death rate did not change significantly between 1954 and the mid-1960s. Another decline in the death rate began after the mid-1960s and has continued with the exception of a slight increase in 1995, with the control of many infectious diseases. As the life expectancy of the population increases, chronic diseases such as heart disease, cancer, chronic lower respiratory disease, and diabetes are now among the leading or contributing causes of death as reported by the Centers for Disease Control and Prevention (CDC) for 2001 (Arias & Smith, 2003).

Despite the progress in conquering infectious diseases, for vulnerable populations, infections are once again among the leading contributors to death in the United States. Diseases that were thought to be under control, such as measles and TB, are resurfacing and a new group of pathogens have emerged. The most effective strategy for eliminating TB is to monitor those infected to ensure completion of treatment by direct observed therapy. Resources are needed at local public health departments to provide follow-up in this typically elusive population. Special strategies have been found to enhance adherence to prescribed care such as cash incentives (five dollars per clinic visit) for the homeless to follow the prescribed isoniazid medication schedule

(Anderson et al., 2007). The national TB surveillance system reports declining TB incidence rates for the native-born United States population (2.3 cases per 100,000 in 2006) but an incidence rate of 21.9 cases per 100,000 of foreign-born individuals residing in the United States. Interventions to eliminate TB include not only adequate resources locally but a need for a collaborative global effort. New strains of extremely drug-resistant TB (XDR-TB) are now emerging (Smith, 2007). Drug-resistant strains of other organisms (*Staphylococcus aureus*, *Streptococcus pneumonia*, and *Salmonella typhimurium*) that cause communicable diseases are also on the rise. Recently, Methicillin-Resistant *Staphylococcus Aureus* (MRSA), previously confined to persons mainly in the hospital and long-term care facilities, gained national attention when the incidence rose in a new population, healthy school-aged children and teens, causing alarm among parents and school officials.

"For continued success in controlling infectious diseases, the U.S. public health system must prepare to address diverse challenges, including the reemergence of old diseases (sometimes in drug-resistant forms), large food borne outbreaks and acts of bioterrorism" (Lee & Estes, 2003, p. 35). Bioterrorism agents (anthrax, plague, smallpox) and chemical agents (ricin and sarin) pose potential threats to the public. Recent global outbreaks of the Hendra virus (1994); Nipah virus (1999); severe acute respiratory syndrome–associated coronavirus (2003); monkey pox, mad cow disease, avian flu (2006); and others (CDC, 2004) pose challenges to global public health. An effective, comprehensive public health system in the United States is imperative if we are to respond to local, national, and global concerns.

Special Population Influences

The second goal of *Healthy People 2010* is to eliminate health disparities among different segments of the populations. Vulnerable populations, especially those living in poverty, are at great risk to experience health disparities (USDHHS, 2007a). For many of these disadvantaged people, the issues of preventing disease and promoting good health are often secondary to the problems associated with everyday survival. Determinants of health in a population are related strongly to socioeconomic status and education level, with populations in the lower strata having worse outcomes. However, individual lifestyle behaviors including dietary choices, level of physical activity, use of alcohol and tobacco, substance abuse, and risky sexual behavior play a significant role in the health status of an individual. Access to health care for prevention, early detection, and treatment are paramount in diminishing health disparities, but programs promoting positive individual lifestyle behaviors are also needed (Lee & Estes, 2003). In addition, minority populations (even when access-related factors such as insurance status and income are controlled for) tend to receive lower quality health care than do nonminorities (IOM, 2003) (Multicultural Awareness box).

Political and Economic Influences

Political and economic considerations are basic to the health care system. **Politics** determines which decision makers negotiate a desired outcome. Economics defines what resources are distributed and how they are distributed. The effect of economics and politics on the delivery of health care is illustrated by the situation in the United States following the Great Depression. Roosevelt's New Deal had an effect on health care, specifically in the passage of the Social Security Act (SSA) in 1935, which authorized grants-in-aid to individual states to improve state and local public health programs. Funds were available for *categorical assistance* programs, with cash grants first given to needy blind and older individuals and later to disabled people. Medical care, through subsequent amendments, was an allowable budget item, but payments often went for food, shelter, or other needs. Later, the SSA developed programs such as Medicaid and Medicare.

Split Between Preventive and Curative Measures

The link between environmental health and personal medical care developed when sanitarians (people who work to maintain a clean environment) realized that their efforts alone were not sufficient to prevent and cure the diseases of the population as a whole; improvement of personal health was also necessary. Early preventive services directed toward individuals originated in medical practice rather than public health but were limited to welfare medicine (caring for individuals through state programs). Community health centers that developed in America before World War I limited their scope to prevention and health education and, with the exception of some prenatal clinics, were generally located in poor neighborhoods. Delivery of preventive services developed separately from clinical medicine and became associated with public health. Most physicians, educated in hospitals, were interested in individuals for whom prevention had failed and whose illnesses brought them to the hospital ward.

Despite the separation of preventive and treatment services, the benefits of prevention eventually were incorporated into clinical medicine for individuals. Preventive and early detection measures became a part of pediatrics and obstetrics during the early part of the twentieth century, when vaccines and vaginal cytology examinations became available and accepted. Later in the twentieth century, internal medicine incorporated early detection of diseases such as diabetes, glaucoma, obesity, and hypertension. A shift to preventive medicine for the individual occurred, but the separate educational programs for public health and medicine still divided these areas. Not until the 1960s did the emphasis begin to turn from individual to societal values (Freyman, 1980).

This new emphasis on societal values parallels another evolution in the role of health in society. Greater governmental involvement in financing the health care delivery

MULTICULTURAL AWARENESS

Transcultural Values and Beliefs about Health Care

WHY DO NURSES NEED TO BE CULTURALLY COMPETENT?

As the demographics of the United States continue to become more diverse, nurses need to be culturally competent as one strategy for eliminating racial and ethnic disparities. The assumption that people are independently oriented and should assume responsibility for caring for themselves is based on Western values of individual autonomy, self-determination, truth telling, self-sufficiency, and personal responsibility for health known as individualism. Some of these Western values are incongruent with non-Western cultural norms. In collectivist societies, the need to maintain individualism is not valued. Instead persons are defined in relation to their family or work group. In a collectivist society (for example ethnic Chinese and Japanese) other norms vary as well with regard to rules about who has decision-making power, cause of illness, and reliance on a higher power for matters of health and healing.

THE NURSE'S ROLE

Nurses need to support rather than interfere with family or group roles, challenge religious beliefs, or cause conflict with established lines of authority. For example, in many Mexican families, collective solidarity relies on the individuals in positions of authority in the family to make decisions for other family members. The older males within the family may make the decisions for other members and hold responsibility and accountability for them. In Western society, autonomy is valued—competent adults are expected to be accountable and responsible for making decisions. Andrews and Boyle (2003) cite an example in which a competent adult Mexican widow was brought to the hospital by her daughter and required immediate surgery for gangrenous toes. The individual and her daughter refused to sign the surgical consent form without consulting the client's oldest son who lived out of state. The son, in turn, contacted his uncle, still living in Mexico. The uncle finally consented to the surgery after several weeks when "He witnessed the client (his sister) suffering from much pain" (p. 516). The family in this example needed to make the decision based on their cultural norms and not on Western values. A nurse's attempt to promote the autonomy of the client in making her own informed decision to consent to surgery would not have been accepted in the collectivist social structure of this family (Andrews & Boyle, 2003).

For nurses to be culturally competent, they must assess cultural values that will enable them to provide culturally congruent nursing care. Unless nurses examine individuals' basic values and beliefs about health and health care, they might assume that all cultures share Western premises and values. Without meaning to impose their values, nurses may unwittingly encourage a behavior that is not culturally congruent for individuals from other-care cultures (see Chapter 2).

Data from Andrews, M., & Boyle, J. (2003). *Transcultural concepts in nursing care* (4th ed.). Philadelphia: Lippincott Williams & Wilkins; and Purnell, L. & Paulanka, B. (2008). *Transcultural health care: A culturally competent approach*. Philadelphia: F.A. Davis.

system has improved access to health care for many populations. Factors that limit a family's access to health care include the availability and location of health care facilities, geographical distance, transportation to these facilities, and the existence or type of health care insurance. Language barriers, hours missed from work or school, availability of child care, and excessively long waits for health care services all influence access to care (Spector, 2004). Each of these factors may be affected by the prevailing public policy of federal, state, and local governments. Technological developments, chronic illness, and the aging population each have an independent and interrelated influence on access to health care and the delivery of health services. Health care reform efforts will need to address health care disparities, especially for vulnerable populations. In 2008, each presidential candidate addressed the issue of health care in his political platform during the election (see discussion later in chapter).

ORGANIZATION OF THE DELIVERY SYSTEM

The health care delivery system in the United States does not consist of a network of interrelated components, designed to work together like one might expect in a system. Instead "it is a kaleidoscope of financing, **insurance**, delivery, and payment mechanisms that remain unstandardized and loosely coordinated" (Shi & Singh, 2004, p. 4). This complex interrelationship involves providers, consumers, and settings, with both private and public sectors providing services. The public sector includes voluntary and nonprofit agencies and official or governmental agencies. Delivery of services is organized on three levels in both sectors: local, state, and national. Each of the three levels consists of private providers combined with official or voluntary public agencies. The nurse is often the professional who assists the health consumer throughout the complex delivery system; therefore, a basic understanding of the system's organization is essential.

Private Sector

Independent Practice

Traditionally, a person enters the health care delivery system by contracting directly with a health care provider for individual care based on **fee-for-service**. Free choice of provider has been the hallmark of the American free market system. However, more recently physicians and other health care providers have been working within managed health care organizations. Although private practice traditionally has been disease oriented, the current emphasis on primary care necessitates a much broader perspective. **Primary care** involves continual and comprehensive care that includes efforts to keep people as healthy as possible and to prevent disease.

Private care may be delivered in numerous settings, from inpatient (hospital or extended care facility) to outpatient (ambulatory) settings. Outpatient care is defined as any health care services that are not provided on the basis of an overnight stay in which room and board costs are incurred. Ambulatory settings include two major categories: (1) care

---

Box 3-2 Types of Ambulatory Care Settings

- *Owner provider:* hospitals, community health agencies, managed care organizations, home health organizations, insurance agencies
- *Service settings:* walk-in clinics, urgent care centers, outpatient surgery centers, chemotherapy and radiation centers, dialysis centers, neighborhood and community health centers, diagnostic and mobile imaging centers, occupational health centers, women's health clinics, wound care centers, fitness-wellness centers, health department clinics, nursing centers

From Shi, L. & Singh, D. (2004). *Delivering Health Care in America: A Systems Approach* (3rd ed.). Sudbury, M.A.: Jones & Bartlett.

---

provided by owners and providers or (2) service settings (Box 3-2). These categories overlap, because many providers practice in their own offices and contract with one or more managed care organizations (see managed care discussion later in this chapter).

Nursing Centers Often situated in strategic locations to serve vulnerable populations, **nursing centers** are nurse-managed health centers that provide primary care to individuals and families (Kinsey & Buchanan, 2004). Nursing centers trace their origin to the Henry Street Settlements, founded by Lillian Wald in 1893 as discussed earlier (Holder, 2004). The modern movement to establish nursing centers began in 1965 when the nurse practitioner (NP) role was created, which allowed nurses to provide primary care to individuals and families. Nursing centers (ambulatory care centers and birthing centers) have provided high-quality nursing care from certified nurse midwives, nurse practitioners, and other APNs. During the 1970s, university-based centers and academic nursing centers were established to provide nursing services to communities, learning experiences for students, and settings for faculty practice and research. The key components of a community nursing center include (1) a nurse as chief manager, (2) a nursing staff that is accountable and responsible for care and professional practice, and (3) nurses as the primary providers of care. Using a multidisciplinary collaboration framework, nurses have the opportunity to provide comprehensive primary care services, including a focus on wellness and health promotion, public health programs, and targeted interventions for populations with special needs. In recent years, more than one half have closed for financial reasons. The Institute for Nursing Centers is an organization whose focus is to promote and enhance the work of nursing centers by providing web casts and other educational programs as well as a national repository of data for nurse-managed health centers funded by the W. K. Kellogg Foundation. Members of the Council for Nursing Centers also provide mentoring and consultation to support colleagues in developing and advancing nursing centers. Nurses can continue to build community support, trust, and skills needed to make the nursing center model part of mainstream health care delivery in the twenty-first century (Kinsey & Buchanan, 2004) (see the Case Study at the end of this chapter).

Advanced practice nurses (APNs), an umbrella term for nurses who practice in the roles of nurse practitioners, clinical nurse specialists, nurse midwives, or nurse anesthetists, are well suited to provide cost-effective, quality care to individuals and families, as well as serve economically disadvantaged and vulnerable populations. APNs not only have specialized clinical knowledge and skills at the masters or doctoral level but their advanced curriculum includes research and theoretical foundations to determine best practices, evaluate health policy issues, and understand the intricacies of health care financial management. Nurse practitioners play a key role within the health care system and often care for vulnerable populations in rural areas and inner cities, as well as practice in primary, acute and long-term care settings (Jansen & Zwygart-Stauffacher, 2006).

Move to Managed Care

Before the 1990s, a person would choose a physician or care provider and receive care, and the provider would bill the individual's insurance company and be paid on a fee-for-service basis. The provider had autonomy to treat the person without oversight from the insurance company. In an effort to control costs, managed care began to regulate the utilization of health care. Physicians contracted with an insurance company for a negotiated fee-for-service, usually at a discounted rate. Today, plans include a network of individual providers, and clients who choose providers within their network usually have full coverage. Individuals who choose providers outside of their network may be uncovered or be covered for a lesser amount and thus face greater out-of-pocket expenses. Within the network, a client has a **primary care provider** (PCP) who serves as a **gatekeeper** and foundation of the **managed care** organization. The PCP may be a physician, physician's assistant, or APN. Physician PCPs are usually general or family practitioners, but they may also be internists, pediatricians, or obstetrician-gynecologists. Physician's assistants are educated and prepared to work under the direct supervision of physicians. APNs who provide primary care are typically nurse practitioners or certified nurse midwives.

In 2002, 95% of workers who carried employer-based health insurance were enrolled in some type of a managed health plan. The principal force behind the growth of managed care is the belief that health care costs can be controlled by "managing" the way in which health care is delivered and controlling costs by controlling utilization (Sultz & Young, 2004).

As a "gatekeeper," the PCP coordinates and oversees individual care. The gatekeeper concept is designed to manage the individual's use of resources, to reduce self-referral to specialists, and to protect the individual from unnecessary procedures and overtreatment (Shi & Singh, 2004). Cost containment is achieved by decreasing hospital admissions and costly procedures as well as limiting referrals to specialists. An oversupply of specialists occur in some areas and

a lack of primary care providers occurs in many rural areas. Specialist salaries typically exceed those of PCPs, and the number of specialists has increased as technology has developed. Box 3-3 provides a glossary of key terms used in managed care.

Health Maintenance Organizations

Health maintenance organizations (HMOs) deliver comprehensive health maintenance and treatment services for a group of enrolled individuals who prepay a fixed fee. The HMO accepts responsibility for the organization, financing, and delivery of health care services for its members. Several models have evolved. The traditional HMO structure was a group or staff model, in which the fiscal agent employed a group of physicians and some specialty services to provide care to its members. Salaried providers generally spent all of their time serving members of the HMO. An example is Kaiser-Permanente Health Care System, which also has its own hospitals. Through a prenegotiated contract, usually based on fee for service, the HMO purchased hospital care and other services for its members. Staff models were described as "closed panel," because employed physicians provided care only for members of the HMO. A community physician could not care for a member of the HMO without prearrangement or authorization by the HMO. As of 1999, less than 1% of individuals were enrolled in this type of HMO, partly due to the lack of flexibility, cost to expand facilities, and competition from independent practice associations (Sultz & Young, 2004).

Medicare Advantage Plans are private health plans that receive payments from Medicare. Enrollees tend to be in better health than the traditional Medicare client and a number of Medicare Advantage Plans fall under the category of HMOs. Recently, 6.2 million beneficiaries were enrolled in a Medical Advantage plan with 92% enrolled in HMO plans. Because of the funding formula, those in Medicare Advantage plans often have extra benefits when compared to the traditional Medicare population (KFF, 2007d).

Independent Practice Associations

Independent practice associations (IPAs) are organizations composed of independent physicians in solo or group practices who provide health care services to members of an HMO in their private offices, eliminating the expense of the staff model HMO, which furnished and owned the facility in which care was provided. Hospital care and specialty services not within the IPA group can be purchased by the HMO for a fee-for-service or prepaid price. Physicians in an IPA contract may be restricted to caring only for members enrolled in the IPA, but some contracts may allow providers to care for nonmembers as well. Other variations of the staff model and IPAs exist. In a group practice model, an HMO contracts with all physicians and specialists needed by the HMO enrollees, but physicians remain independent. Some contracts are exclusive, requiring physicians to restrict care to members of an individual HMO, and other variations

Box **3-3** A Glossary of Managed Care Terms

- *Benefits:* the dollar amount available for the cost of covered medical services
- *Blue Cross/Blue Shield:* a combined medical plan offered through a worker's place of employment that combines both hospital and physician coverage
- *Capitation:* a fixed amount of payment per client, per year, regardless of the volume or cost of services each client requires
- *Copayments:* a fixed dollar payment that is made by the client to the provider at the time of service
- *Cost sharing:* provision of an insurance policy that requires the insured to pay some portion of the covered expenses (does not refer to or include cost of the premium)
- *Deductible:* a fixed dollar amount that the person must pay before reimbursement begins
- *Gatekeeper:* a physician or APN who provides primary care and who makes referrals for emergency services or specialty care
- *Health Maintenance Organization (HMO):* a prepaid health plan delivering comprehensive care to members through designated providers, having a fixed monthly payment for health care services, and requiring members to be in a plan for a specified period of time
- *Indemnity:* monies paid by an insurer to a provider, in a predetermined amount in the event of a covered loss by a beneficiary
- *Independent Practice Association (IPA):* an organization that physicians in private practice can join so that the organization can represent them in the negotiation of managed care contracts
- *Managed Care:* a health care plan that integrates the financing and delivery of health care services by using arrangements with selected health care providers to provide services for covered individuals. Plans are generally financed by capitation fees
- *Out-of-Pocket Expenditures:* the portion of medical expenses a client is responsible for paying
- *Point of Service Plan (POS):* a plan that contains elements of both HMOs and PPOs. They resemble HMOs for in-network services in that they both require copayments and a primary care physician. Services received outside of the network are usually reimbursed on a fee-for-service basis
- *Preferred Provider Organization (PPO):* a health plan generally consisting of hospital and physician providers. The PPO provides health care services to plan members usually at discounted rates in return for expedited claims payment
- *Primary Care:* basic health care that emphasizes general health needs rather than specialized care
- *Primary Care Provider (PCP):* a physician or APN who provides basic and routine health care services usually in an office or clinic
- *Reimbursement:* payment of services. Payment of providers by a third-party insurer or government health program for health care services
- *Self-Insured Plan:* plan offered by employers and other groups who directly assume the major cost of health insurance for their employees or members
- *Third-party payer (carrier):* in health care finance, this is a party (insurance carrier, Medicare and Medicaid or their government-contracted intermediary, managed-care organization, or health plan) that pays for hospital or medical bills instead of the client
- *Underinsured:* refers to people who have some type of health insurance, such as catastrophic care, but not enough insurance to cover all their health care costs
- *Uninsured:* individuals or groups with no or inadequate health insurance coverage
- *Utilization review:* a system used to monitor diagnosis, treatment, and billing practices, the purpose of which is to lower costs by discouraging unnecessary treatment

From United States National Library of Medicine–National Institute of Health. *Health Economics Information Resources: A Self-Study Course.* Available at: *www.nlm.nih.gov/nichsr/edu/healthecon/glossary.html.*

allow physicians to care for members outside the HMO. In a network model, HMOs contract with individual physicians and with physician groups for both primary and specialty services. The HMO maintains control over fee arrangements. As of 2002, approximately 26% of individuals were enrolled in some sort of IPA (Sultz & Young, 2004).

Concierge Medical Practices

According to a U.S. Government Accountability Office report to Congressional Committees, **concierge care** is a type of primary care medical practice in which physicians charge individual clients a membership fee averaging $1500 to $1900 per year (range reported as $60 to $15,000 per year) in return for enhanced health care services or amenities. Only a small number of physicians (estimated to be 114 in 2004) have established concierge care practices but the trend is growing. Amenities most often include same or next-day appointments for nonurgent care, 24-hour telephone access to the physician,

and routine periodic preventive examinations. Some concierge physicians do not accept insurance but 75% report billing client health insurance for covered services and Medicare. Individuals are encouraged to carry health care insurance for services utilized outside of the practice. Although there is wide variation in amenities offered, no–waiting time office visits, access to physicians via cell phones and e-mail, and house calls may be provided and serve as attractive incentives for individuals. Physicians who provide concierge care typically care for fewer persons (800 compared to an average client load of 4000), allowing physicians more time to spend with their clients to provide expanded preventive services and practice amenities that are not available in a traditional practice. Concierge physicians benefit as well, with more time for their own families, research, and professional activities as well as an enhanced income from membership fees (GAO, 2005).

The concept of concierge medical care was originated in Seattle, Washington, by an athletic team physician who realized that the level of service provided to athletes was remarkable and could be expanded to nonathletes. Physicians in this practice provide comprehensive primary care to no more than 100 clients each and currently charge annual membership (or retainer) fees of $13,000 per individual. This group does not bill any form of health insurance (GAO, 2005; Marquis, 2004). Described as *boutique*, *platinum*, *premier*, or *Ritz-Carleton* medical care, this level of health care caters to those who are affluent enough to pay the annual membership fees. The number of concierge medical care practices is growing, but there are those who oppose a form of care that favors the rich (country club elitism) and does not serve the needs of the poor or vulnerable populations (GAO, 2005; Marquis, 2004).

Hospitalist Movement

Responding to the same impetus that spurred managed care in outpatient settings, **Hospitalist** programs—supported by HMOs, hospitals and medical groups—were formed to control hospital costs without compromising quality or satisfaction with client care. Hospitalists are physicians whose professional focus is caring for the hospitalized client. They provide direct inpatient primary, critical, and consultative care to hospitalized clients and are available 24 hours in hospitals with programs. Study findings have found that hospitalist programs reduce length of stay, cost per case, readmission rate, mortality rates, complication rates, and congestion in emergency departments. Hospitalist practices have increased hospital efficiency and improved client satisfaction rates (DiSalvo, 2004; Jeter, 2007). Although reports show improvement in hospitalized client care and a trend to continue and evolve these programs, DiSalvo warns that the programs raise other issues such as long-term funding, physician satisfaction, the rate of physician burnout, and the effects of discontinuity of the care for the client between the outpatient world and the hospital (2004).

Point-of-Service Plans

Point-of-service (POS) plans evolved in response to concern with restrictions of consumer choice in selecting providers and services. POS plans allow members, for an additional fee and higher copayment, to use providers outside of the individual HMO network. Members can choose to pay for this enhanced POS or stay within the HMO network for reduced copayments. In 2002, 18% of HMO members were enrolled in various levels of POS plans (Sultz & Young, 2004).

Preferred Provider Organizations

Preferred provider organizations (PPOs), another delivery model in the private sector, were formed by physicians and hospitals to serve the needs of private, third-party payer, and self-insured firms. Contracted providers in the PPO agree to deliver services to members for a fee-for-service negotiated discount price. To control costs, members must receive care exclusively from providers within the PPO or incur additional cost. "In 2002, PPOs were the most popular managed care plans, with a 52% market share" (Sultz & Young, 2004, p. 280). To control costs, the provider must receive preauthorization from the PPO for a member to be hospitalized, and second opinions are required before major procedures or surgery are performed. PPOs are beneficial to physicians and hospitals because they are assured a certain volume of business (Sultz & Young, 2004).

Public Sector

The public sector contains official and voluntary public health agencies operating at the local, state, federal, and international levels. Before 1900, public health was concerned with problems related to environmental risks and infectious diseases. After the 1900s the public health agenda expanded to address the needs of children and mothers. By midcentury, treating chronic disease had also been added to its agenda. As the century progressed, public health issues came to include substance abuse, mental illness, teen pregnancy, long-term care, epidemics of violence, HIV infections, and most recently bioterrorism and disaster preparedness (Turnock, 2004).

Source of Power

The U.S. Constitution is based on the sharing of sovereign power between federal and state governments. The powers of the federal government in relation to health are not delineated specifically in the Constitution; they are derived from its authority to tax and to spend for the general welfare and from powers delegated to it by the states. The state governor or legislature usually appoints a health commissioner or secretary of health, who directs the health agency (usually the public health department) to protect citizens from communicable diseases and environmental hazards from waste, water, and food (Nies & McEwen, 2007). State health authority is based also on the Tenth Amendment, which reserves for the states, or for the people, those powers not delegated to the federal government by the Constitution. The states then use their powers to create local governments and delegate authority to them in health matters. The United States Public Health Service falls within the larger Department of Health and Human Services (see Box 3-4 for a list of key U.S. Public Health Service Agencies).

Influence of Political Philosophy

The prevailing political philosophy regarding societal health needs affects the relationship among federal, state, and local government. Although the federal government gained power to promote health and welfare in the early twentieth century by the passage of the Sixteenth Amendment (giving it the authority to levy federal taxes), states retained sovereign power as the resources were distributed at the state and local level. Beginning in the 1930s, however, New Deal philosophy began to displace power from the state and local to the federal government. Passage of the Hill-Burton Act of 1946 and establishment of what is now known as the CDC increased

Box **3-4** Key U.S. Public Health Service Agencies

- *Health and Service Administration (HRSA):* provides health resources for medically underserved populations
- *Indian Health Service (IHS):* is responsible for providing federal health services to American Indians and Alaska Natives
- *Centers for Disease Control and Prevention (CDC):* working with states, provides a system of health surveillance to monitor and prevent outbreaks of disease
- *National Institutes of Health (NIH):* provides leadership and direction to programs designed to improve the health of the nation by conducting and supporting research
- *Food and Drug Administration (FDA):* ensures food, medications, medical devices, and radiation-emitting devices (microwaves) are safe. Also oversees feed and

drugs for animals and enforces the Federal Food, Drug, and Cosmetic Act to monitor the manufacture, import, transport, storage, and sale of goods annually
- *Substance Abuse and Mental Health Services Administration (SAMHSA):* strengthens the Nation's health care capacity to provide prevention, diagnosis, and treatment services for substance abuse and mental illness
- *Agency for Toxic Substances and Disease Registry (ATSDR):* seeks to prevent exposure to hazardous substances from waste sites
- *Agency for Health Care Research and Quality (AHRQ):* supports cross-cutting research on health care systems, health care quality and cost issues, and effectiveness of medical treatments

Adapted from Turnock, B. (2004). *Public health: What is it and how does it work?* Sudbury, MA: Jones & Bartlett Publishers. Exhibit 4-1, pp. 139-141.

the federal government's power over state and local affairs. The trend toward increased federal government involvement continued during the Kennedy-Johnson era, when the government focused on societal needs and health care to an unprecedented degree. During the Nixon-Ford era, the trend began to reverse as a New Federalism movement called for less federal encroachment into states' responsibilities and greater state and local responsibility. Clearly, the federal government's role varies according to political philosophy.

During the 1980s the Reagan administration supported free market competition among insurance plans, physicians, and hospitals to offer the best possible services with the lowest price. Reagan was adamant in his opposition to adopting national health insurance legislation for what he labeled "socialized medicine." Reagan's procompetition policies supported a decrease in federal responsibility for health care preferring to give states power by providing block grants and control at the state level.

During the Bush administration (1989-1993), little change occurred in moving new legislation toward health care reform. To avoid increasing taxes, Bush proposed a system of tax deductions or tax credits to reduce the cost of private health insurance for families not covered by Medicaid or Medicare. Bush proposed the creation of large networks of small businesses to purchase group health insurances for their employees, voluntary measures to reduce insurance paperwork, encouragement of enrollment in HMOs, and legislation to reduce medical malpractice suits. Due to an economic recession, many workers employed by small businesses did not have employer health insurance plans and these measures would have assisted in covering working families. However, Congressional Democrats refused to support the proposed reform because it did not include an expansion of federal power with a plan for universal coverage or control over the growing cost of insurance premiums.

In 1993 the Clinton administration proposed the Health Security Act to achieve universal health care coverage in the United States by mandating that all employers provide health insurance to their employees and by giving small businesses and unemployed Americans subsidies with which to purchase insurance. The plan met severe opposition from the insurance industry and the business community. Mass media advertisements by these stakeholders questioned whether HMOs would provide choice and access to health care services. Large segments of the American public, especially the 80% who had employer-based private health insurance, began to fear being forced into HMOs, which would diminish their choice of, access to, and quality of health care. The cost of socialized, universal health care coverage system was estimated to reach trillion-dollar levels. The act was defeated in Congress (Lee & Estes, 2003). A time of political caution followed, stalling any further movement toward universal health care. The portability of health care coverage bill was passed in 1996, allowing persons to access health care throughout the United States, and the focus shifted to balancing the federal budget. Incremental legislation included the Balanced Budget Act (BBA) of 1997, which made significant reforms in Medicare and a new public insurance program and the *State Children's Health Insurance Program* (SCHIP). SCHIP is a public state insurance program supported by federal monies to provide insurance to children of working families that did not have insurance and did not meet state Medicaid requirements (see discussion about Medicaid later in this chapter). A major expansion in the role of the federal government occurred in 2003, when Congress passed the Medicare Prescription Drug Act Part D and in 2007, when legislation was signed to continue funding SCHIP programs.

Due to the rising cost of health care premiums and a growing number of uninsured or underinsured individuals, debate about establishing a socialized national health care program was once again a topic in the 2008 presidential campaign. Concern for rising costs of funding existing federally supported programs for older adults and the poor (Medicare,

research highlights

Community-Based Program for Spanish-Speaking Hispanics with Chronic Disease in Northern California: Taking Control of Your Health

A growing health disparity between Hispanics and non-Hispanics, as well as the increase in the prevalence of chronic disease in the Hispanic population, sparked investigators to study participant outcomes of a 6-week peer-led community-based program for Spanish-speaking Hispanics with known chronic disease. The program, Tomando Control de su Salud (Taking Control of Your Health), was similar to a previously successful English Chronic Disease Self-Management Program. The participants in the study were recruited via community outreach to churches, community centers, and clinics in 4-month cohorts over a 3.5-year period. Participants were eligible for inclusion if they had heart disease, lung disease, or type 2 diabetes. Two and one-half hour class segments focused on exercise, positive thinking, nutrition, relaxation techniques, and problem solving. Disease-specific content was not taught.

Participants were randomized into two groups, intervention and usual care participants. Intervention participants took Tomando immediately, whereas the usual care participants were put on a waiting list for 4 months. Treatment participants in this study numbered 327 and were compared with those placed on the waiting list (224 participants). After 4 months, participants were compared with usual care subjects and demonstrated improved health status, health behavior, and self-efficacy, as well as fewer emergency room visits. After 1 year the improvements were maintained and remained significantly different from the baseline condition. In conclusion, this community-based program has the potential to improve the lives of Hispanics with chronic illness while reducing emergency room use.

From Lorig, K., Ritter, P., Gonzalez, V. (2003). Hispanic chronic disease self-management: A randomized community-based outcome trial. *Nursing Research*, 52(6), 361-369.

Medicaid, and SCHIP) has made Americans aware of the tremendous cost of mandated federal and state programs. Political candidates have discussed health care reform as part of their political platforms. The Democratic Party overall supports expanding existing public programs or adopting new ones. The projected costs of this type of reform are billions of additional dollars. Finance mechanisms would include raising general tax revenues. The Republican Party overall supports a free-market approach to health care reform. Tax cuts and incentives for individuals to purchase health insurance would be put in place as well as the use of health savings accounts.

Future Health Policy

Historically there has been a lack of consensus among the major political parties and stakeholders regarding health care reform. After attempts to implement comprehensive reforms in 1993 and 1994 led to a deadlocked policy process, the focus shifted to making incremental changes in the free market system. Cost, access, and quality continued to be major factors in policy development at all levels of government: local, state, and federal (Lee & Estes, 2003).

A new health insurance paradigm, consumer-driven health plans, surfaced in 2000. These employer-supplied insurance plans are an alternative to managed care health plans and may allow businesses, especially small businesses, an avenue to provide health care coverage to their employees. A health care reimbursement account, a medical savings account (MSA), or a **health savings account** (HSA) is established for the employee. Individual members receive approximately $1000 annually to cover general health care expenditures, and unused monies are rolled over for the next year. Screening and preventive care are generally covered 100%, but higher-cost care (catastrophic, surgery, or hospitalization) has high deductibles. Policy considerations include making health savings accounts tax exempt, which would increase the appeal to both employees and

employers. These plans are expected to grow in number as an alternative to managed care (Herrick, 2004). Other health reform is needed in the area of electronic medical records. The development of a digital health information infrastructure (health IT) where an individual's personal records could be accessed by a provider would streamline paperwork and provide for a more seamless journey for a person through the health care system. A person's medical record would be maintained electronically and could be accessed by region, state, or possible nationally. Details as to privacy issues, control of access, and security measures to ensure that a person's medical information is not exposed to a nonauthorized source would need to be built into the system. Other reform efforts need to address, for example, workforce shortages of health care professionals (nurses, physicians, faculty), medical malpractice issues and costs, safety of the health care delivery system, and funding for the growing needs of the older adult population for long-term and custodial care.

Nursing's Role in the Search for Health Care Reform

Major issues of rising costs, access to care, and accountability for the health care system were addressed in the American Nurses Association (ANA) proposal, "ANA's Health Care Agenda 2005." Developed with the premise that health care is a basic human right, the ANA's plan supports a single-payer mechanism as the most desirable option for financing a reformed healthcare system. The ANA supports the reshaping of the health care delivery system to focus on primary prevention and wellness (primary care) and away from expensive, technology-driven acute hospital care. The first point in nursing's agenda is to provide primary care in convenient, familiar, community settings where individuals live and work, such as schools, work sites, and the home (Research Highlights box) (American Nurses Association [ANA], 2005).

Official Agencies

Official agencies are tax supported and therefore accountable to the citizens through elected or appointed officials or boards. The purpose and duties of official agencies are prescribed or mandated by law. This discussion is from the perspective of the individual gaining knowledge of or access to the health care system.

Local Level The health department of a town, city, county, township, or district is the local health unit and is usually the first line of access and health responsibility for the population that it serves. The chief administrator, the health officer, is appointed by the mayor, the board of health, or some other executive governing body. The local health department's role and functions usually center on providing direct services to the public and depend on the state mandate and community resources. Local governments, but usually not health departments, have the responsibility to provide general health care services for the poor. (See the Medicaid section later in this chapter.)

State Level Public health services are organized by each state, with wide variation from one state to another. The chief administrator is usually a state health officer or commissioner appointed by the governor. One agency, typically the state health department, carries out the primary responsibilities in policy, planning, and coordination of programs and services for local units under its jurisdiction.

Federal Level The federal government assumes overall responsibility for the health protection of its citizens. Although all three branches of the government make health-related decisions, the major policy decisions are made by the president and his staff (executive branch) and Congress (legislative branch). These two branches determine health policy. Once policy is determined, other government agencies are responsible for oversight to ensure implementation.

The USHHS, the main federal body concerned with the health of the nation, consists of a number of separate agencies (see Box 3-4). USHHS agencies that relate directly to nursing include the Health Resources and Services Administration and the National Institutes of Health (NIH). The Bureau of Health Professions, within the Health Resources and Services Administration, contains a division of nursing, which is a source for nursing education and training grants. The National Institute of Nursing Research within the NIH funds nursing research, including health promotion and illness prevention studies.

Chief Nursing Officer The Chief Nursing Officer (CNO) serves in the U.S. Public Health Service (USPHS) and provides advice to and works with the U.S. Surgeon General on policy issues related to nursing and public health. The Commissioned Corps of the USPHS has a nursing division that the CNO represents. In May of 2005, an NP, Teri Mills from Oregon, wrote an editorial to the *New York Times* calling for a National Nurse position to be created by the U.S. Congress to act as a national spokesperson to draw attention to the nursing profession, raise the level of professionalism, and provide public health education. This new federally appointed position would complement the work of the U.S. Surgeon General. A number of organizations supported the cause and federal legislation for the creation of the office was introduced to the 109th Congress. A number of nursing organizations—including The American Association of Colleges of Nursing, American Nurses Association, American Public Health Association, The Quad Council of Public Health Nursing Organizations, and others—oppose the creation of a new office. Since the CNO is the national nurse, they argue, efforts to make the position more visible, expand activities associated with the role, and allocate additional resources to the nursing and public health networks are already in place (Quan, 2008; Wood, 2007).

Military Health Systems At the federal level, the Military Health System (MHS) comprises the entire health system of the Department of Defense and serves approximately 9 million Americans. The Veterans Administration, an independent agency directly under the President, provides health care services for veterans through the Department of Defense, which sponsors health care for military personnel on active duty. For military dependents and retirees, care is covered through the former Civilian Health and Medical Program for the Uniformed Services (CHAMPUS) insurance program, renamed TRICARE.

Wounded Warrior Care When a soldier is severely injured, prolonged care and rehabilitation is often required before a decision can be made whether the soldier should remain on active duty. The MHS is responsible for providing outstanding clinical care to return them to duty or help them make the transition from MHS care to the VA health care system. The MHS and VA have numerous excellence centers dedicated to wounded warrior care. These include the Walter Reed Medical Center Amputee Care Center and Gait Laboratory and National Naval Medical Center's Traumatic Stress and Brain Injury Program. Other specialty centers include burn care, rehabilitation, and combat casualty. Tremendous progress has been made in the rehabilitative care of injured combatants and coordination of MHS care with the VA health system (MHS, 2008). For example, Haben (2008) reports that concussion known as mild traumatic brain injury (TBI) may affect 10 to 20 percent of soldiers and marines engaged in combat in Iraq and Afghanistan. More than 80 percent are treated with complete recovery and are redeployed. Others may need extensive rehabilitation and assistance in returning to civilian life.

Americans with Disabilities Starting in 1992 health care providers, both as employers and as providers of public services, were required to comply with requirements of the Americans With Disabilities Act of 1990. The act is considered the most sweeping civil rights legislation since the Civil Rights Act of 1964. The two parts that apply most directly to health care providers are the prohibitions of employment discrimination and the requirements for provision of services to people with disabilities. An example of health care provider accommodation is to install wheelchair lifts in their shuttle bus systems. Despite their need for health promotion and disease prevention, individuals with disabilities face numerous problems gaining access to health promotion programs and preventive services. The barriers are financial, social, physical, and logistical.

In 1990, President George H. Bush signed the Patient Self-Determination Act, which took effect in December 1991. This law was designed to increase individual involvement in decisions about life-sustaining treatment, ensuring that advance directives for health care are available to physicians at the time that medical decisions are being made and ensuring that individuals who have not prepared such documents are aware of their legal rights. As a condition of Medicare and Medicaid payment, the Patient Self-Determination Act requires health care facilities to comply with the law.

Federal Health Information Privacy Law Developed by the Department of Health and Human Services (HHS), as part of the Health Insurance Portability and Accountability Act of 1996 (HIPAA), federal privacy standards were enacted by Congress requiring new safeguards to protect the security and confidentiality of health information including paper, electronic, and oral communications. Health plans, pharmacies, doctors, nurses, and other health care providers must have a written privacy procedure, provide employee training on HIPAA, and designate a privacy officer to ensure procedures are followed. The privacy law permits disclosures without individual authorization to public health authorities authorized by law to collect and receive information for the purpose of preventing or controlling disease, injury, or disability (USDHHS, 2007c).

International Level WHO, the United Nations' specialized agency for health as previously discussed, was established in 1948. Comprised of membership of more than 190 countries, WHO's core functions include (1) giving worldwide guidance in the field of health; (2) setting global standards for health; (3) cooperating with governments in strengthening national health programs; and (4) developing and transferring appropriate technology, information, and standards (WHO, 2004). WHO also encourages and coordinates international scientific research.

Voluntary Agencies

The voluntary (not-for-profit) health movement, which began in 1882, stems from the goodwill and humanitarian concerns that are part of the nongovernmental, free enterprise heritage of the people of the United States. Nonprofit entities

that maintain a tax-free status are often powerful forces in the health field, voluntary agencies, foundations, and professional associations. The tax-free status of these organizations is challenged at times based on charges that some of them serve only a limited population (e.g., the very rich). Voluntary agencies are influential in promoting health affairs at the national policy level and often have significant influence on health legislation. Their prominent role was demonstrated by the American Cancer Society's early mass media announcements about the health hazards of smoking. The Alzheimer's Association has local chapters that provide resources for families including publications, services, respite for the caregiver, and support groups for clients and families. In 2004, Alzheimer's disease was listed as the fifth-leading cause of death for 65 years and older with a total of 65,313 deaths (NCHS, 2006).

Philanthropic foundations provide valuable stimulation to the health field and operate under fewer constraints than do other sources in supporting research or training projects. Nurses interested in research or advanced clinical study that relates to the special interests of voluntary agencies or foundations may find grant monies available to support their work. For example, The John A. Hartford Institution Trustees awarded a $5 million, 5-year grant to create the John A. Hartford Foundation Institute for Geriatric Nursing at New York University. The Hartford Institute promotes initiatives to improve care of older adults and training projects to prepare faculty to teach care of older adults in baccalaureate nursing programs. The institute has also raised the profile of geriatric nursing by creating nationally recognized awards for excellence in research and practice (Hartford Institute, 2006). Professional associations, organized at the national level with state and local branches, are powerful political forces. Nurses can support their professional organizations in influencing the direction of health policy through membership and active participation.

FINANCING HEALTH CARE
Costs

The health care industry is the largest service industry in the United States today and the most powerful employer in the nation, employing 3% of the total labor force (Shi & Singh, 2004). National health expenditures in the United States were $2 trillion in 2005, a 7% increase from 2004. In 2005, health spending was 16.0% of the gross domestic product and is projected to be 18.4% by 2013. Hospital spending, which accounts for 31% of the national health expenditure, increased by 8% in 2005. The cost of prescription drugs, which accounts for 10% of national health expenditures, increased by 6% in 2005 (NCHS, 2007) (Figure 3-1). In 2005, the per capita expenditure for health care was $6697, the highest of all countries. Table 3-4 lists selective countries with per capita cost comparisons for the years 1980, 1990, 2000, and 2004. Mexico, which borders the United States, is reported to spend $662 per person.

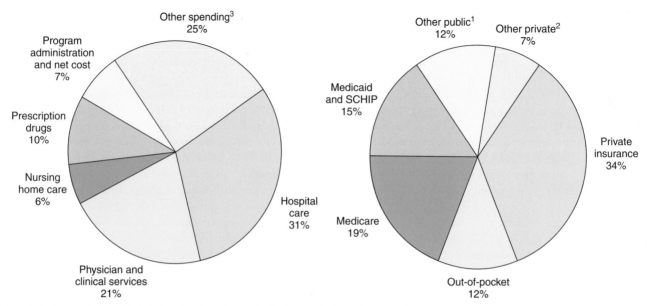

Figure 3-1 The nation's health dollar in 2006. (From Centers for Medicare & Medicaid Services, Office of the Actuary, National Health Statistics Group, 2006.)

[1]"Other public" includes programs such as Worker's Compensation, public health activity, Department of Defense, Department of Veteran's Affairs, Indian Health Services, state and local hospital subsidies, and school health.

[2]"Other private" includes industrial in-plant, privately funded construction, and nonclient revenues, including philanthropy.

[3]"Other spending" includes dentist services, other professional services, home health care, durable medical products, over-the-counter medicines and sundries, public health, research, and construction.

Table 3-4 International Comparisons of Gross Domestic Product and Per Capita Health Expenditures

Country	1980 GDP	1980 Per Capita	1990 GDP	1990 Per Capita	2000 GDP	2000 Per Capita	2004 GDP	2004 Per Capita
Canada	7.1%	$783	9.0%	$1737	8.9%	$2503	9.9%	$3165
France	7.1%	$711	8.6%	$1568	9.3%	$2456	10.1%	$3159
Germany*	8.7%	$965	8.5%	$1748	10.6%	$2671	11.1%	$3043
Japan	6.5%	$580	5.9%	$1115	7.6%	$1971	----	----
Mexico	----	----	4.8%	$293	5.6%	$499	6.2%	$662
Sweden	9.1%	$936	8.4%	$1579	8.4%	$2273	11.6%	$4077
United Kingdom	5.6%	$482	6.0%	$986	7.3%	$1833	8.1%	$2508
United States	8.7%	$1055	11.9%	$2738	13.1%	$4539	15.3%	$6101

*For years prior to 1990, Germany refers to West Germany.

----Data not available.

From U.S. Department of Health and Human Services, National Center for Health. (Nov, 2007). Statistics, United States, 2007. Retrieved January 18, 2008, from *www.cdc.gov/nchs/hus.htm*. Tables 120, 121, pp. 373-5.

In 2005, private health insurance paid 36% of total personal care expenditures, the federal government 34%, state and local governments 11%, and out-of-pocket expenses were 11% (NCHS, 2007).

Health care analysts predict the accelerations in health care cost will continue, putting pressure on public and private payers to finance them. Factors driving costs include: (1) general inflation, (2) health care cost inflation, (3) application of new and more advanced technologies, (4) growth in the proportion of older adults, (5) government financing of health care services, (6) growth of prescription drug usage and costs, (7) misdistribution of health care providers and services, (8) expansion of medical technology and specialty medicine, and (9) the growing number of uninsured and underinsured people (Lee & Estes, 2003; Shi & Singh, 2004). For example, diagnostic and therapeutic techniques—including computer-aided technology and noninvasive imaging (such as magnetic resonance imaging), cardiac surgery, organ transplantation, and operations on joints (particularly hips and knees)—enhance the capabilities of medicine while increasing costs.

| Table 3-5 | National Health Care Expenditures Comparisons: Projections for 1990, 2000, and 2005 |

Type of Service	Total Dollars* 1990	Percent of Total 1990	Total Dollars* 2000	Percent of Total 2000	Total Dollars* 2005	Percentage of Total 2005
National health expenditures	$717.3	100	$1358.5	100	$1988.0	100
Personal health care	607.5	84.7	1139.9	83.9	1860.9	83.6
Hospital care	251.6	35.1	417.0	30.7	611.6	30.8
Physician and clinical services	157.5	22.0	288.6	21.2	421.2	21.2
Dental care	31.5	4.4	62.0	4.6	86.6	4.4
Other professional services	18.2	2.5	39.1	2.9	58.7	2.9
Other personal health care	9.6	1.3	37.1	2.7	57.2	2.9
Home health care	12.6	1.8	30.6	2.2	47.5	2.4
Nursing home care	52.6	7.3	95.3	7.0	121.9	6.1
Prescription drugs	40.3	5.6	120.8	8.9	200.7	10.1
Other medical products	33.7	4.7	49.5	3.6	55.9	2.9

*Total dollars in billions.
Based on data from Centers for Medicare & Medicaid Services, Office of the Actuary, National Health Statistics Group, National Health Expenditures 2005. Retrieved from *www.cms.hhs.gov/NationalHealthExpenData/*.
Note: Numbers are rounded; may not add to totals.

Changes in hospital care and use of hospitalists, increased utilization of outpatient services, shorter inpatient stays, and more care of chronic illness than acute illness—combined, these factors mean that hospitals have less time to offer prevention or health promotion education to individuals. Moreover, workforce shortages, especially in nursing, increase the use of nonprofessional caregivers. Inadequate resources, reimbursement, and numbers of nurses may prevent health care professionals from offering the range of health-promotion educational efforts called for in the original *Healthy People 2010* objectives and revised objectives from the Healthy People Mid Course Review (USDHHS, 2007a).

National health expenditures for 1990, 2000, and 2005 are shown in Table 3-5. In 2005 the largest component was hospital care (30.8%), although its share of total expenditures showed a decline compared to 35.1.7% in 1990. Spending for physician and clinical services totaled 21.2%, dental services 4.4%, and other professionals 2.9%. Another 2.4% went for home health care, 10.0% for prescription drugs, and 6.1% for nursing home care. The Centers for Medicare & Medicaid Services, Office of the Actuary reported spending figures for the calendar year 2006 (see Figure 3-1) that are similar to those of the 2005 reports.

Sources

Ultimately, the American people pay for all health care costs. Money is transferred from consumer to provider by various mechanisms. The major sources are government (federal, state and local monies collected by taxes), third-party payment (private insurance), independent plans, and out-of-pocket support (Sultz & Young, 2004). Also prepared by the same office is where the monies came from. In 2006 (see Figure 3-1) the

largest percentage came from private health insurance, which accounted for 34%. Consumers paid out-of-pocket for 12% of health care costs. The cost of Medicare accounted for 19% of the health care dollar and Medicaid and SCHIP 15%.

Employer Health Benefits

According to the 2007 employer health benefits survey conducted by The Kaiser Family Foundation, the overall inflation rate of employer-sponsored health insurance was 6.1% in 2007 and 7.7% in 2006. In 2006 the average annual total premium cost was $4479 for single coverage and $12,106 for family coverage while the average annual worker contributions for single coverage were $694 and $3281 for family coverage. The majority of covered workers (57%) were enrolled in PPOs followed by 21% in HMOs and 13% in POS plans. High-deductible health plans with a savings option account for 5% of covered workers. Workers also paid general annual deductibles and varying amounts of cost sharing when they were admitted to the hospital, had outpatient surgery, or visited the emergency room or urgent care center. Copayments were required for office visits and for prescription drugs for most workers. The survey also found 60% of employers offered health benefits in 2007 compared to 69% in 2000, with the decrease attributed to the declining number of small firms (3 to 99 workers) offering health coverage (KFF, 2007a).

High-Deductible Health Plans with Savings Option (HDHP/SO)

Large firms (1000 or more workers) are more likely to offer employees a choice of health plans with High-Deductible Health Plans with Savings Options as a choice. About 3.8 million workers are enrolled in some sort of HDHP/SO.

Premiums for this type of health insurance are significantly less, but workers typically have a deductible of at least $1000 for individual coverage and $2000 for family coverage. Employees are permitted to establish and contribute to a health savings account and some plans cover preventive services before the deductible is met. With some plans, employers contribute to the health savings account an average of $806 for individual coverage and $1294 for family coverage. These types of plans may become more readily available in the future (KFF, 2007a).

Federal and state Medicaid spending showed an increasing pattern similar to that discussed earlier in this chapter with Medicaid spending reported to be $5.3 billion in 1970; $207.0 billion in 2000 and in just 4 years, rose an additional $102 billion to $309.0 billion dollars in 2004. In 1996, the Personal Responsibility and Work Opportunity Reconciliation Act with Temporary Assistance for Needy Families (TANF) block grants replaced Aid to Families with Dependent Children (AFDC), requiring Medicaid recipients to go to work. TANF monies were funneled into programs that help recipients find work (Weissert & Weissert, 2006). As a cost savings mechanism, by 2000, 55.8% of Medicaid recipients were enrolled in some form of managed care plan. In fiscal year 2005 the Medicaid program cost taxpayers $329 billion, financing health care for 53 million low-income children, adults, seniors, and people with disabilities. Children make up 50% of individuals in the program but account for only 16% of the spending of Medicaid dollars, while older adults make up 11% of enrollment but account for 30% of the spending. The blind or disabled individuals in the program, representing only 15% of those enrolled, consumed 40% of Medicaid spending. The largest share of Medicaid monies goes for institutional services. Medicaid covers 40% of all costs for long-term care and more than half of all older nursing home residents. With the demographic trends of the nation's baby boomers, Medicaid costs are predicted to grow.

Each state receives from the federal government a matching formula percentage of revenue to run a Medicaid program, leaving state budgets responsible for the remaining cost. Federal tax dollars must fund a minimum of 50% of Medicaid costs. In 2008, New York, California, Colorado, Connecticut, Maryland, Massachusetts, and six other states were funded at the minimum level of 50%, while other states—for example, Arkansas 73.37%, Louisiana 70.47%, Mississippi 76.29%, and West Virginia 74.25%—received a much greater share of the cost of their Medicaid programs from the federal government (KFF, 2007b). The remainder of the cost of Medicaid programs is funded by state and local taxes. For example, New York state tax monies contribute 25% to the cost of Medicaid, and the individual counties must pick up the additional 25%. In 2004, residents saw rising state and county taxes, as well as double-digit increases in property taxes, to meet the needs of the Medicaid population in New York State.

Since Medicaid is an entitlement program, anyone who meets Medicaid's eligibility requirements is entitled to receive benefits; therefore, there is no way to cap the Medicaid budget at the federal or state level under current law. One way to limit the cost of the Medicaid program is to reform the system with the use of block grants. Some Republican and conservative candidates have favored this type of reform. If adopted, an allocation of monies (block grants) would be issued to individual states. Once the state has expended its allocation, any additional services for eligible persons would have to be provided by the individual state (Anderson et al., 2007). In an effort to provide health care to vulnerable populations, many states have more lenient eligibility requirements than those mandated by the federal government and offer more health services.

Mechanisms
Payment

Although some health care providers and other professionals in the private sector are paid on a fee-for-service basis, by third-party private insurance, or by public-supported insurance, most health workers, including nurses in institutional or community agencies and in the military, receive salaries. Since nurses are salaried, the separation of nursing costs from all other health-related costs is difficult. The cost of nursing care typically is incorporated in the room and board charge in the acute care setting. Without documentation of specific nursing costs, validating the need for skilled nursing services is difficult.

In recent years, nurses and Advanced Practice Nurses have entered independent practice to provide direct services. Nurses who are academically prepared for advanced practice represent about 6% of all registered nurses. In March of 2004 there were an estimated 141,209 NPs, 72,521 clinical nurse specialists, 32,523 certified registered nurse anesthetists, and 13,684 certified nurse midwives in the United States (USDHHS, 2004).

Independent nursing practice may be viewed as a logical outgrowth of seeking higher levels of professionalism. The nurse practice acts of some states encourage nurses to use their knowledge more comprehensively than many agencies sanction. In independent practice, the nurse is directly accountable to individuals and is paid either directly or by third parties. The philosophical and realistic issues of private nursing practice range from questions about the equity of fee-for-service to the practical problems of setting up this type of practice. The possibility of independent practice becoming commonplace in nursing's future depends on decisions about reimbursement by third parties in both private and public sectors, because reimbursement continues to be a restriction on practice. Although legislation in 1997 included the reimbursement of APNs by Medicare, not all plans and provider groups include these nurses as primary care practitioners. At the federal level, NPs are encouraging and lobbying lawmakers to allow them to order hospice and home health care (Rollet, 2003). Clearly the nursing practice roles and prescriptive authority of APNs varies state to state. Incremental steps have been taken to advance the APN role at both the federal and state levels. Some states have passed laws for NPs to practice and prescribe without MD oversight.

Alternative forms of payment are salary and capitation. The salary system involves a set amount for services provided in a specified time frame. This system provides the employer with a fixed nursing income that is protected from changes in supply and demand, includes fringe benefits, and obviates fee collection problems. The salary system's flexibility makes it easier to fill unpopular jobs or jobs in underserved areas. Disadvantages of this system include a limit on income and constraints on schedules, vacations, and peer review. The nurse may have to meet goals other than personal ones.

In the **capitation system**, such as in an HMO, each provider receives a flat annual fee for each participant regardless of how often services are used. Individuals who enroll in an HMO pay a fixed amount on a monthly basis whether they use the services or not; prepayment provides an incentive to provide efficient care. The objective is to keep people healthy to prevent costly services. Cost consciousness dictates that illness be treated as early as possible and in the most cost-effective setting. Capitation is simple to administer; no third-party insurance payments are present and the HMO bears the risk of illness. Preventive primary care that avoids costly hospitalization keeps costs down, and the savings revert to the organization. On the negative side, individuals may make unnecessary visits, the increased enrollment necessary to provide more monies may decrease comprehensive care, and there may be limits to quality of care, services, and access to all types of providers.

Cost Containment

The government's interest in hospital treatment cost containment was exemplified by the passage of the Social Security Amendments of 1983 (Public Law 98-21), which mandate the establishment by the Health Care Financing Administration of a prospective payment system for Medicare. This system stipulates that providers be paid at preset rates based on 470 diagnosis-related group categories (DRGs) used to classify the illness of each Medicare-insured person. Rates for each diagnosis are established according to regional and national amounts based on each hospital's urban and rural cost experience. Average hospital occupancy rates in community hospitals declined by 8% between 1980 and 2004. The occupancy rate in community hospitals in 1990 was reported to be 67%, 64% in 2000, and back to 67% in 2004 (NCHS, 2006).

Another piece of legislation that targeted cost containment was the BBA of 1997, which also affected Medicare. This act reduced Medicare spending by limiting provider payments, increased options in the choice of managed care plans, and made Medical Savings Accounts an option. As of 2007, Medical savings accounts were linked to high-deductible **Medicare Advantage** plans (Medicare private health plans) and are currently available in 38 states. An annual deposit is made into an interest-bearing account by Medicare on behalf of enrollees who use the funds to pay for qualified health care expenses until they meet the deductible (between $2500 and $4500 for 2007 plans) at which the plan will pay for all Medicare-covered services. In June 2007, only 2249 beneficiaries were enrolled in MSA plans (KFF, 2007d).

The Medicare Modernization Act of 2003 promotes private managed care plans to reduce the burden on the economy of Medicare entitlements. These HMO plans, called Medicare Advantage (MA) Plans, discussed previously, typically have clients who are healthier than the average. Older adults who are enrolled in these plans pay a monthly premium and are required to choose providers within the network. If care is provided outside of the network of providers, individuals usually must pay out-of-pocket similar to other HMOs discussed earlier. This can be confusing to the older person as there are many MA plans to choose from and they may not realize how an MA plan is different from the traditional Medicare coverage. Provisions have been made for enrollees to change MAs or disembroil during specific time frames. Providers have been lobbying for increased reimbursement as Medicare dictates reimbursement fees based on a predetermined formula. (See further discussion about Medicare later in this chapter.) In 2006, Massachusetts was one of several states who devised plans to provide near universal coverage to state residents. The Massachusetts plan included a mandate for state residents to purchase health insurance by July 1, 2007. Employers with 11 or more employees are required to provide health insurance coverage to workers or pay into a fund that permits workers to purchase health care through a state insurer. The plan relies heavily on Medicaid funds to finance the plans for the poor and near poor. Other states policymakers are debating the feasibility of this type of comprehensive reform (KFF, 2007c).

Care Management Care management began through public programs with nurses in public health departments, social workers in public welfare systems, and caseworkers in mental health departments. In care management, an experienced health care professional, such as a nurse, social worker or gerontologist, helps determine what nursing care is necessary, monitors that care, and arranges for individuals to receive care for the most effective cost and in the most appropriate setting. Care managers are especially effective in meeting the needs of individuals recently discharged from the hospital, older adults, persons with medical conditions that are costly to treat (e.g., spinal cord injuries, or persons with high-volume diseases such as chronic illnesses). Care managers are especially effective in meeting the needs of persons with complex health and social needs, and other cases requiring multiple levels of care (Shi & Singh, 2004). The care manager must achieve a balance between cost and quality and must collaborate effectively with all providers involved, both inside and outside the health plan, and with the person's family to ensure appropriate quality care. Emphasis must be on health management across the continuum of health care services. As Medicaid and Medicare managed care systems continue to develop, demand for nurses to fill the care management role will continue to grow. In addition to working within organizations, care managers can have their own independent practices. Managed care organizations rely on care management to reduce inappropriate use of services, improve quality of care, and control costs (Nies & McEwen, 2007). Basic care management services are described in Box 3-5.

Managed Care Issues

In 2002, 95% of people with employer-based health insurance coverage were in a managed care program (Shi & Singh, 2004). Low copayments and less paperwork are welcomed by individuals, but concerns about the quality of care provided when the overall emphasis is cost control is an issue. Gate keeping by the PCP is not seen by some individuals as a way to maintain or improve quality of care; rather the PCP may be seen as the way managed care attempts to limit health care costs by decreasing the amount of care provided, especially by limiting referrals. Managed care has created new systems, with groups

of providers delivering care in more efficient ways. The Internet has become a valuable resource for informing consumers and employers about health care issues and allowing them to search and compare information on various types of health care plans. The Internet is also a tool nurses can use for their own continuing education needs, as well as to enhance client education within a facility, public library, or home. Nurses can steer clients toward appropriate websites for health promotion and disease-oriented information (Health Teaching box).

Box 3-5 Care Management Services

- *Assessment:* evaluating a person's physical, social, functional, psychological, financial, and spiritual needs, including the family within a specific environment
- *Care planning:* setting goals, identifying specific services to meet individual and family needs, including how to allocate resources, and refer to other resources
- *Service coordination and referral:* facilitating and coordinating access to needed providers
- *Care monitoring and periodic reassessments:* evaluating progress, access to and use of services, and changes in needs

---

HEALTH TEACHING   Access Health Care Information from the Internet

Mary Jones, age 38, and her family are new to a primary care clinic. Mary asks the nurse for advice in choosing a health plan that will best meet the needs of her growing family. Mary is 4 months pregnant with her third child. She and her husband, Joe, work for a state agency that provides multiple health plan choices. Joe, age 48, has many of the symptoms of coronary artery disease. Their son Billy, age 8, has asthma, and their daughter Laurel, age 4, has Down syndrome.

The nurse discusses Mary's family's general health promotion and protection needs and the special needs presented by the diseases that have been identified. She provides some resources for Mary to learn more about the plans available in her area. The Joneses have a computer at home and are eager to access the websites suggested to them.

- From the Agency for Healthcare Research and Quality (AHRQ), a federal government agency with health information for consumers on guidelines to consumers in choosing a health plan: *www.ahrq.gov/consumer/hlthpln1.htm*
- From the U.S. Department of Labor, a federal agency that provides information on health plans, benefits, and has many links: *www.dol.gov/dol/topic/health%2Dplans/*
- For information and links on pregnancy and childbirth with many links: *www.childbirth.org*
- For additional information on pregnancy topics, birth, and tests, with many graphics and links: *http://pregnancy. about.com*

- For information on childhood asthma, care and treatment, news and research with many professional references and links, Ask NOAH About: Asthma, New York Online Access to Health: *http://noah-health.org/en/ lung/conditions/asthma/issues/children/index.htm*
- For information about genetic diseases: Down syndrome, care and treatment, news and research with many professional references and links, Ask NOAH About Genetic Diseases: Down Syndrome, New York Online Access to Health: *www.noah-health.org/genetics/ conditions/downs/what/index.html*
- The National Down Syndrome Society website has information and resources on Down syndrome, advocacy, support groups, education, and links: *www.ndss.org/ content.cfm*
- The American Heart Association website contains information on heart disease, diet, exercise, treatment, news, and links: *www.americanheart.org*
- For information about heart disease, symptoms, cholesterol, prevention, exercise, diet, and links, Ask NOAH About Heart Disease, New York Online Access to Health: *www.noah-health.org/en/blood/disease/causes/ index.html*

Health Insurance

Positive elements of the health care system in America include excellent clinicians, health care facilities, and equipment—all of which are available to people with good health insurance or adequate finances. The U.S. system exhibits a high degree of technological change and innovation and excellent information, quality, and cost-accounting systems. Financial outlays for education of health care workers; products such as drugs, medical equipment, and supplies; and research are second to those of no other country (Shi & Singh, 2004). In 2003, 62.9% of the younger population (ages 0 to 64 years) obtained private health insurance through their own employment or that of a family member, 17.6% were uninsured, 11.0% were on Medicaid, 4.1% had privately-purchased insurance, 1.5% were enrolled in Medicare, 1.4% in SCHIP, and 1.5% received other public health care support. An estimated 45.6 million people, or 16.6% of the younger population, did not have health insurance in 2004 (Anderson et al., 2007). The number of noncitizen foreign-born persons in the United States was estimated to be 21.1 million, comprising both legal and illegal residents. This population is disproportionately low-income and uninsured (NCHS, 2007) and typically delays seeking health care until an urgent problem arises and then utilizes the emergency department, an expensive and inefficient means of receiving health care. (See the discussion of the uninsured later in this chapter.)

Private Health Insurance

In the private sector, the following five types of organizations provide health care insurance:

1. Traditional insurance companies (including the earliest insurer, Blue Cross and Blue Shield, a nonprofit charitable organization) and for-profit commercial insurance companies
2. PPOs acting as "brokers" between insurers and health care providers
3. HMOs, which are independent prepayment plans
4. POS plans, which combine features of classic HMOs with client choice characteristics of PPOs
5. Self-insurance and self-funded plans, in which either the employer takes on the role of insurer or the enrollee sets up a trust account with tax savings

Traditionally, private insurers charged employers or individuals annual premiums and provided services on a fee-for-service basis. Organized at the state and local level, Blue Cross and Blue Shield generally complement each other, with Blue Cross reimbursing hospitals and Blue Shield covering physicians and other providers. After World War II, insurance companies began to provide health insurance plans in competition with Blue Cross and Blue Shield. Today, more than 800 commercial, profit-making insurance companies, such as Metropolitan Life and Aetna, offer policies that cover hospitalization and in-hospital or office-based physician care, and other major medical expenses. Much of the individual insurance sold today is supplementary, such as that designed to supplement Medicare, known as Medigap. These plans reimburse only deductibles and coinsurance payments associated with Medicare.

HMOs attempt to lower health care costs by emphasizing preventive rather than curative care, decreasing the progression and severity of some illnesses. Care is provided in outpatient settings when possible. HMOs tend to use fewer services, with emphasis on the least costly means of providing a service.

POS plans enable enrollees to choose, at the point of service, whether to use the plan's provider network or seek care from non-network providers. Typically, network providers are paid on a capitated or discounted fee basis, and non-network providers are paid on a fee-for-service basis.

Another change in the structure of the insurance industry is the growth of self-insured or self-funded plans. **Self-insurance** means that an employer (or union) assumes the claims risk of its insured employees, whereas self-funding refers to paying insurance claims from an established fund, such as a bank account or trust fund. Self-insurance gives employers a financial advantage, including an Employee Retirement and Income Security Act (ERISA) exemption from state taxes on health insurance premiums and interest earnings on reserves before claims payment (Sultz & Young, 2004). The ERISA exemption, enacted in 1974, has stirred controversy over the years due to the loss of premium revenue taxes for states and the provision of some legal immunity to organizations (Sultz & Young, 2004). Between 1993 and 1997, the percentage of self-insured employers dropped from 19% to 13% (Shi & Singh, 2004).

Public Health Insurance and Assistance

Medicare Medicare is a federal health insurance program that finances medical care for people over 65, disabled individuals who are entitled to Social Security benefits, and people with end-stage renal disease requiring dialysis or a kidney transplant. The Medicare program, also known as Title XVIII of the SSA, went into effect in 1966 after decades of debate and is currently operated under the administrative oversight of the Centers for Medicare and Medicaid Services. Medicare is an entitlement program. "People have contributed to Medicare through taxes, they are 'entitled' to the benefits regardless of the amount of income and assets they have" (Shi & Singh, 2004, p. 205). The intent of Medicare was to protect older adults against the catastrophic financial debts often incurred in managing chronic illness and to assist in the payment of health care. This was the first time that federal legislation was enacted to remove financial barriers to medical care for older adults. In 1983, Medicare added hospice benefits for the last 6 months of life to cover services for the terminally ill. Hospice is based on a philosophy that views death as a normal part of the life cycle and emphasizes living the remainder of life as fully and comfortably as possible. Hospice care accounts for only 1% of the total Medicare expenditures, covering about two thirds of cost, or $2.8 billion per year (Sultz & Young, 2004). See **Website Resource 3A**, which presents Medicare insurance–covered services for 2004.

Medicare, Part A, is financed largely through a mandatory tax of 2.9% of earnings paid by employees and their employers (1.45% each) into the Hospital Insurance Trust Fund. Part A covers inpatient care in hospitals, skilled nursing facilities (not custodial or long-term care), home health services, and hospice care. For those individuals who have contributed to or had a spouse contribute 40 or more quarters of Medicare-covered employment, there is no monthly premium. For those individuals who have not contributed 30 quarters of employment, the monthly premium for Part A in 2008 is $423. Part B is supplementary voluntary medical insurance financed through a combination of general tax revenues and premiums paid by beneficiaries ($96.40 per month in 2008) and accounts for 32% of benefit payments. Part C is not separately financed but a vehicle for providing Part A, Part B (usually), and Part D benefits and accounts for 15% of benefit payments. Part D is financed from beneficiary premiums, general revenues, and state payments if individuals are also in the Medicaid program and accounts for 9% of benefit payments. The cost of Part D increased Medicare spending by 22.1% between 2005 and 2006 and is expected to cost $982 billion over the next decade. Medicare benefit payments totaled $374 billion in 2006 accounting for 12% of the federal budget. Medicare spending averages $5694 per beneficiary except for the last year of life, when the spending is 4 times higher, averaging $22,107. In 2007, Medicare spending was 3.2% of the gross domestic product (GDP). Spending is expected to increase by 7.8% annually through 2016. The Medicare Modernization Act of 2003 assesses the financial status of Medicare funding. It is estimated that by 2016 Medicare's trust fund (HI Trust) will be depleted. Future challenges include increasing price of health care services, increased cost of technology, and increasing volume and utilization of services due to population growth of older adults and increasing life expectancy. By 2030, 79 million people are expected to be enrolled in Medicare compared to 39 million in 2000. Currently there are 4.0 workers to support each beneficiary, but by 2030 that number will drop to 2.4 workers per beneficiary (KFF, 2007f; USDHHS, 2007b). Neither Part A nor Part B of Medicare offers comprehensive coverage. Inherent in the program are deductibles, set amounts that the individual must pay for each type of service before Medicare begins to pay, and coinsurance, a percentage of charges paid by the individual. There are also limitations on the amount of coverage provided. For example, hospital benefits end after 90 days (with a lifetime reserve of an additional 60 days) and extended care facility benefits last a maximum of 100 days.

In 2004, total expenses per beneficiary averaged $12,763 with Medicare paying for 47% of the cost. Direct out-of-pocket expenses averaged 19%, or $2477, which included paying for long-term-care, provider visits, and medical supplies and prescription drugs (KFF, 2007f). Out-of-pocket expenses do not include premium payments for Part B or for supplemental private health insurance, which can add significantly to out-of-pocket expenses. A comprehensive booklet available online or through the Centers for Medicare & Medicaid Services details information on enrollment, costs, and covered and noncovered services. With some exceptions, noncovered services include acupuncture, chiropractic services, custodial care (bathing and toileting), dental care and dentures, routine eye care and glasses, routine foot care, hearing aids, long-term care (if only custodial care is needed), orthopedic shoes, routine or yearly physical exams (except initial when first enrolling), and health care while traveling outside of the United States. Items not covered, especially custodial care, contribute significantly to out-of-pocket expenses. The main population at risk, the older adult, may have limited financial resources to seek preventive health services not covered. Some low-income enrollees may qualify for Medicaid services if income requirements are met and others may have additional benefits through private insurance.

Quality and cost of care have been issues for Medicare for more than 25 years. Numerous pieces of legislation and Medicare amendments have attempted to solve various aspects of the cost and quality concerns.

The case-based reimbursement system established by the Tax Equity and Fiscal Responsibility Act of 1982 (which instituted DRGs) was designed to provide cost-containment incentives. Subsequently, in 1983, Title VI of Public Law 98-21 established a prospective payment system for inpatient services for Medicare clients. This legislation also encouraged growth in the number of HMOs and other comprehensive plans enrolling Medicare beneficiaries. Although the prospective payment system has slowed the growth of inpatient hospital Medicare spending, that of outpatient spending continues to rise. In the Omnibus Reconciliation Act of 1989 (OBRA), Medicare revised its payment scheme for physicians. First, a new payment system that went into effect in 1992 assigned relative values to services based on the time, skill, and intensity required to provide them. Second, a limit was set on the amount that physicians could charge individuals above the amount that Medicare pays. This restriction was designed to limit growth of Medicare costs for physician payments.

The BBA of 1997 included Medicare+ Choice, which offers the option of managed care plans such as HMOs, POS plans, PPOs, or private fee-for-service plans in which the enrollee pays extra when costs for care are higher than Medicare rates. Additionally, Medical Saving Account (MSA) plans are available whereby Medicare pays a health insurance policy, putting money into an MSA. Enrollees use the MSA and their own money for care (up to a certain amount per year); when that amount is reached, the insurance covers all Medicare-approved expenses for the rest of the year. If an enrollee has money in the MSA at the end of the year, that amount is rolled over for the next year (KFF, 2007d; USDHHS, 2007b).

The Balanced Budget Act (BBA) of 1997, the Balanced Budget Refinement Act of 1999, and the Benefits Improvement and Protection Act of 2000 have added services to the Medicare benefits package. These services include coverage for screening tests for breast, cervical, vaginal, prostate, and colorectal cancer; bone mass measurements; diabetes monitoring and diabetes self-management; and influenza, pneumonia, and hepatitis B vaccinations.

The missing Medicare benefit causing great concern was the rising cost and lack of coverage for outpatient prescription drugs. On December 9, 2003, President George W. Bush signed into law the Medicare Prescription Drug, Improvement and Modernization Act of 2003, Public Law 108-173. This lengthy piece of legislation amends Title XVIII of the SSA to provide for a voluntary program for prescription drug coverage and to modernize the Medicare program, including a provision to provide teaching hospitals with increased indirect medical education payments. The new Medicare prescription drug benefit Part D started on January 1, 2006 and is an optional plan to assist older adults in paying for prescription drugs. The Part D drug plan covers some of the costs for certain drugs provided by a private plan that the individual chooses, paying a premium of approximately $20 to $35 a month. Different plans cover different drugs and require older adults to choose a plan that best meets their needs from a plethora of choices. Those with low education or literacy levels, as well as debilitated older adults in long-term care facilities, may have difficulty selecting the best plan for their individual needs. The first $250 in prescription drug costs (called a deductible) is paid by the older adult each year and then Medicare pays 75% of the next $2000 worth of drugs on the Plan's formulary. After that, there is a gap in coverage known as the "donut hole" where individuals pay 100% of drug costs until another $2850 has been spent out-of-pocket. At that point, Medicare will begin paying about 95% of the cost of covered drugs until the end of the calendar year (USDHHS, 2007b). In 2007, 4 in 10 Medicare beneficiaries received subsidies based on low income to reduce out-of- pocket expenses (KFF, 2007e; USDHHS, 2007b). Nine million enrollees did not pay premiums because they receive low-income assistance under Part D. The Centers for Medicare and Medicaid estimate there are 1824 prescription drug plans in 2008 with average premiums of $31.99 and an increase is expected across the next 3 years. Premiums vary widely with approximately 40% of plans costing about $30 per month and 40% of plans with premiums of $40 per month or more. Some premiums are as high as $107.50 per month but typically offer more generous benefits. In 2008, some prescription drug plans will cover generic or brand-name drug costs in the coverage gap (donut hole) but this will lead to higher than average monthly premiums (KFF, 2007e). Much skepticism and debate occurred at the time of enactment of the new law. Some advocates saw the act as a step in the right direction to assist older adults with prescription drug costs and others as a failure in health care reform.

Medicaid Medicaid is a health insurance program available to certain low-income individuals and families who fit into an eligibility group that is recognized by federal and state law. Medicaid pays health care providers directly if they participate in the Medicaid program.

Medicaid is an assistance program, commonly referred to as welfare, managed jointly by the federal and state governments to provide partial or full payment of medical costs for individuals and families of any age who are too poor to pay for the care. Medicaid legislation, Title XIX of the amendments to the SSA, went into effect in 1967. The federal government provides funds to states on a cost-sharing basis, with 50% to more than 80% from the federal government and the remainder from the state, according to the per capita income of each state, to guarantee medical services to eligible Medicaid recipients. In June 2006, a total of 42.7 million persons were enrolled in a Medicaid program (KFF, 2006; USDHHS, 2007b). **Website Resource 3B** presents a comparison of Medicare and Medicaid.

People eligible for Medicaid are those who receive Supplemental Security Income (SSI) and TANF (see discussion of welfare reform). Additionally, Medicaid pays the Medicare premiums, deductibles, and coinsurance for certain low-income Medicare recipients. In 2000, Medicaid consumed 50% of total state health care expenditures. Medicaid plans are open-ended, meaning a state must admit into the program at any time all individuals who meet the criteria. A state is not allowed to cap the Medicaid budget for a particular fiscal year, thus making it difficult to determine exactly how much money needs to be appropriated. The program encourages its own growth and expansion (Lee & Estes, 2003).

States administer Medicaid under broad federal requirements and guidelines. Each state establishes its own eligibility standards; determines the scope, type, duration, and amount of services to be provided; sets the rate of payment; and administers its own program. Programs vary widely from state to state in terms of services covered.

For a list of basic health services mandated, refer to **Website Resource 3B**. Included are inpatient and outpatient care; laboratory and radiology services; prenatal care; family planning services and supplies; rural health clinic services; federally qualified ambulatory and health center services; physician services; nurse midwife, and pediatric and family NP services; home health care for people eligible for skilled nursing services; skilled nursing facility services for people 21 years of age and older; and early and periodic screening, diagnosis, and treatment (EPSDT) of people under 21 years of age. Other services, such as dental care, eyeglasses, or intermediate care facility services, may be added at the state's option.

The EPSDT provision signified the federal government's recognition of the need for primary prevention and health promotion. The emphasis on prevention rather than treatment—the focus of this text—was a positive approach toward health and required development and implementation of new methods of health care delivery. The EPSDT program has five phases: (1) outreach and case findings, (2) screening, (3) testing, (4) compiling and reporting of results, and (5) follow-up and treatment.

State Medicaid programs must cover all pregnant women and children up to 6 years of age with family incomes less than 133% of the federal poverty level and encourages states to voluntarily expand coverage to women up to 185% of the poverty level. The federal government determines the minimal eligibility requirements and health services that must be covered. States can opt to expand enrollment to additional populations and provide enhanced health care (Anderson et al., 2007).

The federal government, in the passage of the Deficit Reduction Act of 2005, made it harder for individuals to qualify for Medicaid nursing home benefits by increasing penalties on individuals who transferred assets for less than fair market value during the previous five years. Since long-term care is expensive (average of $74,095 per individual per year in 2005), purchasing private long-term care insurance to cover nursing home care became an option in four states. Individuals who already have long-term care needs are not eligible and the cost of the premium increases with an individual's age. In 2002 the average cost if purchased at age 50 was $1474 but jumped to $8991 at age 79. For most older persons, the cost of the premium makes long-term care insurance unaffordable (KFF, 2006, 2007d, 2007f).

Several states are participating in the Robert Wood Johnson model program of purchasing long-term care insurance to protect a specific amount of money. Once the insurance monies are paid out up to that amount, the insured individual qualifies for Medicaid. This program is considered an attempt to cut Medicaid costs for long-term care of individuals over the age of 65.

Passage of the welfare reform bill in 1996 (Personal Responsibility and Work Opportunity Reconciliation Act of 1996, Public Law 104-193) revealed a significant philosophical shift in federal thinking about welfare assistance in the United States. For the first time, Medicaid was not linked directly to welfare programs. Ending a 61-year guarantee of federal aid, the TANF program (formerly Aid to Families With Dependent Children) established by this legislation provides temporary financial aid with a 5-year lifetime limit. Legal immigrants who arrive in the United States after the passage of this bill must wait 5 years to become eligible for programs. The aim is to help parents become self-sufficient through welfare-to-work programs. Some states have changed the name of their official department of social services (Family Independence Agency) to reflect the change in philosophy from dependency to temporary assistance (Clemen-Stone et al., 2002). As part of the BBA of 1997, the State Children's Health Insurance (SCHIP) program was enacted to provide health insurance coverage to children whose family's income is below 200% of the Federal Poverty Level or whose family has an income 50% higher than the state's Medicaid eligibility threshold. Some states have expanded SCHIP eligibility to include covering families. The program was approved for funding fiscal years 1998 to 2007. Bush approved reallocation of funding for the program to continue in 2007.

Pharmaceutical Costs

The spiraling cost of prescription drugs continues to add to the complexity of providing adequate health care. Newer drugs cost more than the drugs they replace and contribute 50% of the increased cost. Increased utilization of prescription drugs adds to an increased cost per day of medications. Consumer demand sparked by drug advertisements, new indications for use, and increased consumer knowledge of available drugs has increased the demand for prescription medications. Increased drug cost is attributed to inflation, more days of therapy per user, greater number of drugs per user, cost of research and drug development, and advertising.

The Uninsured: Who Are They?

The United States has the highest proportion of population with no health insurance of all developed countries. Uninsured Americans under the age of 65 ranged from 14.5% in 1984 to 16.4% of the population in 2005. In 2005, 42.1 million persons were uninsured while 68.2% held private insurance and 13% were enrolled in Medicaid programs. The lack of health insurance is greatest for persons of Mexican origin according to the results of the CDC, National Health Interview Survey. In 2005, 40% of Mexican-origin individuals lacked coverage for at least part of the previous 12 months and 29% lacked coverage for more than 12 months. One third of the uninsured are of Hispanic origin and 14% of the uninsured population are non-Hispanic Black (NCHS, 2007). In the 18- to 44-year-old age group, 29.3% of the uninsured were not working. Thirty percent of young adults between the ages of 18 and 24 in 2004 had no health insurance. In 2002 to 2004, the average percent of the population without health insurance ranged from 8.5% in Minnesota to 25% in Texas (NCHS, 2006). Surprisingly, more than 40% of uninsured people had a family income of at least 200% of the federal poverty level (about $42,200 for a family of four) (NCHS, 2007; USDHHS, 2008). The working uninsured are employed in firms that do not offer coverage, are not eligible for coverage, or decline offers of health insurance for financial or other reasons (NCHS, 2007). Another group of the uninsured include young adults who are no longer eligible to be covered on their families' health insurance plan once they turn 19 unless they are full-time college students. Consolidated Omnibus Budget Reconciliation Act (COBRA) plans are available for a fee to cover the gap between reaching age 19 and securing a job with employer-based benefits. Some uninsured adults do not have jobs in which health care is provided, and the cost of individual private health insurance is usually high. Some young adults have employer-based plans but choose not to utilize them due to cost. Other young adults, typically a healthy group, choose not to spend money on a plan due to necessity or personal choice. Instead they seek health care only when necessary and pay out of pocket. For those with acute or chronic health care needs, the price of being uninsured is detrimental to financial solvency. Solutions to providing health care to the uninsured vary, with some success in offering tax breaks or other financial incentives for businesses to offer health insurance plans and in expanding eligibility requirements for Medicaid. Without health insurance, low-income families frequently must rely on a fragmented and difficult-to-use public system of health care. Regular preventive care, including prenatal care, immunization, and well-child care, is sometimes difficult to obtain, and its availability may not be adequately understood.

Illegal Aliens

The National Center for Policy Analysis reports that illegal aliens are straining the American health care system. By federal law, anyone entering an emergency room must be treated regardless of ability to pay or immigration status. United States border hospitals from Brownsville, Texas, to San Diego, California, are especially hard hit with the number of illegal aliens crossing over state lines and then seeking health care. Millions of dollars of uncompensated services are provided to illegal aliens across the country annually. Measures to return illegal aliens to their own countries and steps to control the influx of illegal aliens into America have been ineffective in stopping illegal immigration traffic (National Center for Policy Analysis, 2008).

Another step toward addressing part of the problem for the uninsured and underinsured was the Health Insurance Portability and Accountability Act (HIPAA) (Public Law 104-191), which was passed in 1996 took effect in 1997. The portability provision means that individuals with health insurance who lose or leave their jobs can maintain coverage even when they are sick. However, cost may be a prohibitive factor, because it does not regulate premium costs. Insurers are also prohibited from refusing coverage based on an individual's health status, although limited waiting periods may apply. Additionally, the bill allows individuals in small firms, uninsured individuals, or self-insured individuals with high-deductible plans to set up a tax-exempt MSA (see previous discussion). This MSA allows tax deductions for long-term care insurance premiums and, for those who qualify, unreimbursed home health and long-term care services; it allows the terminally ill earlier access to earnings built up in life insurance policies without tax penalties; it establishes fraud and abuse guidelines; it provides liability coverage for medical volunteers who provide free medical care to low-income individuals in medically underserved areas; and it mandates that USDHHS develop regulations and standards for the electronic transfer of medical information, confidentiality, and a unique health identifier. One of the most costly and complicated changes mandated by HIPAA is that health care companies must design interactive data systems that allow the transfer of health data while maintaining client confidentiality (USDHHS, 2007c).

HEALTH CARE SYSTEMS OF OTHER COUNTRIES

Interest in adopting a socialized system of universal health care makes for a reasonable discussion. By examining the international health care continuum, those interested in reform can find new possibilities for the American system. The United States spends the highest proportion of gross domestic product on health care of all industrialized countries, and has the highest cost per capita. Canada, Germany, and the United Kingdom represent a select sampling of international countries, each having some form of universal health care plan, and these are compared with that of the United States in Table 3-1. Of the countries examined, the United Kingdom spends the least amount on health care and the least per capita.

Canadian Health Care System

The Canadian health care program, called Medicare, is a group of socialized health insurance plans that provide health coverage to all Canadian citizens regardless of medical history, personal income, or job status. The Canada Health Act, legislated at the federal level, determines what services must be provided, similar to the Medicaid program in the United States, but provinces and territories are not obligated to provide services not listed in the Act. The Act specifies basic services including primary care and hospitalizations leaving the individual province or territory responsible for the management, organization, and delivery of health services for their residents. The Canada Health Act does not include services such as physiotherapy, dental coverage, optometrists, corrective lenses, home care, or prescription medicines. The five principles in the Canada Health Act are outlined in Box 3-6. Every Canadian

---

Box 3-6   **Five Principles of the Canada Health Act**

- *Universality:* All insured residents of a province or territory must be entitled to the same level of health care provided by the provincial or territorial health care insurance plan. Excluded persons are tourists, a transient visitor to the province, serving members of the Canadian Forces or Royal Canadian Mounted Police and inmates of federal penitentiaries.
- *Portability:* Residents moving from one province or territory to another must continue to be covered for insured health services by the 'home' jurisdiction during any waiting period which cannot exceed 3 months.
- *Accessibility:* Residents of a providence or territory are entitled to have access on uniform terms and conditions to insured health services at the setting where the services are provided and as the services are available in that setting.
- *Comprehensiveness:* Provincial plans must cover all insured health services provided by hospitals, physicians or dentists (includes only surgical-dental services that require a hospital setting).
- *Public administration:* All administration of provincial health insurance must be carried out by public authority on a non-profit basis and must be accountable to the province or territory.

citizen has the same basic primary health insurance. Each Canadian citizen applies for a provincial health card and, once issued, the card accesses a person's medical information and is used when visiting a physician or health care provider eliminating the need to fill out forms. Canadians pay for health care through a variety of federal and provincial taxes, just as Americans pay for Social Security and Medicare through payroll taxes. The federal government appropriates funds to the provinces and territories through cash and tax transfers. Because the government is the primary payer of medical bills, Canada's health care system is referred to as a single-payer arrangement. Some provinces gain additional funds through sales tax, lottery proceeds, and health premiums. Additional benefits vary among the provinces, but most provide prescription drugs to older adults and low-income clients. Many services are not provided through the public health care provincial plans, so some Canadians have supplemental private insurance either through their employers or purchased insurance packages from private insurance providers to help pay for uncovered services like dental care. In addition to public health care, private clinics offer specialized services not covered by the public health plan. Canadians covered by private health insurance typically have 80% of the costs covered at private clinics and receive specialized services not covered by the public health plan. Higher-income Canadians can pay out of pocket for care received at private clinics, which typically offer services with reduced wait times. For example, obtaining an MRI scan in a hospital may require a waiting period of months, whereas a private clinic could offer the scan much earlier. Canadians with private health insurance and higher incomes have access to greater health care services and more expedient health care.

At one time, the Canadian system seemed to be an ideal model that the United States should adopt; however, increasing health care costs, access issues, delays in treatment, and workforce shortages of health care providers have caused political controversy and debate in Canada. Although all citizens receive the same level of public health care, private insurance allows a two-tiered system favoring Canadians with private health insurance or other financial resources. A major shortage of physicians and nurses in Canada is due in part to lower reimbursement rates by the public health system causing some health care providers to leave Canada and practice in other countries such as the United States. Over the years, the federal government has decreased contributions to the provinces and territories due to large budget deficits and limited fee increases to physicians for services. Regionalization of hospitals has caused access to care issues for those outside of major cities. Canadians can occasionally have longer waiting times than Americans for health care services, diagnostic testing, and surgery. Expansion to offer better access to home care and community-based services is an emerging issue. A greater percentage of physicians are PCPs, not specialists like in

the United States. The Canadian system in 2004 spent $3165 per capita, compared with $6101 in the United States (see Table 3-4 for international comparisons) (NCHS, 2007; Shi & Singh, 2004).

If a Canadian-type system were adopted in the United States, the federal government would determine the level of basic health care and services provided in the basic health plan. States would then be appropriated money through a funding mechanism to provide care similar to the current Medicaid system in the United States. Services not included in the basic health plan would not need to be provided by individual states. Employer insurance would be available for those companies that offered a private plan and workers could choose to purchase private health insurance. Those with private health insurance could utilize private clinics, receiving more expedient care. If a concierge plan were available, those with wealth would receive additional health services (see prior discussion on Concierge Care). Those on the public plan would receive care at public facilities. This two-tiered plan would benefit those with private health insurance and those able to pay for medical care out of pocket. All citizens would be guaranteed to have the same basic level of health care.

German Health Care System

Germany provides near universal access to health care through a decentralized system and use of sickness funds. Over 292 sickness funds provide health coverage for approximately 87% of the population. Approximately 10% of people have private insurers. Private insurers pay physicians higher fees than do sickness funds, allowing preferential treatment to the wealthier. About 0.2% of the population (which is wealthy) has no insurance. If a person retires, changes jobs, or stops working for any reason, that person and the family maintain membership in the sickness fund. Employers and workers pay a percentage into the sickness fund. Employees paid about 14.3% of their annual income into the sickness fund in 2003. The funds are nonprofit and are required to cover hospital costs, physician services, prescription drugs, dental care, prevention, and maternity care with modest copayments. Germans have free choice of physicians, and there is no gate-keeping system from a general practitioner. If hospitalization is needed, usually a referral is needed and care is received from a hospital-based physician. Ambulatory physicians are reimbursed on a fee-for-service basis. Problems include a two-tiered system, with some people who can afford private care bypassing and weakening the public system, as well as increased costs (WHO/Europe, 2007).

INFLUENCING HEALTH POLICY

The primary responsibility of the nurse is to the individual, family, group, or community served. A major portion of the nurse's role is to **advocate** not only for the individual, but also for justice in health care delivery. Nurses need to be aware of issues that have an effect on the health of the American people and to know how to work for needed change.

Health cannot be separated from its environment; therefore, it is essential that nurses become involved in all aspects of planning to maximize the health potential of all Americans. This involvement needs to include attention to policy decisions and political action. Policy affects the broader aspects of environment, the biophysical and socioeconomic conditions of homes, schools, workplaces, communities, and the health care delivery environment. By virtue of their numbers, nurses, who make up the largest group of health care providers in the United States, have tremendous potential to influence decision-making.

Participation in **policy decision-making** requires the nurse take a proactive stance to determine needs before a problem arises. Policy development and change take place on many levels, from within the nurse's agency or work group to the community, state, and national levels. At the institutional level, clinical decisions influence policy, as do management issues. The nurse should examine the rationale behind an existing or planned policy and determine whether or not it is relevant now. Nurses are empowered by their education and experience to use their "people skills" and to apply change theory to influence policy development and change.

Much health-related decision-making is the result of legislation at the local, state, or national level. Laws—rules enforced by a ruling authority by which society is governed—and regulations—agency or department rules developed for the implementation of laws—define what services are being offered to whom and who will pay. Politics influences change and is an arena for nursing's participation that is part of this nation's democratic heritage. The nurse can be politically involved in many ways. Voting, after becoming well informed on current issues and candidates, is an important way for nurses to be actively involved. Getting to know local representatives, informing them about health care issues, and advising them as to the needs of individuals and families within the communities they represent is another way nurses become involved.

The nurse can run for political office (many nurses now represent their local constituencies, and they have increasing visibility at the state and national levels) and support colleagues who represent nursing's interests. Financial contributions to Nurses for Political Action Coalition (N-PAC), ANA's political arm, increase the power base of nurses. Membership in professional and community groups provides the nurse with a collective voice to influence legislators. ANA's Nurses Strategic Action Team (N-STAT) network is an organized grassroots effort by nurses to help elect ANA-PAC–endorsed candidates and to inform members of Congress about policy issues of concern to nurses. When nurses join N-STAT, they receive Action Alert and

Legislative Update, detailing specific legislative issues to keep them adequately informed and enable them to respond to legislators in a timely manner.

Legislators are influenced by the information that they receive and by the sources of that information. Nurses have a wealth of knowledge about health care that legislators need to know. The process of trying to persuade legislators to vote for or against measures important to the interest group represented is called **lobbying**. A **lobbyist** is a registered representative of a special interest group. The ANA, located in Washington, DC, employs nurse lobbyists as do many states.

Communicating with a legislator is essential and can be done by phone, writing a letter, personal visits, or e-mail correspondence. Legislators have staffs of experts in various areas, and each legislator is assigned to committees. To understand the legislative process, the nurse needs to follow the progress of a bill. Thousands of bills are introduced at both the state and federal levels and must be passed within 2 years or die by default. Once a bill is introduced, it is referred to committee, and the committee chairperson determines which bills will be considered. Hearings are then held on the considered bills. When finished in committee, a bill is "reported out" at the federal level to the floor of the Senate or House of Representatives for a vote. Both the Senate and the House must pass identical versions of the bill and, once passed by both chambers, it is forwarded to the President for signing. If signed, it is enacted into law (Milstead, 2008). It is important for nurses to lobby, to inform legislators of new issues, and to give expert testimony on introduced bills. It is essential that nurses become politically aware and active to enable the collective voice of nursing to reach its full potential (Box 3-7).

Unfortunately, the collective voice of nurses is rarely heard. In 2008, of the 2.9 million registered nurses in the United States only 150,000 were members of the ANA or constituent nursing organizations (ANA, 2008). Other health care professionals, like the

---

Box 3-7 Nursing's National Agenda for the Future: Ten Areas of Concern Demanding Action

- Economic value*
- Delivery system*
- Education*
- Work environment*
- Leadership and planning
- Legislation/regulation/policy
- Professional/nursing culture
- Recruitment/retention
- Public relations/communication
- Diversity

*Top priorities of the December 2002 NAF steering committee.
From American Nurses Association Web site. Retrieved January 28, 2005, from *www.nursingworld.org*. Report: *Nursing's agenda for the future.* Retrieved January 28, 2005, from *www.nursingworld.org/naf/*.

NURSING'S AGENDA FOR THE FUTURE

HOT topics

The ANA held a summit in September of 2001 to determine what nursing should look like and where it should be by the year 2010. The summit brought together nurses from many other nursing associations in a collective effort to develop a strategic plan to address the growing nursing shortage and to move the profession forward while providing quality nursing care to consumers. The agenda developed by the steering committee focused on 10 areas of concern derived from an IOM study, *Crossing the Quality Chasm: A New Health System for the 21st Century*, and other evidence-based research (see Box 3-4). The ANA has a history of commitment to the idea that all Americans are entitled to accessible and afford-

able quality health care services. In November 2003, nursing organizations submitted more than 200 proposals to push forward the NAF agenda. As the nation's largest health care profession, nurses can bring about positive changes in both the nursing profession and health care delivery system.

Questions

- How can nurses ensure safe, quality client care?
- What are the root causes of the growing nursing shortage?
- How can nurses work collectively to move the NAF agenda forward?

From ANA Web site 2004. *Report: Nursing's agenda for the future and progress reports on NAF.* Retrieved March 15, 2005, from *www.nursingworld.org/naf/.*

American Medical Association, have a more united professional organization with a large membership base, allowing physicians a united voice and political clout in influencing health care policy and law. With more than 100 professional nursing organizations, the numbers of nurses who are members are divided among the many. Since membership dues can be high, a nurse is not likely to be a member of multiple groups unless the specialty is of personal interest. So although powerful in numbers, the voice of the nurse is diluted as there is no single national nursing organization in which the majority of nurses are members. When an organization takes a stance on an issue, the collective voice of the group sends a more powerful message to influence policy makers. Without a collective voice, the influence of nurses in shaping health care policy is weakened. It is the responsibility of nurses to become and remain well informed. As well-informed, empowered professionals, nurses play a significant role in supporting legislative initiatives that promote and protect the health of the public (Hot Topics box).

SUMMARY

Nurses need to be proactive in shaping policy that affects the health care system. They need to understand the complexity of the system to be able to educate individuals and families about health care resources, to coordinate services, and influence health care policy at the local, state, and national level. To accomplish this task, nurses need to become and remain well-informed citizens and health care consumer advocates.

An historical perspective and a description of the current health care delivery system in the United States provide a framework for the analysis of trends, values, and needs related to health. Comprehensive health services

do exist, but they are fragmented, unequally distributed, and extremely expensive. Although there is more emphasis on health promotion, as evidenced by the broad goals of *Healthy People 2010* and Mid Course Review of *Healthy People 2010* (2007), the current system continues to concentrate on the delivery and financing of illness care. Promotion of health needs to be incorporated into a system that delivers health care to all Americans. The delivery system needs to move beyond a focus on short-term, episodic disease patterns that were predominant during the first half of the twentieth century and conquer the problems facing us today. Chronic health problems require a system that supports long-term continual delivery and financing mechanisms. A change in emphasis and direction is needed.

The U.S. government provides the legal underpinnings for protecting and controlling the environment for health and delivery of health care services through the enactment of laws and the regulation of financing for the system. Social policy, as a reflection of society's values, has changed from a laissez-faire approach during the 1850s to one in which the federal government since the 1970s has had a prominent role in organizing and financing health care. Health care became a major political agenda item in 1991 and has remained a hot topic as health care costs escalate and political debate as to the best solution for health care reform remains muddled. Other industrialized nations provide a variety of types of universal health care to their citizens but none offers an ideal system. Each universal plan has deficiencies and none has been successful in cost containment. The American public is becoming increasingly dissatisfied with the present system and the cost of care. Addressing quality, cost, and access to health care is the challenge for the future.

CASE STUDY

A Nursing Center

A nursing student is completing her clinical experience in a nursing center. She follows a pregnant gestational diabetic adolescent and her family in the home and for visits with a nurse midwife and dietitian in the center. She has the opportunity to participate in holistic nursing care and observe the delivery of a healthy infant during her clinical stay.

Reflective Questions:
1. Compare the philosophy and subsequent care that individuals receive in a nursing center with the illness care they receive in a more traditional outpatient setting.
2. What kind of a role might the nurse pursue within a nursing center after graduation?

CARE PLAN

A Nursing Center

Nursing Diagnosis: Nutrition, Readiness for Enhanced Definition: A pattern of nutrient intake that is sufficient for meeting metabolic needs and can be strengthened.

DEFINING CHARACTERISTICS

- Expresses willingness to enhance nutrition
- Consumes adequate food and fluid intake as prescribed
- Follows appropriate standard for intake

RELATED FACTORS

- Increased nutritional need based on the growth and development needs of adolescence and pregnancy
- Impaired glucose tolerance related to the metabolic changes of pregnancy

EXPECTED OUTCOMES

- The individual demonstrates positive health maintenance behaviors.
- The individual's weight gain throughout her pregnancy will remain within the expected range.
- The teen will deliver a healthy infant with no maternal or fetal complications.

INTERVENTIONS

- The teen will be evaluated by the health care team consisting of her primary care provider, nurse midwife, endocrinologist (if advised), and nurse educator.
- The teen will be evaluated by a registered dietician, who will devise an appropriate dietary plan to meet changing nutritional needs of pregnancy taking into consideration: initial BMI, weight, cultural/religious beliefs and practices, food likes and dislikes. The teen's weight gain pattern will be monitored and dietary plan will be adjusted to meet the needs of pregnancy.
- An initial teaching plan will be developed with mutually agreed on goals and priority needs for learning will be identified, which include: daily dietary requirements, daily intermittent glucose monitoring, periodic glycated hemoglobin (A1C) monitoring, expected weight gains of pregnancy, recognition of early signs and symptoms of any pregnancy-related complications.
- Ongoing education and revision of teaching plan will take place as needed to provide the teen and family with the knowledge and skills necessary for self-management of gestational diabetes.
- Teen will be referred to a high-risk obstetrical team if pregnancy-related complications occur.

- Assessment of family functioning will include the following: adjustment of family to the teen's pregnancy, financial resources, literacy levels, cultural and religious factors, family support, risk for domestic violence, maternal substance use/abuse.
- Refer family to outside support agencies (social services).
- Listen to the teen's concerns: fears related to pregnancy, options for parenting or adopting the infant.
- Counsel the teen to attend prenatal classes with support person to prepare for labor and delivery (possible induction of labor at 38 weeks to avoid complications).
- Support teen's decision to keep or give the infant up for adoption.
- Counsel the teen to attend prenatal parenting/infant care classes with significant other (if involved) if she plans to parent the child.
- Refer teen to a specialized school-based program (if plans are to raise the baby) if available, which provides multidisciplinary services to pregnant and parenting teens while keeping them in school.
- Establish long-term goals with the teen that include: safe and effective contraception/family planning, completion of high school/employment, childcare assistance, and ongoing social support.

REFERENCES

American Academy of Pediatrics. (2007). Policy statement: Contraception and adolescents. *Pediatrics, 120*(5), 1135–1148.

American Academy of Pediatrics: Committee on Adolescence. (1998). Counseling the adolescent about pregnancy options. *Pediatrics, 101*(5), 938–940.

American Academy of Pediatrics: Committee on Adolescence and Committee on Early Childhood, Adoption, and Dependent Care. (2001). Care of adolescent parents and their children. *Pediatrics, 107*(2), 429–434.

Boulvain, M., Stan, C., & Irion, O. (2008). Elective delivery in diabetic pregnant women (review). *Cochrane Database of Systematic Reviews 2001, 2.*

Farrar, D., Tuffnell, D., & West, J. (2007). Continuous subcutaneous insulin infusion versus multiple daily injections of insulin for pregnant women with diabetes. *Cochrane Database of Systematic Reviews 2007, 3,* 1–20.

Muktabhant, B., Lumbiganon, P., & Ngamjarus, C. (2008). Interventions for preventing excessive weight gain during pregnancy (Protocol). *The Cochrane Library,* Issue 4.

NANDA International. (2007). *Nursing diagnoses: Definitions & classification 2-3-2008.* Philadelphia: Author.

Silverstein, J., et al. (2005). Care of children and adolescents with Type I diabetes. *Diabetes Care, 28*(1), 186–193.

REFERENCES

American Nurses Association . (2005). *ANA's health care agenda 2005.* Retrieved October 5, 2007, from *www.nursingworld.org.*

American Nurses Association. (2008). *ANA's statement of purpose.* Retrieved January 25, 2008, from *www.nursingworld.org.*

Anderson, R., Rice, T., & Kominski, G. (2007). *Changing the U.S. health care system* (3rd ed.). San Francisco, CA: John Wiley & Sons, Inc..

Arias, E., & Smith, B. (2003). Deaths: Preliminary data for 2001 (Online). *National Vital Statistics Report, 51*(5), 1–44. Retrieved May 1, 2004, from *www.cdc.gov/nchs/data/nvsr/nvsr51/nvs51r_05.pdf.*

Centers for Disease Control and Prevention, Department of Health and Human Services. (2004). *Health and safety topics A-Z.* Retrieved July 1, 2007, from *www.cdc.gov/az.*

Clemen-Stone, S., McGuire, S., & Eigsti, D. G. (2002). *Comprehensive community health nursing* (6th ed.). St. Louis: Mosby.

DiSalvo, R. (2004). The hospitalist movement. *Quality Matters Newsletter,* Winter 2004/2005.

Freyman, J. G. (1980). *The American health care system: Its genesis and trajectory.* Huntington, NY: Krieger.

Government Accountability Office (GAO). (2005, August). *Physician services: Concierge care characteristics and considerations for Medicare.* GAO-05-929 Retrieved from *www.gao.gov/cgl-bin/getrpt?GAO-05-929.*

Haben, J. (2008, January 17). *Army news releases.* Retrieved from *www.armymedicine.army.mil/news/releases/20080117tbitfrepart.cfm.*

Hartford Institute. (2006). *The John A. Hartford Foundation 2006 Annual Report.* Retrieved from *www.jhartfound.org/ar2006html.*

Herrick, T. (2004). Consumer-driven health care. *Clinical News, 8*(7), 6–7.

Holder, V. (2004). From handmaiden to right hand—The infancy of nursing. *AORN Journal, 79*(2), 374–382, 385–390.

Institute of Medicine, Board on Health Science Policy. (2003). *Summary: Unequal treatment—Confronting racial and ethnic disparities in health care* (pp. 1–28). Retrieved April 28, 2004, from *http://books.nap.edu/books/030908265X/l.html#pagetop.*

Institute of Medicine of the Academies. (2004). In A. Page (Ed.), *Keeping patients safe: Transforming the work environment of nurses.* Washington, DC: The National Academies Press.

Institute of Medicine of the National Academics. (2006). *Preventing medication errors: Quality chasm series.* Retrieved January 8, 2008, from *www.iom.edu/CMS/3809/22526/35939.aspx.*

Jansen, M., & Zwygart-Stauffacher, M. (Eds.). (2006). *Advanced practice nursing: Core concepts for professional role development* (3rd ed.). New York: Springer Publishing Co.

Jeter, L. (2007, November). Hospitalist movement gaining ground. *Medical News Papers, Inc.* Retrieved from *www.medicalnewsinc.com/news.php?viewStory=94.*

Kaiser Family Foundation (KFF). (2006). *Medicaid and the uninsured.* Mento Park, CA: The Henry J. Kaiser Family Foundation KAISER Commission. Retrieved from *www.kff.org/KCMU.*

Kaiser Family Foundation (KFF). (2007a). *Employee health benefits: 2007 Summary of findings.* The Kaiser Family Foundation and Health Research and Education Trust. Retrieved from *www.kff.org* report #7672.

Kaiser Family Foundation (KFF). (2007b). *Federal matching rate (FMAP) for medicaid and multiplier.* The Kaiser Family Foundation. Retrieved from *www.statehealthfacts.org/comparebar.jsp.*

Kaiser Family Foundation (KFF). (2007c). *Massachusetts health care reform plan: An update.* The Kaiser Family Foundation and Health Research and Education Trust. Retrieved from *www.kff.org* report #7494-02.

Kaiser Family Foundation (KFF). (2007d). *Medicare: Medicare advantage.* Menlo Park, CA: The Henry J. Kaiser Family Foundation. Retrieved from *www.kff.org* report #2052-10.

Kaiser Family Foundation (KFF). (2007e). *Medicare Part D 2008 data spotlight: Premiums.* Menlo Park, CA: The Henry J. Kaiser Family Foundation. Retrieved from *www.kff.org* Publication #7706.

Kaiser Family Foundation (KFF). (2007f). *Medicare: Medicare spending and financing.* Menlo Park, CA: The Henry J. Kaiser Family Foundation. Retrieved from *www.kff.org* #7305-12.

Kennedy, M. (2004). Nurses' workplace must change. *American Journal of Nursing, 104*(1), 23–24.

Kinsey, K., & Buchanan, M. (2004). The nursing center: A model of community health nursing practice. In M. Stanhope & J. Lancaster (Eds.), *Public health nursing* (7th ed.). St. Louis: Mosby.

Lee, P., & Estes, C. (2003). *The nation's health* (7th ed.). Sudbury, MA: Jones and Bartlett.

Marquis, J. (2004). *Concierge medical practice expanding across the nation.* Warner, Norcross & Judd. Retrieved from *www.wnj.com/concierge_22004/.*

Military Health System. (2008). *Wounded warrior care.* Washington, DC: The Pentagon. Retrieved from *www.health.mil/woundedwarrior.jsp.*

Milstead, J. (2008). *Health policy & politics: A nurse's guide* (3rd ed.). Sudbury, MA: Jones & Bartlett.

National Center for Health Statistics (NCHS). (2006). *Health, United States, 2006 with chart book on trends in the health of Americans.* Washington, DC: U.S. Government Printing Office.

National Center for Health Statistics (NCHS). (2007). *Health, United States, 2007 with chart book on trends in the health of Americans.* Washington, DC: U.S. Government Printing Office.

National Center for Policy Analysis. (2008). *Illegal aliens straining health-care system.* Retrieved from *www.ncpa.org/sub/dpd/index.php?page=article&Article_ID=5411.*

Neuhauser, D. (2003). Florence Nightingale gets no respect: As a statistician that is. *Quality and Safety in Health Care, 12*(4), 317.

Nies, M., & McEwen, M. (2007). *Community/public health nursing: Promoting the health of populations* (4th ed.). Philadelphia: Saunders.

Quan, K.(2008). *A national nurse for America.* Retrieved from *http://thenursesingsite.com/Articles/national.*

Rollet, J. (2003). Annual legislative update. *Advance for Nurse Practitioners, 11*(12), 37, 40–42.

Schroeder, S. (2007). We can do better—Improving the health of the American people. *The New England Journal of Medicine, 357*(12), 1221–1228.

Shi, L., & Singh, D. (2004). *Delivering health care in America: A systems approach* (3rd ed.). Sudbury, MA: Jones and Bartlett.

Shi, L., & Singh, D. (2005). *Essentials of the US health care system.* Sudbury, MA: Jones & Bartlett.

Shi, L., & Stevens, G. (2005). *Vulnerable populations in the United States.* San Francisco, CA: John Wiley & Sons, Inc.

Smith, M. (2007). *TB incidence rate drops in U.S., but decline slows.* Retrieved from *www.medpagetoday.com/infectiousdisease/Tuberculosis/tb/5308.*

Spector, R. (2004). *Cultural diversity in health and illness* (6th ed.). Upper Saddle River, NJ: Prentice Hall.

Stanhope, M., & Lancaster, J. (2008). *Public health nursing* (7th ed.). St. Louis: Mosby.

Sultz, H., & Young, K. (2004). *Health care USA: Understanding its organization and delivery* (4th ed.). Sudbury, MA: Jones & Bartlett.

Turnock, B. (2004). *Public health: What it is and how it works* (3rd ed.). Sudbury, MA: Jones & Bartlett.

U.S. Department of Health and Human Services. (2007a). *Healthy people 2010: Midcourse review.* Retrieved January 4, 2008, from *http://healthypeople.gov/data/midcourse/html.*

U.S. Department of Health and Human Services. (2007b). *Medicare homepage.* Retrieved from *www.hhs.gov.*

U.S. Department of Health and Human Services. (2007c). *Protecting the privacy of patient's health information.* Retrieved from *www.os.dhhs.gov/news/facts/privacy2007.html.*

U.S. Department of Health and Human Services. (2008). *The 2008 HHS poverty guidelines.* Washington, DC: Federal

Register. Retrieved from *http://aspe.hhs.gov/poverty/08poverty.shtml.*

U.S. Department of Health & Human Services Health Resources and Services (USHHS). (2004). *The Registered nurse population: Findings from the 2004 national sample survey of registered nurses.* Retrieved from *http://bhpr.hrsa.gov/healthworkforce/rnsurvey04.* Appendix-Table 13.

Weissert, C., & Weissert, W. (2006). *Governing health: The politics of health policy* (3rd ed.). Baltimore, MD: The John Hopkins University Press.

Wood, D. (2007, December 3). *National nurse debate fuels concern.* Retrieved from *http://include.nurse.com/apps/pbcs.dll/Article?AID=20071203/NWOZ/3120300026.*

World Health Organization. (2004). *Overview of WHO.* Retrieved May 1, 2004, from *www.who.int/about/overview/en/.*

World Health Organization. (2007). *About WHO.* Retrieved January 20, 2008, from *www.who.int/agenda/en/index.html/.*

Chapter 4

June Andrews Horowitz

The Therapeutic Relationship

objectives

After completing this chapter, the reader will be able to:

- Evaluate values clarification as a prerequisite to effective health promotion.
- Examine the elements and process of communication.
- Analyze differences between functional and dysfunctional communication.
- Develop strategies to promote therapeutic relationships with diverse populations across clinical settings, contexts, and nursing roles.
- Synthesize knowledge of the therapeutic relationship as an essential component of health promotion.

key terms

15-minute interview
Communication process
Countertransference
Empathy
Feedback
Health literacy
Helping or therapeutic relationship
Input
Johari window

Metacommunication
Milieu
Nonverbal communication
Output
Practical reflection
Process
Proxemics
Rapport
Reciprocity
Reflection

Relationship stages
Self-concept
Self-disclosure
Self-esteem
Telehealth
Therapeutic use of self
Transference
Values clarification
Verbal communication

website materials

evolve These materials are located on the book's website at *http://evolve.elsevier.com/Edelman/*.
- WebLinks
- Study Questions
- Glossary

THINK About It

How Does a Nurse Respond When an Individual's Values Conflict with the Nurse's Values of Promoting Healthy Behaviors?

Samantha, a 17-year-old girl, comes into the health clinic at her school to ask the nurse practitioner to prescribe birth control pills for her and to check her for a vaginal discharge. The nurse begins the appointment by asking Samantha about her chief complaint of discharge. Samantha answers these questions until the nurse asks about her relationship with her boyfriend. Samantha comments, "Don't worry about me. We're in love and I just need birth control pills so I won't get pregnant." When the nurse introduces the topic of health risks associated with unprotected sex, Samantha says, "Look, I don't need a lecture. You sound like my mother. I know what I'm doing and I don't need condoms because he's not with anyone else."

1. How can this nurse bridge the apparent gap between the nurse's values and Samantha's values?
2. In this brief encounter, how can the nurse begin to establish a therapeutic relationship?
3. What responsibilities does the nurse need to weigh in responding to Samantha's request?
4. What health risks exist if the nurse does or does not do what Samantha wants at this visit?
5. What does the nurse need to know about policies and care decisions for individuals who are not legal adults? What school health policies might affect the nurse's scope of practice and dialogue with Samantha? How might the nurse use this encounter to promote communication among stakeholders including elected officials, e.g., School Committee members, school administrators, school nurses, parents, and students?
6. What strategies could the nurse use to engage Samantha in a conversation about her sexual behaviors and related health issues?

The therapeutic relationship is the **milieu** in which nursing care occurs. Nursing practice is shaped by the caregiver's ability to focus on the interests, concerns, and needs of the individual (Peplau, 1991). Nurse-person interaction is "a shared process whereby both client and nurse are involved in constructing, interpreting, and defining the actions of the other" (Finch, 2005, p. 14).

Particularly in health promotion, the nurse-person relationship is the context for care. Health promotion requires sensitivity to each person's goals and values—the individual's and the nurse's. Helping a person adopt health-promoting behaviors requires more than giving information. Health promotion also requires effective communication, which is why communication is a focus area of *Healthy People 2010* (U.S. Department of Health and Human Services, 2000) and thus a priority for nursing practice. Successful health promotion involves interpersonal skills, personal insight, accountability, mutual respect, and a supportive working milieu. Essential to this interactional process are values clarification, communication, and the helping relationship. See the *Healthy People 2010* box for the Leading Health Indicators and Priorities for Action.

VALUES CLARIFICATION
Definition

Values are qualities, principles, attitudes, or beliefs about the inherent worth of an object, behavior, or idea. Values guide action by sanctioning certain behaviors and disavowing others. Values and beliefs are essential factors in design and implementation of nursing interventions (Kikuchi, 2005). Cognitive values are those a person ascribes to verbally and intellectually. Active values, in contrast, are those a person physically acts out. Judging the power of a given value by its ability to influence action is important. For example, a nurse may claim to value the worth of all people equally, but

Healthy People 2010

Leading Health Indicators

- Physical activity
- Overweight and obesity
- Tobacco use
- Substance abuse
- Responsible sexual behavior
- Mental health
- Injury and violence
- Environmental quality
- Immunization
- Access to health care

Priorities for Action

- Adopt the 10 Leading Health Indicators as personal and professional guides for choices about how to make health improvements.
- Encourage public health professionals and public officials to adopt the Leading Health Indicators as the basis for public health priority setting and decision-making.
- Urge public and community health systems and our community leadership to use the Leading Health Indicators as measures of local success for investments in health improvements.

From U.S. Department of Health and Human Services. (n.d.). *Healthy People 2010. What are the leading health indicators?* Retrieved October 5, 2007, from *www.healthypeople.gov/LHI/lhiwhat.htm.*

may treat individuals of various races differently and provide the most time and concern for those who are racially similar to the nurse. This cognitive value has little power to shape the nurse's behavior. If the nurse treated people of all races with equal respect, the value would also be active and have great power to motivate behavior.

Box **4-1** The Valuing Process

CHOOSING

1. Choosing freely
2. Choosing from alternatives
3. Choosing after careful consideration of potential outcomes of each alternative

PRIZING

4. Cherishing and being happy with personal beliefs and actions
5. Affirming the choice in public, when appropriate

ACTING

6. Acting out the choice
7. Repeatedly acting in some type of pattern

Box **4-2** Techniques for Assisting Individuals to Clarify Values

IDENTIFY THE INDIVIDUAL'S VALUES

"What is important to you?"
"Which of the following statements sounds most like the way you think?"
"What do you value most in life?"

USE REFLECTION TO RESTATE THE VALUE AND MAKE IT EXPLICIT

"In what you've just told me, I hear that it is very important to you that ..."
"I understand that you value ..."

IDENTIFY VALUE CONFLICTS OR CONFLICTS BETWEEN VALUES AND ACTIONS

"What connection does this value have to your current health or illness and to the healthy behaviors, interventions, or treatments needed to maintain or restore your health?"
"How does this particular value affect your behavior and health?"
"What are some ways that you might put your values into action?"
"Are your actions consistent with your values? If not, then what might you change?"

Many forces shape values. Passed down from one generation to another, values color an individual's identity, goals, and sense of personal meaning. Values are embedded in the culture and taught within a family and social context, giving meaning to the life events and happenings outside the family's boundaries (Wright & Leahey, 2005). To engage in health promotion, the nurse must appreciate that values are culture-bound and explore how culture, traditions, and practices in a multiethnic and multicultural society influence health-related values. Without this understanding, the nurse is likely to relate to individuals with a limited awareness of their assumptions and inadequate sensitivity to the uniqueness and perspective of the person, family, or community.

Values evolve; they are not static. Life events and social processes can spark a reappraisal of personal values. **Values clarification** is a method for discovering one's values and the importance of these values (Raths et al., 1978). Values clarification does not tell a person how to act, but it helps people recognize what values they hold and evaluate how those values influence their actions.

Box 4-1 outlines seven steps in the valuing process. The first three steps of choosing involve a cognitive process, the next two steps involve the affective or emotional domain, and the final steps involve behavior (Raths et al., 1978; Stuart & Laraia, 2005). The nurse uses values clarification to examine personal values and their potential influence on nursing care, and to help people identify their values and reflect on their connection to health-related behaviors. Box 4-2 lists suggestions for putting values clarification into action.

Values clarification becomes a clinical aim when individuals' values lead to behaviors that conflict with the nurse's value of promoting health. For example, a nurse tells a childbirth education class consisting of pregnant women and their coaches that alcohol use poses serious risks to the fetus. After the class, one woman comments, "Do you really think that having a drink once in a while is bad for the baby? I'm sick of being told that I can't do

things because of the baby." In this example, an apparent conflict in values between other women and the individual exists. Intervention is needed to examine how this woman's wish for freedom from restrictions clashes with her desire to have a healthy child. Nurses must consider their own values related to health promotion for the individual and the fetus and must weigh the importance of respecting individuals' rights to make decisions about their own health behaviors. Such value conflicts result in ethical dilemmas. Resolution rests on the nurse's ability to examine conflicting values and available evidence about possible outcomes when fashioning health-promotion interventions.

Values and Therapeutic Use of Self

The self, the most precious and unique of all human endowments, is a personal concept of individuality as distinct from other people and objects. **Therapeutic use of self** is the application of one's cognitions, perceptions, and behaviors to create interpersonal encounters that promote health in another person, family, group, or community. Without self-awareness and clarification of values, therapeutic use of self is impaired. **Self-concept** and **self-esteem** are interrelated components of individuals' judgments and attitudes about themselves. Self-concept is a mental picture of the self—a composite view of personal characteristics, abilities, limitations, and aspirations. Self-esteem, the affective component of self-perception, refers to how individuals feel about the way that they see themselves. Internalized appraisals from others also influence self-concept and self-esteem.

Self-concept evolves throughout life. From birth, family experiences and parental identification mold the child's sense of identity. The classic research studies of Coopersmith (1967) and Sears (1970) demonstrated positive relationships between the self-reliance, self-esteem, and self-confidence of parents and children. Self-esteem is learned from experience (Roth-Herbst et al., 2008). To cultivate children's self-esteem and enable them to have a realistic perception of their strengths and weaknesses, parents should focus on positives, give **feedback** on abilities and limitations, and provide the child with a sense of belonging and realistic confidence. Positive, rewarding, anxiety-free interactions contribute to security, esteem, and positive self-view. Positive but realistic appraisals from significant others, especially the parents, help the young child to develop this healthy self-view (Brown, 2008; Sullivan, 1953).

The self does not develop solely in response to the reflected appraisals of others. Genetic endowment, experiential opportunities, and the individual's action shape self-concept. People can accept or reject the appraisals of others and modify their behavior. The ability to control actions and evaluate outcomes of interactions allows individuals to modify and alter their views of self. As such, the self is dynamic, changing through interaction with the outside world and in response to the various maturational and situational crises of life.

The ability to examine, reflect on, and evaluate the self is a uniquely human talent. Self-awareness involves interactions between the self and the external world and the symbolic connections created by the individual. The self includes an unconscious component that is only partially accessible and influences behavior. Self-awareness is influenced by the degree to which an individual has an accurate concept of all dimensions of the self. The **Johari window** (Luft, 1984) provides a schema for understanding the various components of the self (Figure 4-1). Box 4-3 lists these four components of the self.

Together, these windowpanes represent the total self. Three principles guide an understanding of how the self functions in this representation: (1) change in one portion influences all other portions; (2) the smaller the first portion, the poorer communication will be; and (3) interpersonal learning enlarges the first portion and decreases the size of one or more other portions (Luft, 1969). The goal of self-awareness is to increase the size of the first windowpane while reducing the size of the other three areas (Figure 4-2) (Stuart & Laraia, 2005).

Consider the differences between windows A and B of Figure 4-2. Window A represents an individual with little self-awareness. Windowpane number 4 is large, suggesting that a good deal of the person's experiences, thoughts, and feelings are repressed or suppressed, probably a result of associated anxiety. Additionally, window A suggests a large "not me" portion of the self. In contrast, window B represents a person who is open to the world and is comfortable with his or her self-concept.

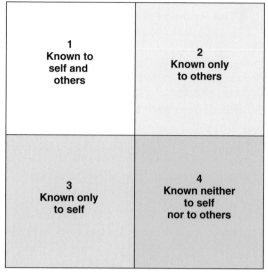

Figure 4-1 Johari window. (From Luft, J. [1984]. *Group processes: An introduction to group dynamics* [3rd ed.]. Palo Alto, CA: Mayfield. Reprinted with permission from Mayfield.)

| Box **4-3** | Components of the Self |

1. The *public self*, which is shown to others
2. The *semipublic self*, which is seen by others but may be outside the individual's awareness
3. The *private self*, which is known to the individual, but not revealed to others
4. The *inner self*, which is the unconscious portion not known even to the individual because it has anxiety-provoking content

The goal of high self-awareness, as illustrated in window B of Figure 4-2, is reached through three steps. The first step is listening to oneself and paying attention to emotions, thoughts, memories, reactions, and impulses. Frequently, people tune out their feelings and thoughts because they are anxious or because they are in a hurry to accomplish some other task. Without self-reflection, people act automatically and lose some of the meaning of living. To improve the ability of self-reflection, ask questions such as the following:

- What am I feeling now?
- What emotions have I experienced today and in the past day or so? What were my thoughts?
- What events led up to these thoughts and feelings?
- What actions did I take? Did my behavior fit with my thoughts and feelings, or was there a lack of harmony?
- Was I aware of my reactions at the time that they took place?
- How have I responded in clinical situations lately?

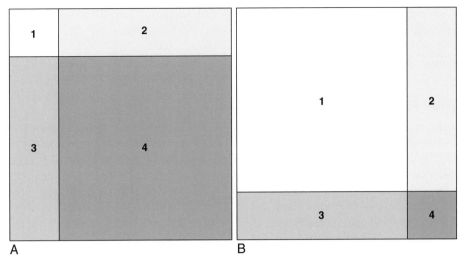

Figure 4-2   Johari windows illustrate varying degrees of self-awareness. **A,** Person has little self-awareness. **B,** Person has great amount of self-awareness. *1,* Public self. *2,* Semipublic self. *3,* Private self. *4,* Inner self. (From Stuart, G. W. [2009]. *Principles and practice of psychiatric nursing* [9th ed.]. St Louis, MO: Mosby.)

- How did I react in response to a particularly happy, sad, or difficult situation? In what way might I alter my actions now? What feelings and reactions did I experience while interacting with this individual?

The second step is listening to and learning from others. Feedback from others that conflicts with self-image can produce anxiety. In response, the feedback is ignored or translated incorrectly to preserve self-image and reduce anxiety. However, this pattern of responding limits knowledge of the self and inhibits the ability to examine the appraisals of others. Limited personal growth results. Asking reflective questions enables the nurse to use feedback effectively. Helpful questions include "What feedback have I received today?" and "What is the other person trying to tell me now?" A person also can ask others directly for feedback. For example, a student nurse might ask another student how he or she comes across. The feedback might be used to alter aspects of behavior that are ineffective or problematic before asking a faculty member for evaluative feedback. Using clinical supervision and consultation with colleagues provides needed opportunity for reflection on practice. How the nurse comes across to the individual or family is crucial to successful health promotion, making self-awareness and sensitivity to feedback essential.

The third step is **self-disclosure**; sharing aspects of the self enriches interpersonal life. Through self-disclosure, people come to know themselves better because they have held thoughts, actions, and feelings up to the light for examination with others. Self-disclosure is an indicator of a healthy personality and a strategy for developing one (Jourard, 1971; Stuart & Laraia, 2005). Self-disclosure by one person tends to trigger self-disclosure by another in a reciprocal pattern of interaction. Therapeutic interactions characterized by reciprocity involve a mutual exchange—a pattern of communication between the nurse and an individual, not a one-way inter-

vention from the nurse to the other person. Traditionally, clinicians have been wary of self-disclosure because it may cross a boundary from a professional to a personal relationship. Additionally, the nurse's self-disclosure might burden the individual and shift the focus of attention from the individual to the nurse. Although these guidelines are kept in mind to prevent excessive or inappropriate self-disclosure, appreciation that self-disclosure occurs within human interactions is needed. Welch (2005) found that experienced psychiatric nurses identified appropriate self-revelation as an effective component of therapeutic relationship. Nurses are not blank screens, robots, or technicians delivering care; individuals value nurses who engage in interactions as real people and who are willing to share information about themselves.

Practical reflection, a thinking process described by Taylor (2004), involves bouncing back one's own thoughts and recollections of events to understand them and to take needed corrective action. The process of practical reflection dovetails with steps toward self-awareness previously described and offers complementary helpful tips. First, the nurse recalls an incident when something went wrong. Then the nurse experiences the incident again by remembering images and by privately retelling events, statements, outcomes, and associated emotions. Next, the nurse interprets the story of communication that failed by examining expectations, ideals, goals, influences, personal actions, and others' actions that occurred during the event. The last step involves honest inspection of the nurse's own role in the story. Insights gained then may be applied in new interactions to prevent things going wrong again in a similar way.

Why is it important for a nurse to clarify personal values and increase self-awareness? The things the nurse values and self-understanding influence behavior. The self is the nurse's greatest tool; to use the self effectively, the nurse must be fully aware of how it functions. Thus, reflection and self-awareness guide the nurse's practice framework. In addition, sensitivity to individuals' perspectives is required to build a collaborative partnership, the cornerstone of the nurse-person relationship (Finch, 2005, 2006; Kikuchi, 2005; Welch, 2005).

THE COMMUNICATION PROCESS

The **communication process** is the forum for all thought and relationships shared among people. In conjunction with the use of scientific and technological advances, communication is an essential tool for the nurse to engage in health-promotion interventions. "Communication between a nurse and a client is a shared process that forms the basis for the professional relationship that is foundational for enhancing client care and affecting outcomes" (Finch, 2006, p. 14). Communication is an information exchange between individuals through shared symbols and signs and commonly understood behavior (Ruesch & Bateson, 1987). This exchange involves all the modes of behavior that an individual uses, consciously or unconsciously, to affect another person. Communication includes the spoken and written word and nonverbal communication (gestures, facial expressions, movement, body messages or signals, and artistic symbols). Increasingly, communication is electronic. **Telehealth**, the use of telecommunications and data technologies to deliver health care services including diagnostic services, treatment, consultation, and health information is rapidly growing as a communication system. Such electronic communication can encompass the spoken and written word, and nonverbal forms of communication. Yet the format and interface differ from the modes of human communication available until the latter part of the twentieth century, and changes will be exponential in the years to come. (For additional discussion, see the Hot Topics box.)

In nursing, communication is the cornerstone of a positive nurse-person relationship. Communication refers to a set of strategies and actions to enhance reciprocity, mutual understanding, and decision-making. Focusing the clinical discussion on the person's story rather than a version reformulated by the provider is essential to person-centered communication. Box 4-4 highlights strategies associated with person-centered communication based on evidence from the research literature.

Considerable evidence supports the effectiveness of these strategies. Research study results showed that nurses communicate effectively when they use a person-centered approach or nurse-person relational approach comprised of being attentive, caring, accepting, empathetic, friendly, comfortable, calm, interested, sincere, and respectful (Finch, 2006; McCabe, 2004; Moyle, 2003). Although these strategies sound simple and basic, such appraisals are noticeably absent in many instances and their presence is essential to quality nursing care (see the Research Highlights box). Furthermore, research findings have indicated that nurses seek communication with individuals

that supports "genuine knowing and understanding that can only evolve from sincere and open interactions" (Finch, 2005, p. 20).

Function and Process

Ruesch and Bateson (1987) have delineated the following functions of communication:

1. To obtain and send messages and to retain information
2. To use the information to arrive at new conclusions, to reconstruct the past, and to look forward to future events
3. To begin and to modify physiological processes
4. To influence others and outside events

Communication transmits information, both interpersonally and intrapersonally, and it provides the basis for action.

The process of communication consists of four components (Watzlawick et al., 1967). Nurses must be able to diagnose communication difficulties in any of these components. **Input** involves taking in information from outside the individual or group. Once taken in, input must be transformed in some manner to be used. For example, symbols must be translated into words to transmit ideas. The flow and transformation of processed input refers to the way information is analyzed and stored within the individual, or the way it is transmitted from person to person within a human system (group or family) before communication with the external environment occurs. The outcome of information processing, **output**, involves further exchange with the environment or other person. A new information exchange is triggered at this point in the cycle by the response called feedback, a monitoring system through which the person or group controls the internal and external responses to behavior (output) and accommodates these responses appropriately. A feedback loop shows the dynamic nature of communication. Each piece of communication is both a stimulus designed to elicit a response and a response to a different stimulus (Figure 4-3).

When interpersonal communication is analyzed, two types of feedback can be identified: positive (encouraging change) and negative (encouraging homeostasis or no change). Parents' commands to a young child illustrate these types of feedback: (1) positive, "Try that again; you almost had it" and (2) negative, "Don't touch that; it's hot." The first statement shows the parent's attempt to encourage the child to continue new behavior; the second illustrates an effort to curtail undesired behavior. Rather than meaning "good" or "bad," positive and negative feedback refer to promotion of system change and stability, which is the process of balancing the direction and magnitude of change. Both types of feedback are needed, depending on the situation.

The situational context of communication is important. The context of communication is the setting's physical, psychosocial, and cultural dimensions. It includes the relationship between sender and receiver; their previous

HOTtopics

TELEHEALTH: THERAPEUTIC RELATIONSHIPS IN THE AGE OF THE INTERNET

Technological advances have produced rapid changes in communication. Automatic teller machines have replaced human tellers at banks for routine transactions. Voicemail rather than a receptionist is likely to answer calls, and messages are recorded electronically. An electronic response to many calls directs the caller to a series of options that may not even include speaking to a person. E-mail, instant messaging, and "texting" are ubiquitous. Information in many areas is now available via access to a computer and an Internet connection. Wireless internet access ("WiFi") increasingly is used as a perk to lure customers to the local coffee spot and to ease passengers' irritation during long flight delays. Nurses use electronic records and communicate updated information via hand-held devices.

Over the past decade, we have witnessed exponential increases in computer penetration (Moore & Primm, 2007). Such technology can speed up work and expand capabilities. Who would prefer to use a traditional typewriter to prepare papers and documents after mastering a word-processing program? Yet many issues deserve examination as we move into the age of telehealth.

Telehealth—the use of telecommunications and data technologies to deliver health care services including diagnostic services, treatment, consultation, and health information—is now omnipresent. Rather than replacing traditional care, telehealth is best understood as a complementary approach to long-distance care delivery, and faster and easily delivered contact. Telehealth has the potential to expand access to care, particularly for individuals receiving home care and those in remote areas, and to contain costs (Coons & Carpenedo, 2007). Moreover, the concept of telehealth also encompasses remote teaching, conferencing, and consulting (Winters & Winters, 2007).

Technological advances have produced benefits; however, technology also can reduce the need for direct interpersonal contact. Barriers to use include the need for financial investment to establish networks, inadequate reimbursement mechanisms, risks to confidentiality with electronic transmission, and licensure issues when care is transmitted across state lines. Challenges include conducting systematic evaluation of outcomes and cost-effectiveness, and ensuring that individuals' economic status and health literacy do not constrain access.

Perhaps the most important threat is that care can become impersonal when face-to-face contact is replaced by electronic interface. Thus, preserving core nursing values as electronic care systems are created, tested, and implemented is a crucial goal. Winters and Winters (2007) identified three strategies to safeguard core professional values in the emerging age of telehealth:

1. Avoid a "one size fits all" approach through individualized or tailored algorithms and design features specific to the system's use.
2. Develop and maintain therapeutic relationships by inviting exchanges between the nurse and person, e.g., by creating a series of layered screens that first introduce the nurse (visually and with a biography) and later invite exchanges, feedback, and sharing of experiences and stories from individuals that may be shared.
3. Foster individual autonomy by building components that encourage decision-making, problem-solving, and knowledge development that is timely and specific to the health problem and stage of treatment or management.

Consider the following questions about telehealth:
- What effects do technological changes have on the therapeutic relationship?
- Will face-to-face interaction become a rare occurrence? In the future, might therapeutic interactions take place primarily via technology, such as voicemail, the Internet, and videotape transmission? What advantages and disadvantages will appear with the increasing use of technology in nursing practice?
- What creative approaches may evolve using technology in therapeutic relationships?
- How can electronic communication systems be used in disaster preparedness to alert people at risk and direct actions to increase safety when a human-caused or natural disaster is suspected, imminent, or in progress?

For additional information about telehealth, see: Coons, C. A., & Carpenedo, D. J. (2007). Research on telehealth in home care: Adoption and models of care. *Home Health Care Nurse, 25,* 477-481; Moore, S. M., & Primm, T. (2007). Designing and testing telehealth interventions to improve outcomes for cardiovascular patients. *Journal of Cardiovascular Nursing, 22,* 43-50; U.S. Department of Health and Human Services, Health Resources and Services Administration. (n.d). *Telehealth.* Retrieved Oct. 9, 2007, from: *www.hrsa.gov/telehealth/*; Winters, J. M., & Winters, J. M. (2007). Videoconferencing and telehealth technologies can provide a reliable approach to remote assessment and teaching without compromising quality. *Journal of Cardiovascular Nursing, 22,* 51-57.

experiences, feelings, values, cultural norms, age and developmental stage; and the physical location (Kasch, 1986; Stuart & Laraia, 2005).

Types of Communication

All human communication occurs in three forms: (1) verbal, (2) nonverbal, and (3) **metacommunication**. Each affects the meaning and influences the interpretation of the message.

Verbal Communication

Verbal communication is the transmission of messages using words, spoken or written. As symbols for ideas, words impart meaning defined by a specific language. Communicating with language is a critical ability.

People who are deaf or hard of hearing often use sign language to communicate. Signs, similar to spoken or written words, are used consistently to represent a particular meaning. Words also may be spelled out through finger spelling in

research highlights

Communication with Nurses: Relational Communications and Preferred Nurse Behaviors

STUDY OVERVIEW

Using both hermeneutical and descriptive methodologies, Finch (2006) examined nurse-person communication dimensions and identified preferred nurse behaviors. A nonrandom convenience sample of 100 participants included 25 older adult residents from an independent living residence, 25 college students who used university health services, and 25 participants recruited initially from a local church with subsequent snowball sampling for final accrual of 50 additional participants. In written and oral instructions, participants were asked to remember a nurse-person interaction from the last 6 months. In addition, several instruments were used to measure demographic characteristics, and participants' views concerning relational behaviors and communications between themselves and nurses.

RESULTS

Results confirmed the importance of relational communication in nurse-person relationships. Across age groups, participants overwhelmingly preferred caring nurses who conveyed concern, compassion, consideration, sincerity, honesty, and kindness. Warm and friendly descriptors of nurses included being cordial, courteous, nice, personable, pleasant, and able to establish rapport. Nursing behaviors defined as professional were being businesslike and straightforward. Competence comprised of being efficient, knowledgeable, and thorough. Nurses who listened were described as attentive and interested. Understanding involved being empathetic, truthful, authentic, and real (i.e., honest and sincere). Findings confirmed outcomes from previous studies concerning nursing competence and interaction style and Peplau's (1991) theoretical perspective.

IMPLICATIONS

Identification of relational communication dimensions and preferred nurse behaviors informs nursing practice and education. Finch summed up the most important implications as follows: "Today's nurse must be a respectful practitioner who goes beyond the mere formality of history-taking and pertinent physical examination. The question is how can today's nurse engage in this depth of communication that obviously requires commitment and effort when nurses are in short supply and patients are more complex than ever?" (p. 20). Findings underscore the necessity of teaching students the fundamentals of relational communication and preferred nurse-person behaviors and supporting nurses to provide evidenced-based practice that reflects optimal communication and behaviors identified in this study. Outcomes from this study and a growing body of research provide evidence for quality indicators of person-preferred nursing communication and behaviors.

Finch, L. P. (2006). Patients' communication with nurses: relational communication and preferred nurse behaviors. *International Journal for Human Caring, 10*, 14-22.

Box 4-4 Strategies Associated with Person-Centered Communication

- Permitting people to tell their stories in their own words and chronology
- Using a conversational interviewing style
- Being friendly through humor and social conversation, and nonverbal cues such as smiling
- Eliciting people's views, perspectives, thoughts, wishes, goals, values, and expectations
- Inquiring about the nature of the person's life
- Attending to the person's needs
- Avoiding overemphasis on technical aspects of care and tasks
- Not being too busy to talk
- Responding to cues concerning emotional issues and problems
- Giving information about self-care and participation in decision-making
- Developing mutual understanding
- Creating collaborative health care plans
- Showing empathy and concern for the individual's well-being
- Connecting with individuals through humor, touch, and selective self-disclosure
- Tuning in to individuals' preferences and style
- Attending to and advocating for individuals' needs
- Maintaining confidentiality

Modified from McCabe, C. (2004). Nurse-patient communication: An exploration of patients' experiences. *Journal of Clinical Nursing, 13,* 41-49; Moyle, W. (2003). Nurse-patient relationship: A dichotomy of expectations. *International Journal of Mental Health Nursing, 12,* 103-109; Welch, M. (2005). Pivotal moments in the therapeutic relationship. *International Journal of Mental Health Nursing, 14,* 161-165.

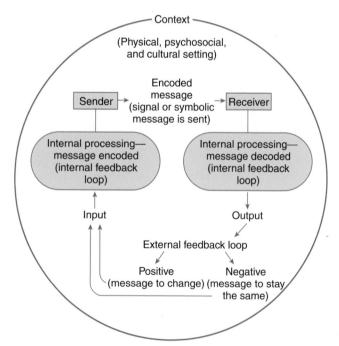

Figure 4-3 Communication system.

a manner parallel to written communication. Braille assists blind and visually challenged people to read. Touch is used to interpret markings that represent letters and words. Sign language and Braille blend aspects of verbal and nonverbal communication, but both forms of communication transmit meaning through a consistent language system.

Verbal communication with people who speak a different language poses a challenge. As societies become increasingly multicultural, assistance from specially trained interpreters is essential to providing culturally competent care. Confidentiality issues, the complexity of health information, and the need to validate understandings and reach mutual decisions make it inappropriate to use untrained personnel or relatives to interpret simply because they are available.

The importance of language development is apparent in its three functions: (1) informing the person of others' thoughts and feelings; (2) stimulating the receiver of a message by triggering a response; and (3) serving a descriptive function by imparting information and sharing observations, ideas, inferences, and memories (Watzlawick et al., 1967). The ability of verbal communication to fulfill these functions is influenced by many factors, including the communicator's social class, culture, age, milieu, and ability to receive and interpret messages.

Nonverbal Communication

Nonverbal communication or language encompasses all messages that are not spoken or written. The channels of nonverbal communication are the five senses. Movement, facial and eye expressions, gestures, touch, appearance, and vocalization or paralanguage all constitute nonverbal modes of communication (Blondis & Jackson, 1982). Although all communication has the potential of being misunderstood, nonverbal communication is particularly subject to misunderstanding because it does not always reflect the sender's conscious intent. Nonverbal messages also tend to be nebulous, without specific beginnings and endings.

Body motion or kinetic behavior includes facial expression (or facies), eye movements, body movements, gestures, and posture (Blondis & Jackson, 1982). When observing facial expression, the nurse notices the affect or emotion that is communicated. Does the person appear happy or sad; alert, distracted, or sleepy; contented, agitated, or anxious? The degree of emotion expressed should also be noted. Does the person's face express what generally is considered an excessive degree of feeling for the situation, too little, or none at all? Eyes, in conjunction with the movement of other facial muscles, move in ways that convey affect. Eye contact conveys messages of interest or trust; lack of eye contact can imply lack of interest or anxiety; constant eye contact can send a message of hostility.

All of these nonverbal messages are culturally and situationally bound. Nonverbal behavior, particularly facial and eye expressions, is contextual. For example, in certain circumstances and cultures, avoidance of direct eye contact between some people can be a sign of respect. Yet, in other situations and cultures, it can be interpreted as indicative of disinterest, avoidance, or disrespect.

Sign language combines features of both nonverbal and verbal communication. Sign language involves nonverbal communication because, although it uses symbols that are communicated through specific signs, these are enhanced by facial expressions and body postures. However, sign language shares many aspects of verbal communication. It has syntax and grammar, words may be spelled out, and a standard meaning is assigned to specific signs to create symbolic language, just as words share common definitions.

Importance of Nonverbal Communication Nonverbal communication has great power to transmit information about another's thoughts and feelings; therefore, careful observation is essential. Even silence can be very revealing. The significance of nonverbal communication is best captured by the axiom, "Actions speak louder than words." Nurses' nonverbal messages that communicate distance from the person, or signal an unfriendly or uncaring attitude, thwart development of a therapeutic relationship (McCabe, 2004) and thereby render health-promotion efforts unproductive.

Metacommunication

Besides verbal and nonverbal communication, a phenomenon called metacommunication refers to a message about the message. Watzlawick, Beavin, and Jackson (1967) described metacommunication as the impossibility of not communicating: that is, "one cannot not communicate. Persons transmit a message about what is being communicated even when words are not spoken" (p. 49). Metacommunication is the relationship aspect of communication. In a sense, metacommunication involves reading between the lines or going past the surface content of the message to glean nuances of meaning. When the content and the relationship aspects, or metacommunication aspects, of a message are incongruent, interpreting the communication accurately may be difficult, leaving the receiver uncomfortable and confused.

Group Process

In group settings, a special type of metacommunication is called **process**. A basic principle of group theory states that all communication has content and process. Content is what is said; process is the relationship aspect of what is communicated. Group process occurs during every group encounter. Staff meetings and clinically oriented psychoeducation, therapy, and counseling groups always involve group process. For example, consider two individuals in a smoking cessation group who always support each other by agreeing with each other and offering comments or criticism to any group member who disagrees. Although this pairing between the individuals offers them some protection from anxiety that may result from self-examination and feedback, it isolates them and curtails feedback from others. Examination of this group process is an essential task. The nurse leader and participants can transform this problematic situation into a learning opportunity by (1) identifying the pattern by pointing out the behavior after it has occurred frequently, (2) helping the pair and other group members to consider what needs are being met through this pattern, (3) looking at each person's role in fostering this process (e.g., why other group members have failed to confront the pair), and (4) discussing potential outcomes of changing the behavior. These steps can be applied in clinical situations when greater self-understanding is a goal.

Effectiveness of Communication

Understanding what makes communication effective improves the nurse's ability to assess needs and to intervene effectively to promote individuals' health. Steps to functional communication include (1) firmly stating the case, (2) clarifying the message, (3) seeking feedback, and (4) being receptive to feedback when it is received.

To state the case firmly, the sender needs to make the content and the metacommunication congruent; when they conflict, the message is confusing. For example, a nurse is angry with a colleague for making statements to an administrator that undermined the nurse's plans for reconfiguring a health-promotion program in their agency. When the nurse had a chance to speak with this colleague, they exchanged pleasantries without mention of what the nurse thought about the colleague's statements to the administrator. When the colleague asked if something was bothering the nurse, the nurse responded that nothing was wrong. The colleague senses that the nurse's verbal and nonverbal communication did not match; in other words, the content of the message and the metacommunication were incongruent. The colleague was left feeling uneasy, and the nurse failed to express his or her thoughts or to take effective action to rectify the perceived problem with the colleague. To make the communication functional, the nurse needed to bring thoughts and feelings into awareness and reflect on the intended message. Once these steps are accomplished, the message's content and metacommunication can be adjusted to match, and the nurse's communication is likely to be effective.

To clarify the message, the sender must give a complete message. Important features should be emphasized and specifics of any request must be stated, not assumed. The message's importance also must be indicated. To illustrate, a woman mentions to her nurse that it is nearly June. The nurse responds that he has noticed how warm the weather is becoming. On the surface, this communication may seem functional until the intent of the woman's message is considered. She meant to imply that June is the 5-year anniversary of her remission from cancer, and she hoped that her nurse would somehow know that she wanted him to comment on the significance of this anniversary. To make this communication functional, the woman needed to expand the message (e.g., "My anniversary after cancer treatment

is coming up") and then clarify her wish for a sensitive response from the nurse (e.g., "This anniversary marks the goal for you to be cancer-free"; "What will you do to celebrate?"). Additionally, she needed to show how important the message was (e.g., "I'd really like to do something special to mark this date"). If the nurse had been attuned to the metacommunication in this exchange, he could have clarified this woman's intent and met her need for recognition and dialogue.

One technique for clarifying and qualifying messages is called the "*I*" *statement*. Use of "I" statements helps the sender state what he or she wants, feels, thinks, or plans (including likes and dislikes). For example, "I felt unimportant when you forgot to recognize this anniversary" is an "I" statement that the person could have used to communicate effectively.

Questions can clarify and qualify, depending on the type of question asked. Open-ended questions tend to elicit descriptive responses rather than one-word answers. For example, the question, "Tell me what you did for exercise this week," is likely to yield a more elaborate description of a health behavior from a person than the question, "Did everything go okay with your exercise plan?" However, direct questions that seek a one-word answer are useful when a specific piece of information is sought. "Did you spend 15 minutes or more walking today?" may be a better approach than "What was your activity like today?" when it is important to discuss and promote minimum exercise requirements. Also, for individuals having trouble expressing more than the simplest thoughts, asking direct questions that call for brief replies can be helpful, such as, "Did you eat breakfast?" This approach is particularly useful with people who are depressed, regressed, cognitively impaired, or unable to handle complex information or communication at a particular time.

Seeking feedback is another element of functional communication. Consensual validation, confirming that both sender and receiver understand the same information, calls for the use of the clarification skills just described. In family communication, the parent, as the sender, should model this behavior for children by asking the child, as the receiver, to explain his or her sense of the message and how to ask the sender for further explanation. For example, "I want you to clean your room" (message from parent) can be followed by, "Tell me how you think you will do that" (validating that child and parent agree about what the task entails). This style of seeking validation can be adapted to nurse–nurse or nurse–other professional exchanges between colleagues and to therapeutic interactions. Such confirmation in communication is essential when providing health-promotion interventions. Without validating that the person understands the information and its importance, and that the person has a behavior plan to follow, health-promotion efforts are likely to fail.

Being open to feedback also is crucial. A "no questions" attitude blocks functional communication, whether in the home, classroom, or clinical setting. Children, students, individuals, and even other nurses may be afraid to question anyone in authority or may assume that the person should magically know what is intended or expected. For example, a person may avoid confronting a nurse who fails to explain the clinical plan and then communicates that the person should know how to follow through. Statements by the sender such as "Tell me what you think" and "What is your understanding of what I said?" are helpful.

Receiving and sending messages involves many of the same processes. Evaluation of the intent of the message, both the content and the metacommunication, is the first step. The receiver frequently needs to seek clarification and validate understanding of the message for communication to be effective. Clarification of expectations, active exchange of information, power sharing, and negotiation will enhance the quality of nurse-person communication. The outcome is a nurse-person relationship based on trust and partnership (Welch, 2005; Yamashita et al., 2005).

Factors in Effective Communication
Listening

Effective listening, an important part of communication, is more than passively taking in information. Effective listening is actively focusing attention on the message. Asking questions to explore what is meant helps the listener reach an accurate assessment of the message's meaning.

Many forms of nonverbal communication have been identified that, from a Western or European perspective, commonly convey that the person is listening. These nonverbal communications include direct gazing and eye contact, head nodding, orienting one's body to maintain interpersonal closeness, leaning forward, facial expressions such as eyebrow animation and smiling, and brief verbal statements that indicate interest, such as "Please go on" or "Tell me more about that ...."

For behavior to communicate that the person is listening also depends on the context and intensity of the activities, and the cultural norms of each person. For example, leaning close to a person might be interpreted as intrusive. Yet, the same behavior could be seen as a sign of support, depending on the context and perspective of those involved. Sensitivity to nuances in communication and validation of meaning can be particularly helpful strategies when the nurse and person come from different cultural backgrounds.

Reciprocity, the patterning of similar activities within the same interval by two people, can help the nurse communicate a listening stance in an effective way. When the nurse matches nuances of the individual's type and style of behavior, the chances that the person will interpret the nurse's behavior as an indication of active listening are increased, and the likelihood of misinterpretation is reduced. Nurses can enhance the quality of their communication, even when encounters are brief, by attending to reciprocity in their interactions and by validating whether or not reciprocity is associated with shared interpretations of meaning.

Poor listening blocks the nurse's understanding of the person. The nurse's failure to listen may be caused by anxiety; lack of experience, which leads to excessive talking by the nurse; preoccupation with personal thoughts; or lack of practice (Stuart & Laraia, 2005). The importance of focusing on the individual's needs and concerns through effective listening is a recurrent theme in research concerning therapeutic interaction (Douglass et al., 2003; McCabe, 2004; Moyle, 2003).

Flexibility

Flexibility is a balance between control and permissiveness. In overcontrol, every message is monitored. In exaggerated permissiveness, anything can be communicated in any way. For communication to be functional, rules are needed about what is appropriate, without rigid prescriptions that inhibit meaningful interchange. For example, the guideline that nurses will not answer questions concerning intimate details of their lives sets an appropriate limit; however, this does not mean that nurses should refuse to answer any question about themselves.

Silence

Silence between people is often uncomfortable for the nurse who is somewhat insecure about what should occur during a therapeutic encounter. However, silence can be beneficial when used carefully. When seeking a verbal response, silence can be perceived as a lack of interest. At other times, silence allows individuals to reflect on what is being discussed or experienced, lets them know that the nurse is willing to wait until they are ready to say more, or simply provides them with comfort and support. Each situation needs evaluation and sensitivity. Rather than asking a flurry of questions to break the silence, the nurse allows the person time to decide when to comment or should make brief comments that do not demand answers, such as "It can be helpful to take time to think about what we've been discussing." Also, comments such as "Try putting your thoughts or feelings into words" can help the person to share these thoughts or feelings when silence is blocking rather than improving the communication.

Humor

Humor is part of being human; it relieves tension, reduces aggression, and creates a climate of sharing. Humor can block communication when it is used to avoid subjects that might be uncomfortable or when it excludes other people. Humor can also inflict emotional pain and communicate negative views or stereotypes about particular individuals or groups through teasing and jokes concerning race, ethnicity, culture, country of origin, occupation, age, gender, sexual activity, or other traits that stand out or are devalued. A direct response to the latent content or message in this type of humor is an effective way to curtail its use and minimize its effect. For example, "That kind of joke makes me very uncomfortable. I don't find it funny to describe [the specific group in question] that way, and I would like you to stop." To be helpful, the meaning of the humor must be understood and its purpose supportive to the individual. Clarification of the meaning should be used when there is doubt or concern.

Touch

Touch is an interesting means of nonverbal communication for nurses, who often touch individuals while administering care. The nurse's concern can be expressed by a gentle or soothing application of touch. Nevertheless, in some instances touch is inappropriate. For example, in interactions with individuals who have trauma histories or acute psychiatric disturbances, touch might be misinterpreted. A woman who has been raped might interpret touch during an examination as an attack. Evaluation of the context and meaning of touch to the individual is based on knowledge of that person and interpretation of feedback. Figure 4-4 illustrates appropriate use of touch.

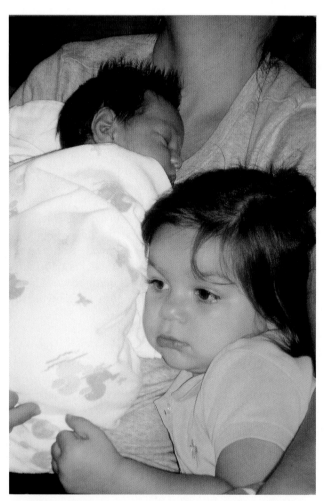

Figure 4-4   Touch is a powerful form of nonverbal communication. (Courtesy Boston College.)

Space

Space between communicators varies according to the type of communication, the setting, and the culture. Hall (1973) researched **proxemics**, the use of space between communicators, and identified four zones of space commonly used in interaction in North America that are presented in Box 4-5 and Figure 4-5.

Understanding the appropriate distance for a given type of interaction helps the nurse to make nonverbal and verbal communication congruent and to avoid violating spatial norms. Awareness of cultural customs concerning distance is important in shaping communication and interpreting the behavior of others. When people from different cultures or groups communicate, there may be discomfort about the acceptable distance between them when speaking. Recognition of differences helps the nurse adjust the distance and interpret the meaning of this nonverbal communication.

Many traits and components discussed in this chapter characterize functional communication. However, communication is a subtle and intricate process. Communication cannot be reduced to a set of parts and principles; its roles and nuances are far more complex and variable. To communicate by language and symbols is a special human ability. Healthy communication enables people to move from being alone to being together—clearly one of the crucial tasks of living. Effective communication is also the foundation for the helping relationship.

THE HELPING OR THERAPEUTIC RELATIONSHIP

A **helping or therapeutic relationship** is a process through which one person promotes the development of another person by fostering the latter's maturation, adaptation, integration, openness, and ability to find meaning in the present situation (Peplau, 1969). The therapeutic relationship emerges from purposeful encounters characterized by effective communication. In this relationship, the nurse respects the individual's values, attends to concerns, and promotes

Box **4-5**	Zones of Space Common to Interaction in North America

1. *Intimate space:* up to 18 inches (45.5 centimeters); used for high interpersonal sensory stimulation (see Figure 4-5, *A*)
2. *Personal space:* 18 inches to 4 feet (45.5 centimeters to 1.2 meters); appropriate for close relationships in which touching may be involved and good visualization is desired (see Figure 4-5, *B*)
3. *Social-consultative space:* 9 to 12 feet (2.7 to 3.6 meters); less intimate and personal, requiring louder verbal communication (see Figure 4-5, *C*)
4. *Public space:* 12 feet (3.6 meters) and over; appropriately used for formal gatherings, such as giving speeches (see Figure 4-5, *D*)

Based on data from Hall, E. (1973). *The silent language.* Garden City, NY: Doubleday/Anchor Press.

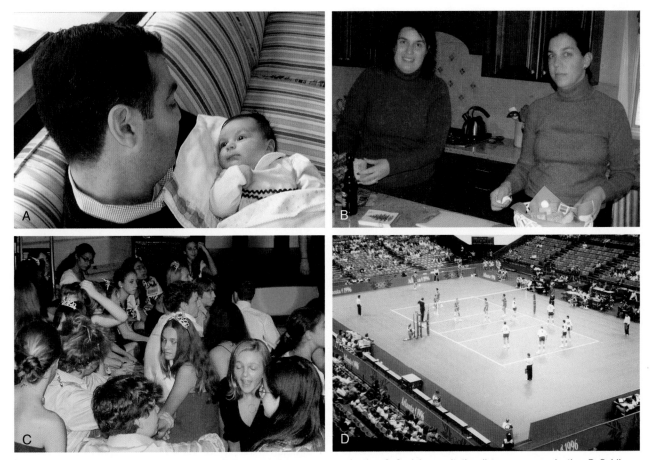

Figure 4-5   A, Intimate distance communication. **B,** Personal distance communication. **C,** Social-consultative distance communication. **D,** Public distance communication. **(B-D** Courtesy Boston College)

positive change by encouraging self-expression, exploring behavior patterns and outcomes, and promoting self-help (Moyle, 2003). This helping relationship is created by the nurse's application of scientific knowledge, his or her understanding of human behavior and communication, and his or her commitment to the individual. The therapeutic relationship is the foundation of clinical nursing practice—the essential element of care with every individual in every situation. Techniques, technology, interventions, and contexts vary, but the relational aspect of nursing practice produces a cohesive unity, allowing each nurse to see people holistically and as unique individuals.

No perfect profile or personality of a helping person exists. However, certain traits can be nurtured without thwarting the nurse's unique personality. These characteristics enable the nurse to be an agent of therapeutic care (Peplau, 1963; Stuart & Laraia, 2005). Box 4-6 lists characteristics associated with therapeutic effectiveness.

Characteristics of the Therapeutic Relationship

No recipe is available for a successful therapeutic relationship. Techniques and concepts serve only as tools. As a nurse develops and evaluates a helping relationship, the following guidelines may be useful.

> **Box 4-6   Characteristics Associated with Therapeutic Effectiveness**
>
> - Self-awareness and self-reflection
> - Openness
> - Self-confidence and strength
> - Genuineness
> - Concern for the individual
> - Respect for the individual
> - Knowledge
> - Ability to empathize
> - Sensitivity
> - Acceptance
> - Creativity
> - Ability to focus and confront

Purposeful Communication

Purposeful communication means that the nurse focuses communication for a particular aim. Social chitchat, communication without a goal, should not make up the bulk of therapeutic interaction. This does not mean that the nurse should never discuss a social topic; nonetheless, there should be some purpose. For example, discussing the weather with a somewhat disoriented older adult individual serves the purpose of orienting that person to the environment. Goals guide the nurse in focusing communication.

Rapport

Rapport is a harmony and an affinity between people in a relationship (Rogers, 1965). By using many of the traits listed for a helping person, the nurse can establish an atmosphere in which rapport can develop. To let the person know that his or her concerns interest the nurse and that working together may alleviate some of his or her difficulties and encourage growth, it is important to be genuine, open, and concerned.

Trust

Trust is a necessary component of any helping relationship. Trust is the reliance on a person to carry out responsibilities and promises, based on a sense of safety, honesty, and reliability. Trust is an important component of partnership (Yamashita et al., 2005). The nurse promotes trust by modeling and structuring the relationship appropriately. Strategies that promote trust include:

- Trusting the individual to do as promised
- Clearly defining the relationship parameters and expectations, particularly the purpose and specifics of time, place, and anticipated behavior
- Being consistent
- Examining behaviors that interfere with trust

Empathy

Empathy is the ability to understand another's feelings without losing personal identity and perspective. Empathic nurses draw on emotions and experiences that enable them to place themselves in the other person's situation. As the person's sense that the nurse is understanding and accepting increases, the individual's distress decreases. Outcome from research studies are building knowledge about the role that empathic nursing care plays in outcomes. For example, Moyle (2003) conducted a phenomenological study to explore the experience of being nurtured while depressed. Interviews with hospitalized participants revealed the importance of nursing presence that included spending time listening and assisting participants to discuss problems, fears, and anxieties. Furthermore, participants described their disappointment when nurses distanced themselves by attending only to physical needs and by limiting contact.

Nurses learn behavioral approaches that enhance empathic relations with people through supervised experiential learning. For example, nurses do not empathize by switching the focus of the interaction to themselves or by sympathizing (e.g., "I know exactly how you feel; that happened to me once"). Rather, they use clinical and personal experience to appreciate the individual's feelings and experiences. Using personal understanding while maintaining boundaries is the essence of empathy in the helping relationship. With empathic understanding, the nurse acknowledges the affective domain of personal experiences and uses this knowledge to appreciate the person's reactions. Empathy enables the listener to share human experiences as the basis for providing care.

Goal Direction

A helping relationship is special in its goal-directed nature. Although most human relationships focus on mutual benefit, a helping relationship exists solely to meet some need or to promote the growth of the recipient. Although the nurse may benefit from the interaction, the relationship is centered on the recipient.

Goals are formulated as desired individual behaviors. Short-term goals are likely to be achieved within 10 days to 2 weeks; all other goals are long term. All goals should be stated in measurable terms and should focus on a positive change or on the decrease of problematic behavior. Ideally, a person works with the nurse to establish goals. However, some individuals, such as those who are seriously ill, depressed, psychotic, or cognitively impaired, are unable to establish goals. When an individual is unable to negotiate appropriate goals, the nurse establishes realistic goals and shares them with the person, who is free to participate or to reject efforts to reach these goals.

Ethics in Communicating and Relating

Ethical decision-making is closely linked with the goal-directed nature of helping relationships. Ethical issues are present in human interactions whenever behavior may affect others, whenever actions involve conscious choices of methods and ends, and whenever actions can be evaluated in reference to standards of right and wrong (Crofts, 2006; Johannesen, 2002). Guidelines that may be adapted as ethical standards for interpersonal communication are highlighted in Box 4-7.

Frequently the nurse may wish to set goals that the individual does not want to reach; the nurse must remember that the problem belongs to the person, as does the choice of care alternatives. The nurse assists the individual in decision-making, with the decision based on the individual's value system. However, the nurse should not take a laissez-faire approach and avoid assisting the person. The nurse's responsibility is to help the individual to examine values, identify conflicts, and prioritize goals and desired health care outcomes. Action follows from understanding values and the best available information. Both the individual and the nurse must bring interpreted facts and personally clarified values to the interaction to establish goals. Recognizing this interplay, the nurse must clarify personal values, subsequently respect the individual's rights, and act to support and protect the integrity of the person and the family.

Therapeutic Techniques

Occasionally, clinicians who are novices in establishing helping relationships assume that they are bound to "say the

Box **4-7** Guidelines for Ethical Interpersonal Communication

---

Ethical interpersonal communication involves:
- Being aware and open to changing concepts of self and others
- Attending to role responsibilities; individual sacrifice, when it is required to make a "good" decision; and emotions, while guarding against letting emotions be the sole guide of our behavior
- Sharing personal views candidly and clearly
- Communicating information accurately, with minimal loss or distortion of intended meaning
- Communicating verbal and nonverbal messages with congruent meanings
- Sharing responsibility for the consequences among communicators
- Recognizing the multicultural context of all communication
- Respecting the dignity of every person
- Avoiding coercion and use of power in communicating
- Being sensitive to gender and cultural contexts of communication and interpretation
- Eliminating any elements of your communication that denigrate, stereotype, or devalue
- Facilitating open and accurate communication among: professional groups, professionals, staff and families, clinical care unit and department staffs or administrators, and clinical care facilities

Unethical communication involves:
- Purposefully deceiving
- Intentionally blocking communication—for example, changing subjects when the other person has not finished communicating, cutting a person off, or distracting others from the subject under discussion
- Scapegoating or unnecessarily condemning others
- Lying or deceiving that causes intentional or unintentional harm
- Verbally "hitting below the belt" by taking advantage of another's vulnerability

---

Modified from Crofts, L. (2006). Learning form critical case reviews: Emergent themes and their impact on practice. *Intensive and Critical Care Nursing, 22*, 362-369; Johannesen, R. L. (2002). Ethics in human communication (5th ed.). Prospect Heights, IL: Waveland Press.

wrong thing" and cause terrible damage to the person, or that they will learn some magical phrases and questions to create instant rapport. No nurse or other professional is so powerful that a "wrong word" will destroy the individual's self-concept or self-esteem. Even people with physical and emotional problems are resilient and have coped, at least to some degree, with a lifetime of stresses. Alternatively, no magical saying exists that the nurse can always plug into an interaction to communicate successfully. Although some techniques are often useful, they must be applied with purpose, skill, and attention to the individuality of each person and to the context of the interaction. The following techniques therefore should be viewed as guidelines, rather than prescriptions, for effective shaping of the therapeutic relationship.

Focus on the Individual

The first step to therapeutic communication is focusing on the individual and why the interaction is occurring. The nurse is not the focus; the person is. Although an overly businesslike style fails to communicate concern and support (Moyle, 2003), delving into one's own personal life to the extent that it diverts attention from the other person's concern also is problematic. Avoiding nurse-directed conversation can be difficult; a useful rule of thumb is to answer or respond to obvious questions and to switch the focus back to clinical concerns when other questions are asked. For example:

Individual (looks at female nurse's wedding ring): "Are you married?"

Nurse: "Yes, I am."

Individual: "What does your husband do for a living?"

Nurse: "Rather than get distracted by a discussion about me, let's get back to planning how you will manage at work."

Keeping focus on the person's concerns includes identifying the portion of the message that is clear and relevant to the purpose of the interaction, seeking validation, and helping the individual to clarify the rest of the message.

Help the Individual to Describe and Clarify Content and Meaning

Too often the nurse rushes to offer an interpretation of the nature of the problem and quickly follows up by suggesting a solution. Solving problems efficiently makes the nurse feel effective, important, and powerful; however, the person's needs may not be met. A crucial step in using the therapeutic relationship effectively is to assist the individual to describe a particular experience or concern. Description is enhanced when the nurse prompts the person to clarify the description and interpret its meaning.

Use of who, what, where, and when questions helps the person to clarify and expand the content and meaning of what is communicated. Phrases such as "tell me," "go on," "describe to me," "explain it to me," and "give me an example" are also likely to elicit description of important content and to diminish distracting generalizations and abstractions. By seeking feedback, the nurse helps the individual to explain the meaning further. In clarifying, the nurse should avoid threatening, detective-like questions. Questions that begin with "why" often increase the person's anxiety because they demand reasons, conclusions, analysis, or causes (Peplau, 1964). Reformulating questions to obtain data first and then helping the individual to analyze links among events, thoughts, feelings, actions, and outcomes is generally a more helpful approach.

A problem-solving approach by the nurse assists the person to describe and clarify the content and meaning of experience. Sequential steps help the individual to explain events, to change circumstances and responses that interfere with health, and to solve problems (O'Toole & Welt, 1989; Peplau, 1963). This problem-solving approach can be adapted for use in health promotion to assist the person in problem solving by working through the steps outlined in the Health Teaching box. These steps are a useful guideline for keeping the focus of concern on the individual and his or her definition of the problem. Rather than telling the person what is wrong and how to fix it, the nurse's primary goal is helping the person to describe the problem and formulate solutions in partnership.

Use Reflection

Reflection is the restatement of what the individual has said in the same or different words. This technique can involve paraphrasing or summarizing the person's main point to indicate interest and to focus the discussion. Effective use of this approach does not include frequent, parrot-like repetition of the individual's statements. Instead, reflection is the selective paraphrasing or literal repetition of the person's words to underscore the importance of what has been said, to summarize a main concern or theme, or to elicit elaborated information. In addition, to verify understanding of health information, the nurse can ask the person to restate what has been communicated. Failure to confirm understanding interferes with desired clinical care outcomes. For example, Penney and Wellard (2007) identified failures in communication, including lack of comprehension of information from providers, as a barrier to older consumers' participation in their care.

Use Constructive Confrontation

Confronting an individual means that the nurse points out a specific behavior and then helps the person to examine the meaning or consequences of the behavior. For example:

> *Nurse:* "You missed your appointment for the consultation we had scheduled."
> *Individual:* "Oh, I didn't notice the date."

> *Nurse:* "You are usually very aware of time and appointments. What do you think was going on with you that you didn't notice the date this time?"

This type of confrontation is not an angry exchange, but a purposeful way of helping the person examine personal actions and their meaning.

Use Nouns and Pronouns Correctly

Some individuals have difficulty separating themselves from others or specifying the object or subject in their language. These individuals misuse pronouns by referring to we, us, they, she, he, him, and her, without clearly identifying the referent, and by making vague statements such as "They don't like me. They told me I was useless." Others may use general nouns, such as everyone, people, doctors, and nurses, to avoid clear communication about specific persons. The nurse can clarify by asking, "Who are they?" or "To whom are you referring?" Additionally, the nurse must be careful to use separate pronouns when speaking of herself or himself and the individual, particularly when the person has disordered thinking. For example, when communicating with an individual who is confused or exhibits disordered thinking, the nurse should say you and I, rather than us or we, to promote clear thinking and communication and to assist the individual to maintain personal boundaries (Peplau, 1963).

Use Silence

Allowing a thoughtful silence at intervals helps the individual to talk at his or her own pace without pressure to perform for the nurse. Silence also permits time for reflection. Particularly helpful to the depressed or physically ill person, silence can reduce pressure and conserve energy. After several moments, the nurse can ask the

---

HEALTH TEACHING   Steps in Promoting Problem Solving

Describe the experience or event of concern.
Helpful Verbal Nursing Strategies: "Tell me what happened." "Describe the experience to me."
Analyze the parts of the experience and see relationships to other events.
Helpful Verbal Nursing Strategies: "What meaning does this have for you?" "What pattern is there?"
Formulate the problem.
Helpful Verbal Nursing Strategies: "In what way is this problematic?" "What do you want to see changed?"
Validate the formulation.
Helpful Verbal Nursing Strategies: "Do you mean … ?" "Let me tell you what I understand you to be saying."

Use the formulation to identify ways to solve or manage the difficulty.
Helpful Verbal Nursing Strategies: "What would you do the next time?" "In what way has your view changed?" "What actions are needed to solve the problem that you've identified?"
Try out the solutions, judge the outcomes, and adjust the plan accordingly.
Helpful Nursing Strategies: Encourage application in new situations through role playing or through practice in appropriate settings; help the individual cycle through the above sequence as needed to evaluate the outcome and make adjustments to the plan.

Modified from Peplau, H. E. (1963). Process and concept of learning. In S. Burd & M. Marshall (Eds.), *Some clinical approaches to psychiatric nursing* (pp. 348-352). New York: Macmillan.

person to share some thoughts. For example, "Try putting your thoughts into words," "Tell me what are you thinking or feeling now," or "I'll be here when you feel ready to talk."

Accept Communication

Acceptance of the person's mode of communication is an important ingredient in a helping relationship. Allowing the person to communicate verbally and nonverbally in a personal fashion promotes feelings of safety and respect. Nevertheless, acceptance of communication does not mean that the nurse always agrees with the individual or tolerates inappropriate behavior, such as verbal or physical abuse, within the established limits of the setting. Rather, accepting communication involves effective use of person-centered communication, as described earlier in this chapter. Box 4-4 presents specific strategies associated with person-centered communication.

Barriers to Effective Communication

Barriers to effective communication can originate with the nurse, the individual, or both. The most obvious barrier is the nurse's failure to use the types of therapeutic techniques just described. Lack of knowledge or experience can limit the nurse's ability to assess the individual's needs and repertoire of skills. Supervision and study can help the nurse apply the steps of the nursing process by using effective intervention approaches.

Communication is also ineffective when some part of the communication-feedback loop breaks down. Failure to send a clear message, receive and interpret the message correctly, or provide useful feedback can interfere with communication. Diagnosing the source of the communication breakdown, taking steps to correct it, and using knowledge of the communication process and appropriate therapeutic techniques are the nurse's responsibility.

Anxiety

When the nurse or individual is highly anxious during an interaction, perception is altered and the ability to communicate effectively is curtailed sharply. Defense mechanisms, such as denial, projection, and displacement, reduce anxiety but block understanding of the true meaning of an interaction. Severe anxiety and defense mechanisms distort reality and lead to disordered communication. To enhance interpersonal communication, the nurse identifies the feeling of anxiety and its source and uses anxiety-reducing interventions.

Attitudes

Biases and stereotypes can limit the nurse's and individual's ability to relate. When the difficulty is the individual's problem, the nurse can assist by examining those views that interfere with the person's relationships. When the problem is the nurse's, openness in the supervisory relationship to examination of personal behavior is crucial. When the nurse fails to examine his or her attitudes toward the person, negativity may be communicated and perceptions of the interaction may be distorted.

Gaps Between Nurse and Individual

Related to attitudinal barriers, differences in gender, age, socioeconomic background, ethnicity, race, religion, or language can block functional communication between the nurse and individual. These factors can cause differences in perception and block mutual understanding. Newly licensed nurses have attributed communication problems to differences in language proficiency among nurses, including English as a second language, as well as to problems in understanding non–English-speaking individuals (Smith & Crawford, 2004). To reduce such gaps, nurses can question unclear verbal or written communications, seek clarification or assistance from translators, and explore how perceptions may be different and how to clarify meanings (see Multicultural Awareness box and Chapter 2).

Resistance

Resistance comprises all phenomena that inhibit the flow of thoughts, feelings, and memories in an interpersonal encounter and behaviors that interfere with therapeutic goals. Resistance arises from anxiety when a person feels threatened. To reduce this anxiety, the person implements resistant behavior, most often in the form of avoidance, such as being late, changing the subject, forgetting, blocking, or becoming angry.

Initially, the nurse should identify the behavior, whether it is the nurse's or the individual's behavior, and then attempt to interpret it in the context of the interaction. Exploration of possible threats in the relationship, goals, or a particular topic can lead to understanding the source of the resistance and finding the ability to handle these difficulties. Anxiety reduction is often a necessary step in dealing with resistant behavior.

Transference and Countertransference

Transference is reacting to another person in an exchange as though that person were someone from the past. Transference may involve a host of feelings that generally are classified as positive (love, affection, or regard) or negative (anger, dislike, or frustration). Typical transference reactions involve an important figure from the past such as a mother or father; however, at times transference may be more general to include all authority figures. Something about another person's characteristics, behavior, or position, in combination with individual dynamics, triggers this response. People in a therapeutic relationship often develop strong transference feelings toward the helping professional, arising from the interaction's intensity and the care provider's authoritative or nurturing role. To work with a person's transference reactions effectively, the nurse first helps the person to examine feelings and thoughts about the nurse.

MULTICULTURAL AWARENESS

Multicultural Context of Communication

As health care providers, nurses might believe that they have expert knowledge about health promotion and the treatment of illness that will be beneficial to others. Therefore it seems logical that nurses would select appropriate information to share with individuals to help them maintain health and manage illness or alterations in health status. However, consider the possible influences of cultural differences between the nurse and individual.

Much of the knowledge generated from nursing-related disciplines and the sciences is rooted in a Western perspective. Particularly in the United States, knowledge is developed and interpreted from the perspective of the dominant cultural group, a White, Anglo-Saxon, Christian point of view. When this perspective remains unexamined, alternative perspectives are ignored and invisible. Nurses who are members of the dominant cultural group may be well-intentioned, but ineffective, when they attempt to engage a person of a different cultural group in a relationship without questioning how culture influences interactions, interpretations of events and information, and beliefs and values concerning health and health care practices. Preconceived ideas about people based on some characteristic or group affiliation, such as racial or ethnic identity, religion, country of origin, gender, or sexual orientation, can interfere with nurses' abilities to relate to people as individuals. At the same time, a lack of knowledge of other cultural groups hampers nurses' understanding of the individual's point of view.

Guidelines for recognizing the multicultural context of communication in therapeutic relationships include the following:

- Make ethnocultural assessment a critical component of every clinical evaluation.
- Allow other people to define themselves.
- Ask the person, and family as appropriate, about cultural health care practices and traditions.
- Respect cultural practices and traditions while providing opportunity for the person to voice preferences and make choices.
- Respect the language of others and do not assume superiority in language.
- Collaborate with trained translators and health promoters (people with the same ethnic or racial background as the individuals).
- Avoid use of racist, sexist, ageist, and other forms of denigrating language.
- Do not perpetuate stereotypes in communication.
- Adapt communication to the uniqueness of the individual.

- Reject humor that degrades members based on gender, race, ethnicity, religion, sexual orientation, country of origin, and so forth.
- Respect the rights of others to have different practices and customs.
- Do not allow injustice to continue through silence.
- Present information clearly to all people to help them make informed choices.
- Do not judge values, traditions, and practices based on their similarity or difference from personal values, traditions, and practices, but based on whether they facilitate human potential.

The following are some issues for the nurse to consider:

- When the nurse works with a person from a different cultural background, what are common barriers to establishing a therapeutic relationship?
- In learning about different cultural groups, is there a risk of creating new stereotypes that interfere with the ability to treat people as unique individuals?
- If the nurse has little or no knowledge about a person's culture, how can the nurse provide meaningful nursing care?
- Are the two previous questions contradictory? How can the nurse meet the different challenges that they imply?
- Research measurements typically are developed from the perspective of the dominant culture. If the nurse wishes to use a standardized instrument to measure clinical or research variables among members of different cultural groups, then what questions about the instrument should the nurse ask, and what problems might the nurse encounter? What would need to be done to determine whether or not an instrument truly measures the same phenomenon across different populations?
- Consider the possible influences of cultural differences between the nurse and the individual. Think of an example of two people from different cultural groups who developed a relationship. Examine how they got to know each other and what differences and similarities they uncovered. Did barriers to understanding each other exist? If so, how did they bridge these barriers? What did they learn about themselves? What did they learn about the ways that culture shapes perspective and interactions? Think about how a nurse can apply these insights to his or her relationships with people from cultural groups that differ from their own.
- How would a multicultural perspective change the practice?

Guidelines developed by the author and modified from information from Johannesen, R. L. (2002). *Ethics in human communication* (5th ed.). Prospect Heights, IL: Waveland Press; Kikuchi, J. F. (2005). Cultural theories of nursing responsive to human needs and values. *Journal of Nursing Scholarship, 37*, 302-307; Posmontier, B., & Horowitz, J. A. (2004). Postpartum practices and depression prevalences: Technocentric and ethnokinship cultural perspectives. *The Journal of Transcultural Nursing, 15*, 34-43.

Then the nurse assists the person to compare and contrast the nurse with people from person's past to remove distortions and comprehend the present reality.

Countertransference basically is the same phenomenon, but it is experienced by the health care professional rather than the person. The nurse experiences many feelings toward the person; these feelings are not problematic, unless they remain unanalyzed and block the nurse's ability to work effectively with the individual. For example, if a nurse has strong feelings for the person and thinks that the person cannot possibly function after discharge without the nurse's aid, the nurse is likely to distort the person's abilities, encourage a childlike dependency, and interfere with the person's progress. This nurse needs to examine such personal feelings to understand their source. Once understood, countertransference reactions generally cease to interfere with the relationship. Consultation with an advanced practice psychiatric nurse is recommended whenever transference or countertransference reactions are persistent and problematic.

Sensory Barriers

When the individual has sensory limitations, the nurse may need to use extra skill in communicating. Use of the other senses to send or receive messages should be attempted. Special help is often available from trained therapists and teachers; for example, many agencies have access to interpreters for deaf people, and visual aides may be useful. Nurses must be as creative as possible, learn from others who are skilled in alternative forms of communication, and make referrals as necessary.

Failure to Address Concerns or Needs

Failure to meet the individual's needs or to recognize the individual's concerns is the most serious barrier to effective interaction. This failure can arise from (1) inadequate assessment; (2) lack of knowledge; (3) inability to separate the nurse's needs from the individual's needs; and (4) confusion between friendship and a helping relationship, including unrecognized or unresolved sexual issues. To correct this problem, the nurse should recognize that a barrier to relating with the person exists. Using the supervisory process to determine the problem's source, the nurse should then take corrective action, such as obtaining more information or knowledge, performing a self-assessment with values clarification, and examining reactions, biases, and expectations.

Setting

The setting of a therapeutic interaction can affect the goals and the nature of the communication. The most important aspect of any setting is that the nurse and individual are able to attend to each other. The nurse's attention to the person helps create this atmosphere. The nurse assesses the influence of factors such as lighting, noise, temperature, comfort, physical distance, and privacy; potentially disturbing factors can be altered or controlled within the limits of the setting. Occasionally the nurse has only minimal control over the setting, as in a busy clinic, health center, inpatient unit, or the individual's home. Although far from the ideal of a quiet, pleasant, well-lit private office, these typical clinical settings can be used effectively by creating a sense of private space. Curtains can be drawn, doors shut, and two chairs pulled to a corner to shape an environment for interaction. When possible, however, nurses seek offices or rooms to establish privacy during significant communication or when imparting important or complex health information. The nurse can also acknowledge verbally that some aspect of the environment, such as an interruption or noise, is bothersome. This strategy shows people that the nurse recognizes possible concentration difficulties and is sharing the environment with them.

Stages

Therapeutic relationships follow sequential phases, which may overlap, vary in length, or involve issues that appear over time rather than in a set sequence. Orientation (introductory), working, and termination phases have been identified by researchers and clinicians (Whittemore, 2000).

Originally these **relationship stages** were identified from clinical interactions that developed over a prolonged period of time. However, they can be observed in brief encounters that are effective; that is, interactions that meet individuals' needs rather than therapeutic interactions that have been reduced to little more than quick question-and-answer sessions. Whether the nurse is engaged in a long-term or short-term relationship with an individual, attention to the relationship stages is important. Brief therapeutic relationships will telescope the stages; therefore, it is particularly important that the nurse focus on meeting the key demands of each relationship phase. It is important to note that individuals may move in and out of direct care episodes while a therapeutic relationship is maintained over a longer period. A relationship exists even when the nurse and individual do not see each other for an extended period, and each encounter takes place within the trajectory of the relationship stages.

Orientation or Introductory Phase

The orientation or introductory phase begins when the nurse and individual meet. This meeting typically involves some feeling of anxiety; neither party knows what to expect. When the therapeutic relationship is primarily a counseling type of relationship, part of the nurse's role is to help structure the interaction by discussing several topics during the initial meeting and sometimes during the first few meetings. Box 4-8 lists topics appropriate to this phase. Discussion of these issues establishes a contract or pact and involves a mutual understanding of the parameters of the relationship and an agreement to work together.

The orientation stage is a critical juncture in any therapeutic relationship. Without successful transition through the orientation phase, no working alliance will exist and treatment goals will remain unmet. Establishing a connection during the orientation phase is facilitated by consistency, sensitive pacing of communication, active listening, conveying concern and warmth, and attention to comfort and control. In contrast, factors that hamper relationships include inconsistency, unavailability, individual factors associated with trust, nurses' feelings about the other person, confrontation of delusions or strongly held views, and unrealistic expectations.

Box **4-8** **Key Topics of Discussion During the Orientation or Introductory Phase of the Therapeutic Relationship**

- What to call each other
- Purpose of meeting
- Location, time, and length of meetings
- Termination date or time for review of progress through follow-up
- Confidentiality (with whom clinical data will be shared)
- Any other limits related to the particular setting

Box **4-9** **Interventions for Use During the Termination Phase of the Therapeutic Relationship**

1. Let the person know why the relationship is to be terminated.
2. Remind the person of the date and how many meetings or appointments are left.
3. Collaborate with other staff so that they are aware of how the person is reacting and any special needs that the person may have.
4. Help the person to identify sources of support and other people with whom a relationship is possible.
5. Review the gains and the remaining goals.
6. Discuss the pros and cons experienced during the relationship to help the person to develop a realistic appraisal.
7. Make referrals for follow-up care as needed.

When the therapeutic relationship is not structured primarily as counseling with a specific number of sessions, the orientation phase may appear less distinct and the topics noted may seem irrelevant. In this case, the nurse can adapt the suggested topics to meet the specific situation. However, except in true emergencies, initial encounters should always include introductions by name, discussion of the purpose, and a plan for ongoing care or specific follow-up.

Working Phase

The working phase of the therapeutic relationship emerges when the nurse and the individual collaborate as partners in promoting the person's health. The working phase may last for an established number of sessions, as in brief psychotherapy, or it may extend over a longer period if the nurse is the primary care provider for an individual or family. During the working phase, the relationship is the context through which change takes place. Goals are set, and the nurse and individual work mutually toward their accomplishment. Interventions are tailored to the specific situation and health needs of the person and family. Solving problems, coping with stressors, and gaining insight are all part of the working phase. The nurse and individual recognize each other's uniqueness. Yamashita et al. (2005) identified trust as the first step in establishing a working relationship. Moreover, these researchers found that the long-term involvement characteristic of successful case management requires realistic expectations and efforts to find flexible ways to persevere over time.

Resistant behaviors may be observed during this phase as the nurse and individual become closer and work on potentially anxiety-producing problems. The person may pull away through the use of defense mechanisms because change can be difficult. Overcoming the resistance becomes an important nursing task.

Termination Phase

Termination marks the end of the relationship established in the therapeutic contract or negotiated in accordance with the limits of the contract. Ending a relationship can cause anxiety for both the individual and the nurse. Termination represents a loss; therefore, it can trigger feelings of sadness, frustration, and anger. Termination in this case is the loss of a relationship and the loss of future involvement, with its attendant realistic expectations or fantasies. Termination also reawakens feelings of previously unresolved losses, such as a death or divorce.

Working through any feelings related to termination is an important part of clinical care. Some individuals require the nurse's assistance to experience the feelings of loss and to connect present reactions to past real or symbolic losses. Box 4-9 lists additional interventions for use during the termination phase.

Both the nurse and the individual can learn much during termination; the process directs both participants to examine problems and progress in the relationship, feelings, and reactions. The experience also helps the nurse and individual gain practice in ending relationships and in exploring reactions, which can be most helpful when future losses occur.

Brief Interactions

Time constraints in practice are unavoidable. Although challenging, brief therapeutic encounters can be meaningful and useful. Limited time is not a valid reason to avoid interviewing or interacting with individuals. Rather, nurses purposefully can structure brief interactions to achieve specific clinical outcomes (Wright & Leahey, 2005). Box 4-10 delineates key ingredients for a **15-minute interview** with a family.

These guidelines for brief interactions with families can be adapted for interviews with individuals. An effective 15-minute interview is feasible if nurses plan to introduce themselves, state the purpose of meeting, validate understanding with the person or family, clarify such parameters as time, focus and listen, and elicit significant individual and family data. Most important, the goal of the interaction must be realistic and clearly defined. For example, the purpose may be to elicit a family's view of the problem

Box 4-10   Key Ingredients for a 15-Minute Family Interview

1. Use manners to engage or reengage. Make an introduction by offering your name and role. Orient family members to the purpose of a brief family interview.
2. Assess significant areas of internal and external structure and function (obtain information from genogram concerning basic family composition and external support data).
3. Ask family members three key questions.
4. Commend the family on one or two strengths.
5. Evaluate usefulness and conclude.

for which the person has sought care or to prioritize problems to be treated. Even when time is limited, the interview is structured to provide an opportunity for the person or family to engage in dialogue as an active participant in care, and the nurse's attention is completely focused on the individual.

Circumstances also can dictate the need for immediate and instructive communications that command specific actions. For example, during a crisis directive clear communication is paramount. Rogers and Lawhorn (2007) demonstrated the importance of preparedness and communication strategies during disaster-related events. Planning in anticipation of human-caused and natural disasters is critical in order to have functional communications systems in place. Such systems increasingly will employ various methods of telecommunication. After tragic events including shootings on college campuses, efforts to communicate more effectively are paramount. Universities, for example, have responded by instituting systems to communicate rapidly with a large campus community. Widely deployed strategies feature instant text messaging and emailing (see Hot Topics box).

Health Literacy

Clear communication improves the quality of health care encounters. **Health literacy**, the capacity to read, comprehend, and follow through on health information, is a critical component of health promotion. Yet, nearly half of American adults do not understand basic health information (Ask me 3. Good questions for your good health, n.d.; Ask me 3. IOM report on health literacy, n.d.; Ask me 3. Tips for clear health communication, n.d.; Health care coalition promotes clear communication, 2004). To

combat low health literacy, nurses can encourage individuals to ask three essential questions at every health visit:

"What is my main problem?"

"What do I need to do?"

"Why is it important for me to do this?" (Ask me 3. Good questions for your good health, n.d.).

Nurses also promote health literacy by creating a safe and comfortable environment, sitting down to establish eye contact rather than standing when communicating, using visual aids and models to illustrate conditions and procedures, and verifying understanding of care instructions by having individuals teach the content back (Health care coalition promotes clear communication, 2004). In the emerging age of telehealth, developing strategies for confirming understanding and individualizing methods of communicating health information is critically important (see the Hot Topics box). The Case Study at the end of this chapter presents a detailed scenario of a home visit and questions related to how the nurse can develop a therapeutic relationship with the person. The Care Plan at the end of this chapter presents a plan of care for the person, including communication interventions.

SUMMARY

Relating to persons offers many challenges and rewards for nurses. Although some aspects of this work are predictable, each person and family is unique and provides a chance for the nurse to learn, grow, and help in new ways. This chapter provides guidelines for developing therapeutic relationships, but these guidelines do not guarantee success or an easy job. The desire and skill of the individual nurse bring this information to life. The blend of the nurse's artistry, humanity, knowledge, skill, and ethics sparks concern and the ability to help another human being communicate effectively—essential components of the nurse-person relationship.

The therapeutic relationship is the primary arena for health promotion. Values clarification, communication, and the helping relationship are its core components. For nurses applying this knowledge to their varied roles is essential to promoting health and providing quality care.

Rising use of technology and mounting pressures for cost-effective care are here to stay. In this climate, the importance of the therapeutic relationship is underscored (see Hot Topics box). Without a relational context, the care dimension in health care is lost, and health promotion is reduced to standardized, recipe-like prescriptions. Effective health promotion directed to the needs of individuals, families, and communities requires reflection on the value of caring, effective communication, and a helping relationship.

CASE STUDY

A Health-Promotion Visit: Maria Sanchez-Smith

As part of a health-promotion visit for Maria Sanchez-Smith and Thomas, her 2-week-old infant, Jessica Mills, a registered nurse, planned to conduct an infant assessment, provide breast-feeding support, teach about normal infant development and care activities, and assess Mrs. Sanchez-Smith's adaptation to motherhood and her postpartum recovery status. Before the visit, Ms. Mills reviewed the clinical information she obtained during Mrs. Sanchez-Smith's hospitalization. Mrs. Sanchez-Smith is a 34-year-old Hispanic, primiparous woman who delivered a 7-pound, 10-ounce healthy boy after a 12-hour labor. The labor had progressed well without complication. Mrs. Sanchez-Smith received epidural anesthesia at 6-cm dilation and the baby was delivered vaginally. Her husband, Mark Smith, provided labor support and was present for the delivery. After a 2-day hospital stay, Mrs. Sanchez-Smith was discharged. At discharge, the infant was breast-feeding, had normal newborn examination findings, and weighed 7 pounds, 5 ounces. Ms. Mills had been impressed by both parents' preparation for the birth. They had attended childbirth classes and read several books about infant development and parenting. Mrs. Sanchez-Smith planned to take an 8-week maternity leave from her position as a lawyer in a large practice and had arranged for a childcare provider to come to the family's home to take care of the infant beginning 2 weeks before the end of her maternity leave. Mr. Smith had not planned to take time off from his job, because he had recently been promoted to a high-level managerial position in his company that required increased travel and time at work. He was able to postpone a business trip to be present at the delivery and had sent a plane ticket to his mother-in-law so she could come and stay at their home during the first week after Mrs. Sanchez-Smith and Thomas were discharged from the hospital.

During the visit, Ms. Mills first assessed the infant. She incorporated teaching concerning normal infant development and concluded that Thomas was a healthy 2-week-old infant who was feeding well. Thomas' circumcision was healing without complication and he had regained his birth weight.

When Ms. Mills asked how Mrs. Sanchez-Smith was doing, Mrs. Sanchez-Smith hesitated and then responded, "I'm not sure. I'm very glad that Thomas is doing well ... but I worry sometimes that I'm not going to be able to do everything right for him. It's funny, but I've spent so many years getting an education and establishing my law career. It was hard work, but I managed to do well. Now a little infant overwhelms me. I don't know how I'll manage this." When Ms. Mills asked Mrs. Sanchez-Smith to talk more about her concerns, Mrs. Sanchez-Smith described how incompetent she felt while her mother was staying with her. "My mother could do everything so easily. I fumbled with every diaper. It felt like she criticized how I did things. When she told me about what she did when she had children, I felt pushed to do things 'her way' and not the way that I had planned. She even wanted to give him a bottle when I was trying so hard to get breast-feeding going. At least the doctor said Thomas had gained enough weight. Thomas' weight gain made me feel like I wasn't a total failure. I couldn't wait for her to go, but I fell apart after she left. I was alone. Mark is out of town until the weekend, and I couldn't get Thomas to stop crying yesterday. I thought I would scream so I put him down in his crib and I just sat there crying. What's wrong with me? I've never felt so out of control before. I want to be a good mother, but I feel like I can't give any more right now."

In response to Ms. Mills' follow-up questions about mental status, Mrs. Sanchez-Smith described frequently feeling irritated and sad, crying a few times over the last several days, difficulty sleeping even when the baby was asleep, feeling fatigued, and being worried about how she would be able to go back to work in only a few weeks. Ms. Mills also inquired about the family's cultural, ethnic, and religious backgrounds. Mrs. Sanchez-Smith responded, "Interesting that you should ask. That's actually another issue right now. I'm from New Mexico and my family is Hispanic and Catholic, but I'm not a practicing Catholic now. You might guess that I'm Latina from my hyphenated name. I added my maiden name to Smith when I got married to honor my family. Mark is Protestant, but not really religious. His family comes from New Jersey. They are very nice and were supportive when we got married. We were lucky that our families accepted us together. I have to admit, though, that we didn't really figure out what we would do about raising the baby. Mark thinks that we'd be hypocrites to have a Catholic christening. Plus my mother told me that I'd be selfish to go back to work so soon. Can you help me? I feel like I'm going out of my mind and I don't know what to do."

This case study raises a variety of clinical concerns. As the nurse in this encounter, Ms. Mills could begin by considering the following questions.

Reflective Questions:

1. What are my feelings as I listen to her story and her distress? Am I aware of how my values and expectations affect my interaction with this person? How can I establish a therapeutic relationship to support Mrs. Sanchez-Smith during this stressful period?
2. What is the significance of the distress symptoms that Mrs. Sanchez-Smith reported? Given that the period during which many women experience postpartum blues has passed, what is the most appropriate action to obtain a thorough mental status examination for postpartum depression?
3. Who is the most appropriate health care provider to evaluate her for postpartum depression, and treat her if it is confirmed? How can I facilitate getting her the care she needs and can I remain available to her? How can I assist Mrs. Sanchez-Smith to meet the infant's developmental needs during this stressful period?
4. In what ways do family dynamics, values, and expectations related to differing cultural and religious heritages contribute to the problems described? What can I do to explore these issues further? What strengths can be harnessed? How can I engage support systems to ameliorate rather than exacerbate the difficulties? What can be done to engage both Mr. Smith and Mrs. Sanchez-Smith in a therapeutic relationship to focus on the couple and parenting concerns, and to involve both partners in treatment strategies?

CARE PLAN

Transition to Parenthood: Maria Sanchez-Smith

Nursing Diagnosis: Potential for Alteration in parenting related to stress involved in transition to parenthood

DEFINING CHARACTERISTICS

- Feeling overwhelmed with responsibilities of new parenthood
- Insecurity about tasks of infant care
- Crying
- Sadness
- Feeling out of control
- Difficulty sleeping even when the baby is asleep
- Worry about going back to work soon

RELATED FACTORS

- Transition from high career achievement to new role as mother
- Differing religious, ethnic, and cultural backgrounds of the two parents and extended families
- Confusion and lack of decisions about religious and cultural traditions to follow for their infant
- Conflicting expectations of extended families, particularly from Mrs. Sanchez-Smith's mother
- Job pressures on Mr. Smith to travel and be away from home
- Unanticipated social isolation for Mrs. Sanchez-Smith during this postpartum period
- Limited social support (particularly from husband due to work-associated travel)

INTERVENTIONS

- Health information is provided about normal newborn and postpartum adjustment.
- Infant care information is provided based on Mrs. Sanchez-Smith's needs.
- Expectations about postpartum adjustment and parenthood are elicited.
- Health information about postpartum depression is provided regarding prevalence and common symptoms.
- Personal and family history is conducted, with a focus on mental health.
- Postpartum depression is evaluated using interview questions and an assessment measure, such as the Edinburgh Postnatal Depression Scale (Cox, Holden, & Sagovsky, 1987), or the Postpartum Depression Screening Scale (Beck & Gable, 2001).
- If symptom levels suggest postpartum depression, a referral for mental health evaluation is made.
- Sources of social support are solicited and specific plans are made to use available support, such as husband, friends, and hired infant care providers.
- Conflicts and areas of shared values, plans, goals for raising the baby are explored.
- Pros and cons of options for raising the baby are examined in relation to religious, ethnic, and cultural considerations.
- A follow-up plan is made to reassess symptoms of postpartum depression and to discuss ongoing concerns about how to raise the baby with Mrs. Sanchez-Smith and Mr. Smith.
- Referral is made to local support and psychoeducational programs for interfaith couples.

EXPECTED OUTCOMES

- Competent mothering and infant care are displayed.
- Mrs. Sanchez-Smith describes her feelings, concerns, and needs.
- Indicators of postpartum depression are evaluated and referral for follow-up made for positive findings.
- Social supports are engaged.
- Mrs. Sanchez-Smith and Mr. Smith successfully negotiate immediate decisions about religious and cultural practice concerning their baby and agree to use counseling services to work out decisions concerning their child's upbringing and involvement of extended family.

REFERENCES

Ask me 3. Good questions for your good health. (n.d.). Retrieved October 11, 2007, from *http://askmethree.org/for_patients.asp*.

Ask me 3. IOM report on health literacy. (n.d.). Retrieved October 11, 2007, from *http://askmethree.org/*.

Ask me 3. Tips for clear health communication. (n.d.). Retrieved October 11, 2007, from *http://askmethree.org/tips.asp*.

Beck, C. T., & Gable, R. K. (2001). *Postpartum depression screening scale.* Los Angeles, CA: Western Psychological Services.

Blondis, M. N., & Jackson, B. E. (1982). *Nonverbal communication with patients: Back to the human touch* (2nd ed.). New York: John Wiley & Sons.

Brown, B. V. (2008). *Key indicators of child and youth well-being: Completing the picture.* New York, NY: Lawrence Erlbaum Associates.

Coons, C. A., & Carpenedo, D. J. (2007). Research on telehealth in home care: Adoption and models of care. *Home Health Care Nurse, 25,* 477–481.

Coopersmith, S. (1967). *The antecedents of self-esteem.* San Francisco: W. H. Freeman.

Cox, J. L., Holden, J. M., & Sagovsky, R. (1987). Detection of postnatal depression: Development of the 10-item Edinburgh Postnatal Depression Scale. *British Journal of Psychiatry, 150,* 782–786.

Crofts, L. (2006). Learning form critical case reviews: Emergent themes and their impact on practice. *Intensive and Critical Care Nursing, 22*(6), 362–369.

Douglass, J. L., Sowell, R. L., & Phillips, K. D. (2003). Using Peplau's theory to examine the psychosocial factors associated with HIV-infected women's difficulty in taking their medications. *The Journal of Theory Construction & Testing 7,* 10–17.

Finch, L. P. (2005). Nurses' communication with patients: Examining relational communication dimensions and relationship satisfaction. *International Journal for Human Caring, 9,* 14–23.

Finch, L. P. (2006). Patients' communication with nurses: Relational communication and preferred nurse behaviors. *International Journal for Human Caring, 10,* 14–22.

Hall, E. (1973). *The silent language.* Garden City, NY: Doubleday/Anchor Press.

Health care coalition promotes clear communication: Patients encouraged to ask "Ask me 3." (2004, July/Aug.). *Clinician News, 4.*

Johannesen, R. L. (2002). *Ethics in human communication.* (5th ed.). Prospect Heights, IL: Waveland Press.

Jourard, S. (1971). *The transparent self* (Rev. ed.). New York: Van Nostrand Reinhold.

Kasch, C. R. (1986). Toward a theory of nursing action: Skills and competency in nurse-patient interaction. *Nursing Research, 35*(4), 226–230.

Kikuchi, J. F. (2005). Cultural theories of nursing responsive to human needs and values. *Journal of Nursing Scholarship, 37*(4), 302–307.

Luft, J. (1969). *Of human interaction.* Palo Alto, CA: National Press Books.

Luft, J. (1984). *Group processes: An introduction to group dynamics* (3rd ed.). Palo Alto, CA: Mayfield.

McCabe, C. (2004). Nurse-patient communication: An exploration of patients' experiences. *Journal of Clinical Nursing, 13*(1), 41–49.

Moore, S. M., & Primm, T. (2007). Designing and testing telehealth interventions to improve outcomes for cardiovascular patients. *Journal of Cardiovascular Nursing, 22*(1), 43–50.

Moyle, W. (2003). Nurse-patient relationship: A dichotomy of expectations. *International Journal of Mental Health Nursing, 12*(2), 103–109.

O'Toole, A., & Welt, S. R. (1989). *Interpersonal theory in nursing practice.* New York: Springer.

Penney, W., & Wellard, S. J. (2007). Hearing what older consumers say about participation in their care. *International Journal of Nursing Practice, 13*(1), 61–68.

Peplau, H. E. (1963). Process and concept of learning. In S. Burd, M. Marshall (Eds.), *Some clinical approaches to psychiatric nursing* (pp. 348–352). New York: Macmillan.

Peplau, H. E. (1964). *Basic principles of patient counseling.* (2nd ed.). Philadelphia: Smith Kline and French Laboratories.

Peplau, H. E. (1969). Professional closeness: As a special kind of involvement with a patient, client, or family group. *Nursing Forum, 8*(4), 342–360.

Peplau, H. E. (1991). *Interpersonal relations in nursing.* New York: Springer.

Posmontier, B., & Horowitz, J. A. (2004). Postpartum practices and depression prevalences: technocentric and ethno-kinship cultural perspectives. *The Journal of Transcultural Nursing, 15*, 34–43.

Raths, L., Harmin, M., & Simon, S. (1978). *Values and teaching.* Columbus, OH: Charles E. Merrill.

Rogers, B., & Lawhorn, E. (2007). Disaster preparedness: Occupational and environmental health professionals' response to hurricanes Katrina and Rita. *AAOHN Journal, 55*(5), 197–207.

Rogers, C. (1965). *Client-centered therapy.* Boston: Houghton Mifflin.

Roth-Herbst, J., Borbely, C. J., & Brooks-Gunn, J. (2008). Developing indicators of confidence, character, and caring in adolescents. In B. V. Brown (Ed.), *Key indicators of child and youth well-being: Completing the picture* (pp. 167–196). New York, NY: Lawrence Erlbaum Associates.

Ruesch, J., & Bateson, G. (1987). *Communication: The social matrix of psychiatry.* New York: W. W. Norton.

Sears, R. R. (1970). Relation of early socialization experiences to self-concepts and gender role in middle childhood. *Child Development, 41*, 267–289.

Smith, J., & Crawford, L. (2004). Issues in communication for newly licensed nurses. *JONA's Healthcare Law, Ethics, and Regulation, 6*(1), 15–16.

Stuart, G. W., & Laraia, M. T. (2005). *Principles and practices of psychiatric nursing.* (8th ed.). St. Louis, MO: Elsevier Mosby.

Sullivan, H. S. (1953). *The interpersonal theory of psychiatry.* New York: W. W. Norton.

Taylor, B. J. (2004). Improving communication through practical reflection. *Reflections on Nursing Leadership, 3*(2), 28–29, 38.

U.S. Department of Health and Human Services. (n.d.). *Healthy People 2010. What are the leading health indicators?* Retrieved October 5, 2007, from *www.healthypeople.gov/LHI/lhiwhat.htm.*

U.S. Department of Health and Human Services, Health Resources and Services Administration (n.d.). *Telehealth.* Retrieved Oct. 9, 2007, from *www.hrsa.gov/telehealth/.*

U.S. Department of Health and Human Services. (2000). *Healthy People 2010: Understanding and improving health.* (2nd ed.). Washington, D.C: U.S. Government Printing Office.

Watzlawick, P., Beavin, J. H., & Jackson, D. D. (1967). *Pragmatics of human communication: A study of interactional patterns, pathologies and paradoxes.* New York: W. W. Norton.

Welch, M. (2005). Pivotal moments in the therapeutic relationship. *International Journal of Mental Health Nursing, 14*(3), 161–165.

Whittemore, R. (2000). Consequences of not "knowing the patient". *Clinical Specialist, 14*(2), 75–81.

Winters, J. M., & Winters, J. M. (2007). Videoconferencing and telehealth technologies can provide a reliable approach to remote assessment and teaching without compromising quality. *Journal of Cardiovascular Nursing, 22*, 51–57.

Wright, L. M., & Leahey, M. (2005). *Nurses and families: A guide to family assessment and intervention.* (4th ed.). Philadelphia: F. A. Davis.

Yamashita, M., Forchuk, C., & Mound, B. (2005). Nurse case management: Negotiating care together within a developing relationship. *Perspectives in Psychiatric Care, 41*(2), 62–70.

Chapter 5

Pamela Grace
Carol Lynn Mandle

Ethical Issues Relevant to Health Promotion

objectives

After completing this chapter, the reader will be able to:

- Discuss the nature and purposes of health care ethics.
- Evaluate the responsibilities of health care professionals (the development and the role of professional codes of ethics, advocacy, political activity, preserving professional integrity).
- Relate the ethical responsibilities of health care professionals to health promotion.
- Contrast the tensions between promoting the health of individuals and that of society.
- Evaluate salient theoretical approaches to ethical problem solving.
- Apply ethical perspectives and principles to health-promotion practice throughout the life span.
- Describe contemporary ethical issues in health promotion (genetics, culture, end-of-life decision-making).
- Analyze problems related to health promotion using an ethical decision-making framework.

key terms

Advocacy	Ethical issues	Moral predictability or certainty
Applied ethics	Ethics	Nonmaleficence
Autonomy	Feminist ethics	Normative theories
Beliefs	Genetic counseling	Paternalism
Beneficence	Informed consent	Preventive ethics
Civil liberties	Justice	Privacy Rule
Codes of ethics	Malfeasance	Self-determination
Confidentiality	Metaethics	Social justice
Consent	Models of ethical care	Trust
Consequentialist	Cultural	Utilitarian theories
Descriptive theories	Feminist	Value theories
Dilemmas	Humanistic	Veracity
Duty-based theories	Moral	
Ethical dilemmas	Moral philosophy	

website materials

evolve These materials are located on the book's website at *http://evolve.elsevier.com/Edelman/*.
- WebLinks
- Study Questions
- Glossary

The Juvenile Interpreter

A Hastings Center Report by Levine, Glajchen, & Cournos (2004) presents the case of a middle-aged Chinese immigrant, Mr. C., who after an emergency admission for chest pain is diagnosed with end-stage heart disease. Neither Mr. C. nor his wife is very fluent in English and the couple's eldest daughter, a 15-year-old girl, is most often relied on to translate for them because an interpreter is not always readily available. Commenting on the case, Myra Glajchen notes that "the U.S. Office of Civil Rights has stated that every Medicare or Medicaid provider must provide language assistance" (p. 11) as needed. This, although a worthy ideal, is often difficult to accomplish because of the multicultural nature of our contemporary society and the diversity of languages spoken. With increasing frequency, health care providers are faced with the problem of assessing the degree to which an interpreter has translated accurately (in either direction) information and thus the extent to which the client is able to make informed decisions.

1. What are the ethical issues associated with asking a minor to translate and impart sensitive, complex, and serious information?
   - From the perspective of the child
   - From the client's perspective
   - From the health care provider perspective
   - From society's perspective
2. What alternatives are possible?
3. What related health care policies should be formulated or supported by health-promotion professionals?

HEALTH PROMOTION AS A MORAL ENDEAVOR

Human health promotion is a moral endeavor. It involves both a critique of arrangements that facilitate or obstruct the well-being of a society overall and of activities that promote, protect, and support health for the individual members of a society. Health is considered a human good because it allows people to live well and achieve their goals. At the level of the individual, health promotion involves providing services that help humans function as well as possible given their particular circumstances. Understanding the contexts of people's lives is crucial to health-promotion endeavors. This entails consideration of a variety of influences on a person's health status such as mental, physical, spiritual, and environmental factors, as well as the person's relationships with others (social factors) (Resnik, 2007). Viewing health promotion as a moral endeavor—some would even call it a moral imperative (Marks & Shive, 2007)—is consistent with the intent and goals of the U.S. government's prevention agenda for the nation as laid out in *Healthy People 2010* (2000, 2005). See *www.healthypeople.gov.*

The two overarching goals of *Healthy People 2010* are:
1. Increase quality and years of healthy life
2. Eliminate health disparities

The purpose of health-promotion efforts, as discussed throughout this book, is to ensure that people have, or have access to, the tools and strategies to live at the highest level of well-being possible. Health-promotion efforts address environmental obstacles to human health, such as pollution, advertising campaigns for harmful products, and economic disparities. Thus health promotion is not the province of a single discipline but involves the collaboration of all professional groups that have the pertinent knowledge and skills to enable or protect health within a society (Parker et al., 2007).

This chapter focuses on understanding the health professional's moral responsibilities toward individuals and society with regard to facilitating health, well-being, or the relief of suffering. Professional responsibilities are obligations incurred by disciplines that provide a service to society.

For example, the American Nurses Association's (ANA, 2001, 2008) Code of Ethics for Nurses with Interpretive Statements (see Box 5-3 later in the chapter) promises that "nursing encompasses the prevention of illness, the alleviation of suffering, and the protection, promotion, and restoration of health in the care of individuals, families, groups and communities" (p. 5). This document, along with the ANA's Nursing's Social Policy Statement (ANA, 2003), an excerpt of which is presented later in the chapter in Box 5-2, lays out the ethical responsibilities of U.S. nurses. The WebLinks for this chapter on the book's Evolve site include a link to the ANA Code of Ethics. The International Council of Nurses (2000) also has a code of ethics, which serves as a standard for nurses worldwide and is easily accessible via the Internet.

Health-promotion ethics is best viewed as a subset of health care ethics that, in turn, has its roots in moral philosophy and value theory. This section of the book discusses the requirements of, as well as obstacles to, health promotion across the life span and in contemporary health care settings. To facilitate this, the development, scope, and limits of ethical theories and perspectives are explored in relation to problem recognition and resolution.

A basic assumption of this chapter is that the anticipation and prevention of ethical problems is a critical component of ethical professional action. Preventive ethics is introduced later in the chapter (see Box 5-4). To illustrate this exploration of ethical issues in health promotion, a variety of real and hypothetical cases are presented. Strategies to aid the health care professional in identifying, anticipating, and addressing ethical issues are provided throughout.

The terms *ethical* and *moral* are used interchangeably throughout the chapter. Although some commentators have distinguished the two concepts from each other, they have the same root meanings. The term ethics is "derived from the Greek ethos . . . meaning customs . . . conduct and character" (Davis et al., 1997, p. 1). The term **moral** is derived from Latin mores and originally meant "to do with custom or habit" (Davis et al., 1997, p. 1).

HEALTH CARE ETHICS
Origins of Applied Ethics in Moral Philosophy

The discipline underlying practice, (or applied) **ethics**, is moral philosophy. **Moral philosophy** is concerned with discovering or proposing what is right or wrong, or good or bad, in human action toward other humans and other entities such as animals and the environment. Singer (1993) confirms that the crucial practical questions of moral philosophy are "What ought I to do? How ought I to live?" (p. vii). Among the tasks of moral philosophy is that of formulating theories or frameworks to guide action. Using a moral theory to propose and implement appropriate actions in troubling situations will most consistently result in good action or the avoidance of harmful actions.

The theories that emerge as a result of philosophical inquiry about good action are called **value theories** because they are concerned either with discovering what humans seem to value (descriptive theories) or proposing what they ought to value (normative theories) given some presupposed philosophy about the nature or purpose of being human, or in order to achieve predetermined goals. What is often called the golden rule is a classic example of a normative principle. The golden rule essentially commits us to treating other people in the manner that we, ourselves, would wish to be treated given similar circumstances. For example, if I were lost in a strange city I would expect that a knowledgeable person would give me directions if asked because I would willingly assist someone who was lost in my city. Normative theories permit judgments about the value of actions based on the extent to which these actions are consistent with the assumptions of the theory.

Types of Ethics
Descriptive Value Theories

These theories are based on observations of human behavior over time and in a variety of settings. **Descriptive theories** do not tell us what actions we ought to take. They are not directive; they merely tell us how people act toward each other and their environments, what they seem to believe are good or moral actions.

Normative Theories

Normative theories, on the other hand, are concerned with ensuring good actions. They are either reasoned and logically explored explanations of the moral purpose of human interactions, or they are divinely "revealed" truths about good action (religious ethics). Actions that are in accord with the foundational principle or principles of the theory will be right or good actions; they are the types of actions we ought to take given that we believe the principles (e.g., fairness and trust are valid). They are key to decision making

and relevant for health promotion, but often overlooked by policy makers (Bennett & Smith, 2007).

Consequentialism The foundational principle of John Stuart Mill's (1861) utilitarian theory proposes that actions are good insofar as they are aimed at yielding the greatest amount of happiness or pleasure or cause the least amount of harm or pain to people and overall within the society. It is often formulated as the greatest good for the greatest number. Pleasure for Mill was a complex concept; he did not mean unthinking pleasure. He defined pleasure in qualitative as well as quantitative terms. The utilitarian perspective is **consequentialist**: it holds that the consequences or intended consequences of actions matter. Therefore from the consequentialist perspective any decision-making about intended actions or interventions must take into account all knowable potential consequences. Among the implications of this type of theory for health care professionals is the imperative that data gathering must be thorough and complete. Additionally, the professional is accountable for possessing the appropriate skills and knowledge to undertake actions that will promote a good for people. The professional's decision can be evaluated as bad or good to the extent that actions are in accord with the theory: in this case "right actions" would be those that are directed toward promoting the greatest good or causing the least harm. The propositions of the theory direct what is needed for moral action or, stated another way, for doing the right thing.

Duty-Based Theories Other normative value theories are not as heavily weighted toward producing good consequences. For example, **duty-based theories** such as that of Immanuel Kant (1724-1804) and those of various religions (Judaism, Christianity, Islam) depend more on adherence to duties than on good consequences. Individuals are viewed as having certain duties that cannot be circumvented, even if deliberately side-stepping the duty would result in good outcomes. For religions these rules are imparted, in some way, by a divine being.

For Kant, our capacity to reason is what permits moral action. Moral reasoning has been proposed as a model for health promotion (Buchanan, 2006). For example, Kant believed that lying is always wrong even if on some occasions it produces a good outcome. It is wrong because it is irrational to lie. If lying were widely practiced, we would lose our ability to trust what others tell us, and this would make effective communication impossible. Kant based his theory on the idea that what separates us from other life forms is our ability to make rules for ourselves using our ability to reason. His main rule, whereby each of us can determine for ourselves a moral course of action, is the categorical imperative. The categorical imperative was framed several different ways by Kant; however, the easiest to understand for current purposes is the following conceptualization, "I ought never to act except in such a way that I can also will that my maxim should become a universal law" (Kant, 1997/1785, p. 318). This could be stated alternatively as a question to ask oneself before acting, "Could any other person in the same or similar circumstances also take this action or refrain from this action?" A variety of philosophical perspectives, including some contemporary ethical positions, are discussed in more detail later in the chapter in relation to individual cases.

Limitations of Moral Theory

It is important to keep in mind that moral theories arise out of a particular perspective or philosophy about the world. They are conceptualized as a result of this perspective and within a historical and political context. The philosophical approach that evaluates value theories or ethical perspectives for their congruence and usefulness in human decision-making across environments is **metaethics**. Philosophers interested in metaethical questions investigate where our ethical principles come from and what they mean. Are they merely social inventions? Do they involve more than expressions of our individual emotions? Metaethics allows us to critique the adequacy of ethical approaches for application across a variety of practice settings and cultural environments. Other sorts of metaethical questions posed by moral philosophers include: Are there such things as absolute ethical truths? If so, how do we go about discovering these? If not, what foundations should we use to guide our actions? What considerations are important? How do we know which actions are good? What is a valid moral theory? Should human values be congruent across settings and cultures?

For example, religiously based moral theories depend on the idea that good actions are those that obey the laws of a supreme being. However, because the foundational tenets of religions do not mirror each other, what constitutes a moral action from a Jewish perspective may well be morally prohibited from a Roman Catholic perspective (Clarfield et al., 2003). Moreover, even within a religion, the tenets of its different sects or branches may not always lead to the same conclusions about good actions. For such reasons, there are equally strongly held but divergent views on what is the good for humans. Many contemporary philosophers have argued that there can be no single approach that permits the identification or resolution of all moral problems (Rachels & Rachels, 2006; Weston, 2005). Even the golden rule can be problematic from a cross-cultural perspective. For example, I might want to be treated as an autonomous being capable of making my own decisions, but a person from Thailand might be more used to family-centered decision-making. Treating my Thai friend as I would wish to be treated would be a mistake. An understanding of cultural beliefs is necessary for good action in such cases (Multicultural Awareness box).

Additionally, **utilitarian theories** emerged out of a particular era and as a result of perceived injustices in societal arrangements in England during the turmoil of the industrial revolution. Utilitarians such as Jeremy Bentham (1748-1832) and John Stuart Mill (1806-1873) sought frameworks that would permit the rectification of unjust policy deci-

MULTICULTURAL AWARENESS
Self-Reflection

The increasingly multicultural nature of contemporary society and the diversity of languages spoken and values held presents health care providers with complex assessment and planning problems. Nurses and allied professionals are charged with facilitating optimal care for all, regardless of "personal attributes" and taking into account "the needs and values of all persons" (ANA, 2001, Provision 1 and interpretive statements). It is not possible to know details about every culture as well as the unique differences of each individual, family community, and group within each culture. However, there are strategies that a health provider or promoter can employ to ensure that an individual's unique values and particular needs are the focus of interventions. When a particular culture is part of your population base, opportunities exist and should be pursued for learning about that culture. Besides asking the client or knowledgeable others generalities about the particular culture, it is important to discover individual differences in beliefs, values, and needs (as they are for any client). To facilitate your assessment, perhaps the most important undertaking is self-reflection (group reflection can help introduce different "takes" on a situation and increase self-awareness). The following are self-reflection and other considerations for providing culturally sensitive care:

1. Commitment to increasing knowledge and skill in sensitivity to cultural differences
2. Self-awareness and awareness of one's own biases, beliefs, and values. Ask yourself:
   - What values and biases you bring to the relationship
   - How your background has influenced your beliefs
   - What knowledge and experience you have to draw on
   - What values you think you share with the client — validate with the client
   - How comfortable you are with who you are
   - What further information you need to facilitate culturally competent care
   - Who or what is the best resource for further information
3. Awareness of the validity of different beliefs and values
4. Attempts to understand the meaning behind client behavior
5. Increased knowledge of the beliefs and values of other cultures
6. Developing cultural skills through encounters with people from other cultures

sions and the vast economic inequities within their society. For this reason such theories have a tendency to privilege the good of the group over the needs of individuals viewed as individuals.

Therefore it is not prudent to adopt one theory to guide actions in every situation related to health promotion. All moral theories have flaws that, when applied indiscriminately, can lead to actions that are problematic, either for an individual or for a group or for a combination of both. Health-promotion activities mandate not only a general understanding of the nature of the problem or potential problem but

Box **5-1** Genetic Counseling

The genome project was completed by the International Human Genome Sequencing Consortium, led in the United States by the National Human Genome Research Institute and the Department of Energy, on April 14, 2003. This represents an important initial step in expanding our potential to understand the genetic contributors to disease and to formulate interventions. However, there are complex ethical issues associated with, and raised by, genetic advances. For health-promotion professionals, a crucial skill is the ability to refer individuals appropriately to specialized genetic counselors. Although many health care professionals have the skills to counsel clients about genetic testing issues, especially in their fields of expertise, genetic counselors are an increasingly important resource.

Genetic counselors are specially trained master's-prepared individuals. These professionals can obtain certification through the American Board of Genetic Counselors. Their professional society is the National Society of Genetic Counselors. Genetic counselors enter the field from a range of backgrounds including biology, genetics, nursing, psychology, public health, and social work.

The goals of the discipline are outlined in society's Code of Ethics (National Society of Genetic Counselors, 2004). Genetic counselors provide counseling services that are nondirective (Andrews et al., 2002), which means that they avoid coercion or persuasion. Although there is controversy about how directive or nondirective advice should be based on the ethical ideals of autonomy, counselors strive to be nondirective while at the same time tailoring information to fit the specific needs of clients. Andrews and colleagues (2002) note that nondirective methodology is a way for the genetic counseling community to avoid association with the eugenics movement. Because advances in embryo preimplantation genetic testing, as well as in utero fetal testing, permit screening for certain superior characteristics or the screening out of certain genetic diseases, the perceived need to distance the profession from this issue is understandable.

Ethical issues related to genetic counseling for screening purposes that apply both for genetic counselors and other health care providers include:

- Understanding the wider context of genetic testing implications (privacy, discrimination, economics, health insurance denials, implications for family members, anxiety and apprehension, and eugenics [striving for perfection] and its associated implications for individuals and society)
- Assisting people to determine the risks and benefits of screening
- Assisting people to prepare for their future needs
- Assisting people with their procreative planning
- Understanding how cultural differences impact counseling needs
- Addressing societal issues related to genetic advances include determining research priorities, justice issues, and discrimination of the genetically disadvantaged

also knowledge of the values, beliefs, needs, and desires of the person who is the recipient of the efforts in question.

It is true that ethical theories are not helpful in many health-related decision-making situations. However, certain principles, derived from a variety of ethical theories, have proved useful in exploring underlying assumptions because they highlight salient aspects of complex problems. "Principles inherent in a variety of ethical theories do serve as useful tools with which to examine the implications of different proposed courses of action; they permit clarification of hidden issues or facets" (Grace, 2004, p. 299) of situations. However, selection of pertinent principles depends both on the context of the problem and the beliefs and values of the individual or group for which action is needed. These tools (principles derived from a variety of ethical theories), although they facilitate communication between professionals in the interests of people, cannot be used effectively in the absence of contextual considerations, because it is often just these contextual considerations that determine which principles are relevant.

For example, a woman seeks assistance in deciding whether to undergo genetic testing for the breast cancer gene BRCA2 because several members of her immediate and antecedent families have been diagnosed with breast or associated cancers. She tells her nurse practitioner that she is not sure whether it would be beneficial to be tested. The nurse practitioner, in facilitating the woman's health-promotion efforts, understands that she must use clinical judgment to facilitate the woman's autonomous choice. Understanding the requirements of the principle of autonomy is important in helping the woman make her decision. However, it is not sufficient to understand the meaning of autonomy and its limits; we also have to know something about the woman's life, values, beliefs, and relationships in order to provide her with the information and resources necessary for her decision. People are contextual beings; therefore, the choices they make affect not only themselves but also others in their lives, sometimes in profound ways. If the woman is screened and the results found positive for the gene, she not only has to decide her next actions, but the results have implications for family members including any children she has. Box 5-1 presents information on **genetic counseling**. Individual principles of importance to decision-making in health care settings are explored in depth later in the chapter. They, along with associated ethical considerations such as professional, feminist, and virtue ethics, underpin a framework of moral decision-making for health promotion that is offered shortly.

Feminist Ethics and Caring
Feminist Ethics

Feminist perspectives on ethics derive from the feminist movement's efforts to expose and rectify injustices to which women historically have been subjected. Nelson (1992) notes that "feminism raised the consciousness of a whole generation to the male-dominated power structures within American society" (p. 8). Feminist thought is not limited in its influence to the United States; it has also influenced societal changes in most other countries. The feminist movement perspectives have broadened to include problems common to all oppressed groups. **Feminist ethics**, emerging as it has out of feminist thought and feminist philosophy, is not another ethical theory as such; rather it presents a viewpoint on moral problems in health care and other areas of life that have been neglected historically.

Feminist scholars have noted that traditional moral theories, and the principles derived from them, when used in health care settings have been unable to adequately capture the nature and origins of health care problems. Feminist critics assert that moral decision-making must include an investigation of both hidden and overt power relationships implicit in ethical problems. Additionally, the importance of understanding both the contexts of situations and the interrelationships of those involved should not be neglected because human beings are not isolated individuals who may be viewed as totally independent of others. Thus moral decision-making must include the illumination of hidden power imbalances in relationships and situations (Donchin & Purdy, 1999; Tong, 1996; Warren, 2001). This additional criterion for exploring the moral content of health care and health-promotion problems permits the underlying causes of complex problems to be uncovered. Feminist ethics, then, can be thought of as contributing a perspective that is mostly missing from traditional ethical approaches. This changes both the way problems are perceived and the way they are explored.

Characteristics of feminist ethics include the following:

1. Understanding that human beings are inseparable from their relationships with others
2. A "focus on care and responsibility in relationships rather than on the application of abstract principles" (Davis et al., 1997, p. 58)
3. A concern with the development of character and attitudes that result in caring actions reflective of a person who is related to rather than detached from context
4. A concern for the rights and the equality of all individuals that is not limited to the oppression of women

Feminist ethics, then, depending on perspective, allows for a critique of the treatment of individuals in the contexts in which they live. The perspective highlights systematic oppressions due to gender, sexual orientation, ethnicity, socioeconomics, politics, and other characteristics (Thorne & Varcoe, 1998; Tong, 1997; Warren, 2001). For example, a punitive approach to perinatal substance abuse is not associated with improved outcomes for the fetus; in fact, the fetus may be at greater risk because it makes women fearful of accessing health services.

For health promotion the feminist ethic of care is an important concept because it permits a focus on the nature of the health care professional–client relationships and the nature of people as inseparable from contexts of the lives. The concept of care has found increasing acceptance in nursing as both a virtue of the nurse and a responsibility of practice in which treatment is more effectively offered on a common ground basis that will support people within their relationships. Carol Gilligan's (1982) research, among that of others, has been instrumental in the acceptance of the concept of care as informing ethics in nursing practice.

The Ethic of Care

The ethic of care entails a responsibility to attend to the individual as individual in all of his or her complexities. In addition to professional knowledge and skills, it requires certain characteristics and attitudes of the nurse or allied provider. These include a predisposition to engage with and focus on a person as a unique and particular individual. The needs of particular unique individuals are uncovered as the result of a focused attention on that person. Benner et al. (1998) define care as "the alleviation of vulnerability; the promotion of growth and health; the facilitation of comfort, dignity or a good and peaceful death" (p. 233). For Benner and colleagues, an ethic of care requires knowledge and experience and is not solely an emotion in the way that care or caring is understood in everyday life. Many of the current conceptualizations of care, viewed as a responsibility of practice, have their origins in the work of Carol Gilligan.

Carol Gilligan (1982) was a graduate student and then colleague of Lawrence Kohlberg, a developmental psychologist. The main focus of Kohlberg's (1981, 1984) body of work was the nature of moral character development. Kohlberg's developmental theory was informed by Piaget's work on the stages of cognitive development in children. Kohlberg's stages of moral development were derived from longitudinal studies of young men. These moral reasoning studies were designed around the idea that an ability to apply conceptions of justice, rules, and principles to difficult situations denoted the highest achievable level of moral development. Gilligan "challenged the male bias in his [Kohlberg's] work" (Liaschenko & Peter, 2003, p. 35). By studying women's experiences, Gilligan (1982) discovered that they had a moral orientation based on the caring and nurturing of others. In this framework, interrelationships and contexts are important and must be included as particularities important to understanding the complexities of a given situation. One way to look at an ethic of care versus an ethic of justice is that justice demands that we treat people fairly and not regard their incidental differences as important in determining what is required. So justice is impartial and nondiscriminatory. Care, however, requires an understanding of situational particularities; it ensures that we understand a given individual's needs in the context of his or her life. Generally justice and care have been viewed as opposing concepts. Liaschenko (1999) presents a compelling argument for them to be viewed as interrelated concepts. Justice is in the interest of particular individuals. In other words, justice issues concern individuals within a society. What is important about people is that they have individual interests that are protected by just policies.

Fry (1990) has identified three **models of ethical care** in contemporary literature: **cultural**, **feminist**, and **humanistic**. She notes that the humanistic model best captures the essence of care viewed as an aspect of nursing practice. Care as a facet of nursing practice requires that the nurse engage with the person in a way that exposes the meaning and context of the person's needs. This requires an understanding of human relationships as complex webs of interdependencies and interrelationships. A person cannot be removed from this complex web and treated as an isolated entity for the purposes of decision-making; to do so would be to miss the point of nursing judgment and the provision of a good for the person. For example, a focus on pathophysiology is liable to miss nonphysiological aspects of illness or ill health (Grace, 2004). A physiological cure does not necessarily remove the factors that made the person vulnerable. It also requires that the nurse is willing to address those needs from the person's perspective where this is possible. Thus in nursing, care is best defined as an engaged knowing of the person. Benner and colleagues (1998) note that care is "the dominant ethic found in [nurses'] stories of everyday practice" (p. 233).

Limits of the Ethic of Care

One problem with using care as an ethic of health-promotion practice has to do with the issue of **moral predictability or certainty** (Nelson, 1992). If the emphasis is on relationships and there are no criteria for right and wrong action, how can one be assured of the morally correct action in a given situation? An answer to this could be that a morally correct action emerges as a result of nursing judgment based on prior knowledge, experience, and an engaged relationship with the person. Thus the process of the interaction, coupled with the character, knowledge, experience, and intent of the moral agent or carrier, is the crucial factor that achieves the moral good for an individual person as individual. The action is right if the nurse possesses the right characteristics and the person's complex needs are met. (For example, see the five semistructured interviews with hospice nurses based on the ethics of "the caring conversation" inspired by the ethical perspective of Ricoeur [Olthuis et al., 2006].) However, when the solution to one person's problems affects others, the rightness of the action depends on more than the one-on-one caring relationship. The problem remains one of choosing between this person's needs and needs of related others who might be affected by the chosen actions. This problem is resistant to resolution via an ethic of care alone. The problem analysis framework described later includes the ethic of care, among

other considerations. Another criticism is that the care ethic does not permit a moral critique of such things as poor institutional practices or poor interprofessional relationships (Nelson, 1992). Both an ethic of care and principles derived from traditional moral theory may be needed for good health-promotion activities.

The purpose of ethical inquiry in health promotion is to gain clarity on actual or potential moral issues arising in the context of health-promotion endeavors and to understand what is expected of the health-promotion agent viewed as moral agent. Ethical inquiry will not permit the resolution of all problems, mainly because the environments in which health-promotion efforts are conceptualized are incredibly complex. It is impossible to foresee all possible consequences of action, but ethical reasoning can facilitate appropriate and in-depth data gathering, permit the uncovering of hidden agendas and interests, and focus us on the most salient aspects of a particular problem, thus enhancing professional judgment.

Professional judgment and ensuing actions have their impetus in the goal to provide a good for the population of concern. Thus health promotion is a moral endeavor requiring morally sensitive and knowledgeable agents. But what are the scopes and limits of a health care professional's obligations to anticipate, identify, and address morally problematic issues related to the promotion and protection of health for individuals, groups, and society? How do health care professionals balance their duties to individuals with a duty to the society? For example, how are individuals' freedoms (autonomy) balanced with the collective responsibilities owed to society and future generations in not knowingly contributing to preventable harms in vaccinations (Wood-Harper, 2005)? The following section addresses these questions.

PROFESSIONAL RESPONSIBILITY
Accountability to Individuals and Society
Professions

Although this section focuses on the nursing discipline's mandate to promote health, the discussion can also be applied to the responsibilities of allied health professions who assume health-promotion responsibilities. Using the term *profession* to denote the status of nursing and other disciplines is controversial. Indeed, the term is ambiguous. This problem has been more throughly explored by Grace (1998, 2001). Nursing is a profession insofar as it provides a service to society, is self-governing, and its members are accountable for their actions. One important facet of professions, perhaps especially of those that provide crucial services to society is that they have codes of ethics outlining what, in essence, are their promises of service to society (Windt, 1989, p. 7). A significant consequence of professional status is that members can be held accountable for their practice formally by professional licensure boards. More importantly, they are morally accountable for practicing according to their discipline's implicit or explicit code of ethics. Codes of ethics provide a normative framework for professional actions. A professional implicitly accepts these codes on acquiring membership in the discipline. Professionals become members of their professions after completing a period of knowledge and skills acquisition and on commencing practice in the professional role (Peter et al., 2004).

Trust

Service professions such as nursing, medicine, and law are in part defined by their relationships to those in need of services. This relationship is one of **trust**. The professional has the knowledge and skills to meet an individual's needs or the needs of a group. The potential recipient of services lacks the knowledge or ability to anticipate or meet his or her own needs or the needs of the group. Indeed, increasingly the individual or group may not have the option of choosing a health care provider. This, in part, makes health care professional–citizen relationships fiduciary ones. Individuals or groups in the position of having to trust that the professional will keep their best interests as the primary goal and will strive to meet those needs. For example, in the current health care environment in the United States, people may have trouble accessing a specialist provider because of their particular insurance coverage or the inability to afford health care insurance or to pay on their own. Newton (1988) argues that professionals' knowledge puts them in the best position to recognize and anticipate obstacles to optimal provision of service. This is an additional aspect of accountability. Newton (1988) asserts that a profession's members are accountable for practices that: are inadequate at any stage of the rendering of the service; make the client (the ultimate consumer) unhappy; provide shabby products or services even when these make an (uninformed) client happy; or provide the client the best available product but the state of the art is not adequate to the client's real needs (p. 49).

Recognizing Barriers

Therefore, health care professionals are responsible not only for promoting health and healing but for recognizing and addressing barriers to health-promotion activities. Nursing's Social Policy Statement (ANA, 2003) provides a detailed account of the nursing discipline's responsibilities and "expresses the social contract between society and the profession of nursing" (p. 1). An excerpt of this statement is presented in Box 5-2. The following definition of professional nursing includes a warrant to advocate for changes when health care services are threatened.

Nursing is the protection, promotion, and optimization of health and abilities, prevention of illness and injury, alleviation of suffering through the diagnosis and treatment of human responses, and advocacy in the care of individuals, families, communities and populations (ANA, 2003, p. 6).

Box **5-2** Social Policy Statement

EXCERPT: KNOWLEDGE BASE FOR NURSING PRACTICE

The knowledge base for nursing practice includes nursing science, philosophy, and ethics.

Nurses partner with individuals, families, communities, and populations to address such issues as:

- Promotion of health and safety
- Care and self-care processes
- Physical, emotional, and spiritual comfort, discomfort, and pain
- Adaptation to physiological and pathophysiological processes
- Emotions related to experiences of birth, growth and development, health, illness, disease, and death
- Meanings ascribed to health and illness
- Decision-making and ability to make choices
- Relationships, role performance, and change processes within relationships
- Social policies and their effects on the health of individuals, families, and communities
- Health care systems and their relationships with access to and quality of health care
- The environment and the prevention of disease

From American Nurses Association. (2003). *Nursing's social policy statement* (2nd ed.). Silver Spring, MD: Author. Retrieved February 25, 2009, from *http://nursesbooks.org*.

Codes of Ethics

Codes of ethics are examples of normative ethics in that they prescribe how members of a profession ought to act given the goals and purposes of the profession related to individuals and society. In this sense the goals and purposes of the profession serve as foundational ethical principles. The provisions of the code provide direction and express "expectations of ethical behavior" (ANA, 2001, p. 5). They represent the profession's promises to society. "A code of ethics makes explicit the primary goals, values and obligations of the profession" (ANA, 2001, p. 5). The *Code of Ethics for Nurses* (ANA, 2001, 2008) is presented in Box 5-3. Although the public is not directly involved in the formulation of such codes and, indeed, is for the most part not even aware of their existence, the profession is responsive to the evolving needs of a given society. It can be said that codes of ethics are the tentative end results of a discipline's political process in that they are not static but result from debate and discussion among the profession's scholars, leaders, and members over time.

When the nurse's strongly held values and beliefs on safety are challenged by a nursing care situation, the nurse has the right to decide whether to participate. Decisions not to participate in a situation cannot be made trivially because of the trust relationship and a nurse's moral accountability for actions. The threat to the nurse's integrity must be serious and the person's well-being must not be jeopardized by the nurse's absence. Other arrangements must be made for care of the person in such circumstances. The nurse who encounters repeated threats to integrity has a responsibility

Box **5-3** *Code of Ethics for Nurses*

1. The nurse, in all professional relationships, practices with compassion and respect for the inherent dignity, worth, and uniqueness of every individual, unrestricted by considerations of social or economic status, personal attributes, or the nature of health problems.
2. The nurse's primary commitment is to the person, whether an individual or part of a family, group, or community.
3. The nurse promotes, advocates for, and strives to protect the health, safety, and rights of the person.
4. The nurse is responsible and accountable for individual nursing practice and determines the appropriate delegation of tasks consistent with the nurse's obligation to provide optimal person care.
5. The nurse owes the same duties to self as to others, including the responsibility to preserve integrity and safety, to maintain competence, and to continue personal and professional growth.
6. The nurse participates in establishing, maintaining, and improving health care environments and conditions of employment conducive to the provision of quality health care and consistent with the values of the profession through individual and collective action.
7. The nurse participates in the advancement of the profession through contributions to practice, education, administration, and knowledge development.
8. The nurse collaborates with other health professionals and the public in promoting community, national, and international efforts to meet health needs.
9. The profession of nursing, as represented by associations and their members, is responsible for articulating nursing values, for maintaining the integrity of the profession and its practice, and for shaping social policy.

From American Nurses Association. (2001). *Code of ethics for nurses with interpretive statements.* Washington, DC: Author. American Nurses Association and American Nurses Association. (2008). *Guide to the code for nurses: Interpretation and application.* Washington, D.C. Author American Nurses Association.

to consider changing the situation in some way. Change efforts may be directed toward institutional policy or may require that an alternative work environment be considered. Some provisions of the ANA Code of Ethics (2001) are discussed in more depth later in the chapter in relation to health-promotion activities.

Codes of ethics tend to offer guidelines not only about responsibilities for ensuring good care but also about responsibilities for recognizing and addressing barriers to service. The nursing profession in the United States, according to the ANA Code of Ethics, proposes that "the nurse promotes, advocates for, and strives to protect the health, safety, and rights of the person" (ANA, 2001, Provision 3). This requires anticipation of future health needs and political activity when necessary to ensure health promotion. Codes of ethics represent the ideals of the profession and thus serve as general guides to action. The ANA Code of

Ethics is nonnegotiable: that is, the goals and intent of the code may not be ignored, diluted, or downplayed by individuals or institutions employing nurses in the United States (ANA, 1994).

Advocacy

Advocacy, as an expectation of nurses, is strongly reinforced both in the code of ethics (ANA, 2001, 2008) and in innumerable scholarly articles. However, advocacy is also a controversial concept. The meaning of advocacy is hard to pin down and, consequently, there is no agreement about the boundaries of a nurse's responsibilities to advocate. The meaning of the term *advocacy* is derived from its use in law. In legal jurisprudence, advocacy is aggressive action taken on behalf of an individual, or perhaps a group viewed as an individual entity, to protect or secure that individual's rights. The term can be traced to the fourteenth-century French *advocacie*, which meant "the function of an advocate; the work of advocating; pleading for or supporting," while advocate is derived from the Latin *advocatus* meaning, "one summoned or 'called to' another, esp. one called in to aid one's cause in a court of justice" (Brown, 1993, p. 194). "Therefore, a lawyer, while defending or representing a client, has this responsibility to the client as a foremost responsibility" (Grace, 2001, p. 154). Thus in law the individual lawyer does not have an opposing obligation to attend to social justice issues. This attention to broader questions of justice is the responsibility of other areas of the justice system.

Unlike advocacy within the justice system, advocacy in health care settings is not a simple concept (Grace, 1998). The adoption of the term *advocacy* to denote professional action in nonlegal settings gives rise to confusion. Nurses (and other health care professionals) have a responsibility to speak up on behalf of people whose rights have been interfered with or endangered in some way. However, that is not the end of their responsibilities. They must also consider that specific actions they undertake in the name of advocacy (regardless of the prevailing definition of advocacy) may pose problems for other people who are relying on them for health care services.

For example, Sally Rimmer, a case manager, is assisting Jim Bailey to apply for services in a rehabilitation facility because he has residual hemiparesis secondary to a cerebrovascular accident. There is a waiting list at the facility, but Sally believes it is a priority for Jim to be treated there, because he lives with his elderly mother who is frail and will not be able to assist him with his activities of daily living. Because Sally represents other people who will also benefit from rehabilitation, her decision to advocate for Jim must be weighed against the needs of these other people. A moral responsibility associated with advocacy in health care settings is that the effect of actions on others is considered. When advocating extra attention or specialized care for a given person, an injustice may be rendered simultaneously to other people in the nurse's care. "Advocacy conceptualized as professional action stemming from the profession's purposes, and more properly termed 'professional advocacy'" . . . requires a balancing of the health needs of the individual with the health needs of the population" (Grace, 2001, p. 159).

Advocacy is an ideal of health care professions that requires attention to individuals and to broader societal concerns. Understanding the interdependent nature of individual and social needs facilitates preventive and health-promotion actions on the part of health care professionals both locally and more globally. Such actions may include political activity in concert with others on behalf of common populations of concern. Preemptive and sociopolitical advocacy permits the source of the ongoing problems to be accurately identified and challenged. Ballou (2000), among others, has strongly argued that nurses have moral obligations related to sociopolitical advocacy on behalf of their populations of concern. Sally Rimmer's obligations include recognizing the problems caused by a chronic shortage of rehabilitation services. Her concerns include discovering the source of this problem and joining with others in an attempt to address it at this level. Strategies for solving seemingly intractable problems of health care or the health care delivery system include collaboration with specialty nursing, medical or client advocacy groups, and publication of the issues in the popular press.

Advocacy at the level of the care of individuals is related to trust. Trust is a necessary part of the health care professional–client relationship. Davis and colleagues (1997) note that an ethical responsibility of the nurse is "to see that the person's rights and interests are protected" (p. 76). This is part of the nurse's role because people may not recognize either what is needed to meet their needs or when the care they are receiving is substandard.

Advocacy for good health care including health promotion is a concept with broader implications. It necessarily includes those activities that are directed toward remedying socially based inequities or inadequacies in the health care delivery system. Gaylord and Grace (1995), among others, note that advocacy should be viewed as an ethic of practice that includes all activities directed toward the person's good. Further, it is proposed that advocacy may be required on an organizational or political level when obstacles to good care are recurrent (Ballou, 2000; Grace, 2001). "So advocacy is an obligation of professional role but not solely in the narrow sense of speaking up for, or acting on behalf of, individuals or groups in specific situations. This is because necessarily included in the nurse's moral decision-making is consideration of which actions will be most supportive of the profession's goals overall" (Gaylord & Grace, 1995, p. 160). Advocacy is often a risky practice in that speaking up, or facilitating the good, for individuals or groups may pit nurses against their peers or against other interested parties (Spenceley et al., 2006). Potential adversaries are those who do not share the same professional goals, or are not as reflective about what these goals entail, or have an economic or other interest in maintaining the status quo.

The health care professional role and its attendant responsibilities (advocacy) require that professional knowledge and judgment be brought to bear on a variety of situations, from the relatively simple to the complex. First, judgment permits the isolation, identification, and analysis of health problems or potential problems, often in collaboration with others. Second, appropriate actions are formulated and their likely consequences considered. Third, obstacles to action are recognized and addressed. Finally, actions are carried out and evaluated. These basic steps are evident whether the object of health care or health promotion is an individual, a group, or society.

Problem Solving: Issues, Dilemmas, and Risks

The nature of health care settings and environments makes it inevitable that some extremely difficult decisions will have to be made. However, many of the ethical problems encountered in health-promotion settings are issues rather than **dilemmas**. Daniel Chambliss (1996), a sociologist who studied nurses in acute care institutional settings, asserts that organizations such as hospitals often give rise to "practical problems, not individual dilemmas" (p. 91). These are nonetheless moral problems because they interfere with the goals of promoting health, well-being, or the relief of suffering. In noninstitutional health care settings obstacles to good care are also caused by health care system arrangements, by interprofessional conflicts, and by the lack of resources. Dilemmas are **ethical issues** of a special sort. The term *dilemma* is a conjoining of *di*, meaning two, coupled with *lemma*, a Greek term meaning assumption or premises (Brown, 1993). In ethics, dilemmas are those situations in which a choice must be made between two (or among more) equally undesirable options. Weston (2005) claims that true dilemmas are actually quite rare and that options often can be found by changing the way the situation is scrutinized.

For the most part ethical problems in health promotion are not dilemmas. However, the goals of health promotion require that both issues and dilemmas be recognized and addressed. Neglected issues can become dilemmas. The situation that Graham Pink faced is an example of an ethical issue that became a dilemma. Mr. Pink was a charge nurse working on a geriatric ward in a British hospital. He had grave concerns about the treatment of people, especially during the night shift, which was chronically understaffed. First Mr. Pink went through the usual channels trying to get changes made. He notified his supervisors verbally and via written documentation but was unsuccessful in achieving change. Indeed, the situation deteriorated further. He went higher in the administrative chain of command with complaints that people were being neglected and endangered by the situation. He was unsuccessful at all levels. Finally, his moral concerns were such that he decided to report the situation to the local newspaper, even though he knew that he might lose his position as a result. He was fired in September 1991 but was eventually exonerated (Wilmot, 2000).

When a nurse is in danger of losing his or her position as a result of advocating for better conditions, one consideration is whether the people are liable to be better served overall by the action. This requires balancing the foreseeable risks of advocating with the likely benefits to the individual or group. A framework for making ethical decisions is offered and discussed later in the chapter. Included in this discussion are considerations for the health-promotion agent related to personal security along with preserving integrity.

Preventive Ethics

Preventive ethics, like preventive health care activities, aims to forestall ethical problems before they develop. Preventive ethics is a requirement of health-promotion endeavors perhaps more specifically than it is of any other area of health-related activities. Preventive ethics requires the health promoter both to envision potential problems and to institute actions that halt their development. For example, it is possible to extend a dying person's life almost indefinitely using available technology, including vasoactive drugs and high-technology devices. It has become the norm (for a variety of reasons) for medical personnel to try to do so. Although a competent person has the right to refuse treatment and this right is legally recognized as a result of the Patient Self-Determination Act (PSDA) of 1991, many people become incapacitated quickly and before they are able to make their wishes known. Although all states recognize and honor advance directives, the legally recognized form varies from state to state (Box 5-4). Most

---

Box 5-4 Preventive Ethics: Patient Self-Determination Act and Advance Directives

One fact that all people face is the uncertainty and fragility of life. Health-promotion endeavors can increase individual capacities to withstand the vagaries of life and even permit humans to flourish while living with chronic illness. However, what often cannot be predicted is whether and when the ability to make our wishes for treatment and care known will be lost. Over the last 2 to 3 decades, great technological and therapeutic advances have been made, with the resulting ability to save the lives of people experiencing catastrophic illnesses and trauma. The side effect of these advances, unfortunately, is that sometimes we are successful only in prolonging the dying process. Although it is now recognized that people have a right to refuse treatment to prolong life, it is not uncommon that critically ill people lose the ability to articulate their wishes for treatment. Advance directives are a way for people to ensure that when they become incapacitated the care and treatment they receive matches their predetermined wishes. At their best, advance directives also have the potential to relieve the strain felt by loved ones as they strive to make the "right" treatment choices for a friend or relative. They also guide health professionals in their decision-making regarding the person in question.

TYPES OF ADVANCE DIRECTIVES

All states have advance directive laws. However, they differ regarding what is the legal form of advance directive and what is required to validate it. For example, in Massachusetts the legal advance directive is a health care proxy. It requires the designation of a person to make one's health care decisions in the event of incapacity. Two people have to witness the signature, neither of whom can be the designee.

1. *Instructional*. A written document, this is also known as a living will or terminal care document. It can be very specific and tailored to order or may be a form document that can be downloaded from the Internet.
2. *Health care proxy*. This is also known as a durable power of attorney for health care. It allows a competent person to designate a decision maker in the event of incapacity.

Fagerlin and Schneider (2004) found that living wills are the least effective advance directive in the absence of a health care proxy. The best advance directive is a combination of proxy and written directions.

The Patient Self-Determination Act (PSDA) of 1991, which was formulated in response to 2 decades of ambiguity and litigation involving right-to-die cases, represented an attempt to ensure that people's rights were honored. The PSDA required changes in public policy, public and professional education, institutional policy, and social awareness (Clarke, 1998). The PSDA was expected to improve communication related to end-of-life care issues and preferences among individuals, health care providers, and proxy decision makers. It requires institutions that receive Medicare and Medicaid funds to:

- Give written information on admission to all (not just the Medicare and Medicaid) clients about their rights under the law to make their own treatment decisions
- Inform people of their rights to complete state-allowed advance directives and provide written policies about those rights
- Document when a client has an advance directive
- Not discriminate or make care conditional on the existence or absence of an advance directive
- Provide staff education about advance directives and personal rights

Although the PSDA has great potential, it serves its purpose only to the extent that it is taken seriously as a responsibility of a given institution. All too frequently institutions fail to ensure that a suitably qualified person is available to impart the information or to request personal preferences. It is important for those involved in health promotion to understand, and therefore address, why people may be reluctant to make an advance directive, why institutions are not diligent in providing information and education, and why even in the presence of the PSDA most people do not have advance directives (Miles et al., 1996).

RESERVATIONS ABOUT, AND IMPEDIMENTS TO THE USE OF, ADVANCE DIRECTIVES

- Discussions with health care providers about the implications of desired choices have been inadequate.

Continued

Box **5-4** Preventive Ethics: Patient Self-Determination Act and Advance Directives—cont'd

- People don't want to talk about future incapacity or death. They may have cultural prohibitions about discussing the possibility of serious illness or death.
- Past encounters with the health care system have led to distrust.
- People can't predict accurately their future preferences and they know too little about what constitutes life support.
- People may change their minds about what they will accept.
- The health care proxy may turn out to be a poor choice or may cause conflicts among other family members or loved ones. The client or family may ask for something that is morally unacceptable.
- Treatments may be specified to which the provider has conscientious objections.

- Documentation may be lost, misplaced, or not accessible in an emergency.
- Written instructions are too vague and open to divergent interpretation to be useful guides.
- Even the most diligent proxy cannot always know what the person would have wanted in the absence of a detailed treatment directive.
- The proxy may make a treatment choice contrary to the person's directive.
- The proxy may make a decision with which the institution or physician disagrees.

Compiled from Fagerlin, A., & Schneider, C. E. (2004). Enough. The failure of the living will. *Hastings Center Report 34*(2), 30-42; Miles, S. H, Koepp, R., & Weber, E. P. (1996). Advance end-of-life treatment planning: A research review. *Archives of Internal Medicine 156*, 1062-1068; and Wolf, S. M. (2001). Sources of concern about the Patient Self-Determination Act. In W. Teays & L. M. Purdy (Eds.), *Bioethics, justice and health care* (pp. 411-419). Belmont, CA: Wadsworth/Thompson Learning.

people have not formulated advance directives. There are many reasons why this is true. Much more work needs to be done on engaging people in discussion and planning for such eventualities while they are still well (Research Highlights box). The work of communication with clients

research highlights

Use of Advance Directives with Adolescents

Scholars of health care ethics have proposed that discussions related to advance directives for care should begin while people are healthy and should take place in an ongoing fashion as part of health maintenance activities (Grace, 2004; May, 2002; McCullough, 1998). McAliley et al. (2000) took this idea one step further, noting that although "The American Academy of Pediatrics (AAP) supports giving children a voice in their health care decision-making, . . . how teens want to be involved in this is not known" (p. 471). To answer this question they conducted an interview study of 107 adolescents between the ages of 15 and 18 years related to having or making a living will.

Results of the study yielded a wide range of information about adolescents and advance directives. Participants were able to pass a test used for demonstrating decision-making competency. They were willing to answer questions related to their own health care treatments as they envisioned themselves in a coma, and those responses are similar to those reported for adults. The vast majority of participants felt it was "somewhat important" or "very important" for someone their age to have a living will. Most of the adolescent participants did not report feeling uncomfortable discussing these issues (McAliley et al., 2000, p. 471).

From McAliley, L. G., Hudson-Barr, D. C., Gunning, R. S., & Rowbottom, L. A. (2000). The use of advance directives with adolescents. *Pediatric Nursing 26*(5), 471-482.

and families can begin before a problem arises. This is often missing both in institutional settings and primary care settings.

Preventive ethics using a feminist ethics perspective would permit addressing institutional practices that make it difficult for high-technology care to be more humanistic or addressing the underlying social issues that lead people to overeat, smoke, or be inclined toward violence. For example, preventive ethics would require investigating why as a society we have trouble discussing death and dying, and why we find it so hard to have a peaceful or good death. Weston (2005) notes that much of the energy used on the polarized abortion debate could be more profitably put to use in determining why people who do not want to be pregnant nevertheless become pregnant. Weston (2005) would reframe the question to ask "why pregnancy, or pregnancy at the wrong time, is so unacceptably burdensome for many women" (p. 43). We need to ask questions about lack of support, lack of education, poor or difficult-to-use birth control methods, resistance from spouses and lovers, lack of child care, and so on. Strategies for identifying potential ethical problems before they occur include examining problematic cases for their antecedents. We should ask fundamental questions about societal arrangements and influences on health trends.

On a local level, nurses and other health promoters need to bring to bear clinical judgment in anticipating and forecasting problems before they arise. For example, when a nurse observes that a person and family either do not understand information that has been given to them or the implications of following a given course of action, the nurse engages in preventive ethics by supplying that information. The nurse acts to prevent negative consequences that can arise as a result of poorly understood information. Many problems in health care occur as a result of poor communication or because information has been provided too late for reasoned decision-making.

Preventive ethics also includes social and political activism, in concert with other nurses or professional nursing organizations, to effect those changes in the health care environment needed to avert potential hazards. Some of these hazards result from inadequate access to health care. "Nursing's Social Policy Statement is clear about the collective responsibility of nursing to influence . . . social and public policy to promote social justice" (ANA, 2003, p. 5).

So far the discussion has traced the origins of moral philosophy and **applied ethics**, along with providing a brief critique of the usefulness of these for guiding professional action. As noted, we cannot use a particular moral theory exclusively to guide health-promotion activities because each theory has flaws that lead to further problems. The principles of duty-based theories can conflict with each other (e.g., I must tell the truth but telling the truth might cause harm). Utilitarian or consequentialist approaches can lead us to neglect the needs of some individuals for the benefit of the larger group. An exclusive emphasis on care gives us no way to evaluate the good of our actual actions. This next section explores certain moral principles, derived from a variety of moral theories, that help clarify problems in health care and locate the essential facets of those problems.

ETHICAL PRINCIPLES IN HEALTH PROMOTION

Although the tenets of nursing's codes of ethics and standards of practice provide some guidance about the nature of practice and the manner in which services will be provided, they tend to be vague and nonspecific, often leaving some ambiguity about the best course of action in morally troubling situations. The use of principles derived from a variety of ethical theories, along with feminist insights or an ethic of care, permits us to get a more nuanced and detailed picture of actual or potential morally problematic health situations. Beauchamp and Walters (2002) note that "principles provide a starting point for moral judgment and policy evaluation, but . . . more content is needed than that supplied by principles alone" (p. 19). In other words, principles such as autonomy, beneficence, and justice often serve as helpful starting points in teasing out the tangled elements of complex issues, but taken alone they are usually insufficient to permit moral problem solving in health care environments. One must decide which principles are important to consider in a given case or situation, and this requires an exploration of the case as discussed in the decision-making framework provided later in the chapter.

Additionally, tenets of the code for nurses (ANA, 2008) and other ANA position statements provide guidance regarding what a nurse's moral responsibilities are in a particular type of situation. Certain tenets (see Box 5-3, provisions 6 to 9) also address the responsibilities of the nurse toward improving the larger health care environment. These obligations include facilitating "community, national, and international efforts to meet health needs" (ANA, 2001, p. 23).

Autonomy as Civil Liberty

In health-promotion settings and endeavors the concept of **autonomy** can be understood from two different perspectives. From the vantage point of public health, the extent of individual autonomy, or freedom of action, may be limited by the duty of protecting the health and safety of the society (Ovrebo, 2001). From this perspective there is an age-old struggle between civil rights and public safety. Moral questions center on the problem of how much liberty the society is justified in regulating in the interests of the health and safety of the society at large (Häyry, 2006). Ovrebo (2001) reminds us that "controversies over coercive health measures" are at least "as old as the quarantining of ships carrying bubonic plague" (p. 23). The first outbreaks of shipborne bubonic plague were noted in ships that had sailed from the Orient to Italy in the 1300s (McGowan, 1995). Sailors on the ships were quarantined and not allowed to disembark; thus their freedom was restricted. There is an inevitable tension associated with curtailing **civil liberties** in the name of safety or health. This tension arises from perceptions that what is important about human life, in most Western contexts, is that some freedom of action is a prerequisite of human flourishing. Additionally, human rights curtailment has permitted control of large populations by small, but powerful, minorities.

Currently there are many indirect threats to the health and safety of our society. Actions to resolve any of these have the potential to impinge on civil liberties including, but by no means limited to, bioterrorism, the spread of HIV-AIDS, drug-resistant tuberculosis, and advances in genetic knowledge. Advances in genetic knowledge present the possibility of discrimination from a variety of sources. It will be difficult to maintain individual privacy. Discrimination based on class or gene profile will be made easier. Genetic enhancement may be used by select individuals who can afford it (Bereano, 2000).

The current managed care environment, while having a stronger focus on inculcating healthy behaviors, can impinge on civil liberties. Prioritizing behavior change or modification in health-promotion endeavors over the need to address underlying social contributors such as poverty and other forms of disadvantage has been criticized by those who feel that a focus on the social determinants of health would permit more effective, less restrictive health promotion and protection (Cribb & Duncan, 2002; Marmot & Wilkinson, 2006; Ovrebo, 2001; Portillo & Waters, 2004).

Autonomy as Self-Determination

A second, related, sense of autonomy has to do with individual choice. In health care and health-promotion settings where individuals are the focus of concern, autonomy means the right to determine what treatments or interventions one will accept. It is perhaps the most powerful moral principle underlying the treatment of individuals, at least in Western societies. This principle asserts that people have the ability to reason, and a consequence of the ability to reason is the capacity to make choices. These choices concern both one's own behavior and how one should act toward others (Atkins, 2006). Although the idea that the essence of being human is our ability to reason originated with Aristotle, Kant (1997/1785) developed this idea in meticulous detail in his work, "Foundations of the Metaphysics of Morals." According to Kant, among all the animals only people are capable of conscious desires and goals. People are free agents capable of making decisions and setting their own goals as guided by their own reason. This principle is still a salient consideration in health care settings: it underpins the health provider and promoter–client relationship and the issue of informed consent. However, there is limited agreement about the scope, limits, and strength of this principle (Beauchamp & Childress, 2008). When describing autonomy in the context of health or treatment choices, it is important to delineate what we mean by autonomy in the context of the problem under discussion. Feminist criticisms of an emphasis on autonomy highlight the problem that our choices necessarily affect others because we are contextual beings inseparable from our relationships with one another.

Generally, respecting autonomy requires that we permit individuals to make their own decisions, even when these decisions seem to others to be ill informed. There are exceptions to this rule. Exceptions include those situations in which there is a high risk of serious injury or death and when it cannot be determined whether the person's judgment is impaired (Box 5-5): that is, we make exceptions to the rule of autonomy when we suspect that an individual is not able to reason

adequately or to reason at the normal level (given that the normal level of functioning is self-sufficient). A person's reasoning ability may be impaired for several reasons. The difficulties may be psychological, physical, or a result of incorrect or incomplete information. Normally respect for people, which is another way of saying respect for human dignity or autonomy, permits individuals to make and learn from their own mistakes and holds them accountable for their actions.

In health care or health-promotion settings, respect for autonomy requires that individuals be given the information they need to make choices. Choices can be considered autonomous only if certain criteria are met. The criteria that determine whether or not a person is actually capable of autonomous (voluntary) choice include cognitive maturity, possession of appropriate information to permit decision-making, intact mental capacities (the ability to reason logically), the absence of internal or external coercive influences, and the ability to appreciate the risks and benefits of alternative choices. This is quite a tall order. It is probably true that nobody acts totally autonomously at any given time because of the influences of entrenched beliefs and values that are derived, for the most part, from our cultural and environmental backgrounds. Some of these are under conscious control in the sense that we can recognize what values we hold and even revise them if they are dissonant with other values. However, some of these influences are not readily recognizable: they lie beneath the surface of consciousness and are hard to access even if we are willing to try. We all have blind spots; autonomy viewed as informed, uncoerced, and reasoned action is therefore an ideal. Many of us, and probably most of the time, fall short of the ideal. Autonomy is the moral principle that underlies the concept of informed consent to treatment, interventions, and health-promotion efforts.

Autonomy and Adolescents

Based on theoretical conceptions and findings from empirical studies related to development and decision-making (Dickey & Deatrick, 2000; Ross, 1997; Weir & Peters, 1997; Weithorn & Campbell, 1982), adolescents 14 to 17 years of age are generally considered capable of meeting these criteria and making decisions as ably as adults. Involving adolescents fully in their own health care facilitates self-care agency (Research Highlights box). For nurse theorist Orem, whose focus on self-care agency includes developmental considerations, there is a relationship between the deliberate self-care activities of mature and maturing people and ongoing optimal development and future functioning. Self-care is learned as a result of membership within family or other social groups. Although for the most part this includes some supervision by responsible adults, respect for an adolescent's developing autonomy facilitates health (Orem, 2001).

Box 5-5 | **Proxy Decision-Making**

I. Autonomy based: person's previously articulated desires
   A. Written
      1. Living will, advance directive
      2. Document details to varying degrees what the person will or will not accept
   B. Substituted judgment
      1. Individual appoints a proxy who is expected to honor previously expressed preferences
      2. Informal (nonappointed significant other)
II. Best interests
   A. Surrogate chooses the actions that will give the highest overall benefit—may or may not be based on a person's previously expressed desires; a quality of life determination based when possible on knowledge about the person (Beauchamp & Childress, 2008)
   B. Best interests may trump the proxy's choice; doubt about the proxy's motives possible
III. Reasonable person standard
   A. Based on the answer to "What would a reasonable person want?"

research highlights

Surrogate Decision-Making

A majority of end-of-life health care decisions are made by surrogate decision makers who are under a great deal of stress over their seriously ill family member. Both surrogate and clinicians have varying degrees of preparation, knowledge, abilities, or comfort in working effectively with another in making very difficult decisions for someone else.

This study surveyed 50 designated surrogates with previous decision-making experience. Through semistructured telephone interviews surrogates were asked to describe and reflect on their experiences of making health care decisions for others.

Four types of factors that made decision-making more or less difficult were identified by surrogates:

1. Surrogate characteristics and life circumstances (e.g., competing responsibilities and coping strategies)
2. Surrogate social networks (e.g., interfamily thoughts and feelings about the "right decision")
3. Surrogate-client relationships (e.g., including communications [or the lack of communications] about difficulties in honoring known preferences)
4. Surrogate-clinician relationships (e.g., surrogate primarily communicating with one clinician "spokesperson")

The results identify areas where clinicians can interfere to facilitate the processes of surrogate "decision-making."

Vig, E. K., Starks, H., Taylor, J. S., Hopely, E. K., Fryer-Edwards, K. (2007). Surviving surrogate decision-making: What helps and hampers the experience of making medical decisions for others. *Journal of General Internal Medicine 22*(9), 1274–1279.

Informed Consent

Informed consent to research, treatments, or health-promotion endeavors is a process of ensuring that a person has all of the appropriate information necessary to come to a decision about participation that facilitates autonomous action. Beauchamp and Childress (2008) note that "informed consent occurs if and only if a person or subject, with substantial understanding and in the absence of substantial control by others, intentionally authorizes a professional to do something" (p. 78). The key phrase is "with substantial understanding." Informed consent may be seen as the (temporary) end result of a process. The consent is temporary because new information may change the balance of risks and benefits of the proposed procedure. Thus even after a consent form is signed, a person has the right to rescind consent in light of changed consequences.

Components of the **consent** process include determining the person's competency to make the decision or to consent: that is, there must be no physical or mental impairments that hinder the person in question from understanding and processing information. For example, a person with pneumonia who is febrile and confused probably is not capable of making an informed decision until the fever is reduced and the confusion has cleared. To be substantially informed a person must be made aware of important details of the proposed intervention, including its nature, purpose, probability of success, and important risks, and must also understand what alternatives (if any) are available. This information must be tailored to meet the specific needs of an individual and thus requires that we know something about the person. In this way an ethic of care is important to our understanding of a person's unique needs. We can check understanding to a certain extent by asking the individual to articulate how the proposed intervention will facilitate his or her own values and goals. There must be no subtle or overt coercion by professionals or others who are significant in the person's life or might otherwise have undue influence (e.g., employer). Finally, appropriate supports must be available to complete the proposed intervention.

Obtaining consent for any interventions, or for involvement in research, is best viewed as a process that entails ongoing assessment of the person's status and evaluation of needs for further information or support. People who are in stressful situations have limited abilities to process information; thus, we should assess for and validate understanding on an ongoing basis. It has been well documented that people do not grasp information well either when they are in stressful situations or when the information is complex.

Most health-promotion activities do not require formal informed consent. However, they do require us to understand both the philosophy behind, and the status and validity of, the supporting research before we assist people to be sure that we use health-promotion strategies that best fit their beliefs and values.

Exceptions to Autonomous Decision-Making

Exceptions to the rule of permitting autonomous decision making exist. In some cases, proxy decision-making on behalf of the individual is required. Nevertheless proxy decision-making must take into account what is known about the person and must follow a path of action that is most likely to respect that individual's previous goals and values when these are knowable. Braun et al. (2008) studied the descriptions of the burdens of end-of-life decision-making by a sample of African American, Caucasian, and Hispanic surrogates. Another study by Vig et al. (2007) described what helps and hampers surrogate decision-making. Certain populations are considered less than fully autonomous for a variety of reasons. People with Alzheimer's disease or other physical or psychological disruptions or deficits that prevent adequate comprehension may require proxy decision makers (see Box 5-5). Incarcerated people are restricted in their choices and may be subject to subtle or not-so-subtle coercion. Children are considered less than fully autonomous because they are not developmentally mature. Additionally, in people with certain mental illnesses, such as psychoses or bipolar disorders, a capacity for decision-making that is in alignment with previous life goals may fluctuate. The President's commission (1982) formed to look at health care decision-making noted that the minimal capacities needed for competent decision-making are: "1. Possession of a set of values and goals, 2. the ability to communicate and to understand information, and 3. the ability to reason and deliberate about one's choice" (p. 57). These criteria are generally accepted as a basic minimum (Beauchamp & Childress, 2008). It can be seen from these criteria that some children would be able to understand the implications of a given course of treatment, and adults with cognitive impairments may be deemed competent to make certain decisions. Buchanan and Brock (1990) have argued persuasively that competency to make autonomous choices is not an all-or-nothing capacity. They remind health care professionals that competency determinations are, as a rule, made for a given decision or task and thus should be task relative. Moreover, they affirm that competency for decision-making occurs along a continuum. Thus, a person may vacillate between competency and noncompetency, depending on either the task at hand (degree of difficulty or risk) or physical or psychological status during the period when a decision must be made.

When advocating decision-making for a cognitively impaired person, it is important to consider the risks of permitting the decision compared with the benefit of allowing the individual to make his or own decision. The benefits in terms of self-esteem may well outweigh the risks of many choices. However, if the risk of injury is high and it is obvious that the person does not grasp this, decision-making should not be allowed. In this case, either we are preserving the person's autonomy so that he or she may engage in decision-making at a future time (and presumably death truncates autonomy) or because severe suffering is likely to occur and the person has not taken this into consideration.

Proxy Decision-Making

When children are involved, it is often the parent or guardian to whom we turn for permission to treat. Nevertheless, in pediatric settings it is incumbent on people involved in health-promotion endeavors or in research with minors to gain assent from the child in addition to consent from the parent or guardian. For the child's assent to be meaningful, an assessment of level of maturity and comprehension is required, and information must be provided in language and terms that are appropriate for the developmental level. Conversely, when there is conflict between the decision of the parent and that of the child, the health care provider has a duty to ensure that the parental choice is in the child's best interest. Where there is serious doubt, it may be necessary to involve the courts.

Limits on Autonomy

Although autonomy remains an important principle for individual decision-making related to interventions of various sorts, curtailments on autonomy are frequent in daily life. We are constrained by our work conditions, by access to information, by unconscious drives, by emotions, and by the impact of our behavior on others. For the sake of societal interests the autonomous actions of individuals may

sometimes be curtailed. This is especially true when the health of other people is put at risk (Shirley, 2007).

Confidentiality

Autonomy is also the principle underlying **confidentiality**. "The ability to maintain privacy in one's life is an expression of autonomy" (Burkhardt & Nathaniel, 2001). People have the right to decide who shall have access to information about them, thus limiting the negative use of personal information by others. In certain situations the status of confidentiality between a person and others, such as clergy, is considered a privilege and as such is shielded from exposure by the legal system. In health care, confidentiality does not carry as strong a status as clergy-supplicant or lawyer-client privilege (Grace, 2004). There may be occasions when health care providers have a duty to warn others who are unknowingly endangered. This duty was highlighted by the landmark Tarasoff case. On October 27, 1969, Prosenjit Poddar killed Tatiana Tarasoff. Poddar was receiving psychiatric care during this period. He had informed his therapist 2 weeks earlier that he was going to kill a certain girl, easily identifiable as Tarasoff, on her return from Brazil. At the time his therapist tried to have him committed. The police detained Poddar briefly but decided he was rational, so they released him. No one warned Tatiana of the danger and Poddar killed her. The courts concluded that "once a therapist does in fact determine, or under applicable professional standards reasonably should have determined, that a person poses a serious danger of violence to others, he bears a duty to exercise reasonable care to protect the foreseeable victim of that danger" (*Tarasoff v. Regents of University of California,* 1976). The court recognized the difficulty of predicting dangerousness and the importance of maintaining confidentiality but determined that when the risk is high, confidentiality should be breached.

Health care professionals must strive to keep the person's personal information confidential so as to enhance trust within the health care professional–client relationship. Therefore, in health care settings there are strong sanctions against breaching confidentiality. In theory the principle of confidentiality may be overridden only in situations in which extreme harm to self or others is imminent. In practice, confidentiality is breached frequently. In hospital settings many people have access to the person's information. Insurance companies demand access to information before payment for services is made. Additionally, there has recently been a push to institute a nationwide medical information bank. The ethical implications of this are many, and such implications are the subject of debates in the ethics literature (Etzioni, 1999; Goldberg, 2000; Gostin, 1997; Hodge, 2000).

In outpatient settings, barriers to privacy may occur when office or other personnel are personally acquainted with the client. This is especially true in the types of settings where health promotion is the focus of practice. In such settings it is important that those supervising the health efforts address confidentiality issues with the staff they supervise. When health professionals are members of the community in which they practice, there may be confidentiality issues associated with the intimate nature of small communities. Nurses and other health-promotion professionals may find themselves being asked by friends and relatives of a client for details about that person's health status. It can be very difficult to respond diplomatically while maintaining the person's privacy.

The Privacy Rule

The **Privacy Rule** (45 Code of Federal Regulations Part 160, 164 subparts A & E) was developed as a result of the Health Insurance Portability and Accountability Act (HIPAA). Its intent was to ensure that individuals' health information is properly protected, while allowing the flow of information needed to provide and promote high-quality care (including using client information for research) and to protect the public's health and well-being. HIPAA was meant to protect the privacy of individually identifiable health information in the face of advances in electronic technology and to limit the ways in which "health plans, pharmacies, hospitals, clinics, nursing homes and other covered entities (any provider that conducts or conveys information in electronic form, e.g., physicians, nurse practitioners)" can use medical information (U.S. Department of Health and Human Services [USDHHS], 2005). Covered entities basically means those covered by the privacy rule. The limitations on use of medical information extend to any identifiable information, written, oral, or computerized. Although there are some legal guidelines about disclosure, nurses and others are responsible for using clinical judgment in deciding what level of detail to share (USDHHS, 2004). It is important to understand that the purpose of the rule is to protect individual rights while still facilitating important public health and epidemiological research. Health-promotion activities include empowering people to exercise these rights when this is necessary. The Privacy Rule ensures that clients are given a copy of the privacy practices at a given institution. Additionally, under the rule individuals have the right:

- To access their own information
- To limit who may receive their information
- To request corrections for errors
- To receive an accounting of how their information has been used
- To request special confidential reporting of their information to them at a location of their choosing (this may be especially important for individuals at risk for intimate partner violence)
- To pursue complaints with the Department of Health and Human Services Office for Civil Rights

A rule of thumb for health professionals related to sharing information with others is to disclose only as much information as is necessary to permit optimal care and only information that is pertinent to the situation. A decision about disclosure of a person's information requires balancing of the risks of information sharing with the benefits of treatment.

Examples are the dual loyalties between employees and employers in occupational health practices. In a survey of the responses to 8 imaginary cases involving an ethical dilemma of privacy, 140 nurses and 94 physicians (practicing in occupational health settings) proposed a variety of strategies (Heikkinen et al., 2007).

Although the privacy rule was meant to help safeguard people's rights, some commentators and researchers are finding the rule overly restrictive and worry that it might discourage important research, perhaps especially genetic research, with its far-reaching implications for individual privacy. As Kulynych and Korn (2002) write:

> Although the rule's drafters wisely opted not to create special standards for genetic information, the limits they have placed upon the use and disclosure of all "identifiable" health information will profoundly affect the conduct of genetic studies and many other forms of research. Research compliance efforts will become more costly and time consuming as institutions and individual providers who use or disclose health information for research confront new procedural requirements and new liability for failures to meet the privacy rule's intricate compliance obligations. Investigators who use health information, as well as the institutional committees that must review human subjects research proposals, will need to familiarize themselves with a confusing array of new terminology, ambiguous standards and burdensome required paperwork. (p. 310)

Adolescents: Special Considerations of Confidentiality

Adolescents often provide health professionals with very tricky confidentiality issues. As Bandman and Bandman (2001) note, the adolescent is torn between wanting to challenge authority and to assert independence while still needing the "help and support of effective parents" (p. 195). The results of risk-taking behavior, such as drug and alcohol experimentation and risky sexual activity, and their normal developmental needs make teenagers a health-promotion challenge. The task of health promotion is to maintain and facilitate the adolescent's emerging autonomy and confidentiality needs, while mediating between the teenager and parental figures who feel that they have a right to information about the child. It is easy to become caught in the tension "between the anger and perceived duties of the parent and the defensiveness and vulnerability of the adolescent" (Bandman & Bandman, 2001, p. 200).

Although federal and state laws, in addition to (and as a result of) ethical considerations, generally serve to protect the privacy and autonomy of adolescents, health promotion involves more than mere protection. It involves facilitating the adolescent's health. Thus responsibilities include helping an adolescent to grasp his or her authentic options and rights, facilitating interaction between the adolescent and parents or guardians, maintaining trust, and conserving confidentiality.

On the other hand, clinical judgment (which includes ethical judgment) is important in determining risk. If the risk of preserving the adolescent's privacy is high, based on all pertinent and available evidence such as the presence of sexual or physical abuse, then it may be necessary to report this information to appropriate authorities. Mandatory reporting laws exist. Such laws are important for the general protection of a society's citizens. However, there may be rare occasions when a judgment must be made about whether upholding the legal obligation would cause more harm than good. In such circumstances there are two separate considerations. First, one must decide whether the risk to professional standing and licensure of not following the legally required path is something that the professional is willing to assume. The second consideration involves assessing the benefits and risks to the client of not reporting. There is no easy resolution for these types of problems. If the situation is not an emergency, it is prudent to solicit appropriate advice from a peer, a counselor, or an ethics expert or resource. In any case, it remains the professional's ethical responsibility to handle the given situation in a manner that preserves trust and provides ongoing support.

Veracity

Veracity, or devotion to the truth, is another principle that supports health-promotion activities. Veracity is important in health care settings, because it involves trust, which is the basis of nurse or health care provider–client relationships. People whose health is in question either do not have the knowledge or skills to address their vulnerability personally, or they rely on the professional to supply this. In most cases they will not have the capacity to assess or access suggested remedies on their own. They are to varying degrees reliant upon the person who does possess the knowledge and skills to bring these to bear on their behalf. The contemporary bioethics literature favors characteristics of "veracity,. . . candor, honesty and truthfulness" (Beauchamp & Childress, 2001, p. 283) as virtues to be nurtured in the development of health professionals. This represents a change from the paternalistic (the physician knows what is best) attitudes that prevailed earlier in this century and up to the late 1960s.

Veracity in giving people information about their health care needs facilitates autonomous choice and enhances personal decision-making. There are times, though, when health care professionals are tempted to withhold certain details from the person when this is seen as in the person's best interests or when family members demand it. In general it is difficult for health care providers to determine how much information and which types of information will best serve a person's needs. Knowledge of the person's beliefs, values, and lifestyle preferences are essential to the process of supplying adequate information to support autonomous decision-making. One way to do this is to give the appropriate information while acknowledging that certain undesirable effects may occur and that these should be reported to the provider. Deliberately withholding information so that a person agrees to a treatment or interventions that the health-promoting agent considers important conflicts with

veracity. It is tempting to avoid the longer route to resolving such problems (e.g., education, understanding people's motives, environmental challenges), but this eventually undermines trust and constitutes a moral problem. Veracity is compromised when the clinician withholds information that a person has a right to know or gives information that is misleading or incomprehensible. Veracity has some cross-cultural implications, in that some cultures have not traditionally valued truth telling in the case of terminal illness. Decision-making about whether to honor veracity in such cases must take into consideration what is known about the culture, the particular person, the strength of his or her personal and cultural beliefs, and whether there is evidence about what sorts of things the person would like to know (see the Multicultural Awareness box).

The absence of veracity may interfere with autonomous action. In the case of terminal illness it may deprive the person of the ability to plan the remainder of his or her life. It is rare, but may be possible, that a person does not want to know a certain diagnosis or a given trajectory. If this is known in advance it may prove an exception to the rule of veracity (e.g., a person may waive the right to certain information in advance).

Veracity can be a problem on a larger scale, for example, in health education endeavors aimed at changing patterns of behavior in social groups or in communities. Should nurses and others just present the facts or should they attempt to persuade? What are the limits of veracity? Is it permissible to exaggerate the dangers of certain behavior in the interests of the health of the society? These questions cannot be answered within the confines of this chapter but are important to keep in mind when assessing the merits of proposed population-based interventions.

Nonmaleficence

Related to autonomy is the principle of **nonmaleficence**, which enjoins people not to harm other people. In general society this principle constrains people from autonomous action when their actions are likely to harm others. In health care settings it prohibits clinicians from harming those for whom they provide services. For health promotion it means that in planning activities either on an individual level or the societal level, possible harms must be minimized. Some harms are acceptable if the overall benefits outweigh the risks of actions. Harms may be intentional or unintentional. It is often impossible to foresee all the risks of a given course of action. However, professionals who engage in health-promotion endeavors are responsible for foreseeing predictable adverse consequences and taking these into consideration. These responsibilities include addressing social or health care policies that are discovered to have unintended effects. Norton (1998) gives an example of a health policy that had unintended negative health effects. This concerned a government initiative in the United Kingdom designed to encourage nurses and midwives to facilitate breast-feeding over bottle feeding.

At first this sounds like a worthy health-promotion strategy because research has shown the advantages to the baby of breast-feeding. However, one health authority proposed that the nurses not discuss formula mixing unless the women themselves broached this subject. The problem is that many women, for a variety of reasons, either choose to or have to bottle feed their babies; therefore, there is "a responsibility for nurses and midwives to ensure that mothers are given accurate information about the safe preparation of these feeds" (Norton, 1998, p. 1273).

The possibility of unintentional harms is a hazard of most actions designed to promote health. One example is the conflict between the promotion of (1) breast-feeding through co-sleeping and (2) the guidelines for the prevention of Sudden Infant Death Syndrome (Pemberton, 2005). Such risks can be minimized by well–thought-out activities for which every effort has been directed toward trying to foresee possible negative effects and to avoid, or control for, these. Professionals are responsible for understanding the limits of their knowledge or the data to which they have access. A synthesis of reflection, critical thinking, and knowledge, along with an understanding of the details and context of a situation, is required before embarking on a course of action aimed at facilitating a person's health or well-being. The overall discomfort encountered by the individual must be the minimum possible to achieve the primary good intended. In other words, the health care provider is accountable for his or her judgment and for providing interventions most likely to bring about the desired result. Thus more than just the intention not to do harm is required.

Nurses and allied professionals can do harm inadvertently through ignorance or incompetence, through referral to another provider who is incompetent or inappropriate, by inadequate supervision or training of those under one's supervision, and so on. A health care professional who genuinely attempts to minimize harms that are necessary to providing a greater good (beneficence) acts with nonmaleficence if what results is more beneficial than it is harmful. Alternatively, even if greater harm than good did actually ensue, if it could not have been anticipated based on available information and the clinician's competent judgment, then the action was not maleficent. For example, a course of exercise is designed for a person subsequent to a thorough physical. The person is educated about proper body mechanics, heart rate parameters, and appropriate exercise maneuvers but during an exercise session faints and fractures his arm. Further testing reveals a previously undetected cardiac anomaly that is subsequently surgically corrected. This is not **malfeasance**; the main objective of the agent was therapeutic and the event was, if not totally unforeseeable, not identified upon routine pre-exercise testing. However, the duty of nonmaleficence does mean that health care professionals are accountable for foreseeing the consequences of their actions when this is possible. This places obligations on the practitioner to evaluate the problem thoroughly in its rich contextual facets. A meticulous and informed evalu-

ation in turn requires professional competence. Thus harm caused through careless, indifferent, or expedient decision-making violates the principle of nonmaleficence. Both deliberate harm and harm caused by indifferent or incompetent decision-making should be considered maleficent and are morally problematic.

Beneficence

Beneficence is the quality or state of doing or producing good. As a moral principle, beneficence presents us with the duty to maximize the benefits of actions while minimizing harms. There are two related senses of the moral principle of beneficence in health-promotion settings. The principle of beneficence may govern actions taken to further the overall health or well-being of the society in general or it may govern actions taken to promote the good of a particular individual.

When society formulates rules designed to protect people against the negative effects of their own actions, these rules are considered beneficent. They are also sometimes described as paternalistic because they override a person's autonomy to disobey them. For example, seat belt laws are paternalistic, as are rules governing the use of therapeutic or so-called recreational drugs. "Paternalism is the interference of a state or an individual with another person, against their will, and justified by a claim that the person interfered with will be better off or protected from harm" (Dworkin, 2002). The term **paternalism** is derived from *parens patrie*, or the interest of the state in protecting the vulnerable in society.

The principle of beneficence, when used to justify overriding an individual's autonomous choice in order to serve that individual's interests, is sometimes justified when a person lacks the capacity to make personal or health care decisions. Thus any of the factors that interfere with autonomy, as discussed previously (coercion, cognitive impairment, lack of understanding), may require the health care provider to beneficently override the individual's decisions. Generally, though, beneficence permits interference only when the risks of the individual's proposed actions are high and we cannot determine how autonomous the decision to act is. This is because autonomy is such a powerful principle in Western societies that a decision to override is not taken lightly. I am justified in preventing a person from taking an overdose of sleeping pills or jumping off a cliff because the risks of not doing so are high and if the person succeeds there is no possibility of future autonomous actions.

Beneficence, unlike nonmaleficence, is not necessarily a moral requirement of action on the part of societal members toward each other (Grace, 2004). Whether beneficence is viewed as a moral requirement of societal members very much depends on philosophical beliefs and the ethical theory or perspective ascribed to (if any): that is, as an ordinary citizen I am not necessarily morally required to go out of my way to help or benefit someone. The exception is when a person is endangered and my assistance would mitigate that danger, in which case failing to offer assistance arguably violates the principle of nonmaleficence. Exceptions to beneficence in everyday life include the actions of parents on behalf of their children and guardians on behalf of their wards. In other words, exceptions exist in which we have responsibility for vulnerable others.

In contrast to ordinary members of society, health care professionals have augmented duties of beneficence because their professional goals involve meeting health care needs and thus are aimed at providing a good. For such reasons, beneficence is a moral expectation of health care professionals. "Beneficence is a requirement to produce net benefit for those on whose behalf health care workers undertake interventions" (Cribb & Duncan, 2002, p. 41).

Beneficence is a difficult principle in health-promotion settings because of the dual nature of health-promotion goals, health for individuals and healthy communities. As noted earlier there is often a tension between the two. Tones (1997) highlights this problem in a discussion of health educators aims. They "need on the one hand to prevent disease and safeguard the public health while, on the other hand, respecting individual freedom of choice—including the freedom to adopt an unhealthy lifestyle" (p. 33). Thus duties of beneficence may be at odds with facilitating autonomy viewed narrowly as freedom of action, even self-destructive action.

A paradox exists when we try to change unhealthy behaviors but don't address the underlying causes of those behaviors. For example, although smoking cessation programs do assist some people to stop smoking, and restricting areas where people may smoke tends to persuade some people that it is just becoming too inconvenient to continue, we ought also to address the advertising campaigns that aim to gather new recruits from among adolescents. Popular press articles note the trend among adolescents to try flavored cigarettes. "Bidis are flavored to taste like strawberry, chocolate, mandarin orange, vanilla, grape, lemon-lime, clove, mint, cinnamon, wild cherry, mango, cardamom, licorice, or raspberry. They are hand rolled into the leaves of an Indian plant, tied with string and attractively and exotically packaged. All in all, it looks like a product that was designed for teens. But these tobacco cigarettes are addictive, dangerous, and rapidly gaining in popularity" (Greater Dallas Council on Alcohol and Drug Abuse, 2002). Norton (1998) notes that a real problem with any education-based health-promotion endeavor is that in the absence of underlying societal changes it is ultimately doomed to fail. This supports the earlier argument about professional obligations to address deep-rooted social problems that jeopardize health or are associated with health disparities. See the Hot Topics and Health Teaching boxes for

DIRECT-TO-CONSUMER MARKETING: DRUGS AND TESTS

HOTtopics

Commercial industries have discovered a novel way to increase profits. Direct-to-consumer marketing (DTCM) can occur via print, the Internet, or television. It impacts health-promotion efforts in a variety of ways and has serious ethical implications. DTCM of genetic testing, interventions for newly discovered diseases, or drugs shifts emphasis away from promoting healthy lifestyles or addressing environmental concerns to quick fixes that are more likely to benefit the commercial enterprise and its stakeholders than the individuals to whom the advertising campaigns are directed. Although similar problems apply to DTCM of drugs, genetic testing is used below as an exemplar of problems.

DTCM: Genetic Testing

In a workshop held in March 2003 sponsored by the National Human Genome Research Institute of the National Institutes of Health, various interested parties, including scientists, ethicists, company spokespersons, and consumers, discussed the pros and cons of this mode of promoting genetic testing. The workshop's summary report notes that "while this DTCM may increase public awareness about the availability of genetic tests, there may also be some risks in adopting this strategy." It was noted that, according to recent research, advertisements could increase consumers' awareness about diseases, but they often fail to accurately convey risk information including the implications of test results on the mental status of test takers and on related others. Additionally, the information may fail to reach those most at

risk. Hull and Prasad (2001), reporting on their research, urge that more research be carried out to better understand consumer responses to advertisements.

Problems Associated with DTCM of Genetic Testing

Note: Some of these problems are also associated with genetic testing in general.

- Resource allocation (in terms of the implications of misdirected testing on consumer and provider time and counseling requirements)
- Lack of utility of available interventions
- Consumer inability to deal with the complexity of the information: confusion, false hope, false anxiety
- Economic harm to consumer
- Missed opportunities to pursue other health interventions
- Professionals with working knowledge of genetic testing not available to advise about testing
- Provider education (or lack thereof) with regard to genetics, nonhealth implications within families, and how to communicate genetic information
- Lack of regulatory oversight for tests, existing oversight is technology driven rather than public health oriented, lack of validated tests, lack of consensus on methods for validating genetic tests
- Scant data about harms or benefits of tests
- Questionable scientific accuracy and validity of the advertisements
- Misinformation in public sector about genetics

Modified from the summary report of the National Human Genome Research Institute, March 23, 2004.

discussions of direct-to-consumer marketing (DTCM) of genetic testing for examples of this.

Beneficence: Conflict with Autonomy

From the previous discussion it can be seen that the principles of beneficence and autonomy sometimes conflict. For example, seat belt rules are ostensibly created to protect people from injury, but they take away autonomous choice. Beneficence may justify overriding the decision of a febrile, confused client who refuses to take her antibiotics for pneumonia. Permitting this client to refuse may risk her life. What is the clinician's responsibility? Duties of beneficence seem to mandate medicating her against her will, ensuring that the good of health is facilitated although violating the principle of autonomy. The justification for this must include an assessment of her status related to capacity for autonomous decision-making for this particular treatment. Preserving the person's life so he or she can make autonomous decisions in the future may be required by beneficence. However, it can be argued that beneficence takes precedence over autonomy only in those cases in which the choice cannot be considered autonomous. Thus we have to explore how autonomous the choice is. First, there has to be evidence that a choice has been made. In this case the choice was between accepting antibiotic treatment versus not accepting antibiotic treatment. Second, the reasonableness (or rationality) of the decision has to be discerned: that is, it must be ascertained whether the person really has grasped the implications of refusing treatment. The reasons given for the treatment refusal, then, should illuminate gaps in information delivery or processing. Finally, it must be determined whether there are any external or internal coercion factors impinging on the decision. Perhaps the person feels she cannot afford the medicine (external) or perhaps she has a mistrust of antibiotics because of a previous experience (internal).

Agich (2003) has noted that competent decision-making requires, among other things, that the person be in possession of adequate information, an understanding of benefits and costs of alternative treatments or plans, and knowledge of personal values and beliefs and the effects of these on the decision. He is expressly discussing decision-making in nursing home settings, but these ideas are applicable to decision-making in all types of settings and perhaps especially in correctional facilities. These criteria can be used to permit clinicians to distinguish informed decisions from those that cannot be considered autonomous or to identify when special measures must be taken to control coercive factors. When a decision cannot be said to be informed, the principle of beneficence directs us to decide treatment based on the person's best interests.

Justice

Justice is an ethical principle of major importance in health-promotion settings. There are various conceptions of justice, and the term is used in a variety of ways. For the purposes of this chapter the discussion is about social justice rather than criminal justice (also known as commutative justice). **Social justice** has to do with any formal or informal systems existing within a given society to determine what will be the distribution of goods such as health, education, food, and shelter (Powers & Faden, 2006). Buchanan (2000) notes that as a result of studying early records, we know "the concept of justice has been central to human understandings of socially significant values" (p. 155).

There are two broad socially oriented ideas regarding justice. One perspective views justice as being based on desert—those who are more worthy of merit, or who contribute more, are viewed as deserving of better social benefits.

HEALTH TEACHING   Helping Clients to Grasp the Health Implications of Direct-to-Consumer Marketing

1. Become educated about genetics, the scope and limits of genetic testing, and related marketing strategies, especially as this relates to your specific area of practice.
   - Thoroughly investigate the merits of any new marketing strategy that your clients bring to your attention.
   - Attend workshops.
   - Keep up to date on the related research and ethics literature (paper or electronic journals, articles, and forums).
   - Be aware of and use local resources for genetic advice (counseling services, ethics services at local hospitals, health care ethics, or bioethics departments of local colleges and universities).
2. Assist clients to make a comprehensive assessment of their own needs and goals and to what extent the publicized testing or other offering is likely to help them meet these.

- Explore with them possible motivations for the particular marketing strategy.
- Formulate a list of pros and cons of using the test, drug, or device.
- Assess the extent to which the particular offering is likely to achieve client goals.
- Explain the possible effects of the test, drug, or device on self, family, and others (psychological, physical, and economic).
- Provide ongoing advice, resources, and support as needed.
3. Refer clients to genetic counselors for further discussion (see Box 5-1 on genetic counseling).

The other perspective views justice as equalizing benefits across society regardless of merit. This latter view is justice as fairness. The tendency when discussing the provision of health care for a society is to focus on justice viewed as fairness and as favoring equality. However, when the discussion turns to allocation of scarce resources, such as organs for transplant, one can detect in the discussion a justice standard that favors merit rather than equality. There are interesting and complex philosophical debates about the use of justice as merit, but they are beyond the scope of this chapter. Instead we will focus on the requirements of justice viewed as fairness, because inequalities in health care exacerbate and are exacerbated by economic disadvantages stemming from a variety of causes.

The social justice arrangements in a society are indicative of what the society values (Crawford, 2006). In democratic societies, the requirements of social justice generally include equitable distribution of the benefits and burdens of societal life. "Justice as fairness" reflects the ideas behind Rawls' (1971, 1999) *A Theory of Justice*. Rawls identifies two "rules of justice that he argues will enable humankind to resolve disputes fairly and justly" (Buchanan, 2000, p. 156). "First: each person is to have an equal right to the most extensive liberty compatible with a similar liberty for others. Second: social and economic inequalities are to be arranged such that they are both (a) reasonably expected to be to everyone's advantage, and (b) attached to positions and offices open to all" (Rawls, 1971, p. 60). Rawls formulates these rules as a result of his hypothetical method for deciding how a society's institutions should be arranged in order to provide for fairness. Rawls proposes that these rules of justice would emerge as a result of an average person's reasoning from behind a "veil of ignorance" (ignorant about their place in society, personal assets, or handicaps) about what social arrangements they would prefer if they did not know what their personal impediments or assets were going to be. Rawls' theory, although respected by ethicists, is subject to criticism on a variety of fronts. The most significant criticism for present purposes is that justice as fairness does not provide much guidance for some common social problems such as abortion, welfare, and the righting of previous wrongs (e.g., affirmative action, the rights of native people) and ignores the problems of those without legal rights such as undocumented workers (Buchanan, 2000; MacIntyre, 2007; Taylor, 1985). However, the standard of equality gives health-promotion professionals a ground to argue the need for just health care provisions and to criticize current conditions of inequity (Kass, 2004).

An emphasis on justice in health care settings is sometimes called the impartialist perspective in that it considers the needs of all who fall under its umbrella. For example, within the prison system, this view of justice would mandate access to care for prisoners in need. Thus it would not permit arbitrary obstacles to access (such as requiring good behavior or favors) that might be presented by prison officers or by other prisoners who wish to exert physical or psychological control. Justice would also require improved access to care for the poor and underprivileged, both in terms of receiving care and transportation or local availability of services.

Although justice might require consideration of the special needs of a disadvantaged group, it does so impartially: that is, it does not distinguish among the particulars of individuals. Each member within the group has an equal right to whatever is proposed. In an economically and profit-driven health care system injustices occur both at the local and societal levels. Because justice viewed as fairness is impartial about individual differences, that moral perspective taken alone is not a perfect tool with which to look at health care disparities and their causes. The combination of justice, feminist concerns about power and oppression, and the acknowledged responsibilities of health care professionals to promote health permit a comprehensive view of problems associated with health protection and promotion. This view incorporates problems both for a society and for individuals within the society. Buchanan (2000) captures this necessary synthesis of perspectives well, noting "the mutually reinforcing relationships among justice, caring and responsibility" which will help health care professionals to "enable people to live well" (p. 167).

STRATEGIES FOR ETHICAL DECISION-MAKING
Locating the Source and Levels of Ethical Problems

Many problems associated with health promotion are not moral or **ethical dilemmas** in the sense described earlier. Although some dilemmas occur and must be addressed, most health-promotion problems are moral or ethical issues in the sense that obstacles exist that prevent an individual from living life well and flourishing, or obstacles exist that prevent or interfere with societal goals related to health. Throughout this chapter discussions of both the larger (societal) and narrower (individual) perspectives have been emphasized and their relationships highlighted. Sometimes tensions between the two require mediation and may force the health promoter to decide which problem must be addressed first. For example, a nurse at a family practice clinic cares for a teenager who is morbidly obese. At the level of the client the nurse is charged with discovering underlying causes of the obesity (e.g., physical, psychological, contextual) and designing strategies in concert with the client to help resolve the problem. However, as a professional who has, both anecdotally and on researching the issue, noted that this is an increasingly prevalent problem, the nurse has responsibilities also to address the issue at the more political level in concert with interested others. As Norton (1998) notes, "health promotion . . . includes a variety of activities such as lobbying to bring about healthy public policy at both government and local levels" (p. 1270).

To address health-promotion issues effectively, professionals need to possess not only their particular disciplinary expertise and an understanding of ethical language, principles, and perspectives, but also a willingness to understand their own values and preconceptions about health and people. Understanding personal philosophy, biases, and values permits one to control for these in the sense of being aware of the influences they have over our interactions with others.

Values Clarification and Reflection

Gaining confidence in moral decision-making is a slow process. The following are suggestions that will permit development related to recognizing and addressing ethical issues.

Examine Beliefs and Values

Cultivate the habit of examining what are your personal values and **beliefs** related to the human condition, justice, and responsibility. Be willing to revise your beliefs in line with your professional knowledge base, experiences, or current research findings. For example, how do beliefs that "people get what they deserve" correlate with what we know—for example, that those of lower socioeconomic status have lower levels of health and that poor health interferes with functioning and is associated with depression? How do our attitudes change when we try to place ourselves in the context of the other person's life?

This is not to say that maintaining personal integrity is not important—it is. Maintaining both personal and professional integrity is essential to good practice. Integrity has to do with a sense of wholeness of the self and consistency of actions with truly examined beliefs and values. "Nurses have both personal and professional identities that are neither entirely separate nor entirely merged, but are integrated" (ANA, 2001, p. 19). Tenet 5 of the ANA (2001) *Code of Ethics for Nurses With Interpretive Statements* validates the nurse's preservation of integrity in those situations in which he or she feels that personal integrity is compromised. It notes that "where a particular treatment, intervention, activity or practice is morally objectionable to the nurse . . . the nurse is justified in refusing to participate on moral grounds" (ANA, 2001, p. 20). When this involves risk to the client, though, other arrangements must be made to safeguard client care.

A true examination of beliefs and values requires a willingness to admit that these may not always be justifiable—they may be remnants from childhood indoctrinations of various sorts. For example, one might believe that certain ethnic groups are inferior in some way, or that one should not question authority. An honest and ongoing examination of one's values and biases permits one to control for these in situations in which personal values and biases are irrelevant to the care of clients.

The Influence of Personal Beliefs and Values

An understanding of how personal beliefs and values are either congruent, or are liable to interfere, with the task at hand is crucial to ethical problem solving. In any given situation, the nurse or allied health professional must ask himself or herself, "What are my beliefs and biases in this situation? How are these likely to influence my actions?" For

example, if the home health nurse believes her below–poverty level, depressed, obese, diabetic client who smokes is responsible for the poor healing of her own leg ulcer, she may be less inclined to work with the client to discover and address the client's goals.

Reflection on Practice

A third helpful strategy is to reflect on situations afterward to discover what worked, what didn't work, and what could be done differently in the future. It is often helpful to interact with peers or other experts after particularly difficult situations to discover alternative perspectives or resources for the purposes of future problem solving.

Decision-Making Considerations

Decision-making in health-promotion settings has inescapable moral components. This is true for the reasons outlined earlier, related to professional responsibility to further the good for individuals and society. Thus the careful exercise of experience, skill, and knowledge is warranted when trying to formulate the best course of action for a given individual or group, or in resolving particular as well as societal health-promotion problems. This framework is offered as a way of ensuring that clarity about a particular case or situation is gained. Because of the diverse nature of health-promotion activities, no straightforward models of decision-making can realistically be applied in all situations. Additionally, it is often true of such issues that decision-making is an ongoing process. Revisions to plans may be required in light of new information. The following are all important facets of decision-making but do not necessarily occur in the order given.

Identify the Main Problem or Issue

What level of problem is this: social, group, or individual? If the location of the problem is societal, it will also impact individuals and groups and a decision has to be made about the order of interventions. Try to determine the main ethical principle involved or whether it is a problem of conflicting principles. For example, in order to provide benefit to the client his autonomy must be overridden. Is this a social justice issue? An autonomy issue? What factors led to the problem? Is there coercion or are there other power imbalances? Who has an interest in maintaining the power imbalances and who gains the most from the imbalance? These are the questions feminist ethics would ask.

Determine Who or What Created the Problem

Who has a stake in the issue and in how it will be resolved? Answering this question will permit a determination of whose input is crucial to the decision-making process. Who or what are important considerations (institutions, individuals, businesses, social policy)? Does this issue result from a failure to predict the consequences of certain social policies?

Determine the Prevalent Values

What are the values held by all the different players? Are there value conflicts? The value conflicts might be individual versus social, as in the case of a client with tuberculosis who refuses to take his medicines, thus putting at risk members of his family or of the community. Values conflicts might also be interpersonal among the health-promotion team or personal versus professional. As a general rule, more weight is assigned to the values of the individual who is most likely to be affected by a decision. It is important to consider the influence of culture on values when the issue has to do with health promotion for culturally diverse groups. It is important to involve people who can help sort out the cultural beliefs, especially when language difficulties are present. A knowledgeable but neutral interpreter may be helpful when liaison between groups is needed.

Identify Information Gaps

This is a good place to reflect upon whether the decision maker(s) are confident about what they do and do not know. This is not always an easy task. Information may exist that has not yet reached our awareness, or we might fail to ask a question that would reveal important information. How can we be confident about the scope and limits of our knowledge? Clinical judgment is a good tool but is not foolproof. When doubts exist or the decision is likely to have serious or risky consequences, we need to involve knowledgeable others or try to determine the best places to gain missing information.

Formulate Possible Courses of Action and Probable Consequences

Courses of action may involve further information gathering, brainstorming, and possibly collaboration with other experts or specialists. Although further data may be needed to resolve problems at the level of individuals or small groups, it is especially necessary to enlist additional help when the issue is one that requires political action to bring about policy changes. It may be necessary to bring in community members and leaders or to enlist the political power of specialty groups. Finally, a determination must be made about which proposed courses of action will be the least harmful and the most beneficial.

Initiate the Selected Course of Action and Evaluate the Outcome

Does the actual outcome match the anticipated outcome? If not, what happened that was unexpected? Would this have been foreseeable given more data? Would you do things differently in another similar situation given what you've learned? Does the problem need to be addressed at a different level (institutional or public policy)?

Engage in Self-Reflection and Peer or Expert Group Reflection

What could you have done differently? Would consulting with others have altered your conception of the problem or your course of action? What insights can you or your peers glean from this that could be appropriate for similar situations in the future? How might continuing education opportunities help you or your peers more appropriately address similar problems in the future? Would an ethics resource (committee or consultant) be helpful in such situations? Could you use this case as a focused learning experience for your peers and collaborators?

ETHICS OF HEALTH PROMOTION: CASES*

Some cases of especial relevance to health-promotion are presented below. They are followed by questions that can be answered by individual readers, but they also provide a good starting point for group discussion. Try using the decision-making strategies suggested throughout the chapter as you explore these problems. It is anticipated that you will want more information than is provided. Deciding what extra information would be helpful is an important part of the exercise.

Case 1 Addressing Health Care System Problems—Elissa Needs Help

Elissa is 38 years old. She recently moved 200 miles from her home to a small town (population 6000) and separated from her abusive husband to escape his continuing threats and to be near her childhood friend. She suffers from chronic, sometimes incapacitating, depression for which she has in the past received antidepressant medications and counseling, with temporary relief. She has been unable to work and has no private health insurance. She is eligible for the state's Medicaid program, however, and has recently discovered that Medicaid will cover her health care needs. Her friend refers her to the only primary care center in the area, where she is seen by Jill, one of the two nurse practitioners. As part of her evaluation, Jill discovers that Elissa was also abused as a child and has very poor self-esteem, although Elissa affirms that her childhood friend is very supportive. Jill believes that longer term psychological counseling would benefit Elissa and facilitate her well-being, but she also knows that none of the counseling services within a 50-mile radius accepts Medicaid payment. Elissa has no transportation.

What are Jill's options? Responsibilities?
What actions might she pursue both on a local level and a political level?
What are her resources?
What is the responsibility of the health-promotion disciplines in cases like this?

Case 2 Assisted Suicide or Emotional Support?—Ana and Victor

A nurse in a clinic is accountable for ongoing assessments of pain management in a population with chronic pain. One of the long-term clients, Ana, has required increasing

*The authors acknowledge the contributions of Carolyn Hayes, who contributed some of these cases.

amounts of narcotics for her pain management over the last year. The nurse has known for over a year that Ana's husband, Victor, has amyotrophic lateral sclerosis, or Lou Gehrig's disease. Victor's disease adds a great deal of stress to both their lives, which has had a negative effect on Ana's physical health. The nurse assesses the emotional toll of Victor's illness as part of Ana's pain assessment. During one of these discussions, Ana asks the nurse how much of her narcotic medication her husband would need to take to end his life.

What does it mean to provide someone with the "means" to commit suicide?

What questions would you have for Ana at this point of the conversation?

What would you do with the answers?

Do you have any obligations to Victor?

Do you collaborate with Victor's physician?

What is in Ana's "best interests"?

Who or what are your resources?

What does nursing as a discipline say about assisted suicide?

What is the law in your state?

What should you do?

Case 3 How Much Money Can One Person Spend?—Joe Does Not Like Taking Pills

A nurse practitioner is caring for people in an economically poor neighborhood. An older woman, Rose, frequently runs out of inhalers for her asthma. The insurance does not pay enough per month for her to be able to use the inhalers as directed. She struggles along as best she can but frequently cancels outings with loved ones because she "can't always catch her breath and it scares the little ones." The nurse practitioner has tried to advocate for more medication. Time and time again, the response of the insurance company is, "There is only so much money to spread around."

Across the street is Joe, who has been a client for nearly 3 years. He needs to take diuretic medications to avoid frequent hospitalizations. He does not like to think of himself as a "man who needs pills." Consequently, he does not take the diuretic medication, resulting in preventable hospitalizations. If he changed his pattern of behavior, there would be money for Rose to receive more medication.

What are the ethical questions in this scenario?

Ethically, can the nurse practitioner tell Joe about Rose's situation to try to persuade him to take his pills?

Is there anything that the nurse practitioner should do individually to resolve this dilemma? Is there anything that nursing as a discipline should do?

What course of action would be in Rose's best interest?

Case 4 She's My Client!—Lilly and "Jake" (a.k.a. Paul)

A nurse practitioner is at a conference when a physician colleague discusses a difficult case. One of his clients, "Jake," is HIV positive but refuses any treatment. The physician explains that Jake fears that his wife will discover and recognize the names of the medications, because he knows "these drug names are discussed on television all the time." He has not told, nor does he ever intend to disclose to his wife, that he is HIV positive. Jake firmly believes his condition is his private information and, for now, the couple uses condoms for birth control. The physician is concerned that Jake will not tell his wife. The physician is presenting this case to colleagues to highlight the public awareness campaigns that, to some extent, have affected client privacy. He argues, "Listen to how they call out your name and the drugs at the pharmacy counter."

The nurse practitioner recognizes bits and pieces of information and comes to the painful realization that Jake is really Paul, and Paul is the husband of one of her clients, Lilly. Lilly has begun to discuss with you that she wants to get pregnant soon. The town is too small for the nurse practitioner to be mistaken. Or is it?

Is it ethical for the nurse practitioner to ask the physician if Jake is Paul?

Is it ethical for her to tell Lilly she suspects Paul is HIV positive?

Should this information change how she counsels Lilly about a pregnancy?

What is in Lilly's best interests?

What resources are available?

SUMMARY

Health promotion is a vast and complex practice area; consequently, the associated ethical challenges are diverse and multileveled. This chapter has outlined the nature and purpose of health care ethics and related this to the responsibilities of health care providers practicing health promotion. Health promotion should be viewed as a moral undertaking of health care professionals. Health care professionals will have gained some of the tools and language needed to explore ethical issues, discuss these with others, and address problematic issues at both the individual and the societal levels. A selection of contemporary issues was used to illustrate points and provide examples. This selection represents a very small portion of potential contemporary problems; nevertheless, the tools and strategies provided are not specific to these problems but can be used to explore issues particular to their specialty settings. Perhaps the most important factor to keep in mind is that practice problems manifesting at the level of the individual almost always have their origins in the broader societal environment.

CASE STUDY

Genetic Screening Programs

Knome, Inc. in Cambridge, Massachusetts, has been sequencing the DNA of 20 individuals. With the individuals' consent, the results will be made available to researchers. Each person will be offered "a guided tour of areas of concern where genetic variations might indicate a higher prosperity to develop" a life-threatening condition.

There are hopes that genetic screenings of large populations will change the practice of health care from a focus on treating diseases to preventing them. Some researchers predict the complete sequencing of each human genome will become routine data available to health care providers, as are the common measurements of blood pressure, pulse, temperature, and blood counts today.

Other research data show, for example, that asking people about their family history of diabetes, their weight, and their age are for better predictors than reading their DNA of whether they will one day develop diabetes.

At present, Knome Inc.'s genetic analyses are done by a laboratory in Beijing, China, take 4 to 6 months to complete, and cost $350,000 for each sequence of DNA.

Reflective Questions:

1. What are your initial thoughts about these DNA analogues?

Apply different concepts and theories of ethics (presented in this chapter) in thinking about the following questions.

2. What are some of the ethical issues of these analyses?
3. What are the responsibilities of health care professionals in the genetic screenings of population?
4. What additional components could a community health nurse add to the following plan of care for participants having their DNA sequenced?

References

Beery, T. A., & Shooner, K. A. (2004). Family history: the first genetic screen. *Nurse Practitioner: American Journal of Primary Health Care, 29*(11), 14–25; Kayton, A. (2007). Newborn screening a literature review. *Neonatal Network—The Journal of Neonatal Nursing, 26*(2), 85–95; Kirsner, S. (2008). Innovation economy: mapping out a nascent market. *Boston Globe.* August 10, 2008 pp. G1 and G5; Lashley, F. R. (2007). *Essentials of clinical genetics in nursing practice.* New York: Springer; Prue, C. E., & Daniel, K. L. (2006). Social marketing: Planning before conceiving preconception care. *Maternal and Child Health Journal, 10*(5), S79–S84; Sheridan, S. L., Harris, R. P., Woolf, S. H. (2004). Shared decision making about screening and chemoprevention. A suggested approach from the U.S. Preventive Services Task Force. *American Journal of Preventive Medicine, 26,* 55–66.

CARE PLAN

Genetic Screening Programs

The use of developments in genetics research, including genetic counseling, testing, and screening, as well as advanced therapeutic and reproduction choices, influence the health of both present and future generations throughout the world.

As previously addressed in several areas of this chapter, health care professionals have many complex ethical responsibilities in the applications of these genetic developments with local, national, and international communities, as well as with individuals and families.

The community health nurse in the case study at the end of this chapter addresses selected aspects of the current ineffective therapeutic management of genetic screenings in a community in the following care plan.

Nursing Diagnosis: Ineffective Community Therapeutic Regimen Management

Definition: Pattern in which a community experiences (or is at risk to experience) difficulty integrating a genetic screening program for the prevention/treatment of illness and reduction of risk situation.

DEFINING CHARACTERISTICS

Major: Community verbalizes desire to manage the genetic screenings and treatment of illness and prevention of sequels.

Community verbalizes difficulty with regulation and integration of prescribed regimens for genetic screening and treatment of illness and its effects or prevention of complications.

Minor: Knowledge of risk factors for illness (expected or unexpected) is accelerated

RELATED FACTORS

Treatment Related

Complexity of genetic screening and therapeutic regimen
Complexity of health care
Financial costs
    Actual cost of procedure
    Potential (e.g., loss of health insurance)
Side effects
    Expected (e.g., anxiety)
    Unexpected (e.g., despair)

Situation/Environment Related

Health and health care needs, multiple and complex, especially for vulnerable population (e.g., unborn children)

Presence of known and unknown environmental (including occupational) health hazards

Availability of community resources for screening for risk factors of diseases

  Less expensive (e.g., family health histories and physical exams)

  More expensive (e.g., genetic screenings)

Overall needs and financial resources

EXPECTED OUTCOMES

With the community health nurses' guidance community members will:

  Evaluate the actual and potential (e.g., significant increases in birth rates) health problems and resources of the community.

  Identify community resources that are needed to promote health and prevent illness, including genetic screenings.

  Participate in program development as needed to improve the effectiveness of the therapeutic regimen management of genetic screening programs.

INTERVENTIONS

1. Complete a community assessment including:
  Actual and potential health problems and needs
  Actual and potential resources for health
2. Develop an overall program plan for genetic screenings
3. Develop a specific program for the genetic screening of an individual, perhaps including the following components:
  Complete initial interview, individual and family histories, and physical exam with appropriate laboratory studies
  Generally discuss the genetic screenings and informed consent, focusing on the concerns of the individual and/or family
4. Assess barriers to learning:
  Physical condition
  Sensory status (e.g., vision, hearing)
  Intelligence, learning abilities/disabilities
  Emotional state(s) (e.g., fears, guilt)
  Stressors, concerns

5. Provide information:
  Explain needed knowledge and perhaps changes (e.g., lifestyle behaviors)
  Discuss and add to individual's knowledge of the pros and cons of genetic screening
  Identify influencing factors to decision-making about individual's genetic
6. Perform screenings (e.g., depression, financial resources)
7. Give time to integrate new information, perhaps having a second appointment to:
  Readdress questions
  Develop informed consent, including policies on privacy
8. Perform actual genetic screening procedure
9. Explain results with genetic and reproductive counseling
10. Repeat and follow-up as necessary

REFERENCES AND SOURCES OF FURTHER INFORMATION

Carpenito-Moyet, L. J. (2007). *Understanding the nursing process: Concept mapping and care planning for students.* Philadelphia: Lippincott. For greater details (including an excellent discussion on knowledge, deficient knowledge, and teaching and learning strategies with human responses, alterations, and patterns of dysfunction) for planning care especially see pp. 302–310.

Carpenito-Moyet, L. J. (2008). *Handbook of nursing diagnosis* (12th ed.). Philadelphia: Lippincott. Compare the diagnostic criteria for Ineffective Therapeutic Regimen Management with other differential diagnosis potentially present in the case study.

Gordan, M. (2008). *Assess notes. Nursing assessment and diagnostic reasoning.* Philadelphia: F.A. Davis.

Grace, P. J., & McLaughlin, M. (2005). When consent isn't informed enough: What's the nurse's role when a patient has given consent but doesn't fully understand the risk? *American Journal of Nursing, 105*(4), 79–84.

Lashley, F. R. (2007). *Essentials of clinical genetics in nursing practice.* New York: Springer.

For more thorough information on planning care with genetic screenings in communities, see pp. 250–295 (Chapter 12, Community and public health nursing and genomics, and Chapter 13, Trends, social policies and ethical issues in genomics).

REFERENCES

Agich, G. J. (2003). *Dependence and autonomy in old age: An ethical framework for long-term care* (2nd ed.). New York: Cambridge University Press.

American Nurses Association. (1994). *Position statement: The nonnegotiable nature of the ANA code for nurses with interpretive statements.* Washington, DC: Author.

American Nurses Association. (2001). *Code of ethics for nurses with interpretive statements.* Washington, DC: Author.

American Nurses Association. (2003). *Nursing's social policy statement* (2nd ed.). Silver Springs, MD: Author.

American Nurses Association. (2008). *Guide to the code of ethics for nurses: Interpretation and application.* Washington, DC: Author.

Andrews, L. B., Mehlman, M. J., & Rothstein, M. A. (2002). *Genetics: Ethics, law and policy.* West Group/Thompson: St. Paul, MN.

Atkins, K. (2006). Autonomy and autonomy competencies: A practical and relational approach. *Nursing and Philosophy, 7*(4), 205–215.

Ballou, K. A. (2000). A historical-philosophical analysis of the professional nurse obligation to participate in sociopolitical activities. *Policy, Politics, & Nursing Practice, 1*(3), 172–184.

Bandman, E. L., & Bandman, B. (2001). *Nursing ethics through the life span* (4th ed.). Upper Saddle River, NJ: Prentice Hall.

Beauchamp, T. L., & Childress, J. F. (2008). *Principles of biomedical ethics* (6th ed.). New York: Oxford University.

Beauchamp, T. L., & Walters, L. (2002). *Contemporary issues in bioethics* (6th ed.). Belmont, CA: Wadsworth.

Benner, P., Tanner, C. A., & Chesla, C. A. (1998). *Expertise in nursing practice: Caring, clinical judgment, and ethics.* New York: Springer.

Bennett, P., & Smith, S. J. (2007). Genetics, insurance and participation: How a Citizen's Jury reached its verdict. *Soc Sci Med, 64*(12), 2487–2498.

Bereano, P. (2000). Does genetic research threaten our civil liberties? Retrieved May 24, 2004, from *www.actionbioscience.org/genomic/bereano.html*.

Braun, U. K., Beyth, R. J., Ford, M. E., & McCullough, L. B. (2008). Voices of African American, Caucasian, and Hispanic surrogates on the burdens of end-of-life decision making. *Journal of General Internal Medicine*, 23(3), 267–274.

Brown, L. (1993). *The new shorter Oxford English dictionary*. New York: Oxford University Press.

Buchanan, A. E., & Brock, D. W. (1990). *Deciding for others: The ethics of surrogate decision making*. New York: Cambridge University.

Buchanan, D. R. (2006). Moral reasoning as a model for health promotion. *Social Science & Medicine*, 63(10), 2715–2726.

Buchanan, D. R. (2000). *An ethic for health promotion: Rethinking the sources of human well-being*. New York: Oxford University.

Burkhardt, M. A., & Nathaniel, A. K. (2001). *Ethics and issues in contemporary nursing* (2nd ed.). Albany, NY: Delmar.

Chambliss, D. F. (1996). *Beyond caring: Hospitals, nurses, and the social organization of ethics*. Chicago: University of Chicago Press.

Clarfield, A. M., Gordon, M., Markwell, H., & Alibhai, S. M. (2003). Ethical issues in end-of-life geriatric care: The approach of three monotheistic religions—Judaism, Catholicism, and Islam. *Journal of the American Geriatrics Society*, 51(8), 1149–1154.

Clarke, D. B. (1998). The Patient Self-Determination Act. In J. F. Monagle & D. C. Thomasma (Eds.), *Health care ethics: Critical issues for the 21st century* (pp. 92–113). Gaithersburg, MD: Aspen.

Crawford, R. (2006). Health as a meaningful social practice. *Health*, 10(4), 401–420.

Cribb, A., & Duncan, P. (2002). *Health promotion and professional ethics*. Malden, MA: Wiley-Blackwell.

Davis, A., Aroskar, M. A., Liaschenko, J., & Drought, T. S. (1997). *Ethical dilemmas & nursing practice* (4th ed.). New York: Prentice Hall.

Dickey, S. B., & Deatrick, J. (2000). Autonomy and decision making for health promotion in adolescence. *Pediatric Nursing*, 26(5), 461–467.

Donchin, A., & Purdy, L. (1999). *Embodying bioethics: Recent feminist advances*. Lanham, MD: Rowman & Littlefield.

Dworkin, G. (2002). Paternalism. In E. N. Zalta (Ed.), *The Stanford encyclopedia of philosophy*. Retrieved June 1, 2004, from *http://plato.stanford.edu/archives/win2002/entries/paternalism/*.

Etzioni, A. (1999). Medical records. Enhancing privacy, preserving the common good. *Hastings Center Report*, 29(2), 14–23.

Fagerlin, A., & Schneider, C. E. (2004). Enough. The failure of the living will. *Hastings Center Report*, 34(2), 30–42.

Fry, S. T. (1990). The philosophical foundations of caring. In M. Leininger (Ed.), *Ethical and moral dimensions of care* (pp. 13–24). Detroit: Wayne State.

Gaylord, N., & Grace, P. (1995). Nursing advocacy: An ethic of practice. *Nursing Ethics*, 2(1), 11–18.

Gilligan, C. (1982). *In a different voice: Psychological theory and women's development*. Cambridge, MA: Harvard University Press.

Goldberg, A. I. (2000). Commentary. *Cambridge Quarterly of Healthcare Ethics*, 9(1), 113–117.

Gostin, L. O. (1997). Personal privacy in the health care system: Employer-sponsored insurance, managed care, and integrated delivery systems. *Kennedy Institute of Ethics Journal*, 7(4), 361–376.

Grace, P. J. (1998). *A philosophical analysis of the concept 'advocacy': Implications for professional-person relationships*. (Doctoral dissertation, University of Tennessee, Knoxville, 1998). Dissertation Abstracts, International, UMI No 9923287.

Grace, P. J. (2001). Professional advocacy: Widening the scope of accountability. *Nursing Philosophy*, 2(2), 151–162.

Grace, P. J. (2004). Ethics in the clinical encounter. In S. Chase (Ed.), *Clinical judgment and communication in nurse practitioner practice* (pp. 295–332). Philadelphia: F. A. Davis.

Greater Dallas Council on Alcohol and Drug Abuse. (2002). *Candy flavored cigarettes gain popularity*. Dallas: Author. Retrieved May 28, 2004, from *www.gdcada.org/stories/print/bidi.pdf*.

Häyry, M. (2006). Public health and human values. *Journal of Medical Ethics*, 32(9), 519–521.

Heikkinen, A. M., Wickström, G. J., Leino-Kilpi, H., & Katajisto, J. (2007). Privacy and dual loyalties in occupational health practice. *Nursing Ethics*, 14(5), 675–690.

Hodge, J. G., Jr. (2000). National Health Information Privacy and New Federalism. *Notre Dame Journal of Law, Ethics and Public Policy*, 14(2), 791–820.

Hull, S. C., & Prasad, K. (2001). Reading between the lines: Direct-to-consumer advertising of genetic testing in the USA. *Reproductive Health Matters*, 9(18), 44–48.

International Council of Nurses. (2000). *The ICN code of ethics for nurses*. Geneva, Switzerland: Author. Retrieved February 8, 2005, from *www.icn.ch/icncode.pdf*.

Kant, I. (1997). *Foundations of the metaphysics of morals* (Trans. L. W. Beck). In A. I. Melden (Ed.), *Ethical theories: A book of readings* (2nd ed., pp. 317–366). Englewood Cliffs, NJ: Prentice Hall (Original work published 1785).

Kass, N. E. (2004). Public health ethics: From foundation and frameworks to justice and global public health. *Journal of Law, Medicine, and Ethics*, 32(2), 232–242.

Kohlberg, L. (1981). *The philosophy of moral development: Moral stages and the idea of justice. Essays on moral development* (Vol. 1). San Francisco: Harper & Row.

Kohlberg, L. (1984). *The psychology of moral development: The nature and validity of moral stages. Essays on moral development* (Vol. 2). San Francisco: Harper & Row.

Kulynych, J., & Korn, D. (2002). Use and disclosure of health information in genetic research: Weighing the impact of the new federal medical privacy rule. *American Journal of Law & Medicine*, 28(2–3), 309–324.

Levine, C., Glajchen, M., & Cournos, F. (2004). A fifteen-year-old translator. *Hastings Center Report*, 34(3), 10–12.

Liaschenko, J. (1999). Can justice coexist with the supremacy of personal values in nursing practice? *Western Journal of Nursing Research*, 21(1), 35–50.

Liaschenko, J., & Peter, E. (2003). Feminist ethics. In V. Tschudin (Ed.), *Approaches to ethics: Nursing beyond boundaries* (pp. 33–43). New York: Butterworth Heinemann.

MacIntyre, A. (2007). *After virtue: A study in moral theory* (3rd ed.). Southbend, IN: Notre Dame University.

Marks, R., & Shive, S. E. (2007). "Health for all": An ethical imperative or unattainable ideal? *Health Promotion Practice*, 8(1), 28–30.

Marmot, M., & Wilkinson, R. G. (2006). *Social determinants of health* (2nd ed.). New York: Oxford University.

May, T. (2002). *Bioethics in a liberal society: The political framework of bioethics decision making*. Baltimore, MD: Johns Hopkins University.

McCullough, L. B. (1998). Preventive ethics, managed practice, and the hospital ethical committee as a resource for physician executives. *HEC Forum*, 10(2), 136–151.

McGowan, T. (1995). *The black death*. New York: Watts Franklin.

Miles, S. H., Koepp, R., & Weber, E. P. (1996). Advance end-of-life treatment planning: A research review. *Archives of Internal Medicine*, 156(10), 1062–1068.

Mill, J. S. (2002). *Utilitarianism* (2nd ed). Indianapolis, IN: Hackett (Originally published 1861).

Morrison, E. E. (2008). *Health care ethics: Critical issues for the 21st century* (2nd ed). Sudbury, MA: Jones & Bartlett.

National Society of Genetic Counselors. (1992). National Society of Genetic Counselors code of ethics. *Journal of Genetic Counseling*, 1(1), 41–43.

National Society of Genetic Counselors. (2004). National Society of Genetic

Counselors *code of ethics*. Retrieved June 3, 2004, from *www.nsgc.org/newsroom/code_of_ethics.asp*.

Nelson, H. L. (1992). Against caring. *The Journal of Clinical Ethics*, 3(1), 8–20.

Newton, L. H. (1988). Lawgiving for professional life: Reflections on the place of the professional code. In A. Flores (Ed.), *Professional ideals* (pp. 47–56). Belmont, CA: Wadsworth.

Norton, L. (1998). Health promotion and health education: What role should the nurse adopt in practice? *Journal of Advanced Nursing*, 28(6), 1269–1275.

Olthuis, G., Dekkers, W., Leget, C., & Vogelaar, P. (2006). The caring relationship in hospice care: An analysis based on the ethics of the caring conversation. *Nursing Ethics*, 13(1), 29–40.

Orem, D. (2001). *Nursing concepts of practice* (6th ed.). St. Louis: Mosby.

Ovrebo, B. (2001). Health promotion and civil liberties: The price of freedom and the price of health. In D. Callahan (Ed.), *Promoting healthy behavior: How much freedom? Whose responsibility* (pp. 23–36). Washington, DC: Georgetown University Press.

Parker, E., Gould, T., & Fleming, M. (2007). Ethics in health promotion—reflections in practice. *Health Promotion Journal of Australia*, 18(1), 69–72.

Pemberton, D. (2005). Breastfeeding, co-sleeping and the prevention of SIDS. *British Journal of Midwifery*, 13(1), 12–18.

Peter, E., Lunardi, V. L., & Macfarlane, A. (2004). Nursing resistance as ethical action: Literature review. *Journal of Advanced Nursing*, 46(4), 403–416.

Portillo, C., & Waters, C. (2004). Community partnerships: The cornerstone of community health research. *Annual Review of Nursing Research*, 22, 315–329.

Powers, M., & Faden, R. (2006). *Social justice: The moral foundations of public health and health policy*. New York: Oxford University Press.

President's Commission for the Study of Ethical Problems in Medicine and Biomedical and Behavioral Research (President's Commission). (1982). *Compensating for Research Injuries: The Ethical and Legal Implications of Programs to Redress Injured Subjects*. Washington, DC: U.S. Government Printing Office.

Rachels, J., & Rachels, S. (2006). *The elements of moral philosophy* (5th ed.). New York: McGraw-Hill.

Rawls, J. (1971 and 1999). *A theory of justice*. Cambridge, MA: Harvard University.

Resnik, D. B. (2007). Responsibility for health: Personal, social, and environmental. *Journal of Medical Ethics*, 33(8), 444–445.

Ross, L. F. (1997). Health care decision making by children. Is it in their best interest? *Hastings Center Report*, 27(6), 41–45.

Shirley, J. L. (2007). Limits of autonomy in nursing's moral discourse. *Advances in Nursing Science*, 30(1), 14–25.

Singer, P. (1993). *A companion to ethics*. Cambridge, MA: Wiley-Blackwell.

Spenceley, S. M., Reutter, L., & Allen, M. N. (2006). The road less traveled: Nursing advocacy at the policy level. *Policy Politics, & Nursing Practice*, 7(3), 180–194.

Tarasoff v. Regents of University of California. (1976, July 1). California Supreme Court 131. California Reporter, *14*.

Taylor, C. (1985). *Philosophy and the human sciences. Philosophical papers* (Vol. 2). Cambridge: Cambridge University.

Thorne, S., & Varcoe, C. (1998). The tyranny of feminist methodology in women's health research. *Health Care for Women International*, 19(6), 481–493.

Tones, K. (1997). Health education as empowerment. In M. Siddell, L. Jones, J. Katz, & A. Peberdy (Eds.), *Debates and dilemmas in promoting health: A reader* (pp. 33–42). Basingstoke, UK: Macmillan/Open University.

Tong, R. (1996). *Feminist approaches to bioethics: Theoretical reflections and practical applications*. Boulder, CO: Westview Press.

U.S. Department of Health and Human Services. (2003). *Fact sheet: Protecting the privacy of patients' health information*. Washington, DC: Author. Retrieved May 24, 2004, from *www.hhs.gov/news/facts/privacy.html*.

U.S. Department of Health and Human Services. Office for Civil Rights. (2004). *HIPAA Privacy Rule*. Retrieved May 24, 2004, from *www.hhs.gov/ocr/hipaa/*.

U.S. Department of Health and Human Services. Public Health Service. (2000). *Healthy people 2010 Understanding and improving health*. Washington, DC: U.S. Government Printing. Retrieved Febraury 25, 2009, from *www.healthypeople.gov*.

U.S. Department of Health and Human Services. Public Health Service. (2005). *Healthy People 2010 Mid-course review*. Washington, DC: U.S. Government Printing. Retrieved Febraury 25, 2009, from *www.healthypeople.gov/Data/midcourse*.

Vig, E. K., Starks, H., Taylor, J. S., Hopely, E. K., & Fryer-Edwards, K. (2007). Surviving surrogate decision-making: What helps and hampers the experience of making medical decisions for others. *Journal of General Internal Medicine*, 22(9), 1274–1279.

Warren, V. L. (2001). From autonomy to empowerment: Health care ethics from a feminist perspective. In W. Teays & L. Purdy (Eds.), *Bioethics, justice, & health care* (pp. 49–53). Belmont, CA: Wadsworth.

Weir, R. F., & Peters, C. (1997). Affirming the decisions adolescents make about life and death. *Hastings Center Report*, 27(6), 29–40.

Weithorn, L. A., & Campbell, S. B. (1982). The competency of children and adolescents to make informed treatment decisions. *Child Development*, 53(6), 1589–1598.

Weston, A. (2005). *A practical companion to ethics* (3rd ed.). New York: Oxford University.

Wilmot, S. (2000). Nurses and whistleblowing: The ethical issues. *Journal of Advanced Nursing*, 32(5), 1051–1057.

Windt, P. Y. (1989). Introductory essay. In P. Y. Windt, P. C. Appleby, M. P. Battin, L. P. Francis, & B. M. Landesman (Eds.), *Ethical issues in the professions* (pp. 1–24). Englewood Cliffs, NJ: Prentice Hall.

Wood-Harper, J. (2005). Informing education policy on MMR: Balancing individual freedoms and collective responsibilities for the promotion of public health. *Nursing Ethics*, 12(1), 43–58.

Unit Two

Assessment for Health Promotion

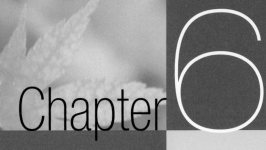

Chapter 6

Anne Rath Rentfro

Health Promotion and the Individual

objectives

After completing this chapter, the reader will be able to:

- Define the framework of functional health patterns as described by Gordon.
- Describe the use of the functional health pattern framework to assess individuals throughout the life span.
- Illustrate health patterns of the functional, potentially dysfunctional, and actually dysfunctional categories of behavior.
- Identify risk factors or etiological aspects of actual or potential dysfunctional health patterns to consider with nursing diagnoses.
- Discuss planning, implementing, and evaluating nursing interventions to promote the health of individuals.
- Develop specific health-promotion plans based on an assessment of individuals.

key terms

Age-developmental focus
Culturally competent care
Expected outcomes
Functional focus

Functional health patterns
Health status
Individual-environmental
 focus

Nursing diagnosis
Nursing interventions
Pattern focus
Risk factors

website materials

evolve These materials are located on the book's website at *http://evolve.elsevier.com/Edelman/*.
- WebLinks
- Study Questions
- Glossary
- Website Resources
  6A: Relationship Between Selected Developmental Tasks and Wellness Tasks for Each Life
     Cycle Stage
  6B: Functional Health Patterns Assessment for an Adult

Sections of this chapter are modified from the curriculum of the Adult Health Nursing, Master of Science Program, Boston College Graduate School of Nursing, Chestnut Hill, MA; Gordon, M. (2008). *Nursing diagnosis: Application to clinical practice* (12th ed.). Philadelphia: Lippincott Williams & Wilkins.

Assessment of Alcohol Consumption

Women have different patterns of alcohol consumption and different thresholds for problem drinking than men. Instruments such as the CAGE detect alcohol dependence and would not be a sensitive enough measure for some women, in particular pregnant women, who are less likely than men to be alcohol dependent. The T-ACE provides a much more sensitive measure of alcohol intake patterns than that derived from the CAGE test (considered Cutting down on drinking, been Annoyed by criticism of drinking, feeling Guilty about drinking, and using alcohol as an Eye opener). Instead, women are better assessed using the T-ACE test. This test, developed for use with women, was the first validated screening tool for assessing drinking risk in pregnant women. A pattern of drinking is established using the following questions:

   T–How many drinks does it **Take** to make you feel high?
   A–Have you ever been **Annoyed** by people criticizing your drinking?

   C–Have you ever felt you ought to **Cut down** your drinking?
   E–Have you ever had a drink first thing in the morning **(Eye opener)** to steady your nerves or get rid of a hangover?

   Scores are calculated as follows:
- A reply of more than two drinks to question T is considered a positive response and scores 2 points, and an affirmative answer to question A, C, or E scores 1 point, respectively.
- A total score of 2 or more points on the T-ACE indicates evidence of problem drinking during pregnancy (McNamara, Orav, WilkinsHaug, & Chang, 2005; McNamara et al., 2006.

1. Why would a nurse tailor the assessments to individual characteristics of a population?
2. How effectively would this screening tool identify alcohol problems in women other than the pregnant women within the population? Why?

Nursing promotes health by encouraging the use of processes in patterns that lead toward wellness. Health and illness within this context reflect changing patterns of the life process. Holistic nursing acts as a central unifying theme to connect pattern recognition to the examination of person-environment relationships throughout the life span. Disorganization or ineffective coping produce fluctuations in patterns that eventually result in illness. Patterns of strength, according to Newman's Theory of Health as Expanding Consciousness, redirect the individual toward more harmonious patterns of health promotion (Fawcett, 2005).

In the United States the health promotion initiative called *Healthy People 2010* has established national goals and provides a framework for prevention (U.S. Department of Health and Human Services, 2000). *Healthy People 2010* established national health objectives that identified the most significant preventable threats to health. A midcourse review of the indicators has been published for communities to use to evaluate progress, and plans for *Healthy People 2020* have begun (U.S. Department of Health and Human Services, 2007). See *www.healthypeople.gov*. Long before the current focus on health promotion with the Healthy People initiatives in the United States (U.S. Department of Health and Human Services, 2000), Florence Nightingale expressed the belief that the laws of both health and nursing are similar and pertinent to both the sick and the well individual (Nightingale, 1992).

The National Council of State Boards of Nursing (NCSBS) defines nursing practice as "assisting individuals or groups to maintain or attain optimal health, implementing a strategy of care to accomplish defined goals and evaluating responses to care and treatment"(National Council of State Boards of Nursing, 2001). Although this broad definition provides a model for state nursing practice acts, the familiar terminology from American Nurses Association's (ANA's) Social Policy statement is more concise. "Nursing is the protection, promotion, and optimization of health and abilities, prevention of illness and injury, alleviation of suffering through the diagnosis and treatment of human response, and advocacy in the care of individuals, families, communities, and populations" (ANA, 2003). Assessment, diagnosis, outcome criteria, process criteria (including planned interventions), implementation, and evaluation provide the framework for the nursing process.

Primary prevention includes generalized health promotion and specific protection from disease, which fall within this scope of nursing practice. The active process of health promotion involves protection (immunizations, occupational safety, and environmental control) along with lifestyle, value, and belief system behaviors that enhance health. Many reference materials describe the medical model of assessment of an individual's biophysical states, including the comprehensive review of systems and physical examination conducted by the nurse, physician, or physician's assistant (Bickley & Szilagyi, 2006). The nurse, however, expands the medical model framework with additional assessment of interactions among a person's biophysical, psychosocial, and spiritual states and patterns with the environment (Fawcett, 2005; Weber & Kelley, 2006). Selected examples of the *Healthy People 2010* (2007) objectives related to individuals are presented in the *Healthy People 2010* box. For the further development of these goals, see the Midcourse Review.

With health promotion serving as the underlying theme, this chapter addresses nursing assessment of individuals. In most areas of nursing, tertiary care and prevention of further disease provide the assessment focus. This focus limits

Healthy People 2010

Selected Examples of National Health-Promotion and Disease Prevention Objectives for Individuals from *Healthy People 2010 Midcourse Review* (2007)

- 13-6a. Increase the proportion of sexually active people who use condoms.
- 22-2. Increase the proportion of adults who engage regularly, preferably daily, in moderate physical activity for at least 30 minutes per session.
- 22-7. Increase the proportion of adolescents who engage in vigorous physical activity that promotes cardiorespiratory fitness 3 or more days per week for 20 or more minutes per occasion.
- 25-11. Increase the proportion of adolescents who abstain from sexual intercourse or use condoms if sexually active.
- 27-1a. Reduce cigarette smoking by adults.

From U.S. Department of Health and Human Services. (2007). *Healthy people 2010 midcourse review.* Retrieved February 5, 2008, from *www.healthypeople.gov/Data/midcourse/.*

reflection to problem solving and thus excludes promotion of overall general health and wellness. Concentrating on strengths in the health-promotion setting provides a foundation to help individuals move toward improved health. Nurses support and enhance the ability of healthy individuals to maintain or strengthen their health. Most nursing diagnoses approved by the North American Nursing Diagnosis Association (NANDA) are problem oriented. The NANDA definition of **nursing diagnosis** includes life processes as well as actual or potential health problems. Although most approved nursing diagnoses reflect a focus on deficit assessment and problem solving, this inclusion of life processes provides a broad base for nursing diagnoses to use strength-based healthy responses or potential for healthy responses (Stolte, 1996). One function of nursing diagnoses in well individuals is to focus on human developmental or maturational tasks.

Current health care systems continue to use deficit assessment rather than the strength-based approach that is more appropriate for health-promotion settings. Mental health, social work, and nursing, however, embrace a strength-based approach to assessment within the health promotion context. From using infant competencies to plan care and person-centered approaches for care of people with dementia, nurses incorporate strength-based assessment into their diagnostic process (Perez et al., 2002; Warchol, 2006). The NANDA approved 11 wellness-oriented definitions for health promotion in 2003 with a call for new nursing diagnosis development for these diagnoses in 2005 (Lavin & Scroggins, 2002; North American Nursing Diagnosis Association—International, 2005). Although the organization calls for work in this area, published material for using wellness diagnoses appears infrequently. In one study

of a small occupational health service (McKeown et al., 2003), a review of 491 employee records revealed the frequent use of wellness-oriented diagnoses such as health-seeking behaviors and knowledge deficit. In that same year NANDA published a poster that described a qualitative study of 51 college students that explored the use of wellness diagnoses. In this study Leiby and Powelson (2003) describe the expression of a desire for improved self-concept, physical health, and athletic performance as a possible criterion for a wellness diagnosis of the potential for enhanced exercise. More work is necessary to develop useful nomenclature for health promotion and wellness diagnoses.

Gordon's (2007) framework, which uses a **functional health patterns** assessment, provides the foundation for most NANDA nursing diagnoses. As NANDA continues to develop wellness diagnoses for health promotion, Gordon's framework will most likely continue to provide the foundation for these diagnoses. This same framework is used throughout this chapter to demonstrate assessment approaches with the family and community (see Chapters 7 and 8). This chapter also discusses components of the nursing process as they relate to health promotion of the individual (Gordon, 2007).

FUNCTIONAL HEALTH PATTERNS: ASSESSMENT OF THE INDIVIDUAL

Nursing assessment determines the **health status** of individuals. Table 6-1 demonstrates aspects of a complete nursing assessment. Assessment, in this case, refers to collection of data that culminates in problem identification or a

Table **6-1**	Aspects of a Nursing Assessment
Definition	**Deliberate and Systematic Data Collection**
Components	Subjective data: Health history, including subjective reports and individual perceptions Objective data: Observations of nurse Physical examination findings Information from health record Results of clinical testing
Function	Description of person's health status
Structure	Organization of interdependent parts describing health, function, or patterns of behavior that reflect the whole individual and environment
Process	Interview, observation, and examination
Format	Systematic but flexible; individualized to each person, nurse, and situation
Goal	Nursing diagnosis or problem identification Identification of areas of strengths, limitations, alterations, responses to alterations and therapies, and risks

diagnostic statement. Determining the deficit or diagnosis stems from judgments about data collected (ANA, 2004). Effective health assessment considers not only physiological parameters, but also how the human being interacts with the whole environment. Behavior patterns, beliefs, perceptions, and values form the essential components of health assessment when maximal health potential of the individual is considered by nurses. Pattern recognition supports our understanding of health of individuals and is reflected in nursing theories such as those initially developed by Newman and Rogers (Fawcett, 2005).

Historically, conceptual models in nursing have employed Gordon's health-related behaviors (Campbell, 2006; Murphy, 2004). Gordon's (2007) 11 functional health patterns interact to depict an individual's lifestyle. Using this framework, nurses combine assessment skills with subjective and objective data to construct patterns reflective of lifestyles.

Functional Health Pattern Framework

Holism and the totality of the person's interactions with the environment form the philosophical foundations of Gordon's functional health patterns. This foundation provides a context for collecting data that provide information about the entire person and most life processes. By examining functional patterns and interactions among patterns, nurses accurately determine and diagnose actual or potential problems, intervene more effectively, and facilitate movement toward outcomes to promote health and well-being (Gordon, 2007). In addition to providing a framework to assess individuals, families, and communities holistically, functional health patterns provide a strong focus for more effective **nursing interventions** and outcomes. This stronger focus provides a solid position from which nurses participate as decision makers in health care systems at organizational, community, national, and international levels.

Definition

Functional health patterns view the individual as a whole being using interrelated behavioral areas. The typology of 11 patterns serves as a useful tool to collect and organize assessment data and to create a structure for validation and communication among the health care providers. Each pattern described in Table 6-2 forms part of the biopsychosocial-spiritual expression of the whole person. Individual reports and nursing observations provide data to differentiate patterns. As a framework for assessment, functional health patterns provide an effective means for nurses to perceive and record complex interactions of individuals' biophysical state, psychological makeup, and relationships to the environment.

Characteristics

Functional health patterns are characterized by their focus. Gordon (2007) uses five areas of focus: (1) pattern, (2) individual-environmental, (3) age-developmental, (4) functional, and (5) cultural.

Pattern focus implies that the nurse explores patterns or sequences of behavior over time. Gordon's term *behavior* encompasses all forms of human behavior, including biophysical, psychological, sociological elements. Pattern recognition, a cognitive process, occurs during information collection. Cues are identified and clustered while gathering information. Patterns emerge that represent historical and current behavior. Quantitative patterns such as blood pressure are readily identified, and pattern recognition is facilitated when baseline data are available. As the nurse incorporates a broader range of data, patterns imbedded within other patterns begin to emerge. Blood pressure, for example, is a pattern within both the activity and exercise patterns. Individual baseline and subsequent readings may present a pattern within expected norms. Erratic blood pressure measurements indicate an absence of pattern. This lack of

Table **6-2**	Typology of 11 Functional Health Patterns
Pattern	**Description**
Health perception–health management pattern	Individual's perceived health and well-being and how health is managed
Nutritional-metabolic pattern	Food and fluid consumption relative to metabolic needs and indicators of local nutrient supply
Elimination pattern	Excretory function (bowel, bladder, and skin)
Activity-exercise pattern	Exercise, activity, leisure, and recreation
Sleep-rest pattern	Sleep, rest, and relaxation
Cognitive-perceptual pattern	Sensory, perceptual, and cognitive patterns
Self-perception–self-concept pattern	Self-concept pattern and perceptions of self (body comfort, body image, and feeling state); self-conception and self-esteem
Roles-relationships pattern	Role engagements and relationships
Sexuality-reproductive pattern	Person's satisfaction and dissatisfaction with sexuality and reproduction
Coping–stress tolerance pattern	General coping pattern and effectiveness in stress tolerance
Values-beliefs pattern	Values, beliefs (including spiritual), or goals that guide choices or decisions

Modified from Gordon, M. (2007) *Manual of nursing diagnosis* (11th ed.). Sudbury, MA: Jones and Bartlett.

pattern forms its own type of pattern. Functional health pattern categories provide structures to analyze factors within a category (blood pressure: activity pattern) and to search for causal explanations, usually outside the category (excessive sodium intake: nutritional pattern) (Gordon, 2007).

Food intake examples illustrate the **individual-environmental focus** of Gordon's framework (Gordon, 2007). Reference to environmental influence occurs within many patterns in the form of physical environments within and external to the individual. Environmental influences in functional health patterns include role relationships, family values, and societal mores. Personal preference, knowledge of food preparation, and ability to consume and retain food govern the individual's intake. Cultural and family habits, financial ability to secure the food, and crop availability also influence food intake. Additionally, the person who secures, prepares, and serves the food, such as the mother or father, controls nutritional intake for children.

Each pattern also reflects a human growth and **age-developmental focus** (Hockenberry & Wilson, 2006). Individual fulfillment of developmental tasks increases complexity. These tasks, however, provide learning opportunities for the individual to maintain and improve health. Over 25 years ago, Bruhn, Cordova, Williams, and Fuentes (1977) proposed a framework to organize specific health tasks for the individual to accomplish at each developmental phase of the life cycle, as identified by Erikson (1994) and Havighurst (1972) (see **Website Resource 6A**). These sources continue to provide the foundation for contemporary assessment of individuals' health status. Developmental tasks begin at birth and continue until death. By considering current epidemiological data and recommended health behaviors, Gordon's framework continues to be useful today for health promotion throughout the life span (Gordon, 2007). Therefore, Unit 4 uses Gordon's framework to explore developmental tasks and their related health behaviors for health promotion.

Functional focus refers to an individual's performance levels. Disciplines other than nursing plan care using functional patterns, but assessment data vary. Physical therapists and occupational therapists, for example, focus on physical ability to perform activities of daily living and rely on assessments of independence of personal activities of daily living to develop their plans (Bottari et al., 2007). For physicians, genitourinary functions refer to frequency or voiding patterns and characteristics of urine, such as color, odor, and laboratory analysis results. In addition to these factors of genitourinary function, nurses assess how the particular voiding pattern affects lifestyle, particularly how urinary frequency affects sleep patterns and the ability to perform activities such as shopping or socializing. Additional concerns might include the individual's ability to walk or climb stairs to the bathroom or to manage these activities safely at night.

Culture, age, developmental, and gender norms, considered during assessment, influence the development of health patterns. Madeline Leininger defines transcultural nursing concepts of cultural care, health, well-being, and illness patterns in different environmental contexts and under different living conditions (Leininger & McFarland, 2006). **Culturally competent care** is delivered with knowledge of and sensitivity to cultural factors influencing health behavior. Complex cultural patterns transmitted from former generations contribute to individuals' health behavior. Culturally competent care respects the underlying personal and cultural reality of individuals. Nurses provide more culturally competent care when they identify and use cultural norms, values, and communication and time patterns in their interpretation of assessment information (Andrews & Boyle, 2008; Berman et al., 2008; Dossey et al., 2004; Leininger & McFarland, 2006).

Functional health patterns form a framework that centers on health. Most nursing assessments use functional pattern assessment as a foundation. Although nursing theoretical and conceptual frameworks vary, the functional health pattern framework is relevant to most conceptual models. In fact, functional health patterns provide the structure used by NANDA to support nursing diagnosis nomenclature. Nursing classification and outcome nomenclature also use Gordon's functional patterns as a foundation (Berman et al., 2007). Advantages of a functional health pattern framework specific to the practice of nursing include the following:

- Provides a consistent nursing focus through a means of collecting, organizing, presenting, and analyzing data to arrive at nursing diagnoses.
- Allows the flexibility to tailor content for individuals and situations.
- Suits diverse practice arenas (e.g., home, clinic, institution) for assessment of individuals (adult/children), families, or communities.
- Supports theoretical components of nursing (education and research) by organizing clinical knowledge using nursing diagnoses, interventions, and outcomes.
- Incorporates medical science data while retaining the focus on nursing knowledge.

The Patterns

Each pattern reflects a biopsychosocial spiritual expression of the individual's lifestyle or life processes from the perspective of both the individual and the nurse. This expression reveals (1) a pattern or sequencing of behaviors, (2) the role of the environment (physical surroundings, family, societal, and cultural influences), and (3) developmental influences. The assessment of each pattern as functional (strengths), dysfunctional (nursing diagnosis), or potentially dysfunctional includes an indication of the individual's level of satisfaction with the pattern. Nurses assess reported problems in more depth to generate an explanation for the problem, remedial actions to take, and the perceived effect of these actions from the individual's perspective. An important goal in assessing each pattern is to determine the individual's knowledge of health promotion, the ability to manage health-promoting activities, and the value that the individual ascribes to health promotion. Each pattern is presented in this chapter, with details for nurses to use to assess individuals and determine diagnoses using a functional health pattern framework along with a discussion of nursing implications for use of the patterns in practice.

Health Perception–Health Management Pattern

The Health Perception–Health Management pattern involves individuals' health status and health practices used to reach current level of health or wellness with a focus on perceived health status and meaning of health (Gordon, 2007). When eliciting this information, nurses discover areas for further exploration under other functional health patterns. For example, when an individual can no longer mow the lawn without suffering shortness of breath or severe back pain, the nurse stores the information to retrieve later when assessing activity and exercise patterns or cognitive-perceptual patterns.

Health perception–health management patterns affect lifestyle and ability to function even when individuals do not perceive actual health problems, are unaware of necessary health promotion in the absence of problems, do not feel capable of managing their health, or believe activity on their part is useless to promote health. Health-promoting activities (adequate nutrition, activity and exercise, sleep and rest), routine professional examinations, self-examinations, immunizations, and safety precautions (auto safety restraints and locked medicine cabinets) provide this pattern's clues to improve or maintain optimal quality of life.

Assessment objectives for health perception–health management consist of obtaining data about perceptions, management, and preventive health practices (Gordon, 2007). Exploring values identifies potential health hazards, such as noncompliance to a prescribed medical or nursing regimen or inability to manage health effectively.* In addition to these kinds of assessment cues, nurses identify unrealistic health and illness perceptions and expectations.

Assessment includes the following parameters:

- Health and safety practices of the individual
- Previous patterns of adherence or compliance
- Use of the health care system
- Knowledge of health service availability
- Health-seeking behavior patterns
- Means to access to health care (e.g., financial resources, health insurance, and transportation)

In addition to methods of health management, nurses explore health perceptions as individuals describe their current health status, past problems, and anticipation of future problems associated with health or health care. These expectations indicate beliefs about health, locus of control, and level of knowledge about their health status of the various ethnic groups emerging in the United States (Wilson & Dorne, 2005) (Multicultural Awareness box). Health and illness perceptions significantly influence overall direction for care planning. Health beliefs, also discussed under the values-beliefs pattern, directly impact participation in care. Individuals are less apt to engage in self-care or preventive measures when they (1) believe it is the responsibility of health team members to keep them healthy, (2) do not recognize or acknowledge their susceptibility to an impending health problem, or (3) believe that they cannot influence their own health status (Callaghan, 2006).

Past health management serves as a predictor of future health management (Daniels, 2006). If adherence to a prescribed regimen has not occurred in the past, recurrence is unlikely unless the nurse is able to identify and remedy the causes of a person's noncompliance. For example, an individual with high blood pressure who has failed to keep follow-up appointments, often forgotten to take medication, and eaten foods with high sodium content should be assessed to determine whether this evident noncompliance is based on a conflict within the value system of the individual (health beliefs), inaccurate information, misunderstanding, inadequate ability to learn, retain, or retrieve information (knowledge deficit), or denial of illness (health perception). Variables such as financial resources, transportation difficulties, nutritional preferences, daily activities (individual and family patterns), and ability to read written instructions (literacy or visual acuity) may affect the individual's behaviors.

Nutritional-Metabolic Pattern

Nutritional-metabolic patterns center on nutrient intake relative to metabolic need (Gordon, 2007). This pattern includes individuals' descriptions of food and fluid consumption (history) as well as evidence of adequate nutrition (physical examination). Nurses ask individuals about their satisfaction with current eating and drinking patterns, including restrictions, and their perceptions of problems associated with eating and drinking, growth and development, skin condition, and healing processes.

Intake and supply of nutrients to tissues and organs influence bodily functions and interact with lifestyle. Sufficient food and fluid intake provides energy for performance of activities, which includes internal physiological functioning of the organs and the external body movements. Interruption in acquisition or retention of food or fluids offsets balance and significantly alters lifestyle. Nutrition and metabolism also govern the growth rates.

*The terms, cues, or clues to problems mentioned within this section refer to defining characteristics identified by NANDA (Gordon, 2007).

MULTICULTURAL AWARENESS

Health Perspectives for Emerging Majority Groups in the United States

Group	Traditional Definitions		Traditional Methods	
	Health	Illness	Maintain/Protect Health	Restore Health
American Indian and Alaska Native population	Total harmony with nature Survive extremely challenging situations	Price paid for past/future Details specific to nations Results from presence of evil spirits Contagious/generalized symptoms Human body considered as whole, with harmony between origins and superficial structures Integration within context of environment Imbalance of ying and yang (Chinese)	Maintain positive relationship with nature Treat body with respect Purification acts using water herbal remedies and rituals	Removal of external causative factor by traditional healer after special ceremony to determine cause Drumming
Asian population	Total physical & spiritual harmony with universe For majority religious traditions pose variations on cultural values Examples respect for life moderation basic relationships balance between evil and good	Human body considered as whole with harmony between organs and superficial structures Integration of human body within context of environment Imbalance of ying and yang	Body is gift from parents/ancestors; must be protected Dietary practices Formal daily exercise (tai chi) Amulets (Chinese)	Acupuncture applying poultices Cupping Bleeding Massage Herbal remedies Other products Use physicians Women treat women Use of immunizations Important to keep the body intact (Chinese) Amulets
African population	Process/energy force rather than a state Consists of body/mind/spirit harmony with nature Older adults held in high esteem	Harmony; illness attributed to demons and evil spirits Pain as sign of illness If no pain then illness is gone	Dietary practices Rest; clean environment Laxatives/cod liver oil taken internally sulfur and molasses on back Protective material of various substances (copper/silver/dried flesh) prayer	Voodoo and magic Cared for the entire community Prayer Use of healers Pictures–Catholic saints/relics Sugar and turpentine herbs, minerals, oral preparations including hot water and lemon garlic, flannel with camphorated oil
Hispanic population	Gift from God	Imbalance in body; punishment for wrong doing Imbalance between hot and cold/wet and dry (definitions vary) Dislocation of body parts Magic or supernatural causes such as evil	Maintain equilibrium in the universe through behavior diet and work	Prayer, dietary practices of hot/cold magic/religious rituals, artifacts Frequently in Catholic and Pentecostal traditions such as offerings, confession, candles, laying of hands Folk holistic healers using herbs, prayer, massage, social rapport, spiritual

Adapted from Wilson, S. H., & Dorne, R. (2005). Impact of culture on the education of the geriatric patient. *Topics in geriatric rehabilitation*, 21(4), 282-294.

Assessment within this pattern includes data about typical patterns of food and fluid consumption, adequacy of consumption patterns, along with perceived problems associated with nutritional intake. Nurses attend to cues to conditions of overweight, underweight, overhydration, dehydration, or difficulties in skin integrity, such as breakdown or delayed healing. Individuals may also be at risk for developing these problems.

Parameters for assessment for this pattern fall into two broad categories of evaluation: (1) nutrient intake and (2) metabolic demand. Intake may be assessed with a 24-hour recall of food and fluid consumption; a listing of dietary restrictions, food allergies, vitamin supplements, and caffeine and alcohol ingestion (when not included in the medication history); and a schedule of eating and drinking patterns. Assessment includes screening for problems associated with swallowing or chewing.

With identified problems, focused assessments include food preferences, feelings about present weight, and eating habits. Intake may be affected when individuals eat alone. Frequent dining out may indicate the need for further exploration within the nutrition area or other functional patterns. Diets may consist of fast food. Consumption patterns may be deficient in essential vitamins or minerals. Food security may also be explored. Who purchases food? Is shopping preplanned with a grocery list? Are financial resources and food budgets adequate? Is food stored properly? Who prepares food? How is food prepared (fried, broiled, steamed, boiled, or baked)?

Metabolic demands vary from individual to individual and within the same individual during times of illness, stress, growth, high or low activity levels, healing, or recovery. Developmental and environmental conditions alter metabolic demands. Appetite and reported changes in weight, skin integrity, and general healing ability are explored during the interview or health history. Individuals may also report decreased tolerances for hot or cold weather.

Nurses' observations and perceptions play a vital role when assessing nutritional and metabolic pattern. Physical examination allows assessment of both nutrient supply to the tissues and metabolic needs of the individual. Objective findings serve as indicators to validate subjective reports concerning nutrient intake. Gross metabolic indicators include temperature, height, and weight. Physical examination focuses on skin, bony prominences, dentition, hair, and mucous membranes. Skin and mucous membranes, in particular, use nutrients rapidly and provide excellent indices of nutritional adequacy. Skin assessment includes color, temperature, turgor, and evaluation of any skin lesions, areas of dryness, scaliness, rashes, pruritus, or edema. Mucous membranes are examined for color, integrity, moisture, and lesions. Dentition is evaluated for structure. Are teeth erupted at normal stages of development? Are teeth firmly implanted? Do dentures fit properly? Additionally, decay and evidence of oral hygiene are evaluated. Healing is assessed when there is evidence of injury.

Although problem identification occurs after assessment of all 11 functional health patterns, a problem in any one area serves as a clue to dysfunction in others. Assessment of one pattern facilitates synthesis and analysis of data collected in other functional health patterns. Nutrition and metabolism influence patterns of health management, elimination, activity, sleep, cognition, roles, and stress tolerance. The values-beliefs pattern may significantly alter all other functional patterns. Sociocultural values and ethnic backgrounds play a major role in the determination of eating patterns. Other areas to consider include eating habits, food preferences, and patterns of nutrient supply and demand across the life span. Raw fruits and vegetables may be fun "finger food" for the toddler, but the older adult, especially one with loose dentures or arthritis of the temporomandibular joint, may find these foods intolerable.

A nutritional pattern focus emphasizes educational needs. Assessment aims to demonstrate strengths in functional patterns along with disclosing dysfunctional or potentially dysfunctional patterns. Nutritional health-promotion activities present a strength that provides impetus for similar activities in the other patterns. For example, if balanced nutritional intake improves functional level, individuals may extend their health-promoting behaviors to stress reduction or other behaviors. Understanding food/fluid intake and balance of body requirements helps individuals adjust caloric intake as growth slows in order to prevent overweight problems during the adult years.

Elimination Pattern

Elimination patterns include bowel, bladder, and skin function. Nurses determine regularity, quality, and quantity of stool and urine through subjective reports about methods used to achieve regularity or control and any pattern changes or perceived problems. Perspiration quantity and quality determine excretory skin function (Gordon, 2007).

Elimination pattern significance varies from individual to individual. Many people view elimination patterns as a measure of health and as a sensitive indicator of proper nutrition and stress level. Individuals' perceptions determine whether patterns become problematic or dysfunctional. Assessment concerns usual patterns. Misconceptions about regularity exist, particularly of bowel function, and self-treatment commonly occurs to correct perceived problems.

Elimination pattern dysfunction affects interpersonal interactions (Berman et al., 2007). Lack of control affects body image (self-perception), activity level, socialization, and sleep patterns. Age, developmental levels, and cultural considerations direct the interview. Pediatric assessment includes toilet training methods, whereas adult assessment may focus on regularity and patterns of dysfunction

(Hockenberry & Wilson, 2006). In addition to constipation, older adults may begin to develop urinary control problems (Berman et al., 2007). Women past childbearing years often develop urinary stress incontinence (Berman et al., 2007; Wong et al., 2005).

Assessment includes data about regularity and control of excreta (Gordon, 2007). Nurses investigate cues suggesting constipation patterns, diarrhea, or incontinence through focused assessment. Elimination pattern changes, pain, discomfort, and perceived problems receive attention. Data collection includes exploration into the individual's explanation of the problem, methods of self-treatment, and perceived results (Gordon, 2007).

Quantity, quality (color, odor, and consistency), frequency and regularity of stool, urine, and perspiration determine the direction of further exploration. Nurses assess excretory mode, time patterns, and control. Nurses encourage discussion about pattern changes, perceived problems, and elimination habits. Examination includes gross screening of specimens, noting amount, consistency, color, and odor. Skin assessment includes careful observation and description of wound/fistula drainage.

Transition from nutrition to elimination pattern assessment can occur seamlessly. Fluid intake affects elimination. Dietary fiber affects bowel elimination patterns. Skin integrity heralds concerns about urinary incontinence, leading to additional discussion of elimination patterns. Direct questions about laxatives may be necessary because of the availability of over-the-counter treatments for constipation. Discrepancies between dietary intake and reported bowel regularity indicate the need for further questioning. Laxative dependency in the form of oral supplements, suppositories, or enemas may indicate knowledge deficits in the area of bowel elimination (Berman et al., 2007). Health education about normal bowel function, nutritional guidelines to assist the individual in elimination, or an exercise program may significantly improve elimination pattern dysfunction. Urinary frequency requires health education as well. Research indicates that prolonged time between urinations is linked to urinary tract infections (Stevens, 2005). Evidence-based practice guides the nurse in establishing a more suitable elimination routine for the individual.

Activity-Exercise Pattern

The activity-exercise pattern centers on activity level, exercise program, and leisure activities. Parameters include movement capability, activity tolerance, self-care abilities, use of assistive devices, changes in pattern, satisfaction with activity and exercise patterns, and any perceived problems (Gordon, 2007). Limitations in movement capabilities or ability to perform activities of daily living significantly alter lifestyle and may affect every other functional health pattern. Movement

and independent functioning in self-care is almost universally valued. Child-rearing practices demonstrate this value: parents boast about their infant who walks early, their toilet-trained toddler, and their preschooler who dresses without assistance.

Activity-exercise patterns provide effective indicators for commitment to health promotion and prevention (Figure 6-1). Exercise's impact on health status has been extensively documented with increased public awareness. Overweight and obesity, linked to sedentary lifestyle, has reached an epidemic state with prevalence of overweight in adults at 66% and projections of overweight as high as 75% of the adult population (Wang & Beydoun, 2007). Obesity prevalence in adolescents has tripled since 1999 (Ogden et al., 2006; U.S. Department of Health and Human Services, 2007). Obesity is currently second only to cigarette smoking in mortality from preventable disease in the United States (Centers for Disease Control and Prevention, 2005). Assessment and planning to prevent obesity has a major impact on the nation's health.

Activity-exercise patterns also indicate energy expenditure and activity tolerance levels. Movement directly affects activities of daily living along with control of the immediate environment. Environment contributes to mobility as well. For example, individuals living alone in high-crime areas may limit activity for fear of harm. Factors such as inclement weather, distance from public transportation, and negotiating stairways with a cane can also influence decisions about activity. Environmental barriers significantly impair exercise-activity patterns for individuals with neuromuscular or perceptual disturbances. Moreover, leisure activities provide clues to individuals' value systems. For example, American work ethic, competitiveness, stage in career, and age influence how individuals perceive leisure and recreational activities (Beatty & Torbert, 2003; Pogson et al., 2003).

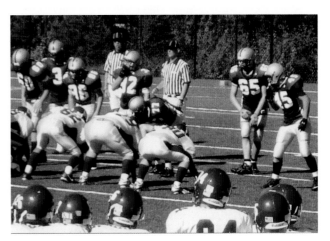

Figure 6-1 The activity of an adolescent provides an indicator of the individual's commitment to health promotion.

The objective of assessment within the activity-exercise pattern is to determine the pattern of activities that require energy expenditure. Components reviewed are exercise, activity, leisure, and recreation (Gordon, 2007). The nurse seeks clues to discover strengths and weaknesses within the pattern. Decreased energy levels, perceived problems, coping strategies, changes within the patterns, and associated explanations for these changes are all important clues that require further exploration. Generally, individuals with respiratory or cardiac disease warrant in-depth assessment, and focused assessment is indicated for individuals with neuromuscular, perceptual, or circulatory impairments.

Dimensions to be described and assessed within the activity-exercise pattern include daily activities, leisure activities, and exercise. Daily activities include (1) occupation (position, hours of work or school, and amount of physical exercise versus cognitive or sedentary activities), (2) self-care abilities (feeding, bathing, grooming, dressing, and toileting), and (3) home-management routines (cooking, cleaning, shopping, laundry, and outdoor activities) (Gordon, 2007). Problems within any of these areas require explanation. Is it a problem of energy expenditure, mobility limitations, or decreased motivation caused by depression, grieving, or incongruent values?

Exercise parameters include type, frequency, duration, and intensity of the individual's regular exercise. Nurses also assess the value the individual places on exercise as a part of determining their feelings about it. A 24-hour recall of the previous day's activities provides an initial picture of the pattern whereas each major component addresses specific elements. Weekly logs provide follow-up assessment for suspected problems. In addition to weekly logs, focused assessments include details about modes of transportation. Is a car used for transportation? If public transportation is used, how far away is the route? Are elevators or stairs used more often? (Gordon, 2007). Factors interfering with exercise or mobility include dyspnea, fatigue, muscle cramping, neuromuscular or perceptual deficits, chest pain, and angina. As with other patterns, feelings of satisfaction and perception of problems provide valuable indications of dysfunctional or potentially dysfunctional patterns.

Nurses evaluate subjective complaints, such as dyspnea, noting difficulty with breathing during the interview and physical examination. Examination includes circulatory, respiratory, and neuromuscular indicators. Assessment also includes skin color, skin temperature, apical heart rate, radial heart rate, and blood pressure, as well as respiratory rate, rhythm, depth of inspiration, and effort involved. Gait, posture, and balance are evaluated during ambulation. Muscle tone, strength, coordination, and range of motion provide useful clues to validate reports of activity and exercise. Assistive devices or prostheses are evaluated for proper use, proper fit, and degree of assistance or support provided (Berman et al., 2007).

Information obtained during the interview is linked closely to the examination. Examination alone may not disclose the invaluable subjective reports of early morning pain and joint stiffness. When appropriate, the nurse may ask the individual to climb stairs or perform self-care activities under observation to assess impairment. Direct observation validates assessment findings. Various instruments have been designed to quantify level of ability or disability. For some individuals, a metabolic activity index, in which each activity is measured according to kilocalories of energy expended per minute, helps to quantify assessment results and plan care.

Developmental norms have been established for infants and toddlers. Milestones such as sitting, crawling, walking, running, and hopping determine a child's development (Hockenberry & Wilson, 2006). Careful assessment of ability, limitations, and interests helps to guide the nurse in a more holistic assessment. Problem identification is reserved for the conclusion of the assessment after all 11 patterns have been constructed. Useful clues within a pattern lead into other pattern areas; however, premature closure of a topic during the exam is avoided. At this point, only tentative diagnoses are possible. Often explanations of problems lie in other functional health patterns. For example, when the individual expresses an inability to perform exercise on a routine basis, barriers may be discovered in another pattern. Barriers may be associated with knowledge deficit, personal or family value system, overriding priorities, or low value placed on exercise. Is the inability to perform activities a result of general fatigue caused by inadequate or decreased sleep time associated with anxiety, nocturia, pain, or an infant waking every 3 hours for feeding? Are responsibilities associated with caring for several preschoolers and inadequate financial resources to secure a babysitter the cause? The assessment's purpose is to narrow the number of possible explanations.

Sleep-Rest Pattern

Perhaps the single most important factor assessed in the sleep-rest pattern is the perception of adequacy of sleep and relaxation. Subjective reports of fatigue or energy levels provide some indication of the individual's satisfaction. People make assumptions about the roles that sleep and rest play in preparing the individual for required or desired daily activities. This pattern becomes extremely important when sleep and rest are perceived as insufficient. Sleep serves a restorative function in most individuals. Sleep deprivation studies provide vivid demonstrations of the need for different types of sleep: light, deep, dream, and rapid eye movement sleep. Again, problems within this pattern may cause problems in other patterns. A person who has difficulty with sleep may be tense and irritable, unable to tolerate stress, more prone to infectious processes, and incapable of making health-promoting relationships. Alterations in appetite, elimination difficulties, and activity intolerance will likely be experienced (Berman et al., 2007). Some degree of cognitive dysfunction generally occurs.

The objective when assessing the sleep-rest pattern is to describe the effectiveness of the pattern from the individual's perspective (Berman et al., 2007; Gordon, 2007). Wide variation in sleep time (from 4 hours to more than 10 hours) does not necessarily affect functional performance; different individuals require different amounts of sleep. Pertinent information includes data suggestive of difficulties with sleep onset, sleep interruptions, and awakening. The nurse also evaluates disturbances such as dreaming and nightmares, sleepwalking, nocturnal enuresis, and penile tumescence. Counseling, institution of safety measures, or medical referral may be necessary. In addition to sleep, the nurse assesses rest and relaxation according to the individual's perceptions. Activities of the sedentary isolate type, such as reading or crocheting, may be relaxing for some individuals. Passive involvement, as with television viewing, may provide the only source of relaxation for the individual. Daily naps or relaxation exercises (meditation, yoga, or breathing exercises) may also be a part of this pattern.

Assessment parameters of the sleep dimension are divided into two parts: (1) sleep quality and (2) sleep quantity. Sleep quality includes the individual's perception of sleep adequacy, performance level, and physical and psychological state on awakening. Sleep quantity, in addition to focusing on the hours slept each day, is used to build a schedule of sleep times. The nurse assesses for regularity the time of retiring, time of awakening, and additional periods of sleep throughout the day. Sleep onset, the number of awakenings, and reasons for them provide clues to problems. The dimensions of rest and relaxation include the parameters of type, frequency or regularity, and duration. The perceived effectiveness of methods used to promote rest is also assessed.

When problems exist, focused assessment that evaluates efficiency of sleep compared with actual sleeping time is warranted. Individuals are conditioned to sleep under certain circumstances, and maintaining bedtime rituals is a distinct advantage in sleep promotion. A person who expects to sleep usually will sleep if such routines are maintained. Nurses should assess schedule and routine changes associated with bedtime. When assessing bedtime routines, rituals along with other aids to sleep such as natural aids (warm milk) or medications (prescription and nonprescription) should be explored. Physical examination includes general appearance, behavior, and performance changes. As with pain, sleep is a subjective experience. Comprehensive examination may be performed (for example, with polysomnography), but discussion of this is beyond the scope of this text. Research indicates that subjective reporting of sleep quality and measures of sleep time closely approximate electroencephalographic findings.

Nursing care focuses on the need to identify evidence of sleep disturbances to design appropriate interventions before sleep deprivation occurs. Frequent awakenings do not necessarily imply sleep interruption. Many individuals awaken numerous times during the night but return to sleep within seconds. These awakenings occur in older adults who generally spend most of the night in stages of light sleep. Normal developmental pattern of aging does not include deep sleep; therefore, awakenings may not affect the sleep cycles. Older individuals, however, more often experience difficulty returning to sleep because they experience discomfort or anxiety. Biological rhythm and peak performance time may be helpful to the nurse when planning health education and return visits. Individuals commonly refer to themselves as morning people or night owls; therefore, patterns of retiring and arising provide clues. Patterns of sleep and rest in conjunction with subjective reports of physical and mental well-being help determine appropriate interventions.

Cognitive-Perceptual Pattern

Cognitive patterns include the ability of the individual to understand and follow directions, retain information, make decisions, solve problems, and use language appropriately. Auditory, visual, olfactory, gustatory, tactile, and kinesthetic sensations and perceptions determine perceptual and sensory patterns. Pain perception and tolerance are analyzed within this pattern area (Gordon, 2007). Capacity for independent functioning is considered a major role of thinking and perceiving. Compensation for cognitive-perceptual difficulties ensures safety. Health requires a balance between individual and environment. Decreased levels of cognition or perception require increased levels of environmental control. For example, mentally or sensory-impaired individuals may require sheltered work environments and supervised group living arrangements.

Interrelationships among the individual, the developmental stage, and the environment contribute to several patterns. For example, the behavior patterns of a 20-year-old high school "dropout" who works in a factory may differ from those of a 20-year-old second-year premedical student. Developmental stage plays a role in cognitive and perceptual abilities as well. Vision and hearing reach full potential when children reach school age with 20/30 vision considered normal in preschoolers. Developmental stage determines the ability to problem solve and conceptualize as described by the theorist Piaget (Hockenberry & Wilson, 2006). As adults mature, visual acuity, hearing, touch, and even taste decline. Cognitive function must be evaluated within the context of the environment (Gordon, 2007). Environmental complexity results in different levels of functioning.

Assessing cognitive-perceptual pattern includes evaluating language capabilities, cognitive skills, and perception related to desired or required activities (Gordon, 2007). Nurses address clues indicating potential problems, particularly sensory deficits, sensory deprivation or overload, and ineffective pain management. Cognitive dysfunction may cause impaired reasoning, judgment, or knowledge deficits related to health practices, as well as memory deficits.

Assessment parameters include hearing and vision test results. Changes in sensation or perception should be noted. In addition to decreased ability or acuity in hearing, vision, smell, and taste, evaluation includes other perceptual disturbances, such as vertigo; increased or decreased sensitivity to heat, cold, or light touch; and visual or auditory hallucinations or illusions. Use and perceived effectiveness of assistive devices, such as hearing aids, glasses, and contact lenses, is also noted.

Discomfort and pain are evaluated further. Useful tools that use pain scales have been designed to record and quantify changes in pain perception (Hadjistavropoulos et al., 2007). Location, type, degree, and duration of pain provide indicators of possible causes or sources. Relief measures used to control pain and their effectiveness provide data and a focus for health education. Medication, heat or cold applications, and relaxation are examples of relief measures that should be explored for their usefulness in a plan of care (Berman et al., 2007; Edwards et al., 2005; McCaffery & Pasero, 1999; McCaffrey et al., 2003). For all individuals, exploring tolerance to pain is appropriate, using questions such as "Do you feel you are particularly sensitive to pain?" and "What level of pain is associated with your (cut, sprain, broken bone, or labor contractions)?"

Other areas of cognitive patterning to be explored include educational level, recent memory changes, ease or difficulty in learning, and preferred method of learning. Even when no problems are apparent or suspected, the nurse may assess these areas in more detail to determine areas of strength for use with health teaching plans.

Objective data are accumulated throughout the interview or assessment process. This data collection begins with the nurse's perception of the individual's general appearance: hygiene and grooming, proper use of clothing, neatness and appropriateness of dress, and indication that these are appropriate to the individual's developmental stage. Language and vocabulary use, the ability to convey an idea with words or with actions when speech is impaired or not yet developed, and grammatical correctness provide clues to cognitive functioning. Amplitude and quality of speech, affect and mood, as well as attention and concentration are all indicative of the individual's mental status. For many individuals, this information is sufficient to relay a sense of the level of understanding, memory, and mentation. Problem-solving abilities usually can be determined when the individual is asked to relate any perceived problems, explanation of the problems, actions taken to solve the problems, and results of the actions taken. Because this is a basic assessment in each functional health pattern, the nurse already has an idea of whether thought processes are logical, coherent, and relevant for this individual.

When problems within the cognitive realm do not surface, the information is recorded as part of the objective data or findings of the physical examination. Data to be noted include language; vocabulary; attention span; grasp of ideas; level of consciousness; orientation to person, place, and time; language spoken (whether primary or secondary); and behavior during the data collection process, including posture, facial expression, and general body movements.

When a problem is apparent or suspected based on age, hereditary factors, or inconsistencies in the assessment data, a focused assessment is essential. Coma scales or functional dementia scales may be appropriate. More commonly, a Folstein Mini Mental status Examination (MMSE) is performed to assess orientation, attention, calculation, language (ability to name objects, repeat abstract ideas, and follow commands), and recall (immediate, short-term, and long-term memory). Abilities to read, write, and copy designs can also be assessed (see Chapter 24: Older Adult). The examination of a sensory-perceptual pattern evaluates hearing, vision, and areas of pain at a screening level; comprehensive examinations are available and may be indicated. A full neurological assessment is warranted when specific sensory deficits are identified during the examination.

Although completing these assessment areas may seem overwhelming, the time required is generally less than in most other pattern areas, perhaps because more information relevant to the cognitive-perceptual patterns becomes available as each pattern is assessed. Transition into the cognitive-perceptual pattern from other patterns may be facilitated by referring to a problem already described, with a question such as "Do you generally find it easy to solve problems effectively?" The self-perception pattern follows the cognitive pattern particularly well, because mental status measures include feelings and perceptions of the individual regarding self. Mood, affect, and responses to the interviewer, such as eye contact, are indications of self-esteem. Cognitive-perceptual ability greatly influences the ability to function (self-care) or manipulate within the environment (activity and exercise).

The placement of each of the patterns in a sequence suitable to each nurse, individual, or situation has been discussed. When the cognitive-perceptual pattern is dysfunctional, however, the individual is most likely unreliable as the historian; therefore, it is wise to consider this pattern early in the assessment process. Approaching this pattern early saves valuable time and permits the identification of patterns that can be assessed more reliably.

Every person has experienced temporary memory lapses at one time or another. These events alone are not sufficient basis for judgments. Sequencing of behaviors and clustering of appropriate signals (defining characteristics) are necessary to determine any nursing diagnosis. Equally important is the need to assess all pattern areas before data analysis and problem identification.

Cognitive and sensory ability data guide the nurse in planning care, which is especially apparent in health teaching. Formulation of health teaching plans ideally reflects each individual's preferred method of learning. The effective plan considers the individual's demonstrated developmental level, the ability to store information, retrieve information, compensate for deficits, as well as the neuromuscular and sensory levels necessary for skills development. An individually tailored plan contains mutually developed goals and short-term objectives. Although self-care might be an outcome for any person newly diagnosed with diabetes mellitus, behaviors expected of an adult with diabetes will differ from those expected of a child.

Self-Perception–Self-Concept Pattern

The self-perception–self-concept pattern encompasses the sense of each individual's personal identity, goals, emotional patterns, and feelings about the self. Self-image and sense of worth stem from the individual's perception of personal appearance, competencies, and limitations, including the individual's self-perception and others' perceptions. The nurse assesses physical, verbal, and nonverbal cues (Gordon, 2007).

The significance of the sense of self to the whole person is best exemplified by personal experiences. Individuals who feel good about themselves look and act differently from those who feel unable to accomplish anything worthwhile.

Patterns of eating, sleeping, and activity usually change if self-concept changes.

The individual's developmental level affects and is affected by this pattern. Erikson (1994) identifies eight stages of human development, proposing that with each stage a central task or crisis must be resolved before healthy growth can continue (Hockenberry & Wilson, 2006). According to Erikson (1998) individuals develop their sense of autonomy in early childhood and struggle with the sense of shame and doubt. When this developmental level is achieved or resolved, the child moves on to develop initiative during the next stage. One of the tasks Havighurst (1972) identifies during this later phase is building wholesome attitudes toward oneself (self-esteem), whereas the model proposed by Bruhn and colleagues (1977) refers specifically to self-concept development. In this model, delays in self-concept development affect progress toward subsequent tasks (Table 6-3) (Hockenberry & Wilson, 2006).

Family climate and relationship patterns provide the environmental impact that influences the self-concept pattern. The family's role in the individual's development is apparent when Erikson's developmental tasks

Table **6-3**	Relationship Between Selected Developmental Tasks and Wellness Tasks for Each Stage of the Life Cycle	
Erikson's Eight Life Stages	**Havighurst's Developmental Tasks**	**Examples of Minimal Wellness Tasks for Each Developmental Stage**
1. Infancy (trust vs. basic mistrust)	Learning to walk Learning to take solid foods Learning to talk Learning to control elimination of body waste	Acquiring the ability to perform psychomotor skills Learning functional definition of health Learning social and emotional responsiveness to others and to physical environment
2. Early childhood (autonomy vs. shame and doubt)	Learning gender difference and sexual modesty Achieving physiological stability Forming simple concepts of social-physical reality Learning to relate emotionally to parents, siblings, and others Learning to distinguish right from wrong and developing a conscience Learning physical skills necessary for ordinary games	Learning about proper foods, exercise, and sleep Learning dental hygiene Learning injury prevention (safety belts and helmets, sunscreen, smoke detectors, poisons, firearms, and swimming) Refining psychomotor and cognitive skills
3. Late childhood (initiative vs. guilt)	Building wholesome attitudes toward self as a growing organism Learning to get along with peers	Developing self-concept Learning attitudes of competition and cooperation with others Learning social, ethical, and moral differences and responsibilities
4. Early adolescence (industry vs. inferiority)	Learning appropriate gender identity: masculine or feminine role Developing fundamental skills in reading, writing, and calculating Developing concepts necessary for everyday living Developing conscience, morality, and scale of values Achieving personal independence Developing attitudes toward social groups and institutions	Learning that health is an important value Learning self-regulation of physiological needs—sleep, rest, food, drink, and exercise Learning risk taking and its consequences (injury prevention)

Continued

Table **6-3** Relationship Between Selected Developmental Tasks and Wellness Tasks for Each Stage of the Life Cycle—cont'd

Erikson's Eight Life Stages	Havighurst's Developmental Tasks	Examples of Minimal Wellness Tasks for Each Developmental Stage
5. Adolescence (identity vs. role confusion)	Achieving new and more mature relations with peers and both sexes Achieving gender identity Accepting physique and using body effectively Achieving emotional independence of parents and other adults Achieving assurance of economic independence Selecting and preparing for occupation Preparing for marriage and family life Developing intellectual skills and concepts necessary for civic competence Desiring and achieving socially responsible behavior	Learning economic responsibility Learning social responsibility for self and others (preventing pregnancy and sexually transmitted diseases) Experiencing social, emotional, and ethical commitments to others Accepting self and physical development Reconciling discrepancies between personal health concepts and observed health behaviors of others (use of alcohol, drugs, tobacco, firearms, and violence) Learning to cope with life events and problems (suicide prevention) Considering life goals and career plans and acquiring necessary skills to reach goals Learning the importance of time to self and world
6. Early adulthood (intimacy vs. isolation) 7. Middle adulthood (generativity vs. stagnation)	Selecting and learning to live with a mate Starting a family; managing a home Taking on civic responsibility Accepting and adjusting to physiological changes Achieving adult social responsibility Maintaining economic standard of living Assisting adolescent children	Committing to mate and family responsibilities Selecting a career Incorporating health habits into lifestyle Accepting aging of self and others Coping with societal pressures Recognizing importance of good health habits Reassessing life goals periodically
8. Maturity (ego integrity vs. despair)	Adjusting to decreasing physical strength and health Adjusting to retirement and reduced income Adjusting to death of spouse Establishing an explicit affiliation with own age group Establishing satisfactory physical living arrangements	Becoming aware of risks to health and adjusting lifestyle and habits to cope with risks Adjusting to loss of job, income, and family and friends through death Redefining self-concept Adjusting to changes in personal time and new physical environment Adjusting previous health habits to current physical and mental capabilities

Modified from Erikson, E. H. (1998). *The life cycle completed.* New York: W. W. Norton. U.S. Department of Health and Human Services. (2007). National health promotion and disease prevention objectives. *Healthy People 2010 Midcourse Review.* Accessed on February 5, 2008 from *www.healthypeople.gov/Data/midcourse/*; and Public Health Service Task Force on Community Preventive Services. (2005). *What works to promote health.* Atlanta, GA: Centers for Disease Control and Prevention.

and the appropriate stages of the family life cycle (see Chapter 7) are analyzed jointly (Erikson, 1998). All people who are closely associated with the individual affect that person's self-esteem. Most people care about what others think of them; therefore, the support of significant others affects the self-perception–self-concept pattern (Bamaca et al., 2005; Schor et al., 2003).

Achieving a sense of "I" versus "we" is vital for the individual. A sense of "I" as a person, apart from the roles that the person may assume, is important. For example, the sense of "me" rather than roles such as mother, father, daughter, son, student, or nurse helps to establish self-perception (Hockenberry & Wilson, 2006).

The assessment objective in this pattern area is to describe each individual's patterns and beliefs about gen-

eral self-worth and feeling states (Gordon, 2007). The nurse looks for clues that indicate identity confusion, altered body image, disturbances in self-esteem, and feelings of powerlessness. Anxiety, fear, and depression states can be identified and are responsive to nursing interventions (Catalano et al., 2004; Dennis & Creedy, 2004; Sword, 2005).

Erikson's framework describes sequential and healthy developmental patterns for each individual. Accomplishment of the wellness tasks may be apparent in other functional health patterns as well, providing additional indications of developmental level (see Unit 4) (Stolte, 1996). Feelings about self contribute additional information for this pattern. Knowledge of individual strengths and limitations along with attitudes toward these strengths and limitations becomes important data when planning care. To elicit this kind of information, questions are asked regarding personal appearance and capabilities in the cognitive, affective, and psychomotor domains. This portrayal provides evidence of a sense of identity and worth, self-image, and body image. A description of emotional patterns or a general feeling state concludes the history when no problems are indicated. A focused assessment may use specific tools, when necessary, to measure body image (Berman et al., 2007; Weber & Kelley, 2006).

The nurse notes general appearance and affect of each individual, which may have been assessed as part of a formal mental status examination. Low self-esteem may be indicated by head and shoulder flexion, lack of eye contact, and mumbled or slurred speech. Anxiety or nervousness might be revealed through extraneous body movements such as foot shuffling or tapping, facial tension or grimace, rapid speech, voice quivering, twitches or tremors, and general restlessness or shifts in body position. Any of these indicators demands further exploration to determine underlying problems for each individual.

Self-concept influences each individual's interaction with others, including the nurse. Because the information in this pattern is personal, sharing the information may actually facilitate the process of goal setting and intervention planning when the nurse possesses strong communication skills and a caring attitude.

Roles-Relationships Pattern

The roles-relationships pattern describes the position assumed and the associations engaged in by the individual that are connected to that position. The individual's perception is a major component of the assessment, and exploration of the pattern includes each individual's level of satisfaction with roles and relationships.

The needs for relationships with other people are universal. Dossey et al. (2004) have identified basic needs for communication, fellowship, and love in high-level wellness. The ability to communicate with other people in a meaningful way greatly affects the whole person (Figure 6-2). The concept of health as the harmonious balance between the individual and the environment indicates the major role that relationships with others play in health status (Dossey et al., 2004). The function development plays in health is apparent in Erikson's stages of ego development (Erikson, 1998). This series of hypotheses about readiness proposes that attainment of each stage is required to progress to the next stage. For example, a person can become immersed in a relationship of genuine intimacy only after self-identity has stabilized. Certain tasks for family development have been identified similarly by Duvall and Miller (Duvall & Miller, 1985; Goldenberg & Goldenberg, 2008) (see Chapter 7). The emphasis within these models is on the individual's relationships within the family and within the larger context of society.

The objective of the roles-relationships pattern assessment is to describe an individual's pattern of family and

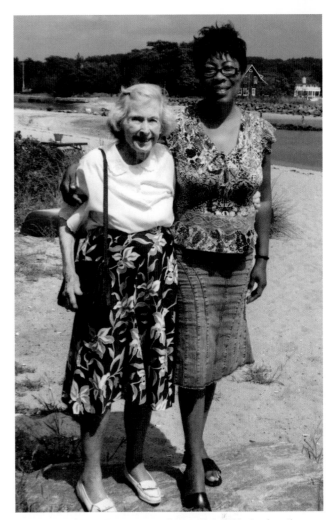

Figure 6-2 The ability to communicate with individuals of another culture greatly affects the development of an individual.

shared circumstances, with the associated responsibilities. The individual's perception of satisfaction with the established relationship contributes to this assessment. Loss, change, and threat produce the major problems within this pattern. Clues indicative of impaired verbal communication, social isolation, alterations in parenting, independence-dependence conflicts, dysfunctional grieving, and potential for violence are pertinent.

Assessment focuses on family, work, and community roles and relationships. Within the family, assessment parameters include the family structure, tasks performed, social support systems, and other dynamics, such as decision-making, power, authority, division of labor, and communication patterns. Parenting or marital difficulties and family violence issues are explored. The roles of student and employee are explored to determine specific occupation or position, along with work responsibilities and work environment. Parameters such as stress, safety, and health factors should be included (see the Case Study and Care Plan and the end of this chapter). Financial concerns, job security, and retirement plans are elicited. Activity-rest patterns elicit information about time commitments, leisure activities, and physical exercise; therefore, the assessment at this point addresses the impact of these factors on the roles-relationships pattern. Community roles and relationships indicate involvement within the neighborhood and other social groups, such as the level of socialization and amount of social support available. Within all three components (family, work or school, and community) the individual is asked to describe the level of satisfaction with the roles and relationships.

Threat of change, actual change, and loss are areas to be explored further. In addition, family or work roles alone may not cause stress, but combining them may cause difficulties, as with the working mother or traveling husband and father.

Objective data for assessment within this pattern are usually unavailable unless the nurse makes a home visit or sees the individual in the company of significant others in some other capacity. Family interaction and communication patterns are noted whenever possible. Cognizant of meaningful relationships within the family, the nurse identifies potential problems, such as those that occur with the college student away from home, the individual who travels or moves frequently, and sole family survivors when older adults outlive their family members and friends (Berman et al., 2007; Hockenberry & Wilson, 2006; Wong et al., 2005). The relationships among the functional health patterns are clearly apparent in light of the developmental stages. Difficulties within the self-concept pattern and difficulties with relationships often appear together (Erikson, 1998). Relationships affect the whole person; therefore, problems in the roles-relationships pattern may be exhibited in other areas such as sleep, appetite, and sexuality.

Sexuality-Reproductive Pattern

The sexuality-reproductive pattern describes the individual's sexual self-concept, sexual functioning, methods of intimacy, and reproductive areas. Data collection combines subjective information, nursing observations, and physical examination. Normal development and perceived satisfaction combine to provide the elements of this pattern (Gordon, 2007).

Sexuality is the behavioral expression of sexual identity. The importance of this pattern area to the individual's life and health is closely related to the self-perception and the relationships patterns. Body image, self-concept, and role and gender identity are linked to sexual identity. This concept of sexual self and the individual's relationships pattern indicate the level and the perceived satisfaction of sexual functioning. Sexual functioning involves, but is not limited to, sexual relations with a partner. Reproductive patterns are equally significant to this pattern assessment, the whole individual, and the family and community (see Chapters 7 and 8).

As discussed, individual development influences reproductive capacities; these include secondary sex characteristics, genital development, ego integrity, and the family life-cycle stage (Duvall & Miller, 1985; Erikson, 1998). Environment also plays a part in expression of the sexuality-reproductive pattern. Cultural and family norms

may contribute to the expression of sexuality and combine with other factors, such as the family's financial stability, to influence reproductive patterns. Norms within society may create issues in expressions of sexuality.

One objective of assessment in this pattern is to describe behavioral problems or difficulties (Gordon, 2007). Equally important is assessing the individual's knowledge of sexual functioning and preventive health practices, such as breast and testicular self-examination, Papanicolaou smears, effective contraceptive use, and avoiding infection. Clues are evaluated for potential or actual sexual dysfunction.

Parameters assessed include (1) sexual self-concept, which may be derived from information collected in the self-perception–self-concept and the roles-relationships patterns; (2) sexual functioning, with the nurse noting evidence of some form of intimacy, the level of sexual activity or libido, and the effect of health or illness on sexual expression; and (3) reproductive patterns in which the nurse collects data pertinent to health-promotion factors, such as feelings related to aging, preventive practices, and knowledge of sexual functioning. For women, reproductive pattern assessment would also include information about menstruation, such as onset, duration, frequency, last menstrual period, discomfort, and menopause, as well as information about reproductive stage, such as pregnancy history and birth control methods.

Level of satisfaction with sexual self-concept, sexual functioning, and reproduction is also explored. Difficulties such as ineffective or inappropriate sexual performance, discharges, infections, venereal disease, discomfort, and history of abuse are evaluated. Focused assessment to collect additional information is warranted with sexual dysfunction or trauma. Physical examination evaluates genital development and secondary sex characteristics. Signs of intimacy between partners, such as holding hands and hugging, are noted.

People may feel threatened by discussion of topics in this pattern; depth of exploration is governed in part by the individual's wishes. Dialogue is encouraged but may be postponed until a firm and trusting relationship is established. A clear representation of the individual's knowledge and use of preventive practices facilitates planning for health promotion. Although sex education usually is associated with school programs, information and discussion about sexuality is just as important for adults of all ages. Sex education is a key element of parenthood classes. Improved understanding of sexuality and sexual function leads to discovery and increased satisfaction (Health Teaching box).

Coping–Stress Tolerance Pattern

Gordon (2007) describes the coping–stress tolerance pattern as a depiction of general coping and the individual's ability to effectively manage stress. This pattern includes the individual's ability to process life crises and to resist disruptive factors that will influence self-integrity of ego, mode of conflict resolution, stress management, and accessibility to necessary resources.

HEALTH TEACHING   Sexuality and Aging Women: Common Myths

- Sexual desire and prowess wane during the climacteric for most women; therefore, menopause is the death of a woman's sexuality.
- Sexual activity is uncommon in older adults, particularly women.
- If the older woman is sexually active, sexual activity generally occurs less than once per month.
- Hysterectomy creates a physical disability that causes the inability to function sexually.
- Sex has no role in the lives of older adults except as perversion or remembrance of times past.
- Masturbation is an immature activity of youngsters and adolescents, not of older women.
- Sexual expression is unacceptable among older women.
- Older women are too frail to engage in sex.
- Sex is unimportant to the older woman.
- Older women do not wish to discuss their sexuality with professionals.
- Medical conditions do not affect sexual expression.

Assessment Guide
- Ask the woman to describe:
  How she expresses her sexuality.
  Concerns she has about fulfilling her sexual needs.
  How her sexual relationship with her partner has changed with her age.
- Use the PLISSIT Model
  P Obtaining **P**ermission from the individual to initiate sexual discussion
  LI Providing the **L**imited **I**nformation needed to function sexually
  SS Giving **S**pecific **S**uggestions for the individual to proceed with sexual relations
  IT Providing **I**ntensive **T**herapy surrounding the issues of sexuality for that individual

Updated with information from Addis, I. B, Van Den Eeden, S. K., Wassel-Fyr, C. L., et al. (2006). Sexual activity and function in middle-aged and older women. *Obstetrics & Gynecology, 107,* 755-764; Wallace. (2005). Try this: Best practices in nursing care to older adults from the Hartford Institute for Geriatric Nursing: Sexuality. *Urologic Nursing, 25*(5), 373-374; and Office on Aging: Aging and human sexuality resource guide. Accessed on February 5, 2008 from *www.apa.org/pi/aging/sexuality.html.*

The ability to manage stress effectively in life is a learned behavior. Stress is a necessary part of life; without it there is no motivation to grow. Stress becomes a problem when tolerance is weak and daily activities are affected (Berman et al., 2007; Dossey et al., 2004). Most stress comes not from great tragedies, but from an accumulation of minor irritations. Stress is not inherent in the event but in the individual's perception of that event. Whereas one individual may experience stress from missing a bus and can think only of being 10 minutes late, another will consider the same event an opportunity to spend 10 minutes reading the newspaper. This difference in perception may represent the different values used to identify sources of stress or it may represent coping strategies.

For purposes of assessing this pattern, coping, which is considered the individual behavioral response to stress, includes both problem-solving ability and use of defense mechanisms. Coping is viewed not as a single act but as a process incorporating many behaviors. The function of coping is to deal with the threat or emotional distress of an event. Coping effectiveness is assessed from the individual's perspective and from the nurse's observation of the individual's ability to function in the presence of actual or potential stressors in the environment.

The perception of stress and the ability to manage it depend on personal development, amount of stress previously experienced, current level of stress within the environment, and sources of social support. For example, an older adult may experience many stresses during life and manage them effectively, but now coping may no longer be possible because too many stressors are present, such as physical incapacitation, fixed income, fear of illness or injury, and lack of transportation. In addition, this person no longer has a social support system (Aday, 2001; Berman et al., 2007).

The objective in assessment is to determine the individual's stress tolerance and past coping patterns. The nurse evaluates clues to difficulties in managing past and current stressors and changes in the effectiveness of a coping pattern in order to determine personal coping capacity.

Assessment parameters include (1) the coping task, including the physical, psychological, and socioeconomic stimuli with which the individual must cope; (2) coping style, or the tendency to use a specific style, such as approach oriented, avoidance oriented, or nonspecific; (3) coping strategies, including specifics; and (4) coping effectiveness. Coping strategy may be divided into information seeking, direct action (fight or flight), inhibition of action, or use of social support. Coping effectiveness is best assessed by eliciting the individual resources and the individual's functional level (Dossey et al., 2004). Individual resources include the variety of coping mechanisms used by the individual, flexibility of these mechanisms, and the health-promotion value associated with each.

Stress tolerance patterns elicit the amount of stress effectively processed in the past. Use of anticipatory coping is assessed along with whether the individual knows how to cope, but does not (production deficit), or simply does not know how to cope (skill deficit). Other indicators of value within this pattern are discussed under the self-perception–self-concept pattern. Objective data of concern include physical signs of restlessness, irritability, and nervousness, such as increased heart rate and blood pressure and perspiration. Evidence of coping ability and tolerance to stress are found in every other functional health pattern. Stress also affects the other patterns, thereby resulting in health problems such as insomnia, weight loss, and poor concentration (Dossey et al., 2004; Gordon, 2007).

Health can be promoted through early intervention to reduce stress. Coping patterns and stress tolerance in the past may uncover unhealthy behavior, such as smoking and drinking, that needs to be replaced by alternative coping strategies. Stress-reduction workshops would be helpful for most of the population because the future undoubtedly holds stressful events, some of which may be overwhelming without coping strategies. The Innovative Practice box includes information about a unique company that offers stress management interventions. Dossey and colleagues (2004) offer categories for stress management: (1) social engineering strategies, such as time management or planned change; (2) personality engineering strategies, such as assertiveness training or cognitive rehearsal; and (3) altered states of consciousness, such as meditation or relaxation. Planning based on the assessment of all functional health patterns to help determine a coping pattern should include these kinds of strategies.

innovative
practice

The Humor Potential, Inc.

The Humor Potential, Inc., is a company that provides resources, products, and seminars for stress management with the use of humor. Company president Loretta LaRoche is an internationally recognized expert on stress management, emphasizing the importance of balancing daily living experiences with humor. The Humor Potential, Inc., offers seminars and lectures to health care professionals, schools, corporations, other organizations, and the general public. The corporation also produces television programs that have been televised nationally in the United States. One television program, *The Joy of Stress*, was nominated for a regional Emmy Award.

Books, prints, audiotapes and videotapes, and other products dealing with humor can be purchased from her website. The collection consists of audiotapes and videotapes that have been developed for corporate meetings and training. An example is *Stressbusters!*, an audiotape and videotape and action guide that increases productivity by reducing stress. Two other tapes, *Not Another Meeting* and *Whoopee! Another Meeting*, are meeting openers for staff development programs given to employees to improve communication, productivity, and outcomes within an organization. A catalog is available for e-mail, fax, phone, and mail orders.

Contact Information:
The Humor Potential, Inc.
Corporate Offices
50 Court Street
Plymouth, MA 02360
Email: inquiries@lorettalaroche.com
Telephone: 800-99-TADAH (800-998-2324)

Based on data from the Humor Potential, Inc. Retrieved February 5, 2008, from *www.lorettalaroche.com*.

Values-Beliefs Pattern

The values-beliefs pattern describes values, including the individual's spiritual values, beliefs, and goals. This pattern also includes perceptions of what is right, what is good, and conflicts that beliefs or values impart. Each of the 11 patterns addresses value systems of individuals, family, and society. Individual beliefs or values develop over time and govern life through personal experiences and family and societal influences (Duvall & Miller, 1985; Wong et al., 2005). The objective in assessing this pattern is to determine the basis for health-related decisions and actions (Gordon, 2007). Rosenstock (1974) suggested that an individual will engage in preventive health behavior when a threat to wellness or health status exists. Several other health belief models expand on this concept by including other motivations, such as personal values and environmental influences. Clues to conflict within the individual's value system or between the person's value system and that of the family or society are explored.

Dimensions of assessment include the individual's values, beliefs, or goals that guide choice or decisions that are related to health. The nurse collects information while exploring each pattern, while summarizing, clarifying, and securing additional information. Specifically, values and beliefs about self, relationships, and society are appraised. Individuals' beliefs, goals, and purposes of life are reviewed, along with any conflicts, perceived philosophies, and those of the family, culture, and society. Sources of strength, such as a higher being or significant individual practices, are explored, including religious beliefs and preferences. Past goals and expectations are assessed through the individual's satisfaction. The nurse must identify the individual's goals and expectations concerning health, clarifying to help the individual achieve them. To be effective, health-promotion interventions are based on the individual's value system and health beliefs (Dossey et al., 2004; Pender et al., 2006). The brevity of this discussion is no indication of the importance that the values-beliefs pattern plays in the assessment of the individual. Individual values play a role in all of the patterns.

INDIVIDUAL HEALTH PROMOTION THROUGH THE NURSING PROCESS

The nursing process—the systematic approach to reduce or eliminate the individual's health problem—is accomplished in several steps, the first being the collection of necessary data. With the individual, the nurse analyzes the data, identifies a nursing diagnosis, projects outcomes, prescribes interventions, and evaluates effectiveness. Reassessment, reordering of priorities, new goal setting, and revising the plan continues as part of the process toward outcome attainment (Carpenito-Moyet, 2008).

Collection and Analysis of Data

Assessment is a systematic technique for learning as much as possible about the individual. The main purpose in collecting data from a new individual is to see whether health problems exist and to identify the individual's health goals. An assessment of an adult based on the functional health patterns is presented in **Website Resource 6B**. Data collection includes biographical data, such as age, sex, and the purpose of the visit. This process is followed by assessment of the previously outlined 11 functional health patterns. Subjective reporting, nursing observations and perceptions, and the physical examination are assessed and recorded. The remaining discussion focuses on nursing diagnosis.

Problem Identification

Although the concept of problem identification has been debated in the past, most nurses now have distinguished *nursing diagnosis* as the problematic label. Diagnosis is a careful examination and analysis of the facts in an attempt to explain something. Nursing diagnosis is the naming of an individual's response to actual or potential health problems or life processes (Carpenito-Moyet, 2008; Gordon, 2007; North American Nursing Diagnosis Association, 2003). Nursing diagnoses provide the basis for selection of nursing interventions to achieve outcomes for which the nurse is accountable (Gordon, 2007). NANDA has provided leadership in developing standardization of the descriptions of human responses that nurses manage. The most recent revision of this taxonomy has been approved for clinical testing and has been endorsed by the ANA (NANDA, 2003).

Gordon (2007) proposed the accepted format of nursing diagnosis that lists the problem, etiology, and signs and symptoms, or defining characteristics, for each diagnosis accepted for clinical testing. At the 1998 NANDA conference a multiaxial framework for nursing diagnoses was proposed but has yet to be completed and approved by the NANDA board. This proposed formation for nursing diagnoses calls for a more detailed clinical language and an improved structure for nursing diagnoses to be included in computerized databases. If approved in the future, nursing diagnoses will be expressed by six axes: (1) diagnostic concept (e.g., parenting); (2) acuity (e.g., altered); (3) unit of care (e.g., individual); (4) developmental stage (e.g., adolescent); (5) potentiality (e.g., at risk for); and (6) descriptor, or creation of the diagnostic statement (NANDA, 2003). The Research Highlights box discusses a study of nursing classification systems.

In discussions of problems, the meaning of problem must be clearly defined and identified. The concept as used in this text refers to Gordon's (2007) proposition that a health problem is defined as a dysfunctional pattern and that nursing's major contribution to health care is in preventing and treating these patterns. A pattern is dysfunctional when it represents a deviation from established norms or from the individual's previous condition or goals. (Normative behavior is further discussed in Unit 4.) A dysfunctional pattern is a problem when it generates therapeutic concern on the

research highlights

Classification Systems

Four nursing diagnosis classification systems were compared. Criteria for classification of nursing diagnosis were identified through review of 50 journal articles. The International Classification of Nursing Practice (ICNP®), the International Classification of Functioning, Disability and Health (ICF), the International Nursing Diagnoses Classification (NANDA), and the Nursing Diagnostic System of the Centre for Nursing Development and Research (ZEFP) were evaluated.

The ICF and NANDA are the only two conceptually driven classification systems. Although ICF and ICNP® describe diagnostic terms, only the NANDA system possesses a description, diagnostic criteria, and related etiologies. There was evidence that the NANDA classification system was the best-researched and most widely implemented classification internationally. The authors concluded that NANDA fulfilled their criteria and that NANDA should be recommended for nursing practice and electronic nursing documentation.

From Mueller-Staub, M., Lavin, M. A., Needham, I., et al. (2007) Meeting the criteria of a nursing diagnosis classification: evaluation of ICNP, ICFR, NANDA and ZEFP. *International Journal of Nursing Studies, 44*(5), 702-713.

part of the individual, others, or the nurse and when it is amenable to nursing therapies.

As patterns are assessed, the nurse proposes several hypotheses regarding functional or dysfunctional labeling. At the completion of the assessment, conclusions must be drawn. The possibility exists that all patterns are functional, that some are functional, and that others are dysfunctional or potentially dysfunctional. Functional refers to wellness and optimal health. Dysfunctional patterns, indicating some health problems, may be present in the absence of disease; that is, nursing care may be needed for health promotion and health maintenance, not health restoration. The case history of Frank Thompson in Chapter 1 effectively illustrates the multiple nursing care needs of an individual who is not ill. In potentially dysfunctional patterns, sufficient evidence exists or enough **risk factors** are present to indicate that a pattern dysfunction will likely occur if interventions are not made. Early identification of potential problems is possible through systematic data collection and analysis.

Contributing Etiological Factors

To plan care, the nurse must first determine what has caused the actual or potential health problem: its contributing etiological factors. The etiological factors of most dysfunctional patterns lie within another pattern or patterns. Although etiology is never an absolute within human sciences, the projection of outcomes or goals must be based on probable causes. Interventions then focus on mediating or resolving the probable causes. Most often, many factors are involved

HEART DISEASE IN WOMEN

Contrary to what many people think, heart disease is the leading cause of death in women. Women generally delay seeking health care perhaps because they believe that cardiovascular disease is uncommon in women. There is also some evidence that women experience different symptomatology. In 2003 in the U.S., 240,000 deaths were attributed to coronary artery disease in women. Older women are particularly susceptible. Cardiovascular disease strikes 1 in 9 women between the ages of 45 and 64 and those rates are expected to increase. There is support for the perspective that women receive substandard treatment compared to men. Although premenopausal women rarely develop coronary artery disease, postmenopausal women's risk increases to that of a man the same age. The vasodilation, antioxidant, and antiproliferation properties of estrogen are thought to protect a woman from cardiovascular disease before menopause.

From Chambers, T. A., Bagai, A., & Ivascu, N. (2007). Current trends in coronary artery disease in women. *Current Opinion in Anesthesiology*, 20(1), 75-82.

and problems are said to relate to rather than be a result of these factors. Potential problems are not actual problems but risk states; therefore, they have no specific cause and are identified when risk factors are present. Nursing intervention is directed toward risk reduction through education (classes or brochures) to improve nutrition, prevent accidents, and so forth. Risk estimate theory and potential health problems are developed further in Chapters 7 and 8 and Unit 4 (Hot Topics box).

Diagnostic Variables

The ability to arrive at an accurate diagnosis, even when comprehensive data isn't available, is governed primarily by the nurse's clinical knowledge. Experience improves the effectiveness when nursing is performed as a scientific process. Nursing requires gathering information, interpreting it based on normative values, organizing, grouping on healthy findings, identifying the problem, and then planning appropriate goals and interventions. Difficulties are encountered when there are no available norms, which occurs frequently in the psychosocial assessment components. Using the 11 interdependent functional health patterns helps to solve these difficulties. By focusing on each of these areas, recognizing whether a problem does or does not exist is easier. Any change within the pattern may be a sign of dysfunction or an unhealthy but stabilized behavior. For example, a sign of dysfunction might be a 2-year-old child who is still not walking; developmental growth is a major factor in activity patterns of infants, toddlers, and children.

The use of physiological parameters clearly demonstrates the idea of a stabilized dysfunctional pattern, but equal attention must be given to psychological development. For instance, a 26-year-old man who lives with his mother and gives no indication of independent decision-

making should be evaluated. It should be apparent that assessment information primarily comes from the initial contact with the individual and the database, which is generally the case in health-promotion activities. However, in any acute situation or emergency, quick assessment of the major problems is given high priority on a hierarchy-of-needs basis and the full nursing assessment is postponed temporarily. For further understanding of the nursing diagnosis, the nurse is referred to books discussing the development of diagnoses, the diagnostic process, and specific details of each accepted diagnosis (Carpenito-Moyet, 2008; Gordon, 2007; North American Nursing Diagnosis Association, 2003).

Planning the Care

In the nursing process, planning is the proposal of diagnosis-specific treatment to assist the individual toward the goal, or expected outcome, of optimal health. The individual's goals and the determined nursing diagnosis provide the basis for planning. Clear goals and diagnoses are critical to development of an effective plan of care. The nursing process identifies the following purposes of the planning phase: (1) to assign priority to the problems diagnosed; (2) to specify the behavioral outcomes or goals with the individual, including the expected time of achievement; (3) to differentiate individual problems that can be resolved by nursing intervention, those that can be handled by the individual or family member, and those that should be handled with or referred to other members of the health team; (4) to designate specific actions, the frequency of these actions, and the short-term, intermediate-term, and long-term results; and (5) to list the individual's problems (nursing diagnosis) and nursing actions (frequency and **expected outcomes**, or goals) on the nursing care plan or blueprint for action (Carpenito-Moyet, 2008). This plan provides the direction for individual and nursing activities and is the guide for the evaluation. There are many research studies involving outcomes from which nurses can draw to improve effectiveness of the care they provide.

Implementing the Plan

Implementation is the completion of the actions necessary to fulfill the goals for optimal health; it is the enactment of the nursing care plan to elicit the behaviors described in the proposed individual outcome. The selection of a nursing intervention depends on several factors: (1) the desired individual outcome; (2) the characteristics of the nursing diagnosis; (3) the research base associated with the intervention; (4) the feasibility of implementing the intervention; (5) the acceptability of the intervention to the individual; and (6) the capability of the nurse (Carpenito-Moyet, 2008). A nursing interventions classification is being developed. As discussed in Unit 1, a critical component of effective communication is the accurate interpretation of the individual's information.

This feedback process continues throughout all phases of the nursing process; the nurse continues to collect data to modify the plan as needed and does not blindly implement the care plan. As discussed in Unit 3, the most frequently used nursing interventions in health promotion are screening, education, counseling, and crisis intervention. All of these interventions require strong communication abilities from the nurse.

Evaluating the Plan

The process of analyzing changes experienced by the individual occurs in the evaluation phase of the nursing process, with the nurse examining the relationships between nursing actions and the individual's goal achievement. Nursing process emphasizes that evaluation is always considered in terms of how the individual responds to the plan of action (Berman et al., 2007; Yura, 1983). As discussed, the nursing diagnosis (or health problems) and the goal (or expected outcome) guide the evaluation of the nursing care plan. Many variables influence outcomes: the interventions prescribed by the health care providers, the health care providers themselves, the environment in which the care is received, the individual's motivation and genetic structure, and the individual's significant others. The task for nursing is to define which outcomes are sensitive to nursing care so as to identify the expected and attainable results of nursing care for each individual (Berman et al., 2007; Yura,

1983). All of these components of the nursing process are documented by the nurse on the individual's health care record (Berman et al., 2007).

SUMMARY

Data relevant to the health-promotion activities of the individual focus primarily on the assessment of the current health status so that the nurse can identify problem areas, or areas of dysfunction, within the individual's health and lifestyle pattern. This process is a fundamental first step and precedes all other components of the nursing process. Without a clear picture of the problem, nursing activities are fruitless. Gordon's functional health pattern framework provides guidance for the individual assessment. The focus of each pattern includes the age-developmental influences exerted, cultural and environmental roles played, functional ability displayed, and behavioral patterns specific to each individual. The interaction between internal mechanisms and the environment is assessed through these 11 functional health patterns. When assessing each pattern, the nurse must understand the pattern definition, the significance of the pattern to the whole individual, the developmental influences, the environmental role, the assessment objectives, the assessment parameters and indicators, and the nursing implications. Assessment is essential to all components of the nursing process in health promotion for the individual.

CASE STUDY

Spiritual Distress: Cindy

Cindy is a single 28-year-old woman. Cindy studies nursing and shares an apartment with two friends. She was having increasing difficulties with her course work and was placed on academic probation. Cindy became concerned about the effect of stress on her ability to finish her studies and on her future career. She grew increasingly nervous and began to ask, "Will I ever be okay?" and "Will I ever be able to finish school and function as a nurse?" Cindy expressed her fear of weakness and feelings of isolation, loneliness, helplessness, and loss of control. These feelings began to find expression in anger related to this major life disruption. She verbalized her anger at God for allowing this to happen to her. Her incapacity deprived her of her normal outlets for expressing and finding support for such concerns. Cindy was unable to

participate in the practices of her faith, in which she previously had found strength in facing life's challenges. Her inability to concentrate and her growing feeling of lethargy added to her frustration. Expressing these fears and concerns was difficult for Cindy. The nurse, however, developed a trusting relationship with Cindy, permitting her to express her fears, anxieties, and concerns. Based on the nurse's assessment, the nursing diagnosis of spiritual distress was formulated.

Reflective Questions:
1. What differential diagnoses should the nurse consider?
2. Describe other individuals you know who have experienced spiritual distress.

Modified from Carpenito-Moyet, L. J. (2008). *Nursing diagnosis: Application to clinical practice*. Philadelphia: Lippincott Williams & Wilkins.

CARE PLAN

Spiritual Distress: Cindy

Nursing Diagnosis: Spiritual Distress Related to a Threat to Well-Being, Loss of Meaningful Role, and Separation From Religious and Family Ties

DEFINING CHARACTERISTICS
- Experiences a disturbance in belief system
- Demonstrates discouragement or despair

Continued

CARE PLAN

Spiritual Distress: Cindy—cont'd

- Chooses not to practice religious rituals
- Shows emotional detachment from self and others
- Expresses concern, anger, resentment, and fear, related to a major life disruption

RELATED FACTORS

- Threat to well-being from change in role as a student and fear of failure
- Loss of meaningful role as a student
- Separation from religious and family ties

EXPECTED OUTCOMES

- Person will verbalize a greater sense of purpose, meaning, and hope.
- Person will express feelings of anger verbally and will discuss anger with another person.

INTERVENTIONS

- Take time to be present and available to listen to the individual.
- Convey a nonjudgmental attitude.
- Encourage the individual to verbalize feelings.
- Engage the individual in values clarification.
- Encourage the individual to acknowledge feelings of anger and to acknowledge and name any other feelings experienced.
- Reassure the individual that it is acceptable to feel anger toward a supreme being.
- Encourage honest dialogue with a peer whom the individual trusts.
- Offer consultation with an appropriate spiritual advisor.
- Inform the individual of religious resources.
- Pray with the individual as indicated.

Modified from Carpenito-Moyet, L. J. (2008). *Nursing diagnosis: Application to clinical practice.* 12th edition. Philadelphia: Lippincott Williams & Wilkins.

REFERENCES

Aday, L. A. (2001). *At risk in America: The health and health care needs of vulnerable populations in the United States* (2nd ed.). San Francisco: Jossey-Bass, A Wiley Company.

American Nurses Association. (2003). *Nursing's social policy statement* (2nd ed.). Washington, DC: American Nurses Association.

American Nurses Association. (2004). *Nursing: Scope and standards of practice.* Washington, DC: American Nurses Association.

Andrews, M. M., & Boyle, J. S. (2008). *Transcultural concepts in nursing care* (5th ed.). New York: Lippincott, Williams & Wilkins.

Bamaca, M. Y., Umana-Taylor, A. J., Shin, N., & Alfaro, E. C. (2005). Latino adolescents' perception of parenting behaviors and self-esteem: Examining the role of neighborhood risk. *Family Relations, 54*(5), 621–632.

Beatty, J. E., & Torbert, W. R. (2003). The false duality of work and leisure. *Journal of Management Inquiry, 12*(3), 239–252.

Berman, A., Snyder, S., Kozier, B., & Erb, G. (2008). *Kozier & Erb's fundamentals of nursing: Concepts, process, and practice* (8th ed.). Upper Saddle River, NJ: Prentice Hall.

Bickley, L., & Szilagyi, P. G. (2006). *Bates' guide to physical examination and history taking* (9th ed.). Philadelphia: Lippincott Williams & Wilkins.

Bottari, C., Swaine, B., & Dutil, E. (2007). Interpreting activity of daily living errors for treatment and discharge planning: The perception of occupational therapists. *Journal of Head Trauma Rehabilitation, 22*(1), 26–30.

Bruhn, J., Cordova, F. D., Williams, J. A., & Fuentes, R. G. (1977). The wellness process. *Journal of Community Health, 2*(3), 209–221.

Callaghan, D. (2006). Basic conditioning factors' influences on adolescents' healthy behaviors, self-efficacy, and self-care. *Issues in Comprehensive Pediatric Nursing, 29*(4), 191–204.

Campbell, M. A. (2006). Development of a clinical pathway for near-term and convalescing premature infants in a Level II Nursery. *Advances in Neonatal Care, 6*(3), 150–164.

Carpenito-Moyet, L. J. (2008). *Nursing diagnosis: Application to clinical practice* (12th ed.). Philadelphia: Lippincott Williams & Wilkins.

Catalano, R. F., Berglund, M. L., Lonczak, H. S., & Hawkins, J. D. (2004). Positive youth development in the United States: Research findings on evaluations of positive youth development programs. *The Annals of the American Academy of Political and Social Science, 591*(1), 98–124.

Centers for Disease Control and Prevention. (2005). *NHANES 1999-2004.* Retrieved January 31, 2006, from *www.cdc.gov/nchs/about/major/nhanes/nhanes99-02.htm.*

Chambers, T. A., Bagai, A., & Ivascu, N. (2007). Current trends in coronary artery disease in women. *Current Opinion in Anesthesiology, 20*(1), 75–82.

Daniels, S. R. (2006). The consequences of childhood overweight and obesity. *The Future of Children, 16*(1), 47–67.

Dennis, C. L., & Creedy, D. (2004). Psychosocial and psychological interventions for preventing postpartum depression. *Cochrane Database of Systematic Reviews, 18*(4), CD001134.

Dossey, B. M., Keegan, L., & Guzzetta, C. E. (2004). *Holistic nursing: A handbook for practice* (4th ed.). Boston: Jones & Bartlett.

Duvall, E., & Miller, B. (1985). *Marriage and family development* (7th ed.). New York: Harper Collins.

Edwards, R. R., Moric, M., Husfeldt, B., Buvanendran, A., & Ivankovich, O. (2005). Ethnic similarities and differences in the chronic pain experience: A comparison of African American, Hispanic, and White patients. *Pain Medicine, 6*(1), 88–98.

Erikson, E. H. (1994). *Identity: Youth in crisis* (Austen Rigg monograph) (Reissue ed.). New York: W. W. Norton.

Erikson, E. H. (1998). *The life cycle completed.* New York: W. W. Norton & Company.

Fawcett, J. (2005). *Contemporary nursing knowledge: Analysis and evaluation of nursing models and theories* (2nd ed.). Philadelphia: F.A. Davis Company.

Goldenberg, H., & Goldenberg, I. (2008). *Family Therapy: An Overview* (7th ed.). Belmont, CA: Brooks Cole.

Gordon, M. (2007). *Manual of nursing diagnosis* (11th ed.). Sudbury, MA: Jones & Bartlett.

Hadjistavropoulos, T., Herr, K., Turk, D. C., Fine, P. G., Dworkin, R. H., Helme, R., et al. (2007). An interdisciplinary expert consensus statement on assessment of pain in older persons. *Clinical Journal of Pain, 23*(1 Suppl), S1–43.

Havighurst, R. J. (1972). *Developmental tasks and education* (3rd ed.). United Kingdom: Longman Group.

Hockenberry, M. J., & Wilson, D. (2006). *Wong's nursing care of infants and children* (8th ed.). St. Louis: Mosby.

Lavin, M. A., & Scroggins, L. (2002). NANDA news. *International Journal of Nursing Terminologies & Classifications, 13*(3), 107.

Leiby, K., & Powelson, S. (2003). Nursing diagnosis. *International Journal of Nursing Terminologies & Classifications, 14*, 46–49.

Leininger, M., & McFarland, M. R. (2006). *Culture care diversity and universality: A worldwide nursing theory* (2nd ed.). Sudbury, MA: Jones & Bartlett.

McCaffery, M., & Pasero, C. (1999). *Pain: Clinical manual* (2nd ed.). St. Louis: Mosby.

McCaffrey, R. L., Frock, T., & Garquilo, H. (2003). Understanding chronic pain and the mind-body connection. *Holistic Nursing Practice, 17*(6), 281–289.

McKeown, E., Barkauskas, V., Quinn, A., & Kresowaty, J. (2003). Occupational nursing service in a small manufacturing plant: Interventions and outcomes. *International Journal of Nursing Terminologies & Classifications, 14*(4), 125–135.

McNamara, T. K., Orav, E. J., Wilkins-Haug, L., & Chang, G. (2005). Risk during pregnancy—Self-report versus medical record. *American Journal of Obstetrics and Gynecology, 193*(6), 1981–1985.

McNamara, T. K., Orav, E. J., Wilkins-Haug, L., & Chang, G. (2006). Social support and prenatal alcohol use. *Journal of Women's Health, 15*(1), 70–76.

Murphy, J. I. (2004). Using focused reflection and articulation to promote clinical reasoning: An evidence-based teaching strategy. *Nursing Education Perspectives, 25*(5), 226–231.

National Council of State Boards of Nursing. (2001). *Nursing practice.* Retrieved September 16, 2007, from *www.nursys.com/public/regulation/nursing_practice.htm.*

Nightingale, F. (1992). *Notes on nursing; what it is, and what it is not; with an introduction by Barbara Stevens Barnum and commentaries by contemporary nursing leaders.* (Commemorative ed.). Philadelphia: Lippincott, Williams & Wilkins.

North American Nursing Diagnosis Association. (2003). In NANDA (Ed.), *NANDA nursing diagnoses 2003-2004: Definitions and classifications.* Chicago, IL: North American Nursing Diagnosis Association.

North American Nursing Diagnosis Association-International. (2005). Call for new nursing diagnoses development. *International Journal of Nursing Terminologies & Classifications, 16*(3), 88.

Ogden, C. L., Carroll, M. D., Curtin, L. R., McDowell, M. A., Tabak, C. J., & Flegal, K. M. (2006). Prevalence of overweight and obesity in the United States, 1999-2004. *JAMA, 295*(13), 1549–1555.

Pender, N. J., Murdaugh, C. L., & Parsons, M. A. (2006). *Health promotion in nursing practice* (5th ed.). Upper Saddle River, NJ: Prentice Hall.

Perez, L. M., Peifer, K. L., & Newman, M. C. (2002). A strength-based and early relationship approach to infant mental health assessment. *Community Mental Health Journal, 38*(5), 375–390.

Pogson, C. E., Cober, A. B., Doverspike, D., & Rogers, J. R. (2003). Differences in self-reported work ethic across three career stages. *Journal of Vocational Behavior, 62*(1), 189–201.

Rosenstock, I. (1974). The health belief model and preventive health behavior. *Health Education Monographs, 2*, 354.

Schor, E. L., Billingsley, M. M., Golden, A. L., McMillan, J. A., Meloy, L. D., Pendarvis Jr., B. C., et al. (2003). Family pediatrics: Report of the task force on the family. *Pediatrics, 111*(6), 1541–1571.

Stevens, E. (2005). Bladder ultrasound: Avoiding unnecessary catheterizations. *MEDSURG Nursing, 14*(4), 249–253.

Stolte, K. (1996). *Wellness: Nursing diagnosis for health promotion.* Philadelphia: Lippincott Williams & Wilkins.

Sword, W. (2005). Review: Some specific preventive psychosocial and psychological interventions reduce risk of postpartum depression. *Evidence-Based Nursing, 8*(3), 76.

U.S. Department of Health and Human Services. (2000). *Healthy people 2010: Understanding and improving health* (Government Report No. Stock Number 017-001-001-00-550-9). Washington, DC: U.S. Government Printing Office, Superintendent of Documents, (HP2010).

U.S. Department of Health and Human Services. (2007). *Healthy people 2010 midcourse review.* Retrieved February 5, 2008, from *www.healthypeople.gov/Data/midcourse/.*

U.S. Department of Health and Human Services. (2007). *The Surgeon General's call to action to prevent and decrease overweight and obesity.* Retrieved June 24, 2007, from *www.surgeongeneral.gov/topics/obesity/callto-action/fact_glance.htm.*

Wallace, M. (2005). Try this: Best practices in nursing care to older adults from the Hartford Institute for Geriatric Nursing: Sexuality. *Urologic Nursing, 25*(5), 373–374.

Wang, Y., & Beydoun, M. A. (2007). The obesity epidemic in the United States—gender, age, socioeconomic, racial/ethnic, and geographic characteristics: A systematic review and meta-regression analysis. *Epidemiologic Reviews, 29*(1), 6–28.

Warchol, K. (2006). Facilitating functional and quality-of-life potential: Strength-based assessment and treatment for all stages of dementia. *Topics in Geriatric Rehabilitation, 22*(3), 213–227.

Weber, J. R., & Kelley, J. (2006). *Health assessment in nursing* (3rd ed.). Philadelphia: Lippincott Williams & Wilkins.

Wilson, S. H., & Dorne, R. (2005). Impact of culture on the education of the geriatric patient. *Topics in Geriatric Rehabilitation, 21*(4), 282–294.

Wong, D. L., Perry, S. E., Hockenberry, M. J., Lowdermilk, D. L., & Wilson, D. (2005). *Maternal child nursing care* (3rd ed.). St. Louis: Mosby.

Yura, H. (1983). *Human needs and the nursing process* (3rd ed.). New York: McGraw Hill Appleton Lange.

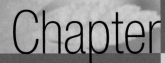

Chapter 7

Anne Rath Rentfro

Health Promotion and the Family

objectives

After completing this chapter, the reader will be able to:

- Assess families throughout the life span using the functional health pattern framework.
- Describe examples of the clinical data to collect in each health pattern during each family developmental phase.
- Provide examples of behavioral changes (functional, potentially dysfunctional, and actually dysfunctional) within the health patterns of families.
- Describe developmental and cultural characteristics of the family to consider when identifying risk factors or etiological factors of potential or actual dysfunctional health patterns.
- Develop planning, implementing, and evaluating nursing interventions in health promotion with families.
- Evaluate a specific health-promotion plan based on family assessment, nursing diagnosis, and contributing risks or etiological factors.

key terms

Cultural competence
Developmental theory
Ecomap
Family
Family developmental tasks
Family function

Family health status
Family nursing diagnosis
Family nursing interventions
Family pattern
Family resilience
Family risk factors

Family strengths
Family structure
Genogram
Risk factor theory
Systems theory

website materials

evolve These materials are located on the book's website at *http://evolve.elsevier.com/Edelman/*.

- WebLinks
- Study Questions
- Glossary
- Website Resources
    - **7A:** Nurse's Roles in Health Promotion and Disease Prevention Through Stages of Family Development
    - **7B:** Developmental Tasks of the Family at Critical Stages
    - **7C:** Eleven Functional Health Pattern Guidelines for Family Assessment
    - **7D:** Newman's Definitions of Family Health
    - **7E:** Examples of Family Nursing Diagnoses

THINK About It

Caring for Older Adults

Adult family members, who may have health problems of their own, find themselves caring for their older adult parents. This type of situation is expected to become more prevalent in the coming years.

1. What are the implications of this growing situation for individuals? Families? Communities? The nation?
2. How will this trend affect individual lives personally and professionally?

A **family** is a set of interacting individuals related by blood, marriage, cohabitation, or adoption who interdependently perform relevant functions by fulfilling expected roles. Relevant functions of the family include values and practices placed on health or family health practice. Health practices, whether effective or ineffective, are activities performed by individuals or families as a whole to promote health and prevent disease. How families complete developmental tasks and how well families, including individuals within a family, generate health-promoting behaviors determine families' potential for enhancement of family health practices.

How family members relate to one another influences the understanding of behavior, which is demonstrated in the family's structural, functional, communicational, and developmental patterns (American Academy of Pediatrics, 2003; Bonell et al., 2006; Friedman et al., 2003). An important consideration, therefore, in appraisal of health promotion and disease prevention is family assessment. Within families, children and adults are nurtured, provided for, and taught about health values by word and by example, and it is within families that members first learn to make choices to promote health. The American Academy of Pediatrics Report of the Task Force on the Family (2003) states that "Families are the most central and enduring influence in children's lives. ... The health and well being of children are inextricably linked to their parents' physical and emotional and social health, social circumstances and childrearing practices." *Healthy People 2010* views families as means of providing important opportunities for health promotion and disease prevention (U.S. Department of Health and Human Services, 2007; U.S. Department of Health and Human Services, 2000). This report asserts that beginning a family should be one of the joys of life. Through family planning, parents assume responsibility of caring for their children. Prenatal care and breast-feeding give infants a healthy start. Nutritious diets support physical growth and development. Children first observe and learn behaviors within their family. Patterns of nutrition, activity, oral hygiene, and coping develop at early ages, supported by family members' example. Patterns of alcohol consumption and tobacco use are similarly established within families. Learning about human development fosters a healthy self-concept, including positive awareness of their sexuality. Promoting self-esteem and reinforcing positive behaviors also strengthens the health of children. Primary care providers support positive behaviors by providing family members with scientifically sound health promotion and clinical preventive services, such as anticipatory guidance for developmental tasks, immunizations, screening for early detection, and appropriate counseling.

Pender claims that family provides the unit of assessment and intervention for health promotion, because families (1) develop self-care and dependent-care competencies; (2) foster resilience among family members; (3) provide resources; and (4) promote healthy individuation within cohesive family structures. Furthermore, fostering health and healthy behaviors becomes a developmental task for functional family process (Pender et al., 2006).

This chapter uses **systems theory**, **developmental theory**, and **risk factor theory** to guide nursing process with families. The 11 functional health patterns described in the previous chapter establish the structure for interview questions during data collection. The analysis phase of the nursing process categorizes these data within stages of family development and, from the analysis, nursing diagnoses are formulated. **Family health status** is considered functional, potentially dysfunctional (potential problem), or dysfunctional (actual problem) (Gordon, 2007). The planning phase begins when family goals and objectives are stated. The family, the nurse, or another health professional facilitates implementation. Later in this chapter, four types of interventions for health promotion and disease prevention are discussed: increasing knowledge and skills; increasing strengths; decreasing exposure to risks; and decreasing susceptibility. Nurses assume various roles throughout the stages of family development, and these roles are also presented. Evaluation of a family plan considers outcomes that are specific, objective, and measurable and that rely on the family's subjective interpretation of concerns and probability of success as well as at the population level (Clark, 2007; Friedman et al., 2003).

THE NURSING PROCESS AND THE FAMILY

Nursing process with families is a two-level process that includes the family as a group and the family member as an individual (Clark, 2007; Friedman et al., 2003). Home is a natural environment for health promotion encounters, although the process may occur in other settings as well. Different age groups (infants, children, and older adults) are likely to be available in the home. Nurses observe physical surroundings firsthand during home visits. For example, household safety hazards are observed directly. Nurses also monitor family unit rituals, roles, and interpersonal interactions. Generally the nurse contacts the family and establishes an appointment time for visiting. Including each family member in the visit provides a broad perspective. During visits, nursing process occurs mutually with families, not for families. Families collaborate with nursing in all phases of the process. Guidelines for home visits are presented in Box 7-1.

| Box 7-1 | Guidelines for Home Visit to Promote Health and Prevent Disease |

PLANNING THE VISIT
- Make arrangements with the family.
- Study information regarding the family from agency records, referral forms, and other sources.
- State the purpose of the visit.
- Obtain appropriate supplies and teaching aids for visits.

MAKING THE VISIT
- Offer an introduction and explain the purpose of the visit.
- Place the nurse's bag in an appropriate location.
- Include all family members in the discussion.
- Identify the family's request for assistance.
- Understand the situation from the family's perspective.
- Identify appropriate activities for health promotion and disease prevention.
- Identify how the home visit is to be financed.
- Make a contract with the family that states specific goals and objectives that the family wants to reach.
- Terminate the visit with specific instructions and information about the next visit: when it will occur, what will happen, who will be present, and what the family must accomplish before then.

Comprehensive family assessment provides the foundation to promote family health (Clark, 2007; Friedman et al., 2003). Several factors influence family assessment, such as nurses' perceptions about family constitution; theoretical knowledge; norms; standards; and communication abilities during visits. In addition to factors that pertain to the nurse, familial factors also influence assessments, such as family cooperation, mutual agreement to work toward goals, and family ability to recognize the relevance of health-promotion plans. Useful health-promotion family assessments involve listening to families, engaging in participatory dialogue, recognizing patterns, and assessing family potential for active, positive change (Clark, 2007; Friedman et al., 2003).

The assessment phase of the nursing process seeks and identifies information from the family about health-promotion and disease-prevention activities. To obtain this information, nurses follow family progress through developmental tasks and identify strengths in the family's ability to generate low risk–taking behaviors associated with disease prevention. The two approaches considered in this chapter are the developmental framework and the risk-factor estimate. Developmental phases as proposed by Duvall and Miller (Clark, 2007; Duvall & Miller, 1985); and risk-factor estimates as proposed in *Healthy People 2010* can be used to guide nurses through the steps of the nursing process when working with families (U.S. Department of Health and Human Services, 2007).

The Nurse's Role

Working with families using a systems perspective helps nurses understand family interaction, family norms and expectations, and effectiveness of family communication, family decision-making, and family coping mechanisms. The nurse's role in health promotion and disease prevention includes the following tasks:

1. Become aware of family attitudes and behaviors toward health promotion and disease prevention
2. Act as role model for the family
3. Collaborate with the family to assess, improve, enhance, and evaluate family health practices
4. Assist the family in growth and development behaviors
5. Assist the family in identifying risk-taking behaviors
6. Assist the family in decision-making about lifestyle choices
7. Provide reinforcement for positive health-behavior practices
8. Provide health information to the family
9. Assist the family in learning behaviors to promote health and prevent disease
10. Assist the family in problem solving and decision-making about health promotion
11. Serve as a liaison for referral or collaboration between community resources and the family

How nurses collaborate with families depends on the frameworks used to guide, observe, and classify situations. Nursing roles for families in various stages of development are presented in **Website Resource 7A**.

THE FAMILY FROM A SYSTEMS PERSPECTIVE

Systems theory explains patterns of living among the individuals who make up family systems. In systems theory, behaviors and family members' responses influence patterns. Meanings and values provide the vital elements of motivation and energy for family systems. Every family has its unique culture, value structure, and history. Values provide a means for interpreting events and information, passing from one generation to the next. Values usually change slowly over time. Families process information and energy exchange with the environment through values. For example, holiday food traditions may be changed slightly by a daughter-in-law whose own daughter may then adjust the traditional recipe within her own nuclear family.

System boundaries separate family systems from their environment and control information flow. This characteristic forms a family internal manager that influences and defines interactions and relationships with one another and with those outside the family system. Family forms a unified whole rather than the sum of its parts—an integrated system of interdependent functions, structures, and relationships. For example, one drug-dependent individual's health behavior influences the entire family unit.

Living systems are open systems. As living systems, families experience constant exchanges of energy and information with the environment. Change in one part or member of the family results in changes in the family as a whole. For example, loss of a family member through death changes roles and relationships among all family members. Change requires adaptation of every family member as roles and functions take on new meanings. Changes families make are incorporated into the system.

Families consist of both structural and functional components. **Family structure** refers to family composition, including roles and relationships, whereas **family function** consists as processes within systems as information and energy exchange occurs between families and their environment.

THE FAMILY FROM A DEVELOPMENTAL PERSPECTIVE

Building on Erikson's (1998) theory of psychosocial development, Duvall and Miller (1985) identified stages of the family life cycle and critical **family developmental tasks**. Although Duvall's classification has been criticized for its middle class homogeneity and lack of diversity in family forms, this conceptual model helps to anticipate family events, and has formed the basis for more contemporary developmental models (Clark, 2007). Knowing a family's composition, interrelationships, and particular life cycle helps nurses predict overall **family pattern**. Box 7-2 lists tasks essential to the family's survival and continuity. From Duvall's perspective, most families complete these basic family tasks. Each family performs these tasks in a unique expression of its personality. Nurses collect data to determine progress toward task attainment (Clark, 2007). In addition to general tasks of survival and continuity, stages of

development exist in this model, with specific tasks related to each stage further developed by Goldenberg and Goldenberg (2008). Specific tasks arise as growth responsibilities during family development. Failure to accomplish a developmental task leads to negative consequences. For example, intimate partner violence, child abuse or neglect may result in intervention by police, welfare, health department, or other agencies (Health Teaching box). Life cycle tasks build upon

---

| Box **7-2** | Tasks for Family Survival and Continuity |

- Providing shelter, food, clothing, health care, and similar needs for its members
- Meeting family costs and allocating resources, such as time, space, and facilities, according to each member's needs
- Determining who does what in the support, management, and care of the home and its members
- Ensuring each member's socialization through the internalization of increasingly mature roles in the family and in society
- Establishing ways of interacting, communicating, and expressing affection, aggression, sexuality, and similar interactions within limits acceptable to society
- Bearing (or adopting) and rearing children, then incorporating and releasing family members appropriately
- Relating to school, church, work, and community life and establishing policies for the inclusion of in-laws, relatives, guests, friends, mass media, and others
- Maintaining morale and motivation, rewarding achievement, meeting personal and family crises, setting attainable goals, and developing family loyalties and values

Modified from Clark, M. J. (2007). *Community health nursing* (5th ed.). Upper Saddle River, NJ: Pearson Education/Prentice Hall.

HEALTH TEACHING   Domestic Violence: Intimate Partner Violence

If the person is still in the relationship:
- Think of a safe place to go if an argument occurs—avoid rooms with no exits (bathroom), or rooms with weapons (kitchen).
- Think about and make a list of safe people to contact.
- Keep a cell phone with you at all times.
- Memorize all important numbers.
- Establish a "code word" or "sign" so that family, friends, teachers, or co-workers know when to call for help.
- Think about what to say to partner if he/she becomes violent.
- Remind the individual that he/she has the right to live without fear and violence.

If the person has left the relationship:
- Change the phone number.
- Screen calls.
- Save and document all contacts, messages, injuries, or other incidents involving the batterer.
- Change locks, if the batterer has a key.
- Avoid staying alone.
- Plan how to get away if confronted by an abusive partner.

- If a meeting is necessary, do it in a public place.
- Vary the routine.
- Notify school and work contacts.
- Call a shelter.

If leaving the relationship or thinking of leaving, the individual should take important papers and documents to facilitate application for benefits or take legal action. Important papers include Social Security cards and birth certificates for self and children, marriage license, leases or deeds, checkbook, charge cards, bank statements and charge account statements, insurance policies, proof of income (pay stubs or W-2s), and any documentation of past incidents of abuse (photos, police reports, medical records, etc.).

The National Coalition Against Domestic Violence provides information to health care providers, a network of shelters, and counseling programs and operates a national hotline: 800-799-SAFE (7233); website: *www.ncadv.org*; address and telephone number: 1120 Lincoln Street, Suite 1603 Denver, CO 80203; Phone: 303-839-1852; Fax: 303-831-9251; Telecommunication Device: TTY - (303) 839-1681.

Adapted from information on the National Coalition Against Domestic Violence. Retrieved from *www.ncadv.org*.

one another. Success at one stage is dependent upon success at an earlier stage. Early failure may lead to developmental difficulties at later stages.

As families enter each new developmental stage, transition occurs. Events such as marriage (heterosexual, homosexual), gay and lesbian relationships, childbirth, single led families, joint custody, or remarried families, releasing members as adolescents and young adults, and continuing through the "empty nest" and aging years move families through new stages.

Each new developmental stage requires adaptation with new responsibilities. Concurrently, developmental stages provide opportunities for families to realize their potential. Nurses anticipate change through analysis of progress through each stage. Each new stage presents opportunities for health promotion and intervention.

Family development stages, although reflective of traditional nuclear families and extended family networks, also apply to nontraditional family configurations (Clark, 2007). For example, couples may marry and bring children from a previous marriage to a blended family that works toward achieving developmental tasks of couples along with family stages for the children. Both the couple and their children bring values and beliefs from the past that must integrate within the present union. Childless couples present developmental tasks that are different from those proposed for couples with children.

Assessment of family developmental stages entails using guidelines to analyze progress toward developmental tasks, family growth, and health-promotion needs. Family developmental task guidelines are summarized in **Website Resource 7B**.

THE FAMILY FROM A RISK-FACTOR PERSPECTIVE

Family risk factors can be inferred from (1) lifestyle; (2) biological factors; (3) environmental factors; (4) social, psychological, cultural, and spiritual dimensions; and (5) the health care system. As outlined in the Frank Thompson case study in Chapter 1, lifestyle habits such as overeating, drug dependency, high sugar and cholesterol intake, and smoking influence health outcomes. Biological risk factors may include the elements of genetic inheritance, congenital malformation, and mental retardation. To fully explore environmental risk factors that influence family function, nurses explore work pressures, stress, anxieties, tensions, and air, noise, or water pollution. Social and psychological dimensions such as crowding, isolation, or rapid and accelerated rates of change are areas to consider when assessing family risk factors. Cultural and spiritual aspects may include traditions of preventing illness such as daily prayer and meditation practices. Finally, health care system factors such as overuse, underuse, inappropriate use, or accessibility are considered in the family risk assessment.

To reduce risk factors, nurses help families focus on influencing health behaviors of their members. Society glamorizes many hazardous behaviors through advertising and mass media that minimizes negative health consequences.

Families influence their members to weigh consequences of risk-taking behavior. Awareness of risk factors may prompt families to reduce modifiable risk factors. Healthy behavior, including use of preventive health care services, is a significant area of family responsibility.

Traditionally, epidemiology has used levels and trends of mortality and morbidity rates as indirect evidence of health. Data such as infant mortality rates, stillbirth rates, and leading causes of death have long been used as indicators of collective community health. Healthy family functioning links the family life cycle stages with specific risk factors. Epidemiology often describes a disease association in terms of risk. Health risks can be physiological or psychological. Physiological risks arise from genetic background, whereas psychological risks include those related to low self-image. Risks also arise from environmental considerations, including physical environment and socioeconomic condition (Barlow et al., 2007; Bauman et al., 2006; Latkin et al., 2007). Risk-factor theory considers families a pivotal part of the environment and also an important support system used to decrease health risks for individuals.

Risk estimates calculate differences between two groups: one with the risk factor and one without. Frequency of deaths, illnesses, or injuries with some specific risk factor compared to another group without the risk factor, or the population as a whole, determines the risk estimate. Some diseases occur more frequently in certain families, such as sickle cell anemia in Black families and Tay-Sachs disease in Ashkenazi (East European) Jewish families (Clark, 2007). Other diseases such as iron deficiency anemia may not be attributed to specific genetic background. The natural history of a chronic disease predisposes family members to greater risk, but specific causes may be difficult to identify. Lubkin and Larsen (2006) describe nine phases that individuals and families may experience as they progress through chronic illness adaptation from the time before the disorder is recognized through a stable adjustment phase to the final relinquishment of life interest and activities.

Probabilities of risk change may also change depending on the family's activities in health promotion and disease prevention. Stages of family development are used to classify risk factors. Age-specific developmental stages, along with their associated age-specific health risks, appear in Table 7-1, which displays periods during which families become most sensitive to certain problems with corresponding key times for health promotion and disease prevention. Risk behaviors highlighted include tobacco and alcohol use, faulty nutrition, overuse of medications, fast driving, stress, and relentless pressure to achieve. Habits learned in family settings help to develop individual lifestyle behaviors. Five habits—(1) diet, (2) smoking, (3) exercise, (4) alcohol use, and (5) stress—affect at least 7 of the 10 leading causes of death listed in the *Healthy People 2010* report (U.S. Department of Health and Human Services, 2007). See the *Healthy People 2010* box for selected objectives related to families.

Table **7-1** Family Stage: Specific Risk Factors and Related Health Problems

Stage	Risk Factors	Health Problems
Beginning childbearing	Lack of knowledge about family planning Adolescent marriage Lack of knowledge concerning sexual and marital roles and adjustments Low–birth-weight infant Lack of prenatal care Inadequate nutrition Poor eating habits Smoking, alcohol, and drug abuse Unmarried status First pregnancy before age 16 or after age 35 History of hypertension and infections during pregnancy Rubella, syphilis, gonorrhea, and AIDS Genetic factors Low socioeconomic and educational levels Lack of safety in the home	Premature baby in family Birth defects Birth injuries Accidents SIDS Respiratory distress syndrome Sterility Pelvic inflammatory disease Fetal alcohol syndrome Mental retardation Child abuse Injuries Birth defects Underweight or overweight
Family with school-aged children	Working parents with inappropriate use of resources for child care Poverty Abuse or neglect of children Generational pattern of using social agencies as way of life Multiple, closely spaced children Low family self-esteem Children used as scapegoats for parental frustration Repeated infections, accidents, or hospitalizations Parents immature, dependent, and unable to handle responsibility Unrecognized or unattended health problems Strong beliefs about physical punishment Toxic substances unguarded in the home Poor nutrition	Behavior disturbances Speech and vision problems Communicable diseases Dental caries School problems Learning disabilities Cancer Injuries Chronic diseases Homicide Violence
Family with adolescents	Racial and ethnic family origin Lifestyle and behavior patterns leading to chronic disease Lack of problem-solving skills Family values of aggressiveness and competition Family values rigid and inflexible Daredevil risk-taking attitudes Denial behavior Conflicts between parents and children Pressure to live up to family expectations	Violent deaths and injuries Alcohol and drug abuse Unwanted pregnancies Sexually transmitted diseases Suicide Depression
Family with middle-aged adults	Hypertension Smoking High cholesterol levels Physical inactivity Genetic predisposition Use of oral contraceptives Sex, race, and other hereditary factors Geographical area, age, and occupational deficiencies Habits (i.e., diet with low fiber, pickling, charcoal use, and broiling) Alcohol abuse Social class Residence	Cardiovascular disease, principally coronary artery disease and cerebrovascular accident (stroke) Diabetes Overweight Cancer Accidents Homicide Suicide Abnormal fetus Mental illness Periodontal disease and loss of teeth Depression
Family with older adults	Age Drug interactions Metabolic disorders Pituitary malfunctions	Mental confusion Reduced vision Hearing impairment Hypertension

Table **7-1** Family Stage: Specific Risk Factors and Related Health Problems—*cont'd*		
Stage	**Risk Factors**	**Health Problems**
	Cushing's syndrome	Acute illness
	Hypercalcemia	Infectious disease
	Chronic illness	Influenza
	Retirement	Pneumonia
	Loss of spouse	Injuries such as burns and falls
	Reduced income	Depression
	Poor nutrition	Chronic disease
	Lack of exercise	Elder abuse
	Past environments and lifestyle	Death without dignity
	Lack of prevention for death	

Modified from U.S. Department of Health and Human Services. (2007). *Healthy People 2010 Midcourse Review*. Washington, DC: U.S. Government Printing Office.

Healthy People 2010

Selected Examples of National Health-Promotion and Disease-Prevention Objectives for Families

- 1-4. Increase the proportion of people who have a specific source of ongoing care.
- 19-2. Reduce the proportion of adults who are obese.
- 19-3. Reduce the proportion of children and adolescents who are overweight or obese.
- 26-9. Increase the age and proportion of adolescents who remain alcohol and drug free.
- 26-10. Reduce past-month use of illicit substances.
- 26-11. Reduce the proportion of persons engaging in binge drinking of alcoholic beverages.

From U.S. Department of Health and Human Services. (2000). *Healthy people 2010: Understanding and improving health* (Government Report No. Stock Number 017-001-001-00-550-9). Washington, DC: U.S. Government Printing Office, Superintendent of Documents (HP2010).

FUNCTIONAL HEALTH PATTERNS: ASSESSMENT OF THE FAMILY

Gordon's 11 functional health patterns (2007) help organize basic family assessment information (Friedman et al., 2003). Patterns form the standardized format for family assessment using a systems approach with emphasis on developmental stages and risk factors. Assessment includes evaluation of dysfunctional patterns within families with corresponding details in one or more of the other interdependent patterns (see Chapter 6).

The presence of risk factors predicts potential dysfunction. Developmental risk and risk arising from dysfunctional health patterns increase whole family risk (see Table 7-1). Gordon (2007) interprets risk states as potential problems. To formulate nursing diagnoses, nurses identify problems along with their associated and etiological factors. Influencing factors may precede or occur concurrently with the problem and are used to plan care. Interventions aim to modify influencing factors to promote positive change.

Family history begins with the health perception–health management pattern. Exploring issues within this pattern first provides an overview to help locate where problems exist in other patterns and to determine which ones may require more thorough assessment. Interviewing from the family's perspective helps families define situations. The roles-relationships pattern defines family structure and function. The remaining nine patterns address lifestyle indicators.

Health Perception–Health Management Pattern

Characteristics of family health perceptions, health management, and preventive practices are revealed with assessment of the Health Perception–Health Management Pattern. The National Survey of Children's Health has been designed to contribute data to identify health-promoting behaviors of families (Van Dyck et al., 2004). Data collected in this survey include information about frequency of family meals together; religious service attendance; characteristics of parental relationship with child; parental coping with raising children; and methods for handling family disagreements (Van Dyck et al., 2004). The intent of the survey is to provide a data source to explore research questions related to *Healthy People 2010* and the variables correlate with drug use (Van Dyck et al., 2004). However, such data has also been associated with eating disorders and risk behaviors other than drug use. These assessment indicators also provide data to guide the remaining functional health pattern assessment. Patterns overlap and findings in one pattern may encourage further assessment in another pattern. Research questions that concern family health promotion may include:

- What are parents' chief concerns regarding their children's development, learning, and behavior?
- How do parents' health practices (physical activity and smoking behavior) relate to children's health status?
- What health-related behaviors, such as eating three meals a day at regular times, eating breakfast every day,

exercising a minimum of 2 or 3 days a week, sleeping 7 to 8 hours each night, and abstaining from smoking does the family practice?

- How safe are homes, schools, and neighborhoods from the perspective of parents (Van Dyck et al., 2004)?

Health practices vary from family to family. Families identify and perform health-maintenance activities based on their beliefs about health. Nurses promote refinement of families' responses to each member as well as to the family environment (Talen et al., 2007). Exploration during the assessment also includes the following areas:

- What is the family's philosophy of health? Does each family member hold similar beliefs? Do family members practice what they believe?
- In what negative behaviors or lifestyle practices, such as smoking, alcohol, and drug abuse, does the family engage?
- What chronic disease risk behaviors are exhibited within the family?
- Are risk factors present for infections, such as lack of immunization, lack of knowledge of transmittable diseases, and poor personal hygiene?
- Are risk factors for bodily injury, accidents, or substance abuse present in the home?
- Do older adult members know what medications they are taking and the reasons for using them?
- Does the family discard outdated medications or those not used?
- What unattended health problems exist?
- Is there a history of repeated infections and hospitalization?
- Is the home understimulating or overstimulating?
- Where does the family obtain health and illness care?
- Is the family engaged in a dental program?
- How does the family describe previous experiences with nurses and other health care professionals?

Nutritional-Metabolic Pattern

The nutritional-metabolic pattern depicts characteristics of the family's typical food and fluid consumption and metabolism (Gordon, 2007). Included are growth and development patterns, pregnancy-related nutritional patterns, and the family's eating patterns. Risk factors for obesity, diabetes, anorexia, and bulimia are identified.

Dietary habits, learned within the family context, involve behavioral patterns central to daily life. Keeping a diary of intake for a week provides a useful strategy for assessing family food and fluid intake patterns. Assessment notes both meals shared with the whole family as well as additional consumption by individuals. Recent research provides evidence that family meal sharing is associated with healthier eating habits (Ayala et al., 2007; Gable et al., 2007). Frequency of family meals has also been inversely associated with other health behaviors and risk factors. For example, Eisenberg et al. (2004) determined that frequency of eating meals together as a family was inversely associated

with use of tobacco, alcohol, and marijuana. Furthermore low grade point average and depressive symptoms such as suicide involvement were likewise associated with fewer meals eaten together.

Exploration during nutrition pattern assessment includes the following areas:

- What kinds of foods are typically consumed?
- Who eats together at mealtimes?
- How is food viewed (reward/punishment)?
- Is there adequate storage and refrigeration?
- How is food purchased?
- How is food prepared?

Elimination Pattern

The elimination pattern describes characteristics of regularity and control of the family's excretory functions (Gordon, 2007). Bowel and bladder function and environmental factors such as waste disposal in the home, neighborhood, and community that influence family life are considered in this pattern.

Questions are phrased according to the age-specific developmental stage of the family. For example, in determining whether there is a problem in the preschool stage, it would be appropriate to ask whether the child is being toilet trained. In families with adolescents, the nurse may ask how often individuals have bowel movements and whether there have been any changes from usual patterns. The nurse may ask older adult members whether they have any problems with constipation. Issues that particularly concern older adults include constipation, diarrhea, polyuria, and incontinence, as well as use of antacids and anticonstipation agents. The nurse evaluates whether use of these agents is appropriate or possibly contributing to poor health.

Activity-Exercise Pattern

The activity-exercise pattern represents family characteristics that require energy expenditure (Gordon, 2007). The nurse reviews daily activities, exercise, and leisure activities. Families create settings for individual members to be physically active, sedentary, or apathetic toward physical activity. The quantity of sedentary activities such as television and video game screen time is explored.

Exploration during assessment of this pattern includes the following areas:

- How does the family exhibit its beliefs about regular exercise and physical fitness being necessary for good health?
- What types of daily activities include physical exercise and who does what with whom?
- What are the television viewing habits of children?
- How are other screen-viewing activities (computers, video games) incorporated into the daily routines?
- How often do children exercise?
- How are these activity and exercise factors related to children's health?
- What does the family do to have fun (Figure 7-1)?

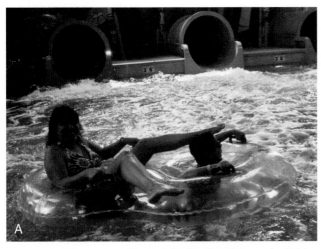 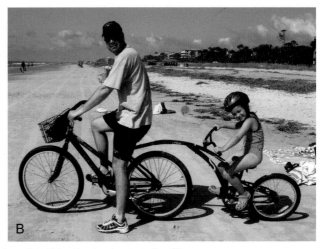

Figure 7-1   Family outings can be **A**, leisurely and restful or **B**, adventurous and exciting.

Sleep-Rest Pattern

Rest habits characterize the sleep-rest pattern (Gordon, 2007). Without the restorative function of sleep, individuals exhibit decreased performance, bad temper, and decreased stress tolerance and may rely on substances such as alcohol or other chemicals to induce sleep. Regular, sufficient sleep patterns are linked to better mental status including learning and decision-making. Most families have sleeping patterns, although in some families these patterns may not be readily apparent. It is important to elicit the data about sleep and rest from the family's perspective.

Assessment of the sleep-rest pattern includes the following:
- What are the usual sleeping habits of the family?
- How suitable are they to the age and health status of the family members?
- What are the usual hours established for sleeping?
- Who decides when and how children go to sleep?
- Do family members take naps or have other regular means of resting or relaxing?
- How early does the family rise? What are the patterns related to bedtime and rising?
- Do all family members have the same general sleep-rest pattern?
- Is there a family member with sleep disruption?

Cognitive-Perceptual Pattern

The cognitive-perceptual pattern identifies characteristics of language, cognitive skills, and perception that influence desired or required family activities (Gordon, 2007). Specifically, this pattern concerns how families access information to make decisions, how concrete or abstract the thought processes are, and whether decisions focus on present or future issues. Decision-making in families is associated with power in family functioning. Highly educated families usually have greater repertoires for problem solving. Power and ability to solve problems are linked to leadership; family leaders must be acknowledged if nursing interventions are to be implemented.

Cognitive-perceptual pattern assessment includes the following:
- How does the family access and interpret information, especially about health (e.g., newspaper, books, computer, television radio)?
- What are the usual family reading patterns and strategies used for ongoing learning, for example, continuing education programs?
- What kinds of materials does the family read to their children?
- How does the family usually make decisions about health promotion and disease prevention?
- How do members contribute to the decision-making process?
- How knowledgeable is the family about risk factors and developmental milestones?
- How are choices made regarding lifestyle?
- How knowledgeable are family members about correct information?
- How do family members acquire information?
- How accurate are the information sources used to make health promotion choices?
- How do family members describe whether their health behavior is constructive or destructive?
- How do family members recognize signs and symptoms of deteriorating health?
- How do family members decide when medical attention is necessary?
- Who makes the decisions about when to seek health care?
- What factors contribute to delays from time of onset to time of treatment?
- How long do families wait before seeking care?
- What are some of the cues that signal to families that care is needed?
- How is professional care accessed?
- What type of health care is generally used (health maintenance for immunizations, well child care or emergency/urgent care facilities)?

- How are decisions made about the use of over-the-counter medications taken or the use of alternative or traditional health practices?

Self-Perception–Self-Concept Pattern

The self-perception–self-concept pattern identifies characteristics that describe the family's self-worth and feeling states (Gordon, 2007). Rapport between the family members and the nurse facilitates disclosure. Families have perceptions and concepts about their image, their status in the community, and their competencies as a family unit. Families manifest these perceptions through shared aspirations, values, expectations, fears, successes, and failures. Relationships in families determine the amount of sharing that occurs. Situations affecting one member influence perceptions of the entire family group. How each member describes the family often gives clues to the family self-concept.

Exploration during assessment includes the following:
- How is this family similar to or different from other families?
- How does this family perceive itself to be similar to and different from other families?
- What special assets does each member contribute to the family?
- What changes would each member like to see occur in the family?
- What kinds of feelings do family members have for each other?
- Describe the general tone of feelings in the family. Is the tone indifferent, secretive, angry, or open?
- How does the family think it assimilates into the neighborhood and community?
- How does the family handle stress and crisis situations?
- How does the family experience changes in the way it feels about itself?
- How does the family describe the events that led to a change?

Roles-Relationships Pattern

The roles-relationships pattern identifies characteristics of family roles and relationships (Gordon, 2007). Both structural and functional aspects of the family are assessed. Structural aspects of families include each member's name, age, sex, education, occupation, and role in the family. Traditionally, families have been described as nuclear and extended. The traditional nuclear family consists of husband, wife, and children, with an extended family that would include aunts, uncles, cousins, and grandparents. Today there are many varieties of nuclear and extended families (Cherlin, 2004; Hamilton et al., 2007). Clark (2007) describes the various contemporary family structures: traditional nuclear family, extended families, single-parent families, stepfamilies, cohabiting families, gay and lesbian families, grandparent-headed families, foster families, and fragmentary families. Traditional nuclear family structure has been influenced by societal changes, such as the women's movement, employment of mothers, divorce, and remarriage. Exploration of family origin and genetic heritage completes family identification data collection. Cultural practices in the home may or may not reflect the family's genetic heritage; therefore, it is important to explore cultural and ethnic practices (Andrews & Boyle, 2008).

The Academy of Pediatrics Task Force on the Family regards family as the most enduring link to health for children (American Academy of Pediatrics, 2003). The U.S. Census Bureau (2007a) released information in 2006 from the annual report of Families and Living Arrangements derived from the Current Population Survey's Annual Social and Economic Supplement. Since 1970, married-couple families with children fell from 40% to 23% in 2005 (U.S. Census Bureau, 2007b). By 2006, families without children comprised the structure for the majority of families (U.S. Census Bureau, 2007b). Whitehead and Popenoe (2006) claim that the combination of increased life expectancy and delayed childbirth in women have contributed to the increase in the numbers of families without children.

Of families with children, 67% have two parents reflecting a decrease from 85% in 1970 (American Academy of Pediatrics, 2003; Bergman, 2007). Many children live with grandparents in the grandparents' home with at least one of the parents present (Bergman, 2007). In 2006, 9% of U.S. households were led by single parents compared to 6% in 1970. Although the number of single male parents has increased (2.5 million), female parents continue to predominate as single parents (10.4 million) (Bergman, 2007). In 2006, 5 times the number of single-mother families lived in poverty (42%) than married couples with families (8%) regardless of race or ethnicity (U.S. Census Bureau, 2007a). These data clearly indicate the need to identify family structure, particularly those at risk (Table 7-2). Family structure and function influence child-rearing and individual development and pose a challenge to the nurse in health promotion and disease prevention.

Divorce and remarriage involve a complex transition that requires the disintegration of one family structure and organization of another (Afifi & Keith, 2004; Clark, 2007). Developmental levels of the children, their individual temperaments, and the quality of their environmental support all contribute to the family response (Borell, 2003; Clark, 2007). Addressing the needs of the children may be difficult for the parents, who are at the same time experiencing an adjustment to each other (Ahrons, 2007). How parents cope during the situational crisis, as well as after the divorce, is a significant variable in long-term individual and family adjustment. See the Case Study at the end of this chapter for presentation of a stepfamily situation.

Table 7-2 Variety of Family Structures

Configuration	Positions in Family
Single parent (separated, divorced, or widowed)	Mother or father Sons(s), daughter(s)
Unmarried single parent (never married)	Mother or father Sons(s), daughter(s)
Unmarried couple	Two adults
Unmarried parents	Mother and father Sons(s), daughter(s)
Commune family	Mothers and fathers Shared son(s), daughters(s)
Stepparents	Son(s), daughter(s) from previous marriage Mother and father
Adoptive	Adopted son(s), daughter(s)
Family of choice	Adults with selected partners and family members
Married couple	Mother and father
Married parents	Mother and father son(s), daughter(s)
Grandparent(s)	Grandmother and/or Grandfather Grandchildren son(s) and/or daughter(s)

In a study conducted by Afifi and Keith (2004), investigators examined the role of loss after divorce. Interviews with 81 stepfamily members revealed loss of previous family structure and parental bonding. A **family resilience** framework may be useful to promote strategies for prevention efforts aimed at strengthening families as they face life challenges. Greeff et al. (2006) explored family resilience in 68 divorced families in Belgium finding positive correlations between components of resilience (commitment, challenge, and control) and family adaptation. Using a family resilience framework may help to address marginalization of families that Jones (2003) describes. Ziffer et al. (2007) describe an innovative counseling program called the "Boomerang Bunch" designed to build on family resilience. The complexity of family structure and function require such innovative strategies to enhance long-term family adjustment to divorce (Kelly, 2003).

Family disruption has been associated with substance abuse and psychosocial maladjustment in adolescents and young adults. For example, Roustit et al. (2007) used data from the Social and Health Survey of Children and Adolescents in Montreal to explore the impact of family function on adolescents' adjustment. Adolescent psychosocial adjustment and family function were associated in their analyses. For example, witnessing violence in the home and psychological disorders were associated. Moreover, family dissolution and family disruption were also both associated with substance abuse, alcohol consumption, and externalizing behaviors such as theft, property destruction, fighting, and assault (Roustit et al., 2007). Dawson et al. (2006) found associations among developmental transitions and alcohol dependence in young adults with their analyses of the U.S. National Epidemiologic Survey on Alcohol and Related conditions. In their analyses, marriage and parenthood were positively associated with recovery from alcohol dependence (Dawson et al., 2006). Both studies provide support for the importance of the role relationship patterns in the development of health-promoting behaviors.

Family organization influences performance of health-promotion and disease-prevention functions. For example, a single parent without an extended family network may be in need of more community resources to help raise the children. A two-parent family living near its extended family may need less support to raise children, but members may need to know about growth and developmental stages and immunization schedules. Individuals may experience a variety of family structures in one lifetime. A person may be part of a nuclear family as an infant, a single-parent family after the parents are divorced, a stepparent family when the mother or father remarries, and an unmarried couple family when the person is one of two adults who share a household. The person brings the values and beliefs about health promotion and disease prevention that were practiced in previous unions to each new family configuration. Divergent values may result in conflicting expectations unless the new union forms a set of integrated values and beliefs. The current trend away from the nuclear family with extended family may influence the general direction of the health care system and the strategies used to promote health with other family configurations.

Certain health-promotion issues are of particular concern to the nurse while assessing family health promotion and disease prevention. Violence is a health problem that threatens the integrity of all families (Bennett et al., 2006). Family violence includes child abuse, spouse abuse, and elder abuse, with women being victimized more often during pregnancy. In fact, mortality in pregnancy is often associated with domestic violence (Asling-Monemi et al., 2003; Chang et al., 2005; Furniss et al., 2007; Webster & Holt, 2004). Health promotion and violence prevention requires a complex set of skills (Bennett et al., 2006; Sege et al., 2006). Nurses use approaches to reduce violence-related injuries and deaths by acquiring the role of advocate and helping to eliminate victim blaming (Gance-Cleveland, 2001; Sege et al., 2006) (Research Highlights box). Explorations to assess families for health promotion and violence prevention may include the following:

- What formal positions and roles does each of the family members fulfill?
- What roles are considered acceptable and consistent within the family's expectations?

research highlights

Intimate Partner Violence (IPV) has Negative Effects on Family Function

This study analyzed behavior of 109 children (18 months to 18 years) to determine if there were differences in behavior between children of mothers who were physically and sexually assaulted compared to those mothers who were not sexually assaulted. Children of mothers experienced both physical and sexual assault scored significantly higher on the Child Behavior Checklist than those children of mothers who experienced physical IPV without sexual IPV. Children with higher scores on CBC had increased nonhealthy behaviors and disorders. Older children exhibited more behavioral disorders, particularly depression and anxiety.

Nurses may use this study to guide referral to community counseling and include child behavior problems in their assessment of IPV.

From McFarlane, J., Malech, A., Watson, K., Gist, J., Batten, E., Hall, I., et al. (2007). Intimate partner physical and sexual assault and child behavior problems. *Maternal Child Health Nursing, 32*(2) 74-80.

- What kind of flexibility in roles takes place when needed?
- What informal roles exist? Who plays informal roles and with what consistency? What purpose do the informal roles serve?
- How are the family social support networks associated with health and development?
- Who were the role models for the couples or single people as parents?
- Who were the role models for marital partners and what were their characteristics?
- How does the family manage daily living? How are the household tasks divided?
- How are problems handled? How are problems with children handled?
- Who is employed outside the home?
- Who takes care of the children when both parents are employed outside the home?
- How does the family care for its ill members? Its older adult members?
- Are behaviors appropriate for family stages of development?
- Is decision-making allocated to the appropriate members?
- Does the family respond appropriately to its members' developmental needs?
- Is there fair distribution of tasks among family members?
- Is the family's emotional climate conducive to growth and development?

When this initial assessment reveals possible neglect, abuse, or violence, further assessment is warranted with a branched assessment that may include the following assessment parameters and questions.

- What cues are present to indicate chemical abuse?
- Who are the significant adult members of the household? (determine presence of boyfriend/girlfriend)

Genogram

A **genogram**, or family diagram, represents the family based on identification data that depicts each member of the family with connections between the generations. This useful technique gathers data on at least three generations, including the current one, their parents, grandparents, aunts, uncles, and their children. The family genogram explores clues within family histories contributing to health problems. Figure 7-2 depicts accepted genogram symbols with a sample genogram of the fictional Graham family portrayed in Figure 7-3 (Stanhope & Lancaster, 2008). The Graham family genogram shows a variety of family structures, including changes resulting from marriage, divorce, death, and childbearing. This information highlights family health patterns to use for anticipatory health guidance, for example in the case of the Graham family, hypertension, type 2 diabetes, cancer, and hypercholesterolemia.

Ecomap

The **ecomap**, which is similar to the genogram, uses pictorial techniques to document family organizational patterns with visual clarity. A genogram is constructed for a family or household. It begins with a circle in the center of the page. Outside the circle, smaller circles are drawn and labeled with the names of significant people, agencies, and institutions in the family's social environment. Lines are drawn from the family-household to each circle. Solid lines indicate strong relationships. Dotted lines reflect fragile or tenuous connections. Slashed lines signify stressful relationships. Arrows can be drawn parallel to the lines to indicate the direction for the energy flow or for resources (Stanhope & Lancaster, 2008). Figure 7-4 shows an ecomap for the fictional Graham family. Both the genogram and the ecomap provide useful information and can be incorporated into any brief family assessment (Martinez et al., 2007).

Sexuality-Reproductive Pattern

Sexuality is the expression of sexual identity. The sexuality-reproductive pattern describes sexuality fulfillment (Gordon, 2007), including behavioral patterns of reproduction. This pattern also includes perceptions of satisfaction or disturbances in sexuality, sexual relationships, reproduction (including contraception), and developmental changes throughout the life span, such as menarche and menopause (Hot Topics box). The sexuality-reproductive pattern addresses transmission of information within the family about sexuality as well as sexuality for the couple, including their sexual relationship, perception of problems, how problems are handled, and actions taken to solve problems (Gordon, 2007). Information transmission during childhood is an

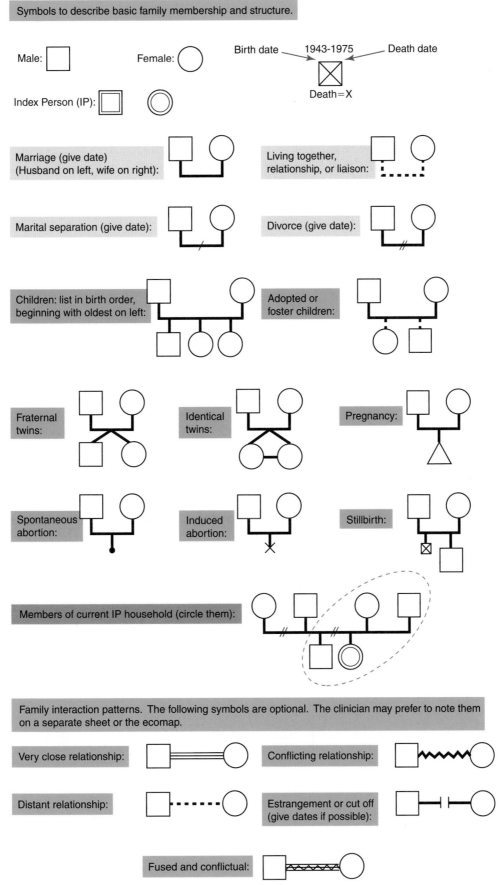

Figure 7-2 Genogram symbols. (Modified from McGoldrick, M., Gerson, R., & Petry, S. [2008]. *Genograms: Assessment and intervention* [3rd ed.]. New York: Norton.)

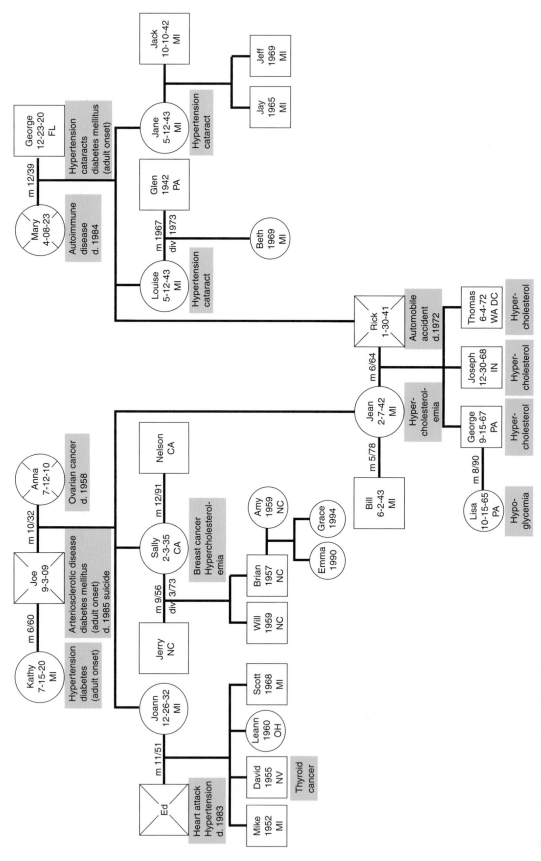

Figure 7-3 Genogram of the Graham family. (From Stanhope, M. & Lancaster, J. [2008]. *Public health nursing: Population-centered health care in the community* [7th ed.]. St. Louis: Mosby, p. 589.)

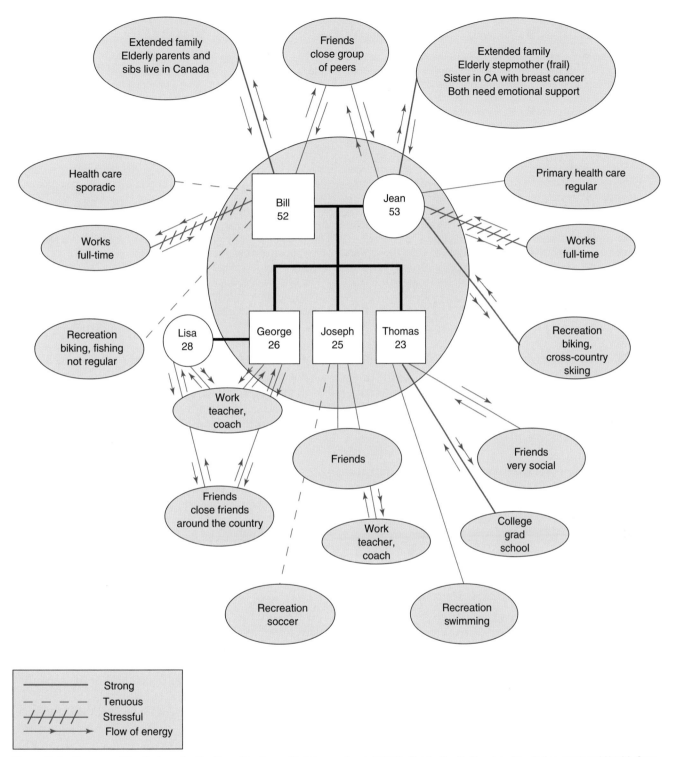

Figure 7-4 Ecomap of the Graham family. (From Stanhope, M. & Lancaster, J. [2008]. *Public Health Nursing: Population-centered Health Care in the Community*, 7th ed. St. Louis: Mosby, p. 591.)

important area to explore to better understand how issues related to sexuality and gender identity are addressed within the family (Gordon, 2007).

Topics to explore during the assessment may include the following areas:
- How do the adults in the family communicate needs to each other?

- How do family members commit to, love, and care for each other, as well as fulfill their obligations and responsibilities toward one another?
- How do the adults in the family view marriage, parenthood, and their relationship as lovers?
- How does the family address family planning and birth control?

HOTtopics

TELEVISION, AGGRESSIVE BEHAVIOR, SEXUALITY, AND OBESITY

Television is one of the most pervasive influences in American society. During formative stages of development, children and adolescents view thousands of hours of television. This sedentary activity involves viewing scenes that depict violence and sexual relationships that are rapid, casual, and frequent. These scenes often convey status without depicting responsibility or consequences of actions. Although more research is needed, evidence shows that mass media influences aggressive behavior as well as beliefs about sexual behavior. In addition, as time viewing television programs increases, physical activity levels decrease.

In a study of more than 2000 children, the relationship between body mass index (BMI) and television habits were explored. Children who were identified as overweight or obese generally viewed more television than those with normal BMI (Atherson & Metcalf, 2005; Bryant, Lucove, Evenson, & Marshall, 2007; Dennison, Erb, & Jenkins, 2002; Wake, Hesketh, & Waters, 2003).

The American Academy of Pediatrics (AAP) has described the negative health effects of television viewing on children and adolescents. Among these effects are aggressive behavior, substance use, sexual activity, obesity, poor body image, and worse school performance. The AAP Committee on Public Education recommends that health professionals remain informed about these issues and use the resources available from AAP, such as the AAP Media Matters campaign and Media History Form. Strategies to ensure appropriate entertainment options should be available in agency waiting rooms and play rooms (American Academy of Pediatrics, 2001).

In addition to the role that television plays with regard to obesity, sedentary activity has been linked to earlier age of menarche. Body fat mass may play a role in accelerating puberty; however, it is clear that prepubertal activity and nutrition contribute to sexual maturation at some level (Wu, Mendola, & Buck, 2002). These issues are essential to consider while evaluating the activity-exercise pattern.

- How do family members participate in choice of family planning and contraceptives used?

When needed, complete pregnancy histories include sexual practices and partners, number and ages of children, number and outcome of pregnancies (including live births, miscarriages, spontaneous/therapeutic abortions, and birth control methods used). Nurses also observe comfort levels the adults demonstrate when discussing their own sexuality, or if an adult seems uninformed when discussing sexual subjects with children. Nurses' responsibilities also include providing appropriate health assessment and information that considers the variety of sexual practices within heterosexual, homosexual, and bisexual relationships with one or more partners (Clark, 2007; Giami, 2002; Knight, 2004).

Coping–Stress Tolerance Pattern

The coping–stress tolerance pattern helps to depict the family's adaptation to both internal and external pressures (Gordon, 2007). On a day-to-day basis family members generate energy to face evolving need. Society continually compels families to adapt to new situations. Survival and growth depend on coping mechanisms as families face external demands required to move from one developmental stage to the next. The family's ability to cope with everyday living demands determines family success. Family relationships support coping or generate more stress. Life events, such as divorce, moving, or developmental stages of the life cycle, and economic hardships, such as loss of a job, provoke stress and mobilize family coping strategies. Exploration of coping and stress tolerance includes the following assessment areas:

- How does the family cope with stressful life events?
- What experiences have family members had with chemical abuse?
- What strengths does the family have and use to counterbalance the stresses?

- What stressful family situations are experienced?
- How does the family view the association between stress and children's health and development?
- How does the family make appraisals of the situations and are they realistic?
- Describe the family's resources? How do family members use knowledge or links to family networks or community resources?
- What kinds of dysfunctional adaptive strategies are used, such as chemical abuse or violence?

Values-Beliefs Pattern

The values-beliefs pattern characterizes the family's perspective and attitudes about life meanings, values, beliefs, spirituality and how these issues affect behavior (Gordon, 2007). Assessment, diagnosis, and intervention are based on these attitudes. Assessment of this pattern enhances the interpretation of family behavior. Exploration of values and beliefs includes the following assessment areas:

- What are the values and beliefs held by the family?
- How flexible are rules?
- How do family members interact (calm, aggressive, competitive, or rigid)?
- How do family members view spirituality?
- Describe the cultural or ethnic group that the family identifies with. What family practices are consistent with the norms of that ethnic group? How are the practices inconsistent with these norms?
- What are the family's traditions and practices?
- How do the significant cultural beliefs affect health or illness?
- Describe the role that religion plays in the family on a regular basis and during times of stress. How does the family rely on religious practices?

- How does the family perceive its competency during crisis?
- What are the family goals and do members perceive that they are attaining these goals?
- How are value conflicts demonstrated within the family?
- How do identified family values affect the health status of the family?

Spirituality, defined as life purpose and connection with others, affects health. The metaphysical and transcendental phenomenon of spirituality as well as the religious and nonreligious systems of belief within families should be assessed (Sessanna et al., 2007). How well families communicate their unconditional love and forgiveness for injury or betrayal may contribute to physical symptoms within families. According to Lawler et al. (2005), spirituality and social skills promote health and prevent disease.

Data collected in the 11 functional patterns reveal ideas about family health-promotion and disease prevention practices. Risks to healthy family functioning may be identified in each pattern. Risk factors may be found in more than one area. For example, passive smoke from one family member's cigarettes may be identified as an environmental risk factor in the home. However, the family's reaction to passive smoking determines their perceived susceptibility, their perceived severity of the problem, and whether they will make a change in the environment to promote family health. The pattern indicates high risk if chronic asthma is described during the family history. In this situation, several other pattern areas support the finding. The nurse determines each risk behavior along with its effects on the others.

ENVIRONMENTAL FACTORS

Environment also influences family health and well-being. Home, neighborhood, and community comprise the family environment. Assessment includes exploration of the following home environment areas:

- What type of dwelling is it (condominium, single dwelling, low-income apartment, or temporary shelter)?
- How has the family acquired their home (purchase, rental)?
- What is the condition of the home (Interior/exterior: glass, trash, broken stairs, peeling paint, inadequate insulation, inadequate lighting on stairs, or broken fixtures)?
- Are the number and type of rooms adequate for the size of the family?
- How satisfactory are the furnishings to meet the needs of the family (enough chairs, beds, and a kitchen table)?
- How comfortable is the temperature (warm in winter and cool in summer, insulated)?
- How adequate is lighting for reading, sewing, and other activities?

- How adequate is the water supply (sufficient/clean/fluoridated/polluted)?
- Does the family have access to a telephone and are emergency numbers available?
- How safe are the kitchen sanitation and refrigeration capabilities?
- How adequate are the bathroom sanitation facilities, water supply, toilet, and towels and soap?
- Are sleeping arrangements adequate for family members, considering age, gender, relationships, and spatial needs?
- How adequate is the plan for escape in an emergency (smoke detectors/escape route/plan inside the home)?
- What are the arrangements and knowledge about first-aid (directions posted for poisons, burns, lacerations, and other first aid needs)?
- What signs of rats, mice, or cockroaches are present inside or outside the home?
- What are the family's impressions about their home? How do they describe the adequacy of their living space for privacy, their own interests, and status?
- How are chemicals stored in the home (out of reach of children)?
- How is safety ensured in the home? What safety issues are evident?

Areas to explore for neighborhood assessment are as follows:

- What is the condition of the dwellings and streets (maintenance/deterioration)?
- How and when is the garbage collected?
- What is the incidence of violent crime, burglaries, and auto accidents?
- What kinds of industry are nearby and do they produce air pollution or toxic waste?
- What are the social class and ethnic characteristics of the neighborhood?
- What are the occupations and interests of the families in the neighborhood?
- What is the population density?
- How available, accessible is public transportation? Why is public transportation not used if it is available?

Exploration during assessment of the community includes the following areas:

- What resources, such as schools, church, transportation, shopping, and recreational facilities, are available for family use?
- How accessible are the health facilities, such as physician's office, clinic, hospital, gym, swimming pool, natural food store, and weight-reduction clinic?

By driving or walking around the area, the nurse can obtain neighborhood and community data. Other sources of information include the family, health professionals, teachers, business people, and others who work in the area. Official resources, such as the reports from the U.S. Census Department (www.census.gov/) or statistics from the city or state health departments and libraries, are also helpful in describing a neighborhood and community.

ANALYSIS AND NURSING DIAGNOSIS

Analyzing Data

After completing the data collection, the nurse and the family analyze it. Several approaches are used to analyze health data, including systems theory, developmental theory, and risk-estimate theory. A systems approach categorizes families as open or closed, with permeable or rigid boundaries determining both structural and functional components of family systems. The 11 functional patterns organize baseline assessment data **(Website Resource 7C)**.

Developmental theory approaches families from the perspective of tasks and progression through cycles. Nurses analyze data to identify accomplishment of family life cycle stages and family tasks needed to function successfully. Family developmental needs are determined considering the wide variety of family structures and functions in society. Although most family models are based on nuclear family structures, additional family structures should be explored as indicated by current population trends (Amato, 2005; Bronte-Tinkew et al., 2006; Fields, 2007; Land & Kitzinger, 2007; Lonczak et al., 2007; Pan & Farrell, 2006; Roy, 2001; Simons et al., 2006; Widmer et al., 2006). Stages of family development guide the baseline data analysis. Identification of gaps, missing data, or conflicting information is obtained and clarified.

Couple Family

The first stage of family development begins when adults define themselves as a family regardless of the legal status. When individuals move from their family of origin to a new couple relationship, adaptation to role expectations of a partner becomes a developmental task for each individual. Establishing a mutually satisfying adult relationship that converges with the kinship network is one family developmental task. Adjustment for couples includes learning how to weave together two personalities, two life histories, and two aspirations of growth. Decisions in this stage include whether adults are gainfully employed, how money is managed, where they live, how they socialize with friends and other family members, patterns of sexual activities, and whether to have children. Determining how to divide household tasks of cooking, washing, cleaning, and shopping occurs either consciously or subconsciously.

Developmental tasks that integrate health practices and habits into the couple's lifestyle require consideration during analysis. Health behavior constitutes particular actions to promote health and prevent disease. Examples of health-promotion and disease-prevention activities may include maintaining well-balanced rest, exercise, diet, contraception; attending smoking-cessation classes; wearing seat belts; and directing activities toward self-actualization. Each individual brings values and beliefs to the relationship. Practices from the family of origin and values from personal experiences combine to form the adult beliefs of the individual. Achieving mutually satisfying relationships depends also on couples' conflict management. Strategies that stem from congruent value systems facilitate couple's adjustment. When couples use divergent strategies, problem solving tends to be less effective.

Childbearing Family

Decisions about adding children to the family commit couples to more complex long-term responsibility. Family development and primary health needs change to focus on additional members. To analyze learning needs of pregnant couples, nurses consider aspects of decisions and motivations involved with the pregnancy. With single-parent families (usually mothers) becoming increasingly common through divorce, death, adoption, or the choice to have a child out of wedlock, analysis addresses these family structures (Amato, 2005; Simons et al., 2006; Widmer et al., 2006).

Attitudes and practices in society regarding sexuality have influenced the incidence of sexually transmitted diseases such as genital herpes, gonorrhea, and syphilis. Acquired immunodeficiency syndrome (AIDS), first described in 1981, poses a threat to the family and society, in addition to affected individuals. Human immunodeficiency virus (HIV) is transmitted through heterosexual, homosexual, or oral sexual intercourse, as well as through direct contact with infected blood, shared needles during intravenous drug use, and perinatal transfer from infected mothers to their infants. Prevention of HIV transmission requires abstinence and modification of relevant behaviors.

Risk factors associated with sexuality include lack of knowledge about safe sexual practices, the reproductive system, and personal hygiene; lack of prenatal care; pregnancy before age 16; pregnancy after age 35; a history of hypertension or infection during pregnancy; and unplanned or unwanted pregnancy.

Risk factors for premature pregnancies and unsatisfying marriage consist of ignorance about, or values regarding, family planning; adolescence; and sexuality and role adjustment. In unplanned pregnancies, adolescent parents put themselves and their developing child at risk. Lack of knowledge about prenatal care, birthing, and child-rearing practices compounds risks for both the mother and the child. Parents who are unable to perform parenting roles risk an unsatisfying relationship and inappropriate developmental growth for this beginning stage of the family life cycle. If couples decide to remain childless, learning needs include information about contraception.

Birth or adoption of a child begins a new family unit. Family members adjust to new roles as the unit expands in function and responsibility. Parents' history as a dyad and their experiences in other groups, particularly their families of origin, influence the development of the triad (Multicultural Awareness box). Accommodating new members disrupts family equilibrium. As a group, families explore ways to meet each others' needs, to minimize differences, and work together. First-time parents often feel a lack of

MULTICULTURAL AWARENESS
Preconception Care

Preconception care is a significant health-promotion opportunity for the whole family. The importance of this care has been recognized by *Healthy People 2010*, the Institute of Medicine, and the Public Health Services Expert Panel on the Content of Prenatal Care.

One important area of preconception care is evaluating a couple's genetic history as documented on the standard family genogram. Further evaluation should be considered for couples who are related outside marriage or who have ethnic backgrounds such as Mediterranean, Black, or Ashkenazi Jew, and for women older than 35 years of age or younger than 16 years of age who have preexisting medical conditions. Couples who have family histories of any of the following health problems should be referred for further genetic testing and counseling: cystic fibrosis, hemophilia, phenylketonuria, Tay-Sachs disease, thalassemia, sickle cell disease or trait, birth defects, or mental retardation.

emotional support during the first several months of parenthood. Some, but not all, new parents have available family leave policies that may facilitate this transition. Without a family network or friends, the first days after the birth or adoption may be difficult. Parents may care for the child proficiently, but may need assistance to grow in the parenting role. If parents are both employed outside the home, they may encounter difficulty with the routines of baby care and being confined to the house more for child care. Anxiety about the adequacy of income may cause parents to increase work hours to increase income. Exhaustion for both parents is common from working full time while providing child care as the infant develops. Single parents, usually mothers, carry these same burdens alone. Emotional support may be limited, particularly if one has not found satisfaction in parenthood. Families of origin or other support systems, such as self-help groups, neighbors, or friends, assist family members as they struggle to adapt to a new member (Clark, 2007; Friedman et al., 2003). Nurses facilitate this process to promote health in the newly formed family unit.

Some parents thrive during the period when an infant needs almost constant care and nurturing. These parents find support in a network of family and friends. Couples who find satisfaction in parenthood seem to realize that parental influence begins at birth and is the single most important factor in the child's physical, emotional, and cognitive development. The parents' ability to assume responsibility depends on a complex array of factors: their own maturity; how they were nurtured as children; their conceptions about self, culture, social class, and religion; their relationship with each other; their values and philosophy of life; their perceptions of and experiences with children and other adults; and the life stresses they have experienced.

In analyzing needs of child-rearing families, nurses consider many factors, including providing for physical health, economic support, and nurturing actions that are vital to learning and social development of children. In analyzing couples' needs during this stage, nurses recognize the importance of interactions among the triad. Observing decision-making helps nurses determine family functioning, member roles, and effectiveness of family members. Risks associated with role relationships include working parents with insufficient resources for child care, abuse or neglect of children, multiple closely spaced children, low family self-esteem, children used as scapegoats for parental frustration, immature parents who are dependent and unable to handle responsibility, and strong beliefs about physical punishment or obedience.

Family with Toddlers/Preschool Children

Families may have more than one child, each growing and developing at an individual pace. Preschool children place great demands on families. Families adjust to each new member with space and equipment for expansion. Needs and interests of preschool children influence home environments. Nurses assess the quality of the home environment for whether children have healthy amounts of stimulation-promoting opportunities. Safety balanced with exploration by the child results in health-promoting home environments. Rather than removing children from the kitchen or garden, finding ways to include them in a cooking or planting activity provides learning experiences. Other environmental influences affecting the child's rate and style of development include religious practices, ethnic background, education, and discipline techniques.

Evidence increasingly demonstrates the link between environment and health. Home environments that contain contaminated air, water, or food increase health risks. For example, lead poisoning, a preventable disease that continues to affect thousands of children, often results from lead paint and other factors in the home. Although restrictions exist in the U.S. to limit lead-based paint to exteriors, many homes have lead within the interior. Both homes and automobiles are considered possible sources of exposure to the poisonous agent carbon monoxide. Nurses also review data for home safety, including storage of dangerous materials, such as detergents, insecticides, and medications.

Health-promotion needs for young children include proper foods, exercise, sleep, and dental hygiene. Parents teach children through modeling and use of positive reinforcement. Family developmental tasks include adjusting to fatigue resulting from parenting demands. Nurses explore alternatives to relieve parents. Parents need time for themselves, individually and as a couple (e.g., to exercise, socialize), while knowing their children are safe with a responsible person. Economic restraints may limit relaxation time away from the children. Sharing child care with friends and family provides one source of support for new parents.

Family with School-Aged Children

A family with children in school may have reached its maximal size in numbers and interrelationships. The parents' major problem during this stage is the dichotomy between self-interest and finding fulfillment in producing the next generation. Family developmental tasks revolve around goals of reorganization to prepare for the expanding world of school-aged children. School achievement becomes a critical task for socialization. Viewing social and educational goals from the perspective of family culture and parents' defined goals becomes particularly important during this developmental stage. For example, many opportunities for health education exist in schools, including influencing healthy beliefs and behaviors. However, school health programs focus on problems such as tobacco and substance abuse with messages aimed at problems and crises rather than healthy behaviors. Families influence health at home and in school by teaching children how to assess situations for risks, how to manage them, and what benefits to expect when practicing healthy behaviors.

As children's activities broaden away from home, another important developmental task for both parent and child becomes letting go. Parents become involved in community groups such as the parent-teacher association, scout groups, sports teams, and other volunteer organizations. Encouraging children to join in family discussions to establish policies and make decisions fosters their positive self-concepts. Children exposed to unsafe home environments are at risk for behavior disturbances, school problems, and learning disabilities. Parents who cannot manage their children in growth-promoting ways soon experience energy depletion and may turn to dysfunctional relief from parenting (e.g., drug and alcohol abuse).

Family with Adolescents

Parents with adolescent children may experience a late pregnancy, resulting in care for an infant while other children in the family are in school. A new family member at this stage may be a source of joy or frustration for the family. The overall goal with adolescent members is to loosen family ties to allow greater responsibility and freedom in preparation for releasing young adults. Although each member of the family strives to achieve individual developmental tasks in the midst of social pressures, the family as a whole has tasks to accomplish. Strengthening the marital relationship to build a foundation for future family stages is a critical task during this time.

Open communication is often difficult during this stage, partly because of the differing developmental tasks of adolescents and adults. Adolescents seek their own identity, and adults attempt to facilitate adolescent decision-making processes. Choices about values and lifestyles may differ. Adolescents may challenge family values and standards. Although parents maintain some authority, adolescents tackle their own desires and needs. Adolescents want to do what their friends do, have their own cars, and make their

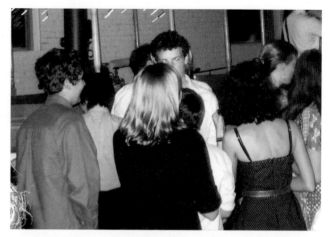

Figure 7-5 Although the parent needs to maintain some responsibility, an adolescent who is given opportunities to experience things with friends will gain an enhanced sense of autonomy and responsibility.

own money to spend in ways that they see fit. Parents who give adolescent members opportunities to experience social, emotional, and ethical situations with others are providing learning opportunities to enhance their sense of autonomy and responsibility (Figure 7-5).

As adolescents become mature and emancipated, families face balancing freedom with responsibility. Health problems in this age group include violent deaths including suicide, injuries, and alcohol and drug abuse. Contributing risk factors involve lack of problem-solving skills, family values of aggressiveness and competition, socioeconomic factors, peer relationships, rigid and inflexible family values, daredevil risk-taking attitudes, and conflicts between parents and children. Environmental risk–related violent deaths and injuries are influenced by the highway system, automobile manufacturers, and the legislation of standards of safety. Families rely on public health officials and nurses' efforts as advocates to reduce environmental risks.

Families support adolescents in this stage of development by including them in decision-making and ensuring that they experience the positive and negative consequences of their choices. Family values of winning at all costs, aggressiveness, and competition may need to be explored during this period. Adolescents may discard these values if they are no longer applicable. Considerable change in adolescent values produces conflict and poses a threat to family cohesiveness. Families may place pressure on adolescents to conform to family values. In matters of life and death—for example, in regard to driving rules—parents must stay firm.

Families with adolescents experience identity crises for the adolescent, the adults, and the family as a whole. Adolescents move from childhood to adulthood while adults progress beyond parenthood. Adolescents struggle to find independent identities that remain connected to their family. Adults, in midlife, must resolve their own adolescent fantasies to move toward an identity for their remaining life.

Family with Young Adults

Families with young adults act as a launching center when children begin to leave home. As children leave home, parents relinquish their parenting roles of many years to return to the marital dyad. The couple builds a new life together while maintaining relationships with aging parents, children, grandchildren, and in-laws. Couples focus on redefining relationships during this stage. For a woman, the role as mother changes, because children no longer need their mother in the same way as during childhood. When mothers devote years to raising children, they must realize a changed role and purpose within the family. Transition from a life with children as the priority to new or renewed interests (e.g., career, community service) may require assistance and support for both parents. Careers for both parents at this stage may become more stable. Developmental tasks at this stage for both adults require focus on future prospects. In addition to individual changes occurring within couples, families with young adults may experience other pressures. Aging parents and adult children may require financial or emotional support. Financial and emotional responsibilities to other family members hinder the couple's ability to focus on the marital relationship during this developmental phase. Health-promoting activities to focus on during this stage include coping with pressures of social roles and occupational responsibilities, maintaining health habits, aging, and reassessing life goals.

Family with Middle-Aged Adults

Families consisting of only two members are able to enhance self-concept and support the marital relationship during middle age. Usually children have left home and parents experience a sense of freedom and well-being. Some marriages, by this stage, have reached a level of security and stability; husband and wife meet each other's needs. Parenting pressures diminish, allowing them to enjoy accomplishments of their children and grandchildren. Couples have acquired a network of friends. Long-time acquaintances seek participation from the couple in neighborhood rituals and events. Economic security and personal self-esteem may be at a peak.

In contrast, some marriages falter at this time. Departed children create a quiet house with less activity, known as the "empty nest." When unprepared for this stage, individuals might seek opportunities to enhance self-concept from outside of the marriage. The couple, thinking that their parenting role is now complete, may develop feelings of inadequacy or begin a new relationship, start a new family, or resort to substance abuse. In addition, this life phase may include becoming grandparents; parenting grandchildren; coping with the needs of middle-aged children; and caring for older adults (children, siblings, or parents).

Health tasks in this developmental stage require new awareness of susceptibility or vulnerability to health problems. Couples adjust their lifestyle and habits to cope with health risks. Losses promote health problems, and at this stage couples begin to cope with deaths among family and friends, along with declining income. If either member has developed physical or mental illness, the other adjusts to resultant physical and mental impairments, redefining self-concept.

Middle-aged families face a host of risk factors leading to three prevalent causes of death: (1) heart disease, (2) cancer, and (3) cerebrovascular accident (stroke). Family lifestyle may decrease risks by placing a high value on physical activity, not smoking, maintaining adequate and sound nutritional habits, and consuming moderate amounts of alcohol. Lifestyle habits that are transmitted through role modeling have a greater influence on the younger members of the family than any verbal edict. Middle-aged members positively influence their health if they are able to choose environments low in water and air pollution and free from crippling stress factors such as excessive noise, traffic, and overcrowding. Family members can also apply pressure on key members of the community to decrease risks in the environment.

Family with Older Adults

Retirement affects many aspects of life for couples and each individual in the family and their relationships with others (Figure 7-6). Besides decreased work hours, retirement also means reduction in income and fixed incomes for most people. Adjusting living standards to retirement income and being able to supplement this income with wage-earning activity is one task of the family with older adults. Other tasks during this stage include ensuring a safe and comfortable home environment, preparing for end of life, and adjusting to the loss of a spouse (Kahana et al., 2004). Surviving spouses often look to their family for support and satisfaction (Kahana et al., 2003, 2004). Illness may create further dependence on family members (Kahana et al., 2003).

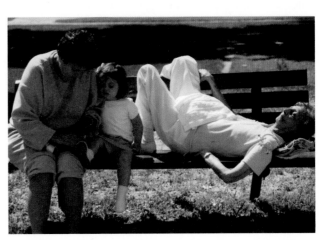

Figure 7-6 Retirement gives the older adult time to relax with his or her family.

Health promotion aims to maintain functional ability, limit effects of disabling conditions, and maintain quality of life. Older adults may fear becoming helpless, feeling useless, and being incapable of caring for themselves. When analyzing risk factors in the aging family, nurses look for the couple's ability to function well enough to carry out normal roles and responsibilities. As with all people, older adults hope for a state of well-being that will allow them to function at their highest capacity physically, psychologically, socially, and spiritually. Many older adults remain in their own homes, and most of these individuals are vigorous and completely independent. According the National Center for Health Statistics, 175 of 1000 adults over 75 years of age reside in nursing homes (National Center for Health Statistics, 2004).

Ego integrity (the union of all previous phases of the life cycle) is the challenge in this stage and demands successful aging through continued activity. Having gone through the various stages of family development, the couple accepts what they have done as their own. At this time, they may need family or professional support to pursue other interests or maintain former activities to feel needed and useful.

The nurse and family jointly analyze the information comparing the family's data to documented norms of health promotion and disease prevention in older adults. Norms or expected values can be derived from the family's baseline information of 11 functional pattern areas, knowledge of growth and development for all age groups and the family as a whole, risk-factor estimates, and population norms. Population norms specify normal ranges for these groups. For example, age is associated with various risk factors; some disorders are so common that they are referred to as diseases of the older person. In certain diseases, such as lung cancer, there is a long period of exposure. Risk increases with cumulative exposure; therefore, the incidence and prevalence of diseases increase with age.

Sexuality In their qualitative study, Gott and Hinchliff (2003) describe the barriers older adults experience in regard to sexual concerns. Because of the popular perception that older adults are asexual, their sexual concerns may be disregarded (Robinson & Molzahn, 2007). Older adults interviewed in this study indicated an inability to share sexual issues with their physician. The paucity of literature about sexuality in older adulthood contributes to providers' inability to offer accurate information and appropriate guidance (Gott & Hinchliff, 2003; Gott, 2006; Robinson & Molzahn, 2007). DeLamater and Sill (2005) found that strength of sexual desire of the older women in their study was more influenced by age, education, and attitude than by biomedical factors.

General population norms for values, beliefs, self-perception, or role relationships may be less available than physical population norms. Cultural, ethnic, and religious factors contribute to values and beliefs about health. Family baseline information provides important comparative criteria for analysis. Family records provide useful information

when available. The first contact assessment provides baseline information for subsequent comparison and evaluation of progress. Whether the family perceives situations to be problematic should also be considered in the analysis phase. Nurse and family perceptions about problems may differ (Denham, 2003). Newman's definitions of family health, presented in **Website Resource 7D**, provide a framework to view increased awareness or consciousness of a family's health (Fawcett, 2005).

Formulating Family Nursing Diagnoses

Writing a **family nursing diagnosis** helps families promote health throughout the life cycle and prevents disease through decreasing risk-taking behaviors. Nurses derive diagnoses from assessed validated data. As a concise summary statement of a problem or potential problem, diagnoses provide direction for outcomes and interventions by identifying negative health states and factors to change to alleviate or prevent the problem (see Chapter 6). Examples of family nursing diagnoses using developmental and risk-factor approaches are presented in **Website Resource 7E**. Describing health and validating potential or actual health problems with families facilitates cooperation. Assessment and negotiation continue until agreement occurs and a plan for resolution develops.

Cultural competence and respect for familial beliefs forms a foundation for nurses. With changing trends in families and shifts in heritage within society, cultural competence becomes a priority within nursing practice (Amato, 2005; Andrews & Boyle, 2008; Lonczak et al., 2007). Cultural competence increases efficacy of health promotion for all families, particularly families from within vulnerable populations.

PLANNING WITH THE FAMILY

Intervention planning stems from complete assessment, analysis, and nursing diagnosis. The plan's purpose aims for behavioral change in families to promote health or prevent dysfunction. As in the assessment phase, family members play an active role in the planning process. Family responsibility for personal health status enhances success of behavioral change outcomes. The planning process involves several steps, with the nurse and family identifying the following:

1. Order of priority for problems or potential problems
2. Items that can be handled by the nurse and the family and items that must be referred to others
3. Actions and expected outcomes

The nursing plan provides direction for implementation and the framework for evaluation (see the Care Plan at the end of this chapter).

As mentioned, a family's health status can be diagnosed as functional, potentially dysfunctional, or dysfunctional. Functional family health status warrants verification by the nurse with a plan for periodic reevaluation that is formulated jointly. Plans to continue healthy living behaviors are reinforced. The nurse provides specific information requested by the family, such as immunization schedules, growth and development milestones, and recommended dietary allowances. In working with healthy families, the nurse controls the assessment and analysis phases of the nursing process. If the health status is judged functional, then planning health education materials, scheduling periodic examinations, and accessibility of the nurse remain professional responsibilities. Implementation and evaluation of health-promotion activities become family responsibilities.

In health promotion and disease prevention settings life-threatening situations rarely occur; however, when such situations do occur they become the highest priority for intervention. For other identified potential or actual problems, the nurse relies on the family to decide which problem or potential problem to approach. After the ordering of priorities is established, the family and nurse determine who will work on the problem. Problems or potential problems to be resolved by the nurse are identified separately from those requiring referral or family intervention. Problems for the family to handle or those the family is already addressing are considered strengths and are acknowledged and supported by the nurse. For example, when there is consistency among values and actions, physical fitness, weight management, and ability to cope with stress, the family is already taking informed and responsible action in these areas. The extent to which family members can provide their own health promotion and disease prevention will depend on their knowledge, skills, motivation, and orientation toward health.

Problems that need medical, legal, or social attention are referred to appropriate agencies. The nurse should have a directory of resources in the community when referrals are needed. Nursing intervention requires clearly stated actions that are purposeful, moral, capable of being accomplished, and adapted to the particular life situation, beliefs, and expectations of the family.

Goals

Goals are statements describing desired outcomes. Family outcome statements include expected family behaviors, circumstances for exhibited behaviors, and criteria for determining performance. Health-promotion goals reflect a desire to function at a higher level of health and to grow beyond maintaining health or preventing disease.

IMPLEMENTATION WITH THE FAMILY

The implementation phase is dynamic. As the nurse and family work together, new information is used to adapt and change the plan as necessary. **Family nursing interventions** aim to assist families in carrying out functions that members cannot perform for themselves. In health promotion and disease prevention, nurses assist families to improve their capacity to act on their own behalf (Amato, 2005).

Families may know that they take risks by smoking, drinking, and engaging in a stressful lifestyle. As the nurse explains the rationale behind proposed changes, families may choose to deny how they jeopardize their future health and continue their risk-taking behaviors. Factors that the nurse has not considered may cause the family's resistance. For example, families may have more pressing basic needs such as food, clothing, and housing. Health promotion and disease prevention may not have been part of the family's life experiences, giving the nurse the educational task to try to change attitudes and values expanding the options for families to consider health promotion.

Four types of nursing interventions appear in health-promotion and disease-prevention planning: (1) increasing knowledge and skills, (2) increasing strengths, (3) decreasing exposure, and (4) decreasing susceptibility. Increasing knowledge and skills to improve family capacity for health-promotion and disease-prevention behavior may be the primary strategy. Use of this strategy helps families make informed choices about healthful lifestyle behaviors and to eliminate harmful environmental influences that affect health. Improved knowledge aims to create awareness as the nurse and family work together to uncover actual or potential problems. Nurses recognize particular families at risk and move toward motivating and supporting behavioral change in these families. The Innovative Practice Box presents an example of one program that provides education and support to people with cancer and their families.

---

innovative practice

The Wellness Community

The Wellness Community, which was founded in the 1980s, has 24 local chapters throughout the U.S., offering free educational and support programs for people with cancer and their families. Weekly support groups help family members support one another, explore new ways of coping with the stresses of cancer, and learn ways to become the most effective partners possible with their health care teams.

Wellness communities offer a wide variety of workshops and programs (Gentle Strength and Stretch, Meditation and Guided Imagery, Nutrition Matters, Nutrition and the Immune System, Nutrition at Midlife: Preventing Heart Disease and Osteoporosis, Tai Chi, Yoga, Mindfulness, and Feng Shui). Social events are organized (Comfort Food Potluck Dinner, Couples Networking Groups, Singles Networking Group, Family and Friends Networking Group).

Although each chapter of The Wellness Community does not charge for its services, donations are appreciated and necessary to help serve the thousands of people living with cancer and their families. The Wellness Community's mission is to provide hope to these individuals and to help them regain a sense of control over their lives.

Contact Information:
The Wellness Community (national office)
919 18th Street, NW Suite 54
Washington, DC 20006
toll-free: 888-793-WELL (-9355)
phone: 202-659-9709
Fax: 202-659-9301
Email: help@thewellnesscommunity.org
Web site: *www.wellness-community.org*

Family strengths or forces that contribute to family unity and solidarity foster the development of inherent family potential (Greeff et al., 2006; Sittner et al., 2007). These factors include the following:

- Physical, emotional, and spiritual factors
- Healthy child-rearing practices and discipline
- Meaningful and clear communication
- Support, security, and encouragement
- Growth-producing relationships and experiences
- Responsible community relationships
- Growth with and through children
- Self-help and acceptance of help
- Flexibility in family functions and roles
- Mutual respect for individuality
- Crisis as a means for growth
- Family unity and loyalty and intrafamily cooperation
- Adaptability of family strengths

In recent years, a shift of family health care from an illness or problem and deficiency focus to a strength-based focus has occurred (Sittner et al., 2007; Stolte, 1996). The McGill model of nursing (Feeley & Gottlieb, 2000) and the Calgary family assessment and intervention model (Wright & Leahey, 2005) each provide a framework for assessment for nurses to plan care using family strengths and resources. Sittner et al. (2007) describe how family members develop and maintain health-promoting behaviors by using commitment, appreciation, affection, positive communication, time together, a sense of spiritual well-being, and ability to cope with stress and crisis. Defrain has developed a tool that is available for nurses to use to generate discussion among family members about their strengths (*www.ianrpubs.unl.edu/epublic/live/nf498/build/nf498.pdf*). Hartrick (2000) identifies corresponding nursing interventions to support and further develop the family dynamics of socialization, support, and nurturance. Additionally, Plager (1999) describes the importance of understanding the significance of family legacy to a family's health and related health practices.

Families with significant strengths may need to learn new, unfamiliar skills for mastering a specific technique such as meditation and to apply new tools for decision-making. These families rarely require ongoing supervision or support of sustained interventions aimed at changing their coping patterns, communication, or role behavior. They may be highly capable of seeking and using information. Assisting functional families may simply involve providing information in terms that can be understood and offering opportunities to ask questions and clarify information.

Decreasing exposure to risk factors may include enhancing parents' ability to assess and adjust their behavior to their child's temperament. Parents with limited literacy may need assistance to learn to respond constructively to their child's communication attempts. Health promotion includes teaching parents to avoid exposure to risks—for example to use adequate restraints in automobiles, to protect their toddler from wandering into dangerous streets, and to supervise children to avoid falls and hazardous materials.

Although no substitute can be found for continuous supervision of a child, homes can be made safer by moving common hazards out of children's reach. This effort includes putting all cleaning solutions and medications beyond their reach; erecting barriers in front of exposed heaters, high windows, and stairways; keeping pots and pans turned inward on the stove; fencing in a yard or a swimming pool; and teaching children to avoid dangerous areas. Becoming aware of peeling paint and toxic chemicals that parents might carry home from the job on their clothing can also protect the child.

Decreasing susceptibility means educating families about prevention principles. Families who realize how diseases are spread are better able to avoid transmission from person to person; through air, water, and food; and by insects and the rodents on which insects live. Health promotion includes emphasizing the role of personal hygiene and cleanliness to avoid infection. Families who know signs and symptoms that require medical attention and how to treat minor illnesses are better able to maintain healthy environments.

Pender et al. (2006) cite research that demonstrates how perceived susceptibility predicts preventive behavior. Perceived susceptibility is the family's estimated subjective probability that a specific health problem will be encountered. Family perceptions of health risks and their susceptibility to them will determine how they change their behavior. If the overweight family believes obesity is a threat to their health the family, they are more likely to react positively to the changes suggested by the nurse than a family who perceives no health threat. Nurses who introduce threat as a motivator to action are morally obligated to reduce the threat by meaningful and purposeful interventions. Table 7-3 lists various nursing roles used in the implementation stage.

EVALUATION WITH THE FAMILY

The purpose of evaluation is to determine how the family has responded to the planned interventions and whether these interventions were successful. Goals and objectives that are stated in specific behavioral terms will make evaluation much easier than when they are given in general terms. Criteria used to evaluate interventions, such as weight change, increased lung capacity from an exercise program, and lower pulse rate as a result of relaxation exercises are simple to measure. Other results of health promotion and disease prevention are not as easy to measure but must be considered in the evaluation step of the nursing process. When considering such factors as values, beliefs, self-perceptions, or role relationships, the nurse may base the evaluation on whether the family indicates that the interventions were successful. Additionally, the family's baseline data are used as comparative criteria in evaluation. The nurse reassesses the situation and compares the new information with that on the original assessment to determine whether change has occurred.

Table 7-3   Possible Nurse's Roles in Health Promotion and Disease Prevention Through Stages of Family Development

Stage	Possible Nursing Role
Couple	Counselor on sexual and role adjustment
	Teacher of and counselor on family planning
	Teacher of parenting skills
	Coordinator for genetic counseling
	Facilitator in interpersonal relationships
Childbearing family	Monitor of prenatal care and referrer for problems of pregnancy
	Counselor on prenatal nutrition
	Counselor on prenatal maternal habits
	Supporter of amniocentesis
	Counselor on breast feeding
	Coordinator with pediatric services
	Supervisor of immunizations
	Referrer to social services
	Assistant in adjustment to prenatal role
Family with preschool or school-age children	Monitor of early childhood development; referrer when indicated
	Teacher of first-aid and emergency measures
	Coordinator with pediatric services
	Counselor on nutrition and exercise
	Teacher of dental hygiene
	Counselor on environmental safety in home
	Facilitator in interpersonal relationships
Family with adolescents	Teacher of risk factors to health
	Teacher of problem-solving issues regarding alcohol, smoking, diet, and exercise
	Facilitator of interpersonal skills with adolescents and parents
	Direct supporter of, counselor on, or referrer to mental health resources
	Counselor on family planning
	Referrer for sexually transmittable disease
Family with young or middle-age adults	Participant in community organizations involved in disease control
	Teacher of problem-solving issues regarding lifestyle and habits
	Participant in community organization involved in environmental control
	Case finder in the home and community
	Screener for hypertension, Pap smear, breast examination, cancer signs, mental health, and dental care
	Counselor on menopausal transition
Family with older adults	Facilitator of interpersonal relationships among family members
	Referrer for work and social activity, nutritional programs, homemakers' services, and nursing home
	Monitor of exercise, nutrition, preventive services, and medications
	Supervisor of immunization
	Counselor on safety in the home
	Counselor on bereavement

The following five measures of family functioning can be used to determine the effectiveness of interventions:

1. Changes in interaction patterns
2. Effective communication
3. Ability to express emotions
4. Responsiveness to needs of members as individuals
5. Problem-solving ability

Using these measures, the nurse returns to the original assessment of the family's functioning and compares current observations with previous data. These characteristics of family functioning continue to provide a useful framework even today, when family structures are becoming more diverse and the nuclear family less prevalent (Amato, 2005).

When, during the planning phase of the nursing process, the nurse has identified the criteria (norms and standards) for the desired outcomes, these outcomes are the basis of evaluation. Data from the family that describe their behavior relative to the desired outcomes determine whether the nursing care was successful. With the criteria stated, the goals and objectives outline how the family can demonstrate a successful outcome and the behavior change expected to result from nursing intervention. The more objective and measurable the desired outcome is, the more reliable the results of evaluation will be.

After the goals and objectives are reached, the problem no longer exists. If evaluation shows the nursing actions did not achieve the goals or objectives, the nurse must review the nursing process to determine whether there were gaps in the assessment data, errors in analysis or nursing diagnosis, or alternative interventions that might have been considered. The nurse also needs to review the process with the family to determine whether they have contributed to outcome failure. Finally, the agency employing the nurse may be another factor; if intervention is costly or a shortage of staff exists, then health promotion and disease prevention may have low priority.

SUMMARY

Learning about health promotion and disease prevention begins at birth, with the family providing the stimulus for incorporating health in the value system of its members. From a systems perspective, the family has both structure and function; relevant functions include values and practices related to health. The effective execution of health-related functions involves the family's progression through its developmental tasks and its ability to generate low risk–producing behaviors associated with disease prevention.

Developmental and risk-estimate theories can be applied effectively to the nursing process with the family. The nurse uses functional patterns (an inherent part of both theories) to collect data for assessment. After organizing information on family life cycle stages for analysis with the family, the nurse writes the nursing diagnosis and plans, implements, and evaluates the interventions used to promote health and prevent disease in the family.

CASE STUDY

Family Member with Alzheimer's Disease: Mark and Jacqueline

Mark and Jacqueline have been married for 30 years. They have grown children who live in another state. Jacqueline's mother has moved in with the couple because she has Alzheimer's disease. Jacqueline is an only child and always promised her mother that she would care for her in her old age. Her mother is unaware of her surroundings and often calls out for her daughter Jackie when Jacqueline is in the room. Jacqueline reassures her mother that she is there to help, but to no avail. Jacqueline is unable to visit her children on holidays because she must attend to her mother's daily needs. She is reluctant to visit friends or even go out to a movie because of her mother's care needs or because she is too tired. Even though she has eliminated most leisure activities with Mark, Jacqueline goes to bed at night with many of her caregiving tasks unfinished. She tries to visit with her mother during the day, but her mother rejects any contact with her daughter. Planning for the upcoming holidays seems impossible to Mark, because of his wife's inability to focus on anything except her mother's care. Jacqueline has difficulty sleeping at night and is unable to discuss plans even a few days in advance. She is unable to visit friends and is reluctant to have friends visit because of the unpredictable behavior of her mother and her need to attend to the daily care.

Reflective Questions:
1. How do you think this situation reflects Jacqueline's sense of role performance?
2. How do you think that Jacqueline may be contributing to her own health?

CARE PLAN

Family Member with Alzheimer's Disease: Mark and Jacqueline

Nursing Diagnosis Risk for Ineffective Role Performance Related to Caring for a Family Member with Alzheimer's Disease

DEFINING CHARACTERISTICS
- Feeling exhausted
- Inability to complete tasks
- Feeling loss of usual or expected relationship with care receiver
- Increased stress or nervousness about the future
- Preoccupation with care routine
- Withdrawal from social contacts or change in leisure activities

RELATED FACTORS
- Illness severity of care receiver
- Increasing needs of care receiver

- Addiction or codependency of caregiver or care receiver
- Conflicting role demands
- Caregiver health impairment
- Unpredictable illness course or instability in the care receiver's health
- Psychological or cognitive problems in the care receiver
- Caregiver not developmentally ready for caregiving role
- Developmental delay or retardation of the care receiver or caregiver
- Marginal family adaptation or dysfunction before caregiving situation began
- Marginal coping patterns of caregiver
- Providing direct, ongoing in-home care
- History of poor relationship between caregiver and care receiver
- Care receiver who exhibits deviant, bizarre behavior
- Incontinence in the care receiver

EXPECTED OUTCOMES

- Caregiver distinguishes obligations that must be fulfilled from those that can be controlled or limited.
- In conjunction with the nurse, the caregiver develops a plan of care for the individual.
- Caregiver receives and accepts appropriate levels of support from family members, friends, and others.
- Caregiver describes help available from informal and formal support systems in the community and takes steps to obtain help.

INTERVENTIONS

- Assess the level of the caregiver's stress.
- Assist the caregiver in developing a realistic plan of care, considering the care receiver's abilities and limitations; the plan will require modification as the person decompensates.
- Instruct the caregiver to encourage the person to participate, to the greatest extent possible, in social and self-care activities such as bathing, dressing, dining out with friends, and playing cards.
- Facilitate a family meeting to help the primary caregiver seek assistance from other family members.
- Support the caregiver and family members as they adjust to the degenerative nature of the disease; be aware that over time the stress associated with caring for the person increases.
- Identify community resources that may offer the caregiver relief from constant supervision of the individual (home health aides, respite care, and adult day care).
- Help the caregiver contact informal sources of support, such as church groups, extended family, and community volunteers.
- Encourage the caregiver to attend an Alzheimer's support group.
- Refer the caregiver to the Alzheimer's Association.

Modified from Carpenito-Moyet, L. J. (2008). *Nursing diagnosis: Application to clinical practice.* (12th ed.) Philadelphia: Lippincott Williams & Wilkins.

REFERENCES

Afifi, T. D., & Keith, S. (2004). A risk and resiliency model of ambiguous loss in post-divorce stepfamilies. *Journal of Family Communication, 4*(2), 65–98.

Ahrons, C. R. (2007). Family ties after divorce: Long-term implications for children. *Family process, 46*(1), 53–65.

Amato, P. R. (2005). The impact of family formation change on the cognitive, social, and emotional well-being of the next generation. *Future of Children, 15*(2), 75–96.

American Academy of Pediatrics. (2001). Children, adolescents, and television. *Pediatrics, 107*(2), 423–426.

American Academy of Pediatrics. (2003). Family pediatrics: Report of the task force on the family. *Pediatrics, 111*(6), 1541–1571.

Andrews, M. M., & Boyle, J. S. (2008). *Transcultural concepts in nursing care* (5th ed.). New York: Lippincott, Williams & Wilkins.

Asling-Monemi, K., Pena, R., Ellsberg, M. C., & Persson, L. A. (2003). Violence against women increases the risk of infant and child mortality: A case-referent study in Nicaragua. *Bulletin of the World Health Organization, 81*(1), 10–16.

Atherson, M. J., & Metcalf, J. (2005). Television watching and risk of obesity in American adolescents. *American Journal of Health Education, 36*(1), 2–7.

Ayala, G. X., Baquero, B., Arredondo, E. M., Campbell, N., Larios, S., & Elder, J. P. (2007). Association between family variables and Mexican American children's dietary behaviors. *Journal of Nutrition Education & Behavior, 39*(2), 62–69.

Barlow, J., Davis, H., McIntosh, E., Jarrett, P., Mockford, C., & Stewart-Brown, S. (2007). Role of home visiting in improving parenting and health in families at risk of abuse and neglect: Results of a multicentre randomised controlled trial and economic evaluation. *Archives of Disease in Childhood, 92*(3), 229–233.

Bauman, L. J., Silver, E. J., & Stein, R. E. (2006). Cumulative social disadvantage and child health. *Pediatrics, 117*(4), 1321–1328.

Bennett, L. R., Shiner, S. K., & Ryan, S. (2006). Using theraplay in shelter settings with mothers & children who have experienced violence in the home. *Journal of psychosocial nursing and mental health services, 44*(10), 38–48.

Bergman, M. (2007). Single-parent households showed little variation since 1994, census bureau reports. *U.S. Census Bureau News.* Retrieved March 27, 2007, from *www.census. gov/Press-Release/www/releases/archives/families.households/009842.html.*

Bonell, C., Allen, E., Strange, V., Oakley, A., Copas, A., Johnson, A., et al. (2006). Influence of family type and parenting behaviours on teenage sexual behaviour and conceptions. *Journal of Epidemiology and Community Health, 60*(6), 502–506.

Borell, K. L. (2003). Family and household. Family research and multi-household families. *International Review of Sociology, 13*(3), 467–480.

Bronte-Tinkew, J., Moore, K. A., & Carrano, J. (2006). The father-child relationship, parenting styles, and adolescent risk behaviors in intact families. *Journal of Family Issues, 27*(6), 850–881.

Bryant, M. J., Lucove, J. C., Evenson, K. R., & Marshall, S. (2007). Measurement of television viewing in children and adolescents: A systematic review. *Obesity Reviews, 8*(3), 197–209.

Carpenito-Moyet, L. J. (2008). *Nursing diagnosis: Application to clinical practice* (12th ed.) Philadelphia: Lippincott Williams & Wilkins.

Chang, J., Berg, C. J., Saltzman, L. E., & Herndon, J. (2005). Homicide: A leading cause of injury deaths among pregnant and postpartum women in the United States, 1991-1999. *American Journal of Public Health, 95*(3), 471–477.

Cherlin, A. J. (2004). The deinstitutionalization of American marriage. *Journal of Marriage and Family, 66*(4), 848–861.

Clark, M. J. (2007). *Community health nursing* (5th ed.). Upper Saddle River, NJ: Pearson Education/Prentice Hall.

Dawson, D. A., Grant, B. F., Stinson, F. S., & Chou, P. S. (2006). Maturing out of alcohol dependence: The impact of transitional life events. *Journal of the Studies on Alcohol, 67*(2), 195–203.

DeLamater, J. D., & Sill, M. (2005). Sexual desire in later life. *Journal of Sex Research, 42*(2), 138–149.

Denham, S. A. (2003). Familial research reveals new practice model. *Holistic Nursing Practice, 17*(3), 143–151.

Dennison, B. A., Erb, T. A., & Jenkins, P. L. (2002). Television viewing and television in bedroom associated with overweight risk among low-income preschool children. *Pediatrics, 109*(6), 1028–1035.

Duvall, E., & Miller, B. (1985). *Marriage and family development* (7th ed.). New York: Harper Collins.

Eisenberg, M. E., Olson, R. E., Neumark-Sztainer, D., Story, M., & Bearinger, L. H. (2004). Correlations between family meals and psychosocial well-being among adolescents. *Archives of Pediatrics Adolescent Medicine, 158*(8), 792–796.

Erikson, E. H. (1998). *The life cycle completed.* New York: W. W. Norton and Company.

Fawcett, J. (2005). *Contemporary nursing knowledge: Analysis and evaluation of nursing models and theories* (2nd ed.). Philadelphia: F. A. Davis Company.

Feeley, N., & Gottlieb, L. N. (2000). Nursing approaches for working with family strengths and resources. *Journal of Family Nursing, 6*(1), 9–24.

Fields, J. (2007). *America's families and living arrangements: 2007.* Retrieved April 7, 2009 from *www.census.gov/population/www/socdemo/hh-fam/cps2007.html.*

Friedman, M. M., Bowden, V. R., & Jones, E. G. (2003). *Family nursing: Research, theory, and practice* (5th ed.). Upper Saddle River, NJ: Prentice Hall.

Furniss, K., McCaffrey, M., Parnell, V., & Rovi, S. (2007). Nurses and barriers to screening for intimate partner violence. *MCN: The American Journal of Maternal Child Nursing, 32*(4), 238–243.

Gable, S., Chang, Y., & Krull, J. L. (2007). Television watching and frequency of family meals are predictive of overweight onset and persistence in a national sample of school-aged children. *Journal of the American Dietetic Association, 107*(1), 53–61.

Gance-Cleveland, B. (2001). Pediatric nurses: Advocates against youth violence. *Journal of the Society of Pediatric Nurses, 6*(3), 133–142.

Giami, A. (2002). Sexual health: The emergence, development, and diversity of a concept. *Annual Review of Sex Research, 13,* 1–35.

Goldenberg, H., & Goldenberg, I. (2008). *Family therapy: An overview* (7th ed.). Belmont, CA: Thompson Brooks/Cole.

Gordon, M. (2007). *Manual of nursing diagnosis* (11th ed.). Sudbury, MA: Jones & Bartlett.

Gott, M. (2006). Sexual health and the new ageing. *Age & Ageing, 35*(2), 106–107.

Gott, M., & Hinchliff, S. (2003). Barriers to seeking treatment for sexual problems in primary care: A qualitative study with older people. *Family Practice, 20*(6), 690–695.

Greeff, A. P., Vansteenwegen, A., & DeMot, L. (2006). Resiliency in divorced families. *Social Work in Mental Health, 4*(4), 67–81.

Hamilton, L., Cheng, S., & Powell, B. (2007). Adoptive parents, adaptive parents: Evaluating the importance of biological ties for parental investment. *American Sociological Review, 72*(1), 95–116.

Hartrick, G. (2000). Developing health-promoting practices with families: One pedagogical experience. *Journal of Advanced Nursing, 31*(1), 27–34.

Jones, A. C. (2003). Reconstructing the stepfamily: Old myths, new stories. *Social work, 48*(2), 228–236.

Kahana, B., Dan, A., Kahana, E., & Kercher, K. (2004). The personal and social context of planning for end-of-life care. *Journal of the American Geriatrics Society, 52*(7), 1163–1167.

Kahana, E., Kahana, B., & Kercher, K. (2003). Emerging lifestyles and proactive options for successful ageing. *Ageing International, 28*(2), 155–180.

Kelly, J. B. (2003). Changing perspectives on children's adjustment following divorce: A view from the United States. *Childhood, 10*(2), 237–254.

Knight, D. (2004). Health care screening for men who have sex with men. *American Family Physician, 69*(9), 2149–2156.

Land, V., & Kitzinger, C. (2007). Contesting same-sex marriage in talk-in-interaction. *Feminism & Psychology, 17*(2), 173–183.

Latkin, C. A., Curry, A. D., Hua, W., & Davey, M. A. (2007). Direct and indirect associations of neighborhood disorder with drug use and high-risk sexual partners. *American Journal of Preventive Medicine, 32*(6 Suppl), S234–S241.

Lawler, K. A., Younger, J. W., Piferi, R. L., Jobe, R. L., Edmondson, K. A., & Jones, W. H. (2005). The unique effects of forgiveness on health: An exploration of pathways. *Journal of Behavioral Medicine, 28*(2), 157–167.

Lonczak, H. S., Fernandez, A., Austin, L., Marlatt, G. A., & Donovan, D. M. (2007). Family structure and substance use among American Indian youth: A preliminary study. *Families, Systems, & Health, 25*(1), 10–22.

Lubkin, I. M., & Larsen, P. D. (2006). *Chronic illness: Impact and interventions* (6th ed.). Sudbury, MA: Jones & Bartlett.

Martinez, A., D'Artois, D., & Rennick, J. E. (2007). Does the 15-minute (or less) family interview influence family nursing practice? *Journal of Family Nursing, 13*(2), 157–178.

National Center for Health Statistics. (2004). *Nursing home residents: Number and annual rate by age, sex, and race. United States, 1977-2004, NNHS (NNR04c).* Retrieved November 24, 2007, from *http://209.217.72.34/aging/TableViewer/tableView.aspx?ReportId=396.*

Pan, E., & Farrell, M. P. (2006). Ethnic differences in the effects of intergenerational relations on adolescent problem behavior in U.S. single-mother families. *Journal of Family Issues, 27*(8), 1137–1158.

Pender, N. J., Murdaugh, C. L., & Parsons, M. A. (2006). *Health promotion in nursing practice* (5th ed.). Upper Saddle River, NJ: Prentice Hall.

Plager, K. A. (1999). Understanding family legacy in family health concerns. *Journal of Family Nursing, 5*(1), 51–71.

Robinson, J. G., & Molzahn, A. E. (2007). Sexuality and quality of life. *Journal of Gerontological Nursing, 33*(3), 19–27.

Roustit, C., Chaix, B., & Chauvin, P. (2007). Family breakup and adolescents' psychosocial maladjustment: Public health implications of family disruptions. *Pediatrics, 120*(4), e984–e991.

Roy, I. (2001). The myth of the nuclear family. *American Journal of Bioethics, 1*(3), 24–25.

Sege, R. D., Hatmaker-Flanigan, E., De Vos, E., Levin-Goodman, R., & Spivak, H. (2006). Anticipatory guidance and violence prevention: Results from family and pediatrician focus groups. *Pediatrics, 117*(2), 455–463.

Sessanna, L., Finnell, D., & Jezewski, M. A. (2007). Spirituality in nursing and health-related literature: A concept analysis. *Journal of Holistic Nursing, 25*(4), 252–262.

Simons, L. G., Chen, Y., Simons, R. L., Brody, G., & Cutrona, C. (2006). Parenting practices and child adjustment in different types of households: A study of African American families. *Journal of Family Issues, 27*(6), 803–825.

Sittner, B. J., Hudson, D. B., & Defrain, J. (2007). Using the concept of family strengths to enhance nursing care. *The American Journal of Maternal Child Nursing, 32*(6), 353–357.

Stanhope, M. & Lancaster, J. (2008) *Public health nursing: Population-centered health care in the community* (7th ed.). St. Louis: Mosby.

Stolte, K. (1996). *Wellness: Nursing diagnosis for health promotion.* Philadelphia: Lippincott, Williams & Wilkins.

Talen, M. R., Stephens, L., Marik, P., & Buchholz, M. (2007). Well-child check-up revised: An efficient protocol for assessing children's social-emotional development. *Families, Systems, & Health, 25*(1), 23–35.

U.S. Census Bureau. (2007a). *Current population survey 2007 annual social and economic supplement, detailed poverty tables POV03 and POV05.* Retrieved February 9, 2008, from *http://pubdb3.census.gov/macro/032007/pov/toc.htm.*

U.S. Census Bureau. (2007b). *Population profile of the United States: Dynamic version.* Retrieved February 9, 2008, from *www.census.gov/population/pop-profile/dynamic/FamiliesLA.pdf.*

U.S. Department of Health and Human Services. (2000). *Healthy people 2010: Understanding and improving health* (Government Report No. Stock Number 017-001-001-00-550-9). Washington, DC: U.S. Government Printing Office, Superintendent of Documents (HP2010).

U.S. Department of Health and Human Services. (2007). *Healthy people 2010 midcourse review.* Retrieved November 29, 2007, from *www.healthypeople.gov/Data/midcourse/.*

Van Dyck, P., Kogan, M. D., Heppel, D., Blumberg, S. J., Cynamon, M. A., & Newacheck, P. W. (2004). The National Survey of Children's Health: A new data resource. *Maternal and Child Health Journal, 8*(3), 183–188.

Wake, M., Hesketh, K., & Waters, E. (2003). Television, computer use and body mass index in Australian primary school children. *Journal of Paediatrics & Child Health, 39*(2), 130–134.

Webster, J., & Holt, V. (2004). Screening for partner violence: Direct questioning or self-report? *Obstetrics Gynecology, 103*(2), 299–303.

Whitehead, B. D., & Popenoe, D. (2006). *The state of our unions 2006 the social health of marriage in America essay life without children.* Retrieved February 9, 2008, from *http://marriage.rutgers.edu/Publications/SOOU/TEXTSOOU2006.htm.*

Widmer, E., Le Goff, J., Levy, R., Hammer, R., & Kellerhals, J. (2006). Embedded parenting? The influence of conjugal networks on parent-child relationships. *Journal of Social and Personal Relationships, 23*(3), 387–406.

Wright, L. M., & Leahey, M. (2005). *Nurses and families: A guide to family assessment and intervention* (4th ed.). Philadelphia: F. A. Davis.

Wu, T., Mendola, P., & Buck, G. M. (2002). Ethnic differences in the presence of secondary sex characteristics and menarche among US girls: The third national health and nutrition examination survey, 1988-1994. *Pediatrics, 110*(4), 752–757.

Ziffer, J. M., Crawford, E., & Penney-Wietor, J. (2007). The Boomerang Bunch: A school-based multifamily group approach for students and their families recovering from parental separation and divorce. *Journal for Specialists in Group Work, 32*(2), 154–164, 202-206.

Chapter 8

Anne Rath Rentfro

Health Promotion and the Community

objectives

After completing this chapter, the reader will be able to:

- Describe the 11 functional health patterns and explain how they are used for data collection to assess communities.
- Evaluate community characteristics that indicate risk.
- Identify developmental aggregates of potential or actual dysfunctional health patterns.
- Explain methods of community data collection and sources of information.
- Describe a method of planned change for the community.
- Discuss planning, implementing, and evaluating nursing interventions in health promotion with communities.
- Develop a health-promotion plan based on community assessment (includes resources), nursing diagnosis, and other contributing factors.

key terms

Ambient
Community
Community diagnosis
Community evaluation
Community health promotion
Community nursing intervention

Community outcomes
Community pattern
Community risk factors
Demography
Developmental theory
Function of a community
Interview data

Measurement data
Observation data
Risk factor theory
Structure of a community
Systems theory
Windshield survey

website materials

evolve These materials are located on the book's website at *http://evolve.elsevier.com/Edelman/*.

- WebLinks
- Study Questions
- Glossary
- Website Resources

    8A: Functional Health Patterns: Data Collection Guide to Community Assessment
    8B: Guidelines for Nursing Interventions for Ethnic Elders

THINK About It

Teenagers: Drinking and Driving

In a small rural community, 7 teenagers have died in alcohol-related car accidents within the past 3 months. Alcohol and drug education is taught during the first year at the local high school, but driver's education classes are not offered because the school cannot afford the program. Parents within this community are extremely concerned.

1. What other information must be acquired before making a diagnosis?
2. What health-promotion ideas could be recommended based on the information provided?

Over the last few decades, several social trends in the United States have increased public interest in health promotion and disease prevention. The landmark project, *Healthy People 2010* documents the U.S. Department of Health and Human Services (2000; 2007) published (see Chapter 1) have been helpful in changing the focus of health care from a reactive stance to a proactive stance that emphasizes prevention of disease and promotion of health. By stating national health objectives as population-specific risks to good health, these documents aim to guide community strategies and to promote health, thereby reducing the risk factors to disease.

Another social trend creating interest in these issues is the changing population of the United States (see Chapter 2). The U.S. Census Bureau estimates that between 2000 and 2030, for example, the population 65 and older will grow faster than the total population doubling this population in 26 of the states (U.S. Census Bureau, 2005). Older people tend to have more chronic diseases and consume larger portions of health care resources than people in other age groups. The aging population, for example, requires more home health care and nursing home services than previous generations, due to increased lifespan and the concurrences of health problems (including altered levels of functioning).

The term **community** is used in various contexts with various meanings, depending on the frame of reference. In this text, the definition of community is the same definition used by *Healthy People 2010* and the Health Promotion Glossary of the World Health Organization (WHO), "A specific group of people, often living in a defined geographical area, who share a common culture, values, and norms and who are arranged in a social structure according to relationships that the community has developed over a period of time" (U.S. Department of Health and Human Services, 2007; World Health Organization, 1998). Using this definition, community encompasses a wide variety of settings. For example, community includes workplaces and schools (U.S. Department of Health and Human Services, 2007).

Nurses in the nation's schools serve youth and provide access to community resources. Linking school nurses with communities can increase access to resources to improve health-promoting behaviors (Frankowski et al., 2006). Results from the School Health Policies Programs Study indicate support for the *Healthy People 2010* Objective 7-4: "Increase the proportion of the Nation's elementary, middle, junior high, and senior high schools that have a nurse-to-student ratio of at least 1:750" (U.S. Department of Health and Human Services, 2007). Since 1998, the percentage of schools who meet this objective has risen from 28% to 53%, with a target of 60% by 2010 (U.S. Department of Health and Human Services, 2007).

People are integral to any concept of community; human beings give each community shape, character, and form. Individual health is reflected in each community through each person's contribution to its statistical rates and cultural and psychological makeup. Conversely, the community is reflected in the individual through similar modes of expression (Aday, 2001).

This chapter focuses on the application of the nursing process to the community with independent, interdependent, and dependent nursing activities. Methods of data collection and sources of information about communities may differ from individual sources. **Systems theory, developmental theory,** and **risk factor theory** guide nursing process. Developmental theory refers to a variety of explanations of phases of human development—physical, psychosocial, cognitive, and spiritual dimensions—based on descriptive research studies. Similarly, risk factor theory identifies human characteristics and behaviors that increase the likelihood of the manifestation of health problems. Gordon's (2007) functional health patterns provide the assessment framework. An example of a data collection guide is presented to facilitate the comprehension, synthesis, and application of **observation data, interview data,** and **measurement data.** An example of data analysis, nursing diagnosis, planning, implementation, and evaluation follows along with a description (also see website materials).

THE NURSING PROCESS AND THE COMMUNITY

Gordon's (2007) health-related patterns provide a useful guide to collect observation, interview and measurement data. Health-related patterns chosen by the nurse for assessment depend on community settings, assessment focus, and preference. Assessing all pattern areas provides a basic data set to analyze and use for comparison during evaluation (see Chapter 6).

Risk factors and development also influence health patterns. For example, a health concern might be identified in one pattern area, such as the increased age-related factor of teenage pregnancy (sexuality-reproductive pattern). Data from other areas may reveal that parental opposition (values-beliefs pattern) tends to restrict sex education to the home (coping–stress tolerance pattern) and thus limit sex education in school. Attempting to restrict sex education to the home and "ignoring" it in school and primary care may place young people of childbearing age in the community at risk for unwanted pregnancies. Factors from several pattern areas may form clusters of risk for certain groups (see Chapter 6).

THE NURSE'S ROLE

Community health nursing combines nursing practice and public health concepts to promote the health of populations. It is not limited to any particular individual or group of individuals (Clark, 2007). Nursing concerns become communities' responses to existing and potential health-related problems, including such health-supporting responses as monitoring and teaching population groups. Nurses supply educational information to at-risk communities to develop health-oriented skills, attitudes, and related behavioral changes.

Community nurses also develop essential relationships aimed to accomplish communities' health-related missions. Complex and dynamic communities, with their increasing public involvement in health and health policy, highlight the importance of human interactions inherent in nurses' responses to potential health problems, needs, and expectations. Community nursing practice, therefore, requires a broad knowledge base derived from the natural, behavioral, and humanistic sciences with application of intellectual, interpersonal, and technical skills using the nursing process.

Community nurses' roles include the interaction of independent, interdependent, and dependent functions. Independent functions include assessing, analyzing, diagnosing, planning, implementing, and evaluating nursing activities such as health promotion and health education. Interdependent functions include collaboration with community members and interdisciplinary teamwork functions that are crucial to effective community health. Dependent functions include implementing the therapeutic plans of team members.

Community health promotion includes all of the following:
- Community participation, with representatives from multiple community sectors including government, education, business, faith organizations, health care, media, voluntary agencies, and the public;
- Assessment guided by a community-planning model to determine health problems, resources, perceptions, and priorities for action;
- Targeted and measurable objectives to address health outcomes, risk factors, public awareness, services, and protection;
- Comprehensive, multifaceted, culturally relevant interventions that have multiple targets for change;
- Monitoring and evaluation of objectives and strategies used (U.S. Department of Health and Human Services, 2007).

METHODS OF DATA COLLECTION

Nurses obtain community assessment data through observation, interviews, and measurement. These three methods are used most frequently in various combinations to ensure the validity of the information. Obtaining data through observation—often referred to as the **windshield survey** approach to assessment—includes the use of the senses (sight, touch, hearing, smell, and taste) to determine community appearances. These appearances include types and condition of residential dwellings, people, and physical and biological characteristics, such as animal and plant life, temperature, transportation, sounds, and odors. Some communities have a characteristic "flavor." Communities' physical characteristics influence health. What type of space is available? Children need space to run and play; young and middle-aged adults require space for recreation and exercise. What spatial barriers exist? Community nurses obtain abundant subjective data by simply walking or riding around a community. Data obtained by observation provides important clues about the community, its actual or potential health problems, and its strengths. Analysis of observation data generates hypotheses to explore further using interview and measurement data.

Interview data, the most common source of information from people, includes verbal statements from community residents, key community officials, health care personnel, and various community agency staff. Interviewing provides a useful way to learn how members perceive their community. Key community leaders often provide important information about community health concerns, necessary health resources, and community strengths along with particular health beliefs and community health goals. Community residents provide useful information about their perceptions of health, health concerns, and needs as well as of the availability, accessibility, and acceptability of health services. Health agency personnel provide data about health resources, population served, availability, and perceptions of concerns and needs. Developing a basic set of questions in advance enhances the relevance of interview data.

Measurement data uses instruments to quantify data during information collection. Measurement data include population statistics, pollution indices, morbidity and mortality rates, census statistics, and epidemiological data. These data can be accessed by Internet or locally in community libraries; health departments; environmental protection agencies; schools; police and fire departments; local health system agencies; and town, city, or state planning offices. Publicly supported agencies share their information, and community nurses readily use such data.

SOURCES OF COMMUNITY INFORMATION

Census information located at *www.census.gov* and also found in libraries and public agencies is the most complete source for population information. Because the U.S. Census is completed once every 10 years at the beginning of a decade, data for most communities become less accurate as the decade progresses. Community agencies and local planning commissions project statistics and developmental trends, which nurses use to understand population patterns and dynamics.

Environmental measurement data can be obtained from the local branch of the U.S. Environmental Protection Agency. Generally local health departments monitor water, food, and sanitation systems. Health departments along with school nurses and administrators provide school health information. Town, city, or county administrations provide information about land use, boundaries, housing conditions, utilities, and community services. Community newspapers supply information about community dynamics, health-related concerns, cultural activities, and community decision-making. Documentation techniques for community observation, interview, and measurement data are similar to those used for individuals and families. A triple-column format that separates the data of each method facilitates recording.

COMMUNITY FROM A SYSTEMS PERSPECTIVE

Systems theory provides an overall framework to connect and integrate community data. Systems consist of interrelated, interacting parts or components within boundaries that filter both the type and rate of input and output (Clark, 2007; McLeroy, 2006; Sterman, 2006). Similar to how families form systems (see Chapter 7), communities viewed as systems have both structure and function. Assessment of communities includes exploration of aspects of populations within specific geographical areas.

Structure

The **structure of a community** system or subsystem consists of a formal or informal arrangement of parts, including both animate and inanimate properties. Nursing, which operates within the context of the health system, can be considered within the context of community systems. Figure 8-1 shows a hierarchical arrangement of a community system. The suprasystem, often a county or state, shapes the larger part of the system that encompasses numerous subsystems. Community structural parts form the subsystems, each of which is in itself a system. Health agencies, schools, fire departments, and governmental bodies are examples of structural parts. Arrangement and organization of a community, such as age distribution and types of health-promotion/protection programs, change over time. Parts fluctuate depending upon environmental processes occurring locally and within the larger environment.

Community leadership provides direction for both health-promotion and health-protection activities; therefore, community assessment includes exploration of various community systems as they relate to health. The practice of viewing the community structure as a population (collection of people) and considering the arrangement of the community's health care parts (existing health services) plays an important role in the assessment process.

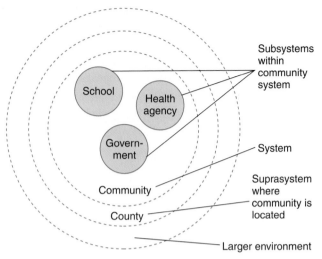

Figure 8-1   Hierarchical nature of a community system.

The study of a population is referred to as **demography**. Demography provides information about population characteristics—such as size and racial composition, along with the distribution of age, gender, marital status, nationality, language, religious affiliations, education, and occupation. Demographic data provide the basis for analysis and a means to identify groups who may have high risk for health concerns. Such information also provides clues for the direction of health strategies. For example, examining age distribution over several years reveals important population shifts with associated needs for additional health-promotion activities. The increase in the number of individuals over age 65 requires changes in community health priorities that reflect this group's needs.

Comparison statistics about population characteristics, which also need to be considered in community structure, enable nurses to make inferences about the community. Comparisons are made among three systems: (1) the town, which is a part of the county; (2) the county, which is a part of the larger system; and (3) the state. Comparisons between communities of similar population size typically occur.

Function

The **function of a community** refers to the process of dynamic change with adaptation in the system's parts and how community systems and subsystems interact. Decision-making and allocation of health-promotion and health-protection resources are important considerations for community assessment. As health educators, nurses interact with the community to promote health. Community health promotion involves a complex array of responsibilities. Nurses act as advocates using proactive planning and collaboration with other disciplines and agencies. As a community liaison, the nurse establishes priorities for programming; matches resources with needs determined by a community needs assessment; empowers community members; and facilitates social, environmental, and political change. These multifaceted functions require expertise in communication and interpersonal relations that involve a deliberate approach. Using such an intentional process, while maintaining the community's vision, can produce effective change.

Interaction

Through dynamic interaction with the environment, systems exchange matter, energy, and information (in such communication forms as verbal and behavioral) to make decisions. Interaction also contributes to the community system's ability to survive, as well as to protect and promote the health of its members. Through environmental interactions, community systems use adaptation mechanisms. Nurses determine how communities apply these mechanisms toward health services.

Various health-related patterns emerge from these interactions. For example, certain human activity patterns negatively alter natural environmental patterns, which in turn influence human health patterns. Gordon's (2007) assessment framework focuses on 11 health-related functional patterns that each assume community and environment interaction from a systems perspective.

COMMUNITY FROM A DEVELOPMENTAL PERSPECTIVE

A framework based on developmental theory can be used to identify existing or potential health problems for particular age groups in communities. A population is a group defined as an aggregate of people who share similar personal or environmental characteristics. Community nurses, focusing on the total community population, use a developmental, age-correlated approach to identify health-promotion and health-protection activities.

Nurses identify age-related risks at each life stage taking steps to maximize wellness and health promotion as a lifelong concern (U.S. Department of Health and Human Services, 2007). For example, adolescent single mothers of infants, at risk both emotionally and physically, require parenting skills. Accidents are the greatest threat to children's health; therefore, accident-prevention activities become a priority for adolescent mothers. Age-related risk factors (see Chapters 6 and 7) associated with individuals and families can be extended to include community groups.

COMMUNITY FROM A RISK FACTOR PERSPECTIVE

Risk factors associated with community disease, illness, and death rates, although not causally associated, play a role in predicting the likelihood of a particular adverse health condition (U.S. Department of Health and Human Services, 2007). Risk factors include a combination of demographic, psychological, physiological, or environmental characteristics (or they may include a single characteristic). For example, age, gender, race, geographical location, consumption pattern, or lack of health services may be considered risk factors, because one or more may contribute to

research highlights

Passenger Safety for Latino Children

The purpose of this research was to demonstrate that the use of a community health worker education program would improve proper use of child automobile safety seats for Latino (primarily of Mexican descent) children in an urban area. Motor vehicle crash injuries are a leading cause of death for Latino children in the United States. In this study, an education intervention was provided by Latino community health workers trained to teach families about proper child safety seat usage. Families who received the intervention were compared to those who did not in regard to proper seat usage. A community participatory approach was used with members of the community participating in both design and implementation of the study. Families that participated in the study were primarily Mexican with low income, education, and acculturation levels. Child safety seats (n = 90) were checked for proper use. The authors concluded that the intervention contributed to proper safety seat usage in this urban low-income Latino community. This study provides some support for nurses to use community-based interventions as appropriate techniques to prevent injuries. The role of the nurse as community advocate and community facilitator is instrumental in promoting positive community change. Effective injury prevention programs need to be analyzed to better describe the patterns of injury, the needs of children in their community, and the interventions that would be most effective to promote more positive outcomes.

From Martin, M., Holden, J., Chen, Z., & Quinlan, K. (2006). Child passenger safety for inner-city Latinos: New approaches from the community. *Injury Prevention, 12*(2), 99–104.

disease or death and place the population sharing them at risk (Research Highlights box). The degree of influence of various risk factors differs from person to person and group to group because of genetic makeup, geographical location, lifestyle patterns, resources, socioeconomic status, level of education, or environmental variation. Some groups may be at high risk from a single risk factor such as insufficient immunizations or exposure to asbestos. A combined potential for adverse health effects exists when many risk factors are present, because they interact in multiple ways and synergistically influence each other (U.S. Department of Health and Human Services, 2007).

Communities, therefore, experience substantial variability in health conditions in regard to both incidence and susceptibility. Risk factor theory views health and disease as multifactorial with etiology attributed to no single risk factor. For example, risk factors such as air pollution, smoking, and forms of radiation in various combinations may be related to high rates of lung cancer, emphysema, and bronchitis in a community. The potential to control risk factors and to make relevant health-related resources available forms the basis for health-promotion and health-protection activities.

Website Resource 8A contains a general description of Gordon's 11 functional health patterns with guidelines for posing questions in interviews and pertinent observations. A variety of functional health pattern assessments are used with communities. Nurses use Gordon's (2007) functional health reference assessment as exemplified in this chapter or other assessments described in the literature (Clark, 2007).

FUNCTIONAL HEALTH PATTERNS: ASSESSMENT OF THE COMMUNITY

Health Perception–Health Management Pattern

The Health Perception–Health Management Pattern identifies data about community health status, health-promotion and disease-prevention practices, and community members' perceptions of health (Gordon, 2007). Residents may perceive a substance abuse problem in adolescents or a high rate of unwanted pregnancies, breast cancer, or sexually transmitted disease as concerns. Valuable information can be elicited from interviewing key community members about their health concerns and issues. Mortality and morbidity statistics and other public health information sources provide measurement data (see Chapter 2).

Nutritional-Metabolic Pattern

The Nutritional-Metabolic Pattern identifies data relevant to community consumption habits as reflected in accessibility and availability of food stores and subsidized food programs for infants, children, and older adults. Community well-being, which depends on adequate dietary habits, food intake, and supply of nutrients, is influenced by culture, the presence or absence of kitchen facilities, and adequate plumbing.

Collecting data by driving or walking through the community while employing all five senses provides information about grocery stores, fast-food establishments, ethnic shopping facilities, and street corner vendors. Government programs, private soup kitchens, and food donations by houses of worship also provide information about nutritional patterns of communities.

Elimination Pattern

The Elimination Pattern identifies environmental factors including exposure to pollutants in the community through contaminated soil, water, air, and the food chain. This pattern further classifies environmental factors into the two broad categories of physical and biological. Alterations in environmental processes threaten health and integrity of communities, necessitating health-promotion and health-protection activities.

Physical agents include geological, geographical, climatic, and meteorological aspects of the community. Certain population groups are particularly susceptible to acute respiratory disease and aggravated asthmatic episodes when the air quality is poor. Geographical locations of communities and major waterways, highways, or mountains located within communities act as barriers to health facilities.

Inaccessibility of health care services also hinders health in at-risk groups. Knowledge of climatic conditions provides clues to susceptibility to illness resulting from temperature or humidity in certain populations.

Biological agents include living things—such as plants, animals and their waste products, disease agents, microbial pathogens, and toxic substances—that can be hazardous to health. For example, Lyme disease, viral hepatitis, pneumonia, influenza, and the large number of diseases associated with childhood continue to be threats to community health. Observation and interviews with key community members reveal information concerning elimination patterns. The Environmental Protection Agency and Centers for Disease Control and Prevention provide excellent resources for community health nurses.

Activity-Exercise Pattern

The Activity-Exercise Pattern identifies physical activities and recreational options within communities. Science and technology have increasingly influenced productivity while simultaneously reducing or eliminating physical work. Consequently, physical activity no longer occurs during the work day for most community members, leaving leisure time as the only time for physical activity. Physical activity reduces the risk of many diseases, including obesity, heart disease, hypertension, cancer, osteoporosis, and diabetes mellitus.

Physiological evidence demonstrates that physical activity improves many biological measures associated with health and psychological functioning. Regular physical activity and musculoskeletal fitness are important to healthy, independent living as people grow older. Observation and interviews provide clues to a community's ability to provide cultural and recreational activities (Figure 8-2).

Sleep-Rest Pattern

The Sleep-Rest Pattern identifies a community's rhythm of sleeping, resting, and relaxing. Some towns never close with stores, traffic flow, and recreational facilities operating during both day and night hours. This ongoing activity produces

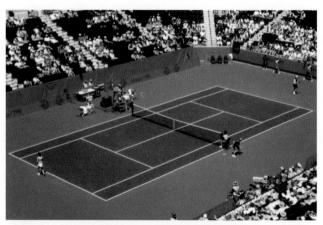

Figure 8-2 The activity-exercise pattern identifies a community's physical activities and recreational options.

unpleasant disturbances, such as unwanted noise that may be harmful to community well-being. Excessive noise from highways or airplanes produces physiological or psychological problems eliciting responses ranging from mild irritation to pain or permanent hearing loss. Although noise cannot be eliminated, efforts to minimize and control it are possible. Observation and interviews provide clues to this pattern.

Cognitive-Perceptual Pattern

The Cognitive-Perceptual Pattern identifies information about problem solving and decision-making within communities. Systems depend on decision-making and resource allocation processes for survival. Communities require functional decision-making bodies to ensure adherence to rules and goals attainment. Individual patterns and environmental patterns connect with important implications for community health. Community assessment includes appraisal of interaction with the environment along with effectiveness of strategies used to meet health concerns and needs (Clark, 2007; McLeroy, 2006).

One strategy, bargaining, offers the community an exchange for health service. For example, a community that owns a mammography machine but has no primary care facility might negotiate with another community to provide mammography for primary care services in return. Strategies using outside authority (legal bureaucratic methods) ensure compliance through rules and structures. In this case, states may mandate that communities maintain certain health standards. For example, a law may require all school children to be immunized against specific diseases before entering public school. Cooperative strategies promote health when members share common goals. For example, community residents may join together to oppose a chemical landfill that is a health hazard.

Convincing people to comply because they hold some loyalty in the situation or relationship is another method that mobilizes communities. For example, community residents might expend a great deal of effort and money to retain a particular health clinic because of loyalty to the agency. Identifying decision-making patterns used by communities provides clues about health priorities and values, as well as matches and mismatches between existing circumstances, health goals, and planning strategies. Data can best be obtained by observation and interviews.

Self-Perception–Self-Concept Pattern

The Self-Perception–Self-Concept Pattern identifies self-worth and personal identity of communities. Characteristics such as image, status, and perceived competency with problem solving indicate community self-concept. Housing conditions, buildings, and cleanliness reflect community image. School systems, crime rates, accidents, and opinions about whether the community is considered a good place to live suggest community perception of self-worth. Competency with social and political issues as well as community spirit creates positive self-evaluation. Community pride facilitates development of innovative health programs. Emotional tone (fear, depression, or positive emotional outlook) relates to findings in other pattern areas. For example, tensions in the cognitive-perceptual pattern (conflict between groups concerning health issues) may explain a general feeling of fear among the residents. Data are obtained through observation and interviews.

Roles-Relationships Pattern

The Roles-Relationships Pattern identifies communication styles along with formal and informal relationships. Of particular concern are roles and relationships affecting community ability to realize health potential. Patterns of crime, racial incidents, and social networks form indices of human relationships in communities. Publicizing health promotion becomes more effective using patterns of official communication. Health program success depends upon support from prominent community members. Community members involved in health programs help identify other key community leaders. Use of media and other mass information programs improves communication, the flow of health information, and the number of community members reached. Interviews, television, the Internet and newspapers are examples of ways to obtain and convey information.

Sexuality-Reproductive Pattern

The Sexuality-Reproductive Pattern identifies reproductive data of communities, which is reflected in live birth statistics, mothers' ages, ethnicity, and marital status. This information provides clues to the health-promotion needs of a particular community group. Premature infant rates, low–birth-weight infants, abortion rates, as well as neonatal, infant, and maternal death rates reflect reproductive patterns of communities. Such information identifies at-risk groups based on particular characteristics associated with these rates. Mismatches between existing health services, health education, and community health statistics also indicate health concerns. Availability of sex education in schools; spouse and child abuse; and sex-related crimes also indicate health-promotion issues. Minutes of meetings, health records, statistical data, and public documents provide sources for these data.

Coping–Stress Tolerance Pattern

The Coping–Stress Tolerance Pattern identifies community ability to cope or adapt. Communities respond to stress in different ways, some of which might threaten their integrity. Community responses reveal the group coping patterns. Communities develop abilities to exchange goods, services, goals, values, and ideals to survive and to promote community health. Community efforts to obtain goods from the environment, contain goods within the environment, retain goods within the community, and dispose of goods play significant roles to influence health. Examples of goods that communities obtain from the environment to promote health include local, state, or federal funding; health services; health-related workforce personnel; new knowledge; and technological advances. Some communities obtain abundant health care services; however, primary services often remain inadequate or nonexistent. Lack of available health services, or lack of ability to obtain them, characterizes community health need. Examples of goods communities may attempt to control include sex-related crimes, diseases, substance abuse, industry, hazardous waste in the water supply, and noxious chemicals in the air.

Community coping patterns aim to retain certain health-protection services, such as immunization services for children and adequate health facilities. Coping efforts may also include strict zoning laws and housing codes or certain values such as sex education within the home. Expendable goods communities include industrial and human wastes. Data can be obtained through minutes of meetings, public documents, health surveys, statistical data, and health records.

Values-Beliefs Pattern

The Values-Beliefs Pattern identifies the community values and beliefs. Such information provides clues for health promotion and protection efforts valued by the community. Values underlie decisions about community health education and tax support for schools, hypertension screening for the public, prevention programs, or well-child clinics. Traditions, norms, and cultural and ethnic groups share values and beliefs in communities. Data can be obtained through interviews with key community members and health-related personnel.

ANALYSIS AND DIAGNOSIS WITH THE COMMUNITY

Analysis refers to data categorization and pattern determination. Data synthesis and organization occur to ascertain patterns of health activities and trends. An example of a clinical scenario about a particular community is presented in the Case Study and Care Plan at the end of this chapter. Decision-making and judgment inherent in the nursing process become most important during the analysis and diagnostic phases. Table 8-1 presents an example of one way to organize community data using Prochaska's stages of change (Clark, 2007; Prochaska & Norcross, 2006).

Table **8-1**	Stages of Change
Stages	**Interventions**
Precontemplation	Provide information (identify risk factors)
	Raise doubts about current behaviors and future outcomes
Contemplation	Discuss risks of not changing
	Discuss benefits of changing
Action	Help plan phases of change
	Help implement phases of change
Maintenance	Help develop strategies to prevent relapse, emphasizing self-efficacy
	Offer encouragement
Relapse	Highlight past successes and future benefits

Modified from Prochaska, J. O. & Norcross, J. C. (2006). *Systems of psychotherapy: A transtheoretical analysis* (6th ed.) Boston: Wadsworth Publishing.

Organization of Data

Charts, figures, and tables graphically display population distributions, morbidity and mortality data, or vital statistics to pinpoint significant community concerns with actual or potential health problems along with health-related responses to these concerns. Another valuable organizational technique, mapping, facilitates data analysis. For example, a series of maps can be used to display data that change over time. Analysis of several variables simultaneously occurs. Overlap of locations of environmental hazards, densely populated areas, health-promotion services, and major highways becomes apparent. Poor environmental conditions; distribution of illness, disease, and death rates; and the accessibility of health-protection and health-promotion activities for the population appear at a glance with dotted scatter maps. Use of maps requires knowledge about the community's population base. Less-populated geographical areas with fewer health facilities or fewer neonatal deaths in a community with fewer women of childbearing age are examples of how population statistics influence interpretation of mapping techniques. Using theoretical frameworks and Gordon's 11 pattern areas facilitates analysis of community data. Several guidelines, presented below, help community nurses analyze population data. Analysis often supports the need for further data collection.

Guidelines for Data Analysis
Check for Missing Data

Complexity, size, and number of community characteristics prohibit gathering all possible facts about the health-related pattern areas; however, missing or insufficient data that indicate areas for further assessment should be identified. Additional assessment may determine specific approaches or a particular **community diagnosis**. Examples of missing data in community assessment include pollution indices, links between health resources and population groups, accessibility to resources, and morbidity statistics. Dates for census data used should be noted.

The nurse examines community data for incongruities and conflicting information. For example, a key community official might deny the existence of pollutants in the water supply, whereas newspaper reports of health department water analysis findings indicate otherwise. The nurse evaluates such inconsistencies before identifying existing or potential health concerns.

Identify Patterns

Clues about a **community pattern** emerge from subjective and objective data gathered. During this stage, community nurses make decisions, begin to formulate diagnostic hypotheses (ideas and tentative judgments about possible health concerns), identify community groups that might be at risk, and establish probable causes or relationships. Ideas generated from this activity direct the search for additional clues in the data to confirm, reject, or revise hypotheses. Judgments about hypotheses continue to support patterns in the data.

To narrow the huge list of possible community health-promotion and health-protection concerns, community nurses formulate broad problem statements based on the health-related pattern areas (Gordon, 2007). For example, the community nurse differentiates among elimination problems (noxious chemicals), coping and stress-tolerance problems, and health perception–health management problems (high teenage mortality rate from motor vehicle accidents). Developing these general categories facilitates analysis.

Apply Theories, Models, Norms, and Standards

Analyzing community data requires extensive knowledge about developmental, age-related risks, theories, concepts of nursing, public health, and epidemiology. Such a broad foundation enables nurses to identify additional clues in health-related patterns that contribute to community nursing diagnoses and intervention. Developmental approaches form a basis to identify groups with potential health concerns. Age groups vary in susceptibility; therefore, nurses examine community resources directed toward highly susceptible groups. For example, community data that indicates increases in live births among older women indicates a need for health-promotion services for this group. If community data show increasing numbers of aging citizens, nurses explore availability and accessibility of existing health services for this older group.

Analysis of data for common personal or environmental characteristics also occurs. For example, select groups may be at risk based on a shared health concern, such as substance abuse, lack of immunizations, unsafe housing conditions, high exposure to asbestos or noxious chemicals, or inadequate health services. Shared characteristics, such as race or ethnicity, provide clues to susceptibility and need for screening activities. For example, Black populations warrant screening for hypertension. Also if fluoridated water supply is unavailable, additional intervention to prevent dental caries in children is justified. In addition, community literacy contributes to health-promotion activity development methods used by nurses to establish educational programs. Literacy level limits the ability to use all available resources.

Environmental information is readily available on the Internet. Databases and search engines provide useful information about environmental hazards and other environmental problems in communities. Prevention of disease worldwide depends on the dissemination of global environmental health information (U.S. Department of Health and Human Services, 2007). Analysis of data relies on standards developed nationally or globally. For example, community data regarding air quality can be compared with state or national ambient air quality standards to determine health (Health Canada, 2006). In this context the term **ambient** refers to outside air in a town, city, or other defined region. Air-monitoring stations are generally located in urban and rural areas within each state (United States Environmental Protection Agency, 2006). One source for air

quality information is the CHARTing Health Information website (*www.sph.uth.tmc.edu/charting/*) maintained by the University of Texas Health Science Center at Houston School of Public Health. The goal of this center is to serve as a resource in Texas for publicly available data to use for analysis and research. Data and links to other sites are continually monitored and updated (The University of Texas Health Science Center at Houston, 2007). Current information about community resources enables more effective strategies to prevent risk factors and avoid health problems. Internet access facilitates identification of gaps in health-promotion and health-protection services.

Identify Strengths and Health Concerns

Interpretation of community data occurs with regard to community concerns, community strengths, and feasibility studies. Community nurses make judgments and inferences about community health, community responses to health situations, and population needs. One approach assumes health concerns exist unless assessment data indicate otherwise (Gordon, 2007). Nurses make diagnoses based on summarized data using the nursing process, which results in one or more of the following determinations:

1. No problem exists, but providing health-promotion or health-protection services may address a potential health concern. For example, providing health education in the high school could offset a potential for increased sexually transmitted disease in the high school population.
2. A problem exists but is recognized by community members or health-related professionals with effective strategies for problem solving; for example, flu immunizations.
3. A problem exists that the community recognizes, but resources are inadequate or the community has not responded. Assistance is needed; for example, highway traffic noise.
4. A problem exists that the community recognizes but cannot cope with at this time, such as a lack of fluoridated water systems. Dentists, nurses, and nutritionists could be assigned to assist the community in resolving actual problems of dental caries.
5. A problem or potential health concern exists that needs further study; for example, lack of sidewalks.

Identifying community strengths integrates plans for health-promotion and health-protection activities. For example, a community may have nutritional feeding programs for older adults, women, and children that are underutilized. Community members may not use them because communication is inadequate. Examples of community strengths and concerns are shown in Table 8-2.

Identify Causes and Risk Factors

Data are examined for factors or characteristics that contribute to identified potential and existing health-related concerns. Nurses make inferences about population groups and identify risk factors. Identifying risk factors guides community

Table **8-2**	Examples of Community Strengths and Concerns

Strengths	Concerns
Well-child clinic available	Unavailable
Feeding program accessible to older adults	Inaccessible
Sex education in schools acceptable	Unacceptable
Family planning services accessible	Inaccessible
Fluoridated water system	Nonfluoridated water system
Open communication	Dysfunctional communication
Interagency cooperation	Dysfunctional transactions
Adequate kitchen and plumbing facilities	Inadequate
High interest of key leaders in health promotion	Lack of interest

MULTICULTURAL AWARENESS

Comparing Poverty Rates by Racial and Ethnic Categories

Comparisons must take into account that racial and ethnic census categories were redefined in 2002. Blacks constitute 12.9 % of the population (reported as Black or African American). This number and those that follow include the 0.6% of the population who reported as Black as well as one or more other races. Although Blacks are represented in every socioeconomic group, 24.1% live in poverty. This is a rate 3 times higher than the non-Hispanic White American rate (8.0%). Among people who reported themselves as being Asian American, 10.3% lived in poverty. Poverty rates have remained the same for non-Hispanic Whites and Asians when compared to the closest available data groupings from 2001. However, the poverty figures among people who reported being Black in 2002 show that there was an increase (U.S. Census Bureau, 2003).

Based on these figures, it seems that poverty is rising in the Black population. Most of the Black population (54%) lived in the South according to Census 2000. The remaining 46% was spread out over the rest of the United States. In areas other than the South, concentrations of the Black population were located in urban areas (McKinnon, 2000).

From McKinnon, J. (2000). *The black population 2000: Census briefs* (No. C2KBR/01-5). Washington, DC: U.S. Census Bureau; and U.S. Census Bureau. (2003). Current population survey: Poverty: 2002 highlights. Retrieved January 6, 2008, from: *www.census.gov/prod/2003pubs/p60-222.pdf*.

nursing actions. Some risk factors signify immediate health concerns, such as polluted water supply, whereas other risk factors indicate potential problems, such as lack of knowledge about childhood disease prevention. Nurses consider whether **community risk factors** can be altered, eliminated, or regulated through nursing actions. Nurses modify factors when possible by using strategies such as health education (Multicultural Awareness box).

Community Diagnosis

Community assessment, as previously described, culminates in nursing diagnoses. The community diagnosis process includes (1) community situations or states within a population or population group; (2) data collection using some combination of observation, interview, and measurement; (3) a framework; (4) existing or potential health concerns; (5) risk factors related to health concerns; and (6) potential solutions through nursing actions. Diagnoses form the basis for planning, implementing, and evaluating solutions to health concerns (Carpenito-Moyet, 2008; Clark, 2007; Gordon, 2007). The Hot Topics and Health Teaching boxes discuss a diagnosis of violence and some recommendations for problem reduction.

Community diagnoses facilitate communication among community health professionals, team members, and laypeople through the use of clear and concise nomenclature with development of diagnostic categories specific to community nursing (Carpenito-Moyet, 2008; Clark, 2007). Diagnoses may be written or stated according to the structural and functional aspects of a community.

Structural aspects include those related to the population, such as the demographic characteristics of groups with similar characteristics (preschool children, adolescents, or a high school population). Functional aspects include those related to the psychosocial, physiological, or spiritual health patterns, such as decision-making (cognitive-perceptual pattern) or communication links among health care resources (roles-relationships pattern). Functional health patterns guide data collection about health concerns and risk factors. Structural and functional aspects of the community provide a framework for diagnostic statements (see Chapter 6).

PLANNING WITH THE COMMUNITY

Community health planning begins with nursing diagnoses. Nurses design goals to resolve existing or potential health concerns. For example, high rates of childhood diseases in the community require goals aimed to decrease rates. Identifying specific or potential health concerns with planned actions to achieve desired **community outcomes** provides the framework and data for **community evaluation**.

Purposes

Major purposes of the planning phase include:
1. Prioritization of problems and diagnoses identified through assessment;
2. Differentiation of problems resolved through nursing actions from those best resolved by others;
3. Identification of immediate, intermediate, and long-term goals, as well as behavioral objectives oriented to the community derived from the goals and specific actions to achieve objectives; and
4. Formalization of a community nursing care plan (see the Care Plan at the end of this chapter) that includes written problems, actions, and expected behavioral outcomes.

HOTtopics

WORKPLACE VIOLENCE

The terrorist attacks on September 11, 2001, or 9/11, were a tragic reminder that targets often chosen by the terrorists are not military in nature. Targets may be places where people work to support their families. Workplace violence was put in a new context that day. Before then, workplace violence was considered as isolated, unplanned incidents that fell under the jurisdiction of the federal Occupational Safety and Health Administration (OSHA). Since 9/11, workplace violence prevention and preparation has included external threats of terrorism. With these new issues in mind, a document called *Workplace Violence: Issues in Response* was prepared to assist in prevention and management of potential workplace violence. The recommendations from this report included the following general categories:

1. Public awareness campaigns
2. Workplace policies and plans
3. Preventive law enforcement
4. Government agencies making workplace violence a priority
5. Training
6. Protection of the abused person when domestic violence or stalking occurs in the workplace
7. Development and distribution of clear and comprehensive legal and legislative guidelines
8. Evaluation of programs and strategies

Suggestions for approaches included the following strategies:

- Educational efforts should reflect cooperative efforts by government agencies, major corporations, unions, and advocacy groups, with OSHA acting as a facilitator and coordinator.
- Put multidisciplinary no-threats–no-violence policies and prevention plans in place.
- Violence prevention training should occur regularly and include practicing the plan.
- Work space and policies should provide a physically secure work environment.
- Preventive measures should be in place including documenting incidents, antiviolence planning, and conducting threat assessments.
- Systems should be developed for monitoring incidents of workplace violence.
- Resource lists should be maintained and include social service, mental health, legal, and other agencies that provide assistance.
- Training programs should extend community policing concepts to workplace violence.
- Government or private organizations should develop training materials for small employers.
- Employers should keep the abuser out of the workplace (e.g., screening telephone calls, making the victim's work space physically more secure, instructing security guards or receptionists).
- Employers should provide resources for emotional, financial, and legal counseling.
- Clear, comprehensive, and uniform legal guidelines should be distributed widely.
- Incentives for employers should be identified and instituted.

From Rugala, E. A., Isaacs, A. R. & Hinojosa, I. (2002). *Workplace violence: Issues in response.* Washington, DC: U.S. Department of Justice, Federal Bureau of Investigation. Retrieved January 6, 2008, from *www.fbi.gov/publications/violence.pdf.*

HEALTH TEACHING   Intervention Techniques to Prevent and Diffuse Workplace Violence

Recognize warning signs, which include changes in mood, personal hardships, mental health issues (e.g., depression, anxiety), negative behavior (e.g., untrustworthy, lying, bad attitude), verbal threats, and history of violence. Do not limit at-risk behavior to a standard profile. Environments should be designed to detect signs of impending violence and to prevent violence with security cameras, key card access, administrative controls, and behavioral strategies. Reporting systems should be confidential and seamless.

- Stay calm; create a relaxed environment and speak calmly.
- Separate the individual from the group, if possible.
- Use nonthreatening body language; build trust and strengthen the relationship.

- Keep your verbal communication simple, clear, and direct; be open and honest.
- Reflect on the person's message to allow time for clarification, allow the person to verbalize, listen attentively, and stop what you are doing and give full attention.
- Ask for examples to help illustrate the points that are being made. Carefully define the problem, exploring with open-ended questions.
- Silence allows the individual time to clarify thoughts.
- Monitor the tone, volume, rate, and rhythm of your speech.
- Seek opportunities for agreement.
- Be creative and open to new ideas.

Compiled from Kohn, C., Henderson, C.W. (2003). Critical warning signs of workplace violence are not what employees expect. *Managed Care Weekly Digest, 22,* 100. DelBel, J. (2003). De-escalating workplace aggression. *Nursing Management, 34*(9); Occupational Safety and Health Administration. (2004). *Preventing workplace violence for health care and social service workers.* Washington, DC: U.S. Department of Labor. Retrieved January 6, 2008, from *www.osha.gov/Publications/osha3148.pdf;* and Crisis Prevention Institute. (2007). Retrieved January 6, 2008, from *www.crisisprevention.com/index.html.*

The planning phase culminates in a nursing plan that provides the framework for evaluation. Once developed, the plan is implemented. Costs associated with delivery of health services and personnel, as well as financial resources available, influence priorities for implementation. Community values and the nurse's philosophy about people, health, the community, and nursing also influence implementation. High-priority issues often include infectious agents, sexually transmitted disease, alcohol and drug use, smoking, inadequate nutrition, inadequate infant and child care, high death rate from motor vehicle accidents, and unwanted teenage pregnancies.

Community participation in health planning facilitates effective assignment of priorities. As health service recipients, community members strive for reasonably priced, high-quality services. Residents aim to acquire appropriate benefits for the needs and concerns of the population. Communication and rationale for designating priorities help to resolve differences in opinion.

During the planning phase, nurses determine those problems most amenable to **community nursing intervention**, behavior implemented by the nurse to fulfill a health goal of the community. Community nurses differentiate problems nursing can resolve from those health concerns that could best be handled by community members, referred to health-related professionals, or handled with community support. Nurses refer problems related to rodents, poor sanitation conditions, or absence of community recreational facilities to appropriate community leaders or agencies.

Community nurses focus on determining goals, developing measurable behavioral objectives and designating actions to achieve expected outcomes. Nurses describe specific behaviors intended to reach projected outcomes. Evaluation includes appraisal of the effectiveness of nursing actions. Health planning emphasizes promoting and protecting population health; therefore, problems, solutions, and actions are defined at the group level. Community nurses plan and implement health plans for groups, such as school-aged children, and facilitate development of health-promotion services for all residents. Nurses frequently act as change agents by taking responsibility for influencing health patterns and behavior. Decisions about health interventions stem from community nurses' appreciation of human behavior and principles of planned change. **Website Resource 8B** offers guidelines for interventions with one population group: ethnic elders.

Planned Change

Planned change results from efforts by individuals or groups and involves fundamental shifts in behavior (Prochaska & Norcross, 2006). Individuals act as agents of their own health conditions. Community health objectives often depend upon active decisions by individuals to change their lifestyles (reducing alcohol consumption or giving up smoking). Efforts to influence and reinforce changes in community health behavior become the central focus of effective risk reduction programs.

Studies attempt to explain why some groups of people effectively participate in certain health programs or make lifestyle changes, whereas others do not. The early health belief model proposed by Rosenstock (Rosenstock, 1974) and more recent models developed by Pender (Pender et al., 2006) and Prochaska (Prochaska & Norcross, 2006), among others, identify critical concepts for understanding how individuals change their health behavior. Rosenstock's model includes the following four steps:

1. Perceiving behavior as a health threat in terms of susceptibility and seriousness;
2. Believing the behavior is a threat to their personal health;
3. Taking action to adopt preventive health behaviors; and
4. Reinforcing the new behavior.

In Rosenstock's model, community members take a passive role at first, then transition from passive to active between steps two and three (belief to action). Ultimately, to improve community health through risk reduction programs, community members assume more responsibility for their own health, become more active in adopting healthy lifestyles, and monitor resources in the community to gain healthy behaviors. In planning health-promotion activities, nurses consider effective strategies to motivate and support community transition from a passive to an active state.

Plans guide nursing actions. Nurses make additions and changes based on community problems, resources, and problem resolution to maintain a viable plan. Table 8-3 provides one example of a community-oriented, health-promotion plan based on the goals recommended by the Surgeon General's report about health promotion and disease prevention. The report's general goal generates several specific objectives. Nursing diagnoses guide the direction of the objectives including risk factors to address. Examples of various rationales in Table 8-3 show how nurses incorporate important concepts of planned change into community-based health-promotion plans.

Communicating plans to other health professionals, community members, and key officials remains an essential aspect of planning. Local newspapers, local bulletins, and school correspondence to parents provide avenues to communicate with the community about health-promotion plans. Other community-based actions for nursing involvement in prevention of alcohol abuse in the community are listed in Box 8-1. The various plans have been categorized according to the health patterns to show that a community problem can be approached from many directions. Feasible plans that are well formulated facilitate implementation (U.S. Department of Health and Human Services, 2005).

Box **8-1** | **Plan Options for Community-Based Action: Alcohol Abuse**

COPING–STRESS TOLERANCE PATTERN
- Identify community alcohol treatment resources.
- Develop local alcohol control laws oriented toward prevention of abuse; develop consistent state regulation and control laws.

ROLES-RELATIONSHIPS PATTERN
- Increase communication among community control agencies, the school, residents, and health-related agencies.
- Restrict community advertisements for alcohol in local newsletters and newspapers.

IMPLEMENTATION WITH THE COMMUNITY

Implementation of the nursing process begins based on the health-promotion and health-protection plans. In collaboration with community members or other health team members, the nurse tests feasibility and implements the plan. Success depends on intellectual, interpersonal, and technical skills as well as on how well the community members accept the plan. Success also depends on overcoming expected resistance to change. Resistance to new health-promotion and health-protection activities, however, provides useful feedback to use to improve planning. People generally resist change to defend values that appear to be threatened by the change. Table 8-4 lists factors that deter community participation. Informed nurses take steps with community members to ensure the successful implementation of plans.

Community nurses implement health-promotion and health-protection plans in multiple community settings (schools, industry, public and private health agencies, and ambulatory care settings) where population groups experience relatively good health. Nursing centers provide nursing faculty, staff, and students unique opportunities to assess health and plan, implement, and evaluate care (including holistic health promotion and primary health care) to individuals, families, and communities with unmet health care needs (Rothman et al., 2005; Wilde et al., 2004). Complexity of health actions varies from one community to another. As plans evolve, nurses learn more about the community and their own responses, strengths, limitations, and abilities to cope or adapt (Baker et al., 2002).

Table **8-3** Implementation of Community Health Plan with Objectives and Rationale		
Nursing Diagnosis: Potential for increasing the incidence of fatal motor vehicle accidents in high school population related to alcohol use and driving. *Goal:* North High School population will have reduced incidence (at least 20%) of fatal motor vehicle accidents related to alcohol use and abuse by December.		
Objective	**Plans**	**Rationale**
1. Community will have access to information about the incidence of fatal motor vehicle accidents and drunken driving arrests of its high school population for the past 5 years by March.	Interview local police about the incidence of fatal auto accidents and substance abuse in the community. Interview parents of deceased high school students, students, teachers, physicians, clergy, and emergency room personnel about the incidence of the problem and suggested measures for decreasing the incidence; suggest that interviews be broadcast over the high school station. Have several people write to the community newspaper commenting on the broadcast and the problem.	*Unfreezing:* For change to occur, the community has to become dissatisfied with status quo and sense a need for change. *Empiric-rational strategy:* People are rational; discussion of facts can bring about support for change. Important elements for preventing the problem include educating the public and having key community leaders discuss their views; concern lends credibility and is necessary for action. People tend to listen to those with informal power. Keeping the issue before the community can raise consciousness.
2. Community will take action to inform the population at risk about responsible drinking and driving by June.	Suggest to school principal and school board the creation of a task force of community residents to plan a health program on individual responsibility and alcohol use in high school. Task force should include teachers, students, parents, clergy, police, nurse, and physician. Task force will examine ways to determine and teach content, integrate it into the curriculum, and recommend that community members, such as a nurse, be involved in teaching content.	*Changing:* Moving to a new level; community involvement will influence acceptability of changes. Community residents like to be involved in decision-making. It is important to establish trust and collaboration between community groups; this opens communication channels between adolescents and the health community. Community involvement facilitates acceptance of change.
3. Community will implement and educational program for its high school population related to the use of alcohol and individual responsibility.	Implement educational plans.	*Refreezing:* Moving to the level of change brought about by community forces. Educational strategies built around the concept of individual responsibility are essential elements in promoting the health of young adults.

Table **8-4**	Potential Sources of Resistance to Health-Promotion Programs, with Agent Responses	

Source of Resistance	Response
Lack of communication about the implementation of the program	Communicate through community newsletter, newspapers, high school radio station, and posters
Misinformation regarding time and place of healthy activity	Disseminate valid information
Fear of the unknown	Inform and encourage
Need for security	Clarify intentions and methods
No desired need to change behaviors	Demonstrate opportunity for change
Cultural or religious beliefs or vested interests threatened	Enlist key community leaders in planning change
Inaccessibility	Focus activities near the largest target population and in an area accessible by public transportation

Although implementation takes an action focus, it also includes assessment, planning, and evaluation activities to monitor actions taken to resolve, reduce, eliminate, or control the health concern.

EVALUATION WITH THE COMMUNITY

During the evaluation phase of the process, community nurses learn whether planned actions achieved desired outcomes. Communities and nurses determine progression toward goal achievement (Clark, 2007). Nurses take responsibility for evaluation, although community members or health team members may participate in the process. For example, if implemented plans intended to reduce the incidence of fatal motor vehicle accidents, nurses take the responsibility to obtain community outcomes data, which should reveal reduced fatalities and the nursing actions that contributed to these outcomes.

Nursing plans, which include nursing diagnoses, expected outcomes, and interventions, provide the evaluation framework. With a community focus, goals and objectives define the evaluation, considering how the community responded to planned actions. For example, if childhood disease rate reduction is expected to result from certain nursing actions, community responses before the actions are compared to those after the actions. This comparison determines the level of effectiveness (complete, partially effective, or ineffective) of the nursing actions to achieve the goal.

The community nurse approaches the dynamic process of evaluation in a purposeful, goal-directed manner (Clark, 2007; U.S. Department of Health and Human Services,

2007). Determining effectiveness of nursing actions evaluates the degree to which goals are achieved. Frequency of evaluation depends on situations, changes expected, and objectives. For example, an individual who is bleeding may need evaluation at frequent intervals, whereas behavioral changes in community groups occur slowly and require less frequent evaluation intervals. Evaluation intervals vary depending upon immediate, intermediate, and long-range goals. The evaluation process is continued until the community realizes the established goals.

Community nursing plan evaluation results indicate needs for reassessment, revision, or modification of plans. Community nurses reassess situations, plan new approaches, then implement and evaluate revised plans creating the continual cycle of the nursing process. Self–evaluation determines strengths and weaknesses as well as ways the nursing plan could have been more effective or efficient. The quality of community health-promotion and health-protection depends on the professional qualities of those providing services along with effective use of the nursing process.

Workable, cost-effective programs of community health promotion are needed. Nurses play an important role in providing evidence to support effective community health plans. Historically documentation of effective health promotion activities has been limited (Tagliareni & King, 2006). Effectiveness is determined through research studies that include analyses and outcome evaluation of home-based and community-centered nursing interventions designed to meet needs of high-risk families, geographical communities, and vulnerable populations. For example, in a study of the implementation of a new protocol for management of leg ulcers by community health nurses, the researchers were able to demonstrate improvement in healing with fewer nursing visits and a statistically significant decrease in cost per case (Harrison et al., 2005). Such evidence-based practice and research help to garner support for community health-promotion programs. The *Healthy People 2010 Toolkit: A Field Guide to Health Planning* (2002) (*www.healthypeople.gov/state/toolkit/ToolkitAll2002.pdf*) includes examples of national and state partnerships setting health objectives and sustaining the initiatives (U.S. Department of Health and Human Services, 2007).

SUMMARY

Risk factors, injury, and disease are not inevitable events experienced equally among a community's members. Effective community nurses understand the dynamic and complex nature of communities. Nurses use various theoretical frameworks to assess health-related patterns, health concerns, and health action potential and to implement the nursing process within communities. Collection and analysis of community data identify at-risk subpopulations. Planning contributes to the development of effective and efficient health-promotion and health-protection services. Nursing process enhances the efficacy of planning activities.

Many communities experience obvious deficiencies in health services that warrant health planning action. Community nurses play a significant role in health planning directed toward reducing risks associated with disease, premature death, and injury as well as health promotion among community members. Nurses use principles of planned change to increase community awareness of health, healthy behavior, and participation in preventive health services. Complexity varies from one community or geographical area to another. Community nurses connect health-promotion actions to specific community phenomena providing scientific evidence that supports the benefits of nursing actions.

CASE STUDY

Community Efforts to Decrease Adolescent Pregnancy Rates

The community health nurse is facilitating a grassroots community group that is determined to decrease the adolescent pregnancy rate in the city. The community population hovers around 100,000. It is a community that lies on the Mexican border of the United States. The population is predominantly Mexican American, and there is a high poverty rate.

The schools offer health courses twice between seventh and twelfth grades. The only formal sex education provided occurs within the context of these two health courses. There is community opposition to increasing the amount of sex education in the curriculum. A community group that has researched the problem has decided to use a social marketing approach because of this community resistance.

Most of the materials reviewed do not address the cultural needs of the region. Many of the Spanish language materials use Spanish from countries other than Mexico. The situations posed in the audiovisual materials show people who the adolescents will perceive as different from themselves.

Reflective Questions:
1. How could the community group approach their goal to decrease the adolescent pregnancy rate in a manner that will be culturally competent?
2. How might the community group approach this issue without the support of the school district?

CARE PLAN

Community Efforts to Decrease Adolescent Pregnancy Rates

Nursing Diagnosis: Risk for Ineffective Community Coping Related to Increased Levels of Teen Pregnancy

DEFINING CHARACTERISTICS
- Absence of education or support for sexually active teenagers
- Absence of programs for pregnancy testing, counseling, or teaching young women to care for infants
- Absence of sex education in the home, school, and community
- Community conflicts over what to teach adolescent and preadolescent children about sex
- Failure of teenagers to perceive long-term effects of having babies
- High incidence of infants who are born prematurely or with health problems
- High rate of teen pregnancy
- Lack of access to birth control pills or devices for teenagers
- Lack of community support for preventive sex education

RELATED FACTORS
- Community members' lack of knowledge about causes and contributing factors in teen pregnancy
- Inadequate community resources for preventing teen pregnancy

- Lack of adequate communication patterns and community cohesiveness regarding strategies to prevent teen pregnancy

EXPECTED OUTCOMES
- Community members express awareness of the seriousness of the high adolescent pregnancy rate in their community.
- Community members express the need for a plan to reduce the prevalence of teen pregnancies.
- Community members develop and implement plans to prevent teen pregnancy.
- Community members evaluate the success of the plan in meeting goals and objectives.
- Community members continue to revise the plan to prevent teen pregnancy as necessary.

INTERVENTIONS
- Assess teenagers' knowledge about sex and sexuality to determine their educational needs.
- Work with schools to develop pregnancy prevention programs that provide adolescents with information about the risks, problems, and complications of early pregnancy.
- Work closely with individual adolescents who are pregnant to assess their needs and provide care.

Continued

CARE PLAN

Community Efforts to Decrease Adolescent Pregnancy Rates—cont'd

- Implement an outreach and health-promotion program to raise community members' awareness of the need to approach teen pregnancy as a community problem. Consider taking the following five steps:
  - Work with teachers, school psychologists, counselors, school nurses, students, and the parent-teacher association to determine the extent of the teen pregnancy problem.
  - Encourage local youth groups, churches, and social service organizations to feature presentations on pregnancy prevention at their meetings.
  - Contact representatives of local corporations to ask for funding for educational programs.
  - Help community members (school nurses, counselors, and teachers) recognize adolescent girls who need counseling regarding such issues as peer pressure to be sexually active and the long-term consequences of pregnancy. Remind community members of the importance of listening attentively and remaining nonjudgmental.
  - Provide education on birth control measures (including abstinence from sex) and make this information available at school.
- Establish clubs for adolescent girls in the community. The goal of these clubs is to foster self-esteem. During club meetings, members should have the opportunity to openly discuss difficult questions, such as why girls consider a baby a status symbol and how to respond to peer pressure to be sexually active. Improved self-esteem has been found the most effective way to reduce teen pregnancy rates.

- Encourage adolescents to participate in peer support networks where they can openly discuss social and dating pressure and other issues related to teen pregnancy, to allow them an opportunity to express their feelings openly and obtain support from peers.
- Encourage community members to establish school-based clinics in which teens can have access to reproductive system models, pregnancy tests, and nonprescription birth control measures to support the teenagers who make the decision to protect themselves from unwanted pregnancies.
- Develop a list of referrals for teenagers, such as hospitals with human sexuality courses, charities that provide prenatal care and childbirth services, women's clinics, and Planned Parenthood, to compensate for restricted access to information in the adolescent's home or school.
- Encourage community members to implement an information campaign to educate adolescents, parents, and community members about the problems associated with teen pregnancy.
- Work with community members to evaluate the effectiveness of the teen pregnancy prevention program and assist in modifying it as needed to ensure its effectiveness and promote the program as a model for preventive health.
- Collect statistical data from the schools to analyze the teen pregnancy rates, to help evaluate the effectiveness of the prevention program.

Modified from Sparks, S. M. and Taylor, C. M. (2007). *Nursing diagnosis reference manual* (7th ed.). Philadelphia: Lippincott Williams & Wilkins.

REFERENCES

Aday, L. A. (2001). *At risk in America: The health and health care needs of vulnerable populations in the United States* (2nd ed.). San Francisco: Jossey-Bass, A Wiley Company.

Baker, S., Conrad, D., Bechamps, M., & Barry, M. (2002). *Healthy people 2010 toolkit.* (Government Report). Washington, DC: Public Health Foundation (HP2010 Toolkit).

Carpenito-Moyet, L. J. (2008). *Nursing diagnosis: Application to clinical practice* (12th ed.). Philadelphia: Lippincott Williams & Wilkins.

Clark, M. J. (2007). *Community health nursing* (5th ed.). Upper Saddle River, NJ: Pearson Education/Prentice Hall.

Crisis Prevention Institute. (2007). *Violence prevention and intervention training.* Retrieved January 6, 2008, from *www.crisisprevention.com/index.html.*

Frankowski, B. L., Keating, K., Rexroad, A., Delaney, T., McEwing, S. M., Wasko, N., et al. (2006). Community collaboration: Concurrent physician and school nurse education and cooperation increases the use of asthma action plans. *Journal of School Health, 76*(6), 303–306.

Gordon, M. (2007). *Manual of nursing diagnosis* (11th ed.). Sudbury, MA: Jones & Bartlett.

Harrison, M. B., Graham, I. D., Lorimer, K., Friedberg, E., Pierscianowski, T., & Brandys, T. (2005). Leg-ulcer care in the community, before and after implementation of an evidence-based service. *Canadian Medical Association Journal, 172*(11), 1447–1452.

Health Canada. (2006). *Regulations related to health and air quality.* Retrieved January 1, 2008, from *www.hc-sc.gc.ca/ewh-semt/air/out-ext/reg_e.html#4.*

McKinnon, J. (2000). *The Black population 2000: Census briefs No. C2KBR/01-5).* Washington, DC: US Census Bureau.

McLeroy, K. (2006). Editor's choice. Thinking of systems. *American Journal of Public Health, 96*(3), 402.

Occupational Safety and Health Administration. (2004). *Preventing workplace violence for health care and social service workers.* (Government Report No. OSHA 3148-01R 2004). Washington, DC: U.S. Department of Labor.

Pender, N. J., Murdaugh, C. L., & Parsons, M. A. (2006). *Health promotion in nursing practice* (5th ed.). Upper Saddle River, NJ: Prentice Hall.

Prochaska, J. O., & Norcross, J. C. (2006). *Systems of psychotherapy: A transtheoretical analysis* (6th ed.). Boston: Wadsworth Publishing.

Rosenstock, I. (1974). The health belief model and preventive behavior. *Health Education Monographs, 2,* 354–386.

Rothman, N. L., Lourie, R. J., Brian, D., & Foley, M. (2005). Temple Health Connection: A successful collaborative model of community-based primary health care. *Journal of Cultural Diversity, 12*(4), 145–151.

Sterman, J. D. (2006). Learning from evidence in a complex world. *American Journal of Public Health, 96*(3), 505–514.

Tagliareni, M. E., & King, E. S. (2006). Documenting health promotion services in community-based nursing centers. *Holistic Nursing Practice, 20*(1), 20–26.

The University of Texas Health Science Center at Houston. (2007). *CHARTing health information for Texas*. Retrieved January 1, 2008, from *www.sph.uth.tmc.edu/charting/*.

U.S. Census Bureau. (2003). *Current population survey: Poverty: 2002 highlights*. Retrieved January 6, 2008, from *www.census.gov/prod/2003pubs/p60–222.pdf*.

U.S. Census Bureau. (2005). *Press release: Florida, California and Texas to dominate future population growth, Census Bureau reports*. Retrieved December 25, 2007, from *www.census.gov/Press-Release/www/releases/archives/population/004704.html*.

U.S. Department of Health and Human Services. (2000). *Healthy people 2010: Understanding and improving health*. (Government Report No. Stock Number 017-001-001-00-550-

9). Washington, DC: U.S. Government Printing Office, Superintendent of Documents (HP2010).

U.S. Department of Health and Human Services. (2005). *Planned approach to community health: Guide for the local coordinator*. (Government Report). Atlanta, GA: U.S. Department of Health and Human Services, Department of Health and Human Services, Centers for Disease Control and Prevention, National Center for Chronic Disease Prevention.

U.S. Department of Health and Human Services. (2007). *Healthy people 2010 midcourse review*. Retrieved 11/29/2007, 2007, from *www.healthypeople.gov/Data/midcourse/*.

United States Environmental Protection Agency. (2006). *Ambient air monitoring QA program—The ambient air monitoring program*. Retrieved January 1, 2008, from *www.epa.gov/air/oaqps/qa/monprog.html*.

Wilde, M. H., Albanese, E. P., Rennells, R., & Bullock, Q. (2004). Development of a student nurses' clinic for homeless men. *Public Health Nursing, 21*(4), 354–360.

World Health Organization. (1998). *Health promotion glossary*. (Conference Resource Document No. WHO/HPR/HEP/98.1). Geneva: World Health Organization (definition: community).

Unit Three

Interventions for Health Promotion

Chapter 9

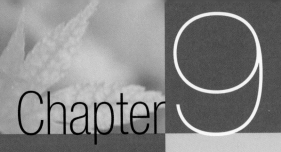

Suzy Harrington*

Screening

objectives

After completing this chapter, the reader will be able to:

- Discuss screening and its relationship to preventive health care intervention.
- Identify the advantages and disadvantages of the screening process.
- Analyze the criteria that determine a screenable disease.
- Discuss the health care and economic issues related to the screening process that result in ethical implications.
- Explain sensitivity and specificity as they relate to the efficacy of screening.
- Identify the broad range of community resources included in and affected by the screening process.
- Describe the nursing role in the screening process.
- Explore critical questions pertaining to culture in relation to screening.
- Discuss how a collaborative partnership may assist a community in the development and implementation of a screening program.

key terms

Asymptomatic pathogenesis
Community assessment
Community resources
Cost-benefit ratio analysis
Cost-effectiveness analysis
Cost-efficiency analysis
Efficacy
Efficiency
False-negative test results
False-positive test results
Group or mass screening

Iatrogenic
Incidence
Individual screening
Interobserver reliability
Intraobserver reliability
Key community individuals
Lead agency
Multiple test screening
One-test disease-specific screening
Prevalence

Quality of life
Quantity of life
Reliability
Secondary prevention
Sensitivity
Significance
Specificity
Stakeholders
Target community
Validity

website materials

evolve

These materials are located on the book's website at *http://evolve.elsevier.com/Edelman/*.
- WebLinks
- Study Questions
- Glossary

*The author acknowledges the work of Marie Truglio-Londrigan and Margaret K. Macali in a prior edition of the chapter.

Screening to Identify Risk Factors

Ms. Lukas is a 55-year-old account executive for a leading advertising firm. This high-power, high-pressure position requires her attention 14 hours a day. There is little time for rest, relaxation, or exercise. Ms. Lukas frequents take-out restaurants because she is unable to find time to cook or shop for healthy food. A recent increase in job pressures has provoked her to resume smoking two to three packs of cigarettes a day.

Ms. Lukas and a colleague visited a health fair one afternoon. Ms. Lukas' blood pressure was 200/110 mm Hg. Her nonfasting serum cholesterol measurement revealed a level of 265 mg/dl. Her colleague, who is 20 years younger and leads a similar lifestyle with similar habits, had a blood pressure reading of 130/82 and a cholesterol level of 215 mg/dl. The counselor evaluated the risk factors for both individuals. This analysis revealed similar risks for both women.

Although Ms. Lukas did benefit from the early identification of hypertension and hypercholesterolemia, she does not reap the benefits of early risk factor analysis like her younger colleague. If counseling and education prove successful, Ms. Lukas' colleague will demonstrate increased wellness through appropriate behavioral changes that could prevent the realization of disease.

1. Research supports the need for screening in an attempt to identify disease at early stages. However, if this is the case, does it not support the notion of screening to identify risk factors that have been associated with disease processes?
2. Will this identification of risk factors dramatically affect the onset of disease?
3. How can nurses use their expertise to help individuals achieve the desired behavioral changes necessary for risk factor reduction?

Screening is a valuable tool for health care professionals, particularly as the paradigm shifts from a medical to a prevention context (Lewis et al., 2007; Medicare, 2007). Although health education about screening comes under the rubric of primary prevention (see Chapter 1), the actual process of screening is a form of **secondary prevention**. The primary objective of screening is to detect a disease in its early stages, to treat it, and deter its progression. The basic assumption guiding this process is that detection during the early asymptomatic period allows treatment at a time when the course of the disease can be altered significantly. The screening concept is based on the principle that frequently disease is preceded by a period of **asymptomatic pathogenesis** (disease development) when risk factors predisposing a person to the pathological condition are building momentum toward manifestation of the disease. Screening takes advantage of the pre-pathogenic state and the early pathogenic state—identifying risks in the earliest and most treatable stages. The administration of tests (often simple in form) during these typically asymptomatic stages identify specific variables that distinguish individuals who most likely have, or have an increased risk to get, the condition from those who do not. Screening is not considered a diagnostic measure; it is seen as a preliminary step to direct a health care provider in assessment of the ostensibly healthy individual's chances of becoming unhealthy. More importantly it is a step towards empowering individuals to make more informed choices about their health and health behaviors. The ultimate goal could be curative, but more often it is to prevent further development of the condition or disease and to ameliorate the possible outcomes. A second, but equally important, objective of screening is to reduce the costs of managing the disease by avoiding the more vigorous interventions required during its later stages. The added attraction of a cost-conscious approach to health care mandates that health care professionals at all levels acquire a basic understanding of the screening process and its application. Screening can be an everyday, in-office activity, or it can be a large community event.

This chapter describes the screening process and the strengths and weaknesses of its implementation, focusing more on a large screening event. The presentation allows the nurse to (1) analyze the screenability of a particular condition and (2) determine the means of implementing a screening program specific to the population, the disease, and the system of health care delivery.

ADVANTAGES AND DISADVANTAGES OF SCREENING

Preclinical illness and previously unrecognized disease in individuals may be detected via screening efforts (Anderson & McFarlane, 2006). Screenings are done by individuals themselves, or they can be performed in clinical, procedural, or lab-based environments. This section will focus on the clinical, procedural, and lab-based test. Screening tests offer several advantages. They are often simple and inexpensive, and frequently a trained technician can administer them. The simplicity of the screening procedure decreases the time and cost of involved health care personnel and enables less-skilled technicians to administer the test. This also reduces cost and permits the more appropriate use of highly skilled, costly professionals at the definitive, diagnostic stage.

A second advantage is the ability to apply the screening process to both individuals and large groups. In an **individual screening** program, one person is tested by a health professional who has designated the individual as high risk. The practitioner can make this selection independently, the health care agency can define a specific policy, or a legislative body can require the screening by law as in the case of phenylketonuria (PKU) or lead-screening programs. **Group or mass screening** occurs when a target population is selected on the basis of an increased **incidence** of a condition or a recognized element of high risk within the group. The target population may be invited to a central location on a designated day to be tested for the selected disorder.

A third advantage is the ability to provide one-test specific screening or multiple test screenings. A **one-test disease-specific screening** is the administration of a single test that searches for a characteristic that indicates a high risk of developing a disorder. An example of this would be blood pressure screening to evaluate the risk of hypertension. **Multiple test screening** is the administration of two or more tests to detect more than one disease. In some cases, one sample can be used to evaluate the possibility of several conditions, saving time and money and making the process efficient and economical. For example, a blood sample can be evaluated for both elevated glucose and cholesterol levels. Ultimately, the combination of the relatively low cost of a screening test and flexibility makes screenings adaptable to all levels of the health care delivery system.

And one final advantage is that screening creates an opportunity for providing health education to a group of individuals who may not otherwise receive it. As noted in Chapter 10, Health Education, the clinical partnership that can be established during screening falls under the Scope and Standards of Practice, which includes "educating people about healthy lifestyles, risk reduction, developmental needs, activities of daily living, and preventive self-care." Many of the chronic illnesses of today are a result of individual health behaviors. Awareness is the first step in prevention. While it requires more than awareness to change behaviors, it is still required to embrace the concept of prevention. If awareness is combined with health education and health promotion tools, individuals would have a better opportunity to manage their own risks. An example is the standard six-month dental screening or "check-up" many insurances cover. While the individual is there to be screened for cavities, the hygienist provides health education in reminders on the correct way and the necessity to brush and floss correctly, while frequently providing a sample toothbrush to be taken home. Another example is the "5As" recommended for successful tobacco intervention: Ask, Advise, Assess, Assist, Arrange. It is not enough to simply screen with the question, "Do you use tobacco?" Readiness to quit should also be determined, as should support on how to quit through "Assist and Advise" (Agency for Healthcare Research and Quality, 2008).

The disadvantages of screening stem largely from the imperfection of modern science, which results in a margin of error for most instruments and tests. When program effectiveness depends on the test's ability to distinguish those who probably do have the disease from those who do not, the margin of error can precipitate serious consequences. Some individuals who do not have the condition will be referred for further tests and some who do have the disease will not. Those incorrectly referred suffer needless anxiety while awaiting more definitive diagnostic procedures. They must also bear the burden of the cost, follow-up visits, lost time, and inconvenience.

The effects on those whose disorders have been missed are even more important. These individuals leave with a false sense of a healthful state that will be shattered eventually, and they lose the opportunity to receive early treatment that could prevent irreversible damage. The difficulty of balancing the benefits to some against the losses to others is an ethical issue of most screening programs. The significance of this disadvantage can vary; therefore, it should be assessed for each project, disease, and population.

SELECTION OF A SCREENABLE DISEASE

The selection of a screenable disease goes beyond examination of the disease alone. The selection process must also encompass less-tangible factors, such as the emotional and financial impact of the disease's detection on the screened population. Even after gathering data and reviewing the critical issues, the final decision to screen or not to screen must often be reached with incomplete evidence or with answers that raise ethical issues. The potential uncertainties confounding the decision emphasize the need to conduct an exhaustive analysis of available material to obtain a decision that is as objective and scientific as possible. The answers to the following three questions provide a basis for designating a disease as screenable or not screenable:

1. Does the significance of the disorder warrant its consideration as a community problem?
2. Can the disease be detected by screening?
3. Should screening for the disease be done?
   A. What are the health benefits?
   B. What are the tangible and intangible costs?

As simplistic as these questions may appear, the answers or lack of answers may expose numerous complex issues that determine whether a well-informed decision can be made on screenability.

Significance

The **significance** of a disease refers to the level of priority assigned to the disease as a public health concern. Although the opinions of political and public interest groups may enter into the evaluation, significance generally is determined by the quantity and quality of life affected by the disorder. The greater the physical and psychological harm experienced by the population, the greater is the need to designate the disease as a priority health problem. The first step in assessing screenability is evaluation of this significance to decide if the disorder warrants the time, effort, and funds that must be allocated.

Estimating the **quality of life** affected by a disease presents problems. The perception of quality of life is subjective and individual evaluations may differ. For example, not all people equally perceive the disability resulting from a disease; some make adjustments and cope, whereas others do not. Those who do not may be more likely to say that the quality of their lives is significantly lower than that of the people around them.

By contrast, measures of the **quantity of life** affected by the disease are more readily obtainable. Disease-specific mortality rates present one picture of this effect, whereas prevalence and incidence rates provide another. **Prevalence** is the proportion of existing cases during a specific time; incidence is the frequency of new cases during a specified period (Lundy & Janes, 2001). Usually chronic conditions are measured by their prevalence (generally existing), whereas acute conditions are assessed by their incidence (rate of occurrence).

In this era of cost-conscious health care, a new dimension has been added to the evaluation of significance: the cost required to treat the disease. In some cases the prevalence of the disorder may not be great, but the problem requires disproportionate amounts spent on maintenance or management after the condition is fully expressed. For example, with PKU the incidence is not significant, but the cost of a case undetected at birth is a lifetime of case management. Given the costly outcome if undetected and the reasonable price of the test itself, the cost of screening all newborns is nominal.

Can the Disease be Detected by Screening?

With the relative significance of the disease established, the next step is to determine if health professionals can screen for the disease. Do well-documented diagnostic criteria for the disorder exist? Is there a valid and reliable screening instrument? Are sufficient community resources and treatment modalities available to support a screening program?

Diagnostic Criteria

Detection of a disease requires knowledge of characteristics that indicate its presence or, as in screening, its early pathogenic, asymptomatic state. Selected diagnostic criteria should be well documented; they should not be merely accepted as commonly used indicators. The impact of uncertainty in detecting disease is amplified when considering the application of the screening design. Some diseases, such as sickle cell anemia, are defined by the presence or absence of a single, isolated factor. Other conditions, such as hypertension, are indicated by the measurement of statistically derived numerical values for which a normal range has been set. Disagreement over the parameters of the normal range, combined with contentions that what is abnormal for one individual may not be abnormal for another, make these conditions more controversial to designate as screenable diseases.

Screening Instruments

The next step is to determine if methods exist to detect the disease during early pathogenesis. If instruments are available, a careful analysis should determine if any of them fulfill the requirements for the screening process: safe, cost-effective, and accurate. Ultimately the question is how well the instrument can distinguish those individuals who probably do not have and will not develop the condition from those who are likely to develop it. The variables that aid in instrument evaluation include reliability and validity.

Reliability Reliability is an assessment of the reproducibility of the test's results when different individuals with the same level of skill perform the test during different periods and under different conditions. If the same result emerges when two individuals perform the test, **interobserver reliability** is shown. If the same individual is able to reproduce the results several times, **intraobserver reliability** is shown. Therefore testing for instrument reliability can yield data on the accuracy and quality of the test (Polit et al., 2001).

From these data, the health professional can determine the amount of training that is required for health care technicians or personnel who administer the test. For example, if interobserver reliability is low, additional training might be required to work toward a more consistent method of delivering the test. This is frequently necessary in hypertension screening. If intraobserver reliability is low, the health professional might surmise that the instrument, and not the individual, is at fault.

Validity Validity reflects the test's ability to distinguish correctly between diseased and nondiseased individuals, or the accuracy of the test (Sackett et al., 2000). In a controlled setting, validity is evaluated by testing the instrument on a group of individuals who have positive or negative results. The ideal result is to have the instrument pick out 100% of the diseased people (positive reactions) and 100% of the nondiseased people (negative reactions). Such accuracy rarely occurs in practice; therefore, the measure of validity has been divided into two components that quantify the margin of error in the screening instrument. **Sensitivity** measures the first component. This refers to the proportion of people with a condition who correctly test positive when screened. A test with poor sensitivity will miss individuals with the condition and there will be a large number of **false-negative test results**; individuals actually have the condition but were told they are disease free. Specificity is the second component. **Specificity** measures the test's ability to recognize negative reactions or nondiseased individuals. A test with poor specificity will result in **false-positive test results**. Individuals with false-positive test results are told that they have a condition when in actuality they do not.

Application of sensitivity and specificity data to the actual outcome of the program raises some interesting points. Consider the issues that a public health nurse must face when given a newly developed screening test with low specificity and moderate sensitivity. Low specificity means few true-negative and more false-positive test results. The nurse and other health professionals must then consider the cost, inconvenience, and psychological stress experienced by the people with false-positive reactions during the period after their incorrect screening test, the unnecessary additional referrals, and the ability of the existing follow-up services to meet these needs. With only moderate sensitivity, a number of false-negative results could occur, which may send away individuals who could benefit from treatment. The issue raised here is ethical: that is, should a screening program be implemented when it is known that the tests deliver false-positive and false-negative results?

A broader issue concerns large health fair screening programs where a targeted population is sought for a mass screening. The **efficiency** and **efficacy** of such programs must be analyzed. Questions that address efficiency and efficacy include: (1) Is the targeted population prepared in an appropriate way before engaging in the screening tests? (2) Are the health care practitioners who are administering the test all educated according to the standard protocols of test administration? and (3) Are follow-up measures instituted in the program? Answers to these questions will challenge the health care providers in the development, implementation, and follow-up processes identified so that efficiency and efficacy will be enhanced.

The issues emerging from investigation of the screening instrument demonstrate the significant influence it has on the entire process. Data on the reliability and validity of the test and screening programs in general provide valuable information to evaluate, anticipate, and ideally control these influences, enabling the program to work effectively toward its goal.

Community Resources

Implementing a screening program depends on availability of appropriate **community resources**, such as funds, health care workers, follow-through, treatment sources, and administrative personnel. Judicious organization of the overall program is key to its success. Knowledge of the disease's characteristics and the screening instrument are useless without financial and organized human support to apply it. The overall approach is complex, requiring intense efforts in the area of partnership development.

A **lead agency** is identified to oversee the development process of the community health program. Origins of the lead agency vary from a community service organization to the local public health department responding to a mandate from the state. Regardless of its origin, the agency must perform a self-evaluation to compare its level of expertise with that required to oversee the process of the screening effort. Early identification of the lead agency, along with potential partnerships, allows for the effective use of talents and the division of labor.

For the lead agency to develop and oversee the development process of the community health program and the delivery of a screening program, partnerships are essential. The agency must contact and organize necessary stakeholders. **Stakeholders** are individuals or groups that have a legitimate interest in the topic. Examples of stakeholders include key community individuals, hospitals, health

and social service agencies such as primary health care centers, and community organizations including houses of worship, community centers, schools, transportation agencies, and volunteer organizations. **Key community individuals** are those people who are considered leaders within the community. The primary rule is to never assume that what is appropriate and effective for one community will be appropriate and effective for another.

The members of the partnership carry out the **community assessment** together. A community assessment is a systematic method of data collection that provides a detailed account regarding the type, quantity, and quality of resources. It includes recreation, physical environment, education, safety and transportation, politics, government, health, social services, communications, and economics, as well as the core components of demographic, vital statistics, and morbidity and mortality data (Anderson & McFarlane, 2000).

After completing the assessment, the data analysis will reveal the **target community** or high-risk population, available health care resources, and the health needs of the high-risk population. The identified partners collaborate, review, and analyze the data leading to the development of health improvement strategies (in this case a screening program), with methods of implementation to move the target population smoothly through the screening process. Finally, monitoring and evaluating outcomes is essential to determine the effectiveness of the program and the achievement of stated goals. Evaluation includes monitoring the entire process, including the successful workings of the partnership. Figure 9-1 presents a model of collaborative partnership: community health program development.

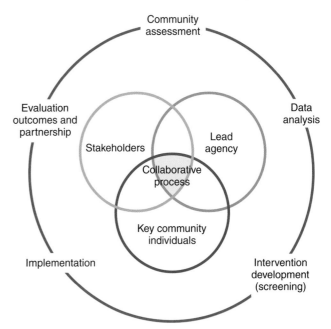

Figure 9-1 Collaborative partnership: community health program development.

Constraints affecting the operation of a screening program include financial concerns, political issues, cultural constraints, follow-up and referral services, and accessible treatment facilities. All partners are aware that responses from the target community are affected partly by their experience with other screening programs, such as the means used to inform them, the accessibility of the location, the availability of transportation, the convenience of the program's hours, and the cultural sensitivity of the delivery and design of the program. A public health nursing approach identifies the necessary community resources and defines how these resources interact and may be mobilized to achieve maximal benefits and positive outcomes. Financial support of the screening program is a constraint that can influence all points in the system. Although some programs are delivered entirely on a voluntary basis, organizers of others must submit grant proposals to local, state, or federal departments when consideration of medical and economic ethics is involved. Planners must look beyond the screening day and investigate financial resources for follow-up care and treatment.

In addition to financial accessibility, follow-up services need to be accessible in terms of convenient locations and open hours. For example, an evening clinic may reach those who are reluctant or financially unable to miss work. An efficient referral system links the follow-up resources to the screening program, providing continuity of care. A method must be devised to encourage the participant to take positive action on the referral. Public health nurses will facilitate this process with a variety of communication techniques, such as telephone or in-person counseling, mailings, and home visits.

Should Screening for the Disease Be Done?

After determining that the disease is significant and can be screened for, establishing whether health professionals should do so is the final step. Screening for a particular disorder and ultimately treating those with the early-identified disorder improves the chances of a favorable outcome in comparison with those whose disorder is not found until signs and symptoms become evident. Therefore, several questions must be considered. If a test accurately identifies a condition in the early stages, is there any benefit to the individual? Are there effective treatment modalities for the condition? The U.S. Preventive Service Task Forces has noted that evidence may be "insufficient to recommend for or against routine screening for" specific conditions due to some of these issues. This may not mean that the disease should not be screened. This depends on other factors as later described. For example, the data do not indicate the necessity of obesity screening in adolescents, yet the easy body mass index test can be a health education tool for adolescents. Those screened may not require a referral, but what they learn from the screening can help them better manage their health.

Interventions and Treatment Modalities

Screening is based on the disease's asymptomatic period; therefore, adequate information must exist concerning (1) the optimal time for screening, (2) specific intervention during this time, and (3) knowledge as to the effect of early detection and treatment on the prognosis. Without this knowledge, health care professionals are unable to explain how the consequences of the detected disease differ from those of the undetected. They can neither evaluate nor explain the health benefits derived from the screening program.

Follow-up is critical to determine if intervention strategies prescribed are in fact taking place. The prescribed regimen may be very broad and include a wide variety of intervention strategies such as diet, exercise, and drug therapy. Follow-up may include an evaluation and review of the literature that discusses evidence-based practice pertaining to a particular drug, as well as the identification of intervention characteristics that impair follow-up, such as cost, inconvenience, or side effects. Consideration must also be given to those factors that enhance follow-up. For example, nurses can provide ongoing counseling and education about a medication and assist individuals in a lifestyle transformation that includes health-promoting behaviors.

Safety of the intervention is a concern when considering the widespread application of a remedy after a screening program. Risks or harmful side effects can be costly in terms of human health and the increased medical care required to correct the **iatrogenic** effects resulting from the intervention. Health care professionals must decide if these risks significantly diminish the success of the treatment and outweigh the benefits derived from the treatment.

The bottom line is that to be effective, a high-quality, cost-effective, research/evidence-based screening tool or technique is needed that identifies a real or potential "problem" and provides a real and workable "solution," in which the tangible and intangible costs of the screening are less than the risk of the disease or condition and the health benefit.

ETHICAL CONSIDERATIONS

A step taken toward improving health usually is deemed a just and moral act within the health care system's values. However, when approaching health care practices with a more critical eye and realizing that not all the results of a well-intended practice are beneficial, the need to balance the benefit against the detriment becomes an issue. The resulting decision process becomes a value judgment and an ethical issue.

Health Care Ethics

A screening program is in a category separate from interventions offered for established disease processes. Rather than receiving those who have performed a self-assessment and elected to enter the system, a screening program invites apparently well individuals to be tested to determine disease risk and the need for follow-up. The request for participation implies that a health benefit will be derived, although at this stage nothing is said about what it will be or what the consumer must do to obtain it. Program planning that attempts to clarify this implication and inform participants of the issues develops the basis for an ethically sound project and enhances the screenability of the disease.

Most screening programs are named by the disease being screened such as hypertension screening or diabetic screening; therefore, it is not surprising that participants enter them assuming the results received are diagnostic and will classify them as disease free or disease laden. This is untrue, because the screening goal is only to identify and refer individuals at risk or who may need further follow-up or evaluation. The initial presentation of and contact with the program implies a benefit not being delivered. To alleviate this problem, the planning committee should develop a method of informing participants of the meaning and limitations of the results. Participants need to know whether the ultimate benefit is preventive, ameliorative, or curative and, most importantly, what responsibility they must assume to secure this outcome.

Misinterpretation caused by the screening instrument is of even greater ethical concern than human misperception. As the information on sensitivity and specificity indicates, false-positive and false-negative results occur with any screening instrument. One of the more difficult ethical issues in screening is to evaluate whether the benefits received by those who receive correct results are worth the problems experienced by those who receive incorrect results. What obligation does the project have to the latter? What is an acceptable number of people with false-negative test results, all of whom will both miss the benefit of early treatment and be misled about the need for tests in the near future? What will be the response of an individual who has a false-positive reaction? Answers to these questions are value judgments that vary according to the disease.

Additional issues that confound the medical ethics of screening are cutoff points for the screening instrument and borderline cases. How precisely do the instrument's numerical values define the high-risk disease state? The goal of a screening program, identifying an individual as high risk or not, depends on this numerical value. When the parameter for this distinction is not clear, a cutoff point is set. Above this point, the person is considered disease positive; below this point, the individual is disease negative. Consequently, readjusting the cutoff point becomes a highly controversial issue, because it controls the percentage of positive and negative results. If the disease were potentially life threatening, an increase in false-positive results (lower cutoff point) would be preferred to missing individuals who may have the disease. In addition, if a disease is relatively benign in terms of potential stigmatization, anxiety, and problems with treatment, lowering the cutoff point could again be safe and ethical.

A problem closely related to the cutoff point is defining a policy for borderline cases. Hypertension is a common disease in which a variance of 5 to 10 mm Hg can make the difference in identifying a person as high risk or not. Guidelines constantly change as new research arrives and new special

interest groups change the definitions, but it is helpful to look at the whole and see it as a great opportunity for health education whether high risk or borderline. A more sophisticated approach may be taken to discriminate between a borderline case that should be referred and one that should not. The health professional can specify other risk factors associated with hypertension, such as family history, diet, and smoking, as criteria for deciding whether to refer an individual. With the increasing interest in and knowledge of risk factors, the effectiveness of this method has improved (see the Case Study and Care Plan at the end of this chapter).

The medical ethics of screening will continue to demand review of the same questions and issues; however, the answers may change as more is discovered about the various conditions and their treatments. An updated literature review is imperative before reviewing these issues in relation to a particular screenable disease.

Economic Ethics

Associating a monetary value with health care outcomes is generally against the nature and ideals of health care professionals. In the past the tendency was to place no limits on the cost of promoting a healthy, disease-free, or disease-controlled status, resulting in a philosophy that all care should be given to all people at all costs. This philosophy has evolved to one of conscious recognition of the costs of screening events. Allocating community funds to a large screening event could result in a lack of funds for other projects. Those benefiting from a screening test will be countered by those suffering from a lack of service for other medical or social needs. These trade-offs result in ethical decisions demanding careful analysis by the screening administration (Hot Topics box).

HOT topics: ECONOMIC ETHICS OF SCREENING

Economic ethics have been discussed within this text to include the consideration of cost-benefit ratio, cost-effectiveness, and cost-efficiency analyses when developing selective screening programs. Those working in the health care system are currently struggling to devise program guidelines that are ethically and economically sound. Questions give way to still more questions as nurses grapple with issues of cost, quality, technological benefits in screening, and service rationing. Managed care models continue to be a key force in important decision-making in health care.

1. How does this affect a health care provider's decision to deliver care?
2. Do health care providers have the autonomy to make decisions that they deem necessary regarding screening and treatment?
3. How does this affect screening protocols?
4. Will the quality of care deteriorate if screening programs are not implemented?

Screening can be a costly project for both organizers and consumers. Initial operational costs must be considered, including buying or renting the screening instruments, renting floor space, engaging professionals or technicians to administer the tests, and interpreting the results.

These costs are encountered again when people are referred for further evaluation. Consumer costs include follow-up visits, treatment, time, and income that is lost while complying with each. Given the combined operational and consumer costs, several questions are raised. Do the costs result in the desired health outcome to the individual, group, or community? Are the benefits reaped worth the expenditures required? The answer is determined partly by what values (other than monetary ones) are attributed to the benefit, such as saving a life. A strictly economic approach, however, generally eliminates the intangible variables, demanding the use of more objective data for decision-making.

When program designs are being considered with screening, three main approaches may be used to evaluate the economic resources affected: (1) cost-benefit ratio, (2) cost-effectiveness, and (3) cost-efficiency analyses. Once far from the thoughts of health care workers, the current relevance and use of such concepts require a basic understanding of their role in the selection of a screenable condition. Although presented here in successive fashion, they are entirely separate methods and most frequently are used independently of one another.

Cost-Benefit Ratio

Cost-benefit ratio analysis is performed first, because it allows the comparison of various outcomes in monetary terms (Sackett et al., 2000). This comparison is necessary in health planning when the initial consideration is which health outcome, such as reduction of cardiovascular disease, decreased infant mortality, or reduction of a visual problem, will be most beneficial to the community at the most reasonable cost.

Cost-Effectiveness

If the reduction of cardiovascular disease is chosen as the desired outcome, the next step is a **cost-effectiveness analysis**, which determines the optimal use of resources to reach a predetermined, constant end point or the desired health outcome (Sackett et al., 2000). The outcome remains the same; the best method of deriving it is the issue. For example, considering the selected health outcome, such as the reduction of cardiovascular disease, various methods might be used. These methods include screening for hypertension, performing electrocardiograms on all individuals aged 25 or older who are admitted to the hospital, beginning an antismoking campaign, or obtaining nutrition counseling. Implementation of all these options would be ideal, but with limited resources a choice must be made.

Cost-Efficiency

The last approach to help bring the economic resources into perspective is **cost-efficiency analysis**. The purpose is to be efficient and budget a limited amount of money toward achieving as much of the desired outcome as possible. The funds are the central issue, not the health benefit.

SELECTION OF A SCREENABLE POPULATION

The selection of a screenable population is as important as the selection of a screenable disease. The objective is to identify a high-risk group that, when tested, will yield a significant number of diseased individuals. With such results, the efforts and cost of screening the population are minimized and the health benefit received is maximized. The main criterion used to define an appropriate population is the definitive presence of risk factors related to the disorder. To ensure a thorough examination of possible risk factors, both person-dependent and environment-dependent factors should be reviewed.

Person-Dependent Factors

The person's age is increasingly important because there are age-dependent changes in levels of risk factors through-out the population (Tables 9-1 and 9-2). Practice has always placed a high priority on screening the vulnerable, at-risk infant population, partly because of the health outcomes that affect the child's growth and development. As the average life span increases, however, the effects of longer-range risk factors are becoming apparent, making certain prevalent and costly chronic conditions equally important to control. Therefore ideal populations for screening can be found in senior citizen housing projects or older adult daycare settings. Middle-aged adults are also being recognized as a screenable group for certain conditions, such as breast cancer, glaucoma, and heart disease, which commonly appear during this period.

Gender has obvious implications for screening programs. For example, women are tested frequently for two conditions, breast cancer and cervical cancer. Men are tested for prostate cancer and testicular cancer.

A population representing a particular ethnic or racial group is also appropriate to consider when planning screening programs (Multicultural Awareness box).

Race refers to a biologically related group of people whose features are inherited (Allender & Spradley, 2005). It is known that some disorders occur more frequently in certain racial or ethnic groups. For example, African Americans have a higher prevalence of and mortality rate from hypertension and cancer of the prostate than Whites, and Native Americans have higher rates of diabetes than do other cultural groups (U.S. Department of Health and Human Services [USDHHS], 2000).

Although these health disparities are of great concern, their cause is not easy to ascertain. It is believed that these differences are actually the result of complex interactions among genetic variations, environmental factors, and health behaviors (USDHHS, 2000). The need to identify the causes of these health disparities has been widely recognized. This is evident by the proliferation of research being

MULTICULTURAL AWARENESS

Eliminating Health Disparities among Ethnic Groups

The United States has been referred to frequently as a melting pot. Diversity has been acknowledged as a strength of the country, but it is apparent that disparities exist among the various racial and ethnic groups in the attainment and maintenance of health. The minority populations of the United States have been categorized as African Americans, Hispanics, Asian-Pacific Islanders, American Indians, and Alaskan Natives. These categories oversimplify the reality of the multicultural nature of assessing health status, screening, and making plans to improve health. These particular racial groupings are not absolute, because there are subgroups within each (U.S. Department of Health and Human Services, 2000).

Over the past decade racial and ethnic health disparities have become increasingly apparent. The second goal of *Healthy People 2010* is to eliminate as many as possible.

These disparities and factors such as access to care need to be taken into consideration when planning screening programs. In order to plan, implement, and evaluate a screening program that targets a specific population, the provider must have an awareness of that population that includes components such as lifestyle, socioeconomic characteristics, education, heredity, environmental factors, values, religious and cultural beliefs, communication style, and language. Partnering with key individuals and organizations in the community through the entire process is important for any screening program to be successful, as the following scenario illustrates.

Hospital administrators in a town located outside a city in the Northeast are concerned about the health status of a new immigrant population. Recent census data indicate that the number of immigrants from Guatemala has grown. The census data also reveal that this population is primarily young adults, male and female. The officials of the town and the hospital are aware that most of the men are day laborers, many of whom gather each morning in the town square to be transported to their jobs. The young women are mothers who work in small, privately owned businesses or are hired by local house-cleaning services.

Based on these data, the hospital officials decide to plan a health and screening day for this population. The hospital sends out flyers into the community in the primary native language of the target population. The day of the screening arrives and the number of participants is very low. The hospital officials are very concerned. They had good intentions. They do not know what to do next.

1. What critical actions did the hospital officials perform that might be considered positive in the planning of the health and screening day?
2. What critical actions did the hospital officials not perform that might have contributed to the poor turnout at the health and screening function?
3. What might the hospital officials consider in their planning for the next health and screening day?
4. How might they engage the community and the target population in planning the health and screening day?
5. What local community agencies and groups might be invited to participate as partners when planning and implementing the health and screening day?
6. Can you identify any creative ways to bring the health and screening day to the targeted population, making the program more accessible?

---

conducted to identify and describe the possible reasons for these differences. When health care professionals have a better understanding as to why these disparities exist, it will be possible to develop effective and efficient plans to counteract them (Research Highlights box).

Income level has been associated repeatedly with the presence or absence of a healthy state, and it underlies many health disparities. Often lower-income groups have the least education. Such differences in both income and education are associated with disparities in the occurrence of disorders, including heart disease, diabetes, obesity, elevated blood lead levels, and low birth weight (USDHHS, 2000). Poverty accompanies poor environmental conditions, inadequate housing, occupational hazards, violence, unemployment, and limited access to health care (Lundy & Janes, 2001).

Personal behavioral characteristics related to lifestyle may suggest the need to screen an individual or group. When health care practitioners consider lifestyle, they are looking at daily habits that affect health and wellness, such as nutrition, fitness, tobacco use, alcohol and drug use, stress management, adequate rest, immunizations, periodic exams, and use of seat belts and other safety factors. Engaging in some of these behaviors while avoiding others is essential for living a healthy life. Therefore screening

research highlights

Differences in Factors Related to Breast Cancer Screening Behavior in Mexican-Born and United States-Born Women of Mexican Descent

A survey was completed by 179 female U.S. residents of Mexican heritage who were born in Mexico (n = 76) or the United States (n = 103). The emphasis of the survey pertained to factors related to breast cancer screening. The women born in the United States had significantly higher levels of income, education, and acculturation. In addition, these women were significantly more likely to be covered by health insurance and to receive health professional interventions and education such as breast self-examination instruction. These factors influenced the women born in the United States to engage in breast self-examination more frequently than did the other group.

In comparison, the Mexican-born women identified significantly more beliefs that breast cancer is a serious illness and that they were relatively more susceptible to the disease than were Americans. The locus of control for these Mexican-born women was geared toward powerful others and chance factors. These factors suggest that Mexican-born women face more breast cancer screening barriers than the U.S.-born women of Mexican descent.

Data from Borrayo, E., & Guarnaccia, C. (2000). Differences in Mexican-born and U.S.-born women of Mexican descent regarding factors related to breast cancer screening behaviors. *Health Care for Women International, 21*(7), 599–613.

Table **9-1**   Screening Tests and Immunizations Guidelines for Women

Screening Tests	Ages 18-39	Ages 40-49	Ages 50-64	Ages 65 and Older
GENERAL HEALTH:				
Full checkup, including weight and height	Discuss with your doctor or nurse.	Discuss with your doctor or nurse.	Discuss with your doctor or nurse.	Discuss with your doctor or nurse.
Thyroid test (TSH)[1]	Start at age 35, then every 5 years.	Every 5 years	Every 5 years	Every 5 years
HEART HEALTH:				
Blood pressure test[2]	At least every 2 years	At least every 2 years	At least every 2 years	At least every 2 years
Cholesterol test[3]	Start at age 20, discuss with your doctor or nurse.	Discuss with your doctor or nurse.	Discuss with your doctor or nurse.	Discuss with your doctor or nurse.
BONE HEALTH:				
Bone mineral density test[4]		Discuss with your doctor or nurse.	Discuss with your doctor or nurse.	Discuss with your doctor or nurse.
DIABETES:				
Blood glucose test[5]	Discuss with your doctor or nurse.	Start at age 45, then every 3 years.	Every 3 years	Every 3 years
BREAST HEALTH:				
Mammogram (x-ray of breast)[6]		Every 1-2 years. Discuss with your doctor or nurse.	Every 1-2 years. Discuss with your doctor or nurse.	Every 1-2 years. Discuss with your doctor or nurse.
REPRODUCTIVE HEALTH:				
Pap test and pelvic exam[7]	Every 1-3 years if you have been sexually active or are older than 21	Every 1-3 years	Every 1-3 years	Discuss with your doctor or nurse.
Chlamydia test[8]	Yearly until age 25 if sexually active. Older than age 25, get this test if you have new or multiple partners.	Get this test if you have new or multiple partners.	Get this test if you have new or multiple partners.	Get this test if you have new or multiple partners.
Sexually transmitted infection (STI) tests[8]	Both partners should get tested for STIs, including HIV, before initiating sexual intercourse.	Both partners should get tested for STIs, including HIV, before initiating sexual intercourse.	Both partners should get tested for STIs, including HIV, before initiating sexual intercourse.	Both partners should get tested for STIs, including HIV, before initiating sexual intercourse.
MENTAL HEALTH SCREENING[9]	Discuss with your doctor or nurse.	Discuss with your doctor or nurse.	Discuss with your doctor or nurse.	Discuss with your doctor or nurse.
COLORECTAL HEALTH:				
Fecal occult blood test[10,11]			Yearly	Yearly
Flexible sigmoidoscopy (with fecal occult blood test is preferred)[10,11]			Every 5 years (if not having a colonoscopy)	Every 5 years (if not having a colonoscopy)
Double contrast barium enema (DCBE)[10,11]			Every 5-10 years (if not having a colonoscopy or sigmoidoscopy)	Every 5-10 years (if not having a colonoscopy or sigmoidoscopy)
Colonoscopy[10,11]			Every 10 years	Every 10 years
Rectal exam[10,11]	Discuss with your doctor or nurse.	Discuss with your doctor or nurse.	Every 5-10 years with each screening (sigmoidoscopy, colonoscopy, or DCBE)	Every 5-10 years with each screening (sigmoidoscopy, colonoscopy, or DCBE)

EYE AND EAR HEALTH:				
Complete eye exam[12]	At least once between the ages 20-29 and at least twice between the ages 30-39, or any time that you have a problem with your eye(s).	Every 2-4 years	Every 2-4 years	Every 1-2 years
Hearing test[13]	Starting at age 18, then every 10 years	Every 10 years	Every 3 years	Every 3 years
SKIN HEALTH:				
Mole exam[14]	Monthly mole self-exam; by a doctor every 3 years, starting at age 20	Monthly mole self-exam; by a doctor every year	Monthly mole self-exam; by a doctor every year	Monthly mole self-exam; by a doctor every year
ORAL HEALTH:				
Dental exam[15]	One to two times every year	One to two times every year	One to two times every year	One to two times every year
IMMUNIZATIONS:				
Influenza vaccine[16]	Discuss with your doctor or nurse.	Discuss with your doctor or nurse.	Yearly	Yearly
Pneumococcal vaccine[16]				One time only
Tetanus-Diphtheria Booster vaccine[16]	Every 10 years	Every 10 years	Every 10 years	Every 10 years
Human papillomavirus vaccine (HPV)[17]	Up to age 26, discuss with your doctor or nurse.			
Meningococcal vaccine[18]	Discuss with your doctor or nurse if attending college.			
Herpes zoster vaccine (to prevent shingles)[19]			Starting at age 60, one time only. Ask your doctor if it is okay for you to get it.	Starting at age 60, one time only. Ask your doctor if it is okay for you to get it.

CITATIONS

[1]Ladenson, P. W., Singer, P. A., Ain, K. B., Bagchi N., et al. (2000). American Thyroid Association Guidelines for Detection of Thyroid Dysfunction, Archives of Internal Medicine. 160,1573–1575.
[2]U.S. Preventive Services Task Force. (2003). Screening for high blood pressure: Recommendations and rationale. Agency for Healthcare Research and Quality, Rockville, MD. www.ahrq.gov/clinic/3rduspstf/highblood/highbloodrr.htm.
[3]Adapted from: National Heart, Lung, and Blood Institute of the National Institutes of Health. (2002). Third Report of the National Cholesterol Education Program Expert Panel on Detection, Evaluation, and Treatment of High Blood Cholesterol in Adults (Adult Treatment Panel III). NIH Publication No. 02-5215.
[4]U.S. Preventive Services Task Force. (2002). Screening for osteoporosis in postmenopausal women: Recommendations and rationale. Agency for Healthcare Research and Quality, Rockville, MD. www.ahrq.gov/clinic/3rduspstf/osteoporosis/osteorr.htm
[5]American Diabetes Association. Frequently asked questions about pre-diabetes. Accessed October 25, 2006, at: www.diabetes.org/pre-diabetes/faq.jsp.
[6]National Cancer Institute. Screening mammograms: Questions and answers. Accessed October 23, 2006, at: www.cancer.gov/cancertopics/factsheet/Detection/screening-mammograms.
[7]National Cancer Institute. The Pap test: Questions and answers. Accessed October 23, 2006, at: www.cancer.gov/cancertopics/factsheet/Detection/Pap-test.
[8]U.S. Preventative Services Task Force. (2007). Screening for Chlamydia infection. Agency for Healthcare Research and Quality, Rockville, MD. www.ahrq.gov/clinic/uspstf/uspschlm.htm.
[9]Adapted from: National Institute of Mental Health. Depression: What every woman should know. Accessed October 25, 2006, at: www.nimh.nih.gov/publicat/depwomenknows.cfm#ptdep8.
[10]Centers for Disease Control and Prevention. Screening Guidelines (Colorectal Cancer). Accessed October 24, 2006, at: www.cdc.gov/cancer/colorectall/basic_info/screening/guidelines.htm.
[11]American Cancer Society. American Cancer society guidelines for the early detection of cancer. Accessed October 24, 2006, at: www.cancer.org/docroot/PED/content/PED_2_3X_ACS_Cancer_Detection_Guidelines_36.asp.
[12]Foundation of the American Academy of Ophthalmology Web site. Eye exams. Accessed March 27, 2008, at: www.eyecareamerica.org/eyecare/treatment/eye-exams.cfm. Reviewed May 2007.
[13]American Speech-Language-Hearing Association. Hearing screening. Accessed October 24, 2006, at: www.asha.org/public/hearing/testing.
[14]American Cancer Society. Monitor your skin for signs of skin cancer. Accessed October 25, 2006, at: www.cancer.org/docroot/nws/content/nws_1_1x_Monitor_Your_Skin_for_Signs_of_Skin_Cancer.asp.
[15]Agency for Healthcare Research and Quality. The pocket guide to good health for adults. Accessed October 24, 2006, at: www.ahrq.gov/ppip/adguide/adguide.pdf.
[16]Centers for Disease Control and Prevention. (2006). Recommended adult immunization schedule—United States, October 2006-September 2007. MMWR, 55, Q1-Q4.
[17]Adapted from: Centers for Disease Control and Prevention. HPV and HPV vaccine: Information for health care providers. Accessed October 25, 2006, at: www.cdc.gov/std/HPV/STDFact-HPV-vaccine-hcp.htm#prohprec.
[18]Centers for Disease Control and Prevention. Meningococcal Disease. Accessed August 23, 2006, at: www.cdc.gov/ncidod/dbmd/diseaseinfo/meningococcal_g.htm.
[19]Centers for Disease Control and Prevention. Recommended adult immunization schedule—United States, October 2007-September 2008. From National Women's Health Information, U.S. Department of Health and Human Services, Office on Women's Health, www.womenshealth.gov/screeningcharts/general/.

Table **9-2** Screening Tests and Immunizations Guidelines for Men

Screening Tests	Ages 18-39	Ages 40-49	Ages 50-64	Ages 65 and Older
GENERAL HEALTH:				
Full checkup, including weight and height	Discuss with your doctor or nurse.	Discuss with your doctor or nurse.	Discuss with your doctor or nurse.	Discuss with your doctor or nurse.
HEART HEALTH:				
Blood pressure test	At least every 2 years	At least every 2 years	At least every 2 years	At least every 2 years
Cholesterol test	Start at age 20, discuss with your doctor or nurse.	Discuss with your doctor or nurse.	Discuss with your doctor or nurse.	Discuss with your doctor or nurse.
DIABETES:				
Blood sugar test	Discuss with your doctor or nurse.	Start at age 45, then every 3 years.	Every 3 years	Every 3 years
PROSTATE HEALTH:				
Digital Rectal Exam (DRE)		Discuss with your doctor or nurse.	Discuss with your doctor or nurse.	Discuss with your doctor or nurse.
Prostate-Specific Antigen (PSA) (blood test)		Discuss with your doctor or nurse.	Discuss with your doctor or nurse.	Discuss with your doctor or nurse.
REPRODUCTIVE HEALTH:				
Testicular exam	Monthly self-exam; and part of a general checkup	Monthly self-exam; and part of a general checkup	Monthly self-exam; and part of a general checkup	Monthly self-exam; and part of a general checkup
Chlamydia test	Discuss with your doctor or nurse.	Discuss with your doctor or nurse.	Discuss with your doctor or nurse.	Discuss with your doctor or nurse.
Sexually Transmitted Disease (STD) tests	Both partners should get tested for STDs, including HIV, before initiating sexual intercourse.	Both partners should get tested for STDs, including HIV, before initiating sexual intercourse.	Both partners should get tested for STDs, including HIV, before initiating sexual intercourse.	Both partners should get tested for STDs, including HIV, before initiating sexual intercourse.
COLORECTAL HEALTH:				
Fecal occult blood test			Yearly	Yearly
Flexible sigmoidoscopy (with fecal occult blood test is preferred)			Every 5 years (if not having a colonoscopy)	Every 5 years (if not having a colonoscopy)
Double Contrast Barium Enema (DCBE)			Every 5-10 years (if not having a colonoscopy or sigmoidoscopy)	Every 5-10 years (if not having a colonoscopy or sigmoidoscopy)
Colonoscopy			Every 10 years	Every 10 years
Rectal exam	Discuss with your doctor or nurse.	Discuss with your doctor or nurse.	Every 5-10 years (if not having a sigmoidoscopy, colonoscopy, or DCBE)	Every 5-10 years (if not having a sigmoidoscopy, colonoscopy, or DCBE)
EYE AND EAR HEALTH:				
Eye exam	Get your eyes checked if you have problems or visual changes.	Every 2-4 years	Every 2-4 years	Every 1-2 years
Hearing test	Starting at age 18, then every 10 years	Every 10 years	Discuss with your doctor or nurse.	Discuss with your doctor or nurse.
SKIN HEALTH:				
Mole exam	Monthly mole self-exam; by a doctor every 3 years, starting at age 20	Monthly mole self-exam; by a doctor every year	Monthly mole self-exam; by a doctor every year	Monthly mole self-exam; by a doctor every year

Table **9-2**   Screening Tests and Immunizations Guidelines for Men—*cont'd*

Screening Tests	Ages 18-39	Ages 40-49	Ages 50-64	Ages 65 and Older
ORAL HEALTH:				
Dental exam	One to two times every year	One to two times every year	One to two times every year	One to two times every year
MENTAL HEALTH SCREENING	Discuss with your doctor or nurse.	Discuss with your doctor or nurse.	Discuss with your doctor or nurse.	Discuss with your doctor or nurse.
IMMUNIZATIONS:				
Influenza vaccine	Discuss with your doctor or nurse.	Discuss with your doctor or nurse.	Yearly	Yearly
Pneumococcal vaccine				One time only
Tetanus-Diphtheria Booster vaccine	Every 10 years	Every 10 years	Every 10 years	Every 10 years

From National Women's Health Information Center, U.S. Department of Health and Human Services, Office on Women's Health. Retrieved from *www.womenshealth.gov/screeningcharts/men/index.cfm.*

HEALTH TEACHING   Pender's Health Promotion Model

A health care provider's responsibility is to assess, plan, implement, and evaluate a screening program. Part of this responsibility includes teaching individuals, families, and populations about the importance of participating in these programs and ultimately engaging in behavior that enhances health. The health promotion model is a useful guide for practice (Pender et al., 2006). The model presents the interrelationship among behavior-specific cognitions and affective factors and individual characteristics and experiences that motivate individuals to engage in behaviors that promote health. The health care provider may find that the application of this model in practice influences the relationship between the provider and the individual in a positive way. The model is a framework that assists the provider in assessing factors believed to influence health behavioral changes. Once the provider has an accurate assessment, obtained via questions, decisions may be made concerning factors that inhibit health-promoting behaviors and, ultimately, potential interventions to assist individuals in achieving positive health outcomes. This information will assist the provider to develop appropriate teaching methods.

Health Promotion Assessment Questions

1. How do you define health?
2. What does health mean to you?
3. How would you describe your health now?
4. Do the choices you make and actions you take affect your health?
5. Can you give examples when choices and actions created a positive change in health for you?
6. Can you give examples when choices and actions created a negative change in health for you?
7. What factors facilitated choices and actions that created a positive change in health?
8. What factors created barriers to choices and actions that led to a negative change in health?
9. Are there any supportive personal influences in your life that would assist you in choices and actions that would create a positive change in your health (i.e., family, friends, and health care providers)?
10. Are there any supportive situational influences, such as more than one plan of action, pertaining to the health change available to you?

Modified from Pender, N., Murdaugh, C., & Parsons, M. A. (2006). *Health promotion in nursing practice* (5th ed.). Upper Saddle River, New Jersey: Prentice Hall.

---

for those personal behavioral characteristics that are considered risky assesses the likelihood of a longer, disease-free life. Once screening suggests those behaviors that are considered risky, the development of healthy behaviors via programming and a conscious transformation in lifestyle is key.

Health care providers bear a responsibility to educate individuals about the next step in the evaluation of their potential condition once a screening is completed. Those being screened bear a responsibility to seek treatment, follow-up, and ultimately engage in behavioral change toward a healthy lifestyle if the screening is to serve a purpose (Health Teaching box).

Environment-Dependent Factors

The area of environmental health and protection has expanded over the years and is becoming more complex. Environmental health and protection has been defined as that science which is concerned with elements of the environment that influence people's health and well-being. These factors include conditions of the workplace, home, and communities including chemical, physical, and psychological forces (Allender & Spradley, 2005). Environment-related risk factors relevant to screening designs are derived from an individual's surroundings. Areas that may be considered include overpopulation; indoor and outdoor air pollution; water pollution; safe drinking water; noise pollution; radiation exposure; biological pollutants; hazardous waste management and disposal of garbage; vector and pesticide control; deforestation, wetlands destruction, and desertification; energy depletion; inadequate housing; contaminated food and foods with toxic additives; safety in the home, worksite, and community; and psychological hazards (Allender & Spradley, 2005).

In occupational health, a legitimate population for screening includes those in high-risk work area, where harmful chemicals, airborne particles, or high-decibel machinery put the workers at risk of cancer, respiratory conditions, or auditory problems. At the other extreme is the sedentary executive work life, lack of exercise are prevalent. The use of an occupational health nurse to provide individual and mass screening for such problems is recognized as an integral role by both the health professions and the business world.

Environment-dependent factors have long been associated with the presence or absence of certain conditions. Primary prevention would be the preferred mode of protection; however, considering the shortsightedness of present society, secondary prevention appears to be the preferred choice. Screening must be focused on the short-term results of certain environmental conditions and on monitoring the long-term trends.

COMMONLY SCREENED CONDITIONS

The following section reviews several commonly screened diseases to demonstrate the complexity of issues that may surround the screening process. Ultimately a systematic approach, in which decision-making is collaborative, will move the targeted population toward health improvement and the attainment of the goals of *Healthy People 2010* (USDHHS, 2000) and the forthcoming *Healthy People 2020* (*www.healthypeople.gov*): (1) Increased quality and years of healthy life and (2) Elimination of health disparities. For more specific objectives related to screening, see the *Healthy People 2010* box.

More specifically, the U.S. Preventive Services Task Force (USPSTF), part of the Department of Health and Human Service's Agency for Healthcare Research and Quality (AHRQ), identifies the following categories in their Guide to Clinical Preventive Services: cancer; heart and vascular disease; injury and violence; infectious diseases; mental health conditions and substance abuse; metabolic, nutrition, and endocrine conditions; musculoskeletal conditions; obstetrics and gynecological conditions; pediatric disorders; and vision and hearing disorders. More information is available at *www.ahrq.gov/clinic/cps3dix.htm*. Table 9-3 summarizes the timelines. The remainder of the chapter will use these categories to identify and describe a small selection of screenable diseases. The availability of Medicare insurance coverage is discussed, to demonstrate that many preventive screenings are covered by insurance. For ongoing changes and recommended screening for cancer, see *www.cancer.org* (American Cancer Society, 2008a).

Healthy People 2010
Objectives Related to Screening

1. Ensure appropriate newborn bloodspot screening, follow-up testing, and referral to services.
2. Increase the proportion of sexually active females aged 25 years and under who are screened annually for genital Chlamydia infections.
3. Increase the proportion of pregnant females screened for sexually transmitted diseases (including HIV infection and bacterial vaginosis) during prenatal health care visits, according to recognized standards.
4. Increase the proportion of women who receive a Pap test.
5. Increase the proportion of newborns who are screened for hearing deficit by age 1 month, have audiologic evaluation by age 3 months, and are enrolled in appropriate intervention services by age 6 months.
6. Increase the proportion of preschool children aged 5 years and under who receive vision screening.
7. Increase the proportion of people who have a dilated eye examination at appropriate intervals.
8. Increase the proportion of adults who receive a colorectal cancer screening examination.
9. Increase the proportion of women aged 40 years and older who have undergone a mammogram within the preceding 2 years.
10. Increase the proportion of people living in pre-1950s housing who have been tested for the presence of lead-based paint.
11. Increase the proportion of adults who have had their blood pressure measured within the preceding 2 years and can state whether their blood pressure was normal or high.
12. Increase the proportion of adults who have had their blood cholesterol levels checked within the preceding 5 years.
13. Increase the proportion of adults with tuberculosis who have been tested for HIV.
14. Increase the proportion of adults in publicly funded HIV counseling and testing sites who are screened for common bacterial STDs (chlamydia, gonorrhea, and syphilis) and are immunized against hepatitis B virus.

From U.S. Department of Health and Human Services. (2000). *Healthy People 2010* (Conference ed.). Washington, DC: The Department.
HIV, Human immunodeficiency virus; *Pap*, Papanicolaou; *STDs*, sexually transmitted diseases.

Breast Cancer

In the United States the most common cancer among women is breast cancer (American Cancer Society, 2008b). A malignant lesion in the breast indicates the disease; severity is based on the size of the lesion and the length of time that it has been present. Screening for asymptomatic cases

Table 9-3 Guide to Clinical Preventive Services, 2007

Recommendation	Adults		Special Populations	
	Men	Women	Pregnant Women	Children
Abdominal Aortic Aneurysm, Screening: One-time screening by ultrasonography in men aged 65-75 who have ever smoked	X			
Alcohol Misuse Screening and Behavioral Counseling Interventions	X	X	X	
Aspirin for the Primary Prevention of Cardiovascular Events: Adults at increased risk for coronary heart disease	X	X		
Bacteriuria, Screening for Asymptomatic			X	
Breast Cancer, Chemoprevention: Discuss with women at high risk for breast cancer and at low risk for adverse effects of chemoprevention		X		
Breast Cancer, Screening: Mammography every 1-2 years for women 40 and older		X		
Breast and Ovarian Cancer Susceptibility, Genetic Risk Assessment and BRCA Mutation Testing: Refer women whose family history is associated with an increased risk for deleterious mutations in BRCA1 or BRCA2 genes for genetic counseling and evaluation for BRCA testing		X		
Breastfeeding, Behavioral Interventions to Promote: Structured education and behavioral counseling programs		X	X	
Cervical Cancer, Screening: Women who have been sexually active and have a cervix		X		
Chlamydial Infection, Screening: Sexually active women 25 and younger and other asymptomatic women at increased risk for infection. Asymptomatic pregnant women 25 and younger and others at increased risk		X	X	
Colorectal Cancer, Screening: Men and women 50 and older	X	X		
Dental Caries in Preschool Children, Prevention: Prescribe oral fluoride supplementation at currently recommended doses to preschool children older than 6 months whose primary water source is deficient in fluoride				X
Depression, Screening: In clinical practices with systems to ensure accurate diagnoses, effective treatment, and follow-up	X	X		
Diabetes Mellitus in Adults, Screening for Type 2: Adults with hypertension or hyperlipidemia	X	X		
Diet, Behavioral Counseling in Primary Care to Promote a Healthy Life: Adults with hyperlipidemia and other known risk factors for cardiovascular and diet-related chronic disease	X	X		
Gonorrhea, Screening: All sexually active women, including those who are pregnant, at increased risk for infection (that is, if they are young or have other individual or population risk factors)		X	X	
Gonorrhea, Prophylactic Medication: Prophylactic ocular topical medication for all newborns against gonococcal ophthalmia neonatorum				X
Hepatitis B Virus Infection, Screening: Pregnant women at first prenatal visit			X	
High Blood Pressure, Screening	X	X		
HIV, Screening: All adolescents and adults at increased risk for HIV infection and all pregnant women	X	X	X	X
Iron Deficiency Anemia, Prevention: Routine iron supplementation for asymptomatic children aged 6-12 months who are at increased risk for iron deficiency anemia				X
Iron Deficiency Anemia, Screening: Routine screening in asymptomatic pregnant women			X	
Lipid Disorders, Screening: Men 35 and older and women 45 and older. Younger adults with other risk factors for coronary disease. Screening for lipid disorders to include measurement of total cholesterol and high-density lipoprotein cholesterol	X	X		

Continued

Table **9-3** Guide to Clinical Preventive Services, 2007—cont'd

Recommendation	Adults		Special Populations	
	Men	Women	Pregnant Women	Children
Obesity in Adults, Screening: Intensive counseling and behavioral interventions to promote sustained weight loss for obese adults	X	X		
Osteoporosis in Postmenopausal Women, Screening: Women 65 and older and women 60 and older at increased risk for osteoporotic fractures		X		
Incompatibility, Screening: Blood typing and antibody testing at first pregnancy-related visit. Repeated antibody testing for unsensitized Rh (D) negative women at 24-28 weeks gestation unless biological father is known to be Rh (D) negative			X	
Syphilis Infection, Screening: Persons at increased risk and all pregnant women	X	X	X	
Tobacco Use and Tobacco-Caused Disease, Counseling to Prevent: Tobacco cessation interventions for those who use tobacco. Augmented pregnancy-tailored counseling to pregnant women who smoke	X	X	X	
Visual Impairment in Children Younger than Age 5 Years, Screening: To detect amblyopia, strabismus, and defects in visual acuity				X

Modified from The Agency for Healthcare Research and Quality, *Guide to clinical preventive services, 2007.* Retrieved from *www.ahrq.gov/clinic/pocketgd07/gcp1.htm.*

and finding unnoticed and presumably smaller masses permit more successful and conservative treatments, because the stage is less severe.

In American women, the incidence of breast cancer increases with age. Nulliparous women, who have never given birth, run a high risk of breast carcinoma; women who had their first child before the age of 20 constitute the lowest-risk group. Women who start menstruating at an earlier age than average and reach menopause at a later age than average also have a somewhat higher risk, as do those who bore their first child in their late 30s. Additional risks may include women with fibrocystic disease of the breast, family history of breast cancer, extended use of estrogen supplements, obesity, and a diet high in fat.

Screening tests that have been considered appropriate for early detection include (1) screening mammography, (2) clinical breast examination (CBE), and (3) breast self-examination.

The USPSTF (2002a) recommends screening mammography every 1 to 2 years, with or without the CBE. The task force report indicated that evidence suggests the benefit is fairly strong, in that screening mammography has a significant impact on reducing breast cancer mortality, and concluded that harms from screening mammography (false-positive results, unnecessary biopsies, cost, and anxiety) tend to decrease in woman aged 40 and over: that is, the benefit-to-harm ratio becomes more favorable to older women. The nurse is often the health care provider who teaches a woman about breast health.

The USPSTF (2002a) has not been able to determine whether there are any screening benefits to the CBE alone,

and although there may be "incremental benefit" of combining CBE with screening mammography, their data are insufficient for specific recommendation. The American Cancer Society recommends:

- For women in good health: yearly mammograms starting at age 40
- Clinical breast exam, as part of periodic health exam
  - Women in their 20's-30's: every 3 years
  - Women over 40: every year
- Monthly self-breast exam starting in their 20's (Women should know how their breasts normally feel and promptly report changes to their health care provider[s].)
- Women with high risk (greater than 20% lifetime risk): mammogram and MRI every year

Medicare pays for one mammogram to women over 40 every 12 months.

Cervical Cancer

The tenth most common cancer among women in the United States is cervical cancer. The principal screening test for cervical cancer is the Papanicolaou (Pap) smear. Although all sexually active women are at risk for cervical cancer, the disease is more common among women of low socioeconomic status, women with a history of multiple sex partners, women with early first sexual intercourse, smokers, and women with certain types of human papilloma virus and human immunodeficiency virus (HIV).

The incidence of invasive cervical cancer has decreased dramatically since the implementation of early detection programs involving the Pap smear. The American Cancer Society guidelines for Pap smear testing include the following:

- Annual screening should be performed on all women, aged 21 years and older, or earlier within 3 years of the onset of vaginal intercourse, or every 2 years using the newer liquid-based Pap test.
- Women beginning at age 30 with three normal Pap smears in a row: every 3 years with conventional or liquid based Pap smear, plus the HPV (human papilloma virus) DNA test
- Women with certain risk factors: annual screenings (diethylstilbestrol [DES] exposure, before birth; HIV infection; weakened immune system—due to transplant[s], chemotherapy or chronic steroid use)
- Women over age 70 may choose to stop Pap smears if they are in good health and have no risk factors (three normal Pap smears in a row and no abnormal ones in the past 10 years)
- Screening is not recommended for women with a history of total hysterectomy as a result of benign disease.

As part of Medicare, a woman may have a Pap test, pelvic exam, and clinical breast exam every 24 months, unless the woman has had an abnormal Pap within the past 36 months, or is at high risk for cervical or vaginal cancer and is of childbearing age, in which case it is covered every 12 months.

Colorectal Cancer

Colorectal cancer is the third-leading cause of cancer deaths for both men and women in the United States (American Cancer Society, 2008a, 2008b). A campaign for early detection of colorectal carcinoma continues to be widely publicized by the American Cancer Society. The USPSTF (2002b) strongly recommends periodic colorectal screening for men and women beginning at age 50. They have concluded that the benefit-to-harm ratio is highly favorable, with the magnitude of each having a different variation with each screening method.

Colon Cancer

The guidelines of the American Cancer Society recommend individuals talk with their physician to determine the screening test, age and frequencies which are most appropriate for them to detect possible signs of colon cancer. For healthy, low-risk individuals the following are possible screenings:

- Colmascopy every 10 years
- Double contrast barium enema every 5 years
- CT scan colonography (virtual colmascopy) every 5 years
- Fecal occult blood test (FOBT), take home sample method or fecal immunochemical test (FIT). "A FOBT or FIT done during a digital rectal exam in the health care provider's office is not adequate" (p. 2).
- Stool DNA test, intervals uncertain at present

More frequent intervals for all of the above tests are recommended for individuals with higher colorectal risk factors including a peremal or family history of colorectal cancer, ladenomaton polyps or chronic bowel disease (Crohn's disease or ulcerative colitis).

The guidelines of the American Cancer Society (2008a) for both men and women who, at the age of 50, should: (1) take an annual take home fecal occult blood test every year, and (2) have a colonoscopy every 10 years or double-contrast barium enema every 5 years. Beginning at age 50, Medicare covers a fecal occult blood test every 12 months, a flexible sigmoidoscopy every 48 months, a screening colonoscopy or a barium enema every 24 months.

Prostate Cancer

Prostate cancer is the most commonly diagnosed cancer in males and the second-leading cause of cancer death among males in the United States (American Cancer Society, 2008b). However, according to the USPSTF (2002c), of the approximately 1 in 6 men who are diagnosed with the disease, only about 1 in 29 will die of it. The risk increases with age, beginning at 50 years, and is considerably higher among Black men.

Screening tests commonly used for prostate cancer include digital rectal exam (DRE) and prostate specific antigen (PSA), the analysis for the serum tumor marker. However, prostate cancer screening continues to be controversial. Although DRE is easily taught and cost-effective, its effectiveness in reducing prostate cancer death rates has not been determined (National Cancer Institute, 2004), and data are inconclusive to prove that early detection actually improves outcome. In addition, there are considerable harms associated with both the screenings and the treatments for some cancers that might never have altered a person's health (USPSTF, 2002c). False-positive results leading to unnecessary biopsies and anxiety are not uncommon, nor are treatment complications of sexual dysfunction or incontinence. A possible exception to the benefit-to-harm ratio may exist among Black men, because both incidence and mortality rates are higher in this group. The best age and intervals for PSA and DRE screenings are not known (National Cancer Institute, 2004). Clinical trials in progress may provide a more definitive answer (USPSTF, 2002c).

The American Cancer Society recommends:

- Discussing with patients these known and unknown factors about the benefits, limitation and risks so they can make informed decisions with their physician
- DRE and PSA annually beginning at age 50 or at age 40-45 in Black men and men with family histories in first degree relatives

Medicare covers a digital rectal examination and a prostate specific antigen test once every 12 months for men age 50 and older.

Cholesterol

One of the major modifiable risk factors for coronary heart disease is elevated blood cholesterol levels (USDHHS, 2000). Extensive research, educational programs, and media attention, and public screenings have increased the knowledge and understanding of the implications of high cholesterol levels and of the role of cholesterol in a healthy lifestyle. Cholesterol screening can identify high-risk individuals who are most likely to benefit from individualized risk factor counseling, dietary instruction, tobacco cessation, weight reduction, physical activity, and drug therapies. Indeed, the strongest support for cholesterol screening is the ability of cholesterol-lowering interventions to reduce the risk of coronary heart disease in those with high cholesterol levels (USPSTF, 1996). Medicare covers this screening every five years.

Screening for total cholesterol (TC) and high-density lipoprotein cholesterol (HDL-C) levels can be obtained in fasting or nonfasting individuals from finger stick or venipuncture samples (USPSTF, 2001). The USPSTF (2001) advises that both TC and HDL-C (less than 40 mg/dL) is a more sensitive measure, but TC of 200 mg/dL or higher alone is acceptable criteria to guide an individual toward modifying lifestyle to reduce risk (American Heart Association, 2008).

Recommendations are for screening for high blood cholesterol levels for all men aged 35 and older and women aged 45 and older. Young adults, beginning at age 20, with other coronary heart disease risk factors such as diabetes, tobacco use, hypertension, or a strong family cardiac history, should also be screened routinely (USPSTF, 2001).

Screening an individual's lipoprotein profile (total cholesterol, HDL cholesterol, and LDL cholesterol and triglycerides) and blood pressure are recommended components every 5 years of each American's overall plan of care (American Heart Association, 2008).

Hypertension

According to the Seventh Report of the Joint National Committee on Prevention, Detection, Evaluation, and Treatment of High Blood Pressure (American Heart Association, 2008), hypertension is a leading risk factor for congestive heart failure, stroke, heart attack, and renal disease. Detecting high blood pressure is a primary prevention strategy for coronary heart disease, cerebrovascular disease, and peripheral vascular disease; it is a secondary prevention strategy for hypertension. Criteria for referral may vary according to the level of elevation and risk factors. Periodic screening is recommended for everyone 18 years of age and older every 2 years with a blood pressure less than 120/80 mm Hg and every year if prehypertensive (USPSTF, 2007). People with systolic blood pressure readings from 120 to 139 mm Hg and diastolic readings from 80 to 89 mm Hg are classified as prehypertensive (USDHHS, National Institutes of Health, 2003). The USPSTF (2007) defined hypertension in adults as a systolic of 140 mm Hg or higher, or a diastolic blood pressure of 90 mm Hg or higher, diagnosed after two or more elevated readings are obtained on at least two visits over a period of 1 to several weeks. However, for people over 50 years of age, the Joint National

Committee, VII (USDHHS, 2003) guidelines indicate that systolic pressure has greater impact on health outcome than the diastolic pressure. Therefore, treatment is recommended when systolic pressure is equal to or greater than 140 mm Hg, regardless of the diastolic readings. Assessment of other cardiovascular risk factors, such as tobacco, diabetes, abnormal blood lipid values, age, sex, sedentary lifestyle, and obesity may modify these guidelines and clinical discretion is always key.

When hypertension is treated effectively, there are important long-term implications for decreased mortality and morbidity from end-organ damage. Therefore it should be a part of any comprehensive screening program.

Human Immunodeficiency Virus

HIV and acquired immunodeficiency syndrome (AIDS) have been reported in every racial and ethnic population, in every age and socioeconomic group, in every state, and in most large cities throughout the United States (USDHHS, 2000). In the United States, AIDS is the fifth-leading cause of death in persons 25 to 44 years and the seventh-leading cause of death in ages 15 to 24. (USPSTF, 2005). *Healthy People 2010* (USDHHS, 2000) reports that infection rates appear to have stabilized to a slower growth rate of approximately 40,000 new infections per year. In addition, recent therapies have reduced the severity of illness and prolonged survival. However, the need for HIV screening to increase the numbers of individuals who know their HIV status continues to be important. An estimated 25% of the 850,000 to 950,000 HIV-infected persons in the United States are unaware of their status. (USPSTF, 2005). The goal is to detect infection at the earliest possible time and decrease transmission when the potential is greatest, and to increase access to early care, prevention, and treatment, including highly active antiretroviral therapy, leading to improved outcomes and reduced mortality (USPSTF, 2005).

Health care providers need to assess the risk factors for HIV infection in all individuals by obtaining a careful sexual history and inquiring about past or present drug use. Periodic screening for HIV should be provided. A person is considered at risk with one or more individual risk factors, which include those who receive care in a high-prevalence or high-risk setting; "men who have had sex with men after 1975; men and women having unprotected sex with multiple partners; past or present injection drug users; men and women who exchange sex for money or drugs or have sex partners who do; individuals whose past or present sex partners were HIV-infected, bisexual, or injection drug users; persons being treated for sexually transmitted disease; and persons with a history of blood transfusion between 1978 and 1985" (USPSTF, 2005). The CDC recommends all individuals between 13 and 64 be screened for HIV regardless of risk factors. All pregnant women should be screened for HIV to reduce rates of mother-to-child transmission through the highly active antiretroviral therapy (HAART), which shows no evidence of an increase in fetal anomalies or other fetal harm (USPSTF, 2007). FDA-approved finger-stick blood spot samples and oral fluid HIV tests are found to be highly accurate and easy to provide (USPSTF, 2005).

Diabetes Mellitus

Diabetes mellitus is a group of disorders that have glucose intolerance as the common factor, characterized by hyperglycemia and other disturbances of carbohydrate, protein, and fat metabolism (Huether & McCance, 2008). Onset of symptoms in type 1 diabetes is acute, and symptoms are detected soon. This type occurs because of the body's failure to produce insulin. A person with type 2 diabetes is often asymptomatic in the early stages, and the disease may remain undiagnosed for many years. This type results from insulin resistance. Undiagnosed type 2 diabetes is associated with long-term damage to multiple organ systems. The risk of developing type 2 diabetes increases with age, obesity, and lack of exercise. Individuals who have a family history of diabetes, hypertension, dyslipidemia; who have had babies weighing more than 9 pounds; or who are members of particular racial or ethnic groups also have increased risk of developing this disease. Other types of diabetes include gestational diabetes and prediabetes (American Diabetes Association, 2009).

The USPSTF (2003b) recommends screening for type 2 diabetes in adults with hypertension or hyperlipidemia. Early detection via screening, in this population, will result in prompt treatment, ultimately reducing the burden of this disease. However, mass screening of all individuals (even all individuals considered at high risk) is not recommended, because there is no evidence to suggest that beginning diabetic management as a result of a mass screening provides an incremental benefit compared with initiating treatment after clinical diagnosis (USPSTF, 2003b). The decision to screen or not to screen should be made based upon expert clinical judgment of the health care practitioner. Screening of high-risk individuals should be considered at 3-year intervals. The fasting plasma glucose test and the oral glucose tolerance test are preferred and recommended tests. High-risk Medicare individuals are eligible for two fasting plasma glucose tests a year (USDHHS, 2008).

Phenylketonuria

PKU is a condition characterized by the genetically determined lack of phenylalanine hydroxylase, an enzyme necessary to metabolize an important amino acid, phenylalanine. In its absence, blood levels of phenylalanine increase, causing irreversible damage to the brain and central nervous system, resulting in severe mental retardation. The significance of PKU screening, therefore, is in its identification of the condition so as to prevent the long-term effects.

The USPSTF (2008) recommends newborn testing after 24 hours of life but before 7 days old, using 1 of 3 approved methods to include the Guthrie Bacterial Inhibition Assay, automated fluorometric assay, and tandem mass spectrometry. Those tested before 24 hours should be retested in 2 weeks.

THE NURSE'S ROLE

The need for nursing involvement exists at all levels of the collaborative partnership process. Being some of the many important stakeholders, nurses play a role in every aspect of the screening program development process, including assessment, data analysis, planning, implementation, evaluation of the health outcomes, and the evaluation of the process (including the workings of the partnership). One aspect of this health process is the development and implementation of screening programs for targeted groups. As nurses become more involved in decision-making, they will be faced with the question, "Should this condition be screened for or not?" In the role of decision maker and planner, the nurse is responsible for reviewing all the issues concerning a screenable disease, including (1) the criteria specific to the disease, (2) the medical and economic ethics, and (3) the community resources that are affected. If the choice is to screen, the participation of nurses and other partnering groups is essential in the development of a care plan. The last step is the planning and development of an efficient referral system to enhance continuity of care and to ensure follow-up.

While these conditions above were highlighted, nurses have long been responsible for screening individuals and educating about healthy lifestyles and decreased risks, in the ordinary office intake assessment process. Questions concerning nutrition, coping, and self-care are all assessment or screening questions, leading to moments of opportunity for health promotion. While these are not evidence-based tools (i.e., proven valid and reliable), these moments are invaluable in assessment. As in any nursing intervention, adequate knowledge of the method of administration and the potential side effects is needed. Teaching individuals the meaning and limitation of the test results is an important element of this role, as is informing them of their part in obtaining the implied benefit.

The combined health educator and screener component means that the nurse continues to educate individuals about risk factors and teach them ways to alter and reduce risks generally through lifestyle changes, such as proper diet, exercise, and stress management, and by limiting the use of alcohol, drugs, and tobacco. The role as educator is essential in the screening process, because nurses provide individuals with the information necessary for choices they will make regarding healthy behavioral change. The nurse is actually practicing primary prevention interventions, but it is in coordination with a secondary preventive role.

SUMMARY

As a method of preclinical secondary prevention, screening is the rapid administration of a simple test to distinguish individuals who may have a condition from those who probably do not have it. It can be an effective, efficient tool in preventive health care if used for conditions applicable to the screening model and directed toward an at-risk population. A unique characteristic and significant advantage of screening is that it can be applied to individuals or groups.

Three questions provide a means of analyzing the screenability of a disease:

1. Is the condition significant?
2. Can screening for the condition be done?
3. Should screening for the condition be done?
   A. What are the health benefits?
   B. What are the tangible and intangible costs?

Screening programs are not appropriate for all conditions or all communities. Alternative methods of reaching the desired health outcome should always be considered. Screening in health care presents numerous roles for nurses and provides them with a valuable preventive tool and health promotion and health education tool in the care of healthy individuals.

CASE STUDY

Women's Health: Mary S.

Mary S. is a 29-year-old seventh grade school teacher who is seeing the GYN nurse practitioner for her annual "women's appointment." Her intake screening identifies her height as 5 foot, 2 inches and weight as 150 pounds (BMI 27.4, classified as "Overweight"). Her TPR are within normal limits but her blood pressure is 145/90. During the assessment interview, she mentions that she has gained "a few pounds" that she needs to lose. She says the teachers have large potlucks and have contests to see who can provide the "best foods." She is proud that she wins at least once a week. She says she stays at school late to grade papers and gets home just in time to watch her favorite prime time television shows. The GYN exam was routine.

Reflective Questions:
1. What risk factors can be identified?
2. What additional screening tests might the nurse practitioner suggest and why?
3. Identify several nursing diagnoses and possible individual and community causes.
4. What questions should be asked to further explore potential interventions?
5. What teaching opportunities are available?

CARE PLAN

Imbalanced Metabolic Intake/Output; Evidence of Cardiac Risk Factors: Mary S.

Nursing Diagnosis: Excessive intake in relation to metabolic need

DEFINING CHARACTERISTICS
- Weight for height is in "Overweight BMI"
- One-time blood pressure above normal limits

RELATED FACTORS
- Verbalizes weight gain and cooking contest
- Verbalizes willingness to lose additional weight

EXPECTED OUTCOMES
Mary S. will:
- Verbalize understanding of cardiac risk factors
- Identify health risk behaviors she can change
- Set appropriate weight reduction goals (1-2 pounds/week to a predetermined weight)
- Design a modification program to meet individual long-term healthy lifestyle goal of healthy eating and increased activity
- Implement modification program and obtain healthy lifestyle goal

INTERVENTIONS
- Promote attitude of openness to new information
- Repeat blood pressure and prescribe a three-day screen if it is still above normal
- Order cholesterol and blood sugar screening lab work and inform individual of the health risks
- Provide weight reduction teaching and assistance
  - Dietitian referral if available
  - Daily food intake log
  - Daily activity log
  - Set acceptable goal
  - Explore nutritional and activity strategies that appeal to individual
  - Offer resources to support goals and strategies
  - Suggest using the summer to build a new health routine
  - Remind to begin new program slowly
  - Suggest shifting the potluck winning focus to healthy, yet "good" dishes
  - Suggest exercising during evening television shows
- Follow-up appointment in 1 month, if possible

REFERENCES

Allender, J., & Spradley, B. (2005). *Community health nursing: Concepts and practice* (6th ed.). New York: Lippincott.

American Cancer Society. (2008a). *Colorectal cancer: Early detection* (On-line). Retrieved December 1, 2008, from *www.cancer.org/docroot/home/index.asp*.

American Cancer Society. (2008b). *Guidelines for the early detection of cancer.* Retrieved December 3, 2008, from *www.cancer.org/docroot/ped/content/ped_2_3x_acs_cancer_detection_guidelines_36.asp*.

American Diabetes Association. (2009). *Diabetes care. (32)*, S1-F97.

American Heart Association. (2008). *Scientific statements and practice guidelines for 2008-2009.* Retrieved March 23, 2009, from *www.americanheart.org*.

Anderson, E. T., & McFarlane, J. M. (2006). *Community as partner: Theory and practice in nursing* (5th ed.). Philadelphia: Lippincott Williams & Wilkins.

Huether, S. E., & McCance, K. L. (2008). *Understanding pathophysiology* (4th ed.). St. Louis: Mosby.

Lewis, S. M., Heitkemper, M. M., & Dirksen, S. R. (2007). *Medical-surgical nursing: Assessment and management of clinical problems* (7th ed.). St. Louis: Mosby.

Lundy, K., & Janes, S. (2001). *Community health nursing: Caring for the public's health.* Boston: Jones and Bartlett.

Medicare. (2007). *Preventive Services: A Healthier US Starts Here.* Retrieved March 11, 2008, from *www.medicare.gov/Health/Overview.asp*.

National Cancer Institute. (2004). *Prostate cancer: Screening and testing.* Retrieved June 4, 2005, from *www.nci.nih.gov/cancerinfo/screening/prostate*.

Pender, N., Murdaugh, C., & Parsons, M. A. (2006). *Health promotion in nursing practice* (5th ed.). Upper Saddle River, NJ: Prentice Hall.

Polit, D., Beck, C., & Hungler, B. (2001). *Essentials of nursing research: Methods, appraisal, and utilization* (5th ed.). Philadelphia: Lippincott.

Sackett, D., Straus, S., Richardson, W., Rosenberg, W., & Haynes, R. (2000). *Evidence-based medicine: How to practice and teach EBM* (2nd ed.). New York: Churchill Livingston.

U.S. Department of Health and Human Services. (2000). *Healthy people 2010* (Conference ed.). Washington, DC: The Department.

U.S. Department of Health and Human Services. National Institutes of Health, National Heart, Lung and Blood Pressure. (2003). *Seventh report of the Joint National Committee: On prevention, detection, evaluation, and treatment of high blood pressure.* Retrieved March 1, 2004, from *http://nhlbi.nih.gov/guidelines/hypertension*.

U.S. Preventive Services Task Force. (1996). *Guide to clinical preventive services* (2nd ed.). Baltimore: Williams & Wilkins.

U.S. Preventive Services Task Force. (2001). *Guide to clinical preventive services: Screening for Lipid Disorders in Adults.* Retrieved March 11, 2008, from *www.ahrq.gov/clinic/uspstf/uspschol.htm*.

U.S. Preventive Services Task Force. (2002a). *Guide to clinical preventive services: Screening for Breast Cancer.* Retrieved March 11, 2008, from *www.ahrq.gov/clinic/uspstf/uspsbrca.htm*.

U.S. Preventive Services Task Force. (2002b). *Guide to clinical preventive services: Screening for Colorectal Cancer.* Retrieved March 11, 2008, from *www.ahrq.gov/clinic/uspstf/uspscolo.htm*.

U.S. Preventive Services Task Force. (2002c). *Guide to clinical preventive services: Screening for Prostate Cancer.* Retrieved March 11, 2008, from *www.ahrq.gov/clinic/uspstf/uspsprca.htm*.

U.S. Preventive Services Task Force. (2003a). *Guide to clinical preventive services: Screening for Cervical Cancer.* Retrieved March 11, 2008, from *www.ahrq.gov/clinic/cps3dizscerv.htm*.

U.S. Preventive Services Task Force. (2003b). *Guide to clinical preventive services: Screening for Diabetes Mellitus, Adult type 2.* Retrieved March 11, 2008, from *www.ahrq.gov/clinic/uspstf/uspsdiab.htm*.

U.S. Preventive Services Task Force. (2005). *Guide to clinical preventive services: Screening for human immunodeficiency virus infection.* Retrieved March 11, 2008, from *www.ahrq.gov/clinic/uspstf/uspshivi.htm*.

U.S. Preventive Services Task Force. (2007). *Guide to clinical preventive services: Screening for High Blood Pressure.* Retrieved March 11, 2008, from *www.ahrq.gov/clinic/uspstf/uspshype.htm*.

U.S. Preventive Services Task Force. (2008). *Guide to clinical preventive services: Screening for phenylketonuria.* Retrieved March 11, 2008, from *www.ahrq.gov/clinic/uspstf/uspsspku.htm*.

U.S. Preventive Services Task Force. (2008). *Guide to clinical preventive service.* AHRQ publication number 0805122. Agency for Healthcare Research and Quality, Rockville, MD. Retrieved April 4, 2009, from *www.ahrq.gov/clinic/nosmoke*.

Health Education

objectives

After completing this chapter, the reader will be able to:

- Analyze the aims of health education.
- Discuss learning principles that affect health education.
- Apply teaching and learning concepts to teaching the family.
- Describe the health belief model and behavior change process.
- Describe the use of the transtheoretical model in planning for health teaching.
- Identify the steps in preparing a health-teaching plan.
- Propose learning strategies appropriate to each learning domain.
- Discuss the importance of evaluating the educational process.

key terms

Behavior change
Empowerment
Health behaviors
Health belief model

Health counseling
Health education
Health promotion
Social cognitive theory

Social learning theory
Social marketing
Transtheoretical (Stages of Change) model

website materials

evolve These materials are located on the book's website at *http://evolve.elsevier.com/Edelman/*.
- WebLinks
- Study Questions
- Glossary

THINK About It

The Challenges of Health Education

An analysis of a nursing assessment often leads to a nursing diagnosis related to the individual's lack of knowledge in the areas of health promotion or health-promotion strategies. The nurse may recognize certain risk factors in a person, such as a lack of knowledge, possession of incorrect knowledge, misinterpretation of information, or reliance on harmful myths and folk medicine. Additionally, the individual may demonstrate little or no interest in learning, a lack of motivation to learn, or a cognitive or perceptual inability to learn.

The success of any health activity or goal will depend on the individual's perception of the situation and responsiveness to teaching. The success of health teaching depends on a person's ability to learn and process information and the motivation to change behaviors to improve the present condition or move toward better health. The nurse assists each person in a process of self-understanding and self-direction, so the individual will experience the desire and motivation to change. Frequently, major life decisions need to be made in the process of learning. If through education and counseling the nurse can elicit logical and clear thinking, then the individual's decision-making abilities and progress in meeting life's needs will be developed further. To encourage critical

Continued

THINK About It

The Challenges of Health Education—cont'd

thinking by an individual, the nurse may pose some of the following questions:

1. What do you know about the health problem or concern?
2. What were you told?
3. What do you think will help you deal with the problem or concern?
4. How do you explain this problem or concern to yourself?
5. How do you see yourself in 6 months?
6. What types of efforts have worked for you in the past with this problem or concern?
7. How does the problem or concern affect your daily life?
8. What one aspect would indicate an improvement in your condition?
9. How much control do you think you have over this situation?
10. What is one goal that you would like to set for yourself?

SCENARIO

Ronald is a successful executive in a local business. In his annual physical examination, an irregular heartbeat was noted on the electrocardiogram. Ronald's father died of a heart attack at age 50; therefore, the physician scheduled Ronald for a thallium stress test. The stress test indicated a need for further evaluation with a cardiac catheterization. A 60% blockage in one artery was detected during this process. Ronald's condition will be handled conservatively at this point. He recognizes that some lifestyle changes are necessary. He is overweight and eats in restaurants frequently. He has not been active in regular exercise. He and his wife live in a condominium. They have grown children and grandchildren. One of their sons has a serious drug problem, so they have not seen him for several years and hear from him only rarely.

1. How might the nurse begin working with Ronald?
2. How likely is he to be motivated to learn and change?
3. What are some barriers to change in his behaviors?

The greatest opportunity to improve the health of the American people lies in addressing unhealthy personal behavioral risk factors. Improvement of the public's health is "more likely to come from behavioral change than from technological innovation" (Schroeder, 2007, p. 1222). Behavior patterns account for 40% to 50% of early deaths among Americans and represent the single most controllable area of influence over the health forecast (McGinnis, 2003).

The current national health objectives, *Healthy People 2010*, and the forthcoming *Healthy People 2020* objectives, emphasize priorities to improve the health of individuals, groups, and communities in the United States (U.S. Department of Health and Human Services, 2000, 2007) (see *www.healthypeople.gov*). Implementation of *Healthy People 2010*, as well as developing of *Healthy People 2020*, seeks to improve life expectancy and quality of life by "helping individuals gain the knowledge, motivation, and opportunities they need to make informed decisions about their health" (Lee & Estes, 2003, p. 58). Achievement of these objectives provides challenges and opportunities for **health promotion**. Although health is influenced significantly by social, economic, physical, and political factors, many health goals are affected by individual lifestyle practices. *Healthy People 2010* objectives related to educational programs appear in the *Healthy People 2010* box.

Nursing, with its unique contributions to health care, represents a professional resource that can help facilitate these changes through health-education strategies. Nurses, in partnership with other health care professionals, can be the link between the philosophy of *Healthy People 2010* and the people who need to hear its messages and act on those messages.

NURSING AND HEALTH EDUCATION

Nurses as educators play a key role in improving the health of the nation. Educating people is an integral part of the nurse's role in every practice setting—schools, communities, work sites, health care delivery sites, and homes. Health education involves not only providing relevant information, but also facilitating health-related **behavior change**. The nurse, using health-education principles, can assist people in achieving their health goals in a way that is consistent with their personal lifestyles, values, and beliefs.

Nursing: Scope and Standards of Practice describes health teaching and health promotion as primary nursing responsibilities. This includes educating people about healthy lifestyles, risk reduction, developmental needs, activities of daily living, and preventive self-care (American Nurses Association, [ANA], 2004). ANA's social policy statement also addresses health teaching and **health counseling** (ANA, 2003). This responsibility to teach individuals is balanced by their right to know about diagnosis, treatment, risks, benefits, costs, and alternatives. The nurse's role is to support the right of individuals to know their health status and to assess and assist a person's physical, psychosocial, and spiritual responses to that knowledge. The nurse also provides health teaching and health counseling based on individual interest and decisions (Bandman & Bandman, 2002).

Healthy People 2010
Selected Health-Promotion and Disease-Prevention Objectives Related to Educational and Community-Based Programs

Goal: To Increase the Quality, Availability, and Effectiveness of Educational and Community-Based Programs Designed to Prevent Disease and Improve Health and Quality of Life

School Setting
- 7-1. Increase the rate of completion of high school.
- 7-2. Increase the proportion of middle, junior high, and senior high schools that provide comprehensive health education to prevent problems in these areas: (1) unintentional injury, violence, and suicide, (2) tobacco use, (3) alcohol and other drug use, (4) unintended pregnancy and sexually transmitted infections, (5) unhealthy dietary patterns, and (6) inadequate physical activity.
- 7-3. Increase the proportion of college and university students who receive information for the institution of each of the six priority health-risk behavior areas listed above.
- 7-4. Increase the proportion of elementary, middle, junior high, and senior high schools that have a nurse-to-student ratio of at least 1:750.

Work Setting
- 7-5. Increase the proportion of work sites that offer a comprehensive employee health-promotion program to their employees.

- 7-6. Increase the proportion of employees who participate in employer-sponsored health-promotion activities.

Health Care Setting
- 7-7. Increase the proportion of health care organizations that provide client and family education.
- 7-8. Increase the proportion of people who report that they are satisfied with the client education that they receive from their health organization.
- 7-9. Increase the proportion of hospitals and managed care organizations that sponsor community disease-prevention and health-promotion activities that address the priority health needs identified by their community.

Community Setting and Select Populations
- 7-10. Increase the proportion of tribal and local health service areas that establish community health-promotion programs.
- 7-11. Increase the proportion of local health departments that establish culturally appropriate and linguistically competent community health-promotion and disease-prevention programs.
- 7-12. Increase the proportion of older adults who have participated during the preceding year in at least one organized health-promotion activity.

Modified from U.S. Department of Health and Human Services. (2000). *Healthy people 2010*. Washington, DC: U.S. Government Printing Office. Retrieved from *www.healthypeople.gov*.

Nurses usually function as health care coordinators for individuals in their care. Depending on the interest and needs of a person, nurses establish a partnership to guide the individual in the selection and use of relevant health services. Principles of health education provide the nurse with strategies and tools for assessing an individual's readiness for health teaching, with technical information, and with help in practicing health care techniques at home. These strategies also help the nurse facilitate behavior change, while satisfying the person's right to relevant health information and the freedom for people to make decisions about their own health. Health education encourages self-care, self-empowerment and, ultimately, less dependence on the health care system.

Nurses have long been involved in public health education, taking on the full-time role of coordinating the educational services provided by a health agency or institution. As a health educator, the nurse may use marketing strategies to enhance the effectiveness of health-education programs that are focused on certain target populations. The health-education specialist helps other nurses and health professionals improve their skills in developing and delivering teaching plans.

Definition

Health education is "any combination of planned learning experiences based on sound theories that provide individuals, groups, and communities the opportunity to acquire the information and the skills needed to make quality health decisions" (Wurzbach, 2004, p. 6). This process involves several key components. First, health education involves the use of teaching-learning strategies. Second, learners maintain voluntary control over the decision to make changes in their actions. Third, health education focuses on behavior changes that have been found to improve health status.

Health education facilitates the development of health knowledge, skills, and attitudes through the application of theories or models. Two commonly used theories, behavioral theory and social learning theory, will be discussed later in this chapter. Generally, health-education strategies help ensure that individuals, as consumers of health services, are satisfied and have received the health care that is most relevant to their problems. From a public health perspective, health-education programs are intended not only to enhance individuals' abilities to make positive lifestyle changes, but also to support social and political actions that promote health and quality of life in communities.

The following scenario is an example of a therapeutic situation in which a health-education approach may be used to meet an individual's health needs.

Sada Thompson, a 21-year-old university senior, visits university health services because she wants to change her method of birth control. She has experienced side effects from the birth control pill that she has been taking for the past year and knows little about other options. She has recently started dating John after breaking up with Steven 3 months ago. Having decided to be sexually active with John, Sada is feeling uncertain about what she needs to do to take care of herself and how to discuss this uncertainty with John. She is aware of all the talk about acquired immunodeficiency syndrome (AIDS) on campus and she knows that John is popular and has dated several other women in school, which concerns her.

Sada needs to learn new information, she may need to acquire new skills, and she needs to clarify any feelings or attitudes that affect her decision to use a new birth control method and ensure her continued safety. After recording her health assessment history and arranging for a gynecological examination and laboratory tests, the nurse develops a teaching plan. Selecting one or more strategies for helping Sada review all the birth control options, the nurse establishes an environment in which Sada can choose to try a new method or request a change in her prescription for oral contraceptives. Together they identify actions that Sada can take to use the method properly. They also anticipate and identify ways that Sada can solve problems of adjusting to the new method.

The nurse answers Sada's immediate questions about safe sex, gives her several pamphlets written for college students about this topic, and suggests that she participate in the peer counseling night on sexually transmitted diseases that will be held on campus in 2 weeks. The peer counseling hotline number and drop-in hours are given to her, and the nurse explains that these students are trained to help other students talk about and deal with this important issue. The nurse invites Sada to call or come back to the office for additional help, information, and problem-solving discussion.

This example illustrates that educational interventions, in addition to direct health services, are necessary to meet the individual's goal. Although health care providers and nurses prefer that people choose to take actions that will promote health and not detract from it, the individual controls the at-home application of health recommendations.

Goals

The goal of health education is to help individuals, families, and communities achieve optimal states of health through their own actions and initiative (Anderson et al., 2008). Health education facilitates voluntary actions to promote health.

Health education encourages positive, informed changes in lifestyle behaviors that prevent acute and chronic disease, decrease disability, and enhance wellness. Another goal of health education that may foster successful changes in health behavior is **empowerment**. People who believe that they can make a difference in health and who are involved in decision-making are more likely to make changes (Anderson et al., 2008).

Changes in health behaviors that are related to health education help prevent disease and disability. Two main objectives of health education and counseling are to change health behaviors and to improve health status. Information alone does not change behavior.

Health education and health counseling are mutually supportive activities. Health educators often use one-to-one and group counseling techniques as strategies for active health learning. Counselors may refer people to health-education resources or assist them in acquiring information pertinent to solving a health problem. The following example helps illustrate the goals of health education.

Kate Hanson, 22 years old, visits the local family health center for fatigue and symptoms similar to influenza. During the assessment with the nurse, Kate discloses that she has missed her last two periods.

The physical examination, the laboratory tests, and the health assessment pattern confirm Kate's suspicions of pregnancy. Psychosocial evaluation reveals that Kate works part time as a secretary for a temporary agency and lives in an apartment with her recently unemployed husband, Jim. Further interviewing reveals that Kate has minimal knowledge of prenatal care; she has a diet of take-out food that is high in fat, sodium, and sugar, with infrequent consumption of fresh fruits or vegetables; and she has three or four beers on the weekends. Kate has never taken vitamins, she leads a sedentary lifestyle, and she obviously is overwhelmed by the news that she is pregnant.

The nurse first takes steps to create a safe and trusting atmosphere in which Kate can feel free to share her concerns and apprehensions. Finding that Kate needs counseling for telling her husband about the pregnancy, the nurse discusses this with her. Kate is then taught the importance of taking a multiple vitamin with an iron supplement daily, discontinuing the use of alcohol, checking with her doctor before taking medications, and making time for more rest during the day. Sensing that this is all that can be accomplished at this time, the nurse gives Kate two pamphlets on prenatal care and makes an appointment for her to return in a week with her husband. Kate acknowledges that she understands the instructions, and the nurse documents the teaching and recommendations in Kate's chart.

During the next visit, the nurse meets with Kate and Jim, explores the meaning of the pregnancy in their lives, and helps them identify actions they will need to take. The recommendations that were made during Kate's first visit are reviewed and reinforced. The nurse then details specifics of dietary changes, the need for proper rest and exercise, and helps them solve problems as they adjust to these new responsibilities. Most importantly, the nurse gives them information on the clinic's weekly prenatal classes and explains that because the classes are partially covered by local community funding, the charge is minimal. The classes include information about physical changes, psychosocial changes, and nutritional needs during the pregnancy, the labor and delivery, and the newborn and postpartum periods. A nurse practitioner conducts the classes at the clinic, which are given in a group format to facilitate social support and problem solving among expectant parents.

The nurse gives them several other pamphlets to read at home, makes an appointment for Kate to see the nurse practitioner in a couple of weeks, and encourages her to call if she has questions or concerns in the interim. A schedule of the prenatal classes is reviewed and a date for the next session is made. The couple is encouraged to meet with the social worker to explore their financial needs and options because Jim was recently laid off. Kate and Jim acknowledge that they understand what they need to do, and the nurse documents what was taught and discussed in Kate's health care record.

This example illustrates the goal of health education: to help individuals achieve optimal health and well-being through their actions and initiative. Through health education, individuals can learn to make informed decisions about personal and family health practices and to use health services in the community. The individual in this example receives educational assistance from the nurse that will promote better health and well-being for herself and her baby.

Learning Assumptions

Individual chapters in this text address the factors to consider when teaching different age groups and the learners' respective characteristics to consider when developing a teaching plan. The general principles of learning that are found in Box 10-1 are fundamental to the planning of successful health-education programs (Wurzbach, 2004).

The nurse considers the developmental stage, cognitive level, and interests of the individual. The level of information to be conveyed and the skills and abilities of the individual will guide the methods and resources used. Children deserve special planning for health teaching (Health Teaching box).

Box 10-1   How to Facilitate Learning

- Use methods that stimulate a variety of senses.
- Involve the person actively in the learning process.
- Establish a comfortable, appropriate learning environment.
- Assess the readiness of the learner, which may be affected by physical and emotional factors.
- Make the information relevant by connecting with the existing needs and interests of the learner.
- Use repetition. Review and reinforce concepts several times in a variety of ways.
- Make the learning encounter positive. Structure it to achieve progress recognizable by the individual and provide frequent, positive feedback.
- Start with what is known and proceed to what is unknown, moving from simple to complex.
- Apply the concepts to several settings to facilitate generalization.
- Pace the learning appropriately for the individual.

HEALTH TEACHING   Teaching Health Promotion to Preschoolers and School-Aged Children

Teaching the principles of health promotion to young children can influence their behaviors now and in the future and may affect family health. Childhood is "an ideal time to help children begin to establish basic behaviors that will promote a healthy lifestyle" (Marotz et al., 2005, p. 4).

Useful Principles for Teaching Children

Children learn best by using all their senses.

- Learning activities are interesting and meaningful.
- Teachers show love and respect for all children.
- Good teaching is based on theory, philosophy, goals, and objectives.
- Children's learning is enhanced through the use of concrete materials.
- Teaching is centered on the child.
- Teaching moves from the concrete to the abstract.
- Teaching is based on the children's interests (Morrison, 2007).

Other Factors

In all planning, the children are considered. When possible, the particular group is observed and the learning experience is as individualized as possible. The approach is planned for the specific group of children with the following factors considered:

- The children's developmental level
- Any special considerations of the children

- The children's attention span
- The children's past experiences, interests, and abilities
- Activities that create enthusiasm and interest
- Activities that stimulate many senses (Bastable & Dart, 2008)

Suggested Teaching Activities

- Games
- Dialogue and interaction with children
- Hands-on practice
- Role playing and dramatic play
- Showing items, objects, and examples
- Puppets, dolls, stories, and books
- Drawing and painting (Bastable & Dart, 2008)

The nurse may wear a costume or a special item of clothing that is related to the topic. The children will enjoy receiving a certificate of completion of a health lesson. Having something to take home to discuss with their parents is also meaningful.

The health teaching emphasizes skills that children can use or develop immediately. Experiences are selected with their cognitive abilities in mind. For example, preschool children cannot understand cause and effect; they cannot anticipate the effects of dangerous situations, poor nutrition, and unsound health practices.

Family Health Teaching

The family plays an important role in health and illness. Since the family is the unit within which health values, health habits, and health risk perceptions are developed, understanding and intervening with the family is essential to promoting health and reducing health risks in individuals and communities (Anderson et al., 2008). Skills in family interviewing and assessment are valuable tools for nurses. Family health assessment and health teaching are closely related. The assessment model in the chapter on family health promotion provides a comprehensive approach to identifying problems, strengths, and health-education needs. The goal is to help the members achieve optimal states of health while guiding them through problem solving and decision-making. This process empowers them. Members believe they can make a difference in their own health.

In clarifying the health teaching needs of a family, the nurse might ask herself, "Who is in this family? What health-related tasks are they performing? How are they functioning and how are they meeting each others' needs? How well are they communicating? What does this family need to know? What do they need to know now? What do they think they need to know? How can they learn what they need to know?"

The nurse sets a broad health-promotion goal for the family but directs the health teaching toward a more specific area. It is essential that the family agrees with the goal and teaching needs. As the family participates in the assessment interview, perhaps members can identify their own health teaching needs. Some broad goals for family teaching include:

- Better family functioning
- Achieving developmental tasks
- Better family communication
- Improved self-concept
- Increased self-esteem
- Reduced health risks
- Healthier lifestyle behaviors (improved diet and health habits)
- Improved energy level within the family
- A sense of control
- Adaptation to change in family structure
- Adaptation to change in family situation or life state

Health teaching includes all family members, with learning activities appropriate for each individual. The general teaching goal will be the same for all members, but the approaches and specific goals for each member or subsystem will be different. Children, adolescents, and older members pose special challenges to the nurse, who may be geared toward teaching young or middle-aged adults.

Health Behavior Change

The process of health education directs people toward voluntary changes of their health behaviors. This section examines (1) the use of the health belief model to analyze the probability that a person will make changes to improve health or prevent disease; (2) the application of social learning theory to clarify environmental and social factors that affect learning of new health behaviors; and (3) the use of the stages of change, or transtheooretical model, in planning health teaching.

Beliefs, attitudes, values, and information contribute to motivation and behavior and are underlying factors in making any decision to change behavior (Richards & Digger, 2008). **Health behaviors** are any activities that an individual undertakes to enhance health, prevent disease, and detect and control the symptoms of a disease. Identifying and teaching people about lifestyle behaviors that need to be changed is only the first step in the process of assisting individuals in moving from knowledge to action. The nurse uses the health belief model and social learning theory as subsequent steps in formulating an action plan that meets the needs and capabilities of each person in making healthy behavior changes.

Health Belief Model

The **health belief model** is a paradigm used to predict and explain health behavior. The health belief model was developed to describe why people failed to participate in programs to detect or prevent disease. The model has been expanded to explain responses to symptoms, disease, prescribed treatments, and potential health problems (Glanz et al., 2003). The health belief model and social learning theory assist the nurse in formulating an action plan that meets the needs and capabilities of the individual making health behavior changes.

The following components of the health belief model provide guidelines for nurses to analyze factors that contribute to a person's perceived state of health or risk of disease and to the individual's probability of making an appropriate plan of action:

- Individual perceptions or readiness for change
- The value of health to the individual compared with other aspects of living
- Perceived susceptibility to a health problem, disease, or complications
- Perceived seriousness of the disease level threatening the achievement of certain goals or aims
- Risk factors to a disease attributed to heredity, race or culture, medical history, or other causes
- Perceived benefits of health action
- Perceived barriers to promotion action (Becker, 1974; Janz & Becker, 1984; Rosenstock et al., 1988)

The health belief model does not specify the interventions that will influence an individual's likelihood of taking action; rather, it explains the role of values and beliefs in predicting treatment outcomes and adherence, while generating data that guide nurses in choosing effective educational strategies. The most appropriate interventions for a particular person need to be negotiated between the individual and the health care professional.

Social Learning Theory

Social learning theory, recently renamed **social cognitive theory**, is another model that adds to the understanding of the determinants of health behavior. Bandura (1997) emphasizes the influence of self-efficacy, or efficacy beliefs, on health behavior. Self-efficacy refers to an individual's belief in being personally capable of performing the behavior required to influence one's own health (see the Case Study and Care Plan at the end of this chapter). Social cognitive theory also describes the roles of reinforcement and observational learning in explaining health behavior change. Modeling, or providing opportunities for imitating the behavior of others, can be used to demonstrate the desired behavior.

Opportunities to observe others performing the behavior in question—such as in a local Young Men's Christian Association (YMCA) risk factor–reduction program in which individuals exercise together and report on health behavior changes of smoking cessation and eating a low-fat diet—can enhance expectations of mastery. To affect a person's self-efficacy, the model provides examples of how to change, increase confidence in ability to change behavior, and convince the person of positive benefits of change (Galavotti et al., 2001).

Transtheoretical Model of Change

The **Transtheoretical Model (TTM), or the stages of change model**, is useful for determining where a person is in relation to making a behavior change. The model, developed by Prochaska and DiClemente (1984), is based on extensive research with smoking cessation. Health-related behavior change is proposed to progress through five stages regardless of whether the change involves quitting or adopting a behavior. The five stages are:

1. Precontemplation: A person is not thinking about or considering quitting or adopting a behavior change within the next 6 months (not intending to make changes)
2. Contemplation: A person is seriously considering making a specific behavior change within the next 6 months (considering a change)
3. Planning or Preparation: An individual who has made a behavior change is seriously thinking about making a change within the next month (making small or sporadic changes)
4. Action: The person has made a behavior change and it has persisted for a period of 6 months (actively engaged in behavior change)
5. Maintenance: The period beginning 6 months after action has started and continuing indefinitely (sustaining the change over time) (Prochaska & DiClemente, 1984)

The TTM is useful in determining the individual's readiness for learning in relation to changing a behavior so that health education or behavior change interventions can be matched to the stage. Self-efficacy is a key construct in this model. The TTM has been used by health professionals in planning interventions with a wide variety of individuals at risk such as women in violent relationships (Anderson, 2003), adolescents at risk for obesity (Mauriello et al., 2006), individuals with heart failure making lifestyle changes (Paul & Sneed, 2004), and breast cancer survivors at risk for osteoporosis (Ott et al., 2004).

Regardless of the quality of nurses' assessment methods and educational strategies, experience in the area of health education indicates that people do not always make the choices recommended to them by health professionals (Rankin et al., 2005). Clinicians often label these people noncompliant, a term that suggests that the individual has not followed his or her instructions. Naturally health professionals want people to choose the recommended course of action, but each individual frequently has the right to choose not to follow advice. Enlisting the individual's partnership or cooperation rather than compliance achieves better results.

Attempts to influence a person's behavior through education are not always successful. Attempting to persuade people to change their behavior to something that might make them, their friends, and their family healthier can be discouraging and sometimes futile. An individual's values, beliefs, and life stresses may present obstacles to these changes. Effective health education requires an understanding of the factors affecting the individual's decision-making (values, beliefs, attitudes, life stresses, religion, previous experiences with the health care system, and life goals).

Many health professionals tend to view a person's cooperation with the medical regimen as a single choice, when this cooperation often involves many choices every day. For example, following a low-fat, low-cholesterol diet involves constant, and often inconvenient, choices throughout the day. The expectation is that people will do this every day for the rest of their lives, even when the nurse cannot guarantee freedom from angina, myocardial infarctions, or other complications.

Ultimately, the nurse needs to respect a person's right to choose. However, nurses can increase an individual's motivation and capabilities to change by involving the individual in planning and goal setting, providing information that is understandable and acceptable, and assisting the person in developing new skills.

After clarifying behaviors that may need to be changed, the nurse can use the following framework based on a cognitive behavioral approach for developing interventions for behavior change:

- Assess the behavior
- Educate about the need for and benefits of change
- Motivate using personalized messages
- Assess and increase self-efficacy
- Decrease barriers to change
- Modify behavior
- Maintain behavior change (Saarmann et al., 2002)

Theories of health behavior change are at the heart of health education. The theories presented in this section help the nurses to assess an individual's stage in the behavior change process and to develop appropriate teaching plans. The goals of the teaching plans and the strategies selected will differ depending on the factors affecting the individual's readiness to learn and to change.

Ethics

The nurse upholds democratic principles such as respect for human dignity and the right to autonomy or self-determination. However, when planning health education to promote health, nurses experience several ethical dilemmas.

Although the focus of health education may be on the behavior change process, the nurse needs to be certain that tactics of coercion, persuasion, and manipulation have not been used (Bandman & Bandman, 2002). Individuals often have priorities different from those of the health care professional, and even what seems like a "bad choice" needs to be respected (Bosek & Savage, 2006). The role of the nurse is to facilitate a communicative environment in which people can exercise their right to make informed free choices. Individuals need to participate in the decision-making process when their lives may be influenced by a change.

Although each person's state of health affects family members and the community, individuals are responsible for their own health maintenance. Health professionals need to accept and welcome individual differences in meeting this responsibility. By selecting interventions that create an environment of open communication and risk taking, individuals can better develop the problem-solving skills to direct their own growth and development.

Cultural Considerations in Health Teaching

Another challenge for health professionals is to apply health-education strategies with people from other cultural backgrounds, people who do not speak English as their native language, and people who cannot read at elementary levels. The health professional needs to take the time to assess cultural beliefs that influence social and health practices and make an effort to analyze educational interventions that are acceptable and satisfying to the individual. Social marketing processes discussed in the next section help identify characteristics, interests, and concerns of target populations.

When teaching people of different cultural, racial, and ethnic groups, the nurse endeavors to provide culturally sensitive client education. Nurses recognize that the person's or group's background, beliefs, and knowledge may differ significantly from their own and seek to understand and show respect for these differences (Degazon, 2008) (Multicultural Awareness box).

MULTICULTURAL AWARENESS
Cultural Aspects of Health Teaching

WHEN THERE IS A LANGUAGE BARRIER
- Use courtesy and a formal approach.
- Address the person by his or her last name.
- Introduce yourself, pointing to yourself as you give your name.
- Project a friendly attitude with a smile and a handshake.
- Speak with a moderate tone and volume.
- Attempt to use words in the person's language, which indicates respect for the individual's culture.
- Use simple, everyday words rather than complex words, medical jargon, or colloquialisms.
- Use hand gestures to help the person understand.
- Instruct the person in small increments.
- Have the person demonstrate understanding of the message.
- Write down the instructions for the person to take home.
- Involve others who can serve as interpreters.
- When available, use flash cards and phrase books in other languages.

AREAS TO CONSIDER IN CULTURAL ASSESSMENT
- Individual's identification with a particular cultural group
- Habits, customs, values, and beliefs
- Language and communication patterns
- Cultural sanctions and restrictions
- Healing beliefs and practices
- Cultural health practices
- Kinship and social networks
- Nutritional beliefs, food preferences, and restrictions
- Religious beliefs and practices related to health
- Attitudes, values, and beliefs about health (Andrews & Boyle, 2008)

SOCIAL MARKETING AND HEALTH EDUCATION

When nurses begin to teach groups of people, they automatically enter a program planning and administrative process. When an organization wants to offer an ongoing health-education program for a target population, social marketing provides a strategy for reaching members of the group and implementing a service that will satisfy these members as consumers. Principles of social marketing and health-education strategies are combined to promote population-based changes in behavior to improve health.

Social marketing is defined as "the application of commercial marketing technologies to the analysis, planning, execution, and evaluation of programs designed to influence the voluntary behavior of target audiences in order to improve their personal welfare and that of their society" (Andreasen, 1995, p. 7). The primary objective of social marketing is to change behavior. Key attributes of a social marketing approach are the offering of benefits and the reduction of barriers to influence market members' behavior. Social marketers attempt to modify the attractiveness of specific behavioral options to favor one choice over competing alternatives. It is a consumer-oriented process that tends to be culturally sensitive (Maibach et al., 2004). For example, social marketing strategies could be used in designing smoking-cessation programs for ethnic minorities. Health-related social marketing offerings may include physical goods such as nutritious lunches, services such as stress management workshops, or ideas and concepts such as encouraging safer sex or preventing heart disease (Bensley & Brookins-Fisher, 2003). Any information about the target population that is generated by social marketing strategies will improve the nurse's ability to develop effective educational interventions.

TEACHING PLAN

Preparation for teaching a group program, such as a seminar or course, begins after the marketing and administrative plans are well underway. These activities ensure that there are enough participants for the program, and they provide the structure for developing the teaching plan—the program objectives, available time, human and material resources, and so on. When the marketing and administrative functions have been provided by others and when educational strategies are developed for one person at a time, the nurse can concentrate efforts on developing the teaching plan.

A health-teaching plan may emphasize a phase of the behavior change process that is related to the individual's health-promotion needs or problems. The written teaching plan represents a package of educational services provided to a consumer or student. The plan is written from the learner's point of view.

The process of generating a teaching plan helps the nurse recognize and use methods of learning that involve the individual as an active participant. The plan includes a list of specific actions or abilities that the person may perform at intervals during and at the end of the educational intervention. Teaching plans help nurses clarify these outcomes. Preparing a teaching plan involves the steps of the teaching-learning process outlined in Box 10-2.

Assessment

Assessment, the first step in the process, involves determining the characteristics of the learner and identifying learning needs. The following characteristics of the learner are important for the nurse to identify and consider in planning:

- Age, developmental stage in the life cycle, and level of education
- Health beliefs
- Motivation and readiness to learn
- Health risks and problems
- Current knowledge and skills
- Barriers and facilitators to learning

The reader is encouraged to refer to the chapters about individual development (see Unit 4).

| Box 10-2 | Steps in the Teaching-Learning Process |

I. Assessment
  A. Learner characteristics
  B. Learning needs
II. Development of expected learning outcomes
III. Development of a teaching plan
  A. Content
  B. Teaching strategies, learning activities
IV. Implementation of the teaching plan
V. Evaluation of expected outcomes
  A. Achievement of learning outcomes
  B. Evaluation of the teaching process

Assessment of the learner can be accomplished by answering the following five questions:

1. What are the characteristics and learning capabilities of the individual?
2. What are the learner's needs for health promotion, risk reduction, or health problems?
3. What does the person already know and what skills can the person already perform that are relevant to the health needs?
4. Is the learner motivated to change any unhealthy behaviors?
5. What are the barriers to and facilitators of health behavior change?

When preparing a teaching plan for one person in a primary care setting, the nurse may learn background information about the individual from that person's record and agency reports that include descriptions of the person's population group. Nurses often agree to teach health classes that others have organized. In this case, the nurse asks for project reports that provide marketing and needs-assessment information about the students who are expected to attend the classes (see the Case Study and Care Plan at the end of this chapter).

Determining Expected Learning Outcomes

To determine the expected learning outcomes of a health-education intervention, the nurse answers the following questions:

1. What broad public health and social goals guide the proposed educational program?
2. What are the participant's learning goals?
3. What does the learner need to know, do, and believe to progress through the behavior change process?

Program Goals

The program goals of a health-education project reflect the desire to facilitate improvement in some health problem or social living condition. Program goals are broad statements on long-range expected accomplishments that provide direction; they do not have to be stated in measurable terms (Porche, 2004).

Learning Goals

Learning goals are best established when the student and the nurse work together. These goals reflect the health behavior or health status change that the person will have achieved by the end of an educational intervention. Learning goals relate to the program goals.

Learning Objectives

Learning objectives indicate the steps to be taken by the individual toward meeting the learning goal and may involve the development of knowledge, skill, or change in attitude. Objectives are most useful when stated in behavioral terms and when they contain these components: (1) the learner and a precise action verb that indicates what the learner will be able to do, (2) the conditions under which the task is performed, and (3) the level of performance expected (Bastable & Doody, 2008). Learning objectives guide the selection of content and methods and help narrow the focus of a teaching plan to more achievable steps; they also aid in setting standards of performance and suggesting evaluation strategies.

Selecting Content

To select appropriate content for a health-education program, the nurse considers what information, skills, and attitudes need to be taught and the level of learning to be achieved.

Three Domains of Learning

Content is commonly divided into three domains: (1) cognitive, (2) psychomotor, and (3) affective. Cognitive learning refers to the development of new facts or concepts, and building on or applying knowledge to new situations. Psychomotor learning involves developing physical skills from simple to complex actions. Affective learning alludes to the recognition of values, religious and spiritual beliefs, family interaction patterns and relationships, and personal attitudes that affect decisions and problem-solving progress.

To learn or change a health behavior, a person may need to acquire new information, practice some physical techniques, and clarify the ways in which the new behavior may affect relationships with others. The nurse's role is to select a combination of content from the three domains that is appropriate to meet the behavioral objective. To find samples of content for a teaching plan, the nurse researches resource materials, such as books, teaching guides, journal articles, pamphlets, and flyers created by nonprofit agencies and professional organizations. The nurse is careful about giving students materials with technical vocabulary that is too complex for the audience.

Examples of Learning Objectives

In writing learning objectives, the nurse selects action verbs from the taxonomies previously mentioned that indicate observable learning. In Table 10-1, examples are given for objectives in each domain of learning. The first objective

Table 10-1 Examples of Objectives that Are Not Measurable Rewritten in Measurable Form

Domain	Objectives
Cognitive	Not Measurable: Dan will understand the correct food choices for following a diabetic diet. Measurable: Dan will correctly **select** food choices based on his diabetic meal plan.
Affective	Not Measurable: Dan will demonstrate the importance of regular blood glucose monitoring by checking his blood glucose before each meal and at bedtime. Measurable: Dan will **verbalize** the importance of checking his blood glucose before each meal and at bedtime.
Psychomotor	Not Measurable: Dan will know how to correctly give himself an insulin injection. Measurable: Dan will **demonstrate** proper technique and dosage when giving an insulin injection to himself.

listed for each domain is incorrect because the verb does not indicate observable learning. The second example for each domain is measurable because the verb used (indicated in bold) allows the learning to be observed.

Levels of Learning

The level of learning to be achieved depends on how the nurse anticipates that the content will be used. Taxonomies developed by Bloom and others (Bloom et al., 1956; Krathwohl et al., 1964) remain widely accepted as the standard tools for arranging levels of learning objectives according to type and complexity. For example, in the cognitive domain, levels of learning include the following:

- Knowledge: person recalls facts and the concept
- Comprehension: person understands the meaning of the concept
- Application: person uses the concept
- Analysis: person can examine or explain the concept
- Synthesis: person integrates the concept with other learning
- Evaluation: person judges or compares the concept

When preparing a teaching plan, the nurse differentiates between information the individual needs to know and information considered helpful to develop appropriate learning objectives. This process provides cues to the nurse for planning effective strategies for the necessary level of learning. As the level of learning to be achieved becomes complex, the educational strategies and methods selected involve the individuals in more active application and analysis of the content.

Designing Learning Strategies

Designing the learning strategies for an educational intervention means selecting the methods and tools and structuring the sequence of activities. The teaching plan to this point provides the foundation on which to base the activity selection and sequence. The following questions guide the design of learning strategies:

1. What are some basic considerations for selecting teaching methods for health-education programs?
2. How does the nurse, as instructor, establish and maintain a learning climate?
3. What actions can the nurse perform to increase the effectiveness of the learning methods?
4. What are the appropriate methods for each learning domain?
5. What methods tend to promote behavior change?

Teaching Strategies

Numerous strategies for teaching are available. A few of those most commonly used are listed and described here. Lecture is a well-known method in which the teacher verbally presents information and instructions to the person or audience. Lecture provides a way to present a large amount of information to a number of people in a nonthreatening way. This can be an effective method if active learning strategies are integrated. Discussion involves interaction between the nurse educator and the individuals. The nurse prepares questions in advance to guide the discussion. This method allows an opportunity for the nurse to gain a better perception of the individuals' understanding of the topic and to clarify the information.

Demonstration and practice is used in learning psychomotor skills such as giving oneself an injection, changing a dressing, or performing exercises. The nurse demonstrates the expected behavior while the person observes. Then the nurse watches and provides feedback and encouragement while the person performs the behavior. Using the actual equipment that the individual will use in their home facilitates successful performance. For complex tasks, teaching a few steps at a time in sequence aids skill development.

Simulation gaming may involve computer learning, board games, or role play. Obviously, the opportunity to use computer learning games depends on the availability of hardware and software appropriate for the individual and the topic. Simple board games can be developed for cognitive learning. An example might be developing a bingo game based on the food pyramid. Role play involves acting out a potential scenario. This allows individuals to practice appropriate responses to challenging situations. For example, a person on a low-fat diet can act out a response to being offered dessert by an insistent family member or friend played by the nurse. Or a grandmother, unsure of what to do when her grandson's blood sugar is high, might practice making calls to the doctor and giving the necessary information.

Considerations for Selecting Methods

The nurse's first consideration is to promote an environment and use methods that foster self-directed learning. An active participant usually learns more.

There will be many learning styles in a group audience; therefore, the nurse varies the teaching methods used in a given session. Taking into consideration the characteristics of the population (developmental stage, age, and knowledge of the topic), the nurse selects teaching methods that best support the goals and theme of the educational program. The order of content proceeds from simple ideas and skills to the more complex concepts, from known material toward lesser-known data. The nurse is sensitive to the energy level and anxiety of the audience when presenting content that requires strong concentration or causes anxiety.

Learning Climate

For group presentations, the nurse addresses several activities when seeking to establish an environment conducive to health behavior change. The first activity is creating a sense of preparedness and organization by providing physical facilities with adequate furnishings and suitable audiovisual materials and handouts. Even the instructor's appearance will lend credibility or distraction to the presentation.

The second activity involves anticipating the needs of the group and communicating information about the schedule and the facilities. This action alleviates the group's apprehension and makes them more comfortable.

The third activity focuses on the nurse's assessment of the individual and group learning needs, possibly through questions and dialogue. Members of the group need to believe that the program will be beneficial and relevant to their situations. The instructor watches for and reinforces signs of motivation to participate in the experience.

Fourth, having established a positive learning climate, the nurse seeks to maintain a high level of motivation, a sense of individualized attention, and a progression. As a reality check, the nurse might ask for periodic feedback from the group about the effectiveness of the program and its relevance to group needs.

Finally, the nurse works with the group to maintain the learning climate. This process involves observing group interactions, helping individuals to participate, intervening to help the group deal with controlling its members, and remaining cognizant of dynamics in the group process that will facilitate or inhibit learning.

Teaching for Each Learning Domain

As mentioned, teaching is directed toward one or more of three learning domains: (1) cognitive, (2) psychomotor, and (3) affective. Examples of appropriate teaching strategies for each domain and the expected outcomes in relation to behavior change are summarized in Table 10-2. Which domain of learning do you think is portrayed by the method of instruction shown in Figure 10-1?

Evaluating the Teaching-Learning Process

The teacher can evaluate the learning, or measure achievement of learning objectives, in all domains through the use of written or oral testing, demonstrations, observation,

Table **10-2**	Domains of Learning, Teaching Strategies, and Examples of Desired Outcomes Related to a Behavior Change	
Domain of Learning	**Teaching Strategies**	**Examples of Desired Outcomes Related to a Behavior Change**
Cognitive (thinking)	Lecture One-to-one instruction Discussion Discovery Audiovisual or printed materials Computer-assisted instruction	Describes and/ or explains information relevant to the behavior change
Affective (feeling)	Role modeling Discussion Role playing Simulation gaming	Expresses positive feeling, attitudes, values toward changing the behavior
Psychomotor (acting)	Demonstration Practice Mental imaging	Demonstrates performance of skills related to the behavior change

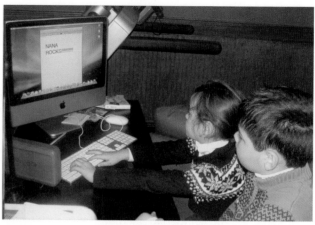

Figure 10-1   School-aged children engaged in computer learning activities.

self-reports, and self-monitoring. Teaching methods for one domain may overlap those for another domain.

The nurse can incorporate written, verbal, and nonverbal techniques into the teaching plan for obtaining feedback about teaching performance. Postprogram questionnaires are the usual method for obtaining written feedback. The nurse may ask for verbal feedback at various times from the group, from individual students, and from observers of the class. Nonverbal communication cues from participants may indicate their satisfaction, fatigue, or frustration with the educational intervention.

The overall process of the teaching-learning experience needs to be evaluated. The procedures used to organize and promote an educational program can affect its ultimate success. The nurse (or a program administration committee) records activities such as advertising, registration, fee collection, and availability and repair of equipment and materials. This evaluative information can then be used to improve subsequent programs. Surveys by telephone or by postprogram questionnaires help obtain the consumer's opinion about these implementation procedures (Research Highlights box). Word-of-mouth referrals to future programs and support from other community agencies and professionals may also indicate approval of the program format.

Occasionally the nurse is asked to justify a health-education program in terms of its effect on the community's public health goals or social problems. Health promotion involves a combination of health-protection activities, preventive health services, and health-education programs; therefore, drawing a direct correlation between an educational intervention and the statistical improvement of the health problem can be difficult.

Nurses often can describe the theoretical influence of an educational intervention on health behaviors, health problems, and social problems. Statistics such as the number of people served each year, the percentage of the target population reached, the number of service providers used, and the number and cost of programs are important and need to be preserved. As these statistics change over time, the data will provide cues to program successes and problems.

Referring Individuals to Other Resources

The end of a teaching plan includes resources for people to use for continuing education, counseling, peer support, and health services. Nurses encourage people to view health education as a lifelong learning process. Each person has different developmental needs and health concerns through the life cycle. Moreover, any one educational intervention may help a person move only from one phase of the behavior change process to the next. Additionally, many variables aside from learning may influence a person's health practices (Hot Topics box).

TEACHING AND ORGANIZING SKILLS

To develop teaching and organizing skills in health education, the nurse often needs to learn new behaviors. A systematic guide can be used for learning these professional skills. To perform these steps, the nurse does the following:

- Seeks self-assessment opportunities
- Identifies, lists, and prioritizes learning needs
- Begins to identify the resources that are available for reading, instructor training, and practice teaching
- Drafts an initial set of learning goals
- Selects the target population and the general topic
- Works through steps of the teaching-learning process, including the development of a teaching plan
- Identifies other people or a project team to help

research highlights

Health Promotion via the Telephone

Telephone interventions have been used by nurses, especially ambulatory care nurses, for many years. Reduced length of hospital stay minimizes the time for individuals' learning and adjustment to their health conditions. Telenursing can bridge this gap by serving as a means to teach individuals and their caregivers. Research documents the effective use of telephone nursing interventions in several areas. These areas include primary, secondary, and tertiary prevention strategies promoting physical and mental health. The specific interventions include:

- Promoting safety of abused women (McFarlane et al., 2004)
- Improving HbA1C levels and adherence to diet and blood glucose testing in people with diabetes (Kim & Oh, 2003)
- Reducing post-discharge anxiety for individuals and their partners recovering from cardiac bypass surgery (Hartford, 2005)
- Providing education and support for self-care practices of older adults who provide care for their spouses with dementia (Teel & Leenerts, 2005)
- Supporting individuals with new ostomies resulting from cancer treatment (Bohnenkamp et al., 2004)
- Monitoring and managing high-risk, older cardiac surgery clients after discharge (Kleinpell & Avitall, 2007)
- Reducing hospital readmission rates among heart failure clients (McManus, 2004)
- Providing post-rehabilitation informational, decision making, and interpersonal support for spinal cord–injured individuals (Lucke et al., 2004)
- Increasing physical activity in sedentary women in the workplace (Purath et al., 2004)
- Reducing unnecessary physician or emergency department visits by giving parents proper advice for home care of febrile children (Light, 2005)
- Providing telephone follow-up for individuals instead of clinic visits after intra-articular knee injection (McGinley & Lucas, 2006)
- Reducing rates of overt heart failure symptoms and hospital readmission of heart failure clients in the community, with telephone interventions by senior nursing students (Wheeler & Waterhouse, 2006)
- Decreasing rehospitalization, decreasing symptoms of heart failure, and increasing quality of life in home care clients (Quinn, 2006)

- Reducing the frequency of home care visits in congestive heart failure clients (Myers et al., 2006)
- Improving systolic blood pressure in urban African Americans with hypertension (Artinian et al., 2007)
- Providing individualized teaching after bone density testing to enhance osteoporosis prevention in women (Sedlack et al., 2005)

Cardiovascular disease affects a tremendous number of people. Telenursing is a low-cost, low-technology intervention that offers a potential means to reduce the risks related to cardiovascular disease. In a study of urban African Americans with hypertension, telemonitoring resulted in clinically and statistically significant reduction of systolic blood pressure over a 12-month period. When compared with the usual care group, the telemonitoring intervention group also had a greater, but not statistically significant, reduction in diastolic blood pressure (Artinian et al., 2007).

Care for persons with heart failure in the community is complex and challenging from many aspects. These challenges include symptom control and prevention of hospital readmission. A study by Wheeler & Waterhouse (2006) reports an effective telephone intervention provided by nursing students for heart failure clients in their homes. Senior nursing students were paired with community nursing staff. Each student was assigned two clients for whom to provide telephone intervention in their homes for 12 to 14 weeks. The individuals who received the telephone follow-up intervention had lower rates of hospital readmissions and fewer overt heart failure symptoms in comparison to the control group (Wheeler & Waterhouse, 2006).

Advantages of telenursing are believed to include decreased cost of therapeutic interactions, increased access to rural and other distant people (including international individuals), and cost savings resulting from direction of individuals to more appropriate use of health care services, such as avoiding unnecessary after-hours visits to the emergency room. With the growth of managed care financing for health care, telephone nursing is expected to increase. Additional research is needed to describe telephone nursing interventions and to evaluate their effectiveness. The current standards of practice for telenursing, developed by the American Academy of Ambulatory Care Nursing in 2007, provide criteria to facilitate studying the outcomes of telephone interventions by nurses.

After implementing the educational intervention, the nurse sets time aside to discuss what took place. Did the program go as planned? What changes were made in the teaching plan? What can be changed for the next program? The nurse reviews the self-developed learning goals and determines new ones.

As additional programs on either an individual or group basis are provided, the nurse will be able to clarify specific instructor teaching and organizing skills that come naturally. These skills tend to improve a program's effectiveness and enable the logistics to run smoothly. The teacher is first a learner; this is true in health education and any other form of education.

SUMMARY

Of all health professionals, nurses spend the most time in direct contact with individuals; they have many opportunities to recognize a need for knowledge and a readiness to learn new information and behaviors. Nurses often coordinate group programs. The more accurate the analysis of the educational aspects of a health-promotion program and the assessment of characteristics and learning needs of the target audience is, the more effective an educational intervention will be in influencing health behaviors.

The principles of health education form a generic basis for implementing a variety of health topics, such as accident prevention and first aid, expectant parent education, hypertension education, nutrition and fitness, stress management, substance abuse, sex education, and client education in areas including diabetes and arthritis. The two scenarios described in this chapter provide insights into the nurse's role in conducting educational interventions about family planning and prenatal care.

Planning to teach one person is different from planning to teach a group. One-to-one interventions tend to follow a counseling or problem-solving approach. Group interventions can range from guided discussions on concerns that evolve from the group to a more structured learning experience involving presentations, skill practice, and attitude-awareness exercises. The range of health education strategies provides nurses and all health care professionals with techniques and methods applicable in health service settings, schools, work sites, and other community facilities.

HOTtopics

THE INTERNET AS A HEALTH EDUCATION TOOL

The availability of health information on the Internet has far-reaching implications for health education. The Internet provides access to information from numerous sources on a broad range of topics to an increasing number of individuals and families. Examples of these topics include well-child care, women's health, nutrition, and information regarding disease treatment and provision of home care for the terminally ill.

Consumers have access to a wealth of valuable information, but they may be overwhelmed by the number and types of resources. Some resources may be useful and accurate; others may be biased, inaccurate, misunderstood, and potentially problematic. Nurses need to develop skill in using the Internet as a client-education tool and in guiding individuals' selection of health information sources.

Guidelines are available for selecting sources. One that is useful is *How to Evaluate Health Information on the Internet: Questions and Answers* from the National Cancer Institute. This can be found on the institute's website at *www.cancer.gov/cancertopics/factsheet/Information/Internet*.

In addition, the Health on the Net Foundation (HON) code on a website indicates that it is a recognized nongovernmental source of "reliable, understandable, relevant, and trustworthy" medical and health information based on eight principles (Health on the Net Foundation, 2008).

Before recommending Internet sources, nurses determine if the source is reputable and reliable and if the information is current, accurate, understandable, and appropriate for the target audience. The nurse identifies sites that may be useful to the target group and checks them before recommending them. Encouraging people to discuss information obtained from Internet resources is essential to establish an opportunity to clarify their understanding and direct them to sources that are more appropriate, when necessary.

Websites that provide access to general health information include:

www.mayoclinic.com
www.healthfinder.gov
www.intelihealth.com
www.medlineplus.gov
www.health.gov
www.aoa.gov
www.nutrition.gov

The Internet may also serve as an avenue of accessibility to an abundance of information for persons from rural areas or who are homebound. Although Internet access is expanding rapidly, it is important to recognize that not everyone has access in their homes. This is particularly true for those with lower levels of income or education.

CASE STUDY

International Travel: Albert

Albert Mitchell is a 36-year-old man who will be traveling to Dubai to give a business presentation in 3 months. Although he has traveled widely in the United States as a consultant, this is his first trip to the Middle East. He requests information regarding immunizations needed prior to his trip. Albert states that since he will only be in Dubai for a few days, he is unlikely to contract a disease in such a short time and does not think that it makes sense to get immunizations. Albert states that he has heard that the side effects of the immunizations might be worse that the diseases they prevent. He is also concerned about leaving his wife at home alone since she is 6-months pregnant.

Reflective Questions:
1. How would you address Albert's beliefs?
2. What learning would be needed in each domain?
3. What learning theories would you consider?
4. How might his family concerns be addressed?

CARE PLAN

Preparing a Teaching Plan: Albert

Nursing Diagnosis: Knowledge Deficit (Specify Area)

DEFINING CHARACTERISTICS

- Verbalization of inadequate information or an inadequate recall of information
- Verbalization of misunderstanding or misconception
- Request for information
- Instructions followed inaccurately
- Inadequate performance on a test
- Inadequate demonstration of a skill

RELATED FACTORS

- Pathophysiological states
- Sensory deficits
- Memory loss
- Intellectual limitations
- Interfering coping strategies (denial or anxiety)
- Lack of exposure to accurate information
- Lack of motivation to learn
- Inattention
- Cultural or language barriers

EXPECTED OUTCOMES

- The individual will express an interest in learning.
- The individual will correctly state the information on the specific topic.
- The individual will correctly demonstrate skills needed to practice health-related behavior.
- The individual and family will explain how to incorporate new information into their lifestyle.
- The individual will modify health behavior based on the acquisition of new knowledge.
- The individual will list resources for more information or support.

INTERVENTIONS

- Provide accurate and culturally relevant information related to the specific topic.
- Select teaching techniques appropriate to the individual's learning needs.
- Explore the individual's interpretation of the information and its meaning in the context of the person's life.
- Demonstrate and then have the individual practice new skills.
- Assist the person in identifying and implementing alternative strategies when initial choices are not successful.
- Include the family or significant others as appropriate.
- Provide names and telephone numbers of resource people or organizations.

REFERENCES

American Nurses Association. (2003). *Nursing's social policy statement.* Washington, DC: The Association.

American Nurses Association. (2004). *Nursing: Scope and standards of practice.* Silver Spring, MD: American Nurses Association.

Anderson, C. (2003). Evolving out of violence: An application of the Transtheoretical Model of Behavioral Change. *Research & Theory for Nursing Practice, 17*(3), 225–240.

Anderson, D. G., Ward, H., & Hatton, D. C. (2008). Family health risks. In M. Stanhope & J. Lancaster (Eds.), *Public health nursing: Population-centered health care in the community* (7th ed.). St. Louis: Mosby.

Andreasen, A. R. (1995). *Marketing social change: Changing behavior to promote health, social development, and the environment.* San Francisco: Jossey-Bass.

Andrews, M. M., & Boyle, J. S. (2008). *Transcultural concepts in nursing care* (5th ed.). Philadelphia: Lippincott Williams & Wilkins.

Artinian, N. T., Flack, J. M., Nordstrom, C. K., Hockman, E. M., Washington, O. G., Jen, K. L., et al. (2007). Effects of nurse-managed telemonitoring on blood pressure at 12-month follow-up among urban African Americans. *Nursing Research, 56*(5), 312–322.

Bandman, E. L., & Bandman, B. (2002). *Nursing ethics through the life span* (4th ed.). Upper Saddle River, NJ: Prentice Hall.

Bandura, A. (1997). *Self-efficacy: The exercise of control.* New York: Worth Publishers.

Bastable, S. B., & Dart, M. A. (2008). Developmental stages of the learner. In S. B. Bastable (Ed.), *Nurse as educator: Principles of teaching and learning for nursing practice* (3rd ed.). Sudbury, MA: Jones & Bartlett.

Bastable, S. B., & Doody, J. A. (2008). Behavioral objectives. In S. B. Bastable (Ed.), *Nurse as educator: Principles of teaching and learning for nursing practice* (3rd ed.). Sudbury, MA: Jones & Bartlett.

Becker, M. H. (1974). *The health belief model and personal health behavior.* Thorofare, NJ: Charles B. Slack.

Bensley, R. J., & Brookins-Fisher, J. (2003). *Community health education methods: A practical guide* (2nd ed.). Sudbury, MA: Jones & Bartlett.

Bloom, B. S., Englehart, M. S., Furst, E. J., Hill, W. H., & Krathwohl, D. J. (1956). *Taxonomy of educational objectives: The classification of educational goals—Handbook 1: Cognitive domain.* White Plains, NY: Longman.

Bohnenkamp, S. K., McDonald, P., Lopez, A. M., Krupinski, E., & Blackett, A. (2004). Traditional versus telenursing outpatient management of patients with cancer with new ostomies. *Oncology Nursing Press, 31*(5), 1005–1010.

Bosek, M. S., & Savage, T. A. (2006). *The ethical component of nursing education: Integrating ethics into clinical experiences.* Philadelphia: Lippincott Williams Wilkins.

Degazon, C. E. (2008). Cultural diversity in the community. In M. Stanhope & J. Lancaster (Eds.), *Public health nursing: Population-centered health care in the community* (7th ed.). St. Louis: Mosby.

Galavotti, C., Pappas-DeLuca, K. A., & Lansky, A. (2001). Modeling and reinforcement to combat HIV: The MARCH approach to behavior change. *American Journal of Public Health, 91*(10), 1602–1607.

Glanz, K., Rimer, B. K., & Lewis, F. M. (2003). *Health behavior and health education: Theory, research, and practice* (3rd ed.). San Francisco: Jossey-Bass.

Hartford, K. (2005). Telenursing and patients' recovery from bypass surgery. *Journal of Advanced Nursing, 50*(5), 459–468.

Health on the Net Foundation. (2008). *www.hon.ch/*

Janz, N. K., & Becker, M. H. (1984). The Health Belief Model: A decade later. *Health Education Quarterly, 11*(1), 1–47.

Kim, H. J., & Oh, J. A. (2003). Adherence to diabetes control recommendations:

Impact of nurse telephone calls. *Journal of Advanced Nursing, 44*(3), 256–261.

Kleinpell, R. M., & Avitall, B. (2007). Integrating telehealth as a strategy for patient management after discharge for cardiac surgery: Results of a pilot study. *Journal of Cardiovascular Nursing, 22*(1), 38–42.

Krathwohl, D. R., Bloom, B. S., & Masia, B. B. (1964). *Taxonomy of educational objectives: The classification of educational goals—Handbook 2: Affective domain.* New York: David McKay.

Lee, P. R., & Estes, C. L. (2003). *The nation's health* (7th ed.). Sudbury, MA: Jones & Bartlett.

Light, P. A. (2005). Nursing telephone triage and its influence on parents' choice of care for febrile children. *Journal of Pediatric Nursing, 20*(6), 424–429.

Lucke, K. T., Lucke, J. F., & Martinez, H. (2004). Evaluation of a peer + professional telephone intervention with spinal-cord-injured individuals following rehabilitation in South Texas. *Journal of Multicultural Nursing & Health, 10*(2), 68–74.

Maibach, E. W., Rothschild, M. L., & Novelli, W. D. (2004). Social marketing. In K. Glanz, B. K. Rimer, & F. M. Lewis (Eds.), *Health behavior and health education: Theory, research, and practice* (3rd ed.). San Francisco: Jossey-Bass.

Marotz, L. R., Cross, M. Z., & Rush, J. M. (2005). *Health, safety, and nutrition for the young child* (6th ed.). Clifton Park, NY: Thomson Delmar Learning.

Mauriello, L. M., Driskell, M. M., Sherman, K. J., Johnson, S. S., Prochaska, J. M., & Prochaska, J. O. (2006). Acceptability of a school-based intervention for the prevention of adolescent obesity. *Journal of School Nursing, 22*(5), 269–277.

McFarlane, J., Malecha, A., Gist, J., Watson, K., Batten, E., Hall, I., et al. (2004). Increasing the safety-promoting behaviors of abused women. *American Journal of Nursing, 104*(3), 40–51.

McGinley, A., & Lucas, B. (2006). Telenursing: A pilot of telephone review after intra-artic-ular knee injection. *Journal of Orthopaedic Nursing, 10*(3), 144–150.

McGinnis, J. M. (2003). A vision for health in our new century. *American Journal of Health Promotion, 18*(2), 146–150.

McManus, S. G. (2004). A telehealth program to reduce readmission rates among heart failure patients: One agency's experience. *Home Health Care Management & Practice, 16*(4), 250–254.

Morrison, G. S. (2007). *Early childhood education today* (10th ed.). Upper Saddle River, NJ: Pearson Education.

Myers, S., Grant, R. W., Lugn, N. E., Holbert, B., & Kvedar, J. C. (2006). Impact of home-based monitoring on the care of patients with congestive heart failure. *Home Health Care Management & Practice, 18*(6), 444–451.

Ott, C. D., Lindsey, A. M., Waltman, N. L., Gross, G. J., Twiss, J. J., Berg, K., et al. (2004). Facilitative strategies, psychosocial factors, and strength/weight training behaviors in breast cancer survivors who are at risk for osteoporosis. *Orthopaedic Nursing, 23*(1), 45–52.

Paul, S., & Sneed, N. V. (2004). Strategies for behavior change in patients with heart failure. *American Journal of Critical Care, 13*(4), 305–313.

Porche, D. J. (2004). *Public and community health nursing practice: A population-based approach.* Thousand Oaks, CA: Sage.

Prochaska, J. O., & DiClemente, C. C. (1984). *The transtheoretical approach: Crossing traditional boundaries of change.* Homewood, NJ: Dow Jones-Irwin.

Purath, J., Miller, A. M., McCabe, G., & Wibur, J. (2004). A brief intervention to increase physical activity in sedentary working women. *Canadian Journal of Nursing Research, 36*(1), 76–91.

Quinn, C. (2006). Low-technology heart failure care in home health: Improving patient outcomes. *Home Healthcare Nurse, 24*(8), 533–540.

Rankin, S. H., Stallings, K. D., & London, F. (2005). *Patient education in health and illness* (5th ed.). Philadelphia: Lippincott Williams & Wilkins.

Richards, E., & Digger, K. (2008). Compliance, motivation, and health behaviors of the learner. In S. B. Bastable (Ed.), *Nurse as educator: Principles of teaching and learning for nursing practice* (3rd ed.). Sudbury, MA: Jones & Bartlett.

Rosenstock, I. M., Strecher, V. J., & Becker, M. H. (1988). The social learning theory and Health Belief Model. *Health Education & Behavior, 15*(2), 175–183.

Saarmann, L., Daugherty, J., & Riegel, B. (2002). Teaching staff a brief cognitive-behavioral intervention. *MEDSURG Nursing, 11*(3), 114–151.

Schroeder, S. A. (2007). We can do better—Improving the health of the American people. *New England Journal of Medicine, 357*(12), 1221–1228.

Sedlack, C. A., Doheny, M. O., Estok, P. J., Zeller, P. J., & Wincehell, J. (2007). DXA, health beliefs, and osteoporosis prevention behaviors. *Journal of Aging and Health, 19*(5), 742–756.

Teel, C. S., & Leenerts, M. H. (2005). Developing and testing a Self-Care intervention for older adults in caregiving roles. *Nursing Research, 54*(3), 193–201.

U.S. Department of Health and Human Services. (2000). *Healthy people 2010* (Vol. 1-2, Conference ed.). Washington, DC: U.S. Department of Health and Human Services.

U.S. Department of Health and Human Services. (2007, November 5). *Healthy people 2020: The road ahead.* Retrieved from *www.healthypeople.gov/hp.*

Wheeler, E. C., & Waterhouse, J. K. (2006). Telephone interventions by nursing students: Improving outcomes for heart failure patients in the community. *Journal of Community Health Nursing, 23*(3), 137–146.

Wurzbach, M. E. (2004). *Community health education and promotion: A guide to program design and evaluation* (2nd ed.). Boston: Jones & Bartlett.

Chapter 11

Lenny Chiang-Hanisko*

Nutrition Counseling for Health Promotion

objectives

After completing this chapter, the reader will be able to:

- Identify *Healthy People 2010* nutrition objectives.

- Analyze the leading nutrition-related causes of illness and death in the United States and identify the dietary factors associated with each cause.

- Summarize the nutrition recommendations contained in the Dietary Guidelines for Americans.

- Compare the number of servings and serving sizes recommended in MyPyramid with serving features currently in the marketplace.

- Compare the current MyPyramid with other suggested versions of daily nutrition requirements.

- Analyze U.S. food aid programs for the poor and older adults.

- Plan a 1-day menu that is consistent with recent dietary guidance for a person at any stage of the life cycle.

key terms

Body Mass Index (BMI)
Bovine spongiform encephalopathy (BSE)
Cancer
Cardiovascular disease
Cholesterol
Coronary heart disease
Creutzfeldt-Jakob disease (nvCJD)
Diabetes mellitus
Dietary guidelines
Dietary Reference Intakes
Dyslipidemia
Fat

Fiber
Heart disease
High-density lipoprotein (HDL)
Human immunodeficiency virus
Hyperglycemia
Hyperlipidemia
Hypertension
Incidence
Low-density lipoprotein (LDL)
Metabolic syndrome
MyPyramid
Nutrition screening

Obesity
Osteoporosis
Overweight
Prevalence
Salmonellosis
Serving sizes
Stroke
Sugar
Teratogenic
Trans fatty acid
Triglyceride
Type 2 diabetes
Underweight

*The author wishes to acknowledge the work of Linda Snetselaar in the previous edition as the foundation of this chapter.

website materials

*e*volve

These materials are located on the book's Website at *http://evolve.elsevier.com/Edelman/.*
- WebLinks
- Study Questions
- Glossary
- Website Resources

  11A: Sodium Content of Foods

  11B: Recommendations for Calcium and Vitamin D Intake

  11C: Healthy Weight, Overweight, and Obesity Among People 20 Years of Age and Older

  11D: Body Weight in Pounds According to Height and Body Mass Index

  11E: Sources of Nutrition Information

THINK About It

Nutritional Self-Assessment

Begin thinking about your food and health and the food and health of people around you. Check each statement that describes the way you usually eat. Add the number of statements that you have checked and compare that number with the scores listed after the questions.

The way I usually eat:
- I eat whole grain or enriched breads, cereals, rice, or pasta daily.
- I eat 2 to 3 pieces or more of fruit daily.
- I eat 2 to 3 cups or more of raw or cooked vegetables daily.
- I drink skim milk and eat low-fat or fat-free dairy products daily.
- I trim fat from meat and take the skin off chicken and turkey or I do not eat meat.
- I eat small servings (no larger than the size of a deck of cards) of meat, poultry, and fish or I do not eat meat.
- Most food and snacks that I eat are not fried or are made with no added fat.
- I add very little fat (butter, margarine, oil, or salad dressing) to my food.

- Most desserts and snacks that I eat contain no added sugar.
- Most of what I drink is made without sugar or contains no added sugar.
- I rarely cook with salt or add salt at the table.
- I do not drink alcohol or I drink no more than 1 to 2 beers, 1 to 2 glasses of wine, or 1 to 2 mixed drinks daily.

Number of statements checked:

Score: 9 to 12. Evaluation: Great job! Recommendation: While reading this chapter, you will be reminded of all the things you are doing that contribute to your healthy lifestyle. You are an excellent role model for others. The best nutrition educators practice what they teach.

Score: 5 to 8. Evaluation: Okay. Recommendation: You do make some good choices, but a number of changes in your food habits would be of great value to you. Hopefully, you will be motivated by some of the ideas presented in this chapter.

Score: 0 to 4. Evaluation: Improvement needed. Recommendation: The first steps toward good eating are the hardest to take, but making healthy choices is worth the investment. Begin investing in your own health.

NUTRITION IN THE UNITED STATES: LOOKING FORWARD FROM THE PAST

Classic Vitamin-Deficiency Diseases

Food and nutrition have always been vitally important to health. Until as recently as the 1940s, many nutrient-deficiency diseases, such as rickets, pellagra, scurvy, beriberi, xerophthalmia, and goiter, were still prevalent in the United States (Carpenter, 2000). Although these conditions still persist in developing countries, they have virtually disappeared from developed areas of the world. Why? An abundant food supply, fortification of some foods with critical nutrients, and better methods of determining and improving the nutrient contents of foods have contributed to the decline of nutrient-deficiency diseases.

The introduction of iodized salt in the 1920s, for example, contributed greatly to eliminating iodine-deficiency goiter as a public health problem. Similarly, pellagra disappeared after the discovery that inadequate niacin levels contribute to the condition. Today, nutrient deficiencies rarely are reported in the United States. The few cases of protein-energy malnutrition that are listed annually as causes of death generally occur as secondary results of severe illness or injury, premature birth, child neglect, problems of the homebound aged, alcoholism, or some combination of these factors. Although undernutrition still occurs in some groups of people in the United States, including isolated or economically deprived people, these once-prevalent diseases of nutritional deficiency have been replaced by diseases of dietary excess and imbalance (Table 11-1).

Table **11-1**	Health Problems Related to Poor Nutrition

A number of health problems are caused or exacerbated by poor nutrition. Health care professionals strive to prevent or delay these health problems.

Health Problem	Questionable Practices
Anemia	Inadequate iron and folate intake
Cancer (breast, cervical, and colon)	Excessive fat intake; low fiber intake
Cirrhosis	Excessive alcohol intake
Constipation	Inadequate fiber or fluid intake; high fat intake; sedentary lifestyle
Dental caries	Excessive, frequent consumption of concentrated sweets; lack of fluoride; poor hygiene
Type 2 diabetes	Excessive energy intake
Hypercholesterolemia	Inadequate fiber intake
Hypertension	Obesity; excessive energy intake; excessive sodium intake in sodium-sensitive individuals
Infection	Malnutrition
Obesity	Excessive energy intake; excessive fat intake; sedentary lifestyle
Osteoporosis	Inadequate calcium intake; inadequate vitamin D intake or inadequate exposure to the sun; sedentary lifestyle
Underweight and growth failure	Inadequate energy intake

Dietary Excess and Imbalance

Problems resulting from overconsumption now rank among the leading causes of illness and death in the United States. The four leading causes of death directly associated with diet are **coronary heart disease** (CHD), some types of **cancer**, **stroke**, and **diabetes mellitus**. In fact, heart disease, cancers, and stroke account for almost two thirds of all deaths every year in America. Four more major causes of death—accidents, cirrhosis of the liver, suicide, and homicide—are associated with excessive alcohol intake.

The number of American children who are **overweight** is currently 17.4% among 12 to 19 year olds, 18.8% among 6 to 11 year olds, and 13.9% among 2 to 5 year olds (total = 50.1%) compared with 10.5%, 11.3%, and 7.2%, respectively from 1988 to 1994 (CDC, National Center for Health Statistics, 2007). Childhood obesity is a critical health issue of our time. Reducing the incidence of **obesity** is an important public health goal (National Institutes of Health, 2004; U.S. Department of Health and Human Services [USDHHS], 2007). Excess weight and obesity is commonly viewed as an imbalance between energy intake and expenditure; however, other factors need to be considered such as how genes are involved in the process of energy balance as well as differences in **fat** distribution by gender and age (Bray & Champagne, 2007). Researchers express concern that overweight or obesity in childhood will lead to health-related problems in adulthood.

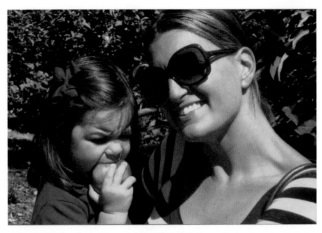

Figure 11-1   Learning nutritional food choices starts at a young age.

Encouraging healthy choices in diet, exercise, and weight control is one of the major themes of *Healthy People 2010* (Figure 11-1). As dietary factors contribute substantially to the burden of preventable illness and premature death, *Healthy People 2010* is aimed at bringing American dietary patterns into line with current dietary recommendations, especially the Dietary Guidelines for Americans (U.S. Department of Agriculture [USDA] and USDHHS, 2005).

HEALTHY PEOPLE 2010: NUTRITION OBJECTIVES

As discussed throughout this text, the 28 focus areas in *Healthy People 2010* contain 467 specific national health-promotion and disease-prevention objectives. Many *Healthy People 2010* nutrition-related objectives target interventions designed to reduce or eliminate illness, disability, and premature death among individuals and communities. Each objective has a target for specific improvements to be achieved by 2010. The topics covered by these objectives reflect the array of critical influences that determine the health of individuals and communities. For example, individual behaviors and environmental factors are responsible for approximately 70% of all premature deaths in the United States. Understanding these influences and how they relate to one another are crucial for achieving *Healthy People 2010* goals and developing 2020 goals.

The report also contains 10 leading health indicators: (1) physical activity, (2) overweight and obesity, (3) tobacco use, (4) substance abuse, (5) mental health, (6) injury and violence, (7) environmental quality, (8) immunization, (9) responsible sexual behavior, and (10) access to health care. By monitoring these measures, states and communities can assess their current health status and follow it over time. Overweight and obesity are supported by two specific measurable objectives:

- 19-3c. Reduce the proportion of children and adolescents who are overweight or obese.
- 19-2. Reduce the proportion of adults who are obese.

The *Healthy People 2010* box presents nutrition-related objectives related to the diseases discussed later in the chapter.

Healthy People 2010
Objectives for Selected Diseases

Heart Disease

Goal: Reduce CHD deaths
- 12-12. Reduce the mean total blood cholesterol levels among adults from 206 mg/dL to 199 mg/dL.
- 12-13. Reduce the proportion of adults with high total blood cholesterol levels.
- 19-8. Increase the proportion of people aged 2 years and older who receive less than 10% of calories from saturated fat.
- 19-9. Increase the proportion of people aged 2 years and older who receive no more than 30% of calories from fat.

Hypertension

- 12-7. Reduce the number of stroke deaths.
- 12-9. Reduce the proportion of adults with high blood pressure.
- 12-11. Increase the proportion of adults with high blood pressure who are taking action (losing weight and reducing sodium intake).
- 19-10. Increase the proportion of people aged 2 years and older who consume 2400 mg or less of sodium daily.

Osteoporosis

Goal: Prevent illness and disability related to arthritis and other rheumatic conditions, osteoporosis, and chronic back conditions
- 2-9. Reduce the overall number of cases of osteoporosis as measured by low total femur BMD.

- 19-11. Increase the proportion of individuals aged 2 years and older who meet dietary recommendations for calcium.

Obesity

Leading health indicators: reduce the proportion of adults who are obese from 23% to 15% and reduce the proportion of children and adolescents who are overweight or obese from 11% and 12% to 5% (objective numbers 19-2 and 19-3).
- 19-1. Increase the proportion of adults who are at a healthy weight from 42% to 60%.

Diabetes

Goal: Through prevention programs, reduce the disease and economic burden of diabetes and improve the quality of life for all people who have or are at risk for diabetes
- 5-1. Increase the proportion of people with diabetes who receive formal diabetes education from 40% in 1998 to 60% in 2010.
- 5-2. Prevent diabetes, from 3.1 new cases per 1000 people in 1994 to 1996 to 2.5 new cases per 1000 in 2010.

Human Immunodeficiency Virus

Goal 13: Prevent HIV infection and its related illness and death
- 13-15. Expand the interval between an initial diagnosis of HIV infection and AIDS diagnosis to increase years of life of an individual with HIV.
- 13-17. Reduce the number of new cases of perinatal-acquired HIV infection.

AIDS, Acquired immunodeficiency virus; *BMD*, Bone mineral density; *HIV*, Human immunodeficiency virus.
Sources: U.S. Department of Health and Human Sources. (2000). *Healthy People 2010*. Retrieved from *www.healthypeople.gov*.
U.S. Department of Health and Human Sources. (2000). *Midcourse Review of Healthy People 2010*. Retrieved from *www.healthypeople.gov*.

Nutrition-Related Health Status

Overweight and high serum **cholesterol** levels, **hypertension** (high blood pressure), and **osteoporosis** (decreased bone mass) increase the risk of CHD, stroke, and bone fracture, respectively. The following statements describe the health status of Americans:

- More Americans are overweight now than in the late 1970s. Many adults also report sedentary lifestyles. Being overweight is associated with many chronic diseases and health outcomes; therefore, its increased prevalence is a cause for public health concern.
- Although the number of adults with desirable serum total cholesterol levels is increasing steadily, many people still have high levels. A high serum cholesterol is a major risk factor for CHD.
- Hypertension remains a major public health problem in middle-aged and older adults. Blacks have a higher age-related prevalence of hypertension than Whites and Hispanic Americans. Hypertension is

the most important risk factor for stroke and a major risk factor for CHD.

Nutrition Objectives for the United States

Although Americans are slowly changing their eating patterns toward more healthful diets, a considerable gap exists between public health recommendations and consumers' practices. The overarching goal for nutrition in the beginning of the millennium is that food intake change in the direction of the targeted goals recommended in *Healthy People 2010*, the **MyPyramid** system, and the Dietary Guidelines for Americans.

FOOD AND NUTRITION RECOMMENDATIONS

Food and nutrition guidelines are introduced in this chapter. A goal of this discussion is to heighten people's interest in the health-promotion power of good nutrition to inspire their gradual adoption of the dietary recommendations presented here.

Box 11-1   Dietary Reference Intakes (DRI) Definition

RECOMMENDED DIETARY ALLOWANCE (RDA)

RDA is the intake that meets the nutrient needs of nearly all (97 to 98 percent) healthy individuals in a specific age and gender group. It should be used to guide individuals in achieving adequate nutrient intake aimed at decreasing the risk of chronic disease. The RDA is based on estimating an average requirement in addition to an increase or decrease to account for variations within a particular group.

ADEQUATE INTAKE (AI)

When sufficient scientific evidence is unavailable to estimate an average requirement, AIs are set. Individuals should use AIs as a goal when no RDAs exist. AI is derived through experimental or observational data that show a mean intake that appears to sustain a desired level of health, such as calcium retention in bone for most members of a population group. For example, AIs have been set for infants through 1 year of age using the average observed nutrient intake of populations of breast-fed infants as the standard.

ESTIMATED AVERAGE REQUIREMENT (EAR)

EAR is the intake that meets the estimated nutrient need of one half of the individuals in a specific group. It is used as a basis for developing the RDA and by nutrition policy makers in evaluating adequacy of nutrient intakes of the group and for planning how much the group should consume.

TOLERABLE UPPER INTAKE LEVEL (UL)

This is the maximum intake by an individual that is unlikely to pose risks of adverse health effects in almost all healthy individuals in a specified group. UL is not intended to be a recommended level of intake, and no established benefit exists for individuals to consume nutrients at levels above the RDA or AI. For most nutrients, this figure refers to total intakes from food, fortified food, and nutrient supplements.

AI, Adequate intake; *EAR,* Estimated average requirement; *RDA,* Recommended dietary allowance; *UL,* Tolerable upper intake level. From International Food Information Council Foundation. (2006). Retrieved from *http://ific.org/publications/other/driupdateom.cfm.*

The kinds and amounts of food that are required to obtain the necessary energy and nutrients are defined in these reports:

- Dietary Reference Intakes (National Research Council [NRC], 2005a), including the Recommended Dietary Allowances (NRC, 2005b, c)
- Dietary Guidelines for Americans, sixth edition (USDA/USDHHS, 2005)
- MyPyramid, a new food guidance system introduced by the USDA in 2005 (USDA/CNPP, 2005).

Dietary Reference Intakes

The **Dietary Reference Intakes** (DRI) is a set of values for the dietary nutrient intakes of healthy people in the United States and Canada. These values are used for planning and assessing diets, including the recommended daily allowance (RDA), adequate intake, estimated average requirement, and Tolerable Upper Intake Level (Box 11-1).

The DRI recommends intake levels for U.S. and Canadian individuals and population groups and sets maximal level guidelines to reduce the risk of adverse health effects from overconsumption of a nutrient. The understanding of the relationship between nutrition and chronic disease has progressed to the extent that intakes can now be recommended that are thought to help people achieve measurable physical indicators of good health. The DRI represents a major leap forward in nutrition science—from a primary concern for the prevention of deficiency to an emphasis on beneficial effects of healthy eating. The new recommendations focus on decreasing the risk of chronic disease through nutrition.

The old RDA, which existed before 1997, established the minimum amounts of nutrients needed to protect against nutrient deficiency. In contrast, the DRI is designed to reflect the latest understanding about nutrient requirements based on optimizing health in individuals and groups. Collectively called the DRI, the new recommendations include four categories of reference intakes that were established by examining the results of hundreds of nutritional studies on both the beneficial aspects of nutrients and the hazards of consuming too much of a nutrient. When the scientific evidence allows, recommendations are made to help individuals at different stages of life to obtain enough of a nutrient to promote health and to maintain normal nutritional status.

Dietary Guidelines for Americans

The influence of the Dietary Guidelines for Americans is wide ranging. First issued in 1980 in response to the public's desire for authoritative, consistent guidance on diet and health, the **dietary guidelines** form the foundation of federal nutrition policy in the United States. Each federally sponsored nutrition program uses these guidelines as a part of its nutrition standard; therefore, every day they directly influence the lives of millions of Americans in food stamp, school lunch, and school breakfast programs and those receiving benefits under the Special Supplemental Nutrition Program for Women, Infants, and Children (WIC). These guidelines also form the basis for nutrition education messages for the general public of adults and children beginning at 2 years of age. The National Nutrition Monitoring and Related Research Act of 1990 mandates that the Dietary Guidelines for Americans be reviewed every 5 years by the U.S. Department of Agriculture (USDA) and the USDHHS.

In the latest report, 2005 Dietary Guidelines for Americans, the principal focus is on health promotion and risk reduction since the general public is now comprised of large numbers of individuals with chronic health problems such as obesity, high blood pressure, and abnormal blood lipid values, as well as a large older population. Topics addressed in detail include recommended nutrient intakes and physical activity; energy balance; relationships of fats, carbohydrates, selected food groups, and alcohol with health; and consumer aspects of food safety.

Box **11-2** Dietary Guidelines for Americans 2005: Key Recommendations for the General Population

ADEQUATE NUTRIENTS WITHIN CALORIE NEEDS

- Consume a variety of nutrient-dense foods and beverages within and among the basic food groups while choosing foods that limit the intake of saturated and trans fats, cholesterol, added sugars, salt, and alcohol.
- Meet recommended intakes within energy needs by adopting a balanced eating pattern, such as the U.S. Department of Agriculture (USDA) Food Guide or the Dietary Approaches to Stop Hypertension (DASH) Eating Plan.

WEIGHT MANAGEMENT

- To maintain body weight in a healthy range, balance calories from foods and beverages with calories expended.
- To prevent gradual weight gain over time, make small decreases in food and beverage calories and increase physical activity.

PHYSICAL ACTIVITY

- Engage in regular physical activity and reduce sedentary activities to promote health, psychological well-being, and a healthy body weight.
- To reduce the risk of chronic disease in adulthood: engage in at least 30 minutes of moderate-intensity physical activity, above usual activity, at work or home on most days of the week.
- For most people, greater health benefits can be obtained by engaging in physical activity of more vigorous intensity or longer duration.
- To help manage body weight and prevent gradual, unhealthy body weight gain in adulthood: engage in approximately 60 minutes of moderate- to vigorous-intensity activity on most days of the week while not exceeding caloric intake requirements.
- To sustain weight loss in adulthood: participate in at least 60 to 90 minutes of daily moderate-intensity physical activity while not exceeding caloric intake requirements. Some people may need to consult with a health care provider before participating in this level of activity.
- Achieve physical fitness by including cardiovascular conditioning, stretching exercises for flexibility, and resistance exercises or calisthenics for muscle strength and endurance.

FOOD GROUPS TO ENCOURAGE

- Consume a sufficient amount of fruits and vegetables while staying within energy needs. Two cups of fruit and 2½ cups of vegetables per day are recommended for a reference 2000-calorie intake, with higher or lower amounts depending on the calorie level.
- Choose a variety of fruits and vegetables each day. In particular, select from all five vegetable subgroups (dark green, orange, legumes, starchy vegetables, and other vegetables) several times a week.
- Consume 3 or more ounce-equivalents of whole-grain products per day, with the rest of the recommended grains coming from enriched or whole-grain products. In general, at least half the grains should come from whole grains.
- Consume 3 cups per day of fat-free or low-fat milk or equivalent milk products.

FATS

- Consume less than 10 percent of calories from saturated fatty acids and less than 300 mg/day of cholesterol, and keep **trans fatty acid** consumption as low as possible.
- Keep total fat intake between 20% to 35% of calories, with most fats coming from sources of polyunsaturated and monounsaturated fatty acids, such as fish, nuts, and vegetable oils.
- When selecting and preparing meat, poultry, dry beans, and milk or milk products, make choices that are lean, low-fat, or fat-free.
- Limit intake of fats and oils high in saturated and/or trans fatty acids, and choose products low in such fats and oils.

CARBOHYDRATES

- Choose fiber-rich fruits, vegetables, and whole grains often.
- Choose and prepare foods and beverages with little added sugars or caloric sweeteners, such as amounts suggested by the USDA Food Guide and the DASH Eating Plan.
- Reduce the incidence of dental caries by practicing good oral hygiene and consuming sugar- and starch-containing foods and beverages less frequently.

SODIUM AND POTASSIUM

- Consume less than 2300 mg (approximately 1 teaspoon of salt) of sodium per day.
- Choose and prepare foods with little salt. At the same time, consume potassium-rich foods, such as fruits and vegetables.

ALCOHOLIC BEVERAGES

- Those who choose to drink alcoholic beverages should do so sensibly and in moderation—defined as the consumption of up to one drink per day for women and up to two drinks per day for men.
- Alcoholic beverages should not be consumed by some individuals, including those who cannot restrict their alcohol intake, women of childbearing age who may become pregnant, pregnant and lactating women, children and adolescents, individuals taking medications that can interact with alcohol, and those with specific medical conditions.
- Alcoholic beverages should be avoided by individuals engaging in activities that require attention, skill, or coordination, such as driving or operating machinery.

FOOD SAFETY

To avoid microbial foodborne illness:
- Clean hands, food contact surfaces, and fruits and vegetables. Meat and poultry should not be washed or rinsed.
- Separate raw, cooked, and ready-to-eat foods while shopping, preparing, or storing foods.
- Cook foods to a safe temperature to kill microorganisms.
- Chill (refrigerate) perishable food promptly and defrost foods properly.
- Avoid raw (unpasteurized) milk or any products made from unpasteurized milk, raw or partially cooked eggs or foods containing raw eggs, raw or undercooked meat and poultry, unpasteurized juices, and raw sprouts.

From U.S. Department of Agriculture. (2005). *Dietary guidelines for Americans 2005: Key recommendations for the general population.* Washington, DC: U.S. Department of Agriculture. Retrieved May 31, 2005, from *www.health.gov/dietaryguidelines/dga2005/recommendations.htm.*

To support these focus areas, key recommendations are grouped under nine interrelated messages and presented in Box 11-2. The principal messages are:

1. Consume a variety of foods within and among the basic food groups while staying within energy needs.
2. Control calorie intake to manage body weight.
3. Be physically active every day.
4. Increase daily intake of fruits and vegetables, whole grains, and nonfat or low-fat milk and milk products.
5. Choose fats wisely for good health.
6. Choose carbohydrates wisely for good health.
7. Choose and prepare foods with little salt.
8. If you drink alcoholic beverages, do so in moderation.
9. Keep food safe to eat.

Nursing professionals play a key role in promoting the guidelines as one component of healthful lifestyles (Multicultural Awareness box). For convenience, the entire dietary guidelines report is available on the Internet (*www.health.gov/dietaryguidelines/dga2005/recommendations.htm*). The report is an excellent source of background information for health care professionals. Individual sections are available to photocopy for use as education materials.

MULTICULTURAL AWARENESS

Food and Culture

The reasons why people eat the way they do are numerous. Although it is true that without food people cannot survive, food is much more than a tool of survival. Food is also a source of pleasure ("Let's eat out tonight"), a source of comfort ("Right now, I could use some of my mother's chicken soup"), a symbol of hospitality ("Please come to my house for brunch on Sunday"), and an indicator of social status (consider an expensive T-bone steak versus a hamburger). Food has ritual significance, also. Drinking champagne to celebrate an important event, the bride and groom saving the top layer of their wedding cake, or people of the Jewish faith sharing challah (braided bread) at their Sabbath (Friday evening) meal are examples.

To a large extent, the environment determines what people typically eat. For example, wheat that is plentiful in the heartland of the United States is the principal grain in North America, whereas rice enjoys a similar status in Asian countries. Typical wheat-based staples in the United States and Canada include a slice of wheat bread, a bowl of wheat cereal, wheat crackers, pastries made from wheat flour, and pasta made from wheat. Rice-based foods form the backbone of the Chinese diet.

Every culture has its particular food ways, or activities related to food. Food ways include the activities that surround procuring, distributing, storing, consuming, and disposing of food, all of which define what is fit to eat, or what is edible. The factors that affect everyone's food choices and factors that affect food selections of new arrivals to a community should be examined.

Food is often believed to promote health, cure disease, or contain other medicinal qualities. Health beliefs, which can have a great influence on food choices, may be beneficial, neutral, and sometimes dangerous. When actions based on these beliefs cause no harm, they should be encouraged. For example, in the United States Americans consume vitamin C in the belief that it might help prevent or cure the common cold. Although large doses (500 to 1000 mg per day) have no significant effect on incidence of the common cold, vitamin C provides a moderate benefit in terms of the duration and severity of cold symptoms in some groups of people. The often-reported improvement in the severity of colds after ingesting vitamin C may be a result of the antihistaminic action of the vitamin at these large doses (National Research Council, 2005a).

Among traditional Chinese people, health and disease are believed to relate to the balance between the forces of yin and yang in the body. Diseases that are caused by yang forces may be treated with yin forces to restore balance. Yin foods include low–caloric density, low-protein foods, such as fresh fruits and vegetables. Yang foods are high in calories, cooked in oil, irritating to the mouth, or are red, orange, or yellow in color. Examples include most meats, chili peppers, tomatoes, garlic, ginger, and alcoholic beverages. The hot-cold theory in Puerto Rico follows the same basic principles as do yin and yang, but the food groupings differ somewhat.

Religious beliefs affect the food choices of millions of people worldwide. Many religions, including Buddhism, Hinduism, Islam, Judaism, and Seventh Day Adventism, specify the foods that may be eaten and how they should be prepared. The following is a summary of the principal dietary practices of these five major world religions (Barer-Stein, 1979; Kittler & Sucher, 2000).

- Many Buddhists practice vegetarianism. Foods of plant origin are viewed as the most appropriate for consumption, except pungent foods (garlic, leeks, scallions, chives, and onions), which are believed to generate lust when eaten cooked and rage when eaten raw. For most Buddhists, however, dietary rules such as these are observed on a voluntary basis. What characterizes all Buddhists is the belief that all forms of life share a common link and are thus sacred. Therefore rather than the specific type of food eaten, more important is the attitude of the person receiving the food and the person's sincere gratitude for the lives of the plants and animals contained in the meal that have served to sustain and further enhance the life of the individual.
- Many Hindus are vegetarians, but those who come from the cold northern areas of India eat meat (except for beef, which is prohibited).
- Islamic food laws prohibit the consumption of foods believed to be unclean, such as carrion or already-dead animals, swine, animals slaughtered without pronouncing the name of Allah on them, carnivorous animals with fangs (dogs, cats, and lions), birds of prey, and land animals without ears (frogs and snakes). Alcohol is also prohibited.
- Judaism prohibits the consumption of swine, carrion, carrion eaters (scavengers), shellfish, animals with a cloven (split) hoof and those that do not chew their cud (horses), and animals not slaughtered by the appropriate ritual method. According to Jewish dietary laws, meat (beef, lamb, veal, and poultry), fish, and meat products (eggs) cannot be served at the same meal or cooked in the same vessels as dairy products.
- The dietary practices of Seventh Day Adventists focus on health, with vegetarianism as the foundation of their dietary standard. Seventh Day Adventists also abstain from alcohol and many do not drink caffeine-containing beverages.

Representing the best and most up-to-date scientific evidence and advice from nutrition experts, these guidelines are intended to reduce the nation's major diet-related health problems such as CHD, high blood pressure, stroke, certain cancers, diabetes and osteoporosis.

MYPYRAMID: A NEW FOOD GUIDANCE SYSTEM
Food Guide Pyramid

The Food Guide Pyramid was introduced in 1992 as a means for the USDA and the USDHHS to translate nutrition recommendations into terms that consumers would understand. As the twentieth-century anthropologist Margaret Mead once said, "People eat food, not nutrition." Nutrition recommendations stated in terms of grams of total fat and saturated fat, or milligrams of vitamin C, are useless unless people are advised as to what types and what quantities of foods should be consumed to obtain the recommended nutrients. The Food Guide Pyramid was a graphic representation of dietary balance and variety. Foods were classified into six food groups, each of which contained a variety of nutritionally similar foods.

MyPyramid

In 2005 the USDA unveiled MyPyramid, a new interactive food guidance system that replaced the 1992 Food Guide Pyramid. MyPyramid, which emphasizes the need for a more personalized approach to improving diet and lifestyle, incorporates the most current information available on nutritional science based upon the new Dietary Guidelines for Americans 2005 (USDA/CNPP, 2005). Figure 11-2 presents the graphic representation of MyPyramid. The new food guidance system remains based on the pyramid approach with food groups represented by a vertical band that corresponds to six food categories: grains, vegetables, fruits, oils, dairy products, and meat and beans (protein sources). The figure ascending the staircase reminds us of the importance of balancing caloric intake with physical activity for a healthy lifestyle.

The new food guidance system includes MyPyramid Tracker, an online assessment tool to evaluate personal diet and physical activity on the basis of age, gender and activity level. Individuals can create a customized diet and exercise plan by calculating food intake and levels of physical activity and then compare their status to recommendations suggested by Dietary Guidelines for Americans, USDA and USDHHS standards. Another feature of MyPyramid, discretionary calories, are the remaining calories in an individual's diet after they have met their nutritional needs and are still below the suggested calorie intake level. These calories are the "extras" that can be used on higher calorie forms of food that contain greater amounts of fats or added sugars or on more food from any food group. Daily discretionary calories allowances are usually very small, between 100 to 300 calories, especially for those who are physically inactive.

Although the USDA's MyPyramid food guidance system reflects general eating patterns of Americans, an important objective has been flexibility in food choice. The USDA developed a Spanish version of MyPyramid incorporating traditional ethnic foods emphasizing eating patterns of this cultural group. Several pictorial representations of the Food Guide Pyramids have also been developed reflecting eating patterns of a variety of ethnic groups including Asian, Mediterranean, and Native American. Food plans can be accessed at the website *http://fnic.nal.usda.gov.*

A child friendly version of MyPyramid called MyPyramid for Kids was developed to provide age-appropriate dietary and physical activity information for children 6 to 11 years old. It was written in a language easily understandable for children to promote healthy food choices and being physically active on a daily basis. MyPyramid for Kids is designed to stem the increase in obesity among children and includes an interactive computer game to support the key concepts of eating right and exercise. Two versions of MyPyramid for Kids have been developed; a simplified graphic for younger children and an advanced rendition for elementary students featuring healthy eating and physical activity messages. MyPyramid for Kids can be accessed at the website *http://teamnutrition.usda.gov/Resources/mpk_poster2.pdf.*

DIETARY SUPPLEMENTS AND HERBAL MEDICINES

The popularity of supplemental vitamins, minerals, proteins, **fiber**, and herbs has, in recent decades, earned a high profile in the health field. A vast array of these products is available without a prescription. All people are entitled to know exactly what they are ingesting, whether it is necessary, and whether it is safe.

Traditionally dietary supplements were products composed of one or more of the essential nutrients (vitamins, minerals, and proteins) that were ingested to enhance the usual diet. Through the 1994 Dietary Supplement Health and Education Act the definition of dietary supplement has been expanded to include any product intended for ingestion as a supplement to the diet, including vitamins, minerals, herbs, botanicals and other plant-derived substances, amino acids (individual building blocks of protein) and concentrates, metabolites, constituents, and extracts of these substances (U.S. Food and Drug Administration, 2004).

Drugs can also be of plant origin. Drugs are used in Western medicine as agents intended to diagnose, cure, mitigate, treat, or prevent diseases. Before marketing, drugs must undergo clinical trials to determine their effectiveness, safety, possible adverse interactions with other substances, and appropriate dosage amounts. The U.S. Food and Drug Administration (FDA) reviews the data collected on a studied drug and, depending on the outcome of the review, officially authorizes it as safe for the general public.

Supplements are sold in the pharmaceutical section of retail stores in a variety of forms (tablets, capsules, powders, soft gels, gel caps, and liquids) that make them resemble drugs. Many people use supplements as if they were drugs, because they are marketed in the same manner as over-the-counter medications. Nevertheless, supplements are unregulated by the FDA.

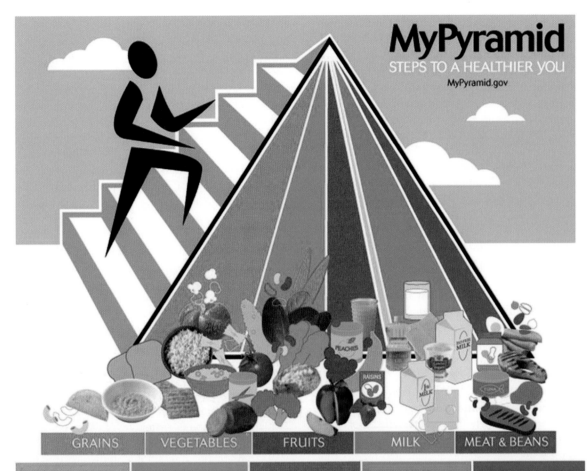

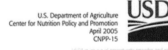

Figure 11-2   MyPyramid, the new food guidance system developed by the USDA. (From U.S. Department of Agriculture, Center for Nutrition Policy and Promotion, April 2005.)

A dietary supplement can be distinguished from an over-the-counter drug by the words *dietary supplement*, which must appear on the product label. A claim that the supplement is formulated to treat or cure a specific disease or condition cannot appear on the label. However, structure-function claims about certain common conditions associated with aging, pregnancy, menopause, and adolescence that do not relate to disease are permitted. These include health maintenance claims ("maintains a healthy circulatory system"), other nondisease claims ("for muscle enhancement" or "helps you relax"), and claims for common, minor symptoms associated with life stages ("for common symptoms of premenstrual syndrome" or "for hot flashes").

Considerable research on the effects of dietary supplements has been conducted in Asia and Europe, where these plant products have a long tradition of use. However, the overwhelming majority of supplements have not been studied scientifically. Therefore the National Institutes of Health (NIH) Office of Alternative Medicine and Office of Dietary Supplements are promoting the scientific study of the benefits and risks of dietary supplements, including medicinal herbs, in health maintenance and disease prevention.

Health care professionals are often asked, "Should I take a nutrient supplement?" Many people in the United States take dietary supplements but not necessarily to meet nutrient requirements. Although the adverse effects of large doses of certain nutrients (such as vitamin A) have been recognized for years, there are no documented reports that daily vitamins and mineral supplements that provide up to the recommended intake for a particular nutrient are either beneficial or harmful for the general population. Low-dose supplements that contain the recommended intakes for micronutrients (vitamins and minerals) appear to be generally safe. Although the desirable way for the general public to obtain recommended levels of nutrients is by eating a variety of foods, when people take dietary supplements they should avoid taking them in excess of the recommended intake on any given day.

Circumstances When Nutrient Supplementation is Indicated

Nutrient supplements and fortified foods are sometimes necessary for specific populations to obtain desirable amounts of particular nutrients (American Dietetic Association, 2005). Some examples follow:

- Folic acid for females who could become pregnant, to help prevent neural tube defects
- Iron during pregnancy
- Calcium for individuals who do not meet the recommended intake
- Vitamin D for older adults who do not drink generous quantities of fortified milk or who do not manufacture sufficient vitamin D from sunlight
- Vitamin B12 for older adults with atrophic gastritis who do not absorb enough from the food they eat

Vitamin Toxicity

An important point of concern for many health professionals is the excessive use of vitamin and mineral supplements. Toxic levels of certain micronutrients may result and can cause a host of health problems. For example, it is important to advise individuals not to overuse vitamins of the fat-soluble class (vitamins A, D, E, and K). Of particular concern is vitamin A, an excess of which may be **teratogenic** during pregnancy. On the other hand, water-soluble vitamins such as vitamin C and the B-complex vitamins pose less danger, because the body is able to excrete them through the urine.

Nutrient imbalances and toxicities are less likely to occur when nutrients are derived from foods. Most nutrient toxicities occur through supplementation. Estimated toxic doses for daily oral consumption of vitamins and minerals by adults are as low as 5 times the recommended intake for selenium, and as high as 25 to 50 times or more the recommended intakes for folic acid and vitamins C and E. The toxicities of high doses of nutrients such as vitamins A, B6, and D, niacin, iron, and selenium are well established. Iron supplements intended for other household members are the most common cause of pediatric poisoning deaths in the United States (National Library of Medicine [NLM] and NIH, 2008).

Large doses of vitamin A may be teratogenic. Because of this risk, supplementation with preformed vitamin A should be avoided during the first trimester of pregnancy unless there is evidence of deficiency. Excess preformed vitamin A (more than 10,000 international units) during the first trimester of pregnancy has been linked to cranial neural crest defects (National Toxicology Program, USDHHS, 2005). Such a risk in early pregnancy raises a need for caution about general vitamin and mineral supplement use by women of childbearing age.

Besides problems with direct toxicity of some individual nutrients, nutrient supplementation can cause problems related to nutrient imbalances or adverse interactions with prescribed medication. Many problems associated with high doses of a single nutrient may reflect interactions that result in a relative deficiency for another nutrient. Some examples follow:

- High doses of vitamin E can interfere with vitamin K action and enhance the effect of Coumadin as one of the anticoagulant drugs.
- Large amounts of calcium inhibit absorption of iron and possibly other trace elements.
- Folic acid can mask hematological signs of vitamin B12 deficiency which, if untreated, can result in irreversible neurological damage. Folic acid can also interact adversely with anticonvulsant medications.
- Zinc supplementation can reduce copper status, impair immune responses, and decrease high-density lipoprotein cholesterol levels (National Research Council, 2005c).

FOOD SAFETY

Food safety is vitally important in promoting health and remains in the limelight as severe food-borne illnesses sweep across the nation. In this section the importance of safeguarding food, the different types of contamination that endanger the food supply, and steps that can be taken to avoid falling victim to food-borne illness are considered.

Every organization and individual connected to the food chain, from food production to the table, share responsibility for the safety and integrity of the food supply. This chain includes people who produce or grow, process, ship, sell, and prepare food and the consumer who makes up the final link in the chain. With the globalization of the food supply, the FDA has developed a comprehensive Food Protection Plan to monitor and prevent the contamination of the nation's food supply. The strategy of the Food Protection Plan is built upon the three elements of prevention, intervention, and response to ensure the safety of both domestic and imported food eaten by American consumers. When the safeguards built into this system fail, however, consumers themselves must serve as the final and sometimes most important guardian against unsafe food. Therefore being informed and educated about the potential dangers of food-borne illness and how to avoid these complications to stay healthy is essential.

Causes of Food-Borne Illness

A food-borne illness is classified according to the source of its contamination (the unintended presence of harmful substances or microorganisms). Food contaminants may be categorized as biological, chemical, or physical. Biological contaminants include bacteria, viruses, parasites, and fungi (yeasts and mold). Chemical contamination refers to the presence of pesticides, kitchen cleaning supplies, and toxic chemicals in food that have been leeched out of worn metal cookware and equipment. Physical contamination includes dirt, glass chips, crockery, wood, splinters, stones, hair, jewelry, and metal shavings from dull can openers.

Mad Cow Disease

The highly active surveillance on beef from Europe and particularly the United Kingdom is a prime example of the effect unsafe food can have on entire populations. The problem known as **bovine spongiform encephalopathy (BSE)**, or more commonly as mad cow disease, is traced back to unsafe practices of certain producers in the meat industry. Cows who eat sheep products and waste meat contaminated with an infectious protein-like particle known as a prion develop a fatal neurological disease. These cows become uncontrollable and wild, much different from their usual docile nature (National Center for Infectious Diseases, 2007). Humans who eat contaminated beef suffer from a similar fatal neurological degeneration called new variant **Creutzfeldt-Jakob disease (nvCJD)**. The prion cannot be destroyed by heat, radiation, or disinfectants. Cooperation among the entire food safety network, especially the consumer, is therefore important for special cases like this one to be controlled. To reduce the risk of acquiring nvCJD, travelers to Europe should be advised to consider either avoiding beef and beef products altogether, or selecting beef or beef products as solid pieces of muscle meat (versus ground products such as burgers and sausages) that have a reduced opportunity for contamination with tissues that might harbor the BSE agent. Milk and milk products from cows are not believed to pose any risk for transmitting the prion (Centers for Disease Control and Prevention [CDC], National Center for Infectious Diseases, 2008).

Escherichia Coli O157:H7 Infection

Escherichia coli bacteria was first discovered in the human colon in 1885 by Theodor Escherich, a German pediatrician. A particularly virulent strain of the bacterium *Escherichia coli* know as *E. coli* O157:H7 was first identified in 1982 as a food-borne pathogen during an investigation of an outbreak of severe bloody diarrhea due to contaminated hamburgers. As a leading cause of food-borne illness, *E. coli* O157:H7 can produce a powerful toxin causing severe illness and damage to intestinal lining. The illness is characterized by severe abdominal cramping, watery to bloody diarrhea, dehydration, nausea, and vomiting with or without low-grade fewer. Hemorrhagic colitis is usually self-limited and lasts for an average of 8 days. The majority of *E. coli* O157:H7 infections are foodborne associated with undercooked or raw ground beef. Outbreaks have also involved unpasteurized fruit juices and milk, alfalfa sprouts, lettuce, spinach and water. Moreover, outbreaks can be caused by secondary person-to-person contamination in homes, daycare centers, nursing homes and hospitals. Another mode of transmission of *E. coli* O157:H7 is by hand to mouth contact with animals or contaminated surfaces at petting zoos and agricultural fairs. Although all people are included in *E. coli* O157:H7 target populations, children and older adults are more susceptible. In cases confirmed in children, infection may develop into hemolytic uremic syndrome (HUS) leading to permanent loss of kidney function. To reduce the risk of *E. coli* O157:H7 infection, avoid eating or serving undercooked ground meat; drink only pasteurized milk, juice, or cider; wash all fruits and vegetables under running water especially if they are not to be cooked; wash hands, utensils, and work areas with hot, soapy water to keep bacteria from spreading after contact with raw meat.

Salmonellosis

According to the USDA, the most frequently reported cause of food-borne illness is *Salmonella* bacteria. Each year in the United States, approximately 40,000 cases of salmonellosis are reported and 600 persons die from acute **salmonellosis** (CDC, 2006). The actual number of infections may be closer to 1.4 million since milder cases are often not diagnosed or reported. Salmonellosis is an infection caused by *Salmonella*, a bacteria discovered over 100 years ago by Dr. Daniel E. Salmon, an American veterinarian-pathologist. *Salmonella* is a gram-negative microscopic germ that passes from the feces of people or animals to other people or other animals. Although the *Salmonella* family includes over 2300 serotypes of bacterium, the most common in the U.S. are *Salmonella Enteritidis* and *Salmonella Typhimurium.*

The most common way humans catch salmonellosis is by eating foods contaminated with animal feces. Foods of animal origin such as beef, poultry, milk, and eggs are often the source of infection, but all foods including seafood from polluted water and vegetables may become contaminated. Contamination may also occur from unsanitary handling of foods and utensils by infected food handlers and contact with the feces of some pets, especially those with diarrhea. Symptoms of salmonellosis include abdominal cramping, mild to severe diarrhea, nausea, vomiting, and fever within 8 to 72 hours after infection. Symptoms may resolve within 4 to 7 days without treatment; however, infections can become life-threatening for people with weakened immune systems as well as infants, young children, pregnant women, and older adults. Antibiotics usually are not necessary unless the infection spreads from the intestines. To prevent the infection of salmonellosis, avoid uncooked egg dishes, undercooked meat, shellfish, and unpasteurized milk and juice. Adherence to sanitary regulations as well as proper food handling is necessary to control salmonellosis outbreaks.

Food Safety Practices

Hand washing is one of the most important practices in the prevention of food-borne illness. Hands should be washed thoroughly before food preparation and before eating. The accepted method of hand washing entails running warm water over the hands, applying soap, and generating friction and agitation for approximately 20 to 30 seconds. Young children should be taught to wash their hands for as long as it takes them to sing the alphabet song twice. Nearly one half of all cases of food-borne illness might be avoided completely if people were to wash their hands more often when preparing and handling food.

Raw, cooked, and ready-to-eat foods should be separated while shopping, preparing, or storing foods. Separating foods prevents cross-contamination, which is the transfer of harmful substances or microorganisms from one location to another. Cross-contamination can occur when unwashed hands come in contact with food, when a microorganism-carrying food comes in contact with another food, or when food comes in contact with a contaminated surface. To prevent cross-contamination, follow these additional safety measures:

- Wash fresh fruits and vegetables thoroughly.
- Drink pasteurized juices.
- Do not consume raw (unpasteurized) milk or cheeses made with raw milk.
- Eat food that has been chilled and refrigerated properly.
- When eating out, make sure that food requiring refrigeration is served chilled.
- When shopping, buy perishable foods last and take them straight home.
- Follow the label. Always read and follow safety instructions on the package, such as, "keep refrigerated" and "safe handling instructions."

- Eat food that is served safely. Keep hot foods hot (140° F or above) and cold foods cold (32-40° F or below). Between these temperatures is the danger zone in which harmful bacteria can grow rapidly, even exponentially.
- Whether raw or cooked, never leave meat, poultry, eggs, fish, or shellfish out at room temperature for more than 2 hours (1 hour in hot weather that is 90° F and above). Be sure to chill leftovers as soon as you finish eating.

These guidelines also apply to carryout meals, restaurant leftovers, and home-packed meals to go. If in doubt, throw it out.

Making a food safe after it has been handled improperly may not always be possible. Therefore the best practice is to discard food when there is a doubt as to the safety of food preparation, service, or storage. For example, certain bacteria found in food that has been left at room temperature too long may produce a heat-resistant toxin that cannot be destroyed by cooking. Therefore the bottom line is to be careful in preparing food, which includes keeping track of the time the food is exposed to certain temperatures and being vigilant when eating out. If there is any doubt about the safety of the food, caution is urged; it is better not to eat it.

Without exception, everyone should exercise their best judgment and care when eating out, when handling their own food, or when handling the food of others. Prevention through education is the key to promoting healthy lives that are unscathed by the potentially severe and life-threatening effects of food-borne illness. People who do not have healthy immune systems (individuals with various health problems and many older adults) and people with immune systems that are not fully developed (infants) are at the greatest risk of developing food-borne illnesses.

Because food is shipped to the United States from all over the world, and because effective antibiotics are not always available to meet the challenge of ever-changing and mutating microbial agents, the Agricultural Research Service (ARS), a division of the USDA, is challenged to develop control strategies and prevent disease transmission. Classical Swine Fever Virus (CSFV), a highly infectious disease from pigs, and highly pathogenic avian influenza (HPAI) from poultry are examples of pathogens resistant to current generations of vaccines and antibiotics (Agricultural Research Services, 2007). When effective vaccines and antibiotics are not available, it is imperative to follow the basic food safety guidelines outlined in this chapter.

On a more positive note, normal healthy adults with healthy immune systems are able to ward off most of the contaminants from the environment and from food without much effort most of the time. Nevertheless, everyone should follow standard safety procedures when eating out and when handling food.

FOOD, NUTRITION, AND POVERTY

Healthy People 2010 Goal: promote health and reduce chronic disease associated with diet.

- 19-18. Increase food security in U.S. households from 88% in 1995 to 94% by 2010. (See progress in midcourse review of 2010 and future developing goals in 2020.)

Poverty and Income Distribution

For most people in the United States, income has risen over time, providing more options for personal consumption expenditures, including expenditures on food. However, growth in income has not increased equally for all households. Poverty still exists in the United States.

According to official 2006 poverty statistics (U.S. Census Bureau, 2006) 12.3% (36.5 million) of people live below the poverty level—a level of income set annually by the government to determine eligibility for various types of government programs as discussed in this section. In 2006, groups with particularly high poverty rates included Hispanics and African Americans, with statistically equivalent poverty rates of 20.6% and 24.3%, respectively. In contrast, the poverty rate was 8.2% for White non-Hispanic people. Children, who make up 35.2% of the poor but only 24.9% of the total population, have a 17.4% poverty rate, which is higher than the rate of any other age group (U.S. Census Bureau, 2006). In 2006, approximately 12.8 million children were poor. Children under 18 living in families headed by single women have a poverty rate of over 16.9%.

Food Assistance for the Poor

For people who are poor, obtaining a nutritious diet without assistance can be a challenge. Federal, state, and local governments and private charitable organizations mitigate this problem by providing billions of dollars annually in food assistance. Overall the bulk of food aid in the United States is financed at the federal level by the USDA. In 2006, federally funded outlays for food assistance programs amounted to almost $52.9 billion (*www.ers.usda.gov/briefing/foodnutritionassistance/*), as detailed below:

- Food Stamps: almost $23.9 billion
- Child nutrition (includes School Breakfast Program, Child and Adult Care Program, and the National School Lunch Program [NSLP]): almost $11.4 billion
- WIC: over $5 billion
- Food donations (e.g., to Native American communities, the Nutrition Service Incentive Program [NSIP], the Emergency Food Distribution Program): almost $500 million

One in six people in the United States receives federally funded food assistance at some point every year. The Food Stamp Program, NSLP, School-Based Partnerships, WIC, and NSIP are the main programs that provide domestic food and nutrition assistance. Table 11-2 contains information on identifying low-income people who need help getting enough food and referring them to the appropriate program.

Food Stamp Program

Food coupons or food stamps are used to supplement the food-buying power of eligible low-income people. The program provides monthly allotments to help low-income families purchase nutritionally adequate foods. Although there is no requirement that food stamps be used to purchase high-quality food, the goal of the food stamp nutrition education program is to increase the likelihood that recipients will make healthy food choices within their limited food budget. Households can use food stamps to buy any

Table 11-2 Referral Guide for Federal Nutrition Assistance Programs

Program	Target Population	Indicators of Need	Where to Call
Child and Adult Care Food Program (CACFP)	Children from low-income family; Adults ages 60 years or older or functionally impaired persons.	Low-income, poor nutritional status	Local social service office
Food Stamp Program	Low-income people and family	Economic stress	Local food stamp offices
School Breakfast Program	Children unlikely to eat before school	Married household, low-income, poor nutritional status	Local school district
School Lunch Program	Children of school age	Poor nutritional status	Local school district
Summer Food Service Program	Children who live in low-income neighborhoods	Economic stress, poor nutritional status	Local social services office
Women, Infants and Children (WIC)	Low-income pregnant, breastfeeding, and non-breastfeeding postpartum women; infants and children up to age 5.	Risk of existing health or nutritional problem	Local health department or community action agency

From USDA Food and Nutrition Service. (2007). Retrieved from *www.fns.usda.gov/fns/*.

food or food product for human consumption and seeds and plants for use in home gardens. Restaurants can be authorized to accept food stamps from qualified homeless, older, or disabled people in exchange for low-cost meals. Among the items that recipients cannot buy with food stamps are alcoholic beverages, tobacco, hot ready-to-eat foods, lunch counter items, foods to be eaten in the store, vitamins, medicines, and pet foods. Food stamps cannot be exchanged for cash. The program is administered nationally by the Food and Nutrition Service (FNS) and locally by state welfare agencies. To qualify, households must meet eligibility criteria, including a gross income at or below 130% of the poverty guidelines issued by the USDHHS. Most able-bodied adult applicants must also meet certain work requirements. Households may own certain resources. In addition to income, the food stamp allotment is also based on family size. In 2006 the Food Stamp Program provided benefits to 26.7 million people: 49% children, 42% adults, and 9% seniors. In 2006 the average monthly benefit per person was approximately $90 and almost $208 per household (USDA, Food and Nutrition Service, 2007).

National School Lunch Program

The federally funded NSLP is administered by FNS, an agency within the USDA. On the state level, the NSLP usually is administered by the U.S. Department of Education, which contracts with local schools to provide balanced, low-cost or free lunches. In 2006, the NSLP reached about 27.8 million children each school day.

- Children from families with incomes at or below 130% of the poverty level are eligible for free school meals.
- Children from families with incomes at 130% to 185% of the poverty level are eligible for reduced-price school meals.
- Children from families with incomes over 185% of the poverty level are eligible for full-price school meals.

Schools that choose to take part in the lunch program are provided with cash subsidies and donated commodities from the USDA. Donated foods include meats, canned and frozen fruits and vegetables, fruit juices, vegetable shortening, vegetable oil, and flour and other grain products. Free or reduced-price lunches must meet these federal minimum pattern requirements:

- Must provide one third of the recommended nutrient intake
- To the extent possible, must be consistent with the Dietary Guidelines for Americans recommendations for reducing **sugar**, salt, and fat intake

To help meet the goal of healthier school meals, the USDA launched Team Nutrition, an initiative designed to help make implementation of the new policy in schools easier and more successful.

School Breakfast Program

Skipping breakfast can adversely affect children's performance in math and reading. A study of low-income elementary school students indicated that children who participated in the School Breakfast Program (SBP) had greater improvements in standardized test scores and reduced rates of absence and tardiness than did children who qualified for the program but did not participate (CDC, 2004). The School Breakfast Program provides assistance to states to initiate, maintain, or expand nonprofit breakfast programs in eligible schools and residential child care institutions. The program is administered by the FNS. Any child attending a participating school may receive a free, reduced-price, or full-price breakfast based on the same income criteria used by the NSLP. In 2006, 9 million daily breakfasts were served (USDA, 2008).

Women, Infants, and Children (WIC)

Food, nutrition counseling, and access to health services are provided to low-income women, infants, and children under the WIC program, which is administered by the FNS. This grant program provides supplemental foods and health care referrals and nutrition education at no cost to the recipient. Low-income pregnant or postpartum women and children younger than 5 years old who are at risk nutritionally are eligible for WIC. The eligibility level is an income less than 185% of the poverty level. Nutritional risk is determined by federal guidelines. Three major types of nutritional risk are recognized: (1) high-priority, medically based risks, such as anemia, being **underweight**, low maternal age, history of pregnancy complications; (2) diet-based risks, such as inadequate dietary patterns; and (3) conditions such as alcoholism or drug addiction that predispose people to medically based or diet-based risks.

WIC participants receive coupons redeemable for foods that are rich in protein, calcium, iron, vitamin A, and vitamin C. Also included are iron-fortified infant formula and infant cereal, iron-fortified adult cereal, fruit, or vegetable juice rich in vitamin C, eggs, milk, cheese, and peanut butter or dried beans. Special therapeutic formulas are provided when prescribed by a physician for a specific medical condition. Each WIC participant is designated to receive one of six different food packages that is specially designed for: (1) infants from birth through 3 months, (2) infants from 4 months through a year, (3) women and children with special dietary needs, (4) children 1 to 5 years of age, (5) pregnant and breast-feeding women, and (6) non–breast-feeding postpartum women. In 2006, of the 8.1 million people who received WIC benefits, approximately 4 million were children, 2.1 million were infants, and 2 million were women (USDA, 2008).

Two major types of nutritional risk are recognized for WIC eligibility:

- Medically based risks, such as anemia, underweight, maternal age, history of pregnancy complications, or poor pregnancy outcome
- Diet-based risks, such as inadequate dietary pattern as determined by 24-hour recall, food frequency questionnaire, or diet history

Financial constraints preclude WIC from serving all eligible people; therefore, a system of priorities has been established for filling program openings. After a local WIC agency has reached its maximum caseload, vacancies generally are filled in the order of the following priority levels:

- Pregnant women, breast-feeding women, and infants determined to be at nutritional risk from serious medical problems
- Infants up to 6 months of age whose mothers participate in WIC or are eligible to participate and have serious medical problems
- Children up to age 5 at nutritional risk from serious medical problems
- Pregnant or breast-feeding women and infants who are at nutritional risk from dietary problems
- Children up to age 5 at nutritional risk from dietary problems
- Non–breast-feeding postpartum women with any nutritional risk
- Individuals at nutritional risk only because they are homeless or migrants and current participants who would likely continue to have medical or dietary problems without WIC assistance

In most WIC state agencies, participants receive checks or vouchers monthly to purchase specific foods to supplement their usual diets. These nutrients frequently are missing in the diets of the program's target population. Food packages are provided for various categories of participants. A few WIC state agencies distribute foods through warehouses; some agencies deliver foods to participants.

The WIC Farmers' Market Nutrition Program, established in 1992, provides additional coupons to WIC participants to use for purchasing fresh fruits and vegetables at participating farmers' markets. The program has two goals: (1) to provide fresh, nutritious, unprepared, locally grown fruits and vegetables from farmers' markets to WIC participants and (2) to expand consumers' awareness and use of farmers' markets. In 1998, this program was offered in 50 states, the District of Columbia, and 33 Indian tribal organizations.

The WIC program is effective in improving the health of its participants. Medicaid costs for women who participate in the program during pregnancy and their infants are lower than those for women who do not participate. WIC participation is also linked to longer gestation periods, higher birth weights, and lower infant mortality rates.

Nutrition Service Incentive Program

Nutrition Service Incentive Program (NSIP) formerly known as the Nutrition Program for the Elderly (NPE) helps provide older adults with nutritionally sound meals. These are provided by Meals on Wheels programs or in senior citizen centers and similar congregate feeding settings, in which meals provide the focal points for activities that have the dual objective of promoting better health and reducing the isolation that may occur in old age. Age is the only factor used in determining eligibility. People 60 years or older and their spouses, regardless of age, are eligible for NSIP benefits. Native American tribal organizations may select an age below 60 for defining an older person for their tribes. Additionally, disabled people who live in elder care housing facilities, people who accompany older participants to congregate feeding sites, and volunteers who assist in the meal service may also receive meals through NSIP.

There is no income requirement for NSIP meals. Each recipient may contribute as much as desired toward the cost of the meal, but they are free to people who cannot make any contribution. In 2004, more than 3.1 million people participated, about one third of whom received home delivery. The NSIP is administered by the Administration on Aging, a component unit of the USDHHS. However, the NSIP receives commodity foods and financial support from the USDA's FNS. This program is administered at the state level; therefore, the local state distribution agency should be contacted for information about local programs.

NUTRITION SCREENING

Nutrition screening is the process of discovering characteristics or risk factors that are known to be associated with dietary or nutrition problems. Its primary purpose is to identify individuals (such as older adults and the poor) who are potentially at high risk from complex and involved problems that relate to nutrition. To serve this purpose, screening criteria must be simple, relatively straightforward, and easy to administer. Screening is also helpful in establishing priorities for the most efficient use of valuable time and money.

The single largest demographic group at disproportionate risk of malnutrition is older Americans. Nutrition screening holds a tremendous preventive health potential for older adults. The nurse should provide nutrition counseling or a referral to a registered dietitian for an older person who has food-related problems. A dietitian or community nutrition program might be appropriate if any of the following are identified in the individual:

- Inappropriate, inadequate, or excessive food intake
- Problems complying with a special diet
- Need for nutrient-specific counseling or counseling related to a disease
- Weight of more than 20% above what is desirable
- Serum cholesterol level of more than 240 mg/dL
- Functional dependency for eating or for food-related activities of daily living

The health care professional should refer the individual to a physician when there has been an involuntary decrease in weight of more than 10 pounds during the previous

6 months. Additional anthropometric measurements suggesting malnutrition include the following:

- Triceps skin-fold thickness less than 10th percentile
- Midarm muscle circumference less than 10th percentile
- Serum albumin level less than 3.5 g/dL
- Evidence of osteoporosis or mineral deficiency (indicated by a history of bone pain or fractures, particularly in housebound older women)
- Evidence of vitamin deficiency (indicated by inadequate fruit and vegetable intake; angular stomatitis, glossitis, or bleeding gums; pressure sores in bedridden individuals)

NUTRITION RISK FACTORS

This section examines the role of nutrition in the etiology and prevention of the leading nutrition-related chronic diseases: **heart disease**, stroke, some forms of cancer, osteoporosis, obesity, and **type 2 diabetes**, and in the early treatment of people who are recently diagnosed with the **human immunodeficiency virus**.

Cardiovascular Diseases

Cardiovascular disease (CVD), principally CHD and stroke, are among the nation's leading killers of both men and women and among all racial and ethnic groups. Approximately one fourth of the nation's population has some form of CVD, including high blood pressure, CHD, and stroke.

Heart Disease
Diet Intervention

In an attempt to reduce CVD, the American Heart Association (AHA) recommends that people over the age of 2 years adopt an overall healthy diet and achieve and maintain an appropriate body weight, cholesterol level, and blood pressure level (Krauss et al., 2000; National Institutes of Health, 2001). (The AHA did not set guidelines for those under 2 years of age.)

To achieve an overall healthy eating pattern, include a variety of fruits, vegetables, grains, low-fat or nonfat dairy products, fish, legumes, poultry, and lean meats. Specifically:

- Choose an overall balanced diet with foods from all major food groups, emphasizing fruits, vegetables, and grains.
- Consume a variety of fruits, vegetables, and grain products.
- Consume at least 5 daily servings of fruits and vegetables.
- Consume at least 6 daily servings of grain products, including whole grains.
- Include fat-free and low-fat dairy products, fish, legumes, poultry, and lean meats.
- Eat at least 2 servings of fish every week.

To achieve and maintain an appropriate body weight, match the energy intake to energy needs, with appropriate changes to achieve weight loss when indicated. Specifically:

- Avoid excess intake of calories.
- Maintain a level of physical activity that achieves fitness and that balances energy expenditure with caloric intake; for weight reduction, expenditure should exceed intake.

- Limit foods that are high in calories and low in nutritional quality, including foods with a large amount of added sugar.

To achieve and maintain a desirable cholesterol level, limit foods high in saturated fat and cholesterol and substitute unsaturated fat from vegetables, fish, legumes, and nuts. Specifically:

- Limit foods with a high content of saturated fat and cholesterol. Substitute these foods with grains and unsaturated fat from vegetables, fish, legumes and nuts.
- Limit cholesterol to 300 mg a day for the general population and 200 mg a day for people with CVD or its risk factors.
- Limit trans-fatty acids. Trans-fatty acids are found in foods containing partially hydrogenated vegetable oils, such as packaged cookies, crackers, and other baked goods, commercially prepared fried foods, and some margarines.

To achieve and maintain a desirable blood pressure level, limit salt and alcohol, maintain a healthy body weight, and enjoy a diet with emphasis on vegetables, fruits, and low-fat or nonfat dairy products. Specifically:

- Limit salt intake to less than 6 g (2400 mg sodium) per day, slightly more than 1 teaspoon a day.
- If you drink, limit alcohol consumption to no more than 1 drink per day for women and 2 drinks per day for men. A drink is defined as 12 ounces of beer, 5 ounces of wine, or 1.5 ounces of distilled spirits.

Many children, adolescents, and adults who already have undesirable levels of lipids in their blood should receive nutrition counseling when their total cholesterol level is elevated. In children ages 2 to 20, an acceptable level of cholesterol is less than 170 mg/dL.

Individuals with **low-density lipoprotein (LDL)** cholesterol levels that are above 2000—the National Cholesterol Education Program (NCEP) targets for primary or secondary prevention—should be advised to reduce their intake of dietary saturated fat and cholesterol to levels below the levels recommended for the general population (Expert Panel on Detection, Evaluation, and Treatment of High Blood Cholesterol in Adults, 2001). The upper limit for these individuals is less than 7% of the total energy for saturated fat and less than 200 mg of cholesterol per day. In both cases, however, even lower intake levels can be of further benefit in reducing LDL cholesterol levels. After the program is outlined, follow-up sessions are scheduled to monitor lipid levels and dietary compliance. After 3 to 6 months, if acceptable lipid levels have not been achieved, then the individual should be referred to a registered dietitian.

The NCEP develops new guidelines periodically, as warranted by research advances. Their first and second guidelines were issued in 1988 and 1993. The most recent set of guidelines was released in 2001, Third Report of the NCEP Expert Panel on Detection, Evaluation, and Treatment of High Blood Cholesterol in Adults, also known as Adult Treatment Panel (ATP) III. The ATP guidelines are

Table 11-3 ATP-III Classification of Serum Lipid Levels* in Adults Age 20 and Older

Classification	LDL-Cholesterol, mg/dL	Total Cholesterol, mg/dL	Triglycerides, mg/dL	HDL-Cholesterol, mg/dL
Optimal/desirable	Less than 100	Less than 200	Less than 150	Greater than or equal to 60
Near optimal/above normal	100-129	—	—	—
Borderline high	103-159	200-239	150-159	—
High	160-189	—	200-499	—
Very high	Greater than or equal to 190	Greater than or equal to 240	Greater than or equal to 500	—
Low	—	—	—	Less than or equal to 40

*Measured in milligrams (mg) of lipid per deciliter (dL) of blood.
ATP, Adult Treatment Panel; HDL, high-density lipoprotein; LDL, low-density lipoprotein.
From Expert Panel on Detection, Evaluation, and Treatment of High Blood Cholesterol in Adults. (2001). Executive summary of the third report of the National Cholesterol Education Program (NCEP) expert panel on detection, evaluation, and treatment of high blood cholesterol in adults (adult treatment panel III). *Journal of the American Medical Association, 285,* 2486-2497.

expected to result in about 6.5 million Americans being treated for high cholesterol through Therapeutic Lifestyle Changes (TLC) (Table 11-3).

The ATP recommends that healthy adults have a lipoprotein analysis once every 5 years. A lipoprotein profile measures levels of LDL, total cholesterol, high-density lipoproteins (HDL), and triglycerides (another fatty substance in the blood). The level at which low HDL becomes a major risk factor for heart disease is less than 40 mg/dL.

In addition to a low **high-density lipoprotein (HDL)**, there are other major risk factors for CHD:

- Clinical forms of atherosclerotic disease (peripheral arterial disease, abdominal aortic aneurysm, and symptomatic carotid artery disease)
- Age (55 for men and above 65 for women)
- Cigarette smoking
- Hypertension (blood pressure [BP] higher than 140/90 mm Hg or taking antihypertensive medication)
- Diabetes (fasting blood glucose higher than 110 mg/dL)
- Family history of premature heart disease (heart disease in a first-degree relative at age less than 55 for men or at age less than 65 for women)

HDL cholesterol above 60 counts as a negative risk factor.

Therapeutic Lifestyle Changes (TLC) Treatment Plan

The TLC treatment plan of nutrition, physical activity, and weight control is recommended for treating people who present with type 2 diabetes, elevated LDL, or metabolic syndrome.

Metabolic syndrome describes the presence of a cluster of risk factors that often occur together, which dramatically increases the risk for coronary events. The syndrome is diagnosed when an individual has three or more of these factors:

- Excessive abdominal fat, as indicated by too large a waist measurement (over 35 inches or 88 centimeters in women and over 40 inches or 102 centimeters in men)

- Elevated blood pressure (higher than 130 mm Hg systolic or 85 mm Hg diastolic)
- Low HDL level (lower than 40 mg/dL)
- Elevated **triglyceride** level (higher than 150 mg/dL), which is significantly linked to the degree of heart disease risk. (The guidelines recommend treating even borderline high triglyceride levels with therapy that includes weight control and physical activity.)

The dietary component of the TLC includes daily intake of:
- Less than 7% of calories from saturated fat
- Less than 200 mg of dietary cholesterol
- Up to 35% of calories from total fat, provided most of the fat is from unsaturated fat, which does not raise cholesterol levels. (A higher fat intake may be needed by some individuals with high triglycerides or a low HDL, or both, to keep their triglyceride levels or HDL status from worsening.)
- Intake of certain foods to boost the diet's LDL-lowering power: 2 g/day of plant stanols and sterols found in cholesterol-lowering margarines and salad dressings, and 10 to 25 g/day of foods high in soluble fiber, such as cereal grains, beans, peas, legumes, and many fruits and vegetables.

A primary treatment goal of the TLC is reducing elevated LDL to:
- Less than 100 mg/dL in the presence of CHD or other forms of atherosclerotic disease
- Less than 130 mg/dL in the presence of two or more risk factors for CHD
- Less than 160 mg/dL in the presence of fewer than two risk factors for CHD

The final goal of the TLC includes weight control (to enhance LDL lowering and raise HDL) and physical activity that lasts at least 30 minutes, expending at least 200 calories per day on most days (to improve HDL and, for some, LDL levels).

Removing Barriers to Compliance

To improve client adherence to ATP-III goals, treatment barriers can be eliminated by developing protocols to encourage long-term client compliance and follow-up, such as establishing clinic policy and developing computerized client databases, establishing management algorithms, reinforcing and rewarding adherence, and enhancing third-party reimbursement. The nurse should use behavioral theories to identify a person's level of readiness to change and focus on counseling strategies to match that level of readiness (Snetselaar, 2004).

Hypertension

Blood pressure, the force of blood against the walls of arteries, is recorded as the systolic pressure (as the heart beats) over the diastolic pressure (as the heart relaxes between beats). The measurement is written one above (or before) the other, with the systolic number on top and the diastolic number on the bottom. For example, a blood pressure measurement of 120/80 mm Hg (millimeters of mercury) is expressed verbally as "120 over 80." Normal blood pressure is less than 130 mm Hg systolic and less than 85 mm Hg diastolic. Optimal blood pressure is less than 120 mm Hg systolic and less than 80 mm Hg diastolic. According to the American Heart Association (2008), hypertension (high blood pressure) for adults is defined as a systolic pressure of 140 mm Hg or higher, or a diastolic pressure of 90 mm Hg or higher. See the Research Highlights box for a summary of the AHA Scientific Statement on how to prevent and treat hypertension.

Epidemiology

In 2002, hypertension contributed to the deaths of approximately 277,000 people in the U.S. (CDC, 2007). Using a definition of hypertension as a BP higher than 140/90 mm Hg, as many as 65 million adult Americans, or nearly 25% of all the adults in the United States have hypertension (Rosendorff et al., 2007). Approximately one third of the people with hypertension do not realize they have high blood pressure. Untreated hypertension can damage arteries and increase the risk of stroke and congestive heart failure. High blood pressure is also responsible for many cases of kidney failure requiring dialysis and increases the risk of kidney failure in diabetics.

---

research highlights

AHA Scientific Statement

DIETARY APPROACHES TO PREVENT AND TREAT HYPERTENSION

The purpose of this scientific statement, which updates prior AHA recommendations, is to summarize evidence on the efficacy of diet-related factors that lower BP and to present recommendations for health care providers, policy makers, and the general public.

DIETARY MODIFICATIONS THAT LOWER BLOOD PRESSURE

Effective strategies that lower blood pressure (BP) include reduced salt intake, weight loss, moderation of alcohol consumption (among those who drink), increased potassium intake, and following dietary patterns based on the "DASH" diet.

DIETARY FACTORS WITH LIMITED OR UNCERTAIN EFFECT ON BP

Inconclusive strategies that lower BP are fish oil supplements, dietary fiber, calcium or magnesium supplements, carbohydrate-rich low-fat diets, intake of fats other than n-3 PUFA, high protein intake, and increased intake of vitamin C.

SPECIAL POPULATIONS

Children

Numerous observational studies have documented that BP tracks with age from childhood into the adult years. At present, direct evidence from rigorous, well-controlled trials in children and adolescents is sparse. Accordingly, the effect of diet on BP in children and adolescents is, in large part, extrapolated from studies of adults.

Older Persons

As a group, older individuals are at high risk for BP-related cardiovascular and renal disease. Because of high attributable risk associated with elevated BP in older adults, the beneficial effects of dietary changes on BP should translate into substantial reductions in cardiovascular risk in older adults. Greater BP reductions from dietary interventions occur as individuals get older.

Blacks

As documented in well-controlled efficacy studies, Blacks as compared with non-Blacks achieve greater BP reduction from nonpharmacological therapies, specifically sodium reduction, increased potassium intake, and the DASH diet. The potential benefits of these dietary approaches are amplified because survey data indicate that Blacks consume high levels of sodium while their potassium intake is less than that of non-Blacks.

CONCLUSION

Dietary modifications that are effective in lowering BP include weight loss, reduced salt intake, increased potassium intake, moderation of alcohol consumption, and consumption of an overall healthy dietary pattern, such as the DASH diet. In view of the increasing levels of high BP in children and adults and the continuing epidemic of BP-related cardiovascular disease, efforts will require individuals to change behavior and society to make substantial environmental changes.

DASH, Dietary Approaches to Stop Hypertension; *NHLBI*, National Heart, Lung, and Blood Institute; *NIH*, National Institutes of Health; *S/D*, systolic/diastolic.
Modified from Appel, L. J., Brands, M. W., Daniels, S. R., Karanja, N., Elmer, P. J. & Sacks, F. M. (2006). Dietary approaches to prevent and treat hypertension: A scientific statement from the American Heart Association, *Hypertension, 47*, 296-308.

African Americans and Hispanic Americans are more likely to suffer from high blood pressure than are White non-Hispanic Americans. Additionally, people with lower educational and income levels tend to have higher blood pressure levels. In 2004 the death rates per 100,000 population from high blood pressure were 15.7 for White non-Hispanic men, 51 for African American men, 14.5 for White non-Hispanic women, and 40.9 for African American women (American Heart Association, 2008).

Diet Intervention

The modifiable nutrition-related risk factors for stroke include obesity, habitual high alcohol intake, and high intake of sodium. No certain method exists for identifying susceptible people or ascertaining how many of them become hypertensive as a result of excessive salt intake; therefore, the conservative preventive health approach recommends a salt intake limited to 6 g or less per day for adults. Sodium chloride is approximately 40% sodium by weight; therefore, a diet with 6 g salt contains about 2.4 g of sodium. This amount is regarded as mild sodium restriction. **Website Resource 11A** lists the approximate sodium content of representative foods.

The three major sources of sodium in the U.S. diet are:

1. Salt added by consumers to food during cooking or at the table
2. Salt added by food processing companies as an ingredient in almost all processed foods (including many foods that do not taste salty, such as baked goods); most processed foods are high in sodium content
3. Salt from all animal products, which are a natural source of sodium

The following recommended food tips are designed to reduce salt and sodium intake:

- Sodium occurs naturally in many foods and is also added to most processed foods; therefore, added salt should be used only sparingly in home cooking and at the table.
- Consume fewer foods that have high sodium levels, such as many cheeses; processed meats; most frozen dinners and entrees; packaged mixes; most canned soups and vegetables; salad dressings; and condiments such as soy sauce, pickles, olives, catsup, and mustard.
- Before warming canned vegetables, rinse them first.
- Salty, highly processed salty, salt-preserved, and salt-pickled foods should be eaten sparingly.
- Check labels for the amount of sodium in foods and choose products lower in sodium.

DASH Eating Plan

Clinical studies show that blood pressure can be lowered by following the "Dietary Approaches to Stop Hypertension" (DASH) eating plan. The National Heart, Lung and Blood Institute (NHLBI), with additional support by the NIH, funded the DASH research with final results appearing in the *New England Journal of Medicine* in 1997. The DASH eating plan makes consuming less salt and sodium easier because the plan includes abundant fruits and vegetables, which are lower in sodium than other foods. The plan also includes more fat-free or low-fat milk and milk products, whole grains, fish, poultry, beans, seeds and nuts, but contains less sweets, added sugars and sugar-containing beverages, fats, and red meats than the average typical American diet.

The plan is rich in magnesium, potassium, calcium, protein and fiber. At approximately 2100 calories a day, the nutrients include 4700 mg of potassium, 500 mg of magnesium, and 1250 mg of calcium. These totals are approximately 2 to 3 times the amounts most Americans receive.

Based on DASH clinical studies, a combination of the eating plan and reduced sodium intake can reduce elevated levels of blood pressure. When blood pressure is normal, the DASH eating plan may help prevent blood pressure problems. If blood pressure is only slightly elevated, then the plan may actually eliminate the need for medication. For more severe high blood pressure, the plan may allow a reduction in medication. Other steps to control or prevent hypertension should continue to be encouraged, including exercising, losing excess weight, not smoking, and limiting alcohol. DASH may improve health in other ways, also. Fruits and vegetables may reduce the risk for some cancers; the calcium in dairy products can lower risk for osteoporosis; and a diet low in saturated fat and cholesterol can reduce CVD risk. The complete DASH eating plan entitled "Your Guide to Lowering Blood Pressure With DASH" (USDHHS, 2006) can be accessed at the website *www.nhlbi.nih.gov/health/public/heart/hbp/dash/index.htm*.

Further evidence supporting the benefits of the DASH eating plan is presented in the AHA Scientific Statement (Research Highlights box).

Cancer
Epidemiology

The American Cancer Society (ACS) estimates that in 2007 approximately 1,444,920 cases of cancer will be diagnosed in the United States. In 2004, approximately 553,888 Americans died of this disease (ACS, 2008). Overall, Blacks were more likely to develop cancer than were people of any other racial or ethnic group. During the period from 1999 to 2003, incidence rates were 1023.6 per 100,000 among Blacks, 976.1 per 100,000 among Whites, 771.3 per 100,000 among Hispanic Americans, 688.8 per 100,000 among Asian Americans, and 664.9 per 100,000 among Native Americans. The incidence of breast cancer in women is highest among White women (132.5 per 100,000) and lowest among Native American women (69.8 per 100,000) (ACS, 2007a). Black women have the highest incidence rates of colon and rectal cancer (23.7 per 100,000) and lung and bronchial cancer (46.2 per 100,000) followed by Whites, Asian Americans, Hispanic Americans, and Native Americans. Blacks are approximately 33% more likely to die of cancer than Whites and are 2 times more likely to die of cancer than Asian Americans, Native Americans, and Hispanic Americans. During the period from 1999 to

2003, cancer mortality rates were 523.4 per 100,000 among Blacks, 402.6 per 100,000 among Whites, 275.2 per 100,000 among Hispanic Americans, 243.7 per 100,000 among Asian Americans, and 265 per 100,000 among Native Americans. Cancer mortality rates for many racial and ethnic groups have begun to decline recently. Black women are more likely to die of breast cancer (34.4 per 100,000) and colon and rectal cancer (23.7 per 100,000) than are women of any other racial or ethnic group (ACS, 2008).

Approximately 40% of cancer incidence among men and 60% among women is related to diet. The introduction of a healthy diet and exercise practices at any time from childhood to old age can promote health and likely reduce cancer risk.

Diet Intervention for Risk Reduction

Many dietary factors can affect cancer risk: types of foods, food preparation methods, portion sizes, food variety, and overall caloric balance. An overall dietary pattern that includes a high proportion of plant foods (fruits, vegetables, grains, and beans), limited amounts of meat, dairy, and other high-fat foods, and a balance of caloric intake and physical activity can reduce the risk of cancer.

Based on its review of the scientific evidence, the ACS updated its nutrition and physical activities guidelines in 2006. The ACS recommendations are consistent in principle with the USDA food guidance system MyPyramid, the Dietary Guidelines for Americans, and dietary recommendations of other agencies for general health promotion and for the prevention of CHD, diabetes, and other diet-related chronic conditions. Although no diet can guarantee full protection against any disease, the ACS believes that the following recommendations offer the best nutrition information currently available to help Americans.

Choose Most of the Foods You Eat From Plant Sources Eat 5 or more servings of fruits and vegetables every day; eat other foods from plant sources, such as breads, cereals, grain products, rice, pasta, or beans several times every day. Many scientific studies show that eating fruits and vegetables (especially green and dark yellow vegetables, foods in the cabbage family, soy products, and legumes) can protect against cancers at many sites, particularly for cancers of the gastrointestinal and respiratory tracts. Grains are an important source of many vitamins and minerals, such as folate, calcium, and selenium, which have been associated with a lower risk of colon cancer in some studies. Beans (legumes) are especially rich in nutrients that may protect against cancer.

Since 1991 the 5 A Day for Better Health Program has raised public awareness about the importance of fruits and vegetables in disease prevention. The program is jointly sponsored by the National Cancer Institute (a division of the USDHHS) and the Produce for Better Health Foundation (a nonprofit consumer education foundation representing the fruit and vegetable industry). Through its unique national public-private partnership, 5 A Day for Better Health Program seeks to increase consumption of fruits and vegetables to 5 or more servings each day. The program gives Americans a simple, positive message: eat 5 or more servings of fruits and vegetables every day for better health.

In The New American Plate, the American Institute for Cancer Research recommends reducing the portion size of meat, fish, or chicken to 3 ounces and filling the rest of the dinner plate with dishes composed of vegetables, fruits, whole grains, and beans. The program urges people to reverse the traditional American plate and think of meat as a side dish or condiment rather than the primary ingredient. In terms that laypeople can understand, this regimen translates into vegetables, fruits, whole grains, and beans covering two thirds (or more) of the plate, with animal-source foods covering one third (or less) (American Institute for Cancer Research, 2000).

The Adequate Intake (AI) for total fiber is expected to reduce the risk of colon cancer, coronary heart disease, type 2 diabetes, diverticular disease, and constipation. The Institute of Medicine (2002) and the Dietary Guidelines for Americans 2005 recommends that children (age 1 and up) and adults should consume 14 grams of fiber for every 1000 calories of food they eat each day. For children over age 1, the recommended intake is at least 19 grams per day. For adults 50 years and younger, the recommended intake is 38 grams for men and 25 grams for women, while for men and women over 50 it is 30 and 21 grams per day, respectively, due to decreased food consumption.

Limit Intake of High-Fat Foods, Particularly From Animal Sources Choose foods low in fat and limit consumption of meats, especially high-fat meats. High-fat diets have been associated with an increased risk of cancers of the colon and rectum, prostate, and endometrium. The association between high-fat diets and the risk of breast cancer is weaker. Two studies funded by NIH are ongoing to identify the causal relationship of low-fat diets and eventual breast cancer. One study, the Women's Health Initiative, focused on primary prevention of breast cancer through low-fat diet in women who currently have no disease. The second, Women's Intervention Nutrition Study, will look at secondary prevention of breast cancer through low-fat diet in women who currently have breast cancer, with the goal being prevention of recurrence of disease. Whether these associations are caused by the total amount of fat, the particular type of fat (saturated, monounsaturated, or polyunsaturated), the calories contributed by fat, or by some other factor in food fats has not been determined. Consumption of meat, particularly red meat, has been associated with an increased risk of cancer at several sites, most notably the colon and prostate.

Be Physically Active: Achieve and Maintain a Healthy Weight Physical activity can help protect against some cancers, either by balancing caloric intake with energy expenditure or by other mechanisms. An imbalance of caloric intake and energy output can lead to being overweight or obese and an increased risk for cancers at several sites, such as the colon and rectum, prostate, endometrium, breast (among postmenopausal women), and kidney. Both physical activity and controlled caloric intake are necessary to achieve or maintain a healthy body weight.

Limit Consumption of Alcoholic Beverages Alcoholic beverages, along with cigarette smoking and the use of snuff and chewing tobacco, cause cancers of the oral cavity, esophagus, and larynx. The combined use of tobacco and alcohol leads to a greatly increased risk of oral and esophageal cancers; the effect of tobacco and alcohol combined is greater than the sum of their individual effects. Studies also have shown an association between alcohol consumption and an increased risk of breast cancer. The mechanism of this effect is not known, but the association may be related to carcinogenic actions of alcohol or its metabolites, to alcohol-induced changes in levels of hormones such as estrogens, or to some other process. Regardless of the mechanism, studies show that the risk of breast cancer increases with an intake beginning at only a few drinks per week. Reducing alcohol consumption is a good way for women who drink regularly to reduce their risk of breast cancer (ACS, 2007b).

Osteoporosis
Epidemiology
In the United States in 2007, 44 million individuals had decreased bone mass, known as osteoporosis, and 34 million more people had low bone mineral density (BMD), placing them at increased risk for osteoporosis. Of the 10 million Americans estimated to have osteoporosis, 80% are women. Of the people with hip fractures, 20% die within a year, and one half of the survivors never walk again. Direct financial expenditures for management of osteoporotic fracture alone are estimated at $15 billion to $17 billion annually. These figures underestimate significantly the true costs of osteoporosis, because they fail to include the costs of treatment for individuals without a history of fractures or the indirect costs of lost wages or productivity of either the individual or the caregiver.

National Osteoporosis Foundation recognized risk factors for osteoporosis:

- Age: As age increases the risk increases.
- Gender: Women have greater risk.
- Race: Caucasian and Asian women are more likely to develop osteoporosis. African American and Hispanic women have lower but significant risk. Among men, Caucasians are at higher risk than others.
- Personal history of fracture as an adult
- History of fragility fracture in a first-degree relative
- Low body weight (less than 127 lb)
- Current smoking
- Use of oral corticosteroid therapy for more than three months
- Impaired vision
- Estrogen deficiency at an early age (less than 45 years)
- Dementia
- Poor health/frailty

- Recent falls
- Low calcium intake (lifelong)
- Low physical activity
- Alcohol intake more than two drinks per day for men, one drink for women

The prevalence of osteoporosis and the incidence of fracture vary by gender and race-ethnicity. The probability that a 50-year-old individual will have a hip fracture during a lifetime is 16% to 18% for a White woman and 5% to 6% for a White man. The risk for Blacks is much lower, at 6% and 3% for a 50-year-old woman and man, respectively.

- White postmenopausal women have a one in seven chance of having a hip fracture during their lifetimes.
- Black women have higher BMD than White women throughout life, and they experience lower hip fracture rates.
- Some Japanese women have lower peak BMD than White women, but they have a lower hip fracture rate, the reasons for which are not fully understood.
- Hispanic American women have bone densities between those of White women and those of Black women.
- Limited information on Native American women suggests they have lower BMD than White women.

Pathophysiology
Osteoporosis is a slowly developing condition that causes loss of bone mass and fractures, especially in the wrist, hip, and spinal areas. Osteoporosis is defined as a skeletal disorder characterized by compromised bone strength predisposing to an increased risk of fracture. Bone strength reflects the integration of two main features: (1) bone density and (2) bone quality. Bone density is expressed as grams of mineral per area or volume and, in any given individual, is determined by peak bone mass and amount of bone loss. Bone quality refers to architecture, turnover, damage accumulation (microfractures), and mineralization. Osteoporotic bone fractures more easily than normal bone; therefore, osteoporosis is a significant risk factor for fracture.

Factors Involved in Building and Maintaining Skeletal Health Throughout Life Growth in bone size and strength occurs during childhood, but bone accumulation is not completed until the third decade of life, after the cessation of linear growth. The bone mass attained early in life is perhaps the most important determinant of lifelong skeletal health. Individuals with the highest peak bone mass after adolescence have the greatest protective advantage when the inevitable declines in bone density associated with increasing age, illness, and diminished sex-steroid production take their toll.

Genetic factors exert a strong and perhaps predominant influence on peak bone mass, but physiological, environmental, and modifiable lifestyle factors can also play a significant role. Among these factors are adequate nutrition and body weight, exposure to sex hormones at puberty, and physical activity. Therefore maximizing BMD early in life presents a critical opportunity to reduce the effect of bone loss related to aging. Childhood is a critical time for development of lifestyle habits conducive to maintaining good bone health throughout life. Additionally, cigarette smoking, which usually starts in adolescence, may have a deleterious effect on bone mass.

Prevention

Once thought to be a natural part of aging among women, osteoporosis is no longer considered age dependent or gender dependent and is largely preventable, thanks to the recent progress in the understanding of its causes, diagnosis, and treatment. Optimization of bone health is a process that must occur throughout the life span in both men and women. Factors that enhance bone health at all ages are essential to prevent osteoporosis and its devastating consequences. Calcium is the nutrient most important for attaining peak bone mass and for preventing and treating osteoporosis.

Good nutrition is essential for normal growth. A balanced diet, adequate calories, and appropriate nutrients are the foundation for developing all tissues, including bone. Adequate and appropriate nutrition is important for all individuals, but not everyone follows a diet that is optimal for bone health.

Table 11-4 suggests dietary calcium intake recommendations for various stages of life. Factors contributing to low calcium intake are restriction of dairy products, a generally low level of fruit and vegetable consumption, and a high intake of low-calcium beverages such as soft drinks. Lactose and vitamin D enhance calcium absorption and exercise enhances calcium balance. Calcium is absorbed best from dairy foods. It is the only source of the disaccharide lactose.

Vitamin D is a fat-soluble vitamin technically encompassing two molecules—vitamin D2 (ergocalciferol) and vitamin D3 (cholecalciferol). Vitamin D3 is the form of vitamin D that best supports bone health. Vitamin D is synthesized in the body when the skin is exposed to the ultraviolet rays of the sun. Commonly added to milk, other food sources of vitamin D include fatty fish (salmon and mackerel); margarine; eggs; and some fortified, ready-to-eat cereals. Most infants and young children in the United States have adequate vitamin D intake from the supplementation and fortification of milk. During adolescence, when consumption of dairy products decreases, vitamin D intake is likely to be inadequate, which may affect calcium absorption adversely. Other nutrients have been evaluated relative to bone health. High dietary protein, caffeine, phosphorus, and sodium can adversely affect calcium balance; however, their effects appear to be unimportant in individuals with adequate calcium intakes.

Food should be selected to provide adequate calcium, paying special attention to that eaten by adolescents, who normally have high mineral requirements, and by women who are susceptible to inadequate dietary calcium because of low caloric intake. Women of all ages should be concerned about adequate calcium intake. A means for increasing individual consumption of calcium includes educating consumers to eat more calcium-rich foods, including calcium-fortified foods such as orange juice, and recommending dietary supplements. Individuals who wish to increase their calcium intake can consume more low-fat or nonfat dairy products or fortified food products. Supplementation with calcium tablets may be appropriate for people at high risk of health problems from inadequate calcium intake.

Although maintaining a proper daily calcium intake through food is preferable, calcium supplements are available for people who do not get enough of the mineral through their regular diets. Calcium carbonate (40% elemental calcium), calcium citrate (24%), calcium lactate (14%), and calcium gluconate (9%) are preferred. (Dolomite and bone meal are not recommended, because they may be contaminated with lead.) Calcium supplement absorption is most efficient for individuals with adequate gastric acid production at individual doses no greater than 500 mg when taken between meals.

Individuals need to be encouraged to increase their consumption of calcium-rich foods. Milk and dairy products deliver the most calcium of any food group, but they are also among the richest sources of fat in the American diet. Low-fat and fat-free milk, yogurt, and low-fat cheeses are the dairy products of choice. Other good sources of calcium include sardines, canned salmon (if the bones are eaten), and some dark green leafy vegetables, especially collard greens. Orange juice and milk fortified with calcium are also good sources. The calcium content of some common foods is summarized in **Website Resource 11B**.

Table **11-4**	Recommendations for Calcium and Vitamin D Intake	
	Calcium (mg/day)	Vitamin D (IU/day)
INFANTS		
0-6 months	210	200
6-12 months	270	200
CHILDREN AND ADOLESCENTS		
1-3 years	500	200
4-8 years	800	200
9-18 years	1300	200
ADULTS		
18-50 years	1000	200
51-70 years	1200	400
Greater than 70 years	1200	600
PREGNANCY		
Less than 18 years	1300	200
19-30 years	1000	200
31-50 years	1000	200
LACTATION		
Less than 18 years	1300	200
19-30 years	1000	200
31-50 years	1000	200

Anyone under 25 years of age who ingests less than the recommended intake of calcium need to be urged to develop strategies for increasing it. Children, particularly preadolescent girls, need to take care to receive the proper amounts. By modeling appropriate behaviors, health care professionals can help prevent or delay the onset of osteoporosis in themselves, their families, and the people who are in their care.

Obesity

As almost everyone in health care in the United States knows, a paradox exists in modern America. On the one hand, many people who do not need to lose weight are trying to do so, and on the other hand, many who actually need to lose weight are not trying; those who are trying are unsuccessful in losing the weight and maintaining their weight loss.

Overweight, defined as about 10% to 20% over healthy weight, can seriously affect health and longevity and is associated with the leading nutrition-related causes of death in the United States: type 2 diabetes, CVD, and some cancers. Obesity, about 20% or more overweight, is also associated with gout and gallbladder disease and may contribute to the development of osteoarthritis in the weight-bearing joints.

Epidemiology

Overweight and obesity are found worldwide and the prevalence of these conditions in the United States ranks high in comparison with that of other developed nations. Approximately 30,000 adult deaths in the United States each year are attributable to obesity. Two thirds of the nation's adults are overweight (including people who are obese) (USDHHS, NIH, National Institute of Diabetes & Digestive & Kidney Diseases, [NIDDK], 2004). **Website Resource 11C** presents a table of healthy weight, overweight, and obesity among people 20 years of age and over.

The prevalence of being overweight has increased steadily over the years among nearly all racial and ethnic groups. From 1960 to 2000 the prevalence of overweight increased from 31.5% to 33.6% in adults in the United States. The prevalence of obesity during this same period increased from 13.3% to 30.9%—a relative increase of more than 50%, with most of this increase occurring during the 1990s. The prevalence of overweight and obesity increases with advancing age until people reach their 60s, when it starts to decline. From 1991 to 1998, obesity increased in every state of the United States, in both genders and across all races and ethnicities, age groups, educational levels, and smoking statuses, with the exception of White non-Hispanic men in their 20s to 40s, in whom the prevalence of obesity decreased from the early 1970s to late 1970s (USDHHS, NIH, NIDDK, 2004).

Obesity is more common in women than in men. Among men there is a modest ethnic variation in the prevalence of being overweight, the greatest difference occurring between Black men (67%) and Hispanic American men (74.6%). Among women, the ethnic variation is substantial. Almost 57.6% of White women are overweight; Hispanic American and Puerto Rican women have a greater prevalence of being overweight (73%) than their White counterparts; and more than 79.6% of Black women are overweight (National Center for Health Statistics, 2007). Potential contributing factors often associated with the greater propensity for adult Black women to become obese include lower level of physical activity, higher energy intake, lower levels of education and social economic status as well as broader acceptance of a larger body size within the African American community (Hawkins, 2007; Sanchez-Johnsen et al., 2006).

Body Mass Index for Adults

Based on an adult's height and weight, **body mass index (BMI)** (wt/ht^2) is a helpful indicator of obesity and being underweight (Garrow & Webster, 1958). A person's BMI can be determined by referring to the table in **Website Resource 11D,** by using a calculator on the Internet (the CDC's online BMI calculator) (*www.cdc.gov/nccdphp/dnpa/bmi/calc-bmi.htm*), or by using a hand-held calculator and the following formulas:

Body Mass Index Formulas
English Formula

$$BMI = \text{weight in pounds} \div \text{height in inches} \div \text{height in inches} \times 703$$

Example: For a 6-foot-tall person weighing 210 pounds: BMI = 210 pounds divided by 72 inches divided by 72 inches multiplied by 703 = 28.5.

Metric Formulas

$$BMI = \text{weight in kilograms} \div (\text{height in meters})^2$$
$$\text{and}$$
$$BMI = (\text{weight in kilograms} \div \text{height in cm} \div \text{height in cm}) \times 10,000$$

Example: For a person who is 182.9 centimeters tall and weighs 95.3 kilograms: BMI = 95.3 kg divided by 182.9 cm multiplied by 10,000 = 28.5.

BMI is a good indicator of body fat, but it cannot be interpreted as a specific percentage of body fat. Age and gender influence the relationship between fat and BMI. For example, women are more likely to have a higher percentage of body fat than men have for the same BMI. At the same BMI, older people have more body fat than do younger adults (Gallagher et al., 1996, 2000). BMI is used to screen and monitor a population to detect the risk of health or nutritional disorders. In an individual, other data must be used to determine whether a high BMI is associated with increased risk of disease and death for that person; BMI alone is not diagnostic.

BMI ranges are based on the effect body weight has on disease and death. A BMI value from 19 to 25 is a healthy target range for adults. BMI values higher than 25 are associated with increasing risks for developing CVD, gallbladder disease, high blood pressure, and non–insulin-dependent diabetes mellitus. A high BMI value is predictive of death from CVD (Calle et al., 1999).

BMI values for adults are expressed with one number, regardless of age or sex, using the following guidelines by World Health Organization Classification of Body Weight (2006):

- Underweight: BMI less than 18.5
- Healthy weight: BMI of 18.5 to 24.9
- Overweight: BMI of 25 to 29.9
- Class 1 obese: BMI of 30 to 34.9
- Class 2 obese: BMI of 35 to 39.9
- Class 3 obese (morbid obesity): BMI of 40 or higher

Body Mass Index Growth Charts for Children

Many parents are familiar with the original growth charts used by pediatric health care providers since 1977. Those charts were used widely by pediatricians, nurses, and nutritionists to track growth and development in children and assist in signaling potential developmental problems. The charts consist of a series of percentile curves that illustrate the distribution in growth of children across the United States.

In 2000 the Centers for Disease Control and Prevention (CDC) released new pediatric growth charts that more accurately reflect the nation's cultural and racial diversity and track children and young people through age 20. These charts are used to monitor children's growth and help identify weight problems earlier in childhood. The charts include an assessment of BMI. The BMI is an early warning signal that is helpful as early as age 2 to help identify children who have the potential to become overweight. Early identification of obesity risk gives parents the opportunity to modify their children's eating habits before a weight problem develops.

The CDC's new charts are based on data gathered through the National Health and Nutrition Examination Survey, the only survey that collects data from actual physical examinations on a cross-section of Americans from all over the country. This survey shows that since the 1980s the number of overweight children and adolescents has doubled. Additionally, it shows that over one half of all American adults are overweight and that the number of obese adults has doubled. It is expected that the new BMI charts will help address this nationwide problem. The growth charts indicate that, in general, children are heavier today than in 1977, but height has remained virtually unchanged. The new charts are available on the CDC website at *www.cdc. gov/growthcharts*.

Diet Intervention

"Please help me lose weight" is one of the most common requests heard in the health field. As discussed, a balanced diet is important and must include the appropriate **serving sizes** for the recommended daily intake of each food group. Additionally, exercise is particularly necessary from the outset, because with exercise there is less need to restrict food. Exercise also favors long-term maintenance of body weight (as described in Chapter 12).

Nurses make referrals to supervised or unsupervised programs as appropriate. People expect this type of advice on maintaining their health. Therefore nurses can play an important role, although not supervising individuals' weight loss efforts directly. (For more information on obesity among adults, see USDHHS, National Heart, Lung, and Blood Institute, 2007.)

There are many positive effects of only relatively small amounts of weight loss (5% to 10% of body weight) for people who are obese:

- Decreased blood pressure (decreased risk of a heart attack and stroke)
- Reduced abnormally high levels of blood glucose associated with diabetes
- Reduced elevated levels of cholesterol and triglycerides associated with CVD
- Reduced sleep apnea (irregular breathing during sleep)
- Decreased risk of osteoarthritis in the weight-bearing joints
- Decreased depression
- Increased self-esteem

The acronym LEARN has been suggested as a mnemonic device for health professionals. LEARN refers to the steps nurses can take to help the person who needs to improve health-related behavior (Brownell, 2000). LEARN is particularly useful as a guideline for communicating with the clinically obese individual who has indicated dissatisfaction with current weight:

L: Listen with sympathy and understanding to the person's perception of the problem.

E: Explain personal perceptions of the problem.

A: Acknowledge and discuss differences and similarities.

R: Recommend treatment.

N: Negotiate an agreement.

In 1992 an NIH-sponsored technical support conference identified the following characteristics of voluntary weight loss and weight control in the United States (USDHHS, 1992):

1. Obesity is a chronic disease.
2. Obesity has many causes.
3. Cure is rare; palliation is realistic.
4. Weight loss is slow.
5. Recidivism is common.
6. Weight regain may be slow, but it is often rapid.
7. Management is often more frustrating than the underlying disease.

The conference noted significant adverse effects for obese dieters who regain lost weight:

- Repeated weight gain and loss may have adverse psychological and physical effects; for example, evidence suggests that mildly to moderately overweight women who are dieting may be at risk for binge eating.
- Although data on the health effects of repeated weight gain and loss (weight cycling) are also inconclusive, weight cycling appears to affect energy metabolism and may cause faster regaining of weight.
- Depression and decreased self-esteem occur.

A new model of health care is needed for people who cannot maintain a BMI under 30. The new paradigm, health at any size, is described in the Hot Topics box. Fad diets do not provide the best way to lose weight and should be avoided (see Health Teaching box).

Two major types of weight-loss pills are lipase inhibitor and appetite suppressant. Lipase inhibitor works by reducing the body's ability to absorb dietary fat. Appetite suppressant medications promote weight loss by acting on appetite centers in the brain to decrease appetite. Table 11-5 provides details of the major medications that promote weight loss.

Diabetes
Prevalence and Incidence

Diabetes is becoming more prevalent. The numbers of existing cases (**prevalence**) and new cases (**incidence**) are increasing, and most of this increase is not a result of aging of the U.S. population. Trends show that minority and older populations

---

HOTtopics

HEALTH AT ANY SIZE: THE SIZE ACCEPTANCE NONDIET MOVEMENT

The new paradigm has replaced the question, "How can fat people lose weight?" with the question, "How can fat people be healthy?" (Spark, 2001). The following tenets are the foundation of the movement:

- Good health is a state of physical, mental, and social well-being. People of all sizes and shapes can reduce their risk of poor health by adopting a healthy lifestyle, which includes (1) eating a variety of healthy foods, (2) being physically active because it is fun and feels good, and (3) appreciating the body as it is.
- Human beings come in a variety of sizes and shapes; size diversity is a positive characteristic of the human race. Respect the bodies of others, although they might be quite different.
- There is no ideal body size, shape, BMI, or body composition that every individual should strive to achieve.
- Self-esteem and body image are strongly linked. Helping people feel good about their bodies and about who they are can help motivate and maintain healthy behaviors.
- People are responsible for care of their own bodies.
- Appearance stereotyping is wrong. Their weight notwithstanding, all people deserve to be treated equally in the job market and on the job, to be treated equally in the media, and to receive competent and respectful treatment by health care professionals.

How to Become a Size-Sensitive Health Professional

- On the intake form, include a question asking whether the person is satisfied with the body size.

If the answer is "yes," then try to avoid the issue in the future.
- When the person asks not to be weighed, the request is acknowledged without complaint and automatically taken into account on follow-up office visits. (There are a few cases in which weighing is necessary, such as when administering certain medications, chemotherapy, or anesthesia.)
- A size-sensitive health care professional does not necessarily avoid mentioning weight but should avoid making an issue of weight, avoid lectures and humiliation, and respect the individual's wishes with regard to weight discussions.
- When weight contributes to a problem, the professional mentions this situation but also considers other diagnoses and recommends tests to determine the actual diagnosis when appropriate. If weight loss is a recommended treatment for a problem, the compassionate professional may mention this, but at minimum, and recommend and prescribe other treatments. Accept the individual's wish not to use weight loss as a treatment.
- Some health care professionals believe that overweight and obesity are not necessarily unhealthy. However, other professionals who believe that fat is unhealthy may acknowledge that weight loss is usually ineffective or that the individuals have the right to direct their own treatment.
- Ideally the waiting area, examining suite, and consultation room are equipped with armless chairs, large blood pressure cuffs, large examination gowns, and other equipment suitable for large people. If this is not the case, then the office staff acknowledges the importance of these items when told.

BMI, Body mass index.

HEALTH TEACHING   Types of Fad Diets

Mediterranean Diet
Main source of fat is healthy monounsaturated fats (e.g., olive oil or canola oil). Dairy foods, low-fat and nonfat dairy or soy products, fruits, vegetables, whole grain breads, cereals, nuts, seeds, and beans. Weekly foods: skinless poultry, fish (high content of omega-3), eggs, lean pork or other lean red meats, lower-fat cheeses, part-skim mozzarella, natural sweeteners (e.g., honey). Monthly foods: high-fat meats, cheeses, desserts, candy, butter, margarine, coconuts, vegetable oils other than olive or canola. Monthly and weekly foods are optional, so vegetarians can follow this diet.

Mayo Clinic Diet
Daily servings of each food group appropriate for your calorie level. Fruits, vegetables with virtually no restrictions. Limited quantities of juice and dried fruit. Carbohydrates, especially unrefined whole grains; lean and low-fat protein and dairy fats. Sweets are limited to approximately 70 calories/day (e.g., one small oatmeal raisin cookie).

The Blood Type Diet
Type O: For weight loss: Kelp, seafood, salt, liver, red meat, spinach, kale, and broccoli. No wheat, corn, navy beans, kidney beans, lentils, cabbage, Brussels sprouts, cauliflower, mustard greens.

Continued

HEALTH TEACHING   Types of Fad Diets—cont'd

Type A: For weight loss: Vegetable, vegetable oil, soy foods, pineapple. No meat, dairy, kidney or lima beans, wheat.

Type B: For weight loss: Greens, eggs, venison, liver licorice, tea. No corn, lentils, peanuts, sesame seeds, buckwheat.

Type AB: For weight loss: Tofu, seafood, dairy, greens, kelp, and pineapple. No red meat, kidney or lima beans, seeds, corn, buckwheat.

Food-Combining Diet

Avoid eating the following foods in the same meal:

1. Carbohydrates and acidic food
2. Concentrated proteins and concentrated carbohydrates together
3. Two concentrated proteins
4. Fats with protein
5. Acidic fruits with proteins
6. Starch and sugars
7. Only one concentrated starch food per meal
8. Eat melons alone
9. Milk is best taken alone or avoided

Sugar Busters Diet

High-fiber vegetables, whole grains, and fruits. Lean and trimmed meats. Low-fat milk and cheese. No saturated fats and trans fats. Six glasses of water a day. No missed meals, eat three regular meals daily and appropriate snacks are allowed. Moderation in portion size. No late-night snacking. No refined sugar, corn syrup, molasses, honey, sugared colas, or beer.

Special K Diet

Two-week regimen of eating Special K cereal for breakfast and later replacing lunch or dinner with cereal. The remaining meal could be any meal that the dieter would normally eat. The cereal is to be eaten with ⅔ cup of skim milk and a piece of fruit.

The Glycemic Index Diet

Foods are rated on the Glycemic Index (GI), which indicates how fast carbohydrates break down and increase blood sugar. Consuming foods on the middle to lower end of the GI should keep you full over a longer period of time, helping you control your appetite and therefore reduce your weight.

The Zone Diet

Fresh vegetables, fruits and nuts, leafy green vegetables, eight glasses of water day. Choose monounsaturated fats over saturated fats. Avoid processed foods and foods high in salt. Proteins (e.g., chicken, fish, beef, turkey, and low-fat pork) should be the size and thickness of your palm. Fats (e.g., olive oil and butter) should equal the size of the tip of your thumb. Avoid breads, pastas, bagels, cereals, sodas, juices, alcohol, caffeine-filled food items, sugary items.

The South Beach Diet

Three Diet Phases:

Phase One: Involves two weeks of strict dieting and is the initial and fastest weight loss period. Nearly all carbohydrates are avoided, but you may still eat normal-sized meals and many people report losing between 8 to 13 lb.

Phase Two: The good carbohydrates are introduced back into your diet; you will continue to lose weight until you reach your target weight.

Phase Three: This is the life-long period, maintaining your desired weight with a healthy balance. If you start to gain weight again, you should return to phase one for a few days. A daily calcium supplement is recommended.

Dr. Atkins Diet

The key to this diet is high-protein foods and consuming no more than 20 grams of carbohydrates per day. By doing this the body will burn stored fat as its energy source rather than carbohydrates. Expectable foods include, but are not limited to, meats, poultry, seafood, eggs, and cheese.

The Cambridge Diet

This diet utilizes four stages to manage weight. First stage is preparation. This stage is the gradual reduction of food intake. The second stage is weight loss. In this stage the Cambridge diet regimen is followed very closely to obtain weight loss. The third stage is stabilization. This is when select regular foods are integrated in with the Cambridge prepared foods. The fourth and final stage is weight maintenance. This is when exercise is added and healthy eating is maintained.

NutriSystem

The system is based on prepackaged meals containing low-glycemic index carbohydrates and calculated amounts of proteins. You eat the provided entrees, snacks, and desserts often throughout the day in order to maintain a stable blood glucose level and achieve a felling of satisfaction and fullness.

The Scarsdale Diet

Low-carbohydrate, low-calorie medical weight loss diet. For 14 days the dieter follows a very structured diet plan, followed by another 14 days of a less structured, but still very specific plan. The cycle is repeated until desired weight loss is achieved. No substitutions can be made to the plan.

---

are disproportionately affected by diabetes. An estimated 21 million Americans had the disease in 2005 (CDC, 2005).

Previously called non–insulin-dependent diabetes mellitus or adult-onset diabetes, type 2 diabetes accounts for 90% to 95% of all diagnosed cases of diabetes. Risk factors include older age, obesity, family history of diabetes, history of gestational diabetes, impaired glucose tolerance, physical inactivity, and race and ethnicity. Blacks, Hispanic Americans, Native Americans, and some Asian Americans are at particularly high risk.

Type 2 diabetes is one of the leading causes of death among Americans and the leading cause of new cases of blindness, kidney failure, and lower extremity amputations; it also greatly increases a person's risk for a heart attack or stroke. In 2005, diabetes accounted for more than $132 billion in direct and indirect medical costs and lost productivity (CDC, 2005). Much of the burden of diabetes can be prevented with early detection, improved delivery of care, and better education on disease self-management (American Diabetes Association, 2008).

Type 2 Diabetes in Children

Although diabetes mellitus in children and adolescents was believed to be exclusively type 1, type 2 diabetes in children and adolescents is now considered a sizeable and growing problem among Native Americans and an emerging

Table **11-5** Medications that Promote Weight Loss

Generic/Trade Name	Drug Type	Side Effects / Potential Risks	Special Precautions	Notes
Orlistat/Xenical, Alli	Lipase inhibitor	Bowel incontinence, abdominal pain, oily spotting on underwear Potential risk: Increased risk of kidney stones in those with history of kidney stones	Not recommended during pregnancy or for nursing mothers. Monitor blood levels and follow timing of medication if taking: Warfarin, Coumadin, Cyclosporin, and Sandimmune	FDA approval 1999 Not established for use beyond two years
Sibutramine/ Meridia	Appetite suppressant	Headache, change in appetite, constipation, heartburn, dry mouth, weakness, back pain, nervousness, difficulty falling or staying asleep, runny nose, flu-like symptoms, flushing, painful menstrual periods. Serious but uncommon side effects: Fast or pounding heart beat, chest pain, shortness of breath, upset stomach, stomach pain, vomiting Potential risk: Can be habit forming, can cause drowsiness and impair judgment	Do not take if you are taking (MAO) inhibitors, including isocarboxazid, phenelzine, selegiline, tranylcypromine. Caffeinated beverages and alcohol use	FDA approval 1997 Not established for use beyond two years
Diethylpropion/ Tenuate, Tenuate dospan	Appetite suppressant	Dry mouth, unpleasant taste, restlessness, anxiety, dizziness, depression, tremors, upset stomach, vomiting, or increased urination Serious but uncommon side effects: Fast or irregular heartbeat, palpations, blurred vision, rash, chest pain Potential risk: May affect blood sugars of diabetic persons	Notify physician if you are taking guanethidine, insulin, MAO inhibitors. If you have heart or blood vessel disease, hypertension, overactive thyroid gland, diabetes, pulmonary hypertension, seizures, or a history of drug abuse.	FDA approval 1959 Short-term use
Phendimetrazine/ Bontril PDM, Phendiet, Plegine, Phenzene, Prelu-2, X-Trozine, Adipost	Appetite suppressant	A false sense of well-being, blurred vision, changes in sexual ability or desire, constipation, diarrhea, difficulty sleeping, dizziness, dry mouth, fatigue, flushing, headache, irritability, nervousness, nausea, sweating, unpleasant taste Serious but uncommon side effects: Breathlessness on exertion, chest pain, depression or severe changes in mood, dry mouth, heart palpitations, increased blood pressure, severe dizziness, problems urinating, vomiting	Notify physician if you are taking linezolid, or medications for hypertension, diabetes, mental depression or herbal products.	FDA approval 1982 Short-term use
Phentermine/ Adipex-P, Obenix, Oby-Trim	Appetite suppressant	Nausea, vomiting, diarrhea, dry mouth, constipation, an unpleasant taste, hives, impotence, palpitations, hypertension, insomnia, restlessness, tremor, and dizziness Potential risk: Phentermine, especially when combined with fenfluramine, has been associated with hypertension in the pulmonary arteries and defects in heart valves, both serious complications. Physical and psychological dependence may occur with long-term use. A withdrawal reaction, which includes excessive drowsiness, fatigue, tremors, and depression, may occur after prolonged use.	Notify physician if you are taking tricyclic antidepressants or MAO inhibitors. Not recommended during pregnancy or for nursing mothers.	FDA approval 1959 Short-term use

public health problem among other North American ethnic groups. The epidemic of obesity among children and adolescents, the decreasing level of physical activity during adolescence, and the increased exposure to diabetes in utero are likely contributors to the increase in type 2 diabetes during childhood and adolescence.

Although some children and adolescents are symptomatic, others do not enter the clinical arena until they are in severe ketoacidosis and may have a transient insulin requirement. Diabetic complications (**dyslipidemia** and hypertension) have been observed among Pima Indians as early as the teenage years. No evidence-based guidelines for treatment of type 2 diabetes in children and adolescents are available, and oral agents have not been tested or approved for this age group. Generally, children and adolescents with type 2 diabetes have poor glycemic control. Population mobility, lack of symptoms, denial, absence of family support, and inadequate health care insurance coverage have all been identified as major barriers to adherence to treatment and follow-up and to successful clinical management. Because of a longer duration of disease (from earlier onset) and because glucose control and compliance are challenging during the teenage years, the lifetime complications (microvascular and macrovascular diseases and decreased quality of life) in this population will probably be considerable (Fagot-Champagna et al., 2000).

Diet Intervention

Medical nutrition therapy (MNT) is the most critical and pivotal component of diabetes care. At the minimum, MNT involves the team efforts of a physician, a registered nurse or registered dietitian, and in some practice settings a mental health professional. The purpose of MNT for people with type 2 diabetes is to delay or prevent the development of diabetic complications (blindness, CHD, nephropathy, and neuropathy). No single diabetic diet or American Diabetes Association diet exists. The recommended diet can be defined only as a nutrition prescription based on assessment and treatment goals and outcomes. Nutrition advice for people with type 2 diabetes is essentially the same as for the general population; they should be following the Dietary Guidelines for Americans. MNT for people with diabetes should be individualized, with consideration given to usual eating habits and other lifestyle factors. Nutrition recommendations are then developed and implemented to meet treatment goals and desired outcomes. Monitoring metabolic parameters, including blood glucose levels, glycosylated hemoglobin levels, lipid values, blood pressure, body weight, renal function (when appropriate), and quality of life is crucial to ensure successful outcomes. The American Diabetes Association further recommends ongoing nutrition self-management education for these individuals.

For people with **hyperglycemia**, **hyperlipidemia**, obesity, or suboptimal nutrition, start with this nonpharmacological management:

1. Recommend an appropriate, tailored meal plan. Determine daily energy needs based on healthy body weight and then use the individual's daily energy needs to determine the appropriate number of choices from the food groups in MyPyramid, the new food guidance system.
2. Encourage regular aerobic exercise.
3. Evaluate the individual using outcome measures in Table 11-6. People who have been counseled regarding diet and exercise but who have not responded satisfactorily after 4 to 6 weeks should be referred to a registered dietitian or nurse who is a registered diabetes educator. Refer to a physician an individual with acute complications of diabetes, such as hypoglycemia, exercise-related problems, renal disease, autonomic neuropathy, hypertension, or CVD.

Nurses learn as much as possible about the individual and the condition of the individual before writing a nutrition prescription. (This requirement is comparable to the physician's need to complete a physical and medical assessment before writing a medication prescription.) The nutrition prescription may be general, but it should reflect the person's therapy goals. The following are some sample orders the nurse might write for the dietitian:

- Diabetic meal plan to achieve clinical goals of diabetes MNT
- MNT to achieve as near-normal blood glucose as possible
- Meal plan to improve diabetes control and blood lipid levels
- Diet for improved glycemia
- Diet for diabetes and hypertension

The prescription may be defined further by the registered dietitian with a summary of the planned nutrition intervention. For example, the dietitian might write:

- Weight-reduction meal plan based on general eating guidelines, 1200 to 1500 calories, 3 meals, and 1 snack
- 2400 mg sodium meal plan with weight maintenance
- Cholesterol-counting meal plan, adjusting cholesterol and meal timing to achieve target glucose goals

Human Immunodeficiency Virus and Acquired Immunodeficiency Syndrome
Epidemiology

In 2005 the estimated number of persons diagnosed with acquired immunodeficiency syndrome (AIDS) was 37,331. CDC has estimated that approximately 40,000 persons in the United States become infected with AIDS/HIV each year. The cumulative estimated number of persons in the United States diagnosed through 2005 with AIDS was 952,629 (CDC, 2007).

Diet Intervention

Attention to nutrition in early HIV intervention is essential for several reasons. AIDS produces nutritional consequences; therefore, good dietary habits early in the disease

Table **11-6**   Goals and Recommendations of Medical Nutrition Therapy (MNT) for Individuals with Type 2 Diabetes

Index	Goal	Recommendation
FPG (fasting plasma glucose)	Greater than 126 mg/dL (7.0 mmol/l). Fasting is defined as no caloric intake for at least 8 hours.	The FPG is the preferred test to diagnose diabetes in children and nonpregnant adults
A1C (also known as glycated hemoglobin or HbA1C)	The A1C goal for people in general is an A1C less than 7%. The A1C goal for the individual client is an A1C as close to normal (less than 6%) as possible without significant hypoglycemia.	Perform the A1C test at least two times a year in individuals who are meeting treatment goals and who have stable glycemic control. Lowering A1C is associated with reduction of microvascular and neuropathic complications of diabetes and possibly macrovascular disease.
Weight change	Modest and gradual weight reduction to achieve target BMI	Modest weight loss has been shown to reduce insulin resistance. Structure program to emphasize life style changes including education and regular physical activity. Reduce energy and fat (≈30% of total energy) intake.
Nutrition	Meet body's daily nutritional needs and minimized risk for chronic disease	Saturated fat intake should be less than 7% of total calories. Intake of trans fat should be minimized. DRI report recommends 45%-65% of total energy from carbohydrate, 20%-30% from fat, and 10%-35% from protein
Physical activity	If no medication limitations, physical activity distributed over at least 3 days per week with no more than 2 consecutive days without physical activity	Physical activity level gradually increased and sustained at target goal. To improve glycemic control, assist with weight maintenance, and reduce risk of CVD, at least 150 min/week of moderate-intensity aerobic physical activity (50%-70% of maximum heart rate) and/or at least 90 min/week of vigorous aerobic exercise (greater than 70% of maximum heart rate).

MNT, Medical nutrition therapy; *DRI*, Dietary reference intake; *CVD*, Cardiovascular disease.
From Standards of Medical Care in Diabetes—2007, (2007). *Diabetes Care*, 30(1), S4-S41. DOI: 10.2337/dc07-S004. *http://care.diabetesjournals.org/cgi/content/full/30/suppl_1/S4.*

may have benefits for end-stage developments such as severe weight loss. The person diagnosed as HIV positive usually becomes depressed. Depression leads to loss of appetite; therefore, attention to nutrition is critical as soon as a diagnosis is made.

An initial nutritional assessment is necessary, suggesting the extent to which nutrition education is needed and providing valuable baseline information for evaluating the disease's progression. The person's significant others are involved in early discussions of optimal nutrition. A nutrient-dense, protein-rich, well-balanced diet that includes a vitamin and mineral supplement should be stressed. Information on food sanitation is provided because people with HIV have altered immune function and will get sicker when exposed to foodborne organisms. The aims of nutrition therapy and counseling specifically for HIV and AIDS follow:

- Determine how the person appeared physically before becoming HIV positive. Was the person obese or heavily muscled? A couch potato or an athlete? Eating a good diet?
- Help meet or exceed the amount of muscle the person had before becoming HIV positive. Introduce the person to proper eating and exercise.

- Help get the person back to the original weight or maintain the current weight.
- Teach about food and water safety.
- Advise on the ability of food to ease some of the gastrointestinal side effects of medications.
- Teach the importance of maintaining eating and medication schedules to ensure maximal absorption of medications.
- When the individual is diabetic or hyperlipidemic, teach about the dietary management of these conditions. Viewing HIV as a terminal illness is no longer appropriate. HIV is now considered a chronic disease, because infected people are living many years (Krales, 2000).

Breastfeeding should be avoided to prevent vertical transmission of HIV from mother to child. This objective is fairly easy to implement in the United States, which has had a long history of safe breast milk substitutes in the form of milk-based and soy-based infant formulas. In many developing countries, however, the risks attached to feeding an infant with something other than breast milk are greater than the 20% risk of vertical transmission of the virus that causes AIDS.

SUMMARY

This chapter introduces a wide range of subjects, including the *Healthy People 2010* and developing *Healthy People 2020* nutrition objectives, the most current diet recommendations to reduce the risks of developing nutrition-related diseases, FDA regulations for food labeling, government food aid programs for the poor and older Americans, and primary and secondary prevention strategies related to the most common nutrition-related chronic diseases. Together these topics form the basis of what is known as preventive nutrition, a requisite for the promotion of the nation's public health. All of the topics examined in this chapter can be studied further using the Internet. High quality, up-to-date materials and continuing nutrition education literature for professionals are free and on-line. **Website Resource 11E** discusses the varied sources of nutrition information. See the WebLinks on the book's website to access live links to numerous Internet resources.

CASE STUDY

Obesity/Overweight: Estella

Estella is a 34-year-old Hispanic, single mother of three sharing a small apartment with her 68-year-old mother in inner-city Los Angeles. She is a full-time laborer in a local manufacturing facility and attends night classes to achieve her Medical Assistant license. She is receiving some government assistance but is raising her children, ages 4, 7, and 10, on a meager income. Most days she arrives home too tired to prepare a well-balanced meal for her family and admits to eating a lot of fast foods. Her mother, despite declining vision, works part time evenings at a local fast food restaurant to help with financial difficulties. Her mother is responsible for most of the preparation of meals. Their diet consists mainly of inexpensive carbohydrates: flour tortillas, breads, pasta, cheese, and potatoes. The family budget does not allow for much fresh fruit or vegetables or expensive meats; therefore, bologna and hot dogs are frequently served.

Estella has recently been hired at a county hospital as a nursing assistant. A required pre-employment physical revealed several health risks. At 5 ft. 4 inches, she weighs 185 lb. Her resting heart rate and blood pressure are also elevated. She has a family history of diabetes and heart disease, her father is deceased due to heart attack at age 55, and her mother is a diabetic requiring insulin injections daily. She was referred to her primary care physician, who recommended immediate lifestyle changes including walking 30 minutes per day, 4 to 5 days per week as well as dietary counseling.

Reflective Questions:

1. What is Estella's understanding of healthy eating?
2. How can learning about simple changes in her eating habits affect her weight and risk for type 2 diabetes?
3. What local resources promote inexpensive programs to help Estella lose weight?

CARE PLAN

Obesity/Overweight: Estella

Nursing Diagnosis: Alteration in current weight related to diet modification and weekly monitoring.

DEFINING CHARACTERISTICS

- Single mother working full time and attending night school. Raising three children and supporting mother on limited income. Income falls into poverty level for family of five.
- Divorced woman with limited support system and resources.
- Current weight is 185 pounds at 5 feet, 4 inches tall (84.1 kg, 162.6 cm). Her body mass index calculates to 31.8 to include her in the category of obesity.
- Resting blood pressure 164/87, pulse 88.
- Father died at age 55 from massive heart attack.
- Mother is overweight, an insulin-dependant diabetic with high blood pressure.
- Diet consists of processed foods and a high-fat diet with little fresh fruit or vegetables.
- Recent job change requiring her to be on her feet, walking, lifting, and transporting clients.
- Inner-city neighborhood unsafe to walk alone or allow children freedom to play outdoors.

- Single mother of three small boys, she realizes the need to improve own health to be able to care for and enjoy her children.

EXPECTED OUTCOMES

- Estella's overall health will improve by reducing her weight, BMI, resting pulse, and blood pressure.
- Establish realistic goals with Estella to improve quality of meals on a limited income.
- Develop realistic exercise plan that is inexpensive and not time consuming.

INTERVENTIONS

- Teach meal planning strategy to include ADA recommendations for a healthy diet.
- Teach easy menus to prepare that substitute more whole grains, fruits, vegetables, and less processed or fast foods.
- Encourage regular exercise program beginning with a walking program of 30 minutes per day four to five times per week. Gradually increase pace and distance to intensify aerobic benefits.
- Investigate safe options such as neighborhood YMCA or park program for family activities.

REFERENCES

Agricultural Research Services. (2007). *Animal Health* (NP 103). Annual Report for 2007. Retrieved from *www.ars.usda.gov/research/programs/program.htm?np_code=103&docid=16469*.

American Cancer Society. (2007a). *Breast Cancer Facts & Figures 2007-2008.* Retrieved from *www.cancer.org/downloads/STT/BCFF-Final.pdf*.

American Cancer Society. (2007b). *Fact sheet; Nutrition and cancer.* Retrieved from *www.cancer.org/docroot/PRO/content/PRO_1_1_220_fact_Sheets.asp?*.

American Cancer Society. (2008). *Cancer Statistics Presentation 2008: Cancer death rates by race and ethnicity.* Retrieved from *www.cancer.org/docroot/PRO/content/PRO_1_1_Cancer_Statistics_2004_presentation.asp?*.

American Diabetes Association. (2008). Standards of medical care in diabetes—2008. *Diabetes Care*, 31, S12–S54.

American Dietetic Association. (2005). Position of the American Dietetic Association: Food fortification and dietary supplements. *Journal of the American Dietetic Association*, 101, 115–125.

American Heart Association. (2008). *High blood pressure statistics.* Retrieved from *www.americanheart.org/presenter.jhtml?identifier=4621*.

American Institute for Cancer Research. (2000). *The new American plate, 2000* (On-line). Retrieved February 26, 2005, from *www.aicr.org/nap2.htm*.

Appel, L. J., Brands, M. W., Daniels, S. R., Karanja, N., Elmer, P. J., & Sacks, F. M. (2006). Dietary approaches to prevent and treat hypertension: A scientific statement from the American Heart Association. *Hypertension*, 47, 296–308.

Barer-Stein, T. (1979). Multiculturalism and nutrition counselling. *Journal of the Canadian Dietetic Association*, 40(2), 112–116.

Bray, G. A., & Champagne, C. M. (2007). The complexity of obesity: Beyond energy balance. In E. D. Schlenker & S. Long (Eds.), *William's essentials of nutrition & diet therapy* (9th ed.). St. Louis: Mosby.

Brownell, K. (2000). *The LEARN program for weight management 2000.* Dallas: American Health Publishing.

Calle, E. E., Thun, M. J., Petrelli, J. M., Rodriguez, C., & Heath, C. W., Jr. (1999). Body-mass index and mortality in a prospective cohort of U.S. adults. *New England Journal of Medicine*, 341(15), 1097–1105.

Carpenter, K. J. (2000). *Beriberi, white rice, and vitamin B: A disease, a cause, and a cure.* Berkeley, CA: University of California Press.

Centers for Disease Control and Prevention. (2004, June). *School Breakfast Program, Child Nutrition and WIC Reauthorization Act of 2004.* Retrieved February 26, 2005, from *www.frac.org/html/federal_food_programs/programs/sbp.html*.

Centers for Disease Control and Prevention. (2005). *National Diabetes Surveillance System: Prevalence of diabetes.* Retrieved July 2, 2005, from *www.cdc.gov/diabetes/statistics/prev/national/index.htm*.

Centers for Disease Control and Prevention. (2006). *Salmonellosis.* Retrieved from *www.cdc.gov/ncidod/dbmd/diseaseinfo/samonellosis_g.html*.

Centers for Disease Control and Prevention. (2007). *Divisions of HIV/AIDS Prevention.* Retrieved from *www.cdc.gov/hiv/stats/htm*.

Centers for Disease Control and Prevention. (2007). *High Blood Pressure Facts.* Retrieved from *www.cdc.gov/bloodpressure/facts.htm*.

Centers for Disease Control and Prevention, National Center for Health Statistics. (2006). *Prevalence of Overweight among Children and Adolescents: United States, 2003-2004.* Retrieved from *www.cdc.gov/nchs/products/pubs/pubd/hestats/overweight/overwght_child_03.htm*.

Centers for Disease Control and Prevention, National Center for Infectious Diseases. (2008). *Bovine spongiform encephalopathy and Creutzfeldt-Jakob disease.* Retrieved from *www.cdc.gov/ncidod/dvrd/cjd/index.htm*.

Expert Panel on Detection, Evaluation, and Treatment of High Blood Cholesterol in Adults. (2001). Executive summary of the third report of the National Cholesterol Education Program (NCEP) Expert Panel on Detection, Evaluation, and Treatment of High Blood Cholesterol in Adults (Adult Treatment Panel III). *Journal of the American Medical Association*, 285(19), 2486–2497.

Fagot-Champagna, A., Pettitt, D. J., Engelgau, M. M., Burrows, N. R., Geiss, L. S., Valdez, R., et al. (2000). Type 2 diabetes among North American children and adolescents: An epidemiologic review and a public health perspective. *Journal of Pediatrics*, 136(5), 664–672.

Fazio, S. (2008). *Mixed dyslipidemia: Using multiple drugs to reduce cardiovascular disease in high risk patients.* Montvale, NJ: Haymarket Medical Education LP.

Gallagher, D., Ruts, E., Visser, M., Heshka, S., Baumgartner, R. N., Wang, J., et al. (2000). Weight stability masks sarcopenia in elderly men and women. *American Journal of Physiology Endocrinology and Metabolism*, 279(2), E366–E375.

Gallagher, D., Ruts, E., Visser, M., Sepulveda, D., Pierson, R. N., Harris, T., et al. (1996). How useful is body-mass index for comparison of body fatness across age, sex, and ethnic groups? *American Journal of Epidemiology*, 143(3), 228–239.

Garrow, J. S., & Webster, J. (1958). Quetelet's index (W/H2) as a measure of fatness. *International Journal of Obesity*, 9, 147–153.

Grundy, S. M., Cleeman, J. I., Merz, C. N., et al. (2004). Implications of recent clinical trials for the National Cholesterol Education Program Adult Treatment Panel III Guidelines. *Circulation*, 110(2), 227–239.

Hawkins, B. (2007). African American women and obesity: From explanations to prevention. *Journal of African American Studies*, 11, 79–93. DOI: 10.1007/s12111-007-9014-5.

Institute of Medicine. (2002). *Dietary reference intakes for energy, carbohydrate, fiber, fat, fatty acids, cholesterol, protein, and amino acids.* Washington DC: The National Academies Press.

Kittler, P. G., & Sucher, K. P. (2000). *Cultural foods: Traditions and trends.* Belmont, CA: Wadsworth.

Krales, E. (2000, April 13). *Setting standards: The expert panel for developing national HIV/AIDS nutrition guidelines. Body positive* (13, On-line). Retrieved February 26, 2005, from *www.thebody.com/bp/apr00/standards.html*.

Krauss, R. K., Eckel, R. H., Howard, B., Appel, L. J., Daniels, S. R., Deckelbaum, R. J., et al. (2000). AHA dietary guidelines. Revision 2000: A statement for healthcare professionals from the Nutrition Committee of the American Heart Association. *Circulation*, 102, 2284–2299. Retrieved February 26, 2005, from *http://circ.ahajournals.org/cgi/content/full/4304635102*.

National Center for Health Statistics. (2007). *Chartbook on trends in the health of Americans. Health, United States, 2007.* Hyattsville, MD.

National Center for Infectious Diseases. (2007). *BSE (Bovine Spongiform Encephalopathy, or Mad Cow Disease).* Retrieved from *www.cdc.gov/ncidod/dvrd/bse/*.

National Institutes of Health. (2001). *NHLBI task force report on research in prevention of cardiovascular disease.* Washington, DC: U.S. Department of Health and Human Services, Retrieved August 25, 2005, from *www.nhlbi.nih.gov/resources/docs/cvdrpt.htm*.

National Institutes of Health. (2004). *Strategic plan for NIH obesity research: A report of the NIH Obesity Research Task Force.* Retrieved from *www.obesityresearch.nih.gov/About/Obesity_EntireDocument.pdf*.

National Library of Health, NIH. (2008). *Iron.* Retrieved from *www.nlm.nih.gov/medlineplus/druginfo/natural/patient-iron.html*.

National Research Council, Institute of Medicine, Food and Nutrition Board. (2005a). *Dietary reference intakes for thiamin, riboflavin, niacin, vitamin B6, vitamin B12, pantothenic acid, biotin, and choline.* Washington, DC: National Academy Press.

National Research Council, Institute of Medicine, Food and Nutrition Board. (2005b). *Dietary reference intakes for vitamin C, vitamin E, selenium, and carotenoids.* Washington, DC: National Academy Press.

National Research Council, Institute of Medicine, Food and Nutrition Board, Standing Committee on the Scientific Evaluation of Dietary Reference Intakes. (2005c). *Dietary reference intakes for calcium, phosphorous, magnesium, vitamin D, and fluoride.* Report of the Subcommittee on Calcium and Related Nutrients. Washington, DC: National Academy Press.

National Toxicology Program, USDHHS. (2005). *Vitamin A. Retrieved from http://cerhr.niehs.nih.gov/common/vitaminA.html.*

Nesto, R. W. (2005). Beyond low-density lipoprotein: Addressing the atherogenic lipid triad in type 2 diabetes mellitus and the metabolic syndrome. *Am. J Cardiovascular Drugs, 5*(6), 379–387.

Rosendorff, C., Black, H. R., Cannon, C. P., Gersh, B. J., Gore, J., Izzo, J. L. Jr., et al. (2007). Treatment of hypertension in the prevention and management of ischemic heart disease: A scientific statement from the American Heart Association council for high blood pressure research and the councils on clinical cardiology and epidemiology and prevention. *Journal of the American Heart Association, 115*(21), 2761–2788. DOI: 10.1161/CIRCULATIONAHA.107.183885.

Sanchez-Johnsen, L. A. P., Fitzgibbon, M. L., Martinovich, Z., Stolley, M. R., Dyer, A. R., & Horn, L. V. (2006). Ethnic differences in correlates of obesity between Latin-American and black women. *Obesity Research, 12*(4), 652–660.

Snetselaar, L. (2004). Counseling for change. In L. K. Mahan, & S. Escott-Stump (Eds.), *Krause's food, nutrition, and diet therapy* (11th ed., pp. 519–532). St. Louis: Elsevier.

Spark, A. (2001). Health at any size: The size-acceptance nondiet movement. *Journal of the American Medical Women's Association, 56*(2), 69–72.

U.S. Census Bureau. (2006). *Income, poverty, and health insurance, coverage in the United States: 2006.* Washington, DC: U.S. Government Printing Office.

U.S. Census Bureau. (2007). *2007 Population Estimates.* Washington, DC: U.S. Government Printing Office.

U.S. Department of Agriculture, Center for Nutrition Policy and Promotion (USDA/CNPP). (2005). *MyPyramid.* Retrieved May 31, 2005, from *www.mypyramid.gov.*

U.S. Department of Agriculture and U.S. Department of Health and Human Services (USDA/USDHHS). (2005). *Dietary guidelines for Americans.* (6th ed.). Washington, DC: U.S. Government Printing Office. Retrieved from *www.health.gov/dietaryguidelines/dga2005/documents/.*

U.S. Department of Agriculture, Food and Nutrition Services. (2007). *Food Stamp Program.* Retrieved from *www.fns.usda.gov/fsp.*

U.S. Department of Agriculture. (2007). *Food and nutrition assistance programs.* Retrieved from *www.ers.usda.gov/briefing/foodnutritionassistance/gallery/programs06.htm.*

U.S. Department of Health and Human Services. (1992). *Methods for voluntary weight loss and control.* Retrieved from *http://consensus.nih.gov/ta/010/010_statement.htm.*

U.S. Department of Health and Human Services. (2001). *The Surgeon General's call to action to prevent and decrease overweight and obesity, 2001.* Rockville, MD: U.S. Department of Health and Human Services, Public Health Service, Office of the Surgeon General.

U.S. Department of Health and Human Services, National Institutes of Health, National Institute of Diabetes & Digestive & Kidney Diseases. (2004). *NIDDK: Recent advances and emerging opportunities.* Retrieved April 14, 2005 from *www.niddk.nih.gov/federal/advances/2004/entire_book.pdf.*

U.S. Department of Health and Human Services, National Institutes of Health, National Heart, Lung, and Blood Institute. (2005). *Your Guide to Lowering Your Blood Pressure With DASH.* Retrieved from *www.nhlbi.nih.gov/health/public/heart/hbp/dash/index.htm.*

U.S. Department of Health and Human Services, National Institutes of Health, National Heart, Lung, and Blood Institute. (2007). *Clinical guidelines on the identification, evaluation, and treatment of overweight and obesity in adults.* Bethesda, MD: U.S. Department of Health and Human Services. Retrieved from *www.nhlbi.nih.gov/guidelines/obesity/ob_home.htm.*

U.S. Department of Health and Human Services. (2007). *HHS launches childhood overweight and obesity prevention initiative.* Retrieved from *www.hhs.gov/press/2007pres/11/pr20071127a.html.*

U.S. Food and Drug Administration, Center for Food Safety and Applied Nutrition. (2004). *Dietary Supplement Health and Education Act of 1994.* Washington, DC: U.S. Food and Drug Administration. Retrieved September 26, 2004, from *www.fda.gov/opacom/laws/dshea.html.*

World Health Organization. (2006). *Global Database on Body Mass Index.* Retrieved from *www.who.int/bmi/index.jsp?introPage=intro_3.html.*

Chapter 12

Kevin Chui
Gary Austin*

Exercise

objectives

After completing this chapter, the reader will be able to:

- Explain the physical activity and fitness goals of *Healthy People 2010* and the progress made toward these goals.
- Describe how physical activity positively influences physical and psychological health.
- Identify the benefits of physical activity throughout the aging process.
- Evaluate the prescriptions for and benefits of daily physical activity, aerobic exercise, and resistance training.
- Discuss how exercise can be combined with mindfulness to facilitate body awareness and self-inquiry.
- Explain the interventions to promote exercise adherence and compliance.

key terms

Aerobic exercise	Fat mass	Physical fitness
Anaerobic exercise	Fibromyalgia syndrome	Relaxation response
Borg Scale	Flexibility	Resistance training
Cardiorespiratory fitness	Muscular fitness	Rheumatoid arthritis
Cool-down period	Obesity	Tai Chi
Cross-training	Osteoporosis	Warm-up period
Exercise	Physical activity	Yoga

website materials

evolve These materials are located on the book's Website at *http://evolve.elsevier.com/Edelman/*.
- WebLinks
- Study Questions
- Glossary
- Website Resource
  12A: Major Coronary Risk Factors

*The authors wish to acknowledge the contributions of James S. Huddleston and Heather O'Brien Gillespie as authors of this chapter in previous editions.

Knowing versus Doing

Having the knowledge about the benefits of exercise does not correlate well with long-term exercise compliance. Confidence in the ability to exercise and a sense of the meaning and purpose (core desire) of exercise in life ensures better success.

1. What motivates putting the effort into developing and maintaining an active lifestyle?
2. Why is being active and physically fit important?

Box 12-1 Health Impact of Physical Activity

- Improves quality of life
- Improves mood and promotes a sense of well-being
- Improves flexibility
- Builds muscle strength
- Increases endurance
- Increases the efficiency of the heart
- Increases bone density
- Helps with weight reduction
- Decreases risk of stroke
- Decreases risk of heart disease
- Decreases risk for diabetes

Regular physical activity and exercise enhance both physical and psychological health. Generally people who exercise regularly, or those who naturally include physical activity in their daily routine, feel better mentally and physically, improve their health profiles, and safeguard their functional independence as they go through the aging process. A holistic approach to physical activity involves exercise for cardiorespiratory health (endurance), exercise for musculoskeletal health (strength, flexibility, and bone density), and body awareness. Body awareness and mindfulness during exercise facilitate self-inquiry and self-acceptance, helping to relieve psychological stress and preventing physical injury (Box 12-1). Not only is an active lifestyle an important component of primary prevention, but regular physical activity is also an essential modality in the treatment of chronic disease, which sets up the potential for benefit in all aspects of the biopsychosocial and spiritual model of health.

DEFINING PHYSICAL ACTIVITY IN HEALTH

To fully understand the *Healthy People 2010* and the developing *Healthy People 2020* objectives regarding exercise, the following definitions will be used:

- **Physical activity**: bodily movement that is produced by the contraction of skeletal muscles and that substantially increases energy expenditure; includes transportation and vocational and leisure-time activity. Leisure-time activity can be further categorized into sports, recreational activities, and exercise training.
- **Exercise** (exercise training): planned, structured, and repetitive bodily movement performed to improve or maintain one or more components of physical fitness.
- **Aerobic exercise**: activity that uses large muscle groups in a repetitive, rhythmic fashion over an extended period to improve the efficiency of the oxidative energy-producing system and improve cardiorespiratory endurance; uses stored adipose tissue as major fuel source.
- **Anaerobic exercise**: high-intensity, short-duration activity that improves the efficiency of the phosphocreatine and glycolytic energy-producing systems and increases muscle strength, power, and speed of reactivity; uses phosphagens and glucose-glycogen as major fuel sources.
- **Physical fitness**: a set of attributes (**cardiorespiratory fitness**, muscular fitness, and flexibility) that people have or achieve that relates to the ability to perform physical activity without undue fatigue or risk of injury.
- **Muscular fitness**: the strength and endurance of muscles that allows for participation in daily activities with low risk of musculoskeletal injury.
- **Flexibility**: adequate muscle length and joint mobility to allow free and painless movement through a wide range of motion (ROM).

HEALTHY PEOPLE 2010 OBJECTIVES

Unfortunately only 23% of the adult population performs enough regular, sustained exercise to gain any significant health benefit, and slightly over 10% of the population exercises at an intensity necessary to promote cardiorespiratory fitness. According to the Physical Activity and Fitness section (focus area) of *Healthy People 2010*, overall 40% of adults 18 years and older report no leisure-time physical activity (U.S. Department of Health and Human Services [USDHHS], 2000). Furthermore, the percentage of adults who report no leisure-time physical activity varies by race and ethnicity, gender, education level, geographic location, disability status, age groups, and whether a person is with or without arthritis symptoms. The tendency to be sedentary, unfortunately, continues to increase with age and affects all of the body's systems such as the cutaneous, cardiovascular, respiratory, gastrointestinal, and urinary systems. As a result of being sedentary, the risk of premature morbidity, mortality, impairment, functional limitation, and disability increases.

The goal of the Physical Activity and Fitness focus area is to "improve health, fitness, and quality of life through physical activity" (USDHHS, 2006). The importance of physical activity in the nation's health is reflected in the 15 physical activity and fitness objectives (USDHHS, 2000), two of which have been revised in the Midcourse Review of *Healthy People 2010* (USDHHS, 2006). These objectives take into account the demonstrated relationship between physical activity and an improvement in the biological markers associated with health, and they identify the reasons for the trend toward a more sedentary lifestyle.

The *Healthy People 2010* box provides a summary of the updated physical activity objectives set for 2010.

Physical Activity Objectives: Making Progress

The Midcourse Review *Healthy People 2010* (USDHHS, 2006) provides evidence of the progress that has been made toward achieving the original objectives. According to the Midcourse Review, none of the physical activity and fitness objectives were met. Seven physical activity and fitness objectives (five for adults and two for adolescents) moved toward their goal. Three of the physical activity and fitness objectives, unfortunately, moved away from their target (all three for adolescents). Data necessary to track five of the physical activity and fitness objectives were not available. As one specific example of progress, the percentage of adults who report no leisure-time physical activity moved toward its target by 15%. The number of people who engage in regular moderate and vigorous physical activity and strength training activities has also increased. However, despite solid gains (indicating that the message regarding the benefits of physical activity is reaching some segments of the population), the improvements fall short of the objectives set for the year 2010. The new goals set for *Healthy People 2010* and *Healthy People 2020* reflect the work that remains (USDHHS, 2006).

The prevalence of overweight children and adolescents and overweight and obese adults has increased in the United States and is considered an epidemic. Children and adolescents are categorized as being overweight if their body mass index (BMI), expressed as weight/height^2, is equal to or greater than the 95th percentile of age and gender specific BMI growth charts. According to results from the 2003-2004 National Health and Nutrition Examination Survey (NHANES), which is conducted by CDC's National Center for Health Statistics, 13.9%, 18.8%, and 17.4% of children and adolescents 2 to 5, 6 to 11, and 12 to 19 years of age, respectively, were overweight (Flegal et al., 2006). Furthermore, the prevalence of overweight children and adolescents has continued to rise since the 1976-1980 NHANES.

Adults, those 20 years of age or older, are considered overweight if their BMI is 25.0 to 29.9, obese if their BMI is 30.0 or higher, and extremely obese if their BMI is 40 or higher. According to age-adjusted results from the 2003-2004 NHANES, 66.3% of adults 20 to 74 years of age were overweight or obese, 32.9% of adults 20 to 74 years of age were obese, and 4.8% of adults 20 to 74 years of age were extremely obese (Ogden et al., 2006). Similar to the trend for children and adolescents, the prevalence of overweight or obese adults has continued to increase since the 1976-1980 NHANES.

The number of adults who combine good dietary practice with regular physical activity in an attempt to attain an appropriate body weight has decreased. This decidedly negative trend may be related to the decline in physical activity in the schools. The number of students involved in daily school physical education (see objective 22-9) decreased from 42% in 1991 to 29% in 1999 (USDHHS, 2000). The Midcourse Review reports that, unfortunately, there was a −5% change (moved away from the target) in

Healthy People 2010

Objectives for Physical Activity and Fitness (Focus Area 22 of 28)

- 22-1. Reduce the proportion of adults who engage in no leisure-time physical activity.
- 22-2. Increase the proportion of adults who engage in moderate physical activity for at least 30 minutes per day 5 or more days per week or vigorous physical activity for at least 20 minutes per day 3 or more days per week.
- 22-3. Increase the proportion of adults who engage in vigorous activity that promotes the development and maintenance of cardiorespiratory fitness for at least 20 minutes per day 3 or more days per week.
- 22-4. Increase the proportion of adults who perform physical activities that enhance and maintain muscular strength and endurance.
- 22-5. Increase the proportion of adults who perform physical activities that enhance and maintain flexibility.
- 22-6. Increase the proportion of adolescents who engage in moderate physical activity for at least 30 minutes per day 5 or more days per week (revised version in Midcourse Review).
- 22-7. Increase the proportion of adolescents who engage in vigorous physical activity that promotes cardiorespiratory fitness 3 or more days per week for 20 or more minutes per occasion.
- 22-8. Increase the proportion of the Nation's public and private schools that require daily physical education for all students.
- 22-9. Increase the proportion of adolescents who participate in daily school physical education.
- 22-10. Increase the proportion of adolescents who spend at least 50 percent of school physical education class time being physically active.
- 22-11. Increase the proportion of adolescents who view television 2 or fewer hours on a school day.
- 22-12. Increase the proportion of the Nation's public and private schools that provide access to their physical activity spaces and facilities for all persons outside of normal school hours (that is, before and after the school day, on weekends, and during summer and other vacations) (revised version in Midcourse Review).
- 22-13. Increase the proportion of worksites offering employer-sponsored physical activity and fitness programs.
- 22-14. Increase the proportion of trips made by walking.
- 22-15. Increase the proportion of trips made by bicycling.

From U.S. Department of Health and Human Services. (2006). Midcourse Review *Healthy People 2010*. Washington, DC.

the number of students involved in daily school physical education (the target is 50%) (USDHHS, 2006). Percent changes away from the targets were also reported for moderate physical activity (−25%, see objective 22-6) and vigorous physical activity (−10%, see objective 22-7) for adolescents.

Physical activity habits tend to track (be consistent) during early childhood, and less active children tend to remain less active over time, increasing their risk of becoming sedentary adults (Pate et al., 1996). If a standard is to be set for the importance of physical activity throughout the life span, it needs to start with children, who have the potential to develop lifelong healthy habits.

As the health care system moves toward a preventive model, primary care providers must facilitate a wellness attitude in their clients, which involves not only encouraging individuals to be physically active, but also leading by example. Recommending regular exercise and espousing the benefits from personal experience can have a significant influence on individual involvement. Health care practitioners are in a position to inquire about and provide counseling for exercise habits of their clients. For example, for each of the practice patterns (musculoskeletal, neuromuscular, cardiovascular/pulmonary, and integumentary), the first corresponding pattern is primary prevention/risk reduction. Although some progress has been made in providing preventive care to reduce risk, data through 1997 indicate a shortfall in reaching the goal set for 2010 of 50% of people (USDHHS, 2006). Although there has been some improvement in some areas, overall the proportion of the population reporting physical activity has remained essentially unchanged and progress is limited. Obviously the progress that has been made toward physical activity objectives for the year 2010 does not reflect a significant shift in the attitude of the general population or the health care profession. There are still populations at risk (Box 12-2).

| Box **12-2** | Populations with Low Rates of Physical Activity |

- Women generally are less active than men at all ages.
- People with lower incomes and less education are typically not as physically active as those with higher incomes and education.
- African Americans and Hispanics are generally less physically active than Whites.
- Adults in northeastern and southern states tend to be less active than adults in north central and western states.
- People with disabilities are less physically active than people without disabilities.
- By age 75, one in three men and one in two women engage in no regular physical activity.

From U.S. Department of Health and Human Services. (2000). *Healthy people 2010.* Washington, DC: Centers for Disease Control and Prevention, President's Council on Physical Fitness and Sports.

AGING

The biological changes attributed to aging closely resemble the effects of physical inactivity. The list for both aging and inactivity includes an increase in body fat and a decrease in aerobic capacity, muscle mass (sarcopenia), metabolic rate, strength and flexibility, bone mass, sexual function, mental performance, immune function, and sleep quality.

Among older adults, exercise can improve health, prevent disability and hospitalizations, improve blood lipid profiles, and reduce body fat.

Exercise is especially important for older women, who make up the majority of the older population, because it may help prevent osteoporosis (Liu-Ambrose et al., 2001; Schneider et al., 2004). In 1991 an estimated 31.8 million older adults resided in the United States, consisting of 19 million older women and 12.8 million older men. In addition it is estimated that by the year 2030, more than 22% of all Americans will be 65 or older (Ourania et al., 2003).

By exercising, older people can improve levels of cardiovascular, cardiopulmonary, and metabolic functions, including muscle performance and aerobic capacity. Several researchers have reported significant improvements in strength, physical performance (functional ability), flexibility, quality of life, balance, continence, and the ability to live independently (Benton & Swan, 2006; Borello-France et al., 2006; Donat & Ozcan, 2007; Galvao & Taaffe, 2005; Lord et al., 2006; Mian et al., 2007; Mandic et al., 2006). Additional resources are available that discuss exercise prescription guidelines for the older adult (American College of Sports Medicine, 2003; McDermott & Mernitz, 2006).

Older adults in particular need to be concerned with their nutritional status since the potential for malnutrition, a common problem for older adults, is associated with a decline in muscle strength and thus poorer outcomes such as decreased function (Asai, 2004; Bales & Ritchie, 2002; Kamel, 2003; Neumann et al., 2005).

The health of the musculoskeletal system depends on movement and activity. Bone is a dynamic tissue, constantly changing and adapting to the stresses to which it is subjected. Bone strength depends on stresses applied by muscular and weight-bearing activity (mechanical stress during active movement). Exercise may improve or maintain bone mineral density (BMD), but recent meta-analytic data suggest that the effects of exercises on BMD may depend on the mode of exercise, body part, and other (e.g., pharmacological) concurrent treatments (Kelly et al., 2000, 2001; Martyn-St James & Carroll, 2006; Palombaro, 2005). To stay healthy, joints must do what they are designed to do—move and bear weight. The health of the cartilage covering the joint surfaces is vital for maintaining proper joint function. The only way the cartilage can receive nourishment is through the manufacture and distribution of synovial fluid, which delivers nutrients, removes waste products, and lubricates joint surfaces. Movement is vital for creating this environment of blood and lymph in and out of joint structures and the adjacent soft tissues. Without the stress of weight-bearing activity, normal bone and cartilage metabolism and repair become dysfunctional, resulting in injury and disease.

Effects of Exercise on the Aging Process

Everyone needs physical activity to be healthy. Human physiology has evolved in preparation for physical exertion. Until recently, survival through the vigor of daily living depended on a moderate degree of physical fitness. However, with mechanization and the style of living in today's society, daily life has become too sedentary. A lifestyle of inactivity places the population at risk for mortality and morbidity, and the literature supports exercise as an essential element of health.

Regular physical activity can help maintain functional independence and improve the quality of life throughout the aging process. Physical and psychological benefits of increased physical activity have been documented widely in healthy and in chronically ill older adults (Geffken et al., 2001; USDHHS, 2000). Only 12% of adults aged 75 and older engage in 30 minutes of moderate physical activity 5 or more days per week, and 65% report no leisure physical activity (USDHHS, 2000). Considerable research has tested interventions to increase activity by younger adults and by populations of all ages. Interventions research with older adults is being reported more frequently. The most common interventions are self-monitoring, general health education, goal setting, supervised center-based exercise, problem solving, feedback reinforcement, and relapse prevention education. A few studies have adapted motivational interventions, used mediated intervention delivery, and integrated multiple theoretical frameworks into the intervention. Lifestyle activity in an older adult recommends the accumulation of minutes of physical activity spread over the entire day. Some evidence suggests potential beneficial effects of lifestyles activity and the probability that some aging adults may be more receptive to lifestyles activity changes that include episodic exercise (Brawley et al., 2000).

CARDIAC RISK FACTORS

The literature strongly demonstrates that the risk of coronary heart disease (CHD) decreases as physical activity increases and that a plausible relationship between the decreased risk and a number of potential physiological and metabolic mechanisms exists:

- Increasing high-density lipoprotein (HDL) cholesterol
- Decreasing serum triglyceride (TRG) levels
- Decreasing high blood pressure
- Improving glucose tolerance and insulin sensitivity
- Decreasing obesity; altering distribution of body fat
- Reducing the sensitivity of the myocardium to the effects of catecholamines, thereby decreasing the risk of ventricular arrhythmias

- Enhancing fibrinolysis and altering platelet function (Berger et al., 2008; Keller et al., 2007)

See **Website Resource 12A** for descriptions of major coronary risk factors.

High-Density Lipoprotein and Serum Triglyceride Levels

Exercise has a major influence on lipoprotein metabolism, primarily affecting plasma levels of HDL and TRG. There is a strong negative correlation between CHD and plasma HDL levels. Increases in HDL lower the total cholesterol-to-HDL ratio, thereby reducing CHD risk. Exercise, a common part of treatment for hypertriglyceridemia, may have a lowering effect on TRG levels (Oh & Lanier, 2007; Pejic & Lee, 2006; Yuan et al., 2007). Exercise training, such as walking and running, increases lipoprotein lipase activity (an enzyme that removes cholesterol and fatty acids from the blood) after exercise (Hamilton et al., 2004; Weise et al., 2005). Furthermore, there is a strong and inverse (negative) relationship between lipoprotein lipase activity and CHD, so as lipoprotein lipase activity increases the risk for CHD decreases (Hamilton et al., 2004). TRG levels are lower and HDL levels are higher in physically active people than in the sedentary population. A dose-response relationship between amounts of physical activity and HDL levels appears to exist, with endurance-trained athletes having 20% to 30% higher HDL levels and lower TRG levels than do healthy, age-matched, sedentary people (Leon, 1991).

The effect of exercise on lipid metabolism may be related more to the volume (duration and frequency) than to the intensity of the exercise. Although single episodes of physical activity result in an improved blood lipid profile that can last for several days (Durstine & Haskell, 1994), regular repeated bouts of activity are needed for long-term benefits. Short periods of exercise training result in modest increases in HDL, but longer periods of training produce larger increases in HDL (Haskell et al., 1992). Exercise's lowering effect on TRG is cumulative; therefore, frequent exercise results in a progressive decrease in TRG. Changes in lipid profiles are most significant with moderate exercise over a prolonged period (1 year). On the average, exercise training has the potential to increase HDL approximately 2 mg/dL. Although this benefit may not appear significant, a 1 mg/dL increase in HDL is associated with a 2% decrease in CHD risk. More exercise may provide even more benefit. In the study by Williams (1996), the 9.6 mg/dL difference in HDL between the groups running the shortest distances and the longest represents a 29% reduction in CHD risk. However, exercise is not a quick fix. At best, exercise appears to involve a commitment to regular, moderately intense physical activity over an extended period—a lifetime commitment to an active lifestyle.

Hypertension

The American College of Sports Medicine (Pescatello et al., 2004) and the American Heart Association (Braith & Stewart, 2006) recommend **resistance training** in the prevention and treatment of HTN. Furthermore, the American College of Sports Medicine (Pescatello et al., 2004) summarizes evidence, of varying degrees, that supports the use of physical activity, dynamic aerobic training, dynamic exercise, and resistance training to decrease blood pressure in adults. Their summary of the evidence supports regular endurance exercise to decrease blood pressure in older adults. There was no evidence to support a different blood pressure response to exercise between genders and different ethnicities.

The evidence summarized by the American College of Sports Medicine thus supports frequent (on most days of the week), primarily aerobic exercise of a moderate intensity for 30 minutes or more supplemented by resistance training (Pescatello et al., 2004).

Low- to moderate-intensity aerobic exercise also appears to be effective in lowering blood pressure (Gordon, 2003; Hass et al., 2001). Mechanisms underlying the exercise-training effect on lowering blood pressure are not completely clear but may involve attenuation of sympathetic nervous system activity. This attenuation results in the dilation of peripheral blood vessels, which decreases systemic vascular resistance. Decreasing sympathetic nervous system activity may have a beneficial effect on the insulin resistance that is often observed in hypertensive people.

Additional mechanisms that may lower blood pressure include decreases in norepinephrine levels, increases in circulation vasodilators, alterations in renal function, and amelioration of hyperinsulinemia (Gordon, 2003).

Hyperinsulinemia and Glucose Intolerance

Hyperinsulinemia and glucose intolerance account for the various types of diabetes. Diabetes mellitus (DM) encompasses a group of metabolic disorders that have in common an increase in blood glucose levels and associated metabolic dysfunction. Insulin-dependent diabetes mellitus (IDDM) involves elevated blood glucose levels that are a result of a deficiency of circulating insulin caused by destruction of the pancreatic ß cells, and non–insulin-dependent diabetes mellitus (NIDDM) involves elevated blood glucose levels from insulin resistance (decreased insulin sensitivity)—largely in skeletal muscles—or impaired insulin secretion. Approximately 90% of those with diabetes have NIDDM.

A recent meta-analysis on the effects of exercise on NIDDM demonstrated significantly improved glycemic control (i.e., significantly decreased glycated hemoglobin levels) and significantly increased insulin response (Thomas & Naughton, 2007). Another recent meta-analysis examined the relationship between physical activity and the relative risk for NIDDM and reported a decrease in relative risk for those who (1) regularly participated in moderate-intensity physical activity compared to being sedentary and (2) regularly walked compared to almost no walking (Joen et al., 2007) (Multicultural Awareness box). In a retrospective population-based cohort study, physical activity (among other variables) was independently related to the risk of diabetes in that being physically active decreased the relative risk for DM (Harding et al., 2006). In another prospective, population-based study, physical activity was strongly inversely associated with mortality (Trichopoulou et al., 2006).

MULTICULTURAL AWARENESS

Walk Away from Ethnic Glucose Intolerance

The Pima Indians of the Gila River Indian Community in Arizona have the highest documented incidence rates of NIDDM in the world. On the island of Mauritius in the southwest Indian Ocean, all four ethnic groups (Hindu and Muslim Asian Indians, African Creoles, and Chinese) have unusually high rates of NIDDM. In the United States, NIDDM is 30% more prevalent in Blacks than in Whites. The presence of NIDDM in each of these ethnic groups provides strong support for the existence of one or more modifiable risk factors in the cause of the disease.

Excessive weight gain is a strong independent predictor of NIDDM. The development of NIDDM (characterized by insulin resistance, hyperinsulinemia, and glucose intolerance) is related to weight gain in adults, particularly in fat accumulation around the waist, abdomen, and upper body (android or apple shape). This type of fat distribution is also associated with a higher risk of developing CHD. Adipose tissue is a major site for insulin insensitivity, and most obese individuals have increased insulin resistance or some degree of glucose intolerance, or both.

Physical activity has an important role in the prevention and treatment of NIDDM. By helping to maintain a proper lean-to-fat body mass, either by losing weight or preventing weight gain, physical activity may indirectly protect against the development of NIDDM. The modulating effect of physical activity on fat stores helps to improve insulin sensitivity and glucose tolerance. Additionally, physical activity may directly affect glucose metabolism. The acute effect of exercise can lower plasma glucose levels by enhancing the effect of insulin; long-term exercise improves insulin action and glucose tolerance.

Epidemiological studies of ethnic groups indicate that physical inactivity is also a risk factor for NIDDM. In the United States, Blacks and Native Americans have a disproportionate number of poor, unemployed, and disadvantaged individuals who lack access to the health care system. The least active individuals within these populations should be given the most attention, because they have the most to gain. The methods and programs that are used to get information on the importance of physical activity out to the public need to be varied, depending on the socioeconomic and cultural factors specific to the ethnic populations. Promotion of physical activity by schools, communities, and government and health agencies, with these factors in mind, will significantly help achieve the goal of improving lifestyles and decreasing the incidence of NIDDM.

During physical activity, contracting skeletal muscles work with insulin to enhance glucose uptake into the cells. Insulin resistance impedes glucose mobilization into cells, increasing plasma glucose levels and setting the potential for developing NIDDM. Although insulin resistance in skeletal muscles may be the primary defect, the development of disease appears to be related to elevated insulin levels, a result of the body's response to the need to mobilize glucose into the cells. Additionally, this syndrome often also involves elevated TRG levels and HTN, which contribute to the potential for disease. Exercise increases insulin sensitivity, improves the inherent effect of endogenous insulin, decreases obesity, and plays a role in lowering TRG levels and blood pressure; therefore, it is recommended in the management of NIDDM. With diet, weight control, and exercise, preventing or decreasing the need for oral antiglycolytic agents and insulin is possible while maintaining normal blood glucose levels. Physical activity may be most beneficial in preventing the progression of NIDDM during the earlier stages of the disease process, before insulin therapy is required. Overall, physical activity has a significant positive effect on a chronic disease that is associated with a high risk of developing CHD. Wei et al. (2000) reveal that cardiorespiratory fitness and physical activity lower mortality rates in men with NIDDM. Low-fitness men are 7.4 times more likely to die from their diabetes and twice as likely to die from CHD.

OBESITY

Overweight and obesity are conditions of excess body fat (adipose tissue). Adults are considered overweight if their BMI is 25.0 to 29.9 and obese if their BMI is 30.0 or higher. Furthermore, the ACSM (Wallace, 2003) considers those with a BMI 40 or higher as being extremely obese.

Obesity may also be defined as weight that is equal to or greater than 120% to 125% of the ideal body weight (Kuczmarski et al., 1994). **Fat mass** (body fat percentage) is also important in determining the ideal body weight. The recommended body fat levels for men and women are approximately 15% to 16% for men and 23% to 24% for women (American College of Sports Medicine, 2003). The average American man and woman tend to exceed the recommended body fat level. An increase in fat mass and the development of obesity occur when energy intake exceeds total daily energy expenditure for a prolonged period. Decreased physical activity may be both a cause and a consequence of weight gain over a lifetime.

The prevalence of obesity, as well as overweight and extreme obesity, is typically reported based on BMI values, as is the case with the NHANES. Unfortunately, the prevalence of obesity in the United States remains high and has been increasing. According to the most recent NHANES (Ogden et al., 2006), the prevalence of adult (age ≥20 years old) overweight or obesity has increased from 64.5% in 1999-2000 to 66.3% in 2003-2004. Furthermore, obesity in adults has increased from 30.5% in 1999-2000 to 32.2% in 2003-2004,

and during these same time periods extreme obesity in adults has increased from 4.7% to 4.8%.

The prevalence of obesity in women exceeds that of men in seven out of nine ethnic groups. Furthermore, the prevalence of obesity differs by racial/ethnic group for female adults only (Ogden et al., 2006). That is, adult females of Mexican American, and non-Hispanic Black racial/ethnic backgrounds have greater odds of being obese than do those of non-Hispanic White background. In contrast, the odds of overweight and obesity are comparable for males of non-Hispanic White, Mexican American, and non-Hispanic Black racial/ethnic backgrounds.

Obesity also increases in prevalence with aging and is associated with an increased risk of HTN, type 2 diabetes, cardiovascular disease, certain types of cancer, and other illness (Dennis, 2004). Obesity is not often considered an independent risk factor for CHD, because its effects are exerted through other risk factors such as HTN, hyperlipidemia, and DM. Nevertheless obesity should be considered an independent target for intervention in health promotion. Being overweight and obese are major contributors to many preventable causes of death. On average, higher body weights are associated with higher death rates (USDHHS, 2000).

Maintaining fitness and health is closely related to controlling weight. Literature supports the positive influence that physical activity has on body weight and obesity. A recent meta-analysis concluded that exercise produced weight loss in people who were overweight or obese (Shaw et al., 2006). In fact, when compared to a control group (no treatment), the meta-analytic data show that exercise alone produced favorable changes in body weight, BMI, diastolic blood pressure, serum triglycerides, serum HDL, and fasting serum glucose. Physical activity does the following:

- Promotes a negative energy balance (burns calories)
- Increases metabolic rate for an extended period after the activity
- Increases metabolic efficiency for burning calories by increasing lean body mass
- Helps counteract the decrease in metabolic rate associated with low-calorie diets by preserving lean body mass
- Is a good alternative to eating when eating is a response to stress rather than to hunger

Unfortunately most overweight people ignore exercise as a means of weight loss or they exercise at rates below federal health guidelines (Centers for Disease Control and Prevention, 2007).

Management of obesity involves a comprehensive program of nutrition management, behavior modification, and physical activity or exercise. The key to normalizing body fatness is long-term adherence and permanent lifestyle changes, not dieting or short-term exercise trials.

Increasingly sophisticated obesity treatments that demonstrate the best outcomes emphasize five components: behavioral techniques, cognitive strategies, social support, nutrition, and exercise. The effectiveness of physical activity is related to the frequency and duration of each activity session and the longevity of the activity program. Recommended ACSM guidelines for exercise include the following (Wallace, 2003):

- A program of low-impact aerobic exercise, increase in daily activities, and resistance training
- A frequency of 5 to 7 times a week
- A length of 40 to 60 minutes a day or 20 to 30 minutes twice daily

As long as calorie expenditure is similar, moderate lifestyle activity may be as effective as structured exercise. Moderate intensity appears to be most effective for total and fat calorie consumption during the activity (Health Teaching box).

Women tend to have a 5% to 10% lower resting metabolic rate than men and a higher percentage of body fat than men of similar weight. Consequently, women have a lower percentage of lean body mass and may not be as metabolically active as are men during exercise. Women may expend up to 40% fewer calories than do men during the same exercise protocol at the same relative intensity (Tremblay et al., 1985).

Fat in men is stored primarily in the upper body or upper abdominal region. Fat in women is primarily stored in the lower half of the abdomen, the hips, and the thighs. Adipose tissue metabolism tends to be different in various regions. The fat-metabolism response to exercise appears to be less in the femoral-gluteal region than in the upper body–abdominal region. Femoral-gluteal adipose tissue serves as an important source of energy during lactation. Women may not lose fat as easily as do men in response to exercise, because genetic differences are related to where and how fat is stored and metabolized. Consequently women who need to lose weight may need to be more diligent about increasing

the duration of their exercise training sessions and to make resistance training a priority to facilitate maximal energy expenditure.

In the April 2004 issue of *Obesity in Children and Teens*, the American Academy of Child and Adolescent Psychiatry reported on a survey of 83 parents, 23% of whom had overweight children. Only 10.5% of parents with overweight children perceived their children's weight accurately compared with 59.4% of other parents. "Focus on healthy lifestyles and on the person's strength. Talk about the advantages of exercise: improved strength, athletic abilities," suggests Daniel Bronfin, MD, Vice Chairman of Pediatrics at New Orleans Ochsner Clinic.

OSTEOPOROSIS

Osteoporosis, or porous bone, is the most common bone disease. It is characterized by low bone mass and structural weakness of bone tissue, leading to bone fragility and increased risk of fractures (National Institute of Health, Osteoporosis and Related Bone Disease—National Resource Center, 2006; Bloomfield & Smith, 2003). Osteoporosis is a major health threat for 44 million Americans, or 55% of those older than 50 years of age (National Osteoporosis Foundation—Fast Facts, 2008). In the United States, an estimated 10 million people have osteoporosis and 34 million more, given their low bone density, have an increased risk for developing osteoporosis (National Osteoporosis Foundation—Fast Facts, 2008). Eighty percent of those affected are women (Berarducci et al., 2000).

Some loss of bone occurs naturally after age 30. Twenty to thirty percent of bone mass development is regulated by environmental factors, such as nutrition and physical activity. In addition to the importance of optimizing physiological intake of calcium and vitamin D, and maintaining normal menstrual cycles for maximizing peak bone mass, physical activity plays a significant role in developing bone mass during childhood and

---

HEALTH TEACHING Prevalence of No Leisure-Time Physical Activity: Report from 35 States and the District of Columbia, 1988 to 2002

Fact: Physical inactivity is associated with obesity and increased risk for chronic diseases (e.g., cardiovascular disease, certain cancers, and diabetes mellitus) and premature mortality. A national health objective for 2010 is to reduce the prevalence of no leisure-time physical activity to 20% (see objective 22.1).

Fact: Women, older adults, and most racial-ethnic minority populations have the greatest prevalence of leisure-time physical inactivity.

Fact: The findings in this report indicate that, in 2002, the overall prevalence of no leisure-time physical activity in 35 states and Washington, DC, was at the lowest level in 15 years.

Fact: Despite the recent decline in no leisure-time physical activity, the prevalence of overweight and obese people has increased (Mokdad et al., 2003). This disparity might be explained, in part, by nationally representative

data indicating an increase in the caloric intake of the overall U.S. population (Centers for Disease Control and Prevention, 2004). In addition, the declines in leisure-time physical inactivity might not have been accompanied by increases in physical activity sufficient to maintain or lose weight.

State and local public health departments and other organizations are encouraged to promote physical activity by teaching evidence-based strategies recommended by the Task Force on Community Preventive Services: (1) community-wide campaigns, (2) signs near elevators and escalators encouraging stair use, (3) individually adapted health-behavior change programs, (4) school physical education, (5) social support interventions in community settings, and (6) creation of, or enhanced access to, physical activity sites combined with informational outreach activities.

Data from Centers for Disease Control and Prevention. (2004). *Trends in intake of energy and macronutrients—United States, 1971-2000. Morbidity and Mortality Weekly Report, 53,* 80-82; Mokdad, A. H., Ford, E. S., Bowman, B. A., Dietz, W. H., Vinicor, F., Bales, V. S., et al. (2003). Prevalence of obesity, diabetes, and obesity-related health factors, 2001. *Physical activity and health: A report of the surgeon general.* Atlanta, GA: U.S. Department of Health and Human Services, Centers for Disease Control and Prevention.

adolescence and in maintaining skeletal mass into adulthood and old age. Using environmental changes and lifestyle modification during the third and fourth decades of life, women can increase their bone mass and effectively retard osteoporosis (Berarducci et al., 2000). Physical activities, those that involve running and jumping in particular, increase bone mineral density (Borer, 2005) and provide for a stronger skeletal foundation throughout aging (USDHHS, 2000). Several empirical referents support the belief that adequate intake of calcium from dietary sources during the developmental years of skeletal growth is imperative for achieving peak bone mass (Packard & Hearney, 1997). Unfortunately, Caucasian females in North America aged 4 to 8, 9 to 18, 19 to 50, and older than 51 years intake 105%, 64%, 74%, and 55% of the recommended amount of calcium, respectively (Borer, 2005). Although dietary sources are the preferred means of achieving adequate calcium intake, foods fortified with calcium are becoming more prevalent and are manufactured to provide approximately 300 mg of calcium in each serving (see Chapter 11).

Bone mass increases during childhood and adolescence and peaks during the third decade of life. When a person reaches approximately age 30, age-related bone loss occurs throughout the skeletal system, in all races, and in both sexes. However, there are significant differences in bone loss patterns between the sexes, with the female gender being a risk factor for osteoporosis. Women have less bone mass than men at all ages and by their mid-30s can expect age-related bone loss at approximately 1% annually. The rate of bone loss accelerates rapidly during the first 5 postmenopausal years, with annual losses of 3% to 5% common. By the fifth decade, or during their 40s, women can anticipate a 10% loss of vertebral bone mass. Cumulative bone loss can approach 40% of peak bone mass over a woman's lifetime. Unfortunately, a loss of at least 30% in bone mass is required for detection on plain film radiographs (McKinnis, 2005). Therefore it is important to detect women at risk early in the natural course of the disease and to target interventions toward lifestyle-oriented health promotion. Additional risk factors for osteoporosis include Caucasian/Asian race, family history, low body weight for height, premature menopause, lack of physical activity, chronic smoking, and excessive alcohol consumption among others (Bloomfield & Smith, 2003).

Maintenance of bone mass may be related to the intensity of the physical activity and the degree to which the activity stresses the bone. Weight-bearing actions that stress the skeleton (walking, stair climbing, floor calisthenics, and aerobic dance) have a positive effect on bone density. Weight-bearing exercise, which increases mechanical stresses on the skeleton, is an important component of reducing osteoporosis risk. These exercises should be performed for 20 to 30 minutes or more, at least 3 to 5 times per week (Bloomfield & Smith, 2003). Aerobic exercise and resistance training have also been advocated for people with osteoporosis (Hass et al., 2001). In fact, a meta-analysis showed that weight-bearing, aerobic, and resistance training were all effective in increasing bone mineral density of the spine in postmenopausal women (Bonaiuti et al., 2002). In younger women the goal of exercise is to increase bone density; in older women who are already 30 to 40 years past menopause a more realistic goal would be to decrease the risk of fractures through fall prevention (Research Highlights box).

research highlights

Resistance and Agility Training Reduce Fall Risk in Women Aged 75 to 85

Objectives: To compare the effectiveness of group resistance- and agility-training programs in reducing fall risk in community-dwelling older women with low bone mass.

Design: A randomized, controlled, single-blind 25-week prospective study with assessments at baseline, midpoint, and trial completion.

Setting: Community center.

Participants: Community-dwelling women aged 75 to 85 with low bone mass.

Intervention: Participants were randomly assigned to one of three groups: resistance training (n = 32), agility training (n = 34), and stretching (sham) exercises (n = 32). The exercise classes for each study arm were held twice weekly.

Measurements: The primary outcome measure was fall risk (derived from weighted scores from tests of postural sway, reaction time, strength, proprioception, and vision), as measured using a Physiological Profile Assessment. Secondary outcome measures were ankle dorsiflexion strength, foot reaction time, and Community Balance and Mobility Scale Score.

Results: Attendance at the exercise sessions for all three groups was excellent: resistance training (85.4%), agility training (87.3%), and stretching program (78.8%). At the end of the trial, Physiological Profile Assessment fall-risk scores were reduced by 57.3% and 47.5% in the resistance and agility training groups, respectively, but by only 20.2% in the stretching group. In the resistance and agility groups, the reduction in fall risk was mediated primarily by improved postural stability, where sway was reduced by 30.6% and 29.2%, respectively. There were no significant differences between the groups for the secondary outcomes measures. Within the resistance-training group, reductions in sway were significantly associated with improved strength, as assessed using increased squat load used in the exercise sessions.

Conclusion: These findings support the implementation of community-based resistance- and agility-training programs to reduce fall risk in older women with low bone mass. Such programs may have particular public health benefits because it has been shown that this group is at increased risk of falling and sustaining fall-related fractures.

Liu-Ambrose, T., Khan, K. M., Eng, J. J., Janssen, P. A., Lord, S. R., McKay, H. A. (2004). Resistance and agility training reduce fall risk in women aged 75 to 85 with low bone mass: A 6-month randomized, controlled trial. *Journal of the American Geriatric Society, 52*, 657-665.

ARTHRITIS

Arthritis upsets the balance of joint health. Although rheumatoid arthritis and osteoarthritis have different causes and attack different parts of the joint, impaired joint function is the result. Cartilage is worn away and irregularities occur in the bone ends. As proper joint alignment changes, normal ROM is decreased, normal muscle balance and activity are altered, disfigurement and dysfunction occur, and ultimately normal movement patterns are altered. Although there is an ongoing progression in arthritis that cannot be reversed by exercise, physical activity nevertheless helps to restore health to synovium and cartilage, improve strength and flexibility, decrease joint vulnerability, and delay the onset of dysfunction. Most importantly, exercise has been shown to decrease pain and disability and to increase function. Exercise should, however, be postponed when there is an exacerbation of rheumatoid arthritis.

One of the chief goals of exercise and physical activity for the individual with arthritis is to counter the effects of inactivity (ACSM, 2003). Although researchers have concluded that regular exercise cannot improve or cure arthritis, exercise has quality-of-life benefits for people with arthritis:

- Improvement in joint function and ROM
- Increase in muscle strength and aerobic fitness that enhance daily activities of living
- Improvement in psychological state
- Decrease in loss of bone mass
- Decrease in the risk of chronic disease (Nieman, 2000)

Consequently, exercise programs based on individual needs and interests should emphasize exercises to develop joint ROM and flexibility (daily) and should also include muscle strengthening (2 to 3 times per week), aerobic exercise (30 to 45 minutes most days of the week), and recreational activities that are enjoyable (ACSM, 2003).

The collective evidence strongly and consistently suggests that exercise is beneficial for persons with osteoarthritis. The specific aspects of exercise prescription for persons with osteoarthritis have been studied to differing extents. In terms of the different modes of exercise, various forms of exercise have been shown to be effective for osteoarthritis. A systematic review of studies of the effect of aquatic exercise on osteoarthritis concluded that the current best evidence consistently demonstrates short-term beneficial effects on function and quality of life and, to a lesser extent, pain (Bartels et al., 2007). Likewise, a systematic review of the effects of land-based exercise in persons with osteoarthritis of the knee concluded that this mode of exercise improved function and reduced pain (Fransen et al., 2001). Similarly, an umbrella review found high-quality evidence supporting the beneficial effects of exercise on pain and function in persons with osteoarthritis of the knee (Jamtvedt et al., 2008). Lastly, an 18-week trial comparing aquatic exercise with land-based exercise found that while both modes of exercise improved both function and pain, the aquatic exercise group demonstrated a significantly greater reduction in pain (Silva et al., 2008). Long-term effects have not been shown to date; thus we suggest aquatic exercise either be

incorporated into a broader exercise program or modified and progressed regularly to promote adaptation to and avoid accommodation to the training stimulus.

Exercise intensity is another important consideration for exercise prescription in persons with osteoarthritis; however, unlike mode of exercise, intensity has received little attention. Research into the effect of intensity of exercise on persons with osteoarthritis, including a systematic review, failed to find a difference in fitness level, function, gait, or pain due to exercise intensity (Brosseau et al., 2003; Mangione et al., 1999). The research in this area has focused disproportionately on persons with knee osteoarthritis, as opposed to hip osteoarthritis. An umbrella review of the few studies of the effect of exercise on persons with hip osteoarthritis has shown that, although the studies demonstrate a reduction in pain, there is insufficient quantity and low-quality evidence to draw conclusions regarding pain, function, or disability (Moe et al., 2007).

Two related arthritic conditions that have begun to be studied more are **rheumatoid arthritis** and **fibromyalgia syndrome**. Preliminary evidence suggests that exercise in various forms may be beneficial for persons with rheumatoid arthritis or fibromyalgia; however, this evidence is sparse and low quality (Christie et al., 2007). In particular, two forms of exercise, Tai Chi and aerobic exercise, have been studied in persons with rheumatoid arthritis. The current best evidence, while low level (Christie et al., 2007), suggests that Tai Chi may improve range of motion in the lower extremity. Importantly, although the evidence has not shown that Tai Chi reduces pain or other symptoms of RA, it does not appear to exacerbate these symptoms (Han et al., 2004). Similarly, aerobic exercise has been shown to increase aerobic capacity, muscle strength, and joint mobility without increasing disease activity, joint damage, or pain (Van den Ende et al., 1998). Again, exercise should be postponed when there is an exacerbation of rheumatoid arthritis. A review of the studies of the effects of aerobic exercise and strength training on individuals with fibromyalgia syndrome concluded there is high-level evidence for the benefits of exercise in this population (Busch et al., 2007). In the studies reviewed, exercise training included aerobics such as stepping and walking, strengthening exercises such as lifting weights or using resistance exercise machines, and stretching for flexibility. Although exercise is part of the overall management of fibromyalgia syndrome, this review examined the effects of exercise when used separately or combined with other strategies such as education programs, biofeedback, and medications. In the studies, aerobic exercises were done for at least 20 minutes once a day (or twice for 10 minutes), 2 days a week. Strength training was done 2 to 3 times a week and with at least 8 to 12 repetitions per exercise. The exercise programs lasted between 2½ to 24 weeks (Busch et al., 2007).

LOW BACK PAIN

Low back pain is a common medical and social problem frequently associated with disability and absence from work. Traditionally, most causes of low back pain are believed to be related to lifelong histories of poor posture, weak muscles, poor body mechanics, and a sedentary lifestyle. However, exercise can have a positive influence on back pain. Staal et al. (2004) concluded that graded activity was more effective than usual care in reducing the number of days of absence from work because of low back pain. Hilde et al. (2007) concluded in their systematic review that although the best current evidence suggests that activity alone has minimal benefits for individuals with low back pain, the risk of harm is small. Given the acknowledged detriments of bed rest, staying active is good advice for individuals with low back pain.

The spinal column is composed of 24 vertebrae stacked vertically, forming natural curves that allow the bony column to function with the resiliency of a spring. The intervertebral disks help with mobility and shock absorption. The health of the bony vertebrae and the cartilaginous disks depends on movement. The cartilage gets its nutrients from cyclical compression and decompression as a function of weight-bearing and non–weight-bearing movement. Similarly, repeated weight-bearing and non–weight-bearing activity stimulates vertebral bone integrity.

Muscles are intimately involved in the support and function of the spinal column. Maintaining the proper curves (anterior and posterior convexities) of lordosis in the cervical and lumbar vertebrae and kyphosis in the thoracic vertebrae is vital for sustaining the spring and shock-absorption qualities of the spine. The lumbar curve is especially influenced by three sets of muscles that are attached to the pelvis and the lumbar vertebrae. By altering the tilt of the pelvis, these muscles can increase (iliopsoas muscle) or decrease (abdominal and hamstring muscles) the lumbar curve. In addition, the deep muscles of the back (paraspinal muscles) work in controlled synergistic and antagonistic fashions to control spinal planes of motion; they are also influential in supporting the spinal curves in posture. Weakness or shortening of any of these muscles can adversely impact posture and increase stress on the back. The result can be back pain from muscle strain, altered joint function (facet joints), and abnormal force on the intervertebral disks.

In a systematic review, Hayden et al. (2005) concluded that in persons with various levels of low back pain exercise was beneficial in terms of reducing pain, improving function, and improving absenteeism. The American Pain Society and American College of Physicians have also jointly stated that there is good evidence for the effectiveness of exercise in reducing chronic low back pain (Chou & Huffman, 2007). Specific types of exercise that have been shown to be effective in persons with low back pain include training of the deep and superficial paraspinal muscles as well as unweighted or suspended exercise. The only systematic review of the effects of unweighted movement on persons with chronic low back pain concluded that there was consistent and strong evidence to support unweighted exercise to decrease pain and improve function (Slade & Keating, 2007). Exercise targeting specific lumbar paraspinal muscles

has been shown to substantially reduce pain and restore function (Hides et al., 2001; Shaughnessy & Caulfield, 2004; Koumantakis et al., 2005).

The goal of exercise programs for individuals with low back pain is to prevent debilitation as a result of inactivity and to improve endurance, strength, and flexibility, allowing for a return to usual functional activities. Exercise recommendations and progression of activity are highly individualized based on origin, duration, and severity of pain. Strengthening exercises for trunk and extremity musculature have been demonstrated to benefit people with low back pain. Aerobic conditioning, such as walking, swimming, and stationary bicycling, is recommended to maintain endurance and prevent debilitation from inactivity (American College of Sports Medicine, 2003).

Advanced age, osteoporosis, arthritis, and low back pain are not reasons to exclude exercise from anyone's lifestyle. In fact, the opposite is true. These conditions are reasons to remain as physically active as possible to facilitate the ability to function throughout the aging process.

IMMUNE FUNCTION

The relationship between exercise and immune function has a fairly long history of study, but renewed interest has grown out of the human immunodeficiency virus (HIV) epidemic. Several studies demonstrate that people with impaired immune function can exercise safely without risk to their health status and can enhance their physiological and psychological well-being with regular exercise (Fillipas et al., 2006; Galantino et al., 2005; Sax, 2006; Terry et al., 2006). In fact, two recent meta-analyses found that aerobic exercise, progressive resistance exercise, or a combination of both can be safely performed by adults living with HIV/AIDS and may be beneficial by improving fitness and well-being (Nixon et al., 2005; O'Brien et al., 2004).

The effect of exercise on immune system markers (e.g., CD4 levels, CD4/CD8 ration, or viral load) of people with HIV/AIDS is unclear. Recent reviews discuss the effects of exercise on immune function in individuals with HIV/AIDS and reports conflicting findings (Anderson, 2006; Dudgeon et al., 2004). A recent meta-analysis compared aerobic exercise groups with nonexercising groups and found no significant differences in CD4 count, CD4 percentage, or viral load (Nixon et al., 2005). Similarly, recent meta-analytic data compared the combination of aerobic and progressive resistance exercise groups with nonexercising groups and found no significant differences in CD4 count (O'Brien et al., 2004). Despite the fact that the CD4 count did not differ between exercising and nonexercising groups, there were significant beneficial changes in depressive symptoms, mean body weight, mean arm and thigh girth, and maximum heart rate for those in the exercising groups (Nixon et al., 2005; O'Brien et al., 2004).

Evidence suggests that regular exercisers and athletes do not get sick as often as sedentary women (Nieman, 1994) and middle-aged men and women (Matthews et al., 2002).

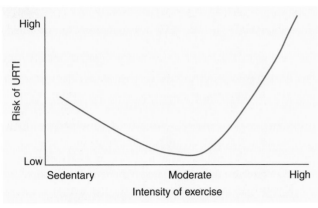

Figure 12-1   Relationship between exercise and the risk of upper respiratory tract infection (URTI). This relationship is often referred to as a J curve. (Modified from Nieman, D. [1994]. Exercise, upper respiratory tract infection, and the immune system. *Medicine and Science in Sports and Exercise, 26*, 128-139.)

In direct contrast, evidence also suggests that athletes are also at increased risk for infection during increased periods of training or after competition (Nieman, 1994; Nieman et al., 1990; Pedersen & Bruunsgaard, 1995; Peters-Futre, 1997).

Epidemiological studies indicate that a J-curve relationship may exist between the intensity of exercise and the risk of upper respiratory tract infection (URTI) (modified from Nieman, 1994; Pedersen et al., 1998) (Figure 12-1). That is, in theory moderate exercise may decrease the risk of URTI below that of a sedentary individual, but high-intensity exercise may raise the risk above average. In direct contrast, Lee et al. (1992) concluded that immune function was not linked to the risk for URTI in a group of cadets during basic training and Pyne et al. (1995) reported similar rates of URTI between elite swimmers under intense training and age- and gender-matched sedentary controls. Factors that confound studies on the relationship between exercise and URTI include: (1) failing to distinguish between new infection and the clinical manifestations of a dormant infection (Gleeson et al., 2002) and (2) failing to distinguish between airway hyper-responsiveness and URTI (Langdeau & Boulet, 2001).

Immune system changes that are apparently related to the intensity of exercise have been identified. Moderate-endurance exercise stimulates the neuroendocrine system, which causes changes in the function and numbers of various immune system cells, such as the NK, CD4, and CD8 cells as mentioned. Evidence also indicates that moderate exercise is associated with a prolonged improvement in the killing capacity of neutrophils (one of the most efficient phagocytes). Several immune marker changes suggest increased risk for illness in those who engage in high-intensity exercise, including low level of salivary immunoglobulin (antibodies), low serum complement levels, low lymphocyte count, depressed NK cell activity, low helper and suppressor T-cell ratio, and decreased neutrophil phagocytic capacity (Mackinnon, 1992; Nieman, 1994; Pedersen & Ullum, 1994).

Changes in immune cell counts and activity may be related to hormonal immunoregulation. Moderate exercise increases the release of immunostimulatory hormones, such as growth hormone and endogenous opiates (β-endorphin and methionine-enkephalin). The increase in β-endorphins with exercise seems to have a positive effect on NK cell activity. Conversely, intense exercise is associated with increases in catecholamine and corticosteroid (cortisol) levels, which have immunosuppressive characteristics (Mackinnon, 1992). High-intensity exercise is also associated with muscle cell damage and inflammation. The immune system is involved in tissue repair. It is theorized that while immune cells are busy with the repair process, host protection may suffer. A window of opportunity for infection during recovery from high-intensity exercise appears to exist. Accordingly, rest is recommended after vigorous exercise to allow the body to recover, and moderate exercise may be the better choice for enhancing health and well-being.

Research examining if physical activity has a protective effect against colon cancer, and if this effect is influenced by gender, is inconclusive and conflicting (Harriss et al., 2007). Evidence does, however, suggest that physical activity is a modifiable risk factor for breast cancer (Bardi, 2007). Physical activity appears to lower the risk for many conditions, in particular breast cancer (Warburton et al., 2007). Unfortunately, physical activity during adolescence does not appear to play a protective role for the risk of breast cancer later in life (Gammon et al., 1998). A large prospective study of over 12,000 men suggests that cardiorespiratory fitness and higher levels of physical activity may protect against prostate cancer (Oliveria et al., 1996). A synthesis of clinical practice guidelines, systematic reviews, meta-analyses, and individual studies suggest that exercise may minimize or prevent adverse physiological effects of cancer and its treatment (Ingram & Visovsky, 2007).

MENTAL HEALTH

People who exercise regularly generally state that they feel better, have increased self-esteem, and have a more positive outlook on life. Not only do they feel better physically, they also feel better mentally. Epidemiological research with both men and women suggests that physical activity may be associated with reduced symptoms of depression and anxiety and improvements in positive affect and general sense of well-being (USDHHS, 2000).

Evidence from a review of the literature (prospective studies, randomized controlled trials, and meta-analyses) found that exercise protects against and is an intervention for mild to moderate depression (Donaghy, 2007). Research of the National College Health Assessment examined the association between vigorous/moderate or strength-training exercise and mental health in a national sample of college females (Adams et al., 2007). Both vigorous/moderate and strength-training exercise were positively associated with perceived health. Furthermore, both vigorous/moderate and strength-training exercise were negatively associated with several indicators of mental health (e.g., depression, anxiety, and suicidal ideation). Similarly, research of the Aerobics Center Longitudinal Study examined the association between physical activity and mental health (Galper et al., 2006). Increases in cardiorespiratory fitness and regular physical activity were associated with lower depressive symptomatology and greater emotional well-being. The mental health benefits of physical activity, as an intervention, have been summarized elsewhere and include: (1) promoting mental health and well-being, (2) preventing and treating mental disorders, and (3) supporting psychosocial rehabilitation (Saxena et al., 2005). As an example of one such intervention, Tai Chi significantly improved both psychological (perceived well-being) and physical

(functional capacity, knee extension strength, and flexibility) health over baseline levels (Macfarlane et al., 2005).

EXERCISE PRESCRIPTION

Literature certainly reflects both the physiological and psychological benefits that can be experienced with commitment to an active lifestyle. In short, regular physical activity or exercise can help people feel better, look better, and perform better. Unfortunately, as discussed, Americans have failed to embrace the concept and health value of an active lifestyle. Many have been overwhelmed by the misperception that to gain health benefits they must perform vigorous, continual exercise. The result has been discouragement in getting started and poor compliance in staying with it. "No pain, no gain" has been an unfortunate, common refrain (Hot Topics box).

HOTtopics

LESS PAIN, MORE GAIN

In an attempt to encourage increased participation in physical activity, a panel of scientists from the Centers for Disease Control and Prevention and the American College of Sports Medicine came together to review the evidence related to physical activity and to issue a public health message concerning the recommended types and amounts of physical activity. The evidence clearly indicates that the protective effects of exercise can be achieved at more moderate levels of intensity than had been recommended previously. The health and fitness benefits of exercise appear to be related more to the total amount of exercise accomplished (calories expended) rather than to the specific exercise intensity, frequency, and duration. The recommendations are as follows:

- Adults should accumulate 30 minutes or more of moderate-intensity (brisk) physical activity on most (or all) days of the week, for a weekly total of 3 to 4 hours.
- The activity need not be continuous; benefits can be realized with short bouts of activity (a minimum of 10 minutes) over the course of the day.
- This amount of activity will expend about 150 to 200 calories per day (the equivalent of walking 2 miles briskly) or 1000 to 1400 calories per week.
- All types of activity can be applied to the daily total (raking leaves, dancing, or gardening).
- Lower-intensity activities should be performed more often, or for longer periods, or both. More vigorous activities should be performed for shorter periods or less frequently.

Because most adults do not meet these standards, they have the most to gain by incorporating a few minutes of increased activity into their day, gradually building up to 30 minutes a day. People who are active on an irregular basis should strive to be more consistent. People who prefer more formal exercise can choose to participate in more vigorous, organized exercise regimens, sports, and recreational activities. A dose-response curve best represents

the relationship between physical activity (dose) and health benefit (response).

Sedentary individuals gain the most by increasing their activity to the recommended level. However, any person who already meets the standards can derive some additional benefit by becoming more active.

People who do a little bit of exercise are better off than those...
who do none and those who do a little more are better off still.
(Franklin, 1993, p. 476)

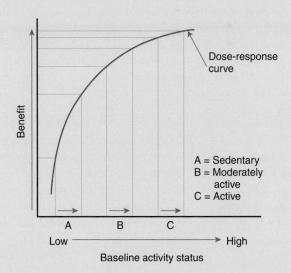

The dose-response curve represents the best estimate of the relationship between physical activity (dose) and health benefit (response). The lower the baseline physical activity status, the greater the health benefit associated with a given increase in physical activity (arrows *A*, *B*, and *C*).

From Pate, R. R., Pratt, M., Blair, S. N., Haskell, W. L., Macera, C. A., Bouchard, C. et al. [1995]. Physical activity and public health: A recommendation from the CDC and the ACSM. *Journal of the American Medical Association, 273*, 402-407.

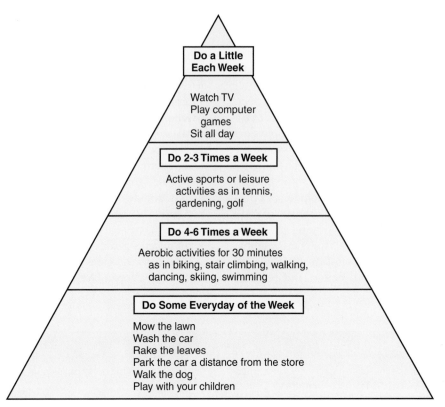

Figure 12-2   Physical activity pyramid.

People need to be reminded that many of their daily physical activities are actually forms of exercise (Figure 12-2). This approach to physical activity serves as a good foundation to a healthy lifestyle. However, when possible, individuals should also be encouraged to include more formal exercise training in their overall activities to promote optimal cardiorespiratory fitness and significantly improve muscle strength and endurance. How much exercise is required to achieve these goals is determined by the parameters of an exercise prescription:

F (Frequency)	3 to 5 times a week of aerobic exercise 2 to 3 times a week of resistance training
I (Intensity)	Moderate to vigorous, by heart rate and perceived exertion Able to complete each resistance exercise, 8 to 12 repetitions, without strain
T (Time)	20 to 60 minutes, plus warm-up and cool-down periods 15 to 30 minutes to complete a series of 8 to 10 resistance exercises
T (Type)	Aerobic (walking, jogging, biking, swimming, rowing, cross-country skiing, NordicTrack, StairMaster, aerobics, dancing, skating, or rollerblading) Resistance training (weight machines, free weights, and calisthenics such as push-ups, sit-ups, or pull-ups) (ACSM, 2005).

Aerobic Exercise

The benefits of aerobic exercise are cumulative; therefore, a frequency of three to five times a week is recommended. Every other day is a good frame of reference. The benefits of exercising more than five times a week are outweighed by the risk of injury, especially with higher-impact activities. When more frequent exercising is a goal, cross-training is recommended. **Cross-training** means performing different types of exercise on different days of the week or performing different types of exercise within one session. The benefits of cross-training include a decreased risk of musculoskeletal injury, an increased potential for total body conditioning, and improved long-term compliance because variety decreases boredom and eliminates the exercise barrier of limited choices.

The intensity of exercise that results in health and fitness benefits ranges from moderate to vigorous and is comfortable, but challenging (brisk). Intensity is defined by the objective measure of heart rate (HR) and the subjective measure of perceived exertion.

The increase in HR during exercise has a strong linear relationship with exercise intensity and aerobic capacity. Resting heart rate (RHR) is the HR measured at rest. Maximum heart rate (MHR) is the rate measured at the highest workload tolerated during exercise. MHR also decreases with age; therefore, a generic formula for determining MHR is 220 minus age. Formulas for determining appropriate exercise HRs have been developed that take RHR and MHR into consideration.

The **Borg Scale** for rating perceived exertion (RPE) is a psychophysical category scale for the subjective rating of

6	No exertion at all
7	Extremely light
8	
9	Very light
10	
11	Light
12	
13	Somewhat hard
14	
15	Hard (heavy)
16	
17	Very hard
18	
19	Extremely hard
20	Maximal exertion

Borg RPE Scale®
© Gunnar Borg, 1970, 1985, 1998.

Figure 12-3 Borg RPE Scale ®. Copyright © Gunnar Borg, 1970, 1985, 1998. (From Borg, G. [1998]. *Borg's Perceived Exertion and Pain Scales*, Champaign, IL: Human Kinetics, USA; Borg, G. [2004]. Principles in Scaling Pain and the Borg CR Scales ®, *Psychologica*, *37*, 35–47; and Borg, G. and Borg, E. [2001]. A new generation of scaling methods: Level-anchored ratio scaling, *Psychologica*, *28*, 15–45. For basic information about scale construction, metric properties, correct administration, etc., it's necessary to read the book [Borg, G. 1998, *Borg's Perceived Exertion and Pain Scales*, Human Kinetics]. Scales and instructions can be obtained for a minor fee from Dr. G. Borg and his company, Borg Perception, Stockholm, Sweden. Email: borgperception@telia.com.)

sensations associated with the intensity of physical work (Borg, 1973, 1982) (Figure 12-3). The scale uses ratings based on the individual's overall feeling of exertion and physical fatigue. These ratings correspond well with metabolic responses to exercise, such as HR and oxygen consumption. The strong linear relationship between HR and RPE was originally suggested by Borg and has been verified by subsequent studies. Correlation coefficients from 80% to 90% have been reported consistently using a variety of work tasks and exercise conditions (Borg, 1973, 1982; Skinner et al., 1973). However, perceptions of exertion and the relationship to HR are influenced by both physiological and psychological factors (aches, cramps, pain, fatigue, shortness of breath, anxiety, depression, and introversion or extroversion). Smutok et al. (1980) noted that some subjects are more accurate in regulating exercise intensity by RPE than are others and that this variability may be more the result of psychological than physiological factors. Other factors that may alter the strong relationship between HR and RPE are drug-related situations (β-blockers), age, and disease states.

Despite this potential for variability in perception, RPE correlates well with HR clinically, and together they form a complementary means of helping individuals determine a comfortable, beneficial level of exercise intensity. An RPE of

11 to 14 corresponds well with 50% to 85% MHR. Subjective parameters include being slightly short of breath, but not out of breath; able to talk without difficulty, but unable to sing a song easily; being pleasantly fatigued, but not exhausted; and having mild musculoskeletal discomfort, but no pain.

Attention to RPE helps a person develop a sense of body awareness and an appreciation for the body's response to the stress of activity. Awareness of RPE helps people listen to their bodies and to become aware of how it feels to move, where they carry tension, and where they have discomfort. With this increased awareness, individuals can choose how they want to respond, adjusting their exercise practice on a day-to-day basis, making the activity more enjoyable, decreasing the risk of injury, and improving long-term exercise compliance.

The recommendation for the duration of aerobic conditioning exercise is generally 20 to 60 minutes. Less than 20 minutes usually provides minimal benefit. However, for people who are unaccustomed to exercising or for those who are greatly deconditioned, short durations are permissible, gradually increasing to a beneficial, comfortable level as tolerance and confidence improve. Everyone has to start somewhere and doing a little is much better than doing nothing at all.

The benefit of sessions longer than 45 to 60 minutes is again outweighed by the potential for injury. Exercising more than 60 minutes on occasion is certainly not wrong, but a person who increases duration should consider decreasing intensity. Improvements in cardiorespiratory fitness can also be accrued from intermittent bouts of moderate to vigorous exercise (10-minute segments) on a workout day. As discussed, longer bouts of exercise are more beneficial for weight loss. The range of acceptable duration allows for greater flexibility, giving reassurance of benefit to the individual who varies exercise choices daily based on capability, interests, and life demands.

As mentioned, many different choices for aerobic exercise are available. The question is often asked, "What is the best aerobic exercise?" The answer is, "the one that the individual is willing to do on a regular basis." Different aerobic exercises have different benefits; they all have their advantages and disadvantages. From a cardiovascular point of view, with relative intensity, frequency, and duration being equal, the benefit is about the same for all modes. Probably the best scenario is cross-training, which results in the best all-around benefits. However, the most important recommendation is that people get out and start moving. The type of exercise they prefer and will continue doing is the best one for them to do.

Walking is probably the most accessible and popular form of aerobic exercise. Done briskly, walking provides a good cardiorespiratory challenge in 60% to 80% of the adult population. Walking is also an activity that nearly everyone can do, requires little equipment or cost, can be done almost anywhere, and can be a social or a solitary activity, depending on individual needs. For people who are unaccustomed to exercising, walking is a great place to start.

Walking is often the recommended exercise of choice for people who are greatly deconditioned or for those who have physical limitations. Considered a low-impact activity, walking can be easily regulated to accommodate a wide range of fitness levels and motor abilities. Cycling, rowing, and swimming (or water walking or other water aerobics) are non–weight-bearing to low–weight-bearing activities that may be good choices for individuals with physical limitations. Water activities are a good exercise alternative for individuals with musculoskeletal limitations who need some weight relief with exercise. Although the buoyancy of the water provides this weight relief, the water also provides resistance to the limbs as they move, encouraging an increase in intensity and conditioning. Individuals should be encouraged to do the types of aerobic exercise that best fit their needs, interests, and lifestyles while providing reasonable benefits.

Warm-Up and Cool-Down Periods

In addition to the endurance phase of exercise, warm-up and cool-down periods should be a regular part of the exercise session. The **warm-up period** usually lasts 5 to 10 minutes and may include light stretching, calisthenics, or performance of the chosen aerobic activity at a low intensity. This approach prepares both the musculoskeletal and cardiorespiratory systems for the transition from rest to exercise by increasing blood flow, respiration, body temperature, and muscle flexibility. The warm-up period decreases the risks of injury and heart irregularities.

The **cool-down period** follows the endurance phase and usually lasts 5 to 10 minutes. This phase allows the body to readjust gradually from the demands of exercise back to baseline. Stretching and slow, rhythmical movement help to increase muscle elasticity, prevent blood pooling and hypotension, and facilitate dissipation of body heat and removal of lactic acid. The result is the prevention of injury, light-headedness, fatigue, and muscle soreness.

Yoga is an excellent example of one form of exercise to use during warm-up and cool-down periods. The word yoga means union or "established in being," which implies a mind-body connection. Simply defined, yoga is mindful stretching. The mind is quiet and awareness is focused on feeling the body as it moves. Movement into and out of yoga postures (called asanas) provides the necessary stimulation of weight-bearing activity to help keep bones strong, provides the movement to increase joint ROM, and stretches and tones muscles. The sun salute (surya namaskar), a series of 12 flexion-extension yoga postures linked together as one fluid movement by the breath rhythm, is a wonderful practice to include in the warm-up and cool-down phases of exercise, providing both physiological and mind-body benefits.

Yoga also helps develop an appreciation for the experience of the basic resting state, a mindfulness of how it feels to be relaxed physically and mentally during the activity. In this form, exercise becomes an inner experience: that is, quiet and settled on the inside, dynamic and lively on the outside. The yoga philosophy encourages an appreciation of bodily sensations, slow stretching, and maintenance of proper posture, all of which help to prevent injury and promote health.

Flexibility

Flexibility is a basic component of physical fitness. Warm-up and cool-down periods provide the opportunity to work on stretching muscles and increasing joint ROM. A safe stretch is one that is gentle and relaxing; a little discomfort may be felt as the muscle stretches, but the discomfort should never reach the point of pain. Stretching mindfully, as in yoga, will ensure a safe stretch. Holding the position for 10 to 20 seconds and repeating the stretch 3 to 5 times will encourage optimal flexibility (ACSM, 2005).

Resistance Training

Studies suggest that people who maintain or improve their flexibility and strength are better able to perform daily activities and avoid injury and disability (Pate et al., 1995). Resistance training increases muscle strength and endurance, increases muscle mass, improves metabolic efficiency, maintains or increases bone density, prevents limitations in performance of everyday tasks, decreases the effort required to perform these tasks, and decreases the potential for injury during physical activity.

On the average, after their early 20s people lose about one half a pound of muscle every year through lack of use. This reduction in muscle mass is largely responsible for a decrease in resting metabolic rate, which may translate into weight gain. Resistance training is recommended for the general population because it has a positive effect on many of the degenerative problems associated with the aging process.

Every individual should try to perform activities throughout the day that stimulate muscle strength and endurance. Activities that involve lifting, carrying, or performing repetitive movement against a resistance (vacuuming, raking, shoveling, or baking bread) help preserve lean body mass. If these types of activities are not performed on a regular basis, then the guidelines for resistance training provided in Box 12-3 are suggested. These guidelines are not meant to represent workouts performed by bodybuilders and competitive weight lifters; they are not meant to result in "bulking up." The purpose of weight training from a health perspective is (1) to develop toned, healthy muscles that provide the strength to do daily activities without risk of injury and (2) to stimulate bone health.

The figures in Box 12-3 demonstrate several suggested resistance exercises for upper body strengthening. Resistance training for all major muscle groups is appropriate, but individuals often choose to concentrate on the upper body, because these muscles tend to be neglected in daily activity and other exercise regimens. Although many people believe that they need to do three sets of each exercise, excellent results can be attained by doing one set (Hass et al., 2000). The weight that is lifted should result in near muscle fatigue at the end of each set (8 to 12 repetitions) and should be performed without strain and while maintaining proper form. Once 12 repetitions can be completed easily, the resistance can be increased (by 5% or less), or the same weight can be used to do another set of

Box **12-3** Resistive Training Exercises

CHEST PRESS (FIGURES 1 AND 2)

a. Lie on bench with feet flat on bench, or lie on the floor with knees bent, feet flat, whichever is more comfortable.
b. Hold weights near shoulders with elbows out and palms facing away from body.
c. Exhale while extending arms straight up, following an "A" pattern with weights touching at peak.
d. Slowly lower weights back to original position while inhaling.
e. Repeat 8 to 12 times.

BENT OVER ROW (FIGURES 5 AND 6)

a. Bend at waist while supporting body with one hand (on table, bench, etc.) and holding weight with other in an overhand grip.
b. Keep knees bent while weight is hanging perpendicular to torso.
c. Slowly pull weight up to chest as if starting a lawn mower, exhaling and keeping elbow away from body.
d. Slowly lower weight back to starting position while inhaling.
e. Repeat 8 to 12 times on each side.

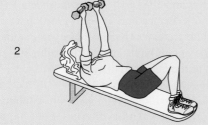

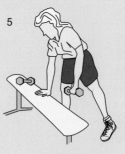

CHEST FLY (FIGURES 3 AND 4)

a. Lie on bench with feet flat on bench, or lie on the floor with knees bent, feet flat, whichever is more comfortable.
b. With palms facing each other, extend arms above chest, keeping elbows slightly bent at all times.
c. Inhale and lower arms perpendicularly away from body until arms are out of peripheral vision.
d. Exhale while returning to starting position by visualizing arms hugging a barrel that is lying on the chest.
e. Repeat 8 to 12 times.

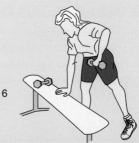

DUMBBELL CURL (FIGURES 7 AND 8)

a. Stand or sit with weights held at sides in an underhand grip, keeping elbows close to body and upper arms stationary.
b. Curl weight to chin or upper chest while exhaling.
c. Inhale while slowly lowering weights.
d. Keep back straight through duration of motion.
e. Repeat 8 to 12 times.

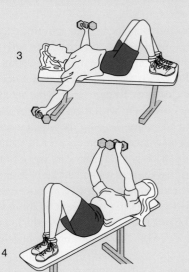

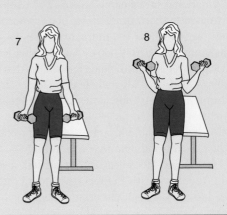

Continued

Box **12-3** Resistive Training Exercises—cont'd

TRICEPS EXTENSION (FIGURES 9 AND 10)
a. While seated or standing in neutral back position, lift hand holding weight straight above head and in alignment with ear.
b. Keeping upper arm tight, slowly bend elbow to lower weight between shoulder blades.
c. Use free hand to support elbow and to prevent movement in upper arm.
d. Raise weight back to its original position by straightening arm and exhaling.
e. Repeat 8 to 12 times on each side.

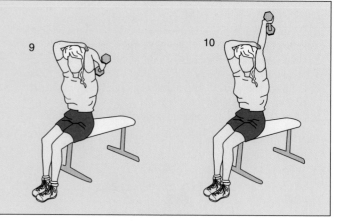

8 to 12 repetitions (ACSM, 2005). The movements should be made slowly, preferably coordinated with the breath. Slow, controlled movements result in greater benefits, lower risk of injury, and an appreciation of how the body feels as its muscles are challenged.

EXERCISE THE SPIRIT: RELAXATION RESPONSE

Exercise should not be considered merely a physical regimen with objective outcomes (calories burned and repetitions completed). Exercise is also a process of challenging the body and the mind to gain a sense of well-being and a feeling of accomplishment, an opportunity to learn about who we really are.

Most people understand the physical benefits of exercise and some people enjoy the challenge of being physically active, but few realize the learning potential inherent in physical activity. Success in embracing a physically active lifestyle may involve a change in focus from the mechanics of exercise to an appreciation for how it feels and what it means to move. Physical activity can be time spent in meditation that fuels both the body and the spirit.

The **relaxation response** (RR) is an inborn set of physiological changes that offset those of the fight-or-flight (stress) response. When elicited, the RR results in a "letting go" of physical, emotional, and mental tension. The RR is a physiological response inborn in everyone and, although it can sometimes occur without the individual being aware of it, people generally need to develop techniques that help them let go on a more regular basis. Some techniques that are used commonly to elicit the RR include diaphragmatic breathing, meditation, imagery, mindfulness, yoga stretching, and repetitive exercise.

The RR can be combined with exercise to facilitate the release of tension and improve self-awareness and the feeling of well-being. However, a shift in attitude about exercise is also involved, with the focus becoming the process and awareness of movement. Successful elicitation of the RR involves two basic components: (1) a repetitive focus (the breath, a mantra, and the cadence or rhythm of physical activity) and (2) a nonjudgmental attitude (about everyday thoughts and the quality of performance) (Benson & Stuart, 1992). Berger and Owen (1988) have developed exercise characteristics that facilitate stress reduction and support an exercise environment that allows the successful elicitation of the RR. Activities must:

- Be pleasant and enjoyable
- Be noncompetitive (Competition implies judgment about the self and others.)
- Be predictable (Elicitation of the RR involves a shift in awareness from the external to the internal environment that will take place only with a sense of safety and reliability.)
- Be repetitive and rhythmical (The cadence of activity provides a focus for awareness.)
- Facilitate abdominal breathing (Watching the breath serves to anchor thoughts in the moment; in combination with cadence, it provides a focused awareness.)
- Continue for 20 to 30 minutes at a comfortable intensity on most days of the week (This continuity restores a sense of serenity.)

All forms of exercise can be used to gain this experience. As discussed, yoga involves mindful stretching with a breathing focus, providing an environment for successful elicitation of the RR. **Tai Chi** is another exercise practice with roots in Eastern philosophy. Known as moving meditation, Tai Chi combines movement with focused awareness, involving a physical and cognitive focus for moving in choreographed forms that become a meditation.

The quality of body awareness can also be brought into a more traditional exercise practice. Aerobic exercise lends itself well to the elicitation of the RR, because it has rhythmical and repetitive form and because it facilitates abdominal breathing. The practitioner can focus on the breath rhythm, the step cadence of walking or jogging, the pedaling cadence of bicycling, or the stroke cadence of swimming. Mantras can be used to create a positive mindset and to focus the mind in the present moment as the experience unfolds. Resistance training takes on new meaning when coordinated with the breath. Focusing on the muscles and how it feels to move through the ROM enhances the knowledge of what feels good and what does not, providing feedback on accepting physical challenge.

Exercise focus can and should vary on a day-to-day basis depending on need, mood, and intent. Some days it feels right to focus on the more physical aspects of the activity, appreciating the challenge of working harder or longer. Other exercise sessions may be more contemplative, letting creativity run, working through the tension of a lingering stressor, quieting the mind for relaxation, listening to music, or appreciating nature. Focusing on the process rather than the outcomes brings meaning and purpose to the activity and helps achieve something more valuable than mere physical outcomes.

When exercise integrates mind and body, it stops being something that has to be done and instead becomes something desired. Being mindful during physical activity and exercising in the moment increases awareness. With awareness comes choices in the possibilities of self-care. Exercise for fitness of the spirit, walk for the soul, and just let the body do the work.

MONITORING THE INNER AND OUTER ENVIRONMENT

The primary purpose of exercise is to enhance health. However, because exercise involves stress to the body, the potential to cause or exacerbate health problems is inherent. When a person is not feeling well, the exercise effort should be decreased or stopped until the individual is feeling better. With an infection, a cold, or influenza, the body is under stress and overexertion will only increase that stress and possibly lengthen the healing time. The level of activity should be adjusted to accommodate how the individual feels, slowly progressing to normal workout levels until strength and energy return. This philosophy also holds true for chronic diseases such as arthritis and HIV. During an acute exacerbation, activity should be limited to necessary activities of daily living (ADLs), but on a regular basis staying active is important, adjusting activity levels as tolerated. Exercise can be a useful tool in coping with chronic illness.

Missing an occasional workout will not affect the fitness level; choosing to stop or cut back on exercise when not feeling well is the right choice. However, after missing workouts for 2 weeks, a decline in fitness is inevitable. When starting up again, resuming the activity should be slow, gradually working back to the usual level of activity. Inactivity for 3 to 5 months results in the loss of all conditioning benefits gained, and resumption of exercise involves starting over (ACSM, 2005). Being aware of the external exercise environment is also important. Extremes of heat and cold affect performance as the body adjusts to different temperatures and wind conditions. Changing the time of day for exercise (early morning or later evening are better choices for humid days), adjusting fluid intake, and varying the length of warm-up and cool-down periods will improve tolerance for environmental conditions and enhance exercise safety.

Fluid News

Proper hydration is an important component of a good fitness program. Extra fluid is needed to support physiological homeostasis during exercise, especially during hot weather. Drinking a cup of water 15 to 30 minutes before exercise is recommended. If the weather is hot or the indoor exercise area is very warm, then 5 to 12 ounces of fluid should be taken in every 15 or 20 minutes during exercise.

Under certain circumstances, the American College of Sports Medicine recommends consuming beverages containing electrolytes and carbohydrates during exercise over water alone (American College of Sports Medicine et al., 2007). For exercise routines lasting longer than 1 hour, a sports drink with carbohydrates and electrolytes enhances performance and is recommended. This type of liquid provides muscles with energy and helps delay fatigue while meeting fluid needs. Sports drinks containing a 4% to 6% carbohydrate concentration are designed to replace carbohydrates at the proper rate during exercise. They also contain sodium, which promotes fluid retention, enhances flavor, and protects against hyponatremia, which can occur with lengthy exercise sessions. Most sports drinks provide 14 to 20 grams of carbohydrate per 8-ounce serving. The recommended intake is 5 to 12 ounces every 15 to 20 minutes. Which sports drink is the best? Several brands should be tried to determine personal preference in taste, but one should be chosen that contains approximately 50 to 80 calories per 8-ounce serving; any more and the carbohydrate concentration will inhibit fluid absorption. Table 12-1 provides choices for sports drinks that both hydrate and energize.

SPECIAL CONSIDERATIONS

Most adults do not need to consult a physician before starting a moderate-intensity physical activity program. However, men older than 40 years of age and women older than 50 years of age who plan a vigorous program (intensity more than 60% of MHR or VO_2 maximum) or who have either chronic disease or risk factors for chronic disease should consult an appropriate health care provider before starting exercise (Table 12-2 and Box 12-4).

Table 12-1	Sports Drinks That Hydrate and Energize	
Brand	Calories	Carbohydrate (grams)
All Sport	70	19
Cytomax	80	19
Endura	62	16
Gatorade	50	14
Hydra Fuel	70	17
Isostar	70	16
Met-Rx ORS	75	19
Perform	60	16
Powerade	70	19
PowerSurge	80	20
Race Day	63	15
XLRB	62	15

| Table **12-2** | ACSM Recommendation for Medical Examination and Exercise Testing Before Beginning an Exercise Program |

Medical Examination and Clinical Exercise Test Recommended Before					
	Apparently Healthy			Increased Risk*	
	Younger†	Older	No Symptoms	Symptoms	Known Disease‡
Moderate exercise§	No	No	No	Yes	Yes
Vigorous exercise¶	No	Yes	Yes	Yes	Yes

*Persons with two or more risk factors or one or more signs or symptoms (see Box 12-4).
†Persons with known cardiac, pulmonary, or metabolic disease.
‡Younger implies ≤40 years of age for men, ≤50 years of age for women.
§Moderate exercise defined by an intensity of 40% to 60% of VO_2 maximum, or if intensity uncertain, an effort well within the individual's current capacity and that can be comfortably sustained for a prolonged period (60 minutes), slow progression, and generally noncompetitive.
¶Vigorous exercise is defined by an intensity >60% of VO_2 maximum, or if intensity is uncertain, exercise intense enough to represent a substantial cardiorespiratory challenge or result in fatigue within 20 minutes.
ACSM, American College of Sports Medicine.
From American College of Sports Medicine. (2006). *Guidelines for exercise testing and prescription* (7th ed.). Philadelphia: Lippincott, Williams & Wilkins.

| Box **12-4** | Symptoms and Signs Suggestive of Cardiopulmonary Disease |

1. Pain, discomfort (or other anginal equivalent) in the chest, neck, jaw, arm, or other areas that may be ischemic in nature
2. Shortness of breath at rest or with mild exertion
3. Dizziness or syncope
4. Orthopnea or paroxysmal nocturnal dyspnea
5. Ankle edema
6. Palpitations or tachycardia
7. Intermittent claudication
8. Known heart murmur
9. Unusual fatigue or shortness of breath with usual activities

   These symptoms must be interpreted in the clinical context in which they appear, because they are not all specific for cardiopulmonary or metabolic disease.

From American College of Sports Medicine. (2006). *Guidelines for exercise testing and prescription* (7th ed.). Philadelphia: Lippincott, Williams & Wilkins.

People with CHD or diabetes have special exercise needs. Earlier in this chapter the ways in which exercise and physical activity positively affect primary and secondary prevention in both disease processes were discussed. Limitations in the ability to exercise are related to the severity of the disease and the signs and symptoms of intolerance. For people with CHD and DM, safety with starting a new exercise program requires supervision and guidance from knowledgeable health care providers. Before starting, these individuals should have a medical evaluation, including an exercise tolerance test (ETT), to determine functional capacity and severity of disease.

Coronary Heart Disease

Exercise plays a strong role in rehabilitation after a cardiac event such as MI, coronary artery bypass surgery, percutaneous transluminal coronary angioplasty or stent placement, and angina. Increased physical activity appears to benefit individuals from all of these groups. Benefits include the following:

- Reduction in cardiovascular mortality
- Reduction of symptoms
- Improvement in exercise tolerance and functional capacity
- Increase in the confidence and ability to carry out usual ADLs
- Improvement in psychological well-being and quality of life (Schneider et al., 2003; Rees et al., 2004; USDHHS, 2000)

Generally, people with CHD demonstrate a reduction in VO_2 maximum and the ability to do submaximal levels of work. With exercise training, the increase in VO_2 maximum in persons with CHD averages approximately 20% after 3 months. This improvement in conditioning is the result of both central (cardiac) and peripheral (muscular) changes (American College of Sports Medicine, 2003). Some of the most significant improvements in exercise tolerance have been noted in individuals with angina. With a decrease in submaximal HR or a decrease in systolic blood pressure (SBP) resulting from conditioning, myocardial oxygen demand is decreased and individuals are able to do a greater amount of work before reaching the anginal threshold. This boost is reflected in an observed increase in rate pressure product (RPP: HR × SBP) at the anginal threshold (American College of Sports Medicine, 2003). An increase in functional capacity allows for progression of exercise tolerance and progression with daily activities and leisure or vocational activities.

Appropriately prescribed and conducted exercise training programs improve exercise tolerance and physical fitness in persons with CHD. Moderate and vigorous regimens are of value, but care must be taken to determine safe exercise parameters for each individual. The parameters of the exercise prescriptions are the same as those for the general population, including frequency, intensity, duration, and mode of exercise.

Aerobic exercise improves cardiorespiratory fitness and functional capacity. Any of the aforementioned aerobic exercises are acceptable for this population, depending on the level of fitness and musculoskeletal limitations. Traditionally, resistance training was not commonly recommended for persons with CHD. The belief was that lifting weights resulted in a disproportionate rise in blood pressure, increased the myocardial oxygen demand, and increased risk of angina and MI. However, data from several studies indicate that moderate, supervised weight training is feasible, tolerable, and beneficial for individuals with HTN and CHD. Strength training can keep the heart healthy by helping to control body weight, reduce cholesterol levels, and control blood sugar levels. Guidelines for determination of appropriate individual training include an aerobic capacity of at least 4 to 5 metabolic equivalents, or METS, an ejection fraction of greater than 30%, and no severe, symptomatic aortic stenosis. However, clinical experience demonstrates that people with more severe disease can use small hand weights to increase muscle tone without risk of cardiovascular compromise.

The exercise intensity for persons who have had a cardiac event but who have not had a symptom-limited ETT should be kept at a low level based on an elevated heart rate (EHR) of 20 to 30 beats per minute above the RHR and an RPE rating of less than 12. After an ETT has been performed, intensity should then be prescribed based on 50% to 85% MHR, an RPE of 11 to 14 or below the ischemic, anginal, or arrhythmic threshold. Duration and frequency recommendations are similar to those for the general population. People who are the most deconditioned may need to exercise at lower intensities, for short durations, and more frequently throughout the day. Generally, a reasonable goal is 3 to 5 times per week for 20 to 40 minutes, plus 5 to 10 minutes each for warm-up and cool-down (American College of Sports Medicine, 2007).

Diabetes

Exercise has long been regarded as part of the triad in the management of diabetes in conjunction with diet and medication (insulin or oral medication). In the early 1900s it was determined that exercise lowers the blood glucose concentration of people with diabetes. After the introduction of insulin, studies revealed that exercise can potentiate the hypoglycemic effect of injected insulin. More recently, findings suggest that in individuals who are in poor control (excessive blood glucose levels), exercise may induce a further increase in blood glucose levels, resulting in ketosis. On the average, people with diabetes have a lower MHR, achieve a lower cardiac output at maximal exercise, and have a higher blood pressure during exercise, resulting in lower maximal oxygen consumption. However, these individuals can improve their exercise capacity with training and can experience the benefits related to overall fitness and cardiorespiratory training similar to the benefits gained by people without diabetes.

Apparently, both benefits and risks from exercise exist for people with diabetes. The overall goals regarding physical activity should be to teach individuals to incorporate activity into their daily life, pursue an exercise program if they wish, and develop strategies to avoid the complications of exercise.

As discussed, in addition to diet and weight loss, regular physical activity is an important modality in the prevention and treatment of NIDDM. People with NIDDM should monitor their blood glucose levels and determine their responses to exercise. However, individuals with NIDDM usually can follow the same exercise prescription parameters as those of the general population. Although the same exercise benefits can be achieved by people with IDDM, the inherent behavior and function of endogenous insulin makes exercising a more difficult proposition for them. The major functions of insulin are to promote glucose uptake into the cells and control metabolic homeostasis during exercise, working in synergy with the counter-regulatory hormones. With exercise, insulin secretion decreases slightly and the concentration of counter-regulatory hormones increases. This increase stimulates hepatic glucose production, which balances the increased use of glucose by the working muscles, maintaining normoglycemia. However, with injected insulin the plasma insulin concentration does not decrease with exercise, hepatic glucose production does not keep up with glucose use, and a decrease in blood glucose results. In contrast, people who have poorly controlled diabetes with decreased plasma insulin concentrations already have elevated blood glucose levels, because there is insufficient insulin to assist glucose transport into cells. During exercise the liver is stimulated to produce more glucose, which causes a further elevation in blood glucose levels, worsening the hyperglycemic condition. Ketosis may also result from increased mobilization and incomplete combustion of free fatty acids in muscle cells and accelerated ketone body formation in the liver (Federici & Benedetti, 2006).

Although each person with diabetes should be evaluated and given individual exercise recommendations, the goals of an exercise program are universal:

1. Maintain or improve cardiovascular fitness to prevent or minimize long-term cardiovascular complications
2. Improve flexibility that is impaired as muscle collagen becomes glycosylated
3. Improve muscle strength, which may deteriorate as a result of neuropathy
4. Allow people with IDDM to safely participate in and enjoy physical activities or sports
5. Assist with weight control for people with NIDDM
6. Allow people with diabetes to experience and gain the same benefits and enjoyment from regular exercise as do people without diabetes

Box 12-5 presents a list of recommendations and precautions for people with diabetes who are interested in regular physical activity and exercise.

BUILDING A RHYTHM OF PHYSICAL ACTIVITY

Participation in regular physical activity increased gradually from the 1960s to the 1980s but seems to have plateaued in

| Box **12-5** | Recommendations and Precautions for People With Diabetes Who Are Interested in Regular Physical Activity and Exercise |

1. Notify primary care physician, ophthalmologist, and podiatrist of intent to exercise.
2. Monitor blood glucose level before and 20 to 30 minutes after exercise to determine the response to exercise.
3. Be sure blood glucose level is less than 300 mg/dL in those with IDDM or less than 400 mg/dL in those with NIDDM, and urine test results are negative for ketones (if blood glucose level is greater than 240 mg/dL). If blood glucose level is consistently equal to or greater than 250 mg/dL, improved control must be established before continuing exercise.
4. If possible, exercise approximately 1 hour after meals when blood glucose level is highest. This plan helps with weight loss, because extra food will not have to be eaten to ward off hypoglycemia. When exercising before meals, a snack may be necessary. (See Table 12-3 for suggestions on food adjustments to maintain blood glucose balance with exercise.)
5. Know the action and peak times of insulin dosage and avoid exercising at peak. (Table 12-4 shows the peak action of insulin preparations.)
6. Consider adjusting oral medication or insulin dosage to prevent low blood glucose level during exercise. The adjustment will depend on the intensity of the exercise, how long the exercise session lasts, and the type of insulin that is acting during exercise.
7. Watch out for the hypoglycemic lag effect that may occur 12 to 24 hours after vigorous exercise; an extra snack after exercise will help.
8. Avoid injecting insulin into a muscle area that will be active during exercise; the pumping action of the muscle may speed up absorption of the insulin and cause a rapid decrease of blood glucose.
9. Use proper footwear and make frequent foot inspections.
10. Avoid high-impact activity when prone to neuropathy in the legs or feet or when there is a history of neuropathy.
11. Keep SBP below 180 to 200 mm Hg in the presence of eye or kidney disease.
12. Exercising every day is best, but at least 3 to 4 times per week. Start with 10 to 20 minutes and gradually increase to 30 to 40 minutes at 50% to 75% MHR. Continuous aerobic activity helps maintain good blood glucose control better than stop-and-go activities. Do not forget the 5-minute to 10-minute warm-up and cool-down periods.
13. Avoid high-intensity anaerobic exercise, but low- to moderate-intensity resistance training is acceptable.
14. Carry a concentrated form of carbohydrate (sugar packets, glucose tablets, or hard candy) when exercising.
15. Wear some form of diabetes identification.
16. People with NIDDM need to test blood glucose levels with exercise and potentially adjust oral medications. Consider decreasing medication if blood glucose level is less than 80 mg/dL after exercise. For weight loss, plan the best time to exercise so that snacks can be avoided.

IDDM, Insulin-dependent diabetes mellitus; *MHR,* maximum heart rate; *NIDDM,* non–insulin-dependent diabetes mellitus; *SBP,* systolic blood pressure.

| Table **12-3** | Food Adjustments |

Duration and Intensity	Blood Glucose (mg/dl)	Suggested Food Adjustment
<30 min of moderate activity Examples: walking a mile or bicycling <30 min	Less than 100 100 to 180 >180	1 Fruit + 1 bread + 1 meat 1 Bread or 1 fruit May not need snack
30 to 60 min of moderate activity Examples: tennis, swimming, jogging, bicycling, yard work, or housework	Less than 100 100 to 180 >180 to 240 >240	1 Fruit + 1 bread + 1 meat 1 Bread or 1 meat 1 Bread or 1 fruit May not need snack
60 min of moderate- to high-intensity activity Examples: sports, strenuous bicycling, long-distance running, heavy shoveling	If doing strenuous activity or playing sports, consult a physician or exercise physiologist for advice on blood glucose management. Insulin adjustment may be required in addition to food adjustments (see Table 12-4). Blood glucose should be tested hourly: 1 bread or 1 fruit per hour unless blood glucose is ≥180 (snack may not be needed for that hour).	

Modified from Beaser, R. S., & Campbell, A. (2005). *The Joslin guide to diabetes,* 2nd ed. New York: Simon & Schuster.

recent years. The progress made toward *Healthy People 2010* physical activity goals indicates that most of the population has not embraced a physically active lifestyle (USDHHS, 2006). Although the benefits of physical activity are common to all people, patterns of physical activity vary among population subgroups defined by gender, age, racial background, income, and body fat. The following generalities are true:

- Men are more active than are women.
- Physical activity declines with age.
- Ethnic minorities are less active than are White Americans.
- Higher education and income are associated with more leisure-time activity.
- People who are obese are usually less active than their leaner counterparts.

Table 12-4	Peak Action of Insulin Preparations	
Rapid-Acting	**Intermediate-Acting**	**Long-Acting**
Regular insulin peak action = 2 to 4 hr	Isophane insulin peak action = 6 to 12 hr	Glargine peak action = 5 to 24 hr
Aspart peak action 0.6-0.8 hr	Insulin zinc peak action 8-12 hr	Extended insulin zinc 18-24 hr
Lispro peak action 0.5-1.5 hr		
Glulisine peak action 0.5-1.5 hr		

From Ciccone, C. D. (2007). *Pharmacology in rehabilitation*, 4th ed. Philadelphia: F. A. Davis.

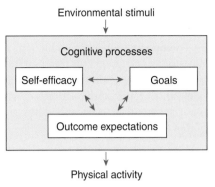

Figure 12-4 Three interacting cognitive processes of Bandura's social cognitive theory. (Modified from Dzewaltowski, D. A. [1995]. Physical activity determinants: A social-cognitive approach. *Medicine and Science in Sports and Exercise, 26*, 1395-1399.)

Adherence and Compliance

Physiological, behavioral, and psychological variables all influence the decision to be physically active. Each person is unique, and success with exercise over the long term comes from recognition of personal motivation or core desire and support from the social environment. Core desire defines the purpose behind putting the effort into developing and maintaining an active lifestyle; it is what motivates the individual to exercise. People should be encouraged to spend some quiet time meditating on why being physically fit is important to them.

Finding meaning and purpose in an active lifestyle can enhance behavior. Biopsychosocial and spiritual variables need to be considered in promoting physical activity. An individual's biopsychosocial factors and spiritual beliefs affect the behavioral and attitudinal factors that influence the motivation and ability to adhere to an active lifestyle. Generally, however, physical activity is more likely to be initiated and maintained if the individual:

- Perceives a net benefit
- Chooses an enjoyable activity
- Feels competent doing the activity
- Feels confident in overcoming barriers that may interfere with the activity
- Feels safe doing the activity
- Can access the activity easily on a regular basis
- Perceives no significant negative financial or social cost
- Experiences minimal musculoskeletal discomfort
- Is able to address competing time demands
- Is readily able to fit the activity into the daily schedule
- Balances the use of labor-saving devices with activities that involve physical exertion (NIH, 1998)

Educating the public about physical activity helps to provide guidelines for safe and effective exercise, to reinforce potential benefits, and to alleviate misperceptions that may interfere with the decision to change behavior. However, knowledge about exercise and the intent to exercise do not correlate well with long-term compliance. Confidence in the ability to be physically active—and the confidence that overcoming barriers produces positive benefits that are related to personal goals (self-efficacy)—is strongly related to participation and compliance (Figure 12-4). Exercise self-efficacy is increased when people perform exercise successfully, receive positive feedback about success, view exercise role models, and learn more about the relationships among exercise, health, and body awareness (see the Case Study and Care Plan at the end of this chapter).

Creating a Climate that Supports Exercise

Clearly exercise and fitness need to be social norms. A climate that supports and encourages physical activity should be fostered. Other people and organizations in the individual's social environment can influence the adoption and maintenance of physical activity.

Health Care Professionals

People are more likely to increase physical activity if counseled to do so by clinicians. Clinicians inquire about exercise habits, communicate the benefits of increased activity, assist the person in initiating activity, and provide adequate follow-up. Challenging perceived individual barriers to exercise and offering alternative viewpoints can help create new exercise paradigms. Clinicians also serve as role models by demonstrating enthusiasm and the health benefits for being physically active.

Recognizing the stages of behavioral change helps in meeting people at their stage of readiness to change behavior. Providing information on physical activity designed for specific stages of readiness enables people to move from stages of contemplation and preparation into action. An individual in precontemplation is not ready to actively change behavior. This person may respond better to support and information about the benefits of changing behavior rather than being placed in an action environment. The decision to change may come gradually. After a person has made the commitment to change, the action phase lasts about 6 months. Continued follow-up throughout the action phase into maintenance is valuable in helping the individual stay committed until the termination phase is reached and the behavior is secure.

Family and Friends

Social support can be a valuable resource for behavioral change. Significant others or friends can serve as buddies, providing a source of companionship and motivation. These people can offer to share daily responsibilities to free up time for exercise, i.e., child care. Parents can support their children's activity by having family outings and providing transportation, praise, and encouragement. Joining a fitness club or an exercise group at work provides various forms of stimulation and socialization, which increases the potential for new friendships grounded in an appreciation of the rewards of exercise.

Schools

Schools are one of the most important resources for increasing physical activity. Strategies must be developed to facilitate increased activity in children because it is clear that children are becoming less active and more obese. Schools are providing less opportunity and poorer quality time for physical activity during school hours. All schools should provide opportunities for physical activity that:

- Are appropriate and enjoyable for children of all skill levels and are not limited to competitive sports or physical education classes
- Appeal to girls and boys and to children from diverse backgrounds
- Are offered daily
- Can serve as a foundation for activities throughout life

Schools can also serve as a resource for the community. Expanding operating hours at either end of the school day creates a safe, indoor environment for hall walking.

Communities

Participation in regular physical activity at the community level depends in large part on the availability and proximity of facilities and safe environments. Community government agencies, local health agencies, schools, and places of worship have the potential to provide activity resources to the population at large. Churches seem to be particularly successful in reaching ethnic minorities and older adults. Making neighborhoods safe for outdoor activities can have a major effect on improving activity habits, especially among low socioeconomic and disadvantaged populations, who report lower levels of daily physical activity.

Recognizing that many of the previous recommendations require a financial commitment, government agencies must respond to reports by health agencies and establish public policies that support the importance of physical activity for the general population. Individuals should make a personal commitment to be physically active, but that commitment needs to be supported by a social and political environment that values this type of lifestyle choice.

SUMMARY

It is important that people incorporate increased activity into their lifestyles on a long-term basis; exercise in the short term is of little overall benefit. Helping them gain the knowledge (benefits of exercise and recommended parameters for exercise), skills (self-monitoring), and attitude (core desire) improves compliance. People need to be motivated enough to start, enjoy the activity enough to want to continue, and appreciate the value enough to start again if they lapse. Lapses should be anticipated to avoid the unrealistic sense of total success or total failure. Behavioral change is cyclical rather than linear; success often comes with repeated movement through stages of change and it helps to explore the reasons for the lapse and to view the lapse as a learning experience rather than a failure. The goal is to prevent a relapse that results in a more permanent noncompliance.

The benefits and enjoyment derived from a physically active lifestyle have a significant effect on the quality of life. However, this lifestyle is successful only when it is supported by a degree of self-awareness and self-care. People must realize that they are worth the effort of doing something good for themselves, that they have the right to be happy and healthy, and that exercise can help them achieve that end. By adding a mind-body component to physical activity and not regarding it solely as a physical regimen, people can experience true health rather than mere fitness. A great deal of bodily exercise is not required; 30 minutes a day can make a significant difference. Success comes with building a rhythm of physical activity into everyday life. Suggestions for a lifestyle approach to exercise include:

- Something is better than nothing.
- Attempt small changes over time (gradualism).
- Emphasize moderate intensity.
- Make activity an integral part of life.
- Focus on the process rather than the outcome.
- Clinicians can provide a knowledgeable, supportive, and enthusiastic environment to encourage the change to a healthier, more active way of life.

CASE STUDY

Exercise Self-Efficacy: Sharon G.

Sharon G. is a 53-year-old account executive who is 2 years post-menopause, complains of insomnia, and has chronic LBP and knee pain.

History: Motor vehicle accident (2000), resulting in bone graft to left leg (her left leg is shorter than her right leg). As part of rehabilitation, Sharon started jogging, which was more comfortable than walking with chronic right-sided sacroiliac joint pain.

She started running marathons in 2002 and continued until 2003. In 2003, she began to add more variety into exercise and decreased her running, but she still identified herself as being an athlete.

In 2004, she suffered a fall that resulted in chronic LBP and was unable to continue aerobic exercise. She began to experience depression and insomnia; exercise had been a significant coping mechanism in the past and now her whole sense of well-being was being affected. As Sharon attempted to rebuild her exercise practice, she would alternate between doing too much, exacerbating symptoms, and then having to stop and recuperate, reinforcing her negative self-image.

MRI showed mild arthritis in her knees.

Reflexive Questions:

1. What are some of her barriers to exercise?
2. How will a regular practice of mindfulness and the RR benefit her exercise practice?
3. How would she benefit from cross-training?
4. What exercise is she doing that is beneficial for helping to prevent osteoporosis?

Answers to Questions:

1. Barriers to exercise:
   - Past image of self as high-level exerciser
   - Current negative self-image
   - Musculoskeletal limitations
   - Exacerbation of symptoms with excessive exercise
   - Outcome oriented versus process oriented
2. With practice of RR, mindful stretching (yoga), and being more mindful with regular exercise, Sharon is able to gradually accept herself in the present and let go of expectations related to past experiences. She is able to accept decreased level of exercise intensity and to adopt the idea of "less is more," listening to her body and not to mental messages. She is now enjoying the experience of being physically active rather than focusing on specific accomplishments.
3. Cross-training provides overall body conditioning and decreases risk of injury (or exacerbating existing conditions) by decreasing repetitive stress to body parts. Cross-training also provides a greater variety of choices, eliminating barriers and improving enjoyment and compliance.
4. Weight-bearing activities, such as walking, low-impact aerobics, and weight training, stress the skeleton and help stimulate bone density preservation.

After a 3-month period, Sharon demonstrates the following improvements:

- Frequency of low back and knee pain has decreased from constant to 2 to 4 times per week; although she still has some discomfort, the intensity is less and it interferes less with her life.
- Insomnia is decreased from 2 to 3 times per week to once per month; she has stopped taking sleep medications.
- She experiences decreased depression and anxiety.
- She is less unhappy about weight gain and more accepting of who she is.

LBP, Low back pain; *MRI*, magnetic resonance imaging.

CARE PLAN

Exercise Self-Efficacy: Sharon G.

Nursing Diagnosis: Altered Sleep Pattern related to low back pain, depression, and recent weight gain.

Medications

- Serax (oxazepam) 30 mg, 4 to 6 times a week; Ginkgo biloba

DEFINING CHARACTERISTICS

- Insomnia
- Chronic low back and knee pain
- Depression
- Upset about recent weight gain of 10 lb (61½ inches, 118 lb); sees ideal body weight as 108 lb

EXPECTED OUTCOMES

- Walking, treadmill, bicycling, and low-impact aerobics (30 minutes, 3 to 4 times per week)
- Weights 3 to 4 times per week
- Stretching 3 to 4 times per week
- Daily RR
- Build mindfulness into exercise practice

EXERCISE PRACTICE

- Treadmill and walking daily for 30 minutes
- Weights 2 to 3 times per week
- Yoga and stretching daily

RR, Relaxation response.

REFERENCES

Adams, T. B., Moore, M. T., & Dye, J. (2007). The relationship between physical activity and mental health in a national sample of college females. *Women & Health, 45*(1), 69–85.

American Academy of Child and Adolescent Psychiatry. (2004). *Obesity in Children and Teens, No. 79.* Retrieved April 18, 2005, from *www.aacap.org/publications/factsfam/79.htm*

American College of Sports Medicine. (2003). *ACSM's exercise management for persons with chronic diseases and disabilities* (2nd ed.). Champaign, Il: Human Kinetics.

American College of Sports Medicine. (2006). *ACSM's guidelines for exercise testing and prescription* (7th ed.). Philadelphia: Lippincott, Williams & Wilkins.

American College of Sports Medicine & American Heart Association. (2007). Exercise and acute cardiovascular events: Placing the risks into perspective. *Medicine and Science in Sports and Exercise, 39*(5), 886–897.

American College of Sports Medicine, Sawka, M. N., Burke, L. M., Eicher, E. R., Maughan, R. J., & Stachenfeld, N. S. (2007). American College of Sports Medicine position stand: Exercise and fluid replacement. *Medicine and Science in Sports and Exercise, 39*(2), 377–390.

Anderson, S. L. (2006). Physical therapy for patients with HIV/AIDS. *Cardiopulmonary Physical Therapy Journal, 17*(3), 103–109.

Asai, J. L. (2004). Nutrition and the geriatric rehabilitation patient: Challenges and solutions. *Topics in Geriatric Rehabilitation, 20*(1), 34–45.

Bales, C. W., & Ritchie, C. S. (2002). Sarcopenia, weight loss, and nutritional frailty in the elderly. *Annual Review of Nutrition, 22*, 309–323.

Bandura, A. (1997). *Self-efficacy: The exercise of control.* New York: Worth Publishers.

Bardi, A. (2007). Can physical activity reduce the risk of breast cancer? *Clinical Nutrition Insight, 33*, 1–3.

Bartels, E. M., Lund, H., Hagen, K. B., Dagfinrud, H., Christensen, R., & Danneskiold-Samsøe, B. (2007). Aquatic exercise for the treatment of knee and hip osteoarthritis. *Cochrane Database of Systematic Reviews*, Issue 4.

Beaser, R. S. & Campbell, A. (2005). *The Joslin guide to diabetes.* (2nd ed.). New York: Simon & Schuster.

Benson, H., & Stuart, E. (1992). *The wellness book: The comprehensive guide to maintaining health and treating stress-related illness.* New York: Simon & Schuster.

Benton, M. J., & Swan, P. D. (2006). Addition of resistance training to pulmonary rehabilitation programs: An evidence-based rationale and guidelines for use of resistance training with elderly patients with COPD. *Cardiopulmonary Physical Therapy Journal, 17*, 127–133.

Berarducci, A., Burns, P. A., Lengacher, C. A., & Sellers, E. (2000). Health-promoting educational practices related to osteoporosis. *Applied Nursing Research, 13*(4), 173–180.

Berger, B., & Owen, D. (1988). Stress reduction and mood enhancement in four exercise modes: Swimming, body conditioning, hatha yoga, and fencing. *Research Quarterly for Exercise and Sport, 59*(2), 148–159.

Berger, J. S., Brown, D. L., & Becker, R. C. (2008). Low-dose aspirin in patients with stable cardiovascular disease: A meta-analysis. *American Journal of Medicine, 121*(1), 43–49.

Bloomfield, S. A., & Smith, S. S. (2003). Osteoporosis. In *ACSM's exercise management for persons with chronic diseases and disabilities.* (2nd ed.). Champaign, IL: Human Kinetics, pp. 222–229.

Bonaiuti, D., Shea, B., Iovine, R., Negrini, S., Welch, V., Kemper, H. H. C. G., et al. (2002). Exercise for preventing and treating osteoporosis in postmenopausal women. *Cochrane Database of Systematic Reviews*, Issue 2.

Borello-France, D. F., Zyczynski, H. M., Downey, P. A., Rause, C. R., & Wister, J. A. (2006). Effect of pelvic-floor muscle exercise position on continence and quality-of-life outcomes in women with stress urinary incontinence. *Physical Therapy, 86*(7), 974–986.

Borer, K. T. (2005). Physical activity in the prevention and amelioration of osteoporosis in women: Interaction of mechanical, hormonal, and dietary factors. *Sports Medicine, 35*(9), 779–830.

Borg, G. A. (1973). Perceived exertion: A note on "history" and methods. *Medicine and Science in Sports, 5*(2), 90–93.

Borg, G. A. (1982). Psychophysical bases of perceived exertion. *Medicine and Science in Sports and Exercise, 14*(5), 377–381.

Braith, R. W., & Stewart, K. J. (2006). Resistance exercise training: Its role in the prevention of cardiovascular disease. *Circulation, 113*(22), 2642–2650.

Brawley, L., Rejeski, W., & Lutes, L. (2000). A group-mediated cognitive-behavioral intervention for increasing adherence to physical activity in older adults. *Journal of Applied Biobehavioral Research, 5*(1), 47–65.

Brosseau, L., MacLeay, L., Robinson, V. A., Wells, G., & Tugwell, P. (2003). Intensity of exercise for the treatment of osteoarthritis. *Cochrane Database of Systematic Reviews*, Issue 2.

Busch, A. J., Barber, K. A., Overend, T. J., Peloso, P. M., & Schachter, C. L. (2007). Exercise for treating fibromyalgia syndrome. *Cochrane Database of Systematic Reviews*, Issue 4.

Centers for Disease Control and Prevention. (2007). *Physical activity and good nutrition: Essential elements to prevent chronic diseases and obesity 2007.*

Chambers, T. A., Bagai, A., & Ivascu, N. (2007). Current trends in coronary artery disease in women. *Current Opinion in Anesthesiology, 20*(1), 75–82.

Chou, R., & Huffman, L. H. (2007). Nonpharmacologic therapies for acute and chronic low back pain: A review of the evidence for an American Pain Society/American College of Physicians clinical practice guideline. *Annals of Internal Medicine, 147*(7), 492–504.

Christie, A., Jamtvedt, G., Dahm, K., Moe, R. H., Haavardsholm, E. A., & Hagen, K. (2007). Effectiveness of nonpharmacological and nonsurgical interventions for patients with rheumatoid arthritis: An overview of systematic reviews. *Physical Therapy, 87*(12), 1697–1715.

Dennis, K. E. (2004). Weight management in women. *Nursing Clinics of North America, 39*(1), 231–241.

Donaghy, M. E. (2007). Exercise can seriously improve your mental health: Fact or fiction? *Advances in Physiotherapy, 9*(2), 76–88.

Donat, H., & Ozcan, A. (2007). Comparison of the effectiveness of two programmes on older adults at risk of falling: Unsupervised home exercise and supervised group exercise. *Clinical Rehabilitation, 21*(3), 273–283.

Dudgeon, W. D., Phillips, K. D., Bopp, C. M., & Hand, G. A. (2004). Physiological and psychological effects of exercise interventions in HIV disease. *AIDS Patient Care and STDs, 18*(2), 81–98.

Durstine, J. L., & Haskell, W. L. (1994). Effects of exercise training on plasma lipids and lipoproteins. *Exercise and Sport Sciences Reviews, 22*(2), 477–521.

Federici, M. O., & Benedetti, M. M. (2006). Ketone bodies monitoring. *Diabetes Research & Clinical Practice, 74*, S77–S81.

Fillipas, S., Oldmeadow, L. B., Bailey, M. J., & Cherry, C. L. (2006). A six-month, supervised, aerobic and resistance exercise program improves self-efficacy in people with human immunodeficiency virus: A random-

ized controlled trial. *Australian Journal of Physiotherapy, 52*(3), 185–190.

Flegal, K. M., Tabak, C. J., & Ogden, C. L. (2006). Overweight in children: Definitions and interpretations. *Health Education Research, 21*(6), 755–760.

Franklin, B. (1993). How much exercise is enough? *Encyclopedia Britannica.* Los Angeles: Encyclopedia Britannica Inc., pp. 471–476.

Fransen, M., McConnell, S., & Bell, M. (2001). Exercise for osteoarthritis of the hip or knee. *Cochrane Database of Systematic Reviews*, Issue 2.

Galantino, M. L., Shepard, K., Krafft, L., Laperriere, A., Ducette, J., Sorbello, A., et al. (2005). The effect of group aerobic exercise and t'ai chi on functional outcomes and quality of life for persons living with acquired immunodeficiency syndrome. *Journal of Alternative and Complementary Medicine, 11*(6), 1085–1092.

Galper, D. I., Trivedi, M. H., Barlow, C. E., Dunn, A. L., & Kampert, J. B. (2006). Inverse association between physical inactivity and mental health in men and women. *Medicine and Science in Sports and Exercise, 38*(1), 173–178.

Galvao, D. A., & Taaffe, D. R. (2005). Resistance exercise dosage in older adults: Single versus multiset effects on physical performance and body composition. *Journal of the American Geriatric Society, 53*(12), 2090–2097.

Gammon, M. D., Schoenberg, J. B., Britton, J. A., Kelsey, J. L., Coates, R. J., Brogan, D., et al. (1998). Recreational physical activity and breast cancer risk among women under age 45 years. *American Journal of Epidemiology, 147*(3), 273–280.

Geffken, D., Cushman, M., Burke, G., Polak, J., Sakkinen, P., & Tracy, R. (2001). Association between physical activity and markers of inflammation in a healthy elderly population. *American Journal Epidemiology, 153*(3), 242–250.

Gleeson, M., Pyne, D. B., Austin, J. P., Francis, J. L., Clancy, R. L., McDonald, W. A., et al. (2002). Epstein-Barr virus reactivation and upper-respiratory illness in elite swimmers. *Medicine and Science in Sports and Exercise, 34*(3), 411–417.

Gordon, N. F. (2003). Hypertension. *ACSM's exercise management for persons with chronic diseases and disabilities.* (2nd ed.). Champaign, IL: Human Kinetics. 76–80.

Hamilton, M. T., Hamilton, D. G., & Zderic, T. W. (2004). Exercise physiology versus inactivity physiology: An essential concept for understanding lipoprotein lipase regulation. *Exercise and Sport Sciences Review, 32*(4), 161–166.

Han, A., Robinson, V. A., Judd, M. G., Taixiang, W., Wells, G., & Tugwell, P. (2004). Tai chi for treating rheumatoid arthritis. *Cochrane Database of Systematic Reviews*, Issue 3.

Harding, A., Griffin, S. J., & Wareham, N. J. (2006). Population impact of strategies for identifying groups at high risk of type 2 diabetes. *Preventive Medicine, 42*(5), 364–368.

Harriss, D. J., Cable, N. T., George, K., Reilly, T., Renehan, A. G., & Haboubi, N. (2007). Physical activity before and after diagnosis of colorectal cancer: Disease risk, clinical outcomes, response pathways and biomarkers. *Sports Medicine, 37*(11), 947–960.

Haskell, W. L., Leon, A. S., Caspersen, C. J., Froelicher, V. F., Hagberg, J. M., Harlan, W., et al. (1992). Cardiovascular benefits and assessment of physical activity and physical fitness in adults. *Medicine and Science in Sports and Exercise, 24*(6 Suppl), S201–S220.

Hass, C. J., Feigenbaum, M. S., & Franklin, B. A. (2001). Prescription of resistance training for healthy populations. *Sports Medicine, 31*(14), 953–964.

Hass, C. J., Garzarella, L., de Hoyos, D., & Polloch, M. (2000). Single versus multiple sets in long-term recreational weightlifters. *Medicine and Science in Sports and Exercise, 32*(1), 235–242.

Hayden, J. A., van Tulder, M. W., Malmivaara, A., & Koes, B. W. (2005). Exercise therapy for treatment of non-specific low back pain. *Cochrane Database of Systematic Reviews*, Issue 3.

Hides, J. A., Jull, G. A., & Richardson, C. A. (2001). Long-term effects of specific stabilizing exercises for first-episode low back pain. *Spine, 26*(11), E243–E248.

Hilde, G., Hagen, K. B., Jamtvedt, G., & Winnem, M. (2007). Advice to stay active as a single treatment for low back pain and sciatica. *Cochrane Database of Systematic Reviews*, Issue 6.

Ingram, C., & Visovsky, C. (2007). Exercise intervention to modify physiologic risk factors in cancer survivors. *Seminars in Oncology Nursing, 23*(4), 275–284.

Jamtvedt, G., Damm, K. T., Christie, A., Moe, R. H., Haavardsholm, E. A., Holm, I., et al. (2008). Physical therapy interventions for patients with osteoarthritis of the knee: An overview of systematic reviews. *Physical Therapy, 88*(1), 123–136.

Joen, C. Y., Lokken, R. P., Hu, F. B., & van Dam, R. M. (2007). Physical activity of moderate intensity and risk of type 2 diabetes: A systematic review. *Diabetes Care, 30*(3), 744–752.

Kamel, H. K. (2003). Sarcopenia and aging. *Nutrition Reviews, 61*(5 Pt 1), 157–167.

Keller, T. T., Squizzato, A., & Middeldorp, S. (2007). Clopidogrel plus aspirin versus aspirin alone for preventing cardiovascular disease. *Cochrane Database of Systematic Reviews*, Issue 3.

Kelley, G. A., Kelley, K. S., & Tran, Z. V. (2000). Exercise and bone mineral density in men: A meta-analysis. *Journal of Applied Physiology, 88*(5), 1730–1736.

Kelley, G. A., Kelley, K. S., & Tran, Z. V. (2001). Resistance training and bone mineral density in women: A meta-analysis of controlled trials. *American Journal of Physical Medicine and Rehabilitation, 80*(1), 65–77.

Koumantakis, G. A., Watson, P. J., & Oldham, J. A. (2005). Trunk muscle stabilization training plus general exercise versus general exercise only: Randomized controlled trial of patients with recurrent low back pain. *Physical Therapy, 85*(3), 209–225.

Kuczmarski, R. J., Flegal, K. M., Campbell, S. M., & Johnson, C. L. (1994). Increasing prevalence of overweight among U.S. adults. The National Health and Nutrition Examination Surveys, 1960 to 1991. *Journal of the American Medical Association, 272*(3), 205–211.

Langdeau, J. B., & Boulet, L. P. (2001). Prevalence and mechanisms of development of asthma and airway hyperresponsiveness in athletes. *Journal of Sports Medicine, 31*(8), 601–616.

Lee, D. J., Meehan, R. T., Robinson, C., Mabry, T. R., & Smith, M. L. (1992). Immune responsiveness and risk of illness in US Air Force Academy cadets during basic cadet training. *Aviation, Space, and Environmental Medicine, 63*(6), 517–523.

Leon, A. S. (1991). Effects of exercise conditioning on physiologic precursors of coronary heart disease. *Journal of Cardiopulmonary Rehabilitation and Prevention, 11*(1), 46–57.

Liu-Ambrose, T., Khan, K. M., & McKay, H. A. (2001). The role of exercise in the prevention and treatment of osteoporosis. *International SportMed Journal, 2*(4), 1–14.

Lord, S. R., Matters, B., St George, R., Thomas, M., Bindon, J., Chan, D. K., et al. (2006). The effects of water exercise on physical functioning in older people. *Australian Journal on Ageing, 25*(1), 36–41.

Macfarlane, D. J., Chou, K., & Cheng, W. (2005). The effect of tai chi on the physical and psychological well-being of Chinese older women. *Journal of Exercise Science & Fitness, 3*(2), 87–94.

Mackinnon, L. T. (1992). *Exercise and immunology*. Champaign, IL: Human Kinetics.

Mandic, S., Riess, K., & Haykowsky, M. J. (2006). Exercise training for individuals with coronary artery disease or heart failure. *Physiotherapy Canada, 58*(1), 21–29.

Mangione, K. K., McCully, K., Gloviak, A., Lefebvre, I., Hofmann, M., & Craik, R. (1999). The effects of high-intensity and low-intensity cycle ergometry in older adults with knee osteoarthritis. *The Journals of Gerontology, 54*(4), M184–M190.

Martyn-St James, M., & Carroll, S. (2006). High-intensity resistance training and postmenopausal bone loss: A meta-analysis. *Osteoporosis International, 17*(8), 1225–1240.

Matthews, C. E., Ockene, I. S., Freedson, P. S., Rosal, M. C., Merriam, P. A., & Hebert, J. R. (2002). Moderate to vigorous physical activity and risk of upper-respiratory tract infection. *Medicine and Science in Sports and Exercise, 34*(8), 1242–1248.

McDermott, A. Y., & Mernitz, H. (2006). Exercise and older patients: Prescribing guidelines. *American Family Physician, 74*(3), 437–444.

McGill, S. M. (2001). Low back stability: From formal description to issues for performance and rehabilitation. *Exercise and Sport Sciences Reviews, 29*(1), 26–31.

McGill, S. M., & Cholewicki, J. (2001). Biomechanical basis for stability: An explanation to enhance clinical utility. *Journal of Orthopaedic and Sports Physical Therapy, 31*(2), 96–100.

McGill, S. M., Grenier, S., Kavcic, N., & Cholewicki, J. (2003). Coordination of muscle activity to assure stability of the lumbar spine. *Journal of Electromyography and Kinesiology, 13*(4), 353–359.

McKinnis, L. N. (2005). *Fundamentals of orthopedic radiology* (2nd ed.). Philadelphia: F. A. Davis.

Mian, O. S., Baltzopoulos, V., Minetti, A. E., & Narici, M. (2007). The impact of physical training on locomotor function in older people. *Sports Medicine, 37*(8), 683–701.

Moe, R. H., Haavardsholm, E. A., Christie, A., Jamtvedt, G., Damm, K. T., & Hagen, K. B. (2007). Effectiveness of nonpharmacological and nonsurgical interventions for hip osteoarthritis: An umbrella review of high-quality systematic reviews. *Physical Therapy, 87*(12), 1716–1727.

Morganti, C. M., Nelson, M. E., Fiatarone, M. A., Dallal, G. E., Economos, C. D., Crawford, B. M., et al. (1995). Strength improvements with 1 yr of progressive resistance training in older women. *Medicine and Science in Sports and Exercise, 27*(6), 906–912.

National Institutes of Health. (1998). *Clinical guidelines on the identification, evaluation, and treatment of overweight and obesity in adults* (Vol. 8), Pub. No. 98-4083. Bethesda, MD: Dept of Health and Human Services, National Institutes of Health, National Heart, Lung, and Blood Institute.

National Institute of Health, Osteoporosis and Related Bone Disease—National Resource Center. (2006). *Osteoporosis*. Retrieved January 5, 2008, from *www.niams.nih.gov/Health_Info/Bone/Osteoporosis*

National Osteoporosis Foundation. (2008). *Fast Facts*. Retrieved January 5, 2008, from *www.nof.org/osteoporosis/disease*

Neumann, S. A., Miller, M. D., Daniels, L., & Crotty, M. (2005). Nutritional status and clinical outcomes of older patients in rehabilitation. *Journal of Human Nutrition and Dietetics, 18*(2), 129–136.

Nieman, D. (1994). Exercise, upper respiratory tract infection, and the immune system. *Medicine and Science in Sports and Exercise, 26*(2), 128–139.

Nieman, D. (2000). Exercise soothes arthritis: Joint effects. *ACSM's Health & Fitness Journal, 4*(3), 20–28.

Nieman, D. C., Johanssen, L. M., Lee, J. W., & Arabatzis, K. (1990). Infectious episodes in runners before and after the Los Angeles Marathon. *The Journal of Sports Medicine and Physical Fitness, 30*(3), 316–328.

Nixon, S., O'Brien, K., Glazier, R. H., & Tynan, A. M. (2005). Aerobic exercise interventions for adults living with HIV/AIDS. *Cochrane Database of Systematic Reviews*, Issue 2.

O'Brien, K., Nixon, S., Glazier, R. H., & Tynan, A. M. (2004). Progressive resistive exercise interventions for adults living with HIV/AIDS. *Cochrane Database of Systematic Reviews*, Issue 4.

Ogden, C. L., Carroll, M. D., Curtin, L. R., McDowell, M. A., Tabak, C. J., & Flegal, K. M. (2006). Prevalence of overweight and obesity in the United States, 1999–2004. *JAMA*, 295(13), 1549–1555.

Oh, R. C., & Lanier, J. B. (2007). Management of hypertriglyceridemia. *American Family Physician*, 75(9), 1365–1371.

Oliveria, S. A., Kohl, H., Trichopoulos, D., & Blair, S. (1996). The association between cardiorespiratory fitness and prostate cancer. *Medicine and Science in Sports and Exercise*, 28(1), 97–104.

Ourania, M., Yvoni, H., Christos, K., & Ioannis, T. (2003). Effects of a physical activity program. The study of selected physical abilities among elderly women. *Journal of Gerontological Nursing*, 29(7), 50–55.

Packard, P. T., & Hearney, R. P. (1997). Medical nutrition therapy for patients with osteoporosis. *Journal of the American Dietetic Association*, 97(4), 414–417.

Palombaro, K. M. (2005). Effects of walking-only intervention on bone mineral density at various skeletal sites: A meta-analysis. *Journal of Geriatric Physical Therapy*, 28(3), 102–107.

Pate, R. R., Baranowski, T., Dowda, M., & Trost, S. G. (1996). Tracking of physical activity in young children. *Medicine and Science in Sports and Exercise*, 28(1), 92–96.

Pate, R. R., Pratt, M., Blair, S. N., Haskell, W. L., Macera, C. A., Bouchard, C., et al. (1995). Physical activity and public health. A recommendation for the Centers for Disease Control and Prevention and the American College of Sports Medicine. *Journal of the American Medical Association*, 273(5), 402–407.

Pedersen, B. K., & Bruunsgaard, H. (1995). How physical exercise influences the establishment of infections. *Sports Medicine*, 19(6), 393–400.

Pedersen, B., Rohde, T., & Ostrowski, K. (1998). Recovery of the immune system after exercise. *Acta Physiologica Scandinavica*, 162(3), 325–332.

Pedersen, B., & Ullum, H. (1994). NK cell response to physical activity: Possible mechanisms of action. *Medicine and Science in Sports and Exercise*, 26(2), 140–146.

Pejic, R. N., & Lee, D. T. (2006). Hypertriglyceridemia. *Journal of the American Board of Family Medicine*, 19(3), 310–316.

Pereira, M. A., Kriska, A. M., Joswiak, M. L., Dowse, G. K., Collins, V. R., Zimmet, P. Z., et al. (1995). Physical inactivity and glucose intolerance in the multiethnic island of Mauritius. *Medicine and Science in Sports and Exercise*, 27(12), 1626–1634.

Pescatello, L. S., Franklin, B. A., Fagard, R., Farquhar, W. B., Kelley, G. A, & Ray, C. A. (2004). American College of Sports Medicine position standard. Exercise and hypertension. *Medical Science in Sports and Exercise*, 36(3), 533–553.

Peters-Futre, E. M. (1997). Vitamin C, neutrophil function, and upper respiratory tract infection risk in distance runners: The missing link. *Exercise Immunology Review*, 3, 32–52.

Pyne, D. B., Baker, M. S., Fricker, P. A., McDonald, W. A., Telford, R. D., & Weidemann, M. J. (1995). Effects of an intensive 12-wk training program by elite swimmers on neutrophil oxidative activity. *Medicine and Science in Sports and Exercise*, 27(4), 536–542.

Rees, K., Taylor, R. S., Singh, S., Coats, A. J. S., & Ebrahim, S. (2004). Exercise based rehabilitation for heart failure. *Cochrane Database of Systematic Reviews*, Issue 3.

Sax, P. E. (2006). Strategies for management and treatment of dyslipidemia in HIV/AIDS. *AIDS Care*, 18(2), 149–157.

Saxena, S., Van Ommeren, M., Tang, K. C., & Armstrong, T. P. (2005). Mental health benefits of physical activity. *Journal of Mental Health*, 14(5), 445–451.

Schneider, J. K., Eveker, A., Bronder, D. R., Meiner, S. E., & Binder, E. F. (2003). Exercise training program for older adults. Incentives and disincentives for participation. *Journal of Gerontological Nursing*, 29(9), 21–31.

Schneider, J. K., Mercer, G., Herning, M., Smith, C., & Prysak, M. D. (2004). Promoting exercise behavior in older adults: Using a cognitive behavioral intervention. *Journal of Gerontological Nursing*, 30(4), 45–53.

Shaughnessy, M., & Caulfield, B. (2004). A pilot study to investigate the effect of lumbar stabilisation exercise training on functional ability and quality of life in patients with chronic low back pain. *International Journal of Rehabilitation Research*, 27(4), 297–301.

Shaw, K., Gennat, H., O'Rourke, P., & Del Mar, C. (2006). Exercise for overweight or obesity. *Cochrane Database of Systematic Reviews*, October, 18(4), CD003817.

Silva, L. E., Valim, V., Pessanha, A. P. C., Oliviera, L. M., Myamoto, S., Jones, A., et al. (2008). Hydrotherapy versus conventional land-based exercise for the management of patients with osteoarthritis of the knee: A randomized clinical trial. *Physical Therapy*, 88(1), 12–21.

Skinner, J. S., Hustler, R., Bergsteinova, V., & Buskirk, R. (1973). The validity and reliability of a rating scale of perceived exertion. *Medicine and Science in Sports*, 5(2), 94–96.

Slade, S. C., & Keating, J. L. (2007). Unloaded movement facilitation exercise compared to no exercise or alternative therapy on outcomes for people with nonspecific chronic low back pain: A systematic review. *Journal of Manipulative and Physiological Therapeutics*, 30(4), 301–311.

Smutok, M., Skrinar, G., & Pandolf, K. (1980). Exercise intensity: Subjective regulation by perceived exertion. *Archives of Physical Medicine and Rehabilitation*, 61(12), 569–574.

Staal, J. B., Hlobil, H., Twisk, J. W., Smid, T., Koke, A. J., & van Mechelen, W. (2004). Graded activity for low back pain in occupational health care: A randomized, controlled trial. *Annals of Internal Medicine*, 140(2), 77–84.

Terry, L., Sprinz, E., Medeiros, N. B., Oliveira, J., & Ribeiro, J. P. (2006). Exercise training in HIV-1-infected individuals with dyslipidemia and lipodystrophy. *Medicine and Science in Sports and Exercise*, 38(3), 411–417.

Thomas, D. E., Elliot, E. J., & Naughton, G. A. (2006). Exercise for type 2 diabetes mellitus. *Cochrane Database of Systematic Reviews*, Issue 4.

Tremblay, A., Després, J. P., & Bouchard, C. (1985). The effects of exercise-training on energy balance and adipose tissue morphology and metabolism. *Sports Medicine*, 2(3), 223–233.

Trichopoulou, A., Psaltopoulou, T., Orfanos, P., & Trichopoulos, D. (2006). Diet and physical activity in relation to overall mortality amongst adult diabetics in a general population cohort. *Journal of Internal Medicine*, 259(6), 583–591.

U.S. Department of Health and Human Services. (2000, Jan.). *Healthy people 2010.* (Vol. 1 and 2, Conference ed.). Washington, DC.

U.S. Department of Health and Human Services. (2006, Dec.). *Midcourse Review. Healthy people 2010.* Washington, DC.

Van den Ende, C. H. M., Vliet Vlieland, T. P. M., Munneke, M., & Hazes, J. M. W. (1998). Dynamic exercise therapy for treating rheumatoid arthritis. *Cochrane Database of Systematic Reviews*, Issue 4.

Wallace, J. P. (2003). Obesity. In *ACSM's Exercise Management for Persons with Chronic Diseases and Disabilities.* (2nd ed.). Champaign, IL: Human Kinetic, pp. 149–156.

Warburton, D. E., Katzmarzyk, P. T., Rhodes, R. E., & Shephard, R. J. (2007). Evidence-informed physical activity guidelines for Canadian adults. *Canadian Journal of Public Health*, 98(Suppl 2), S16–S68.

Wei, M., Gibbons, L. W., Kampert, J. B., Nichaman, M. Z., & Blair, S. N. (2000). Low cardiorespiratory fitness and physical activity as predictors of mortality in men with type 2 diabetes. *Annals of Internal Medicine*, 132(8), 605–611.

Weise, S. D., Grandjean, P. W., Rohack, J. J., Womack, J. W., & Crouse, S. F. (2005). Acute changes in blood lipids and enzymes in postmenopausal women after exercise. *Journal of Applied Physiology*, 99(2), 609–615.

Williams, P. T. (1996). High-density lipoprotein cholesterol and other risk factors for coronary heart disease in female runners. *New England Journal of Medicine*, 334(20), 1298–1303.

Yuan, G., Al-Shali, K. Z., & Hegele, R. A. (2007). Hypertriglyceridemia: Its etiology, effects and treatment. *Canadian Medical Association Journal*, 176(8), 1113–1120.

Stress Management

objectives

After completing this chapter, the reader will be able to:

- Analyze concepts of stress, stressor, eustress, and distress.
- Evaluate potential physical, psychological, social, and behavioral stressors.
- Analyze the pathophysiology of the stress response and effects on health and illness.
- Examine primary and secondary appraisals of stress.
- Develop evidenced-based stress management interventions that can be used in clinical practice.
- Explain the nurse's role in stress management.

key terms

Active listening
Acupuncture
Affirmation
Anxiety sensitivity
Aromatherapy
Assertive communication
Cognitive restructuring
Coping
Distress
Empathy
Eustress
Exercise
Expressive writing

Fight-or-flight response
Goal setting
Healthy diet
Healthy pleasures
Humor
Hypnosis
Journal writing
Meridian
Mini-relaxations
Presence
Primary appraisal
Reflexology
Reiki

Relaxation response
Secondary appraisal
Self-awareness
Sleep hygiene
Social support
Spiritual practice
Stress
Stress management
Stress response
Stress warning signs
Stressor
Values clarification

website materials

evolve These materials are located on the book's Website at *http://evolve.elsevier.com/Edelman/*.
- WebLinks
- Study Questions
- Glossary

THINK About It

Do We Live to Work or Work to Live?

When asked about yourself, what is your first response? Do you say what you do for work or do you describe your characteristics? For most of us, our work roles, including being students, define us to a great extent. For most adults in the United States and many other societies, employment is a primary source of income and social connection; working also contributes to a personal sense of accomplishment. However, how much work is too much? Americans take fewer yearly vacation days than their counterparts in other industrial countries, and workplace pressures can increase risk for a variety of disorders. Work-related stress can be a real problem.

1. What aspects of work typically create stress?
2. How do people manage work-related stress? Which strategies are effective and which strategies increase health risks?
3. What health-promotion strategies could you implement to reduce your own work-related stress?
4. What could you do to promote workers' health in your own practice?

Stress is an excellent paradigm for understanding the relationships among the determinants of health, the leading health indicators, and health outcomes. Stress has been shown to cause or exacerbate many of the leading health problems in the United States today, such as those related to obesity, alcohol and drug abuse, and sexually transmitted diseases (U.S. Department of Health and Human Services [USDHHS], n.d.). Consequently, helping individuals, families, and communities to find more effective ways to respond to stress is an important health-promotion goal.

Stress management has been an effective intervention for health promotion, disease prevention, and symptom management. Stress management strategies such as relaxation and imagery, self-monitoring, **goal setting**, cognitive restructuring, and problem solving have long been the staple of community health promotion programs, including Alcoholics Anonymous, Smoke Enders, and Weight Watchers. These strategies help people to modify health risk behaviors and thereby improve quality of life. However, current national health data indicate the need for continued and expanded use of these modalities across the life span. Unfortunately, although the United States health care system provides excellent, expensive, heroic care, it provides poor quality low-cost health promotion/preventive care, including stress management. Moreover, to ameliorate many harmful effects of stress, community-level health promotion is essential. Although shifting focus from providing acute care for individuals to enhancing health of communities requires a revolution in our health care delivery systems and outlook, successful community health-promotion initiatives hold promise for the future (Butterfoss, 2007).

The goal of stress management is to improve quality of life by increasing healthy, effective **coping**, thereby reducing unhealthy consequences of distress. This process produces a dynamic interaction of mind, body, and spirit, which affects not only physical health and well-being, but also cognitive and emotional states and behavior. Stress management is thus an essential tool for expert nursing practice, which recognizes the interface of mind, body, and spirit. The use of critical reasoning to examine multiple factors contributing to symptom development provides a valuable contribution

to meeting the goals of *Healthy People 2010* and developing *Healthy People 2020*. Stress management can have a significant impact on the following leading health indicators in *Healthy People 2010*: physical activity, obesity, tobacco use, substance abuse, responsible sexual behavior, mental health, injury and violence, environmental quality, immunization, and access to health care (USDHHS, n.d.). (See Chapter 1 for additional discussion of *Healthy People 2010*.) This chapter outlines the psychophysiological aspects of stress, examines strategies shown to mediate its harmful effects, reviews clinical situations in which stress management has been effective, and explores the unique perspective nurses bring that helps individuals identify healthy stress management strategies.

SOURCES OF STRESS

A **stressor** is any psychological, social, environmental, physiological, or spiritual stimulus that disrupts homeostasis thereby requiring change or adaptation (Bartol & Courts, 2005). Stress is a defined as "a state of threatened homeostasis or disharmony and is counteracted by a complex repertoire of physiologic and behavioral responses that reestablish homeostasis" (Tsigos et al., 2005, p. 101). These definitions underscore important ideas: even welcome events are stressors because they precipitate change, stress is not intrinsically bad or unhealthy, and stress is experienced psychophysiologically. Stress is an essential component of being alive.

Individuals encounter a variety of physical, psychological, social, spiritual, and environmental stressors. Stressors range from health and illness experiences such as childbirth, physical illness, trauma, or blood loss; to activities of daily living such as caring for children, meeting work deadlines, and cleaning or repairing the house; to less common events such as taking a critical examination, experiencing the death of a relative, losing possessions in a fire, losing a job, getting a divorce, or getting married. Stressors can be organized into three categories: (1) stressors over which people have no control (extrinsic factors), such as the weather, a traffic jam, or the death of a spouse; (2) stressors that individuals can modify by changing their environment,

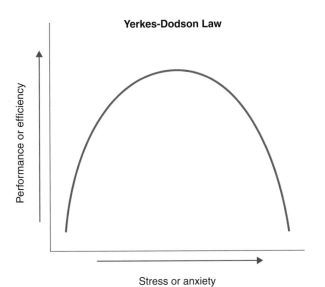

Yerkes-Dodson Law

Performance or efficiency

Stress or anxiety

Figure 13-1 Yerkes Dodson law. (Modified from *Your Maximum Mind* by Herbert Benson, M.D., copyright © 1987 by Random House, Inc. Used by permission of Crown Publishers, a division of Random House, Inc.)

---

social interactions, or behaviors; and (3) stressors created or exacerbated (intrinsic factors) by poor time management, procrastination, poor communication, catastrophic negative thinking (expecting the worst), or struggling with self-defeating behaviors. Stress is a person-environment process in which the person appraises a situation as taxing or as exceeding his or her resources and endangering well-being (Carver, 2007; Lazarus & Folkman, 1984). Appraisal is an important concept that helps to explain why two people react in different ways to the same situation.

The example of Ms. Smith and Ms. Jones is a case in point. Both individuals are about to become residents at an assisted living facility in their hometown. Ms. Smith perceives this move as an opportunity to increase the ease of her socializations and activities of daily living, and is looking forward to making new friends and participating in new recreational activities. In contrast, Ms. Jones views this move as abandonment by her family and fears that available care will be inadequate. Although the event is virtually the same for both Ms. Smith and Ms. Jones, the physiological and psychosocial consequences are likely to be different because of the way that each woman perceives her situation.

Stress is the physical, psychological, social, or spiritual effect of life's pressures and events. Stress is an interactive process that involves appraisal and response to loss or the threat of loss of the person's homeostasis or well-being (Carver, 2007). Canadian physiologist Dr. Hans Selye (1982) demonstrated that, to a certain extent, stress can be challenging and useful, which he identified as **eustress**. Selye also observed that when stress becomes chronic or excessive, the body is unable to adapt and maintain homeostasis and thus **distress**. Stress can be both useful and harmful. As stress increases, efficiency and performance also increase, but not endlessly. As illustrated in Figure 13-1, at a certain point performance and efficiency start to decrease

significantly if stress continues unabated. It is important to understand the many causes of stress and the negative physical, psychosocial, and spiritual consequences of distress. Understanding the many-sided sources of stress provides the rationale for a multifaceted approach to its management (Hot Topics Box).

PHYSICAL, PSYCHOLOGICAL, SOCIOBEHAVIORAL, AND SPIRITUAL CONSEQUENCES OF STRESS

Physiological Effects of Stress

An individual's response to stress provides a model to examine changes across biopsychosocial-spiritual domains. In response to a perceived threat (i.e., stressor), the body prepares to meet the challenge. Perception of threat stimulates a physiological pattern of neuroendocrine activation and behavioral changes mediated by the central nervous system (Figure 13-2) (Bartol & Courts, 2005; Carver, 2007). In most cases this reaction is an adaptive, short-term, acute response to a stressor. First termed the **fight-or-flight response**

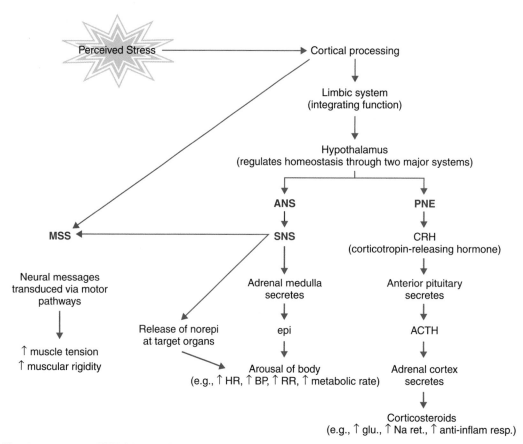

Figure 13-2 The stress response. *ACTH,* Adrenocorticotropic hormone; *ANS,* autonomic nervous system; *anti-inflam resp.,* anti-inflammatory response; *BP,* blood pressure; *CRH,* corticotropin-releasing hormone; *epi,* epinephrine; *glu.,* blood glucose level; *HR,* heart rate; *MSS,* musculoskeletal system; *Na ret.,* sodium retention; *norepi,* norepinephrine; *PNE,* pituitary-neuroendocrine system; *RR,* respiratory rate; *SNS,* sympathetic nervous system. (From Wells-Federman, C., Stuart-Shor, E., Deckro, J., Mandle, C. L., Baim, M., & Medich, C. [1995]. The mind/body connection: The psychophysiology of many traditional nursing interventions. *Clinical Nurse Specialist, 9,* 60.)

(Cannon, 1914) and later called the **stress response** (Selye, 1982), the individual's reaction to a real or imagined threat prepares the body for emergency reaction and fosters survival in circumstances of immediate, time-limited threat. The hypothalamus signals the sympathetic nervous system to release epinephrine and norepinephrine, along with other related hormones. A resultant state of arousal is characterized by increased metabolism, pulse, blood pressure, respiration, and muscle tension. This physiological arousal proceeds along three main pathways: (1) the musculoskeletal system, (2) the autonomic nervous system, and (3) the psychoneuroendocrine system.

The musculoskeletal system responds by increasing tension and tone. At the same time, the autonomic nervous system, via the sympathetic branch, orchestrates a generalized arousal that includes increases in heart rate, blood pressure, and respiratory rate. Additionally, a heightened awareness of the environment is triggered, and blood shifts from the visceral organs to the large muscle groups. Concurrently the psychoneuroendocrine system stimulates the hypothalamic-pituitary-adrenal axis and the secretion of corticosteroids (primarily cortisol) and other neuroendocrine substances

into the systemic circulation, increasing blood glucose levels, influencing sodium retention and, in the acute phase, increasing the anti-inflammatory response.

Study findings have shown that maladaptive stress can cause or exacerbate disease or symptoms of diseases. Proinflammation associated with stress is emerging as a common pathway in a variety of diseases such as asthma, angina, cardiac arrhythmias, pain, tension headaches, insomnia, and gastrointestinal complaints (Bartol & Courts, 2005; Fitzpatrick et al., 2007). Additionally, stress can produce hyper- or hyporeactivity of hormones regulated by the psychoneuroendocrine system (Semmer et al., 2005).

As mentioned, in most cases the stress response is a beneficial adaptive pattern that increases efficiency and quality of performance, but it can prove maladaptive when a stressor continues indefinitely. Maladaptive stress is an enduring and sometimes self-sustaining cascade of responses that degenerate physical, psychosocial, and spiritual well-being. Not surprisingly, stress and specifically depression have been associated with increased susceptibility to cardiovascular disease, as well as to poor response to its treatment. However, indirect influences of stress and depression on self-care health behaviors might explain these associations. Needless to say, further investigation is needed to demonstrate direct causal links as well as effectiveness of psychological interventions for persons with cardiovascular disease (Lane et al., 2007; Rees et al., 2004).

Psychological Effects of Stress

The psychological effects of stress are best illustrated by its contributory role in negative mood states, including anxiety, depression, hostility, and anger. "With respect to the link between stress and distress, the path is unquestionable. There is no doubt that stressful events produce emotional distress" (Carver, 2007, p. 131). Exposure to stressful stimuli is associated with elevated cortisol levels and resultant effects on the immune system. Duration, intensity, and timing of a stressor have been shown to affect immune responses in animals. Although systematic studies to explain different patterns of immune response have not yet been conducted with humans, the interactive nature of the mind and immune system is an exciting area of investigation that may contribute to future evidence-based practice (Kemeny, 2007).

The interplay of stress, emotional distress, and various health outcomes is illustrated by a growing body of clinical research outcomes. For example, research results concerning health effects of stress on frail older adults and on terminally ill individuals and family members demonstrate the influence of stress on quality of life. Loeher et al. (2004) found that transition from rehabilitation care to a nursing home was associated with significantly more depression symptoms than transition back to living alone or with others. Qualitative research with individuals who had terminal cancer defined suffering as experiences of violence, feeling deprived and overwhelmed, and apprehension (Daneault et al., 2004). Family members of decedents reported the following sources of stress in relation to changes in their loved ones prior to death: loss of bodily functions, being dependent, and being a burden. Findings indicate that worries about loss of quality of life, independent of level of symptom severity of loved ones, contributed to suffering (Hickman et al., 2004). Thus stressful aspects of illness experiences and life transitions are associated with negative health effects for ill individuals and their family members.

Sociobehavioral Effects of Stress

In response to stress, individuals often revert to or increase their reliance on less healthy behaviors, such as overeating, excessive use of alcohol or drugs, and smoking. Recognizing that such behaviors are inconsistent with the healthy behaviors needed to cope with stress is easy; however, stopping these behaviors and using health-promoting strategies is not. Risky behaviors and traits such as a sedentary lifestyle, obesity, overeating high-fat foods, smoking, drug use, and social isolation have been linked to morbidity and mortality (USDHHS, n.d.). Conversely, **exercise**, **healthy diet**, smoking cessation, healthy weight maintenance, and social interaction have been identified as leading indicators of

health in this country (USDHHS, n.d.). Encouraging these health behaviors supports goals of *Healthy People 2010*. However, without understanding how psychosocial factors affect health behaviors, promoting effective self-care is an unrealistic goal (Weinger, 2007).

Spiritual Effects of Stress

Interest in the connection between spirituality and health is significant. Spirituality can be defined as: "The feelings, thoughts, experiences, and behaviors that arise from a search for meaning.... The essence of being and relatedness that permeates all of life and is manifested in one's knowing, doing, and being. The interconnectedness with self, others, nature, and God/LifeForce/Absolute/Transcendent" (American Holistic Nurses Association & American Nurses Association, 2007, p. 71). Spirituality and religion intersect for many, yet they are not synonymous.

In response to stress, people often feel disconnected from life's meaning and purpose; harmful effects on their health and well-being can result. Finding meaning and connection through spirituality, including religion, can protect against negative outcomes of stress, at least to some extent. After large-scale community disasters such as Hurricanes Katrina and Rita in 2005, September 11th in 2001, and the Oklahoma City bombing in 1995, turning to spirituality and religion, as well as engaging in open discussion and community activities, helped people to cope with their reactions to these events (Wainrib, 2006). Research outcomes have demonstrated a variety of associations between spirituality or religious activity and stress reduction. For example, religiosity among a sample of women with fibromyalgia had protective effects against stress (Dedert et al., 2004). Difficulty forgiving oneself and negative religious coping were related to depression, anxiety, and posttraumatic stress disorder symptom severity among a sample of veterans (Witvliet et al., 2004). Among a group of African American heterosexuals with human immunodeficiency virus infection, religious and existential well-being explained 32% of variance in depression (Coleman, 2004). Thus research now affirms what nurses have long known: that is, helping people use interventions that influence or restore connection with life meaning and purpose has important health-promoting benefits (Nightingale, 1859, 1992).

The previous section discussed how stress can adversely affect biological activity, cognition, emotions, behavior, and spiritual well-being. This understanding of the psychophysiology of the mind-body-spirit connection is fundamental to the application of stress management in nursing and provides an obvious rationale for a multifaceted approach. Further support is provided from research endorsing the health-promoting effects of managing stress. The Research Highlights box presents a study of effects of guided imagery with relaxation on health-related quality of life in older women with osteoarthritis that illustrates many ideas presented in this chapter.

research highlights

Effect of Guided Imagery with Relaxation on Health-Related Quality of Life in Older Women with Osteoarthritis

Osteoarthritis, a common cause of disability among older adults, negatively affects quality of life due to joint degeneration and pain. A randomized pilot study was conducted to test the effectiveness of guided imagery with relaxation to increase quality of life. Researchers assigned 28 women to an intervention group and a control group. The intervention group received guided imagery with relaxation consisting of listening to a 12-minute audiotape twice a day for 12 weeks. The intervention group experienced significantly increased health-related quality of life in comparison to the control group, even after adjusting for changes in pain and mobility. Findings suggested that guided imagery with relaxation shows promise as an effective, easy-to-use, cost-effective self-management intervention to improve quality of life of older women with osteoarthritis.

From: Baird, C. L., & Sands, L. P. (2006). Effect of guided imagery with relaxation on health-related quality of life in older women with osteoarthritis. *Research in Nursing & Health, 29,* 442-451.

HEALTH BENEFITS OF MANAGING STRESS

A growing body of evidence underscores the importance of controlling stress to promote health and quality of life for people with a variety of health problems. Immune system diseases have responded to interventions that reduce the stress response. For example, continuous labor support reduces the stress response during childbirth, promotes a woman's positive memory of the experience, and affects various desired health outcomes (Pascali-Bonaro & Kroeger, 2004). Psychotherapeutic approaches, such as interpersonal and cognitive-behavioral psychotherapies that focus on perception and management of life stressors, are effective treatments for depression and related mental health disorders (Markowitz, 2004; Power, 2004).

Promoting a positive attitude and development of skills to cope with stress is foundational to many stress management interventions. Kobasa et al. (1982) made a groundbreaking contribution to understating the stress-illness relationship when they identified characteristics of hardiness. They described individuals with stress-hardy characteristics who, when exercising and accessing **social support**, were less vulnerable to stress-related symptoms and diseases. The characteristics of stress hardiness are control, challenge, and commitment. For stress-hardy individuals, stress is viewed as a challenge rather than a threat; they feel in control of situations in their lives, and they are committed to rather than alienated from work, home, and family.

Research outcomes support the value of promoting stress management as a key to better health outcomes. For example, Pâquet et al. (2005) found that men and women who had been hospitalized for myocardial infarction, angina, or percutaneous angioplasty focused on the importance of stress management rather than managing health habits

as important to their recovery and future health. Support groups were identified as helping participants accept their condition and understand their limits and improving continuity of care.

Investigators also have found links between health and explanatory style. For example, in a study of people undergoing cardiac rehabilitation, optimism contributed to positive health outcomes directly, as well as indirectly, because it led to fewer harmful coping strategies and fewer symptoms of depression (Shen et al., 2004). Recognizing the influence of explanatory style on health and well-being furthers the understanding of how thoughts, feelings, behaviors, and physiological activity interact. Furthermore, nurses can identify people with high stressors and unhealthy personality traits that increase their risk for stress-related illnesses and assist them to modify these factors to enhance their health.

The previous section described the interrelationships among thoughts, feelings, behaviors, beliefs, and biological activity and offered a systematic way to understand these interactions. Evidence was presented that perceptions, or the way individuals view situations, can lead to stress and, in turn, adversely affect biological activity, emotions, behavior, and the connection with life meaning and purpose. This interaction among perceptions, stress, and multifaceted effects, in turn, increases stress and fosters a negative stress cycle. The remainder of this chapter presents assessment of stress relating to the physical, psychosocial, and spiritual health and well-being of individuals, and describes application of a variety of strategies shown to help break the negative stress cycle and mitigate its harmful effects across the biological, psychosocial, and spiritual domains.

ASSESSMENT OF STRESS

Assessment of the stress-coping abilities of an individual, family, or community is part of comprehensive health assessment that includes past and present subjective and objective data. Collecting these data enables the individual and nurse to determine the status of the person's stress-coping pattern, and actual and potential strengths and weaknesses.

The nurse thoroughly collects data during the history, physical examination, and health patterns assessment (see Chapter 7, 8, and 9). Identifying the stress-coping pattern is especially important. Each individual is the primary data source; no other person can explain accurately the individual's perceptions of the stressors, stress responses, and resources to prevent or alleviate the stress.

Stress is experienced across biological, psychosocial, and spiritual domains; therefore, all perceptions are important to the assessment. Throughout the assessment process, individuals may become aware of information of which they were previously unaware, or they may identify information related to their perceived problems. For example, a man may be aware of the stress of his job but may be unaware that his high blood pressure was brought about at least in part by this stress.

Lazarus and Folkman (1984) proposed a theory comprising primary and secondary appraisals of stressful events, situations, or demands and the effectiveness of an individual's coping skills. **Primary appraisal** of coping includes descriptions of perceived actual and potential positive and negative outcomes. Negative outcomes refer to harm, whereas positive outcomes refer to the challenges resulting from stressors that an individual perceives can be overcome. Examples of negative outcomes are physical injury, disease, loss of a cherished relationship, position or possession, and death. Positive outcomes include graduation, promotion, and development of important relationships (see the Case Study and Care Plan at the end of this chapter).

Secondary appraisal follows primary appraisal. Secondary appraisal consists of the individual's identification of choices to cope with the actual or potential harm, threat, or challenge. The choices may be internal or external resources and responses. For example, a social resource in coping with the needs of a toddler might be learning strategies in a parent-effectiveness training course. A coping response to the challenges of parenting a toddler might be restructuring the toddler's and parent's schedules to allow for more frequent cycles of activities and rest.

The individual's primary and secondary appraisals of stress provide opportunities to consider the stress experiences in different ways. Resources that had been forgotten may be remembered, or a threat may be newly viewed as a challenge and an opportunity for enhanced development and status. Stress responses are mediated by the appraisal process.

By using measurement instruments with established reliability and validity, nurses can improve assessment of an individual's stress and coping. Tools can help nurses distinguish between diagnoses that have many signs and symptoms in common. For example, disturbances in thinking and feeling processes can be difficult to distinguish and may have confounding clinical pictures. These disturbances can occur separately or simultaneously in the same person. An example of this complexity is the overlapping symptomatology of depression and dementia. The nurse determines whether one health problem is actually the cause of the other in order to develop an effective plan of care (see the Case Study and Care Plan at the end of the chapter).

A wide variety of instruments are available to help nurses assess orientation, attention, cognitive skills and patterns, traits and states of emotions, symptoms of mental health distress and disorders, and overall quality of life. For example, The Schedule of Recent Experiences (Holmes, 1981) and The Impact of Event Scale (Horowitz et al., 1979) are two well-established instruments used widely in clinical assessment and research to measure stress associated with life changes and events. Before using any instrument, clinicians and researchers need to check training requirements and copyright restrictions (e.g., purchase requirements) that can affect access to it.

Use of standardized instruments promotes accuracy in developing diagnoses and plans of care, and assists in evaluating the effectiveness of care. For example, a nurse may compare an individual's self-evaluation scores before intervention with postintervention scores and revise the plan of care accordingly. Additionally, nurses may analyze population baseline scores for relevant characteristics and develop programs of research and quality improvements aimed at improving outcomes.

STRESS MANAGEMENT INTERVENTIONS

Stress management strategies are beneficial to people across a broad spectrum of chronological, gender, cultural, and ethnic characteristics. Men and women, young and old, from divergent socioeconomic, cultural, and ethnic backgrounds can benefit from stress management interventions. Sensitivity to needs and values of individuals and communities, particularly for high-risk groups, guides assessment and intervention techniques. The language, belief system, and cultural distinctions of individuals guide the choice and adaptation of stress management strategies.

Developing Self-Awareness

Self-awareness is one of the most effective stress management tools. Self-awareness helps people learn about interactions among mind, body, and spirit; increases a sense of control; and counters self-defeating perceptions. Interventions that promote self-awareness help people make sense of life events and circumstances that may be bewildering or discomforting. Many experiences in life lead to feelings of emptiness and disharmony, because people are unable to connect the experience with thoughts, feelings, actions, and physiological responses. Self-awareness helps individuals recognize stress that they create through negative, exaggerated, unrealistic thinking. This recognition affords an opportunity to change these negative thought patterns, thereby decreasing stress and increasing control. Strategies that increase self-awareness can empower individuals to make new connections and to reframe and reinterpret their experiences in light of their own inner strengths and wisdom.

Techniques for Developing Self-Awareness

Monitoring Stress Warning Signs The negative stress cycle can be difficult to interrupt. Recognizing warning signs of stress is a necessary first step. Often individuals have long ignored physical, emotional, or behavioral cues or reactions to a stressor that are **stress warning signs**. A man suffering from chronic intermittent backaches, who ignores the daily muscle tension caused by poor posture that precedes the backaches, provides an example. If he had attended to his early stress warning signs of poor posture and muscle tension, he might have avoided the backache that kept him from exercising and socializing. Becoming aware of these stress warning signs is the first step. Attending to these cues is the next step. After this connection is made, developing skills to reduce negative mood states, unhealthy behaviors, and physical symptoms becomes much easier. Furthermore, some people misinterpret physiological signs of anxiety (e.g., shortness of breath, racing heartbeat) as indicative of serious physical danger (e.g., suffocation, myocardial infarction). This tendency to misinterpret physical anxiety cues is referred to as **anxiety sensitivity**, a belief that bodily sensations associated with anxiety indicate imminent and dangerous outcomes, and is associated with various anxiety disorders and health anxiety (Deacon & Abramowitz, 2006). By assisting individuals who are prone to anxiety sensitivity to interpret bodily sensations accurately, nurses help to reduce individuals' misinterpretations, as well as the likelihood of escalation of anxiety symptoms and possibly even development of anxiety disorders.

To continue with the previous example, preventing a backache from becoming disabling is easier when the man notices muscle tension and then stops, takes a few deep breaths, corrects his posture, and gently stretches the area, rather than waiting for the backache to become incapacitating before acting.

Nurses teach people to identify their warning signals of stress and to stop, take a few breaths, and break the cycle. Figure 13-3 is a sample form for identifying and recording this information. These signals or cues differ from individual to individual and can be physical, emotional, behavioral, cognitive, relational, or spiritual. When asked to monitor their responses to a particular event, individuals become more consciously aware of these cues. Although this heightened awareness initially may increase an individual's consciousness of physical pain or emotional discomfort, awareness is a necessary first step in recognizing the negative effects of stress and the relationship of thoughts, feelings, behavior, and biological processes. In addition, nurses and other clinicians have a responsibility to screen for emotional distress to help people to recognize and monitor their own physical and mood states. For individuals with health conditions such as coronary artery disease known to have high comorbidity with emotional distress and specifically depression, routine screening should be the standard of care (Ketterer et al., 2007).

Try this: ask an individual to identify a stressful experience and the physical or emotional reactions (stress warning signals) to that particular experience. For example, after being instructed to stop, take a breath, and notice the physical and emotional response to a stressful situation, one woman related the following:

> On my way to work yesterday, I sat in a huge traffic jam. I noticed that my heart was racing, my breathing had changed, and my hands were gripping the steering wheel. I felt angry and frustrated because I was going to be late for work.

Although these responses seem quite obvious, most people are unaware of the effects of stress on their minds and bodies. After individuals become aware of these effects, they may be able to release tension more easily, countering the negative effects of stress and increasing a sense of control. Techniques that help to reduce negative effects of stress include using distraction by purposefully shifting focus to pleasant thoughts or engaging in a diversional activity, and using a **relaxation response** technique, as described below.

Learning and Practicing a Relaxation Response Technique Eliciting the relaxation response is another technique to help people develop awareness and counter the negative effects of stress (Figure 13-4). Relaxation response techniques counter the stress response by reducing sympathetic arousal (Benson, 1975). The immediate physiological effects of relaxation are decreases in heart rate, blood pressure, respiratory rate, and muscle tension. The long-term physiological effect is a decrease in central nervous system arousal with a concomitant decrease in musculoskeletal system, autonomic nervous system, and psychoneuroendocrine system arousal. To the extent that stress causes or exacerbates a symptom, eliciting the relaxation response can break this stress-symptom cycle. In addition to these physiological changes, psychological changes such as improved mood and behavioral changes, including a reduction in risky behaviors, can occur. The relaxation response can counteract stress-related disease processes, particularly processes associated with immunological, cardiovascular, and neurodegenerative disorders (Nelson & Simmons, 2005).

The relaxation response is an innate physiological response (Benson, 1975); therefore, a number of techniques that involve mental focusing can be used. Details on these techniques and guidelines for clinical applications can be found in Chapter 14. All of these techniques have two basic components:

1. The repetition of a word, sound, phrase, prayer, image, or physical activity
2. The passive disregard of everyday thoughts when they occur

Audiotapes can be used to help guide this process of focusing, especially during the initial learning phase.

Nurses often can introduce individuals to the immediate calming effects of the relaxation response in less than 5 minutes. One effective way is to have the person make a fist and notice what happens to the breathing pattern. Most people have a tendency to hold their breath while tensing a body part. Now ask the person to take a few deep diaphragmatic breaths while making a fist. Most people will notice that the tension is much harder to maintain while taking a deep breath. This awareness helps to recognize the relationship between breath and tension. Lamaze techniques for helping mothers manage pain during delivery are based on this connection between breathing and relaxation. Most people hold their breath when they perceive a threat (stress), feel anxious, or become angry. By stopping and taking a few deep breaths when they become aware of physical changes (holding the breath or clenching the jaw) or emotional changes (feeling anxious or angry), individuals can elicit the relaxation response, reduce sympathetic arousal, calm negative mood states, and gain a sense of control.

Using Mini-Relaxations Mini-relaxations can be taught quickly and used throughout the day to help develop awareness and to counter the negative effects of stress on the

STRESS WARNING SIGNALS

Physical Symptoms

____ Headaches	____ Back pain
____ Indigestion	____ Tight neck and shoulders
____ Stomachaches	____ Racing heart
____ Sweaty palms	____ Restlessness
____ Sleep difficulties	____ Tiredness
____ Dizziness	____ Ringing in ears

Behavioral Symptoms

____ Excess smoking	____ Grinding of teeth at night
____ Bossiness	____ Overuse of alcohol
____ Compulsive gum chewing	____ Compulsive eating
____ Attitude critical of others	____ Inability to get things done

Emotional Symptoms

____ Crying	____ Overwhelming sense of pressure
____ Nervousness and anxiety	____ Anger
____ Boredom (no meaning to things)	____ Loneliness
____ Edginess (ready to explode)	____ Unhappiness for no reason
____ Feeling powerless to change things	____ Easily upset

Cognitive Symptoms

____ Trouble thinking clearly	____ Inability to make decisions
____ Lack of creativity	____ Thoughts of running away
____ Memory loss	____ Constant worry
____ Forgetfulness	____ Loss of sense of humor

Spiritual Symptoms / Relational Symptoms

Spiritual Symptoms	Relational Symptoms
____ Emptiness	____ Isolation
____ Loss of meaning	____ Intolerance
____ Doubt	____ Resentment
____ Unforgiving	____ Loneliness
____ Martyrdom	____ Lashing out
____ Looking for magic	____ Hiding
____ Loss of direction	____ Clamming up
____ Cynicism	____ Lowered sex drive
____ Apathy	____ Nagging
____ Needing to "prove" self	____ Distrust
	____ Lack of intimacy
	____ Using people

Figure 13-3   Stress warning signals. (From *Medical symptom reduction clinic patient notebook.* Boston: The Benson-Henry Institute for Mind Body Medicine of Massachusetts General Hospital, Harvard Medical School.)

mind, body, and spirit. Individuals can be taught to monitor minor stress warning signs (jaw and shoulder tension) and to use a mini-relaxation to keep these initial symptoms of stress from developing into an incapacitating tension headache. A mini-relaxation exercise can be anything from a few conscious, deep diaphragmatic breaths to several minutes of sitting quietly (Health Teaching box).

Alternative and Complementary Therapies A variety of alternative and complementary therapies can prevent and reduce harmful effects of stress (Snyder & Lindquist,

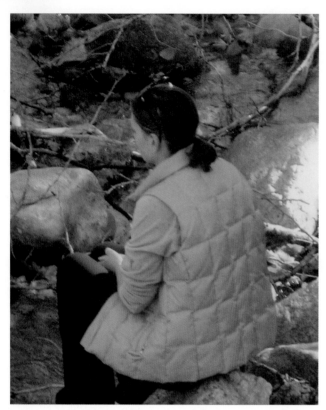

Figure 13-4 Relaxation techniques counter the stress response by reducing sympathetic arousal.

HEALTH TEACHING Mini-Relaxation

Nurses teach individuals to perform a mini-relaxation exercise through a variety of suggestions, including:
- Count slowly up to 4 as you inhale and slowly back down again as you exhale.
- Change your breathing to diaphragmatic breathing. Try inhaling through your nose and exhaling through your mouth. You should feel your stomach rising about 1 inch as you inhale and falling about 1 inch as you exhale.
- Take a few deep diaphragmatic breaths. As you do so, begin to recall something that would bring a smile to your face, which might be the image of your child's face, your favorite pet, or another loved one; or it could be the memory of a favorite place, food, or event in your life.

Nurses remind people to notice how quickly "minis" help to relieve tension and worry. People are advised to practice often throughout the day to counter the harmful effects of arousal from the stress response.

Modified from The Benson-Henry Institute for Mind Body Medicine of Massachusetts General Hospital. (n.d.b). *Stress.* Retrieved December 30, 2007, from: *www.mbmi.org/basics/whatis_stress.asp*; The Benson-Henry Institute for Mind Body Medicine of Massachusetts General Hospital. (n.d.a). *The relaxation response.* Retrieved December 30, 2007, from *www.mbmi.org/basics/whatis_rresponse.asp*.

2006). These include **acupuncture**, **hypnosis**, **aromatherapy**, **reflexology**, **Reiki**, chiropractic, and herbal therapies. These approaches have developed outside the mainstream of traditional Western medicine; however, developing evidence of efficacy has promoted growing acceptance of some of these approaches. People increasingly are using alternative and complementary practices as self-help measures, and research to study their effects has exploded in recent years (American Holistic Nurses Association & American Nurses Association, 2007; Dossey et al., 2004; Wainrib, 2006). Nurses can help individuals evaluate the safety and efficacy of various alternative and complementary therapies. In particular, herbal remedies require cautious use because they can have harmful, as well as beneficial, effects, and they sometimes interfere with other treatments and medications. Among the alternative therapies available, there is strong evidence of effectiveness of acupuncture and hypnosis, and they are becoming widely accepted within mainstream health care.

Acupuncture is an ancient Chinese technique used to reduce pain and to prevent and manage various disorders by placement of fine needles at specific **meridian** points on the body. Acupuncture is not a self-help approach, so seeking treatment from an experienced acupuncturist is required. The Western scientific community cannot explain why acupuncture works but acknowledges its effectiveness. Even the World Health Organization has listed illnesses that can be managed with acupuncture (Killeen, 2005), and some health insurance plans cover it.

Hypnosis comes from a Greek word meaning sleep. Hypnosis narrows consciousness and elicits relaxation, inertia, and passivity, like sleep, yet awareness is never lost completely and the hypnotized person can respond (Heap & Kirsch, 2006). The exact mechanisms through which hypnosis works are not known, although perhaps its ability to induce deep relaxation and its possible action in shifting brain activity from the "analytical" left side to the "nonanalytical" right side might be explanatory. Nevertheless, its effectiveness in managing a variety of conditions, notably smoking and anxiety-related problems, and managing pain is well recognized. Trained therapists provide hypnotherapy to manage stress and various mental health problems, including phobias, addictions, and posttraumatic stress disorder. Self-hypnosis, a form of deep relaxation similar to relaxation techniques described in this chapter, can be a useful stress-reduction tool. Self-help guides provide safe and easy-to-follow guidelines. One note of caution is warranted: hypnosis is not recommended for people with organic brain disorders, psychotic disorders, or other severe mental disorders.

Reiki (pronounced ray-kee), is made up of two Japanese words: *Rei*, or universal spirit (sometimes thought of as a supreme being), and *ki*. Thus, the word Reiki means universal life energy. Reiki is a therapy that uses energy fields with the intent to affect health. To transmit ki, believed to be a life-force energy, the Reiki practitioner places hands on or near the person receiving treatment. In the United States, Reiki is designated as a form of complementary and alternative medicine (CAM) (National Center for Complementary and Alternative Medicine, n.d.).

Expressive Writing Transforming thoughts and emotions related to stressful experiences into written language has demonstrated positive effects on health (Pennebaker & Chung, 2007). In its therapeutic meaning, **expressive writing** involves telling a "story" about traumatic, emotionally charged, or stressful events and personal reactions. **Journal writing**—more specifically, self-confessional writing—is a form of expressive writing that typically is done via entries in a journal over time that describe unfolding personal responses to life events. Expressive writing is useful in disclosing and processing emotions, and in measurably improving physical and mental health.

Expressive writing, including journaling, can help people reflect on stressful events and their reactions to these events. Such reflection is an opportunity to reform perceptions and to consider alternative ways to manage stress. Individuals may find resolutions to conflicts that work uniquely for them. These resolutions then may increase a sense of control and mediate negative consequences of stress. This self-reflective process shares elements of cognitive-behavioral therapy—an intervention effective in reducing harmful effects of stress.

Nurses can advise people to get a special notebook for a journal and write about a stressful event for 15 minutes a day, in a setting in which they will not be interrupted. From a health perspective, people will be more effective when making themselves the only audience. The nurse should warn that the individual may feel sad or depressed immediately after the writing session, but these feelings usually dissipate within an hour. Nonetheless, exploring deep thoughts and feelings on paper is not a panacea. When an individual is coping with death, divorce, or some other major stressor, feeling better instantly after writing cannot be expected. A person can, however, develop a clearer understanding of feelings and of the situation through journal writing. In other words, journal writing helps people objectify experiences, identify the influence of stress on symptoms, and develop insights into more effective problem solving. Some individuals may recognize the need for psychotherapeutic support through journal writing, and an appropriate referral can then be made.

Healthy Diet

Countering negative effects of stress requires caring for physical health and well-being. The mind and body are connected; therefore, paying attention to one while ignoring the other does not promote overall health. The body requires rest, a healthy diet of balanced food choices and exercise. Over the last few decades, nutrition has moved to the forefront as a major component of health promotion, disease prevention, and symptom management. Food is now viewed as a positive influence on health, physical performance, and state of mind, rather than simply a fuel

needed to prevent disease and sustain life. Adaptive eating is characterized by "balanced eating patterns, appropriate caloric intake, and body weight that is appropriate for height" (Cochrane, 2005, p. 517). Nutrition is an important component of early intervention strategies to improve physical, cognitive, emotional, social, and spiritual functioning (Luck, 2005).

However, the American lifestyle has made practicing healthy eating habits increasingly difficult. Americans frequently replace nutritionally balanced meals with readily available high-fat, high-calorie foods. Many times this course of action is an attempt to find immediate gratification to counter feelings of anxiety and depression caused by stress (stress-disinhibition). One of the frustrations that nurses experience is trying to help children and adults develop healthy eating habits. This effort takes planning and correctly choosing a variety of foods, and choosing a diet low in fat, saturated fat, and cholesterol, with plenty of vegetables, fruits, and grain products. The current U.S. dietary guidelines presented in the Food Guide Pyramid (O.D.P.H.P, 2005; U.S. Department of Agriculture [USDA], n.d.) emphasize that daily food choices should be made from the five food groups. The pyramid is under ongoing review, and updated government guidelines may be issued. Yet regardless of adjustments to specific recommendations that may be forthcoming, the pyramid will continue to serve as an outline of what to eat each day, not a rigid prescription, and represents a general guide that helps individuals choose a healthful diet. A detailed discussion of the health benefits of balanced nutrition and guidelines throughout the life span can be found in Chapter 11.

Encouraging healthier dietary choices helps people to recognize that control over their health and well-being is possible. This knowledge, in turn, helps counter the negative effects of stress and lower the stress-disinhibition effect that can influence poor dietary choices. Nurses encourage people to monitor their daily dietary patterns to gain awareness of how they use food in times of stress. Tools like food diaries help people to monitor the amount and quality of what they eat and drink and to set realistic goals.

Physical Activity

Combining a healthy diet with a regular exercise routine has many health benefits and can positively affect quality of life. For example, one of the most effective ways to lose weight and improve self-esteem is to combine exercise with nutritious eating. Exercise (physical activity that improves strength, flexibility, and conditioning) and balanced nutrition serve as protective factors against several major chronic diseases. Regular physical activity decreases the risk of death from heart disease, lowers the risk of developing diabetes, and is associated with a decreased risk of colon cancer (USDHHS, n.d.). Exercise helps prevent high blood pressure and helps lower blood pressure in people with elevated levels. Regular physical activity, even at moderate levels, is associated with lower death rates for adults of any age. Psychological well-being is enhanced and the risk of developing depression can be reduced; regular physical activity appears to reduce symptoms of depression and anxiety and to improve mood.

Additionally, children and adolescents need weight-bearing exercise for normal skeletal development, and young adults need this type of exercise to achieve and maintain peak bone mass (USDHHS, n.d.). Regular physical activity also increases the ability of older people, and those with certain chronic, disabling conditions, to perform activities of daily living. Nevertheless, high stress could increase injury risk for athletes, and injured athletes may experience greater stress than noninjured peers when they are sidelined from competition. Chapter 12 provides a comprehensive discussion of the benefits of exercise and clinical application throughout the life span.

Regular physical activity helps people adopt a more active lifestyle as they begin to feel better physically and emotionally, thereby breaking the negative stress cycle. These positive effects can be obtained with exercise of only moderate intensity. For example, a brisk walk of 30 to 60 minutes, 3 to 5 times a week, promotes fitness and decreases risk of disease. Being physically active on a daily basis is extremely important; therefore, nurses can help individuals increase physical activity by suggesting a variety of activities in which they might engage each day (Box 13-1). An exercise diary can generate a baseline for usual activity to set realistic goals and monitor progress. By simply changing a few daily routines, individuals can gain enormous physical, psychosocial, and spiritual rewards that promote health and break the negative stress cycle.

Sleep Hygiene

Good health and the ability to meet life's many demands and manage stress effectively require proper rest. Many people suffer from sleep deprivation that can cause or

---

Box **13-1**	Helping Individuals Increase Physical Activity

Nurses can suggest ways for individuals to increase physical activity throughout the day, including:
- Have fun and play active games with children.
- Engage in a sport.
- Find a friend with whom to walk or jog.
- Take a class in yoga or Tai Chi.
- Get and walk a dog.
- Garden on the weekends.
- Walk or bicycle to school or work.
- Take the stairs, never the elevator.
- Park the car at the farthest point in the parking lot at work, school, or when shopping.

By simply changing a few daily routines, a person can gain enormous physical, psychosocial, and spiritual rewards that promote health and break the negative stress cycle.

---

exacerbate conditions such as depression and fatigue and contribute to poor concentration and ineffective problem solving. Insomnia can be induced by stress or other cognitive-behavioral factors, such as unrealistic expectations, inappropriate scheduling of sleep, trying too hard to sleep, consuming caffeine, getting inadequate exercise, and a number of other factors including illness, alcohol use, or drug use (Stuart, 2005b; Wainrib, 2006). Determining the extent to which sleep disturbance is the result of behavior or stress-related issues is a necessary assessment. Overcoming sleep disturbances cannot be done quickly. Changing these behaviors requires patience and persistence. Once factors associated with sleep disturbance are identified, nurses can help individuals improve their sleep patterns by counseling them to follow several **sleep hygiene** or behavior guidelines (keeping a sleep diary, having a regular sleep-wake cycle, and making prudent dietary changes). Assisting people to make healthy behavior changes in their sleep habits provides another opportunity for them to increase self-regulation, confidence, and control, thereby reducing stress and improving quality of life. Box 13-2 presents several sleep hygiene strategies.

Cognitive-Behavioral Restructuring

Many stressful situations can be created or exacerbated by negative, exaggerated, catastrophic thinking. Cognitive-behavioral therapy is a conceptually based short-term intervention to modify this thinking and related behaviors, and thereby reduce stress. In the context of therapy, cognitive-behavioral restructuring is a technique or series of strategies that help people evaluate their thoughts, challenge them, and replace them with more rational cognitive and behavioral responses. Appraisal, or the way in which a situation is viewed, can be a major cause of stress. When situations are viewed in a negative, distorted, or illogical manner, such perceptions can adversely affect emotions, behaviors, beliefs, and physiological parameters. Cognitive-behavioral restructuring teaches people to recognize that negative thinking often causes emotional distress and associated behaviors. This recognition, in turn, alters problematic thinking and behavior, reduces the negative consequences of stress, and enhances health (Stuart, 2005a; Stuart & Wells-Federman, 2005).

Cognitive-behavioral restructuring does not gloss over or deny misfortune, suffering, or negative feelings. Many circumstances exist in peoples' lives for which it is appropriate to feel sad, anxious, angry, or depressed. More accurately, cognitive-behavioral restructuring is a technique that helps some people become unstuck from these moods so that they can experience a broader range of feelings and try out new behaviors (Stuart, 2005a). In this structured method, individuals are asked to consider their cognitive appraisal of a situation and how this assessment affects feelings, behaviors, and physiological processes. Reframing, or cognitive reappraisal, educates individuals in monitoring thoughts

Box **13-2** Sleep Hygiene Strategies

Nurses find the following suggestions to be helpful for individuals with sleep disturbance resulting from behavioral or stress-related issues:
- Keep a sleep diary, which helps determine sleep patterns more accurately, assess progress, and reinforce behavior change.
- Challenge irrational beliefs.
- Reduce consumption of alcohol and caffeine. (Chapter 11 gives some tips.)
- Avoid use of sleeping pills.
- Have a regular sleep-wake schedule, even on the weekends.
- If unable to fall asleep within 20 to 30 minutes or if waking up and unable to fall back to sleep within that time, get out of bed and do something until groggy and sleepy again.
- Focus on relaxation, not sleep. Use a relaxation tape, practice diaphragmatic breathing. Limit naps during the day to less than 45 minutes. Longer naps reset the biological clock and disturb nighttime sleep.
- Exercise within 3 to 6 hours of bedtime. Exercise improves sleep by producing a significant rise in body temperature, followed by a compensatory drop a few hours later, making it easier to fall asleep and stay asleep. Furthermore, because exercise is a physical stressor, the brain compensates by increasing the amount of deep sleep.
- Take a hot bath 2 hours before bedtime. The temperature drop after the bath helps to induce sleep.
- Sleep in a cool room. Individuals grow sleepier and become less active when body temperature falls.

Modified from Stuart, G. W. (2005b). Psychophysiological responses and somatoform and sleep disorders. In G. W. Stuart & M. T. Laraia (Eds.), *Principles and practice of psychiatric nursing* (8th ed., pp. 285-302). St. Louis: Mosby; Wainrib, B. R. (2006). *Healing crisis and trauma with mind, body, and spirit.* New York: Springer Publishing Co.

Box **13-3** The Four-Step Approach to Cognitive Restructuring

To help individuals develop the skill of cognitive restructuring, nurses can teach them to examine a stressful situation using a four-step approach.
1. *Stop* (break the cycle of escalating, negative thoughts).
2. *Breathe deeply* (elicit the relaxation response and release tension).
3. *Reflect* (ask, "What is going on here? What am I thinking? Is the thought true? Is the thought helpful? Am I jumping to conclusions or magnifying the situation?").
4. *Choose* a more realistic, rational response.

From Stuart, G. W. (2005b). Psychophysiological responses and somatoform and sleep disorders. In G. W. Stuart & M. T. Laraia (Eds.), *Principles and practice of psychiatric nursing* (8th ed., pp. 285-302). St. Louis: Mosby.

and replacing those that are negative and irrational with those that are more realistic and helpful. Adding behaviors that are consistent with reframed thinking follows.

For example, a woman may have had plans to meet a friend for lunch on a day she woke up with a migraine headache. She might begin to think such thoughts as "This always happens to me when I have plans," "This headache will never go away," "I shouldn't have to deal with this," or "My day is ruined." The result of this negative, irrational self-talk is disappointment, frustration, and anger. This emotional arousal will, in turn, increase muscle tension and a variety of other stress-related symptoms, which may exacerbate the headache. To help individuals develop the skill of cognitive-behavioral restructuring, nurses can teach them to examine a stressful situation using the four-step approach highlighted in Box 13-3.

In the previous example, the woman may reflect that "I am having a migraine headache and I hate that it is on a day that I had made plans, but I will take my medication, listen to my relaxation tapes, and rest. I'll call my friend and see if we can change our plans. Perhaps she can come over to visit me for tea this afternoon if I feel better." Although it is understandable that anyone would be disappointed and upset over this situation, applying the four-step cognitive restructuring technique can help identify healthy choices and gain a sense of control.

Based on the work of pioneers such as Aaron Beck (e.g., 1976, 1979) and Albert Ellis (e.g., Ellis, 1962; Ellis & Dryden, 1987), cognitive therapy has emerged during the past five decades as a treatment designed to alter dysfunctional beliefs and thoughts associated with depression, anxiety disorders, and other emotional problems. Over time, theorists, clinical researchers, and clinicians recognized the effectiveness of this approach for many persons, as well as the value of linking helpful alterations in thinking to complementary behavioral changes. As a result, cognitive-behavioral therapy (CBT) emerged. CBT is an efficacious treatment approach for many stress-related and mental health disorders. For example, researchers have shown that CBT is as effective as antidepressant medications in treating postpartum depression (Highet & Drummond, 2004). Intervention strategies derived from CBT have been shown to have widespread applicability in ameliorating symptoms associated with stress and illness. In a study to test the effectiveness of a cognitive-behavioral intervention in decreasing symptom severity among individuals with advanced cancer, Sherwood et al. (2005) found that the intervention was effective for symptom self-management. The researchers recommended that problem-solving strategies be included in educational programs for persons with advanced cancer. Thus evidence provides strong support for use of cognitive-behavioral restructuring as a stress management approach. The Multicultural Awareness box presents relevant information related to the effects of racial/ethnic discrimination on cognitive appraisals of interactions as threatening and harmful resulting in increased overall stress burden.

MULTICULTURAL AWARENESS

Examining Links Among Discrimination, Stress, and Health Disparities

Racial/ethnic discrimination is a stressor that has been identified as a contributing factor to health disparities, although precise mechanisms of action remain unclear. Experiences of racial discrimination typically lead a person to appraise future interactions and experiences as threatening and harmful resulting in increased overall stress burden. To examine links among discrimination, stress, and health disparities, researchers recruited a sample of 113 multiethnic participants, primarily composed of Blacks and Latinos, who completed a diary page every 30 minutes for a day. The diary entries concerned moods and perceptions of social interactions. After controlling for personal characteristics, analyses indicated that perceptions of discrimination were positively associated with anger and ratings of social interactions as "harassing, exclusionary, and unfair." The researchers concluded that the diary data support accumulating evidence that measuring daily experiences, including perceived discrimination, adds to knowledge of psychosocial stress assessment beyond information provided from use of traditional personality measures. Identifying pathways through which discrimination influences mood and possibly undercuts social interactions is an important area for future research.

The take-home message for nurses and other health care clinicians is that perceptions of discrimination during daily social encounters can be expected to exacerbate stress and negatively affect health outcomes. Recognizing the importance of individuals' perceptions of discrimination during social interactions is critically important in establishing rapport and assisting individuals to identify specific experiences that contribute to their overall stress and affect their health. Stress management strategies may be helpful in reducing negative effects for individuals; however, social change is needed to address racial/ethnic discrimination as a factor contributing to health disparities.

From: Broudy, R., Brondolo, E., Coakley, V., Brady, N., Cassells, A., Tobin, J. N., & Sweeney, M. (2007). Perceived ethnic discrimination in relation to daily moods and negative social interactions. *Journal of Behavioral Medicine, 30,* 31-43.

Affirmations

Affirmations can be an effective stress management and cognitive-behavioral restructuring skill, because they are a method of countering self-defeating negative thoughts and attitudes in addition to being helpful in addressing spiritual needs. An **affirmation** is a positive thought, in the form of a short phrase or saying, which has meaning for the individual. By reinforcing new ways of thinking or behaving in the present moment, affirmations are statements that people can use to reaffirm new intentions and to clarify goals.

Nurses coach individuals to create an affirmation as a way of developing a more helpful, realistic belief system. For example, thoughts such as "I can't handle this" and "My day is ruined" can be countered with "I can handle this" and "I know ways to increase my comfort." Repeating an affirmation often throughout the day, perhaps after eliciting the relaxation response or as part of a breathing exercise, can become second nature and can help to enhance self-esteem and reduce stress.

Social Support

Having supportive family, friends, and co-workers is for many individuals an important contributor to effective coping and stress hardiness (Kobasa et al., 1982; Taylor, 2007). Many people believe that confiding in others and talking out problems can be a helpful way to get good advice or uncritical support. Social support comprises a network of close family, friends, co-workers, and professionals. Social support literature notes that both the number of supports and the quality of the relationships are important (Taylor, 2007).

Research outcomes demonstrate the protective health effects of social support. Among people participating in a cardiac rehabilitation program, social support contributed to desired health outcomes (Shen et al., 2004). Emotional support during labor and delivery appears to affect positive health outcomes. Delivery by cesarean (C-section), the most common surgical procedure performed in the United States, increases the risk of complications to mother and child and extends hospital stay (USDHHS, n.d.). Researchers found that the presence of a supportive woman (doula) during labor and delivery reduced the need for many medical procedures, including C-sections, and enhanced breastfeeding success, mother-infant bonding, and mothers' memories of the experience (Pascali-Bonaro & Kroeger, 2004).

Nurses do much to facilitate social support to promote effective coping and reduce stress. Using information available in their local communities or through national organizations, nurses suggest support groups (see Chapter 8), Website chat rooms, educational classes, and exercise facilities, to name a few. Individuals and their families are often referred to organizations such as the American Lung Association, American Heart Association, American Cancer Society, and the Arthritis Foundation for resources related to specific health-promotion needs.

Assertive Communication

Effective communication is an important stress-management skill. An important coping and problem-solving skill, communication can be adversely affected by exaggerated negative thoughts and deeply held negative beliefs and assumptions (Stuart, 2005a). (See Chapter 4 for additional discussion of communication.) People who have difficulty with communication usually have one or all of the following problems:

- Disparity between what they say (statement) and what they want (intent)
- Confusion about or resistance to stating clearly how they feel, what they want, or what they need (assertiveness), with either a tendency to deny their own feelings (passiveness) or indifference toward the feelings of others (aggressiveness)
- Difficulty listening to others

The importance of matching the statement with intention is illustrated by the following example:

As David is leaving for his basketball game on a Saturday afternoon, his mother tells him, "Remember to be home early tonight." When David arrives home at 9:00 PM, his mother, who is waiting at the front door, yells, "Where were you? Is this your idea of early? You know your father and I had plans tonight. We were counting on you. You think only of yourself. This always happens. You'll never change. You'll always be irresponsible and selfish."

The first guideline for effective communication is that people need to be clear about what they want and what they need (intent) in statements to others. Although it would be wonderful if a son or daughter, spouse, friend, or others were great mind readers, assuming that people automatically know what is meant does little to help with communication. Nurses help individuals match statements with intentions. This process requires that individuals recognize distorted, exaggerated thoughts and emotions and take responsibility for their part of the conversation. Communicating effectively is a learned art and skill.

Reviewing the previous example, if the mother's intention was to have her son home before 8:00 PM, then her statement needed to indicate this. She could have said, "I hope you enjoy the game, but remember your father and I are going out tonight. We need to have you home before 8:00 PM to take care of your sister." It is important that the person understands that the other person in the conversation is not obligated to respond as one would wish. However, a request can be much clearer when the statement reflects the intent.

The next guideline for effective communication is to be assertive. **Assertive communication**, in most cases, is the most effective way to communicate. An assertive statement is nonjudgmental, expresses feelings and opinions, and reaffirms perceived rights. The general format of an assertive statement is: *I feel* [emotion], *when you* [the behavior], *because* [explanation].

The formula requires that all three elements be included. **Cognitive restructuring**, as described earlier, facilitates assertive communication, because it requires individuals to identify their thoughts and feelings. In the previous example, David's mother could:

1. *Stop* (breaking the cycle of escalating, negative thoughts)
2. *Breathe deeply* (releasing physical tension; promoting relaxation)
3. *Reflect*:
   How do I feel emotionally? (frustrated)
   What are my automatic thoughts? ("If he cared about us, then he would have been home on time. He's always selfish and irresponsible. He's never going to change.")
4. *Choose*:
   A more realistic, helpful way of thinking ("He's not always selfish and irresponsible. Even though it feels like he doesn't care about us when he does this, I know he cares.")

Becoming aware of her automatic thoughts and feelings would help David's mother plan an assertive statement when David comes home. She could then say, "I feel frustrated [emotion] when you are late [behavior], because I expected you would be home in time to care for your sister while your father and I went out, or that you would have called if you were going to be late [explanation]." This statement makes both her feelings clear and explains why she feels this way, which in turn provides a better opportunity to work on problem solving. When people cannot verbalize both their feelings and their needs, others are forced to figure out what they are. When others fail to do so correctly, individuals may feel victimized and blame the others for not understanding. Nurses help people recognize that they have a right and a responsibility to speak up and to do so in an assertive manner. The nurse helps individuals in matching their emotion with the explanation (frustration equals unmet expectation). It is important to remind them that this way of communicating may feel awkward and uncomfortable at first. Practicing this technique many times will be required before communication improves. Other people need time to become accustomed to the changes. Effective communication takes both practice and patience with everyone involved.

Empathy

Empathy is an effective stress management intervention because it helps communication. Empathy is the ability to consider another person's perspective and to communicate this understanding back to that person. Empathy helps individuals become better listeners.

Empathy can be facilitated through the technique of active listening. **Active listening** requires conscious, empathic, nonjudgmental awareness. Listening also helps clarify the issues involved and can deescalate many emotional exchanges. For example, during a situation in which a spouse announces, "I'm fed up with you always being late," the response may be important to resolving the issues without promoting further miscommunications and increasing problems. Rather than being caught by a defensive, emotional reaction, individuals can learn to communicate empathetically using the four-step approach:

1. *Stop* (breaking the cycle of escalating, negative thoughts)
2. *Breathe deeply* (releasing physical tension; promoting relaxation)
3. *Reflect*:
   How do I feel emotionally? (hurt, angry)
   What are my automatic thoughts? ("How could [person] say that? It's not my fault. I have things to do. [Person] always accuses me. This is never going to change.")
   What are the thoughts and emotions being expressed by the other person?
   The practice of asking this question will provide a different view. The individual can then begin to plan a response.

4. *Choose:*

"My feelings are hurt, but I don't have to react defensively."

"I'm going to try to understand [person's] perspective using this phrase: 'You sound _____ about _____' and listen to [person's] response."

By using this phrase, an individual can gain awareness from another person's perspective (Rogers, 1951). Continuing with the scenario, the response might be, "You sound upset about my being late." Possible responses to this empathetic statement might include, "It's not just about that. Everything went wrong today and this was just one more thing," or, "You're right. I hate having to wait. It feels like you don't respect or value my time."

When one uses active listening, the other person often feels heard. An opportunity to clarify any misunderstanding becomes available. This exercise may help reduce emotional arousal, defensive behavior, and conflict. Active listening allows the individual to buy time and to get a better perspective on what the other person is thinking and feeling. Individuals can then make a choice as to how they want to respond. They may choose to use assertive communication or to step away from the interaction. Active listening promotes empathic, objective, and nonjudgmental communication. Nurses recommend use of stress management skills that include active listening techniques to facilitate effective communication which, in turn, reduces conflict and stress.

Healthy Pleasures

Engaging in **healthy pleasures** (activities that bring feelings of peace, joy, and happiness) is, for most individuals, an important part of life. However, for individuals who are feeling overwhelmed with daily hassles, illness, or loss, this practice may have been lost. Individuals may feel that they do not deserve to have pleasure or that they are waiting for happiness until they feel better, until the stressors are resolved or until they go away. This belief makes breaking the stress cycle even more challenging; however, rewards motivate behavior (Stuart, 2005a). By asking people to pursue a healthy and pleasurable activity every week, motivating them to become more involved in their lives and break this cycle is often easier. The activity can be simple and it need not cost money. For example, people often find pleasure in nature, spending time with a friend, reading a book, or watching a movie. Hobbies are purposeful leisure activities that can balance hectic, stressful lives. A hobby should be chosen from interest and/or talent. Many hobbies have added benefits of increasing activity (e.g., gardening) or promoting social engagement (e.g., a book club or chorus). Nurses advise individuals to make leisure activities a regular part of the week as a purposeful and conscious plan to break the stress cycle.

Spiritual Practice

In response to stress, people can feel disconnected from life's meaning and purpose, which in turn affects spiritual health and well-being. Meeting spiritual needs may be facilitated by **spiritual practice** or activities that help people find meaning, purpose, and connection. For example, individuals may choose to elicit the relaxation response through prayer. This focused, relaxed state of mind might help them develop a spiritual perspective that can engender a shift in values and beliefs to help cope with a stressor they cannot change, such as chronic illness or loss of a loved one. Expression of anger or confusion in the face of difficulties, trauma, or tragedy also can provide a therapeutic outlet, but conversely may engender spiritual or religious doubt, or a sense of alienation from one's beliefs. Nurses suggest a referral to a chaplain or clergy member, provide spiritual music or art work, recommend spiritual reading material, and provide personal presence (Box 13-4).

Box **13-4**	**A Stress Management Strategy for Nurses**

Develop the skill of personal presence. **Presence** is the gift of self through availability and attention to needs. Presence means "being there" for another person. To be available to others in this way, first practice the skill of being present with yourself. One effective way of developing this skill is through mindfulness, which is the ability to focus attention on what you are experiencing from moment to moment. Mindfulness encompasses the abilities of slowing down and bringing your full attention (thoughts, feelings, and bodily sensations) to the action in which you are engaged at the moment. The practice can be particularly useful in allowing yourself to extend the benefits of eliciting the relaxation response in more areas of your daily life.

Some ideas for practicing personal presence (mindfulness) are:

- When you awaken each morning, bring your full attention to your breathing. Allow your awareness to expand gradually into the room and then slowly begin to listen to the sounds of the outdoors.
- On your way to work, focus on how you walk, drive, or ride the transit. Take some deep diaphragmatic breaths and relax your body as you travel.
- Take a moment to attend to your breath, relax your body, and focus your mind before entering a client's room.
- As you eat a meal, carefully examine it through all of your senses, the sight, smell, touch, taste, and the sound of each bite. Mindfully enjoy this new experience.
- Recurring events of the day can become cues for a mini-relaxation (the ringing telephone; auscultating a heart beat; answering a call light, before, during, and after rounds or report).
- Make the transition home from work mindful. Leave thoughts and worries of work at work and be conscious of your home environment each day.
- Once again, focus on your breathing and become completely aware of your surroundings as you go to sleep. Practice mindfully letting go of today and tomorrow as you allow your mind and body to get some much needed rest.

Modified from The Benson-Henry Institute for Mind Body Medicine of Massachusetts General Hospital. (n.d.). *Stress.* Retrieved December 30, 2007, from: *www.mbmi.org/basics/whatis_stress.asp*; The Benson-Henry Institute for Mind Body Medicine of the Massachusetts General Hospital. (n.d.). *The relaxation response.* Retrieved December 30, 2007, from *www.mbmi.org/basics/whatis_rresponse.asp*.

Nurses propose activities that provide a sense of meaning and purpose. Keeping a journal can be an important strategy to help individuals focus on aspects of life that are more positive and that become clouded from view when feeling overwhelmed by stress. Finding ways of helping others (tutoring children, reading to the blind, or visiting an older adult) can have a positive influence on spiritual health and well-being. Altruism, generosity, kindness, and service to others are more than moral virtues. These attributes not only help to make the world a better place, they also help people find meaning and purpose in life. Religious and existential well-being has provided some defense against depression for people living with chronic and life-threatening conditions (Coleman, 2004). Older, chronically ill, and homebound people can be encouraged to produce written or oral histories that can be a legacy or, when able, to contact others needing care or to make telephone calls to raise funds for a favorite charity.

Clarifying Values and Beliefs

To manage stress and develop a balanced lifestyle, people must recognize the things that are important to them, reflect on where they are in life, evaluate what needs to be changed, and generate an action plan for that change (Gaydos, 2005) (see Chapter 4). This process is known as **values clarification**. The first step is to identify what is important, meaningful, and valuable so as to assess whether actions are consistent with beliefs. What people believe and value guides their actions by endorsing certain behaviors and changing others. When people assess their values and beliefs, they employ the ability to make their own choices rather than relying on beliefs and values dictated to them by others.

One method nurses use to help people identify what they value and, ultimately, to help them clarify the relationship between their beliefs and actions is to ask them to identify what is important or meaningful to them. The form in Figure 13-5 is an example of questions used in the Medical Symptom Reduction Program at the Benson-Henry Institute for Mind Body Medicine at Massachusetts General Hospital in Boston. Individuals are asked to identify what is important and meaningful to them in eight domains. Nurses change the domains to reflect more accurately the values and beliefs of the individuals they are counseling. After reviewing the results, individuals may find that they have not been doing certain things that are important to them (becoming more physically active, eating a healthier diet, volunteering, or spending time with their children). When people detect inconsistencies between their values and their actual living habits, they can begin to develop a working plan for correcting these inconsistencies. This process enables them to make conscious choices and to have more control.

Setting Realistic Goals

Developing an action plan for change to work toward a more balanced health-promoting lifestyle that is consistent with a person's values and beliefs is an important stress management strategy. Setting realistic, attainable goals facilitates this exercise. Goal setting is a dynamic process that involves both the individual and the nurse. Goals should be specific, concrete, measurable, and achievable. Nurses facilitate this process by respecting the individual's input, using a values clarification exercise (such as the one mentioned) to facilitate a more complete database to guide individuals to identify and prioritize problems to be addressed, and set mutually agreed on long-term and short-term goals. Nurses encourage individuals to challenge themselves when their behaviors are not consistent with what they identified as important and meaningful to them. For example, when an overweight man with hypertension and high cholesterol levels continues to smoke and eat high-fat foods, nurses help him to look at these behaviors relative to what is meaningful to him, such as his family. The cost and benefit are usually clear and the responsibility for the change is with the individual, not the nurse. Nurses ask the following questions to help individuals clarify long-term goals:

- What is important to you?
- What would you like to change about your life?
- What can you do to start that change?
- When will you take that action?
- How will you measure success?
- How will you maintain the desired change?
- How can I help you to reach your goal?

Setting realistic, attainable goals helps to create a sense of confidence and achievement and to build enthusiasm to set future goals. This process, in turn, increases a sense of control and mitigates the negative effects of stress.

Humor

Humor is an enjoyable and effective antidote to stress for many people. Humor can have health-promoting properties (Stuart, 2005c; Wooten, 2005), although effects of a sense of humor on health generally have been weak and inconsistent across various research outcomes (Beehr & Bowling, 2005). When acting as a stress reducer, humor produces laughter. Laughter creates predictable physiological changes in the body. Similar to how it behaves with other forms of exercise, the body responds in two stages: (1) an arousal phase with an increase in physiological parameters and (2) a resolution phase, during which these parameters return to resting values or lower values (Wooten, 2005).

Humor can open different perspectives on problems and facilitate objectivity, which increases a sense of self-protection and control. Finding humor in a stressful situation can help people to reframe perceptions of the event. Some hospital staffs are using laughter libraries, humor rooms, comedy carts that can be wheeled into an individual's hospital room, and clowns

"What Is Important and Meaningful to You in Life?"

In each of the following areas, what do you want for yourself, today, next week, a year from now?

Under each of the following categories, please ask yourself these important questions.

Professional, educational, and intellectual
Today _____
Next week _____
A year from now _____

Relationships
Today _____
Next week _____
A year from now _____

Creative things
Today _____
Next week _____
A year from now _____

Spiritual
Today _____
Next week _____
A year from now _____

Volunteer and altruistic
Today _____
Next week _____
A year from now _____

Health
Today _____
Next week _____
A year from now _____

Fun and play
Today _____
Next week _____
A year from now _____

Material objects
Today _____
Next week _____
A year from now _____

Figure 13-5 What is important and meaningful in life? (From *Medical symptom reduction program patient notebook.* Boston: The Benson-Henry Institute for Mind Body Medicine of Massachusetts General Hospital, Harvard Medical School.)

to bring laughter and joy to the bedside. Humor has potential as an accessible, enjoyable, and inexpensive stress reduction strategy that can offer people new perspectives on their world and themselves. Nevertheless, recognizing that humor can mask conflict or be hurtful is critically important in judging when and how to use it in clinical encounters (Box 13-5).

EFFECTIVE COPING

When people believe that they can cope effectively, the harmful effects of stress can be minimized. The stressful situation is perceived as a challenge rather than a threat. This often elusive difference has vital mind, body, and spirit effects. When people believe that their lives are more

Box **13-5**   **Humor Strategies for Stress Reduction***

Nurses help individuals use humor for health promotion and stress reduction in a variety of ways, including:
- Keeping a humor journal: looking for the unintentional amusing remark, watching for funny things young children say or do, and looking in the newspaper for humorous grammatical errors or an inappropriate choice of words and writing them down in a journal
- Looking on the Internet for humorous resources
- Creating a scrapbook of humorous cartoons, pictures, stickers, poems, and songs
- Reading a cartoon or joke in the newspaper every day and sharing it with a friend
- Watching funny movies or reruns of old television programs
- Finding and spending time with funny, light-hearted people

*For more information about using humor to reduce stress, see p. 164 in Chapter 6.

balanced and under control, they are productive, but not driven; aroused, but not anxious; and may even be physically or mentally tired, but not exhausted.

Effective coping is what helps people face great adversity (such as illness) and recognize the opportunity that the situation often presents (Beehr & Bowling, 2005). First and foremost, individuals must recognize that coping is the ability to find a balance between acceptance and action, between letting go and taking control. Many stress management strategies help individuals distinguish these differences by providing a format for observing or objectifying their experiences. Other strategies such as exercise and balanced nutrition help individuals promote physical health and well-being to counter the harmful effects of stress.

Nurses help individuals improve effective coping by guiding them in the art of choosing the right strategy at the right time. In doing so, people gain a sense of control that minimizes or buffers harmful effects of stress. Nurses use the interventions described in this chapter to assist individuals to manage extrinsic and intrinsic stressors.

When individuals cannot control or influence the situation (extrinsic stressors), nurses advise them to:
- Take care of physical health and well-being: exercise; eat healthy, balanced meals; and practice sleep hygiene.
- Accept: learn to accept that some situations or people cannot be changed or avoided. Forgiveness and letting go of resentment are often a part of acceptance.
- Use distraction: distraction involves putting a worry aside, when necessary, until the situation can be dealt with directly. This prioritizing is quite different from procrastinating or denial, because it is a necessary delay rather than avoidance.
- Reduce emotional arousal: practice mini-relaxations, listen to a relaxation tape, use the four-step cognitive-behavioral restructuring technique, exercise, seek

social support, pray, use humor and affirmations, write in a journal, or engage in a healthy pleasure.

When individuals can alter or influence the situation, or when they are contributing to or creating the stress (intrinsic stressors), nurses advise them to:
- Take care of physical health and well-being: exercise; eat healthy, balanced meals; and practice sleep hygiene.
- Reduce emotional arousal: practice mini-relaxations, listen to a relaxation tape, exercise, seek social support, pray, use humor and affirmations, write in a journal, engage in a healthy pleasure, or use the four-step cognitive-behavioral restructuring strategy:
  1. *Stop* (breaking the cycle of escalating, negative thoughts)
  2. *Breathe deeply* (eliciting the relaxation response and releasing tension)
  3. *Reflect* (asking, "What is going on here? What am I thinking? Is the thought true? Is the thought helpful? Am I jumping to conclusions or magnifying the situation?")
  4. *Choose* a more realistic, rational response and related behavioral reaction.
- Problem-solve:
  1. Clarify values and beliefs.
  2. Gather information.
  3. Seek advice, support, assistance, or information.
  4. Use assertive communication and empathy.
  5. Set realistic goals, design action strategies, and determine the best steps to handle the problem.
  6. Take action.

See the Care Plan for John R. for an example of a plan for effective coping.

SUMMARY

Good health and the ability to meet effectively the many demands of life require managing stress. Combining careful assessment and choice of strategies, thoughtful and honest feedback, and continued support, nurses assist people to cope more effectively with the innumerable stressors they encounter. Research to discern the interplay of physiological, psychological, social, and spiritual responses to stress has yielded important knowledge for practice. However, uncovering the intricate workings of the brain within the context of human stress and coping experiences is a daunting and critical challenge for today's health researchers.

Stress management strategies provide an opportunity for individuals to acquire the necessary skills to cope more successfully and become confident in self-management. Such awareness enables the individual to challenge and change perceptions, decrease stress reactivity, improve self-management skills, and minimize the harmful consequences of stress. This process positively influences health promotion, disease prevention, and symptom management. Understanding influences of stress on health and illness is essential to all nursing practice.

CASE STUDY

Health Assessment: John R.

John R., a 29-year-old man separated from his wife, walked into the health maintenance organization (HMO) stating he had a severe sore throat, could not eat, had not worked for a day, and was feeling "awful." He wanted to see the doctor and get a prescription for an antibiotic. The medical record revealed two episodes within the last 9 months of complaints of a sore throat, culture of organism, and antibiotic treatment. The separation from his wife occurred 1 year ago. He had not had a physical in 2 years. During the assessment interview, the nurse gathered the following information: John R. appeared tired, he presented his problem in short, terse statements, he was irritable about the clinic's slow service, and he expressed a need to get back to work. Within the last 3 weeks, he had been required to work overtime because he faced deadline penalties, and his boss said that John R.'s promotion, due in 2 months, depended on his performance now. John R. said that, in general, things were fine. His wife was apparently happy without him and he was too busy to care or to think about that relationship. He made one remark about his boss, "What do you do with a nervous boss?" He described his diet as fast food "taken on the run." He said he gets about 6 hours of sleep per night and awakens one to two times near morning. He has infrequent contact with family members, who live in the area.

Reflective Questions:

1. Describe how John R.'s nurse will comprehensively assess his health.
2. Discuss several different diagnoses and possible individual, family, and community causes.

CARE PLAN

Plan for Effective Coping: John R.

Nursing Diagnosis: Ineffective Individual Coping related to increased stress at work and limited coping strategies.

DEFINING CHARACTERISTICS

- Physiological disturbances
- Abuse of alcohol or drugs
- Participation in potentially dangerous activities
- Engaging in lifestyle with risk to health
- Impairment of social role functioning:
  - Nonproductive lifestyle
  - Failure to function in usual social roles
  - Nonperformance of activities of daily living
  - Inappropriate behaviors in social situations
  - Self-absorption
  - Lack of concern for or detachment from usual social supports
- Poor morale:
  - Unhappiness
  - Lack of future orientation
  - Hopelessness
  - Unacceptable quality of life
  - Pessimism
- Defensive patterns:
  - Inflexibility
  - Hypervigilance

- Avoidance
- Inertia
- Refusal or rejection of help

EXPECTED OUTCOMES

John R. will:
- Report increased information on and consequences to himself of stressors experienced
- Practice the relaxation response for 20 to 30 minutes every day through prayer or contemplation; use multiple mini-relaxations throughout each day
- Report increasing weekly exercise or activity and healthy changes in nutrition and sleep or rest patterns
- Develop effective coping and problem-solving abilities to manage stress, beginning with the stress at work

INTERVENTIONS

- Promote an attitude of openness to new information.
- Enroll him in a cognitive behavioral group program to learn stress management strategies and health promotion.
- Monitor his daily practice of relaxation response.
- Monitor his changes in exercise or activity, nutrition, sleep or rest patterns, and mood.
- Guide him to develop two coping strategies through cognitive-behavioral restructuring.

REFERENCES

American Holistic Nurses Association & American Nurses Association. (2007). *Holistic nursing: Scope & standards of practice.* Silver Springs, MD: *www.nursesbooks.org,* The Publishing Program of ANA.

Baird, C. L., & Sands, L. P. (2006). Effect of guided imagery with relaxation on health-related quality of life in older women with osteoarthritis. *Research in Nursing & Health,* 29(5), 442–451.

Bartol, G. M., & Courts, N. F. (2005). The psychophysiology of body mind healing. In B. Dossey, C. Guzetta, & L. Keegan (Eds.), *Holistic nursing: A handbook for practice* (4th ed., pp. 111–134). Sudbury, MA: Jones & Bartlett.

Beck, A. T. (1976). *Cognitive therapy and the emotional disorders.* New York: International Universities Press.

Beck, A. T. (1979). *Cognitive therapy of depression.* New York: Guilford Press.

Beehr, T. A., & Bowling, N. A. (2005). Hardy personality, stress, and health. In C. L. Cooper (Ed.), *Handbook of stress medicine and health* (2nd ed., pp. 193–211). Boca Raton, FL: CRC Press.

Benson, H. (1975). *The relaxation response.* New York: William Morrow & Co.

Butterfoss, F. D. (2007). *Coalitions and partnerships in community health.* San Francisco: Jossey-Bass.

Cannon, W. (1914). The emergency function of the adrenal medulla in pain and the major emotions. *American Journal of Physiology, 33,* 356–372.

Carver, C. S. (2007). Stress, coping, and health. In H. S. Friedman, & R. C. Silver (Eds.), *Foundations of health psychology* (pp. 117–144). New York: Oxford University Press.

Cochrane, C. E. (2005). Eating regulation responses and eating disorders. In G. W. Stuart & M. T. Laraia (Eds.), *Principles and practice of psychiatric nursing* (8th ed., pp. 517–537). St. Louis: Mosby.

Coleman, C. L. (2004). The contribution of religious and existential well-being to depression among African American heterosexuals with HIV infection. *Issues in Mental Health Nursing, 25*(1), 103–110.

Daneault, S., Lussier, V., Mongeau, S., Paillé, P., Hudon, E., Dion, D., et al. (2004). The nature of suffering and its relief in the terminally ill: A qualitative study. *Journal of Palliative Care, 20*(7), 7–11.

Deacon, B. J., & Abramowitz, J. S. (2006). Anxiety sensitivity and its dimensions across the anxiety disorders. *Journal of Anxiety Disorders, 20,* 837–857.

Dedert, E. A., Studts, J. L., Weissbecker, I., Salmon, P. G., Banis, P. L., & Sephton, S. E. (2004). Religiosity may help preserve the cortisol rhythm in women with stress-related illness. *International Journal of Psychiatry in Medicine, 34,* 61–77.

Dossey, B., Keegan, L., & Guzetta, C. (2004). *Holistic nursing: A handbook for practice* (4th ed.). Sudbury, MA: Jones and Bartlett.

Ellis, A. (1962). *Reason and emotion in psychotherapy.* New York: L. Stuart.

Ellis, A., & Dryden, W. (1987). *The practice of rational emotive therapy (RET).* New York: Springer Pub. Co.

Fitzpatrick, A. L., Kronmal, R. A., Gardner, J. P., Psaty, B. M., Jenny, N. S., Tracy, R. P., et al. (2007). Leukocyte telomere length and cardiovascular disease in the cardiovascular health study. *American Journal of Epidemiology, 165,* 14–21.

Gaydos, H. L. B. (2005). The art of holistic nursing and the human health experience. In B. Dossey, C. Guzetta, & L. Keegan (Eds.), *Holistic nursing: A handbook for practice* (4th ed., pp. 57–76). Gaithersburg, MD: Aspen.

Gill, K. M., Mishel, M. H., Belyea, M., Germino, B., Germino, L. S., Porter, L. S., et al. (2004). Triggers of uncertainty about recurrence and long-term treatment side effects in older African American and Caucasian breast cancer survivors. *Oncology Nursing Forum, 31*(3), 633–639.

Heap, M., & Kirsch, I. (Eds.). (2006). *Hypnosis: Theory, research and application.* Burlington, VT: Ashgate.

Hickman, S. E., Tilden, V. P., & Tolle, S. W. (2004). Family perceptions of worry, symptoms, and suffering in the dying. *Journal of Palliative Care, 20,* 20–27.

Highet, N., & Drummond, P. (2004). A comparative evaluation of community treatments for post-partum depression: Implications for treatment and management practices. *Australian and New Zealand Journal of Psychiatry, 38,* 212–218.

Holmes, T. H. (1981). *The schedule of recent experience.* Seattle: University of Washington Press.

Horowitz, M., Wilner, N., & Alvarez, W. (1979). Impact of event scale: A measure of subjective stress. *Psychosomatic Medicine, 41*(3), 209–218.

Kemeny, M. E. (2007). Psychoneuroimmunology. In H. S. Friedman, & R. C. Silver (Eds.), *Foundations of health psychology* (pp. 92–116). New York: Oxford University Press.

Ketterer, M. W., Brawner, C. A., Van Zant, M., Keteyian, W., Ehrman, J. K., Knysz, W., et al. (2007). Empirically derived psychometric screening for emotional distress in coronary artery disease patients: Efficiency, efficacy, and source. *Journal of Cardiovascular Nursing, 22*(4), 320–325.

Killeen, T. K. (2005). In G. W. Stuart & M. T. Laraia (Eds.), *Principles and practice of psychiatric nursing* (8th ed., pp. 618–629). St. Louis: Mosby.

Kobasa, S. C., Maddi, S. R., & Kahn, S. (1982). Hardiness and health: A prospective study. *Journal of Personality and Social Psychology, 42,* 391–404.

Lane, D. A., Chong, A. Y., & Lip, G. Y. H. (2007). Psychological interventions for depression in heart failure (Review). *The Cochrane Library,* Issue 3.

Lazarus, R., & Folkman, S. (1984). *Stress, appraisal, and coping.* New York: Springer.

Loeher, K. E., Bank, A. L., MacNeill, S. E., & Lichtenberg, P. A. (2004). Nursing home transition and depressive symptoms in older medical rehabilitation patients. *Clinical Gerontologist, 27,* 59–70.

Luck, S. (2005). Nutrition. In B. Dossey, C. Guzetta, & L. Keegan (Eds.), *Holistic nursing: A handbook for practice* (4th ed., pp. 451–476). Gaithersburg, MD: Aspen.

Markowitz, J. C. (2004). Interpersonal psychotherapy of depression. In M. Power (Ed.), *Mood disorders: A handbook of science and practice* (pp. 183–200). West Sussex, England: John Wiley & Sons.

National Center for Complementary and Alternative Medicine. (n.d.). *Backgrounder: An introduction to Reiki.* Retrieved June 29, 2008, from http://nccam.nih.gov/health/reiki/#.

Nelson, D. L., & Simmons, B. L. (2005). Gender differences in the management of work stress: Preventing distress and savoring eustress. In C. L. Cooper (Ed.), *Handbook of stress medi-*

cine and health (2nd ed., pp. 309–329). Boca Raton, FL: CRC Press.

Nightingale, F. (1859, 1992). *Notes on nursing: What it is and what it is not* (Commemorative ed.). Philadelphia: J. B. Lippincott.

O.D.P.H.P. (2005). *The dietary guidelines for Americans 2005.* Retrieved February 29, 2008, from *www.health.gov/dietaryguidelines/ dga2005/recommendations.htm.*

Pâquet, M., Bolduc, N., Xhignesse, M., & Vanasse, A. (2005). Re-engineering cardiac rehabilitation programmes: Considering the patient's point of view. *Journal of Advanced Nursing, 51*(6), 567–576.

Pascali-Bonaro, D., & Kroeger, M. (2004). Continuous female companionship during childbirth: A crucial resource in times of stress or calm. *Journal of Midwifery and Women's Health, 49*(4 Suppl 1), 19–27.

Pennebaker, J. W., & Chung, C. K. (2007). Expressive writing, emotional upheavals, and health. In H. S. Friedman, & R. C. Silver (Eds.), *Foundations of health psychology* (pp. 263–284). New York, NY: Oxford University Press.

Power, M. (2004). Cognitive behavioral therapy for depression. In M. Power (Ed.), *Mood disorders: A handbook of science and practice* (pp. 167–181). West Sussex, England: John Wiley & Sons.

Rees, K., Bennett, P., West, R., Davey, S. G., & Ebrahim, S. (2004). Psychological interventions for coronary heart disease (Review). *Cochrane Database of Systematic Reviews,* Issue 3.

Rogers, C. (1951). *Client-centered therapy.* Boston: Houghton Mifflin.

Selye, H. (1982). History and present status of the stress concept. In L. Goldberger & S. Breznitz (Eds.), *Handbook of stress: Theoretical and clinical aspects* (pp. 7–17). New York: Free Press.

Semmer, N. K., McGrath, J. E., & Beehr, T. A. (2005). Conceptual issues in research on stress and health. In C. L. Cooper (Ed.), *Handbook of stress medicine and health* (2nd. ed., pp. 2–43). Boca Raton, FL: CRC Press.

Shen, B. J., McCreary, C. P., & Myers, H. F. (2004). Independent and mediated contributions of personality, coping, social support, and depressive symptoms to physical functioning outcome among patients in cardiac rehabilitation. *Journal of Behavioral Medicine, 27,* 39–62.

Sherwood, P., Given, B. A., Given, C. W., Champion, V. L., Doorenbos, A. Z., Azzouz, F., et al. (2005). A cognitive behavioral intervention for symptom management in patients with advanced cancer. *Oncology Nursing Forum, 32*(6), 1190–1198.

Snyder, M., & Lindquist, R. (Eds.). (2006). *Complementary/alternative therapies in nursing* (5th ed.). New York: Springer.

Stuart, E., & Wells-Federman, C. L. (2005). Cognitive therapy. In B. Dossey, L. Keegan, & C. Guzetta (Eds.), *Holistic nursing: A handbook for practice* (4th ed., pp. 377–426). Gaithersburg, MD: Aspen.

Stuart, G. W. (2005a). Cognitive behavioral treatment strategies. In G. W. Stuart & M. T. Laraia (Eds.), *Principles and practice of psychiatric nursing* (8th ed., pp. 364–385). St. Louis: Mosby.

Stuart, G. W. (2005b). Psychophysiological responses and somatoform and sleep disorders. In G. W. Stuart & M. T. Laraia (Eds.), *Principles and practice of psychiatric nursing* (8th ed., pp. 285–302). St. Louis: Mosby.

Stuart, G. W. (2005c). Therapeutic nurse-patient relationship. In G. W. Stuart & M. T. Laraia (Eds.), *Principles and practice of psychiatric nursing* (8th ed., pp. 15–49). St. Louis: Mosby.

Taylor, S. E. (2007). Social support. In H. S. Friedman & R. C. Silver (Eds.), *Foundations of health psychology* (pp. 145–171). New York, NY: Oxford University Press.

The Benson-Henry Institute for Mind Body Medicine. (n.d.a). *The relaxation response.* Retrieved December 30, 2007, from *www.mbmi.org/basics/whatis_rresponse.asp.*

The Benson-Henry Institute for Mind Body Medicine. (n.d.b). *Stress.* Retrieved December 30, 2007, from *www.mbmi.org/basics/whatis_stress.asp.*

Tsigos, C., Kyrou, I., & Chrousos, G. P. (2005). Stress, endocrine manifestations, and diseases. In C. L. Cooper (Ed.), *Handbook of stress medicine and health* (2nd ed., pp. 101–129). Boca Raton, FL: CRC Press.

U.S. Department of Agriculture. (n.d.). *The Food Guide Pyramid.* Retrieved December 30, 2007, from *www.mypyramid.gov/.*

U.S. Department of Health and Human Services. (n.d.). *Healthy People 2010.* Retrieved December 30, 2007, from *www.healthypeople.gov/publications.*

Wainrib, B. R. (2006). *Healing crisis and trauma with mind, body, and spirit.* New York: Springer Publishing.

Weinger, K. (2007). Psychosocial issues and self-care. *American Journal of Nursing, 107,* 34–38.

Wells-Federman, C., Stuart, E., Deckro, J., Mandle, C. L., Baim, M., & Medich, C. (1995). The mind-body connection: The psychophysiology of many traditional nursing interventions. *Clinical Nurse Specialist, 9,* 59–66.

Witvliet, C. V., Phipps, K. A., Feldman, M. E., & Beckham, J. C. (2004). Posttraumatic mental and physical health correlates of forgiveness and religious coping in military veterans. *Journal of Traumatic Stress, 17*(3), 269–273.

Wooten, P. (2005). Humor, laughter, and play: Maintaining balance in a serious world. In B. Dossey, L. Keegan & C. Guzzetta (Eds.), *Holistic nursing: A handbook for practice* (4th ed., pp. 497–520). Sudbury, MA: Jones & Bartlett.

Chapter 14

Gina Lowry

Holistic Health Strategies

objectives

After completing this chapter, the reader will be able to:

- Define holistic health.
- Compare holistic health care and conventional health care.
- Describe the philosophical base of energy medicine.
- Explain the origin and practice of selected holistic health strategies.
- Contrast the importance of self-exploration for individuals and health care professionals.

key terms

Acupressure	Holism	Qi
Acupuncture	Imagery	Qi Gong
Allopathic medicine	Ki	Reflexology
Alternative/complementary therapies	Massage	Reiki
Aromatherapy	Meditation	Subtle energy
Asana	Meridians	Tai Chi
Centering	Moxibustion	Therapeutic touch
Chi	Polarity	Touch therapies
Curandero	Prana	Yoga
Energy	Prayer	
	Presence	

website materials

*e*volve These materials are located on the book's website at *http://www.evolve.elsevier.com/Edelman/*.

- WebLinks
- Study Questions
- Glossary
- Website Resources
  14A: Proportions of U.S. Adults Using Holistic Therapies in 2001 and 2002
  14B: Example of a Personal Health Workbook
  14C: Holistic Practitioners' Specialties and Definitions of Their Practice

Please Answer the Following Questions:

- When you wake up, does the idea of the day to come excite you?
- Does a lack of energy keep you from doing what you want to do?
- What makes you laugh? Can you laugh at yourself? Do you laugh often?
- Are you confident about the decisions you make?
- Do the choices you make have the outcomes you expect?
- Are you valued and appreciated at home, on the job?
- Are there people you appreciate? Do you tell them so?
- Do you have friends who offer you love, companionship, and support?

  If you answered "no" to any of these questions, you may have identified areas in your life that you want to change. Knowing yourself—the good and not so good—is the first step toward holistic health.

Modified from the American Holistic Health Association. (2003). *Wellness from within: The first step.* Anaheim, CA: Author. Retrieved April, 20, 2005, from *http://ahha.org/ahhastep.htm.*

HOLISM

Too often in health care practice, an individual seeking care has been viewed as the sick part (the gallbladder) or characterized by the sick function (the insomniac). Consumers are often dissatisfied with conventional health care and perceive that, within the conventional model, they are viewed as machines with parts and pieces. Consumers are seeking an alternative style of health care that will focus on increasing well-being and giving consumers greater control over self-care (Cassileth & Deng, 2004). Behind the idea of **holism** is the understanding that people are not just physical bodies; people have emotions, spirits, and relationships that combine with the physical body to make a whole person. People have relationships with the earth and their environment, with other people, and with themselves as they attempt to find the meaning and purpose in life. The meaning of life, in short, is found in connection (Ventegodt et al., 2003). The holistic movement in the healing arts reflects the theory of holism and recognizes that all these aspects of the person must be considered when planning and delivering care.

Holistic practitioners believe that health is more than the absence of disease; health is optimal wellness in all aspects of one's being—emotional, environmental, intellectual, physical, social, and spiritual. Gaydos (2005) defines wellness as "integrated, congruent functioning aimed toward reaching one's highest potential" (p. 58). The individual seeking health defines health. Working toward health and wellness is an ongoing process that includes self-knowledge and self-care. When disease occurs, holistic practitioners seek to support the person's natural healing systems, to consider the whole person, and to consider the environment (both physical and mental) surrounding the person. Many

of the interventions used in holistic health care practice are backed by centuries of tradition, but they are often considered complementary or alternative practices and are not currently incorporated into most conventional health care practices.

This view is changing; alternative and complementary practices are moving into the mainstream. Many medical and nursing schools are adding courses on **alternative/ complementary therapies** to their curricula (Innovative Practice box). Dr. Dean Ornish's Program for Reversing Heart Disease, which originally incorporated diet, yoga or other mild exercise, and meditation/relaxation (Ornish, 1990), is now available in many areas of the country (BlueCross/BlueShield Association, 2007); current research based on this original work is discussed in the section of this chapter about yoga practice on p. 350. Alternative/ complementary therapies can also be used as an adjunct to conventional medical care. Rapidly increasing numbers of managed care groups, insurers, and hospitals are including holistic health practices. **Website Resource 14A** presents a table depicting how many adults in the United States use holistic therapies. The Van Elslander Cancer Center at St. John Hospital in Detroit, Michigan, has a clinic that also offers Qi Gong, Tai Chi, yoga classes, hypnotherapy, and guided imagery (Van Elslander Cancer Center, 2007). With a vision "to promote health and healing of body, mind, and spirit," the Woodwinds Health Campus located in Woodbury Minnesota, offers complementary therapies including the use of essential oils, energy-based therapies, imagery, music, acupuncture, acupressure, and massage (Woodwinds Health Campus, n.d.). The Veterans Affairs Hospital in Salt Lake City, Utah, offers 13 complementary therapies (herbal and nutritional supplement education, acupuncture, hypnosis, Qi Gong, meditation, yoga, and **prayer**) as an adjunct to

Innovative practice

Repar and Patton (2007) report on a program to assist nurses to "reconnect emotionally and spiritually with themselves, their clients, and fellow healthcare workers" (p. 182). Noting that nursing has become a more difficult career during this time of nursing shortages and hoping to avoid nurse burnout, a program at the University of New Mexico Hospitals developed an Arts-in-Medicine (AIM) program.

This program offers a 10-minute chair massage and allows nurses time to make art and to relax and be introspective during 1½-hour sessions during the work day on their units where they work. Each unit is visited by artists, massage therapists, and movement therapists approximately twice a semester. In addition, three longer sessions called Afternoon Delights (p. 184) help nurses relax and learn to practice self-care.

Repar, P. A., & Patton, D. (2007). Stress reduction for nurses through Arts-in-Medicine at the University of New Mexico Hospitals. *Holistic Nursing Practice, 21*(4), 182-186.

conventional healthcare (Smeeding & Osguthorpe, 2005). Franklin Memorial Hospital, in western Maine, offers Reiki services to inpatients (Kendall, 2007). This integration of holistic practices with standard **allopathic medicine** will serve to introduce more people to complementary therapies and may give these practices more credibility with those who currently question the value of the practices.

Holistic interventions are used to promote wellness. Holistic interventions are used to manage illness and reduce pain and can help meet the goals of *Healthy People 2010*, including increasing quality and years of healthy life, increasing physical activity and flexibility in all age groups, decreasing pain, and reducing substance abuse (USDHHS, 2007). See the *Healthy People 2010* box for selected objectives that relate to holistic interventions. Holistic practices are moving into the mainstream; therefore, nurses understand the interventions that constitute holistic practice in order to discuss these practices with individuals who are using them. Nurses who understand holistic practices may make referrals to alternative/complementary practitioners. Nurses also find that holistic interventions such as energy work, bodywork, aromatherapy, prayer, meditation, massage, imagery, music therapy, and the movement arts of yoga, Tai Chi, and Qi Gong provide a useful adjunct to current nursing practice. Nurses interested in certification as holistic practitioners or training in various holistic interventions will find the American Holistic Nurses Association (*www.ahna.org/*) a useful resource.

INTERVENTIONS
Energy Work

People are animate beings with **energy**, a life force present in all living and nonliving elements of the universe. This energy is the animating force that flows through the body and extends beyond the body to interact with the energy in the environment (Pierce, 2007). The human energy field may be detected, assessed, and manipulated by an energy practitioner. Certain types of body energy are well known. Electrical energy in the body is reflected in diagnostic studies including electrocardiogram and electroencephalographic tracings.

People can be affected by the energy of their environments, including the energy of other people. For example, anxiety is contagious and moves readily and quickly from person to person (Bowman, 2004). There are medical uses for energy that comes from the environment. The energy of radiation is used to shrink tumors; sound energy, in the form of ultrasound waves, is used to break up kidney stones (Gray, 2004). Music, a form of sound energy, can be relaxing or stimulating and has been used to decrease the anxiety of persons who are being mechanically ventilated (Thomas, 2003) and to decrease pain, depression, and disability (Siedliecki & Good, 2006). Light energy is useful in treating seasonal affective disorder (Lam et al., 2006; Srinivasan et al., 2006). Color, another form of light energy, may have an effect on emotions and behaviors (Stone, 2003). Lasers, focused light energy, are used in many types of surgery and to treat other disorders (Frech & Adler, 2007; Kujawa et al., 2004).

Other energies can affect healing. Many cultures believe that an energy flows through the body that nourishes organs and promotes optimal functioning. Chinese call this energy **chi** (or **qi**), Japanese call it **ki**, and East Indians call it **prana**. In the West, this energy is often called **subtle energy**, *life energy*, or *universal energy*. Most of the detailed information on this energy system originally came from ancient practices and texts, including descriptions by people who have the exceptional ability to see the energy as it affects people. Personal experience may reveal the subtle energy in the body, as demonstrated by the exercise in Box 14-1.

Illness, stress, emotional upset, or spiritual distress can affect the flow of life energy; the flow can become blocked, unbalanced, or chaotic. These disruptions in the flow of life energy can cause or exacerbate illness in the physical body and can increase emotional and spiritual distress.

Healthy People 2010
Selected National Health-Promotion and Disease Prevention Goals and Objectives

- Increase quality and years of healthy life (p. 8)
- Quality of life reflects a general sense of happiness and satisfaction with our lives and environment (p. 10)
- Reduce the proportion of adults who engage in no leisure-time physical activity (p. 22-8)
- Increase the proportion of adults who engage regularly, preferably daily, in moderate physical activity for at least 30 minutes per day (p. 22-9); adolescents for at least 30 minutes on 5 or more of the previous 7 days (p. 22-17)
- Increase the proportion of adults [and adolescents, p. 22-19] who engage in vigorous physical activity that promotes development and maintenance of cardiorespiratory fitness 3 or more days per week for 20 or more minutes per occasion (p. 22-11)
- Increase the proportion of adults who perform physical activities that enhance and maintain muscular strength and endurance (p. 22-11)
- Increase the proportion of adults who perform physical activities that enhance and maintain flexibility (p. 22-15)
- Reduce substance abuse to protect the health, safety, and quality of life for all (p. 26-3)
- Increase the mean number of days without severe pain among adults who have chronic joint symptoms (p. 2-11)
- Reduce the proportion of adults with chronic joint symptoms who experience a limitation in activity due to arthritis (p. 2-11)

From U.S. Department of Health and Human Services. (2000). *Healthy people 2010: Understanding and improving health and objectives for improving health* (2nd ed.). Washington, DC: U.S. Government Printing Office.

Box **14-1** Feel Your Own Energy

This exercise will help you feel your own energy, or chi.
- Sit quietly, back straight, feet touching the floor.
- Place your hands in your lap.
- Take a few deep breaths. Become quiet and still.
- Breathe slowly in and out for a few minutes.
- Slowly raise your hands in front of you, palms facing, hands about 15 inches apart. Cup your fingers as though you are holding a basketball between your hands.
- Concentrate on the space between your hands. What is there? Can you feel anything?
- Slowly bring your palms closer together, focusing on the space between your hands.
- Can you feel warmth? Does it feel spongy? Can you move your hands around a shape?
- What you are feeling is the energy coming from the energy centers in your hands. Focus on the energy. Try to increase the sensation of fullness in the space between your hands.
- If you do not feel anything right away, bring your hands back out to 15 inches apart and slowly move your hands together again. Try no more than 3 times each time you attempt the exercise.

The basic goal behind the various modalities of energy work is to release blockages to energy flow, stimulate deficient life energy, and rebalance life energy.

Acupuncture, Acupressure, and Reflexology

Acupuncture Acupuncture manipulates life energy (chi or qi) by stimulating precisely mapped points on the skin surface. The points overlie the channels, called **meridians**, through which chi travels (Figure 14-1). The channels are named for the organs they affect, such as the lung meridian, heart meridian, and kidney meridian. Acupuncture may be used to diagnose disharmony; the points become tender to palpation in the presence of a disturbance in energy flow. The acupuncture points act as valves in the meridian system. When the points are stimulated, acupuncture becomes a treatment modality to correct disturbances in flow. When stimulated, the valve may open to release blocked or excess chi or close to allow chi to collect if chi is deficient. Stimulation of the points may be accomplished in several ways: by inserting fine needles into the points, by electrostimulation, by laser, and by light stimulation. Burning herbs can be used on or over the points to increase point stimulation; this technique is known as **moxibustion**. See *www. nlm.gov/medlineplus/acupuncture* for more information.

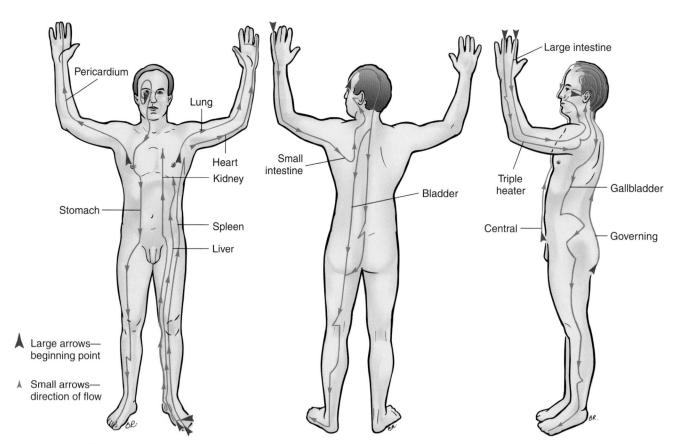

Figure 14-1 Typical locations of meridians. (From Anderson S. K. [2008]: *The practice of shiatsu.* St. Louis: Mosby).

Acupuncture is a useful treatment for substance abuse; the treatments may stand alone or be combined with other forms of therapy. The National Acupuncture Detoxification Association (NADA) protocol for addiction involves general stimulation of five points in each ear. Using a similar treatment protocol, Courbasson et al. (2007) found less depression, anger, and anxiety, and reduced cravings among the women who received acupuncture plus standard therapy during withdrawal (n=185) than among those women who had standard therapy with no acupuncture. Auricular acupuncture has also been demonstrated as an effective treatment for insomnia (Chen et al., 2007). Information on training in auricular acupuncture can be found at the NADA website (*http://acudetox.com/index.php?page_name=training*).

Acupuncture is also an effective adjunctive treatment for musculoskeletal pain of the knee (Berman et al., 2004; Witt et al., 2005). The National Center for Complementary and Alternative Medicine (NCCAM) also reports that acupuncture "reduces nausea and vomiting after surgery and chemotherapy" (*www.nccam.nih.gov/health/acupuncture*). Acupuncture education is available through many schools of traditional Chinese medicine and other sources; a Web search of acupuncture schools provides several sources for education.

Acupressure The meridian points may also be stimulated by hand pressure. **Acupressure** involves stimulation of the acupuncture points by pressing, knuckling, rubbing, squeezing, and stretching. No oil is used for acupressure, and the treatments may be performed with the person fully clothed. Both shiatsu and Amma therapy use acupressure along with massage to move and balance the body's energies. Education in these methods may be acquired through massage schools. Ezzo et al. (2005) found that acupressure was effective in reducing chemotherapy-induced nausea and vomiting. Maa et al. (2007) found acupressure was effective in improving both symptoms and quality of life for individuals with bronchiectasis. Tian and Krishnan (2006) found that auricular acupressure reduced cravings more than placebo acupressure treatment among a group of Hispanic individuals with a history of substance abuse.

Reflexology **Reflexology** is another method of moving energy by using hand pressure. Rather than to acupuncture points, the reflexologist applies pressure to mapped points on the feet or hands or both. Pressure is applied with the thumbs, pressing deeply into the point to release tension and stimulate circulation of blood, lymph, and energy. Reflexology is more than massage; practitioners believe that the points correspond to the organs of the body and that stimulating the points will stimulate the organs (Wynn, 2006). There are many websites related to reflexology. The Association of Reflexologists home page (*www.aor.org.uk*) provides information on reflexology history, training, and research.

Touch Therapies

In the **touch therapies** (therapeutic touch, healing touch, Reiki, pranic healing, Qi Gong healing, and polarity therapy, among others), practitioners use their hands to direct life energies drawn from the environment to the individual in an effort to restore balance and harmony within the human energy system (Fritz, 2004). The mechanism of action for the touch therapies is, at this time, unknown. Knowledge of the mechanisms continues to be studied. An actual exchange of physical energy may take place between practitioner and individual (Bruyere, 1994); others believe that the intent and consciousness of the practitioner is the mechanism that causes the effect of the intervention. During these therapies, the hands can be placed directly on the person's body (contact) or at a distance from the body (no contact).

Therapeutic Touch Therapeutic Touch (TT) may be the best known of the touch therapies. In the early 1970s, at about the same time that influential nursing theorist Martha Rogers conceptualized the idea that humans were composed of energy fields that interacted with the energy fields of their environments (Wright, 2007), Delores Krieger and her friend Dora Kunz, a lay healer, began the development of TT. Krieger, a registered nurse and professor of nursing, observed Kunz and others healing by laying on of hands, analyzed their techniques, trained herself in the technique, and began treating individuals. Krieger (1979) believed that the ability to transmit universal energy is a natural ability of all humans; she taught a small group of nursing students to perform laying-on-of-hands therapy. This small group became the basis for TT and, since this modest beginning, approximately 200,000 persons from all over the world have been trained in the techniques.

TT practice comprises three essential elements. The first element is centering by the practitioner. **Centering** is a process of becoming calm, present in the moment, and connected with the individual being treated, allowing the practitioner to give the person undivided attention. The centered practitioner is able to let go of personal feelings and emotions and is more open to inner perceptions (Krieger, 1998). The practitioner remains centered throughout the treatment. During assessment, the second element, the practitioner's hands move over the individual's body at a height of about 3 inches above the skin in an attempt to sense disturbances or imbalances in the person's energy field (Figure 14-2).

Assessment is performed before treatment begins and continues throughout treatment. Krieger (1993) describes the treatment techniques, the third element of TT practice. These techniques consist of methods to change the patterns in the human energy field (unruffling), to direct energy to the person to replenish depleted energy (modulation), and to balance or redistribute the individual's energies (modulation). The Case Study and Care Plan at the end of this chapter present the treatment of one person using TT for neck pain and additional information on the techniques of TT; please note that the way this nursing diagnosis is written, there is an implicit requirement that the nurse be trained to assess and recognize the energy field disturbance.

Much of the research on touch therapies has examined TT, and not everyone agrees that current research is scientifically valid (Hot Topics box). Many of the studies have small sample sizes, reducing their power. In many of the studies, the results are not statistically significant; this, too, could be the result of small sample sizes. Denison (2004) found that individuals with fibromyalgia who received TT treatments had a decrease in pain after each treatment and an improvement in quality of life scores following a series of six treatments. Pregnant women hospitalized for chemical

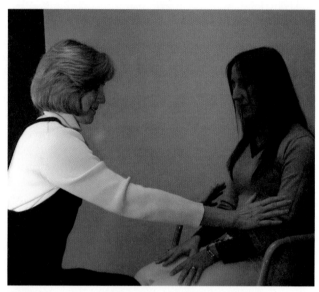

Figure 14-2 The assessment phase of therapeutic touch. The practitioner is attempting to sense disturbances or imbalances in the person's energy field.

dependency who received daily TT treatments for seven days had decreased anxiety (Larden et al., 2004). Newshan and Schuller-Civitella (2003) report that a "majority of hospitalized individuals who receive TT have a positive outcome" (p. 191). Information on becoming a Therapeutic Touch practitioner is available from Nurse Healers–Professional Associates International (*www.therapeutic-touch.org*).

Healing Touch A technique known as healing touch (HT) is a modality similar to TT, developed by Janet Mentgen. HT adds full-body techniques for moving energy and disorder-specific energetic interventions to the modulation phase of TT (Hover-Kramer, 1996). Wardell and Weymouth (2004) reviewed studies of HT and found that the studies indicated "results in reducing stress, anxiety, and pain; accelerated healing … and a greater sense of well-being" (p. 154). Healing Touch International (*www.healingtouch.net*) provides information on training programs.

Other Touch Therapies Qi Gong healing, pranic healing, and Reiki are similar modalities from the Chinese, East Indian, and Japanese traditions, respectively. Yoga practitioners may offer training in pranic healing during 1-day workshops. Qi Gong healing is provided primarily by Qi Gong masters and some traditional doctors of Chinese medicine, but others who practice Qi Gong regularly may also use the Qi Gong energy to heal (Cohen, as reported in Horrigan, 2003). Lee et al. (2003) found decreases in anxiety (p = 0.014), depression, fatigue, pain, and blood pressure in a group receiving Qi therapy.

Reiki healing, from the Japanese tradition, requires training by a Reiki master. In addition to teaching the hand placements and symbolic gestures used in Reiki, the master attunes the student. Attunement opens the energy channel,

---

HOTtopics
HOW SHOULD ALTERNATIVE/COMPLEMENTARY THERAPIES BE EVALUATED?

Those who use Therapeutic Touch (TT) believe strongly that it is an effective intervention because they have seen it work. Despite an impressive body of research, TT continues to be attacked in the media by people who do not believe that scientific evidence of the effectiveness of the practice exists (Fish, 2005). Much of the research on TT has attempted to test efficacy using a version of the randomized controlled clinical trial (RCT) study design to conform to current scientific paradigms concerning the acceptability of research evidence. Many of the study findings have been statistically nonsignificant. Although this lack of statistical significance could have been due solely to small sample size, it added fuel to the fire of those who question the validity of the practice.

Many complementary and alternative therapies, including TT, are tailored specifically to the individual and produce treatment plans that are therefore nonstandardized, which does not fit the requirements of the RCT design. A TT treatment is dictated by the needs of the individual and is finished when the practitioner

believes that it is finished, not within a rigid time limit imposed by a study protocol. A TT practitioner cannot participate in a blind trial, because intentionality is a large part of the practice. Additionally, healers may be unable to perform identically from day to day, and psychological and physical changes within the healer may affect the ability to heal. Herman et al. (2006) suggest using health services research designs, which include pragmatic trials rather than RCTs, to study alternative/complementary therapies.

1. What standards of proof should the nurse require before adopting an alternative/complementary therapy in clinical practice?
2. Have all (or even most) of the alternative/complementary therapies commonly used by nurses today been subjected to these standards?
3. Have all (or even most) of the standard therapies commonly used by nurses and medicine today been subjected to these standards?

Compiled from Fish, S. (2005). *Therapeutic touch: Healing science or psychic midwife?* Retrieved November 3, 2007, from *www.equip.org/site/c.muI1LAMNJrE/b.2739771/k.BB29/DN105.htm*; and Herman, P. M., D'Huyvetter, K.D., and Mohler, M. J. (2006). Are health services research methods a match for CAM? *Alternative Therapies in Health and Medicine, 12*(3), 78-83.

enabling the student to bring universal energy through the body and to the recipient (Vitale & O'Connor, 2006). Research involving Reiki is increasing. Olson et al. (2003) found that individuals with advanced cancer who received standard care and Reiki treatments had improved pain control and improved quality of life compared to a control group who received only standard care. Vitale and O'Connor (2006) found Reiki to be effective in reducing pain and anxiety in women who had undergone hysterectomy. Further information on Reiki research is available at the website for The International Center for Reiki Training (*www.reiki.org*). Johrei, also from the Japanese tradition, is a similar healing modality. Johrei has been shown to reduce laboratory-induced stress (Laidlaw et al., 2006) and to be helpful in the recovery from substance abuse (Brooks et al., 2006).

Polarity therapy was created by Randolph Stone, D.C., D.O., as a combination of energy work, caring intention, movement exercises, and dietary regimens. Polarity therapy is aimed at clearing energy blockages and building health (American Polarity Therapy Association, 2003). Information regarding training and treatment may be found at the American Polarity Therapy Association website (*www.polaritytherapy.org*) as well as other websites.

Other skilled people have developed healing schools and training programs. Rosalyn Bruyere and Barbara Brennan are skilled at reading auras (the extension of the energy field beyond the physical body) and the energy flow through the body (Brennan, 1987; Bruyere, 1994). The Brennan school appears to be formally structured; classes, tuition, and other information can be found on the school's website (*www.barbarabrennan.com*). Rosalyn L. Bruyere, an ordained minister, teaches healing through a series of workshops. Rev. Bruyere also has a website (*www.rosalynlbruyere.org*).

Energy healing takes place in many cultures. There are other types of healing and healers. Shamanism has existed in many parts of the world for centuries. As the population of Hispanic Americans increases in the United States, the **curandero** (healer) of Mexican, Central American, and South American cultures, who often treats diseases with heat and cold (Multicultural Awareness Box), is becoming more familiar. Faith healers are associated with many different religions.

The Movement Arts

The movement arts of Qi Gong, Tai Chi, and yoga have also been found to be helpful for body, mind, and spirit. Similar to energy work practices, the movement arts manipulate life energies.

Qi Gong

Qi Gong (pronounced chee gung), a part of traditional Chinese medicine, combines relaxed movements with a meditative aspect and controlled breathing to move qi energy through the energy channels and increase vital energy. Many books and videos explain Qi Gong practice. Lee et al. (2003) found decreases in blood pressure and

MULTICULTURAL AWARENESS
Hot/Cold Diseases

Hispanic culture considers disease causation as an imbalance between hot and cold. Specific diseases are classified by their causation, and the treatments (food, home remedies, and medications) used to treat the diseases are generally the converse; e.g., a cold treatment is used for a hot disease. Some hot diseases are constipation, diarrhea, fever, pregnancy, ulcers, and rashes. Examples of cold diseases include arthritis, a cold, indigestion, menstrual cramps, stomach aches, and muscle spasms.

Hispanic use of complementary and alternative therapies is substantial; these therapies are often used to support chronic conditions. Hypertension, which is considered to be caused by anger, fear, nervousness, and thick blood, is a hot disease. It is treated by the cold treatments of lemon juice and various teas. Asthma is a cold disease, treated by traditional herbal mixtures and by massage. Diabetes is a hot disease. Home treatments traditionally complement traditional therapies and include cactus, aloe vera, and bitter gourd. If home treatments, which are generally initiated by an influential female in the home, are not successful, family and friends are consulted for advice. A spiritual leader (curanderismo) may also be consulted to perform a healing ritual for an especially recalcitrant problem. If this treatment fails to resolve the problem, an allopathic physician may be consulted.

Since there is potential for drug interactions between allopathic medicines and the traditional medicines of the Hispanic population, it is especially important that allopathic providers understand the home treatments that this population is using. One way to ease the assessment of the use of home treatments is an open mind and acceptance of folk practices.

From Ortiz, B. I., Shields, K. M., Clauson, K. A., & Clay, P. G. (2007). Complementary and alternative medicine use among Hispanics in the United States. *Annals of Pharmacotherapy, 41,* 994–1004.

improved ventilatory function in hypertensive middle-aged individuals who practiced Qi Gong for 10 weeks. Pippa et al. (2007) found that persons with cardiac problems who participated in a 16-week Qi Gong training problem had greater functional capacity than those in the control group.

Tai Chi

Tai Chi (pronounced tie chee) began as a Chinese martial art. Tai Chi combines physical movement, breath control, and meditation in a dancelike sequence of poses based on the movements of animals. One pose flows into the next in a slow, relaxed, gentle, unbroken rhythm. The slowness of movement and focus on breathing brings an awareness of the moment-to-moment state of the body and produces a meditative state. Tsai et al. (2003) found that Tai Chi had beneficial effects on blood pressure, lipid profiles values, and anxiety status when subjects participated in a 12-week program. Wang et al. (2004) present a systematic review of the research literature on the effects of Tai Chi in individuals with chronic conditions and conclude that "Tai Chi appears to have physiological and psychosocial benefits … [and promotes] balance control, flexibility and cardiovascular fitness" (p. 493).

Yoga

Yoga, from the Hindu tradition, originated as a form of spiritual practice. The word *yoga* means union, and the system of yoga teaches the methods by which the individual can be joined with the Supreme Being and achieve liberation (Sivananda, 2005). There are several types of yoga—several paths to liberation. Karma yoga is the yoga of right action and good works; bhakti yoga, the yoga of devotional practices; raja yoga is the yoga of meditative practices; jnana yoga, the yoga of the study of spiritual texts; mantra yoga is the yoga of repetition of a sacred phrase; laya yoga is the yoga of blending self with the Supreme (Sivananda, 2005). Hatha yoga, the yoga of physical practice of various postures called asanas and of breath control, is most familiar to Western cultures. **Asana** practice is simply the beginning of one's spiritual quest, allowing us to understand better body, mind, and spirit (Iyengar, 2005).

Yoga asanas often have evocative, descriptive names, such as proud warrior, waterfall, runner's pose, downward-facing dog, mountain pose, and eagle pose. Other asana names are simple descriptions of what the body is doing during the posture, such as standing forward bend and spinal twist. Some of the poses are restful and restorative; some require strength and flexibility, which comes with regular practice. Asana practice is a process of gentle effort that often involves a letting go and relaxing into the pose rather than forcing the body into the pose. Asana practice is noncompetitive. The practice is not about how the person looks in the pose, but rather is about how the person feels in the pose from the inside out. During asana practice, the breath flows easily in and out through the nostrils. The body is active, but the mind is restful and watching, a witness to your actions. The energies of the body should extend equally through all the limbs and in all directions. Relaxation pose follows the active asanas and allows the body to incorporate the work that has been done.

Hatha yoga also includes breathing exercises known as pranayama. Prana means vital energy and is synonymous with breath (Iyengar, 2005). Control of the breath helps the yogi to control the mind and keep it focused on the present moment or the Supreme Being or both. Breath control also helps move the subtle energy (prana) through channels in the body (nadis) to nourish the body organs and the spirit (Iyengar, 2005). Iyengar states:

> one must do asana not merely as a physical exercise but as a means to understand and then integrate our body with our breath, with our mind, with our intelligence, with our consciousness, with our conscience, and with our core (2005, p. 23).

Yoga practitioners will recognize that many well-researched techniques are derived from yoga, including various relaxation techniques, Lamaze breathing techniques, physical therapy stretches, and athletic stretches. Yoga has been used to help people stop smoking (McIver et al., 2004). It improved balance and flexibility while decreasing disability and depression in a small sample of persons with low back pain (Galantino et al., 2004), improved functional ability in persons with back pain (Jacobs et al., 2006), and decreased self-reported symptoms of depression and anxiety in mildly depressed young adults (Woolery et al., 2004). Building on the work of Dr. Dean Ornish, Yogendra et al. (2004) found that individuals with proven coronary artery disease who participated in a year-long yoga program and dietary modification had decreased cholesterol, regression of their disease, and improved anxiety scores. Daubenmier et al. (2007) examined Ornish's Multisite Cardiac Lifestyle Intervention Program and noted that the yoga and meditation components of the program were linked to a reduction in hostile attitudes, reduced depression, and increased metabolic functioning. Streeter et al. (2007) found yoga practice to increase GABA levels, indicating a possible benefit for persons with anxiety disorder or depression. Carson et al. (2007) found that women with metastatic breast cancer had (a) less pain and fatigue and (b) higher levels of energy, relaxation and acceptance, on the day following yoga sessions. Morone and Greco (2007) found that both yoga and tai chi were associated with pain reduction in older adults with chronic nonmalignant pain.

Self-instructional videos in the movement arts are available from many sources; however, a well-trained teacher can help refine practice. Qi Gong, Tai Chi, and yoga classes are available at many fitness centers and community settings. There are different styles of practice within each discipline; therefore, experience with different teachers might be necessary to find one whose practice corresponds to the needs of the student.

Meditation

Meditation involves the focusing of concentration on a single point. When the mind wanders, the individual consciously brings the mind back to the point of concentration. The focus of concentration can be a burning candle, a word, a phrase, the breath, or simply a quiet awareness of what is happening in the present moment. During meditation, one becomes "still, so that you can discover who you are" (Tigunait, 2003, p. 30). A part of the religious life of many cultures, meditation has become prevalent in the West as a tool to improve physical and mental well-being. Centering prayer can be considered a form of meditation as practitioners focus on a sacred word. Meditation can be practiced while sitting, walking, or moving. There are many techniques for meditating. One of the best known is Transcendental Meditation (TM). There are an estimated 6 million TM practitioners worldwide (Maharishi Vedic Education Development Corporation, 2007). The Indian spiritual leader Maharishi Mahesh Yogi brought TM to the

United States during the 1960s. The TM technique is repetition of a mantra (a word, sound, or phrase). Practitioners repeat the mantra silently over and over again (for 20 minutes, morning and evening). When other thoughts arise during mantra repetition, the practitioner should notice the thought, let the thought go, and return to the mantra.

Mindfulness meditation is a way of paying attention; the point of focus varies. The individual can choose to focus on thoughts, on actions, or the environment. Hendricks (2007) speaks of a mindfulness exercise used by Amy Connolly. Students take "as many as eight minutes to eat a raisin, noticing along the way every groove and wrinkle, the way the raisin smells and feels [in the hand and in the mouth], its color and shape" (p. 16).

Walking meditation is another form of mindfulness practice; with each step, the person is aware of the movements of the body that make the step possible and of both the external environment and the internal environment. Carlson and Garland (2005) found that mindfulness meditation (body scan meditation, sitting and walking meditation, and yoga) improved sleep quality and reduced stress, mood disturbance, and fatigue in a group of individuals with cancer. (See the Research Highlights Box for another study involving mindfulness meditation.)

One of the simplest methods of meditation is concentration on breathing. With breath meditation, there is no need for a special room, a special mat, or a cushion. The breath is an ever-present tool. Breath meditation can evoke the relaxation response. Breath meditation was used, along with yoga and body scanning, in a study by Robert-McComb et al. (2004) that examined the effects of mindfulness on stress hormones and physical functioning. Breath meditation was found to reduce heart rate and blood pressure in a group of young people with essential hypertension (Barnes et al., 2004). This technique can be taught easily (Health Teaching box) and is useful for anyone who is having a bad day.

The Website for TM (*www.tm.org*) states that more than 600 studies have been completed on the technique; the studies can be viewed on the site. Paul-Labrador et al. (2006) found TM improved blood pressure and insulin resistance in individuals with heart disease.

Bonadonna (2003) presents a literature review summarizing various studies involving both TM and other types of meditation.

research highlights

Mindfulness Meditation versus Relaxation Training

Stress levels are high for students in the health professions. Jain et al. (2007) compared mindfulness meditation (MM), somatic relaxation (SR), and a control group. The researchers hypothesized that both intervention groups would experience decreased stress; they also hypothesized that the MM group would experience a decrease in distractive thoughts and behaviors, increased reports of spiritual experiences, and increased positive mood states when compared to the SR and control groups.

Eighty-one students from the health professions were randomly assigned to one of the three groups; 15 men and 66 women took part in the study. The MM intervention focused on body scan meditation, hatha yoga, walking meditation, and loving-kindness meditation. The SR intervention consisted of progressive muscle relaxation, simple breathing techniques, and guided imagery focused on relaxation of the body. Both the MM group and the SR group were given tapes and homework during the one-month intervention. The control group had no interaction with researchers during the study; instead, following the final data collection, they were given manuals or tapes from their choice of MM or SR techniques and one class on stress reduction.

The researchers measured "psychological distress, positive states of mind, distractive and ruminative thoughts and behaviors, and spiritual experiences" (p. 11) preintervention and postintervention. This study found that both MM and SR reduced distress and improved positive mood states in the participants. Only MM was effective in reducing distractive and ruminative thoughts, and the researchers speculate that this may be why MM is so effective in reducing distress.

Data from Jain, S., Shapiro, S., Swanick, S., Roesch, S. C., Mills, P. J., Bell, I., et al. (2007). A randomized controlled trial of mindfulness medication versus relaxation training: Effects on distress, positive states of mind, rumination, and distraction. *Annals of Behavioral Medicine, 33*(1), 11-21.

HEALTH TEACHING   Teaching the Technique of Breath Meditation

- You may stand, sit, or lie quietly as you begin to focus on your breath.
- Inhale and feel the air come into your nostrils, move down your throat, and into your lungs. Do not try to control the breath. Just observe it.
- Exhale and feel the air move up from your lungs and into your throat. Feel the warmth of the exhaled air in your nostrils.
- Breathe. Feeling the air move in and out. Concentrate on the breath. Do not try to control the breath. Just observe it.

- Continue watching the breath for 5 to 10 minutes. As other thoughts come into focus, notice them and let them go. Focus again on the breath.
- As you become comfortable with breath meditation, you may easily add simple imagery to this technique.
- As you inhale, imagine breathing in peace or love or wellness.
- As you exhale, imagine breathing out pain or sorrow or grief.
- As you inhale, breathe in whatever it is that you need.
- As you exhale, breathe out whatever you wish to be free of in your life.

Prayer

It is a common belief that prayer aids in recovery from illness (Benson et al., 2006). People pray for themselves, and they pray for others. Prayer has different meanings to different people; a prayer may be a request for divine intervention, a type of meditation (centering prayer), or a form of intentionality that is useful in healing. Prayer is the basis for Christian Science healing practices (The Church of Christ Scientist, 2007); prayer facilitates healing by causing changes in consciousness that help individuals recognize their innate wholeness.

The research evidence of the effect of prayer on health conditions is mixed. One of the earliest research studies involving prayer (Byrd, 1997) indicated that prayer had a positive effect on study participants in a cardiac care unit; this study was replicated by Harris et al. (1999) with similar results. While in an earlier pilot study, prayer produced a reduction in postprocedure distress in participants undergoing cardiac catheterization, Krucoff et al. (2005) found no significant impact of distant prayer in a larger study. Masters and Spielmans (2007) also found no discernable effects achieved following distant intercessory prayer; they did find that prayer may be useful as a coping mechanism. Benson et al. (2006) found that intercessory prayers had no effect on whether complications arose following coronary artery bypass graft surgery.

Distant Healing

Praying for others may be a form of distant healing. While the results of recent research on distant healing have not shown significant results, many who practice energy work believe that their efforts are effective over long distances. One method of participating in distance healing is the healing circle. The members of the healing circle join hands. Each member sends healing energy to his or her neighbor on the right until the energy is flowing around the circle. When the energy is flowing readily, each member of the group focuses the energy on one group member, who acts to send the energy to someone they know in need of healing. Each member of the circle may, in turn, receive energy from the group and send it to an individual in need of healing.

Guided Imagery

The body may react to sensory images in the mind the same way it responds to an actual stimulus; the body does not know the difference between "what one is thinking and what is actually happening" (Reed, 2007, p. 262). Reed proposes that the mechanism for this response is explained by psychoneuroimmunology; a cascade of chemical agents floods the body in response to thoughts and emotions. Persons can turn on their "inner pharmacy," releasing adrenalin with their thoughts. For example, the threat of losing one's employment can create the fight or flight response (Reed) with increased anxiety and autonomic nervous system changes. This is an example of the negative effect of imagination.

Imagination can also have a positive influence on health. **Imagery** can be used to turn on the "inner pharmacy" to

release endorphins to promote a sense of well-being and to help people relax (Toth et al., 2006). During imagery practice, the person relaxes and focuses attention on the images chosen or presented. Generally the images are presented verbally but are designed to evoke all the senses. Guided imagery scripts are available from several sources, but individuals may also develop their own script that is specific to their need. For example, imagery for distraction during a painful procedure might involve asking the individual to identify a special place as a retreat. If the person's special place is a beach, the practitioner might ask the individual to hear the water softly lapping at the shore, to see the white sand (senses of hearing and sight), and to feel the warm sun falling softly on skin (sense of touch) as the smell of orange blossoms drifts through the air (sense of smell).

When people learn and understand some basic principles of anatomy and physiology, imagery can be used to affect physiological functioning. Research on imagery has shown improvements in chronic pain (Lewandowski, 2004), sleep (Richardson, 2003), limb performance in hemiparesis (Stevens & Stoykov, 2003), asthma symptoms (Epstein et al., 2004), and recurrent abdominal pain in children (Ball et al., 2003), as well as improvement of hand function in participants who had experienced a stroke (Dijkerman et al., 2004) and reduced anxiety and heart rate in a group of people recently admitted to a general medical unit (Toth et al., 2006).

Music Therapy

Music therapy is the use of specific kinds of music (or sounds) to produce desired changes in behaviors, emotions, and physiological processes. Music influences the limbic system, the area of the brain involved with emotions and feelings (Brown et al., 2004). Various types of music may be used therapeutically, and some music is composed specifically for therapeutic effect. This music is called designer music, which may include sound frequencies that alter brainwave frequencies to achieve a particular brain state or emotion. When using music as therapy, the music choice should be tailored to the individual. People's musical tastes vary widely; the music that some find relaxing may be grating to others. Music can serve as a reminder of past events and be useful in opening communication. It is worth noting that some of the events remembered can be unpleasant. While listening to Gregorian chants during an energy therapy session, one person reported "I feel like I'm at a mass." This was not something she found soothing, and the feelings that arose while listening to the music interfered with her relaxation.

McRee et al. (2003) write of several studies in which music therapy decreased anxiety and increased pain thresholds in individuals who had undergone surgical procedures; Brunges and Avigne (2003) found decreased anxiety and shorter lengths of postoperative stays when study participants listened to music before and during surgery; and Sendelbach et al. (2006) found that music was more effective than uninterrupted rest at reducing pain and opioid consumption after cardiac surgery. Ulrich et al. (2007) examined the effects of group music-making in a study with 21 hospitalized participants diagnosed with schizophrenia. Using a pretest-posttest design, the authors report that the participants had greater psychosocial orientation and fewer negative symptoms following the intervention. Gallagher et al. (2006) studied the effects of music therapy on persons with advanced cancer and report that individuals reported significant (p<0.001) improvements in symptoms. Family members also had significant improvements in mood and verbalizations. Although music therapy can be used by anyone, the American Music Therapy Association (*www.musictherapy.org*) offers training in music therapy and certifies music therapists who have completed formal education programs.

Bodywork
Massage

Massage is the manipulation of soft tissues of the body. Formal massage techniques are variations of rubbing a sore spot after bumping your head or rubbing a friend's back as consolation after a loss. Nurses are taught to give massage (back rubs) to promote sleep and relaxation and are taught that massage is a useful adjunct therapy for pain control and stress reduction (Shaw, 2007). Massage may involve stroking, kneading, pulling, or pinching the skin (Figure 14-3). Skin lubrication with oil, lotion, or powder reduces friction, pinching, and hair pulling during the massage.

Massage has been found to reduce systolic blood pressure in individuals going for cardiac catheterization (McNamara et al., 2003), to increase weight in neonates (Arora et al., 2005), to lessen the frequency and severity of migraine (Lawler & Cameron, 2006), and to lessen anxiety and improve sleep (Hanley et al., 2003). Huth et al. (2005) report that a review of the literature indicates preliminary support for the use of massage in children with cystic fibrosis. When combined

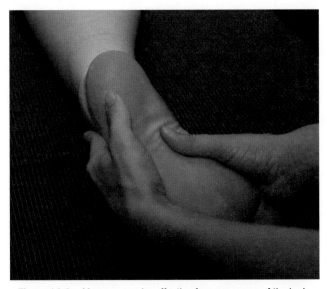

Figure 14-3 Massage can be effective for many areas of the body.

with acupuncture, massage was determined to decrease pain and depressive mood postoperatively in individuals diagnosed with cancer (Mehling et al., 2007). Many massage therapists, who may be certified by the American Massage Therapy Association after their training, practice a variety of bodywork modalities and may also include forms of energy work in their practices. A brief overview of several additional modalities follows.

Trager Therapy

Trager Psychophysical Integration involves tissue manipulation, relaxation, and movement reeducation. Practitioners work from a meditative state while they rock, jiggle, vibrate, and stretch the person's body in an effort to set off waves of motion that will lead to deep relaxation and greater mobility. This relaxation and mobility can release long-standing physical and mental patterns. Following treatment, the person is taught a series of exercises and stretches that will reinforce the treatment. Training in Trager therapy is available through schools of massage. A Web search for the topic "Trager therapy" yields a multitude of sites.

Craniosacral Therapy

Craniosacral therapy originated in osteopathy, a medical practice that adds manipulation of the bones of the body to conventional medical education. Craniosacral therapists believe that the bones of the cranium, spine, and sacrum are moveable and connected and that the cerebrospinal fluid has a pulse that can be felt. The therapist uses gentle pressure to restore free movement of cerebrospinal fluid, allowing for normal functioning. The therapist also believes that emotions are stored in musculoskeletal tissue and can be released through manipulation of the craniosacral system. Craniosacral therapy training is provided through the Upledger Institute (*www.upledger.com*).

Bowenwork

Bowenwork is based on the work of Tom Bowen, an Australian natural healer. The therapy involves gentle, precisely placed, rolling moves across physical structures of the body (muscles, tendons, and neurovascular bundles). Treatments may be performed with the person fully clothed. Bowenwork is helpful for a variety of conditions: pain or numbness from accidents, whiplash, sports injuries, muscular and skeletal problems, scoliosis, neck and shoulder problems, tennis elbow, restricted joints, arthritis, temporomandibular joint (TMJ) problems, stress, tension, emotional depression, respiratory problems, asthma, allergies, fibromyalgia, and chronic fatigue (Further information on treatable conditions and training may be found at *www.bowtech.com*.

Aromatherapy

Aromatherapy uses aromatic plant materials and the essential oils of plants. There is a long history of the use of plant materials in both ayurvedic medicine and traditional Chinese medicine. The use of aromatherapy without professional clinical training is strongly discouraged; people must have this training to know the specific warnings and contraindications for each oil, to know how to handle the oils, and to be aware of possible allergic reactions to oils (Buckle, 2003). The essential oils have a pharmacological, a physiological, and a psychological effect on the human body. Essential oils may be added to the bath or used in a douche, mixed with carrier oils and used during massage, placed on a cloth and applied as a compress, applied directly to minor injuries to speed healing, or inhaled (Buckle, 2003). Buckle (2003) presents several case studies that demonstrate the use of essential oils to help with the healing of herpetic lesions (eucalyptus oil), reduce the itching of psoriasis (lavender oil), reduce vaginal yeast infection (tea tree oil), and reduce pain in persons with cancer and bony metastases (rose oil). Aromatherapy research has demonstrated decreased agitation behaviors in participants with dementia (Thorgrimsen et al., 2004). Soden et al. (2004) found improvement in sleep and reductions in depression when aromatherapy (lavender oil) was combined with massage in a hospice setting. Shin and Lee (2007) combined a mixture of lavender, rosemary, and peppermint oils with accupressure. While both the aromatherapy plus accupressure group and the accupressure only group had decreased pain following treatment, the aromatherapy group had a significantly (p<0.01) greater decrease in pain. Han et al. (2006) found that abdominal massage using a mixture of lavender oil, clary sage, and rose in almond oil reduced symptoms of dysmenorrhea in college-age women. Buckle (2007) conducted a literature review of studies undertaken by nurses in U.S. hospitals that subsequently led to changes in hospital protocols (Table 14-1).

Presence

The way people interact with one another can cause pain or promote healing. A classic study by Halldorsdottir (1991) examined individuals' perceptions of their interactions with nurses. Subjects maintained that nurse interactions followed a continuum from life-destroying to life-sustaining to life-giving. Individuals perceived life-giving nurses as a healing force; they were perceived as "being present with," rather than simply being there for, the individuals.

As described by Fredriksson (1999), "being there" (Table 14-2) would normally be considered acceptable nursing behavior. However, the individuals in the Halldorsdottir (1991) study demonstrate that nurses can be much more than acceptable; the nurse's presence can actually contribute to healing. In examining the differences in "being there" and "being with," Fredriksson (1999) found that when nurses are "being with" subjects, the nurses' attention was focused rather than merely attentive, their touch was caring rather than task oriented, and nurses did not merely hear, they listened.

When using **presence** as a holistic intervention and establishing a whole person–to–whole person relationship, the nurse becomes vulnerable to the pain of the individual. Nurses may choose to avoid this pain by walking away, maintaining a professional distance, and being too busy with other tasks to be fully present. The key to overcoming these barriers to using presence in nursing practice is self-knowledge and self-care.

SELF-KNOWLEDGE

Holistic health involves knowing the physical self, the emotional self, the mental self, and the spiritual self, seeking a comfortable balance among these aspects of being, and knowing what changes need to be made to achieve this balance (American Holistic Health Association, 2003). This knowledge is vital to both the nurse attempting holistic practice and the individual interested in pursuing holistic health. The Think About It questions at the beginning of

Table **14-1** Studies Developed by Nurses Using Aromatherapy with Positive Results		
Authors, Date	**Symptom**	**Oils**
Hartman & Coetzee, 2002	Wound	Chamomile & lavender
Unpublished	Pressure ulcer/ MRSA	Tea Tree & aloe vera gel
Geiger, 2005	Postoperative nausea	Ginger
Piotrowski, 2006	Nausea	Peppermint
Curran, 2003	Agitation	French Lavender
Quate, 2002	Agitation	Not specified
Denert, 2005	Agitation	Bergamot
Fowler, 2006	Agitation	Ylang Ylang, Sweet marjoram & bergamot
Ballard, 2004	Pre-phlebotomy	Piper nigrum
Anderson, 2004	Terminal agitation	Lavender, sandalwood, & frankincense
Unpublished	Terminal agitation	Lavender
Ocampo, 2001	Terminal agitation	Frankincense

Summarized from Buckle, J. (2007). Literature review: Should nursing take aromatherapy more seriously. *British Journal of Nursing, 16*(2), 116-120.

Table **14-2** BEING THERE versus BEING WITH	
The Nurse Who Is BEING THERE	**The Nurse Who is BEING WITH**
Is attentive	Is available with whole self
Is task oriented	Enters the person's world
Does the right thing	Becomes vulnerable
Fulfills a role	Is present as a whole person
Assists with coping	Alleviates suffering
Provides security	Enables growth

this chapter can assist both nurse and individual in the exploration of self that begins the process of self-care. An example of a more detailed assessment instrument, a personal health workbook, is presented in **Website Resource 14B**.

Self-exploration is valuable to the nurse who wants to use presence in her practice because presence requires authenticity (Anderson, 2007). The more that is known about oneself, the more there is of oneself to offer to another, and "the only thing you ever have to offer to another human being, ever, is your own state of being" (Dass, 1976, p. 6).

When self-knowledge is gained, one or more of the holistic health strategies mentioned in this chapter can be useful in helping people achieve optimal wellness. In addition to the strategies mentioned, many other holistic interventions can be helpful. These strategies include homeopathy, flower essences, crystals, and additional forms of bodywork and movement therapies. Every person is a whole, unique being; therefore, each person needs to explore the possible strategies and decide which modalities are the best methods to achieve an improved state of wellness.

People beginning this self-exploration and the practice of holistic health strategies may find that the practice changes their lives. Using presence and giving the gift of self both enhance personal growth in the giver by helping the giver find meaning in relationship (Covington, 2005). Whelan and Wishnia (2003) found that Reiki practice benefits the nurse by reducing daily stress and burnout and increasing intuition, insight, and time spent with individuals; after all, the nurse who gives a Reiki treatment is moving positive energy through his/her body, thereby receiving a treatment as she/he gives a treatment.

SUMMARY

Holistic health strategies are designed to view the individual as a biopsychosocial-spiritual whole being. Many holistic health strategies have been practiced in other cultures for many years; some began as religious practices. As these practices moved to the West, the health-promoting nature of these therapies came to the forefront and the emphasis on religion waned. Many of these strategies can be used to help nurses and those they serve reach the *Healthy People 2010* goals of increasing physical activity and flexibility, decreasing substance abuse, reducing pain, and improving quality of life. A body of research already exists supporting the use of these therapies and more research is being performed. Although the studies to date have been unsuccessful in persuading some health care practitioners of the utility of the practices, holistic health practitioners are convinced that these practices help promote and maintain health.

Every person is a unique, individual being; therefore, some exploration of self, the various strategies, and the practitioner will be necessary before determining which strategy is the right fit for the individual. The right-fit strategy will increase both physical and mental well-being. **Website Resource 14C** presents a summary list of definitions of many holistic strategies, most of which were discussed in the chapter. Nurses need to understand holistic health strategies because individuals are using them in increasing numbers. Nurses who begin to practice holistic interventions may find them a useful adjunct to their nursing practice.

CASE STUDY

Use of Therapeutic Touch: George P.

George P., an 82-year-old White man, came to the clinic reporting neck pain and stiffness of approximately 4-months duration. He was previously treated with ibuprofen (Motrin), acetaminophen, and oxycodone (Percocet), and physical therapy. At the time of the initial clinic visit, Mr. P. was still taking Motrin but had stopped taking Percocet because the pain "isn't bad enough to take drugs [narcotics]." He rated his neck pain as 5 on a scale of 1 to 10. Neck range of motion (ROM) had improved, but it still caused problems for him when driving. Mr. P. lives next to a very busy street and did not feel that he could turn his neck well enough to see the traffic coming. He was afraid to pull out into the street. His daughter had driven him to the clinic. She said, "Pop is still in pain. He has little interest in doing anything. He walks like an old man and he can't work in his garden because of the pain." The goal of treatment for George P. is pain relief and increased ROM.

Reflective Questions:

1. What holistic health strategies might be used to relieve George's pain and to help him increase his ROM?

2. After the treatment goals are reached, what holistic health strategies would you recommend to assist George P. in maintaining and improving his health?

Therapeutic Touch (TT) was offered to George P. Although he was skeptical that this treatment would be effective, he agreed to treatment to please his daughter. Increased heat was noted in the neck and shoulder areas. A 30-minute TT treatment was performed, with special attention given to the neck and shoulder area. Immediately following the TT treatment, Mr. P. rated his pain as 0 on a scale of 1 to 10 and reported that he "couldn't remember when he'd been so relaxed"; the excess heat had dissipated. Mr. P. was also given some simple yoga exercises for the neck and advised to perform the exercises twice a day, five gentle repetitions each time. Mr. P. was seen in the clinic a total of 8 times for TT and was given increasingly difficult yoga stretches for the neck and shoulders. His pain rating at the end of treatment remained at 0 on the 10 scale. He had stopped taking Motrin, saying, "I don't need it anymore." His neck ROM had improved, and he was driving and working in his garden again. He continues his yoga stretches and has started performing daily Qi Gong exercises.

CARE PLAN

Use of Therapeutic Touch: George P.

Nursing Diagnosis: Energy Field Disturbance Related to Slowing or Blocking of Energy Flow Secondary to Repetitive Motion Injury

DEFINING CHARACTERISTICS

- Perceptions of changes in patterns of the energy flow, such as:
  - Temperature change: warmth, coolness
  - Visual changes: image, color
  - Disruption of the field: vacant, hole, spike, bulge
  - Movement: wave, spike, tingling, dense, flowing
  - Sounds: tone, words

RELATED FACTORS

- Pathophysiological: illness, injury
- Treatment-related: immobility, perioperative experience, labor and delivery
- Situational: pain, fear, anxiety, grieving
- Maturational: age-related developmental difficulties or crises

EXPECTED OUTCOMES

- The person will report increased sense of relaxation.
- The person will report decreased anxiety and tension.
- The person will demonstrate evidence of physical relaxation (e.g., decreased blood pressure, pulse, respiratory rate, muscle tension).

- The person will report an increased sense of well-being.

INTERVENTIONS

- Provide privacy if possible.
- Explain energy therapy (therapeutic touch, Reiki, healing touch) and obtain permission to treat.
- Position the person comfortably.
- Become quiet and still (centered) and bring the focus to the person.
- Assess (scan) the energy field for openness and flow.
- Clear the exterior energy field by combing through the field from head to toe (unruffling).
- Move the palms of the hands toward the person, 2 to 4 inches over the person's body, from head to feet in a smooth, light movement.
- Sense the cues to energy imbalance (i.e., warmth, coolness, tightness, heaviness, tingling, emptiness).
- Focus on perceived areas of imbalance to repattern the energy flow.
- Reassess and smooth the exterior energy field, ensuring that the energy flow is open in the feet.
- Gently stop the treatment and provide the person time to rest.
- Encourage the person to discuss the experience.

Modified from Carpenito-Moyet, L. J. (2004). *Nursing diagnosis: Application to clinical practice* (10th ed.). Philadelphia: Lippincott.

REFERENCES

American Holistic Health Association. (2003). *Wellness from within: The first step (booklet).* Anaheim, CA: Author. Retrieved April 20, 2005, from *http://ahha.org/ahhastep.htm.*

American Polarity Therapy Association. (2003). *About polarity therapy.* Retrieved March 20, 2004, from *www.polaritytherapy.org/polarity/index.html.*

Anderson, J. H. (2007). The impact of using nursing presence in a community heart failure program. *Journal of Cardiovascular Nursing, 22*(2), 89–94.

Arora, J., Kumar, A., & Ramji, S. (2005). Effect of oil massage on growth and neurobehavior in very low birth weight preterm neonates. *Indian Pediatrics, 42*(11), 1092–1100.

Ball, T. M., Shapiro, D. E., Monheim, C. J., & Weydert, J. A. (2003). A pilot study of the use of guided imagery for the treatment of recurrent abdominal pain in children. *Clinical Pediatrics, 42*(6), 527–532.

Barnes, V. A., Davis, H. C., Murzynowski, J. B., & Treiber, F. A. (2004). Impact of meditation on resting and ambulatory blood pressure and heart rate in youth. *Psychosomatic Medicine, 66*(6), 909–914.

Benson, H., Dusek, J. A., Sherwood, J. B., Lam, P., Bethea, C. F., Carpenter, W., et al. (2006). Study of the Therapeutic Effects of Intercessory Prayer (STEP) in cardiac bypass patients: A multicenter randomized trial of uncertainty and certainty of receiving intercessory prayer. *American Heart Journal, 151*(4), 934–942.

Berman, B. M., Lao, L., Langenberg, P., Lee, W. L., Gilpin, A. M. K., & Hochberg, M. (2004). Effectiveness of acupuncture as adjunctive therapy in osteoarthritis of the knee: A randomized, controlled trial. *Annals of Internal Medicine, 141*(12), 901–910.

BlueCross BlueShield Association. (2007). *Dr. Dean Ornish's program for reversing heart disease improves lives.* Retrieved January 18, 2008, from *www.bcbs.com/innovations/blueworks/consumer/dr-ornish-program.html.*

Bonadonna, R. (2003). Meditation's impact on chronic illness [Electronic Version]. *Holistic Nursing Practice, 17*(6), 309–319.

Bowman, G. (2004). *Test anxiety.* Retrieved March 19, 2004, from *www.hsc.edu/counseling/selfhelp/test_anxiety.html.*

Brennan, B. A. (1987). *Hands of light: A guide to healing through the human energy field.* New York: Bantam.

Brooks, A. J., Schwartz, G. E., Reece, K., & Nangle, G. (2006). The effect of Johrei healing on substance abuse recovery: A pilot study. *The Journal of Alternative and Complementary Medicine, 12*(7), 625–631.

Brown, S., Martinez, M. J., & Parsons, L. M. (2004). Passive music listening spontaneously engages limbic and paralimbic systems. *Neuroreport, 15*(13), 2033–2037.

Brunges, M., & Avigne, G. (2003). Music therapy for reducing surgical anxiety. *AORN Journal, 78*(5), 816–818.

Bruyere, R. L. (1994). *Wheels of light: Chakras, auras, and the healing energy of the body.* New York: Simon & Schuster.

Buckle, J. (2003). *Clinical aromatherapy: Essential oils in practice* (2nd ed.). New York: Churchill Livingstone.

Buckle, J. (2007). Literature review: Should nursing take aromatherapy more seriously? *British Journal of Nursing, 16*(2), 116–120.

Byrd, R. (1997). Positive therapeutic effects of intercessory prayer in a coronary care unit population. *Alternative Therapies in Health and Medicine, 3*(6), 87–90.

Carlson, L. E., & Garland, S. N. (2005). Impact of mindfulness-based stress reduction (MBSR) on sleep, mood, stress and fatigue symptoms in cancer outpatients. *International Journal of Behavioral Medicine, 12*(4), 278–285.

Carpenito-Moyet, L. J. (2004). *Nursing diagnosis: Application to clinical practice* (10th ed.). Philadelphia: Lippincott.

Carson, J. W., Carson, K. M., Porter, L. S., Keefe, F. J., Shaw, H., & Miller, J. M. (2007). Yoga for women with metastatic breast cancer: Results from a pilot study. *Journal of Pain and Symptom Management, 33*(3), 331–341.

Cassileth, B. R., & Deng, G. (2004). Complementary and alternative therapies for cancer. *The Oncologist, 9*, 80–89.

Chen, H. Y., Shi, Y., Ng, C. S., Chan, S. M., Yung, K. K., Zhang, Q. L. (2007). Auricular acupuncture treatment for insomnia: A systematic review. *The Journal of Alternative and Complementary Medicine, 13*(6), 669–676.

Courbasson, C. M., de Sorkin, A. A., Dullerud, B., & Van Wyk, L. (2007). Acupuncture treatment for women with concurrent substance use and anxiety/depression: An effective alternative therapy? *Family & Community Health, 30*(2), 112–120.

Covington, H. (2005). Caring presence: Providing a safe space for patients. *Holistic Nursing Practice, 19*(4), 169–172.

Dass, R. (1976). *The only dance there is.* New York: Jason Aronson.

Daubenmier, J. J., Weidner, G., Summer, M., Mendell, N., Merritt-Worden, T., Studley, J., et al. (2007). The contribution of changes in diet, exercise, and stress management to changes in coronary risk in women and men in the Multisite Cardiac Lifestyle Intervention Program. *Annals of Behavioral Medicine, 33*(1), 57–68.

Denison, B. (2004). Touch the pain away: New research on therapeutic touch and persons with fibromyalgia syndrome. *Holistic Nursing Practice, 18*(3), 142–151.

Dijkerman, H. C., Ietswaart, M., Johnston, M., & MacWalter, R. S. (2004). Does motor imagery training improve hand function in chronic stroke patients? A pilot study. *Clinical Rehabilitation, 18*(5), 538–549.

Epstein, G. N., Halper, J. P., Barrett, E. A., Birdsall, C., McGee, M., Baron, K. P., et al. (2004). A pilot study of mind-body changes in adults with asthma who practice mental imagery. *Alternative Therapies in Health and Medicine, 10*(4), 66–71.

Ezzo, J., Vickers, A., Richardson, M. A., Allen, C., Dibble, S. L., et al. (2005). Acupuncture point stimulation for chemotherapy-induced nausea and vomiting. *Journal of Clinical Oncology, 12*(28), 7188–7198.

Fish, S. (2005). *Therapeutic touch: Healing science or psychic midwife.* Retrieved April 21, 2005, from *www.equip.org/free/DN105.htm.*

Frech, E. J., & Adler, D. G. (2007). Endoscopic therapy for malignant bowel obstruction. *Journal of Supportive Oncology, 5*(7), 303–310.

Fredriksson, L. (1999). Modes of relating in a caring conversation: A research synthesis on presence, touch and listening. *Journal of Advanced Nursing, 30*(5), 1167–1176.

Fritz, S. (2004). *Mosby's fundamentals of therapeutic massage* (3rd ed.). St. Louis: Mosby.

Galantino, M. L., Bzdewka, T. M., Eissler-Russo, J. L., Holbrook, M. L., Mogck, E. P., Geigle, P., et al. (2004). The impact of modified Hatha yoga on chronic low back pain: A pilot study. *Alternative Therapies in Health and Medicine, 10*(2), 56–59.

Gallagher, L. M., Lagman, R., Walsh, D., Davis, M. P., & Legrand, S. B. (2006). The clinical effects of music therapy in palliative medicine. *Supportive Care in Cancer, 14*(8), 859–866.

Gaydos, H. L. B. (2005). The art of holistic nursing and the human health experience. In B. M. Dossey, L. Keegan, & C. E. Guzzetta (Eds.), *Holistic nursing: A handbook for practice* (4th ed., pp. 57–76). New York: Jones and Bartlett.

Gray, M. (2004). Renal and urologic problems. In S. M. Lewis, M. M. Heitkemper, & S. R. Dirksen (Eds.), *Medical-surgical nursing: Assessment and management of clinical problems* (6th ed., pp. 1172–1209). St. Louis: Mosby.

Halldorsdottir, S. (1991). Five basic modes of being with another. In D. A. Gaut & M. M. Leininger (Eds.), *Caring: The compassionate healer* (NLN Publication No. 15-2401, pp. 37–49). New York: National League for Nursing Press.

Han, S. H., Hur, M. H., Buckle, J., Choi, J., & Lee, M. S. (2006). Effect of aromatherapy on symptoms of dysmenorrhea in college students: A randomized placebo-controlled clinical trial. *Journal of Alternative and Complementary Medicine, 12*(6), 535–541.

Hanley, J., Stirling, P., & Brown, C. (January, 2003). Randomised controlled trial of therapeutic massage in the management of stress. *British Journal of General Practice, 20*–25.

Harris, W. S., Gowda, M., Kolb, J. W., Strychacz, C. P., Vacek, J. L., Jones, P. G. et al. (1999). A randomized, controlled trial of the effects of remote, intercessory prayer on outcomes in patients admitted to the coronary care unit. *Archives of Internal Medicine, 159*(19), 2273–2278.

Hendricks, M. (2007). Nursing the whole patient [Electronic version]. *John Hopkins Nursing Magazine, V*(1), Retrieved January 18, 2008, from *www.son.jhmi.edu/jhnmagazine/ spring2007/pages/fea_nrsgwholept.htm.*

Herman, P. M., D'Huyvetter, K., & Mohler, M. J. (2006). Are health services research methods a match for CAM? *Alternative*

Therapies in Health and Medicine, 12(3), 78–83.

Horrigan, B. (2003). Ken Cohen, MA, MSTH. Healing through ancient traditions: Qigong and Native American medicine (Interview). *Alternative Therapies in Health and Medicine, 9*(3), 83–91.

Hover-Kramer, D. (1995). *Healing touch: A resource for health care professionals.* Albany, NY: Delmar.

Huth, M. M., Zink, K. A., & Van Horn, N. R. (2005). The effects of massage therapy in improving outcomes for youth with cystic fibrosis: An evidence review. *Pediatric Nursing, 31*(4), 328–332.

Iyengar, B. K. S. (2005). *Light on life: The yoga journey to wholeness, inner peace, and ultimate freedom.* Emmaus, PA: Rodale.

Jacobs, B., Avins, A., Epel, E., Acree, M., Maurer, S., et al. (2006). Iyengar yoga for the treatment of chronic low back pain: A randomized controlled pilot study [Abstract]. *Alternative Therapies in Health and Medicine, 12*(3), 52.

Jain, S., Shapiro, S., Swanick, S., Roesch, S. C., Mills, P. J., Bell, I., et al. (2007). A randomized controlled trial of mindfulness meditation versus relaxation training: Effects on distress, positive states of mind, rumination, and distraction. *Annals of Behavioral Medicine, 33*(1), 11–21.

Kendall, M. (2007). Ancient wisdom, modern care. *Advance for Nurses, 13*, 24.

Krieger, D. (1979). *The therapeutic touch: How to use your hands to help or to heal.* New York: Simon & Schuster.

Krieger, D. (1993). *Accepting your power to heal: The personal practice of therapeutic touch.* Santa Fe, NM: Bear & Company.

Krieger, D. (1998). Healing with therapeutic touch (Interview). *Alternative Therapies in Health and Medicine, 4*(1), 87–92.

Krucoff, M. W., Crater, S. W., Gallup, D., Blankenship, J. C., Cuffe, M., Guarneri, M., et al. (July, 2005). Music, imagery, touch, and prayer as adjuncts to interventional cardiac care: The Monitoring and Actualisation of Noetic Trainings (MANTRA) II randomised study. *The Lancet, 366*, 211–217.

Kujawa, J., Talar, J., Gworys, K., Gworys, P., Pieszynski, I., & Janiszewski, M. (2004). The analgesic effectiveness of laser therapy in patients with gonarthrosis: An evaluation. *Ortopedia, Traumatologie, Rehabilitacja, 6*(3), 356–366.

Laidlaw, T. M., Naito, A., Dwivedi, P., Hansi, N. K., Henderson, D. C. & Gruzelier, J. H. (2006). The influence of 10 min of the Johrei healing method on laboratory stress. *Complementary Therapies in Medicine, 14*(2), 127–132.

Lam, R. W., Levitt, A. J., Levitan, R. D., Enns, M. W., Morehouse, R., Michalak, E. E., et al. (2006). The Can-SAD study: A randomized controlled trial of the effectiveness of light therapy and fluoxetine in patients with winter seasonal affective disorder.

American Journal of Psychiatry, 163(5), 805–812.

Larden, C. N., Palmer, M. L., & Janssen, P. (2004). Efficacy of therapeutic touch in treating pregnant inpatients who have a chemical dependency. *Journal of Holistic Nursing, 22*(4), 320–332.

Lawler, S. P., & Cameron, L. D. (2006). A randomized, controlled trial of massage therapy as a treatment for migraine. *Annals of Behavioral Medicine, 32*(1), 50–59.

Lee, M. S., Jang, J., Jang, H., & Moon, S. (2003). Effects of Qi-therapy on blood pressure, pain and psychological symptoms in the elderly: A randomized controlled pilot trial. *Complementary Therapies in Medicine, 11*(3), 159–164.

Lee, M. S., Lee, M. S., Choi, E., & Chung, H. (2003). Effects of Qigong on blood pressure, blood pressure determinants and ventilatory function in middle-aged patients with essential hypertension. *American Journal of Chinese Medicine, 31*(3), 489–497.

Lewandowski, W. A. (2004). Patterning of pain and power with guided imagery. *Nursing Science Quarterly, 17*(3), 233–241.

Maa, S. H., Tsou, T. S., Wang, K. Y., Wang, C. H., Lin, H. C., & Huang, Y. H. (2007). Self-administered acupressure reduces the symptoms that limit daily activities in bronchiectasis patients: Pilot study findings. *Journal of Clinical Nursing, 16*(4), 794–804.

Maharishi Vedic Education Development Corporation. (2007). *The Transcendental Meditation Program*. Retrieved January 18, 2008, from *www.tm.org*.

Masters, K. S., & Spielmans, G. I. (2007). Prayer and health: Review, meta-analysis, and research agenda. *Journal of Behavioral Medicine, 30*, 329–338.

McIver, S., O'Halloran, P., & McGartland, M. (2004). The impact of Hatha yoga on smoking behavior. *Alternative Therapies in Health & Medicine, 10*(2), 22–23.

McNamara, M. E., Burnham, D. C., Smith, C., & Carroll, D. L. (2003). The effects of back massage before diagnostic cardiac catheterization. *Alternative Therapies in Health and Medicine, 9*(1), 50–57.

McRee, L. D., Noble, S., & Pasvogel, A. (2003). Using massage and music therapy to improve postoperative outcomes. *AORN Journal, 78*(3), 433–442.

Mehling, W. E., Jacobs, B., Acree, M., Wilson, L., Bostrom, A., West, J., et al. (2007). Symptom management with massage and acupuncture in postoperative cancer patients: A randomized controlled trial. *Journal of Pain and Symptom Management, 33*(3), 258–266.

Morone, N. E., & Greco, C. M. (2007). Mind-body interventions for chronic pain in older adults: A structured review. *Pain Medicine, 8*(4), 359–375.

Newshan, G., & Schuller-Civitella, D. (2003). Large clinical study shows value of

therapeutic touch program. *Holistic Nursing Practice, 17*(4), 189–192.

Olson, K., Hanson, J., & Michaud, M. (2003). A phase II trial of Reiki for the management of pain in advanced cancer patients. *Journal of Pain and Symptom Management, 26*(5), 990–997.

Ornish, D. (1990). *Dr. Dean Ornish's program for reversing heart disease*. New York: Ballantine.

Paul-Labrador, M., Polk, D., Dwyer, J. H., Velasquez, I., Nidich, S., Rainforth, M., et al. (2006). Effects of a randomized controlled trial of transcendental meditation on components of the metabolic syndrome in subjects with coronary heart disease. *Archives of Internal Medicine, 166*, 1218–1224.

Pierce, B. (2007). The use of biofield therapies in cancer care. *Clinical Journal of Oncology Nursing, 11*(2), 253–258.

Pippa, L., Manzoli, L., Corti, I., Congedo, G., Romanazzi, L., & Parruti, G. (2007). Functional capacity after traditional Chinese medicine (Qi Gong) training in patients with chronic atrial fibrillation: A randomized controlled trial. *Preventive Cardiology, 10*(1), 22–25.

Reed, T. (2007). Imagery in the clinical setting: A tool for healing. *Nursing Clinics of North America, 42*, 261–277.

Repar, P. A., & Patton, D. (2007). Stress reduction for nurses through Arts-In-Medicine at the University of New Mexico Hospitals. *Holistic Nursing Practice, 21*(4), 182–186.

Richardson, S. (2003). Effects of relaxation and imagery on the sleep of critically ill adults. *Dimensions of Critical Care Nursing, 22*(4), 182–190.

Robert-McComb, J. J., Tacon, A., Randolph, P., & Caldera, Y. (2004). A pilot study to examine the effects of a mindfulness-based stress-reduction and relaxation program on levels of stress hormones, physical functioning, and submaximal exercise responses. *The Journal of Alternative and Complementary Medicine, 10*(5), 819–827.

Sendelbach, S. E., Halm, M. A., Doran, K. A., Miller, E. H., & Gaillard, P. (2006). Effects of music therapy on physiological and psychological outcomes for patients undergoing cardiac surgery. *Journal of Cardiovascular Nursing, 21*(3), 194–200.

Shaw, V. (2007). Complementary and alternative therapies. In S. M. Lewis, M. M. Heitkemper, S. R. Dirksen, P. G. O'Brien, & L. Bucher (Eds.), *Medical-surgical nursing: Assessment and management of clinical problems* (7th ed., pp. 94–109). St. Louis: Mosby.

Shin, B. C., & Lee, M. S. (2007). Effects of aromatherapy acupressure on hemiplegic shoulder pain and motor power in stroke patients: A pilot study. *Journal of Alternative and Complementary Medicine, 13*(2), 247–251.

Siedliecki, S. L., & Good, M. (2006). Effect of music on power, pain, depression and

disability. *Journal of Advanced Nursing, 54*(5), 553–562.

Sivananda, S. S. (2005). *Practice of yoga* (8th ed.). Shivanandanagar, India: The Divine Life Society.

Smeeding, S., & Osguthorpe, S. (2005). The development of an integrative healthcare model in the Salt Lake City Veterans Affairs Healthcare System. *Alternative Therapies in Health and Medicine, 11*(6), 46–51.

Soden, K., Vincent, K., Craske, S., Lucas, C., & Ashley, S. (2004). A randomized controlled trial of aromatherapy massage in a hospice setting. *Palliative Medicine, 18*(2), 87–92.

Srinivasan, V., Smits, M., Spence, W., Lowe, A. D., Kayumov, L., Pandi-Perumal, S. R., et al. (2006). Melatonin in mood disorders. *World Journal of Biological Psychiatry, 7*(3), 138–151.

Stevens, J. A., & Stoykov, M. E. (2003). Using motor imagery in the rehabilitation of hemiparesis. *Archives of Physical Medicine and Rehabilitation, 84*(7), 1090–1092.

Stone, N. J. (2003). Environmental view and color for a simulated telemarketing task. *Journal of Environmental Psychology, 23*, 63–78.

Streeter, C. C., Jensen, J. E., Perlmutter, R. M., Cabral, H. J., Tian, H., Terhune, D. B., et al. (2007). Yoga Asana sessions increase brain GABA levels: A pilot study. *The Journal of Alternative and Complementary Medicine, 13*(4), 419–426.

The Church of Christ, Scientist. (2007). About Christian Science. Retrieved September 3, 2007 from *www.tfccs.com/aboutchristianscience/index.jhtml*.

Thomas, L. A. (2003). Clinical management of stressors perceived by patients on mechanical ventilation. *AACN Clinical Issues, 14*(1), 73–81.

Thorgrimsen, L., Spector, A., Wiles, A., & Orrell, M. (2004). Aroma therapy for dementia (Cochrane Review). In *The Cochrane Library*, Issue 3. Chichester, UK: John Wiley & Sons.

Tian, X., & Krishnan, S. (2006). Efficacy of auricular acupressure as an adjuvant therapy in substance abuse treatment: A pilot study. *Alternative Therapies in Health and Medicine, 12*(1), 66–69.

Tigunait, P. R. (2003, Nov.). Dialogue with Pandit Rajmani Tigunait. *Yoga International, 74*, 30–34.

Toth, M., Wolsko, P. M., Foreman, J., Davis, R. B., Delbanco, T., & Philllips, R. S. (2006). A pilot study for a randomized, controlled trial on the effect of guided imagery in hospitalized medical patients [Letter to the editor]. *Journal of Alternative and Complementary Medicine, 13*(2), 194–197.

Tsai, J. C., Wang, W. H., Chan, P., Lin, L. J., Wang, C. H., Tomlinson, B., et al. (2003). The beneficial effects of Tai Chi Chuan on blood pressure and lipid profile and anxiety status in a randomized controlled trial.

Journal of Alternative & Complementary Medicine, 9(5), 747–754.

Ulrich, G., Houtmans, T., & Gold, C. (2007). The additional therapeutic effect of group music therapy for schizophrenic patients: A randomized study. *Acta Psychiatica Scandinavica, 116,* 362–370.

U.S. Department of Health and Human Services. Office of Disease Prevention and Health Promotion. (2007). *Midcourse review: Healthy People 2010.* Retrieved January 21, 2008, from *www.healthypeople. gov/data/midcourse/html/default.htm.*

Van Elslander Cancer Center. (2007). *Services.* Retrieved October 21, 2007, from *www.stjohn.org/VanElslander.*

Ventegodt, S., Anderson, N. J., & Merrick, J. (2003). Quality of life philosophy I. Quality of life, happiness, and meaning in life. *The Scientific World Journal, 3,* 1164–1175.

Vitale, A. T., & O'Connor, P. C. (2006). The effect of Reiki on pain and anxiety in women with abdominal hysterectomies: A quasi-experimental pilot study. *Holistic Nursing Practice, 20*(6), 263–272.

Wang, C., Collet, J. P., & Lau, J. (2004). The effect of Tai Chi on health outcomes in patients with chronic conditions: A systematic review. *Archives of Internal Medicine, 164,* 493–501.

Wardell, D. W., & Weymouth, K. F. (2004). Review of studies of healing touch. *Image: The Journal of Nursing Scholarship, 36*(2), 147–154.

Whelan, K. M., & Wishnia, G. S. (2003). Reiki therapy: The benefits to a nurse/Reiki practitioner. *Holistic Nursing Practice, 17*(4), 209–217.

Witt, C., Brinkhaus, B., Jena, S., Linde, K., Streng, A., Wagenpfeil, S., et al. (July, 2005). Acupuncture in patients with osteoarthritis of the knee: A randomised trial. *The Lancet, 366,* 136–143.

Woodwinds Health Campus. (n.d.) *Healing arts therapy.* Retrieved on August 29, 2007, from *www.woodwinds.org/CareService/ 4_Healing_Arts/index.cfm.*

Woolery, A., Myers, H., Sternlieb, B., & Zeltzer, L. (2004). A yoga intervention for young adults with elevated symptoms of depression. *Alternative Therapies in Health & Medicine, 10*(2), 60–63.

Wright, B. W. (2007). The evolution of Rogers' science of unitary human beings: 21st century reflections. *Nursing Science Quarterly, 20*(1), 64–67.

Wynn, C. (2006). *Simply reflexology.* Heatherton Victoria, AU: Hinkler Books.

Yogendra, J., Yogendra, H. J., Ambardekar, S., Shetty, S., Dave, M., Lele, R. D., et al. (April, 2004). Beneficial effects of yoga lifestyle on reversibility of ischaemic heart disease: Caring heart project of International Board of Yoga. *Journal of Association of Physicians of India, 52,* 283–289.

Unit Four

Application of Health Promotion

15

Martha Driessnack*

Overview of Growth and Development Framework

objectives

After completing this chapter, the reader will be able to:

- Explain the importance of growth and development as a framework for assessing and promoting health.
- Define the terms growth, development, and maturation.
- Discuss factors that influence growth, in an individual.
- Describe Erikson's theory of psychosocial development.
- Contrast Piaget's and Vygotsky's theories of cognitive development.
- Compare Kohlberg's and Gilligan's theories of moral development.

key terms

Denver Developmental Screening Test
Development
Developmental patterns
Erikson's theory of psychosocial development
Gilligan's theory of moral development

Growth
Growth charts
Growth patterns
Kohlberg's theory of moral development
Learning
Maturation

Piaget's theory of cognitive development
Scaffolding
Vygotsky's theory of cognitive development
Zone of proximal development

website materials

evolve These materials are located on the book's Website at *http://evolve.elsevier.com/Edelman/.*
- WebLinks
- Study Questions
- Glossary

*The author acknowledges the work of Marinda Allender in a prior edition of the chapter.

THINK About It

Vaccine Issues and Controversies

A 4½-year-old child begins to scream as the nurse approaches with her "kindergarten shots." Her mother tries to comfort the child, as she turns anxiously to the nurse saying "I've heard shots can be dangerous. No wonder she's frightened. Are they really necessary?"

1. What influence might the mother's anxiety have on the child's behavior?
2. What approaches and information can the nurse have for the mother?
3. What approaches can the nurse take to gain the child's cooperation?

Unit 4 introduces **growth** and **development** as a framework for health assessment and promotion throughout the life span. Understanding human growth and development facilitates nursing assessment of health knowledge and behavior. Further, health education is more effective when the nurse acknowledges and incorporates growth and developmental needs as well as the individual's prior understanding of and beliefs about health and health-related concepts.

This chapter focuses on the study of health promotion at individual developmental levels by exploring basic concepts of growth and development as well as providing an overview of representative theories of development. Each of the following nine chapters provides health assessment and promotion strategies appropriate for selected age groups across the life span. The age groups described are prenatal; infant; toddler; preschool child; school-age child; adolescent; and young, middle, and older adult (Table 15-1).

OVERVIEW OF GROWTH AND DEVELOPMENT

Understanding of growth and development has continued to expand with advances in science. Today we find ourselves at the intersection of the genomic era and the age of technology. We are only just beginning to appreciate the long-term impact of early interactions on later health and health-related behavior.

Individuals continue to evolve throughout the lifespan, and developmental transitions occur beyond childhood and adolescence, extending into the young, middle, and older adult years. Today, aging adults are receiving increased attention as the average life expectancy increases and adults over 85 years old become the fastest growing age group, providing new challenges for health assessment and promotion.

Growth

Growth refers to a quantifiable change in structure. In the body, this change means an increase in the number and/or size of the cells, resulting in an increase in the size and weight of the whole, or any of its parts. During childhood, physical changes in height, weight, and head circumference, or growth parameters, are measured and charted regularly. While growth refers to these obvious changes to the whole individual, it also refers to the increases (and as we age, decreases) in the size of specific organs and systems. The health history and physical assessment of an individual should include all body systems, but should also emphasize systems undergoing the most change. Table 15-2 outlines growth as it takes place throughout the body systems and life span. The growth of some systems, such as the skeletal and muscular systems, is influenced by gender, whereas the growth of others, such as the nervous and respiratory

Text continued on p. 370

Growth and Development | Table 15-1

Overview of Developmental Periods

Period	Age	Characteristics
Infant	0 to 12 months	Fully dependent on others for basic needs Ends as infant begins to explore environment, walking alone, and develops basic communication skills
Toddler	12 months to 3 years	Motor development progresses significantly Child achieves a degree of physical and emotional autonomy while maintaining a close identity with the primary family unit
Preschool child	3 to 6 years	Child has increased interest and involvement with peers and may have social interactions with many people
School-age child	6 to 10 years	Marked by entrance into elementary school Interests turn away from family toward peers
Adolescent	11 to 18 years	A period of transition, adjustment, and personal exploration Ends when adolescent demonstrates readiness to assume full adult responsibilities of financial, emotional, and social independence
Young adult	18 to 35 years	Getting started in an occupation or career, finding and learning how to live with a partner, and starting and rearing a family
Middle adult	35 to 65 years	Being established in a marriage, an occupation or career, and a community May continue to be a time of transition Adjusts to physiological changes of middle age
Older adult	Over 65 years	May be a time of continued involvement in work and active socializing Adjusts to decreased physical strength and health; retirement; reduced income; decreasing independence; and deaths of spouses, friends, and self

Growth and Development | **Table 15-2**

Flowchart Showing Directions of Growth Changes Throughout Life Cycle*

Overview of Developmental Changes	Prenatal→	Infancy→	Childhood→	Puberty and Adolescence→	Adulthood→	Middle Age→	Old Age
HEART AND CIRCULATORY SYSTEM							
Action of heart and circulatory system is under control of autonomic nervous system. Throughout life cardiac rate is responsive to organ needs and emotional states (fear, anxiety, tension, depression).	Heart formed and begins to beat about third week	Heart grows somewhat more slowly than rest of body (weight doubled by 1 yr, body weight tripled) Grows steadily during childhood With birth, considerable change in paths and relative volumes of blood flow, reflected in loss of certain fetal structures and changes in heart and major vessels		At puberty, heart takes part in rapid growth, reaching mature size with rest of body	Heart weight remains relatively constant after age 25 (only organ other than prostate that does not decrease in weight with age) Cardiac output decreases 30% to 40% between age 25 and 65 Cardiac strength lessens with age, whereas expenditure of energy is more than in youth Capacity to increase rate and strength of beat during physical work is diminished After maturity, women have slightly higher pulse rate than men, 65 beats/min (girls' temperature remains stationary, higher than boys'); men maintain same pulse rate in maturity (slightly lower body temperature than women)		
	Heart rate high, approx. 150 beats/min	Heart rate falls steadily throughout childhood					
		130 beats/min	70 to 80 beats/ min	60 beats/min in adolescence, rate differs with gender			
		Heart rate more variable during childhood—regular Not until middle childhood does peripheral blood picture become same as adult					
URINARY SYSTEM							
Parallels growth as a whole. Proportion of bodily water and solids follows pattern related to growth—tendency for human organism to dry out as life progresses. Function of kidneys, with other organ systems, is to help in regulation of internal environment of body.	Young fetus is about 90% water Urinary system begins in first month	Newborn is about 70% water Urinary system does not complete full development until end of first year All renal units immature at birth; thus fluid and electrolyte imbalance occurs readily Kidney function adequate at birth if not subjected to undue stress	Composition of urine in healthy child (after age 2) changes very little as child matures; thus renal function and urinalysis can be used as monitor of well-being		Adult is about 58% water Glomerular filtration rate decreases about 47% from age 20 to 90		

*This chart indicates only general trends and directions of growth and development; it is not all inclusive. No distinct ages, absolute values, or ranges of normal variations are intended in this flowchart. Modified from the format originally developed in Sutterly, D., & Donneley, G. (1973). *Perspectives in human development: Nursing throughout the life cycle.* Philadelphia: J. B. Lippincott. Modified from Papalia, D.E., Olds, S.W., & Seldmaw, R.D. (2007). *Human Development.* New York: McGraw Hill.
CNS, Central nervous system; GI, gastrointestinal.

Continued

Growth and Development   Table 15-2

Flowchart Showing Directions of Growth Changes Throughout Life Cycle—cont'd

Overview of Developmental Changes	Prenatal→	Infancy→	Childhood→	Puberty and Adolescence→	Adulthood→	Middle Age→	Old Age
DIGESTIVE SYSTEM							
As a whole, grows as total body grows, although evidence suggests that various parts of gastrointestinal system undergo separate periods of growth, maturity, and senescence.	Before birth nutrients are supplied through placental circulation; digestion and absorption do not occur in the GI tract	Stomach size increases rapidly first months, then grows steadily throughout childhood			All actions of the GI tract (food intake, digestion, absorption, elimination) not only respond to physiological needs but from birth to old age are sensitive to tensions and anxiety		
		Digestive apparatus immature at birth (food passes through rapidly, reverse peristalsis common) Acidity of gastric juices varies over life span; low during infancy, rises during childhood, plateaus about age 10, rises during puberty Free gastric acid (HCl) more marked in boys		Spurt of growth at puberty	Data suggest generalized atrophy of entire GI tract with advancing age Nutritional needs vary according to individual variation—decreasing metabolism → enzyme production ↓ HCl ↓ stomach volume—tone of large intestine may become impaired until decrease with senescence (also diminished taste)		
SPECIAL SENSES							
Most are well developed at birth, although their association with higher centers comes about gradually during early life and diminishes with advancing age.	Begin very early in embryonic development—3 to 6 wk	Increase rapidly during first 3 mo; reach relative adult proportions by age 2					
		Sense of touch is developed first, then hearing and vision Vision: infant can perceive simple differences in shape but not complex patterns (greater proportion of total growth before birth); various dimensions of vision develop at various ages, eye muscles function at mature level first year, fusion begins 9 mo until 6 yr; refractive power changes over life cycle—hyperopia increases until eyeball reaches adult size (approx. 8 yr), then reverses trend toward emmetropia—postpubertal years—toward myopia until 30 yr when myopia decreases and hyperopia increases					

ADIPOSE TISSUE

Although adipose tissue varies greatly from individual to individual, overall lifetime pattern exists. Fat accumulation varies greatly with body build and constitution. Relationship between caloric intake, amount of exercise, and utilization or accumulation of fat is not yet fully understood but is basis of much interrelated research.

Accumulates rapidly before birth; peak at seventh gestational month. Premature infant may look wrinkled and scrawny because of lack of adipose tissue	Decreases from first to seventh year in both genders	Then begins to increase slowly to puberty. Fat begins to accumulate slowly and continues uninterrupted in girls, producing feminine curves, and accounts for much of weight gain	Some girls slim down after full maturation; many maintain about the same amount of adipose as at puberty	Typically both sexes tend to gain weight in 50s and 60s but do not maintain same body contours of earlier years at same weight (increase deposit on abdomen and hips)	Usually fat stores are lost after seventh decade in both genders. Sharpness in contours, increasingly prominent bony landmarks
Increases rapidly during first 6 mo	(Gender differences are not noted in the body shape of prepubescent children)	Deposition of fat differs in body—amount decreases sharply at time of maximum growth spurt (increased weight caused by increase in muscle mass and bones)	After full maturation, fat accumulation begins→		

LYMPHOID TISSUE

Lymphoid tissue is scattered widely throughout body and includes lymph nodes, tonsils, adenoids, thymus, spleen, and lymphocytes of the blood; follows unique pattern of growth, rapid in infancy and begins to atrophy at puberty.

Begins during last month of uterine life—cross placenta at levels equal to mother's and remain for several months after delivery	Grows most rapidly during infancy and childhood, reaching maximum size a few years before puberty; parallels development of immunity	Then atrophies and is smaller in volume at full maturity than during childhood
	Thus increased incidence of disease with increasing age of child	Thymus so small that it is difficult to locate in older people

Continued

Growth and Development | **Table 15-2**

Flowchart Showing Directions of Growth Changes Throughout Life Cycle—cont'd

Overview of Developmental Changes	Prenatal→	Infancy→	Childhood→	Puberty and Adolescence→	Adulthood→	Middle Age→	Old Age
RESPIRATORY SYSTEM Growth parallels that of total body growth. Respiratory apparatus is a highly organized system of organs under nervous and hormonal regulation, which functions in coordination with rest of body. Gender difference in gas exchange becomes apparent during puberty.	Before birth, air sacs do not contain air; oxygen supplied through maternal circulation	When umbilical cord is cut, infant must use own breathing apparatus—breathing irregular at first both in rate and depth—fast in infancy—gradually slowing through childhood until maturity is reached		Respiratory exchange gradually becomes more efficient as life advances. Actual volume of air inhaled with each breath increases as lung size expands with general body growth. Vital capacity and maximum breathing capacity rise gradually in both genders, increasing more in boys during puberty; adult men have more efficient respiratory exchange, are capable of greater feats of muscular exertion without exhaustion than women.	No gender difference in respiratory rate at anytime of life	Basal metabolic rate declines (rate higher in men than women)	
SKELETAL SYSTEM Bone growth passes through successive stages of development from connective tissue to cartilage to osseous tissue; completion of calcification indicates end of growing period and is thus a useful measure of growth rate and physiological maturity. Most growth ceases during adolescence.	Follows cephalocaudal law of development 70% of head growth before birth; bones of hands and wrist laid down in cartilage	After first year, legs fastest growing, 66% of total increase in height; longer puberty is delayed, greater the leg length Trunk fastest growing, 60% of total increase		Length of trunk and depth of chest reach peak growth Reserved during growth spurt	Maximum height in early 20s to 30s	Then gradual decline until onset of senescence Thinning of vertebral disks beginning in middle years; most rapid in last decade	

System	Prenatal	Infancy	Childhood	Adolescence/Puberty	Adulthood	Older Adulthood
MUSCLE SYSTEM	Number of striated muscle fibers is roughly same in all human beings. Tremendous difference in size, not only from fetus to adult, but among adults, is caused by ability of individual muscle fibers to increase in size. Muscle formation begins early, assuming final shape by end of second month.	At birth, shafts of metacarpals are ossified (and visible by radiography); carpal bones begin to ossify. Increases rapidly during infancy but slowly during childhood	Growth in both genders is same in childhood. Increase in muscle size means increasing strength in children; increase in skill is more intimately related to maturation of nervous system	With onset of puberty, muscle strength is greater in boys (when muscle growth is stimulated by testosterone). Greatest increase begins in puberty; muscle size precedes muscle strength in boys. Growth of both genders nearly even until onset of puberty in girls first (approx. 10 yr); Boys begin approx. 2 yr later, but markedly greater; Peak in height comes before peak in weight	Muscle mass continues to increase gradually—maximum strength in early adulthood—then declines slightly—according to use and genetic constitution. Will increase in bulk and strength as used until onset of senescence	Spinal column shortens (osteoporosis) with thinning vertebrae—shortening of trunk with long extremities—reversal of growth proportions in infancy. Atrophy and loss of muscle tone
NERVOUS SYSTEM	Growth and maturation of central and peripheral nervous system (brain, cord, peripheral nerves, many sense organs) reflected by changing size of head. Growth very rapid during intrauterine development; head grows at greater rate than rest of body.	Has all the brain cells in first year, which will continue to increase in size; number and complexity of axons, dendrites, and synapses will continue to increase			Function continues with use	Depletion of fully functioning brain cells, whether they are lost, shrink, or lose connections

Continued

Growth and Development   Table 15-2

Flowchart Showing Directions of Growth Changes Throughout Life Cycle—cont'd

Overview of Developmental Changes	Prenatal→	Infancy→	Childhood→	Puberty and Adolescence→	Adulthood→	Middle Age→	Old Age
NERVOUS SYSTEM, CONT'D							
		All neural tissues grow rapidly during infancy and early childhood.		(No neural growth spurt at puberty)			Decrease in myelin sheath, impulses decrease; slow down speed of action and reaction
		Brain grows rapidly after birth, reaching 90% of total size by age 2.	By middle childhood almost reaches adult size	Then slow increase to full maturity	Brain weight decreases with age		
	Segmented spinal nerves are mature, fully myelinated, and functioning at term (e.g., knee jerk), but acquisition of myelin in cortex, brainstem, and cord is closely correlated with observed behavior (myelination of this tract follows cephalocaudal, proximodistal law). Equipment for sense of taste and smell present at birth and perhaps most acute at that time					Taste less acute, less discriminatory with advancing age. Structural changes in CNS result in impaired perception	
REPRODUCTIVE SYSTEM							
Organs of reproductive system show little increase during early life but rapid development just before and coincident with puberty. Maturation and fulfillment of reproductive functions of maturity (in female) are followed by involution in later years.	Genital organs form during uterine life; uterus undergoes growth spurt before birth (hormonal stimulation from mother).	Female sex organs well formed but not functioning at birth (but have full quota of sensory nerves)	Quiescent during childhood →	Maturation at puberty (menstruation) →			Involution after menopause
		Uterus undergoes involution to half its birth weight. In male—testes, as with ovaries, remain dormant and small, not even growing in proportion to rest of body (with sensory nerves)	Regained size by age 10 to 11 →. Until puberty, interstitial cells of Leydig reappear and secrete testosterone, so testes and penis continue to increase in size; pubic hair appears	Adult size at puberty→		Maximum increase with pregnancy →	Begin to atrophy with advancing age

System	Prenatal	Infancy (birth)	Childhood	Adolescence (puberty)	Adulthood	Old age
INTEGUMENTARY SYSTEM Includes skin and its appendages and adnexa (nails, hair, sebaceous glands, eccrine and apocrine sweat glands). Although all skin is similar, this organ shows considerable variability in different parts of body (and from individual to individual) and varies greatly during the life span.	Mammary glands develop in both sexes during fetal life. Sex hormones: until puberty girls and boys produce male hormones (androgens) and female hormones (chiefly estrogens) in small and roughly equal amounts	Enlargement of breasts at birth (both sexes)→	Nonsecretory during childhood until puberty→	Development rapid→	Enlarge during pregnancy, developing alveoli→	Atrophy with advanced age
	Hair, skin, and sebaceous glands fully formed in utero	Skin contains all its adult structures at birth but immature in function	Matures slowly until puberty (children prone to rashes)	Rapid spurt in maturation of skin and all its structures		Changes in skin most obvious sign of aging (exposure and environmental conditions)
	Lanugo begins to decrease before birth and continues regression few weeks postnatally→			Replaced by body hair, less extensive distribution; marked difference in type and distribution of hair at puberty→		Regenerative and growth power decreases and skin loses elasticity
		Activity of sebaceous glands decreases after birth→		Increases rapidly at puberty (more prone to acne)		
ENDOCRINE SYSTEM Consists of number of glandular structures scattered throughout the body. Although small in size, their hormones influence all growth and development of whole organism.	Immaturity of entire endocrine system puts infant at disadvantage if required to adjust to wide fluctuations in concentration of water, electrolytes, glucose, amino acids. All are interrelated, but each organ develops at own rate: Thyroid—increases from midfetal life to maturity; slightly larger in boys than girls; growth spurt at adolescence Adrenals—after birth decrease in size and continue throughout first year, increase again during childhood (but smaller than birth); spurt at puberty, reaching maturity with rest of body; greater increase in male gonads and testes and female ovaries (endocrine glands as well as reproductive organs), follow genital type of growth pattern Hypophysis, or pituitary gland—produces or stimulates hormones that influence growth Parathyroid—produce hormones that maintain homeostasis of calcium and phosphorus Islets of Langerhans—dispersed through pancreas; produce insulin and glucagon					With age, decline occurs in all endocrine gland functions

MULTICULTURAL AWARENESS

Childhood Lead Poisoning in Hispanic Children

While the U.S. has made tremendous progress in eliminating some of the more significant sources of lead (lead paint was banned in 1978; the use of leaded gasoline was phased out during the early 1990s), lead poisoning remains a significant threat to today's children. Chronic low-level lead exposure results in learning disabilities, impaired growth, poor eye-hand coordination, antisocial behavior, dental decay, and hearing loss. The National Safety Council (NSC) emphasizes that, while lead exposure continues to affect large numbers of children, lead poisoning is a totally preventable disease. During the past two decades, public health and provider efforts have resulted in a 90% decline in the overall number of children affected. However, the risk for children of Hispanic families has remained steady.

In 1997 the Centers for Disease Control and Prevention (CDC, 1997) issued new guidelines for blood lead screening. Children were to be screened if they met any of the following criteria:

1. Receives services from public assistance programs for the poor
2. Lives in an area where more than 27% of the housing was built before 1950
3. Parent or guardian answers yes to any of the following:
   a. Does your child live in or regularly visit a house that was built before 1950?
   b. Does your child live in or regularly visit a house that was built before 1978 with recent or ongoing renovations or remodeling?
   c. Does your child have a sibling or playmate who has or did have lead poisoning?

These screening questions primarily target those children whose exposure is through lead-based paint. However, this is not the primary source of lead exposure for the majority of children in Hispanic families. Food and culturally defined health practices bring additional risk to this population. Foods packaged or canned outside the United States, especially in Mexico or South America; foods cooked, stored, eaten, or drunk using ceramic containers or pottery made outside the United States, especially in Mexico or South America, Mexican or South American raisins, and wrapped Mexican candies (specifically tamarind fruit candies and lollipops), all increase lead exposure (MMWR, 2002).

Empacho, a common Hispanic term for stomach or intestinal upset or obstruction, is often treated with a folk remedy that coincidently is 70% to 90% lead. It is known by many names, including *Alarcon, Azarcon, Coral, Greta, Liga, Maria Luisa,* and *Rueda.* Another common Hispanic folk remedy containing lead is *Pay looah.*

Further, an often-overlooked risk is the use of warm, hot, or boiled tap water from contaminated pipes. Many Hispanics feel that heating the water rids it of contaminants, although any heat mobilizes the lead and makes it easier to absorb. This is also true of pottery that is heated by cooking in it, placing heated fluids in it, or heating it in the microwave. While typical instruction pamphlets teach that tap water should be run for a full minute before it is consumed, it fails to state that the water consumed should come from the cold tap if it is to be consumed.

When screening for lead poisoning in Hispanic children, the nurse remembers to include questions about the use of folk remedies, pottery, imported foods and candies, as well as the use of boiled or hot tap water. In addition, the nurse should include dietary education that encourages decreasing fat intake, because lead is retained in fat, and increasing vitamin C, calcium, and iron intake, all of which reduce the amount of lead in the body.

For more information about the health effects of lead on children, how to identify children with elevated lead levels, or obtain a lead dust test kit, visit the following websites:

National Safety Council (NSC)
www.nsc.org/resources/issues/lead.aspx
Centers for Disease Control and Prevention: General Lead Information
www.cdc.gov/nceh/lead/faq/about.htm
Environmental Protection Agency: Protect Your Child From Lead Poisoning
www.epa.gov/lead
Environmental Protection Agency: Eliminating Child Lead Poisoning
http://yosemite.epa.gov/OCHP/OCHPWEB.nsf/content/leadhaz.htm/$file/leadhaz.pdf
Mayo Clinic: Lead Poisoning
www.mayoclinic.com/health/lead-poisoning/FL00068

---

systems, is independent of gender. Changes that take place in young, middle-aged, and older adults should be noted. People who think of growth only as it applies to infants, children, and adolescents are missing important changes from conception throughout adulthood.

Influences on an individual's potential for growth include genetic factors, prenatal and postnatal exposures, nutrition, and environmental factors (see the Case Study and Care Plan at the end of this chapter). Other influences include emotional health as well as ethnic and cultural practices that influence child-rearing, life style, and health care practices (Multicultural Awareness box). Although growth potential is primarily determined by individual genetics, health and environmental exposures influence the attainment of that potential. The timing of exposure to environmental hazards may determine to a great extent the amount and

kind of effects of these influences. For example, if a pregnant mother is exposed to the rubella virus, the developing fetus is much more vulnerable than either the mother or an older child, especially during the first trimester, when all organs systems are in a stage of rapid growth and development. Teens who fracture a limb at the bone's growth plate are also more affected than older teens and young adults who have completed their growth spurt.

Growth Patterns

Expected **growth patterns** exist for all people. Growth is not steady throughout life. The periods of extremely rapid growth—prenatal, infancy, and adolescence—are contrasted with slower rates of growth during the toddler, preschool, and school-age periods. Infants typically double their birth weight by 6 months of age and triple their birth weight by

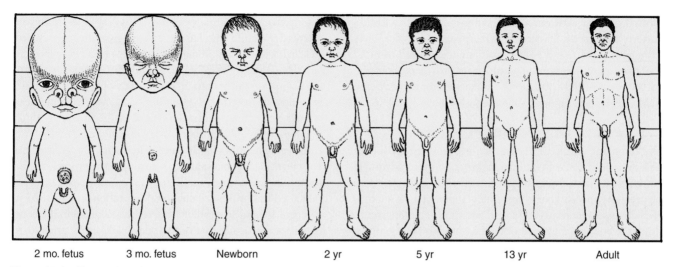

Figure 15-1 Changes in body proportions from birth to adulthood. (Redrawn from Crouch, J. E., & McClintic, J. R. [1976]. *Human anatomy and physiology* [2nd ed.]. New York: John Wiley & Sons.)

1 year of age. The well known "growth spurt" in height typically occurs early in adolescence for girls and later in adolescence for boys.

Different parts of the body increase in size at different rates. For example, during early life the head is the fastest growing section, followed by the trunk, and then the arms and legs. Newborns' heads account for one quarter of their overall length, as opposed to adults' heads which account for one ninth of their overall height. The changes in proportion of body parts from infancy to adulthood are demonstrated in Figure 15-1.

Growth Charts

Growth is one of the most important indications of a child's overall health and well-being. Accurate growth assessment depends on precise measurement of growth parameters using proper equipment, correct and consistent techniques, careful plotting of measurements, and thoughtful interpretation of the data (Winch, 2002).

The Centers for Disease Control and Prevention (CDC) **growth charts**, released in May 2000, consist of both revised versions of the old growth charts developed by the National Center for Health Statistics (NCHS) in 1977 and the addition of body mass index (BMI)-for-age charts. The BMI is an anthropometric index of weight and height combined with age. These charts are used to identify children and adolescents as underweight, overweight, or at risk of overweight. The CDC recommends that the BMI-for-age charts be used for all children and adolescents 2 to 20 years of age. The revised growth charts are more reflective of ethnic diversity and current feeding practices and also include percentile curves up to 20 years of age, as well as the addition of a 3rd and 97th percentile (Winch, 2002). See the Research Highlights box for more details on the changes.

A single measurement, although helpful, does not allow for the best assessment of a child's growth. Serial measurements,

research highlights

New Centers for Disease Control and Prevention Growth Charts

In a policy statement issued in 2003, the American Academy of Pediatrics outlined the need for widespread, comprehensive prevention efforts to address the increased prevalence of overweight in children and adolescents, identifying the sequential assessment of Body Mass Index (BMI) as an important strategy in addressing the problem. The CDC growth charts (2000) consist of revised growth charts and the newly introduced BMI-for-age charts. Use of BMI-for-age allows significant changes in growth patterns to be recognized and addressed before children become severely overweight. It also facilitates anticipatory guidance for children and adolescents at risk of overweight or for those who are underweight.

An appropriate reference population, accurate measurements, and age calculations are important factors when assessing childhood growth. Comparing body measurements with the appropriate age-specific and gender-specific growth chart enables pediatric health care providers to monitor growth and identify potential problems related to health or nutrition. When the 1977 National Center for Health Statistics growth charts were developed, they were based on a sample consisting primarily of White, middle-class, formula-fed infants and children from southwestern Ohio. The new charts, on the other hand, are based on data that include a nationally referenced population reflective of age, sex, and racial and ethnic composition, as well as breast-fed and formula-fed infants.

The new CDC growth charts furnish health care providers and researchers with an improved tool to assess and track the growth of infants, children, and adolescents up to 20 years of age. They provide one set of growth charts for all racial and ethnic groups that can be used for both breast-fed and formula-fed infants. Condition-specific growth charts are also available for children with special health care needs such as Turner syndrome, achondroplasia, Down syndrome, Marfan syndrome, sickle cell anemia, and myelomeningocele. All growth charts and instructions for their use are available at the CDC website (*www.cdc.gov/growthcharts*).

plotted on a growth chart over time, best reflect a child's pattern of growth. Slowed growth, plateaus, or decreases in height, weight, and head circumference, as well as rapid increases, raise questions for health care providers about the adequacy of a child's nutritional intake, syndromes or disease states, neglect, or emotional problems (Winch, 2002).

Concept of Development

Development refers to gradual change and expansion of ability and advance in skill from lower to more-advanced complexity. In contrast to growth, which is a quantitative or precisely measurable change, development is a qualitative change. Qualitative changes are more challenging to describe, because they cannot be measured in precise units. Development has best been conceptualized as a process that can be assessed as it follows certain sequencing or patterns, although the timing of this advancement is individual.

Developmental Patterns

All individuals follow similar **developmental patterns**, with one stage of development building on and leading to the next. Early development proceeds as follows:

Pattern of Development:
1. Cephalocaudal: head to toe
2. Proximodistal: midline to periphery
3. Differentiation: simple to complex; general to specific

Examples:
1. Infants gain neck and head control before controlling the movements of the extremities.
2. Infant central nervous systems develop before the peripheral nervous system.
3. Infants use a whole-hand grasp before learning the finer control of the pincer grasp, and they coo or babble before they speak.

Although the sequence of development is predictable, the exact timing of the sequencing is individual. Individuals develop at their own rate, on their own schedule. For example, infants creep and crawl before they walk and their primary teeth erupt in a predictable sequence, but each will walk and teethe on an individual schedule. However, there are guidelines or parameters that assist parents and health care providers in assessing whether children are progressing in an acceptable developmental sequence within a reasonable time frame. Areas of assessment usually focus on personal and social, gross and fine motor, and language development. The **Denver Developmental Screening Test**, which was revised in 1992 (now known as Denver II), is a screening tool that assists health care providers in monitoring children's development in each of these areas from birth to 6 years of age. The Denver II is presented in **Website Resource 17A.**

Social expectations can influence developmental tasks with expectations that an individual achieve certain landmarks during each period of development. However, the age at which a child is expected to master certain developmental tasks is determined partly by cultural expectations. Some cultures are comfortable with breast-feeding their children well into childhood, while others expect the transition to self-feeding with a cup much earlier. When assessing a child's abilities, nurses are aware that a child who has never been given the opportunity to learn or master a skill may be developmentally capable, but fails when tested. For example, a child who is capable of learning colors or numbers can do so only if taught, just as the child who was breast-fed well into childhood, never having been offered a cup, may well be developmentally capable of drinking from a cup but probably will fail at early tries.

Development is closely interrelated with the concepts of both learning and maturation. **Learning** is the process of gaining specific knowledge or skills that results from exposure, experience, education, and evaluation. **Maturation** is an increase in competence and adaptability that reflects changes in the complexity of a structure that make it possible for that structure to begin to function or to function at a higher level. Maturation of a structure, system, or individual refers to the emergence of the genetic potential of that structure, system, or individual. Learning cannot occur unless the individual is mature enough to understand and control behavior. Children can be toilet trained only when their bodies have matured to the point of developing internal and external sphincter control. Earlier attempts will be frustrating for both child and parent.

Growth and development are complex, interrelated processes that are influenced by and, in turn, influence the health of an individual. The nurse who understands this relationship is aware of the need for age-specific health assessment and promotion strategies (Health Teaching box).

HEALTH TEACHING Anticipatory Guidance

The nurse is often in a position to provide anticipatory guidance to parents, which involves teaching them ways to handle a situation before it becomes an issue or problem. Knowledge of normal growth and development provides a foundation for this teaching. For example, the toddler period is one of intense exploration of the environment, when locomotion is the major gross motor skill acquired. The nurse, knowing the number one cause of death in toddlers is accidents, provides the following teaching to the parents of a child who is entering the toddler period:
- Always use a federally approved car restraint and check for proper installation and placement.
- Supervise child closely near any source of water, including buckets, bathtubs, and toilets.
- Turn pot handles toward the back of the stove and use the back burners whenever possible.
- Place all toxic substances in a locked cabinet and have the poison control contact number easily accessible. Avoid the use of syrup of ipecac unless advised by a poison control representative to do so.
- Move toddler from the crib to a bed.
- Provide barriers on open windows.
- Decrease the water heater temperature to avoid scald burns from tap water.
- Avoid foods that pose a choking hazard such as nuts, hard candies, raisins, fresh carrots, whole grapes, chewing gum, hot dogs, and fish with bones.

THEORIES OF DEVELOPMENT

Specific aspects of development of the person have been studied for centuries. Many theories of development are used in the study of individuals throughout the life span; the nurse may wish to refer to a text on developmental psychology to become familiar with some of these theories. Five theories are introduced in this unit to gain a holistic view of the progression of individual development throughout the life span. These theories were originally developed by Erikson, Piaget, Vygotsky, Kohlberg, and Gilligan.

Psychosocial Development: Erikson's Theory

Erik Erikson described the development of identity of the self through successive stages that unfold throughout the life span (Erikson, 1968, 1995; Erikson & Erikson, 1998). Although he studied with Freud and supported the psychosexual theory of development, **Erikson's theory of psychosocial development** is based on the need of each person to develop a sense of trust in self and others and a sense of personal worth. Erikson described a healthy personality in positive terms, not merely through the absence of disease.

Psychosocial development is based on critical stages, each requiring resolution of a conflict between two opposing forces (e.g., intimacy vs. isolation). Each stage depends on the stage before it and must be accomplished successfully for the person to proceed. Erikson's use of a psychosocial framework acknowledges the influence of other people and the environment but maintains that it is ultimately the individual who must master each of the conflicts. Although each of the conflicts is predominant at a certain stage in life, it is important to recognize that all the conflicts exist in each person, to some extent, at all times and that a conflict, once resolved, may emerge again in appropriate situations. These stages are summarized in Table 15-3 and discussed more fully in the chapters on each developmental age group. See the Case Study at the end of this chapter about an infant girl and how hospitalization could affect her psychosocial development.

Cognitive Development

Another aspect of development is cognitive development. Jean Piaget, a Swiss psychologist, also trained in biology and philosophy, is well known for his theory of cognitive development. He viewed children as biological organisms interacting with their environment, and his theory contends that cognitive development reflects children's attempts to make sense of their worlds. The major criticism of his work is that he underestimated children's capabilities and gave little or no consideration for cultural differences. Lev Vygotsky, a Russian contemporary, was also trained in both the physical sciences and psychology. He presented his theory of cognitive development stating that a child's development could not be separated from the social and cultural context in which it occurs. He also credited children with more innate

Growth and Development	Table 15-3	
Erikson's Eight Stages of Human Development		
Age Group	Psychosocial Stage	Lasting Outcomes
1. Infancy	Basic trust versus basic mistrust	Faith and hope
2. Toddler stage	Autonomy versus shame and doubt	Self-control and willpower
3. Preschool stage	Initiative versus guilt	Direction and purpose
4. School age	Industry versus inferiority	Method and competence
5. Adolescence	Identity versus role confusion	Devotion and fidelity
6. Young adulthood	Intimacy versus isolation	Affiliation and love
7. Middle adulthood	Generativity versus stagnation	Production and care
8. Older adulthood	Ego integrity versus despair	Renunciation and wisdom

Modified from Erikson, E. H. (1995). *Childhood and society (35th anniversary ed.)*. New York: W. W. Norton; Erikson, E. H., & Erikson, J. M. (1998). *Life cycle completed*. New York: Norton.

ability to learn and emphasized the importance of language (Vygotsky, 1986). Both Piaget and Vygotsky are presented in more detail below.

Cognitive Development: Piaget's Theory

Jean **Piaget's theory of cognitive development** is concerned primarily with structure rather than content, with how the mind works rather than with what it does. Piaget uses the word scheme to describe a pattern of action or thought. A scheme is used to take in or assimilate new experiences or may be modified or accommodated by new experiences. Each person is striving to maintain a balance, or equilibrium, between assimilation and accommodation (Phillips, 1969; Piaget, 1950).

Piaget described the stages of cognitive development throughout the developmental years. Through a natural unfolding of ability, the child acquires sequentially predictable cognitive abilities. Given adequate environmental stimuli and an intact neurological system, the child gradually matures toward full ability to conceptualize. Piaget's theory of cognitive development encompasses the time from birth to approximately 15 years of age. Each of the four distinct stages is summarized in Table 15-4 and discussed more fully in the specific chapters on each developmental age. Piaget suggests that quantitative, but no further qualitative, changes in cognitive function take place after about age 15.

Cognitive Development: Vygotsky's Theory

One of the significant differences between the cognitive theories of Piaget and Vygotsky is that Piaget believed that development preceded learning. Piaget proposed that

Growth and Development	Table 15-4

Piaget's Stages of Cognitive Development

Stage	Age	Characteristics
Sensorimotor	Birth to 2 years	Begins with a predominance and reliance on reflexes that set the body up to learn
		Reflexes decrease and voluntary acts develop
		Imitation predominates
		Thought is dominated by physical manipulation of objects and events
		Develops the concept of object permanence and the ability to form mental representations
Preoperational	2 to 7 years	Advancing use of language and movement
		Development of egocentric, animistic, and magical thinking
		Uses representational thought to interpret and learn, not in terms of general properties, but in terms of the relationship or use to them
		No cause-and-effect reasoning
		Thought is dominated by the senses—what is seen, heard, or experienced
Concrete operations	7 to 11 years	Mental reasoning processes assume logical approaches to solving concrete problems, including cause and effect
		Collecting; mastering facts
		Can consider other points of view
		Thought influenced by social contacts
		Language is perfected
Formal operations	11 to 15 years	True logical thought and manipulation of abstract concepts emerge
		Morality

Modified from Schuster, C., & Ashburn, S. (1992). *The process of human development: A holistic life span approach.* Boston: Lippincott; Piaget, J. & Inhelder, B. (2000). *The psychology of the child.* New York: Basic Books; Piaget J. (1959). *Language and thought of the child.* New York: Routledge.

Growth and Development	Table 15-5

Kohlberg's Stages of Moral Development

Stage	Goal
Preconventional	Avoiding punishment
	Gaining reward
Conventional	Gaining approval
	Avoiding disapproval
Postconventional	Agree upon rights
	Personal moral standards
	Justice

Compiled from Kohlberg, L. (1981). *The philosophy of moral development, Vol. 1.* San Francisco: Harper & Row.

a level of cognitive development must be reached *before* learning could take place. Vygotsky thought that by viewing development and learning in this way, adults will teach to the lowest ability, aiming instruction at those mental functions or intellectual operations that have already matured in the child (Wink & Putney, 2002). In contrast, Vygotsky proposed that learning precedes development (Table 15-5). He states that learning pulls development, which is in stark contrast to Piaget, who felt children were not able to learn something until they were developmentally ready.

Vygotsky argued that, while learning may be similar among children at certain times or phases of development, it is not identical in all children because of their differing social and cultural experiences (Vygotsky, 1978). He felt Piaget overemphasized the intellectual and biological universality of developmental stages. Vygotsky was more interested in the cultural and social influences on learning and development as well as how individual children actively internalize what they learn from others. For Vygotsky, development begins as an interpersonal process of meaning making and then becomes an individualized process of making sense. There are no predetermined levels of development; rather, experience is in the front—leading and expanding development in unlimited ways.

While **Vygotsky's theory of cognitive development** is less known to health care professionals, educators have embraced his theory, especially what he refers to as the zone of proximal development. The **zone of proximal development** is the distance between the actual and potential developmental level (Wink & Putney, 2002). In this zone, children are pulled toward new learning through their interaction with others and the environment. The guidance given by others in this zone is referred to as **scaffolding**. According to Vygotsky, all people need to understand not only how an individual learns and develops but also the social, cultural, and political context in which that learning and development takes place. This difference has the potential for profound impact on how the nurse approaches teaching and learning.

Moral Development: Kohlberg's Theory

One aspect of cognitive development is the development of moral thinking and judgment. Lawrence **Kohlberg's theory of moral development** is based on interviews that focused on hypothetical moral dilemmas such as: Should a man steal an expensive drug that would save his dying wife? From these interviews, Kohlberg developed his theory, which is outlined in Table 15-5 (Kohlberg, 1981; Kohlberg & Kramer, 1969). The three stages of moral development, preconventional, conventional, and post-conventional, are based on Piaget's theory of cognitive development and emphasize an ethic of justice. Progression through the successive stages of moral development generally takes place during the school-age, adolescent, and young-adult years. Beyond the young-adult years, stabilization or increased consistency of thought and perhaps an increased correlation between moral judgment and moral action occurs (Kohlberg, 1981).

Moral Development: Gilligan's Theory

Carol **Gilligan's theory of moral development** (1982, 1993) suggests that there is a different process of moral development in women in society. While a doctoral student, Gilligan did research with Lawrence Kohlberg at Harvard University. She discovered that Kohlberg's original research was conducted using only men and that women often scored lower in Kohlberg's subsequent investigations. She asserted that women were not inferior in their moral development, just different. In developing her own research with female subjects, she proposed her own theory of moral development which, like Kohlberg's, has three stages (Table 15-6). However, Gilligan concluded that the transitions between stages are based on changes in one's sense of self rather than on changes in cognitive development, as Kohlberg proposed. She also reported that women

think more in terms of caring and relationships than men do, who are more inclined to think in terms of rules and justice. The Hot Topics box discusses self-esteem in males versus females.

SUMMARY

Individuals make many choices that affect their health each day, and a number of factors influence how these choices are made. The stage of growth and development, as well as the context in which learning takes place, influences how individuals experience different situations and the choices available to us in them. Knowing theories of the concepts of human growth and development, nurses have a clear understanding of what challenges an individual is likely to encounter as well as what skills the individual is likely to have and/or need for successful growth and development, and maturation throughout the life span. Theories provide nurses with frameworks for health assessment, promotion, and intervention.

Growth and Development Table 15-6		
Gilligan's Stages of Moral Development (for Women)		
Stage	**Characteristics**	**Goal**
Preconventional	What is practical to others and best for self, realizing connection to others	Individual survival
Conventional	Sacrifices wants and needs to fulfill others' wants and needs	Self-sacrifice is goodness
Postconventional	Moral equal of self and others	Principle of nonviolence, do not hurt self or others

Compiled from Gilligan, C. (1982). *In a different voice: Psychological theory and women's development*. Cambridge, MA: Harvard University Press; Gilligan, C., Ward, J. V., & Taylor, J. M. (Eds.) (1990). *Mapping the moral domain: A contribution of women's thinking to psychology and education*. Cambridge, MA: Harvard University Press.

HOTtopics   HOW TO RAISE A GENIUS

It is clear that the American Academy of Pediatrics (AAP) recommendation of *no (television/video) screen time for children younger than 2 years* has not been widely heeded. Recent studies have found that 64% to 100% of infants and toddlers watch TV. Further, popular educational videos, such as the *Baby Einstein* series, have attracted millions of parents eager to provide their babies with an intellectual boost. In a recent study conducted at the University of Washington, 40% of infants are regularly watching educational TV or DVD/videos, and this percentage increases to 90% of regular screen time by 24 months. Only a third of the parents reported watching the shows with their child. This finding is noteworthy in the context that the goal of the content is to promote parent-child interaction. The assumption is that increased stimulation for babies is good and that the more stimulation a baby gets the better. However, the study suggests that these products may be doing more harm than good. The research team found that for every hour each day that infants watched educational DVDs, they understood an average of seven fewer words (10% less) than those babies who did not view them. Previous studies report that infants and toddlers learn faster and better when they are able to interact, rather than just watch and listen. Children who interact with their parents through reading or games showed an increase in language skills.

- How can nurses use the results of this study when teaching parents that face-to-face interaction with their children promotes development more than the children watching TV or videos?
- Could baby videos be producing a generation of overstimulated children?
- Should videos be used in childcare?

Birth of a Disabled/Chronically Ill Child: Avery

Avery is a 33-year-old female who has been trying to become pregnant for a number of years. Now, at 30 weeks gestation, she and her partner just learned that the baby has a congenital malformation called spina bifida with an associated meningomyelocele. As the perinatologist leaves the room, Avery turns to the nurse and starts to cry.

Reflective Questions:

1. What is the nurse's role when parents learn a child has a chronic disease and/or disability?
2. What can the nurse anticipate for these new parents for the remainder of the pregnancy? At the birth of the baby? In the first two weeks after birth? Over the baby's first year of life?
3. How will this child's growth, development, and goals for health promotion be affected? How about those of the parents?
4. What factors might contribute to Avery's development of chronic sorrow?
5. If Avery becomes depressed, how might this affect the growth and development of the new baby?
6. How might the nurse intervene to lessen the effects of chronic sorrow?

CARE PLAN

Birth of a Disabled/Chronically Ill Child: Avery

Nursing Diagnosis: Chronic sorrow (parental) related to missed opportunities and unending care-giving for a new child

Definition: Cyclical, recurring, and potentially progressive pattern of pervasive sadness experienced (by a parent, caregiver, individual with chronic illness or disability) in response to continual loss, throughout the trajectory of an illness or disability.

DEFINING CHARACTERISTICS
- Parental expression of disparity between preconceived notions of parenting and reality.
- Parental expression of an ongoing or recurrent sense of sadness or loss.
- Parental expressions of negative feelings (e.g., anger, depression, disappointment, emptiness, frustration, self-blame, helplessness, hopelessness, loneliness, overwhelmed) that are often triggered by health care crises or conflict with expected social norms for child or family.

RELATED FACTORS
- Change in family structure
- Change in parental role expectation
- Parental coping styles
- Goal: Assist family unit to attain, maintain, or regain optimal health

EXPECTED OUTCOMES
- Grief resolution: *Adjustment to actual or impending loss.* For example: Parents verbalize reality of loss, progress through stages of grief, decreasing preoccupation with loss, verbalize acceptance of loss and resolve feelings about loss.
- Hope: *Optimism that is personally satisfying and life-supporting.* For example: Parents express inner peace, expectation of a positive future.
- Psychosocial adjustment: *Adaptive psychosocial response of an individual to a significant life change.* For example: Parents set realistic goals, maintain productivity, verbalize optimism about present, use effective coping strategies, report feeling socially engaged.

NURSING INTERVENTIONS
- Grief work facilitation: *Helping another cope with painful feelings of actual or perceived responsibility.* For example: Listen to expression of grief, Encourage identification of fears, Assist in identifying needed modifications in lifestyle.
- Hope inspiration: *Enhancing the belief in one's capacity to initiate and sustain actions.* For example: Help identify areas of hope in their lives, Demonstrate hope by recognizing the disability or illness as only one facet of the child, Provide parents opportunities to be involved with support groups, especially with other parents of children who are disabled/chronically ill who have transcended.
- Coping enhancement: *Assisting a person to adapt to perceived stressors, changes, or threats that interfere with meeting life demands and roles.* For example: Provide an atmosphere of acceptance, Seek to understand each parent's perspective of the situation, Appraise and discuss alternate responses to situation, Foster constructive outlets for negative feelings, Assist the parents to identify positive strategies to deal with limitations and mage need lifestyle changes.
- Resiliency promotion: *Assisting individual, families, and communities in development, use, and strengthening of protective factors to be used in coping with environmental and societal stressors.* For example: Encourage positive health-seeking behavior, Facilitate development and use of neighborhood resources.

REFERENCES
Bulechek, G. M., Butcher, H. K., & Dochterman, J. M. (Eds.). (2008). *Nursing interventions classification (NIC).* (5th Ed.) St. Louis: Mosby.

Hobdell, E. (2004). Chronic sorrow and depression in parents of children with neural tube defects. *Journal of Neuroscience Nursing;* 94, 82–88.

Johnson, M., Bulechek, G., Butcher, H., Dochterman, J. M., Maas, M., Moorhead, S., & Swanson, E. (2006). *NANDA, NOC, and NIC linkages.* (2nd Ed). St Louis: Mosby.

Kearney, P. M., & Griffen, T. (2001). Between joy and sorrow: Being parents of a child with developmental disability. *Journal of Advanced Nursing,* 34(5), 582–592.

Langridge, P. (2002). Reduction of chronic sorrow: A health promotion role for children's community nurses. *Journal of Child Health Care,* 6(3), 157–170.

Moorhead, S., Johnson, M., & Maas, M. (Eds.). (2004). *Nursing outcomes classification (NOC).* (3rd Ed.) St. Louis: Mosby.

Neal, M. (Ed.). (2007). *Nursing diagnosis: Definitions & Classification 2007-2008.* NANDA International: Philadelphia.

Russell, F. (2003). The expectations of parents of disabled children. *British Journal of Special Education,* 30(3), 144–149.

REFERENCES

Centers for Disease Control and Prevention. (1997). *Screening young children for lead poisoning.* Atlanta: CDC.

Erikson, E. H. (1968). *Identity. Youth and crisis.* New York: Norton.

Erikson, E. H. (1995). *Childhood and society* (35th anniversary ed.). New York: Norton.

Erikson, E. H., & Erikson, J. M. (1998). *Lifecycle completed.* New York: Norton.

Gilligan, C. (1982). *In a different voice: Psychological theory and women's development.* Cambridge, MA: Harvard University Press.

Gilligan, C., Ward, J. V., & Taylor, J. M. (Eds.). (1993). *Mapping the moral domain: A contribution of women's thinking to psychology theory and education.* Cambridge, MA: Harvard University Press.

Kohlberg, L. (1981). *The philosophy of moral development* (Vol. 1). San Francisco: Harper & Row.

Kohlberg, L., & Kramer, R. (1969). Continuities and discontinuities in childhood and adult moral development. *Human Development, 12,* 93–120.

Lindeke, L., Rogers, S., & Finley, L. (2002). An update on growth charts, old and new. *Pediatric Nursing, 28*(138), 140–141.

MMWR. (2002). Childhood lead poisoning associated with tamarind candy and folk remedies—California, 1999-2000. *MMWR Morbidity and Mortality Weekly Report, 51*(31), 684–686.

Phillips, J. L. (1969). *The origins of intellect: Piaget's theory.* San Francisco: W. H. Freeman.

Piaget, J. (1950). *The psychology of intelligence.* London: Routledge and Kegan Paul.

Taylor, J. M., Gilligan, C., & Sullivan, A. (1997). *Between voice and silence: Women and girls, race and relationship.* Cambridge, MA: Harvard University Press.

Vygotsky, L. S. (1978). *Mind in society: The development of higher psychological processes.* Cambridge, MA: Harvard University Press.

Vygotsky, L. S. (1986). *Thought and language.* Cambridge, MA: MIT Press.

Winch, A. E. (2002). Obtaining accurate growth measurements in children. *Journal for Specialists in Pediatric Nursing, 7*(4), 166–169.

Wink, J., & Putney, L. (2001). *A vision of Vygotsky.* Boston: Allyn & Bacon.

Zimmerman, F. J., Christakis, D. A., & Meltzoff, A. N. (2007). Associations between media viewing and language development in children under age 2 years. *The Journal of Pediatrics, 151*(4), 364–368.

Zimmerman, F. J., Christakis, D. A., & Meltzoff, A. N. (2007). Television and DVD/video viewing in children younger than 2 years. *Archives of Pediatric and Adolescent Medicine, 161,* 473–479.

Susan Scott Ricci

The Prenatal Period

- Differentiate fetal development and the newborn transition to extrauterine life.

- Analyze changes in the maternal system during pregnancy based on their influences on pregnancy adaptation.

- Interpret the role of the nurse in promoting the physical, mental, and spiritual health of the childbearing family.

- Compare fetal problems caused by maternal drinking, smoking, drug use, and viral exposure during pregnancy.

- Outline the nursing role during labor and birth with a focus on the physical, emotional, spiritual, and educational needs of the woman giving birth and her family.

- Analyze the influence of factors such as ethnicity, legislative priorities, and the sociopolitical context of the health care delivery system on prenatal and childbirth care and the needs of families.

key terms

Acquired immunodeficiency syndrome (AIDS)
Amniocentesis
Amniotic membranes
Apgar scoring system
Bacterial vaginosis
Bradycardia
Candida albicans
Chlamydia
Chloasma
Chorionic membranes
Chorionic villi
Colostrum
Conception
Congenital defect
Cytomegalovirus
Dilation
Down syndrome
Effacement of the cervix
Embryo
Endometrium
Estrogen
Fertilization
Fetal alcohol syndrome
Fetal heart monitor

Fetus
First stage of labor
Fourth stage of labor
Fundus
Gestation
Gestational hypertension
Gonococcus
Group B Streptococcus
Hepatitis B
Herpes simplex
Human chorionic gonadotropin
Human immunodeficiency virus (HIV)
Infant mortality rate
Infertility
Labor
Lamaze
Linea nigra
Meconium
Miscarriage
Pica
Placenta
Polyhydramnios
Positive signs of pregnancy

Premature delivery
Probable signs of pregnancy
Progesterone
Quickening
Rh blood group incompatibility
Rubella
Second stage of labor
Sexually transmitted infections (STIs)
Spontaneous abortion
Stages of labor
Station
Stillbirth
Striae gravidarum
Syphilis
Tachycardia
Teratogen
Third stage of labor
Toxoplasmosis
Trimesters
Ultrasound
Zygotic cells

website materials

THINK About It

First Pregnancy Labor

Laura, currently 41 weeks into her first pregnancy, is admitted at 2:00 AM to St. Jude's Medical Center with uterine contractions occurring every 8 minutes since midnight. Her cervix is dilated to 2 cm and is 80% effaced, and station is –3. Her husband is out of town on a business trip, and Laura's neighbor has accompanied her to the hospital. Although Laura attended Lamaze classes with her husband, she is anxious about the labor. She says to the nurse, "My back is about to break, I have so much bottom pressure, and I wanted to go natural, without medication and all this high-technology stuff, including the monitor."

1. Based on your knowledge of ethical and legal principles of care, how would you as a caregiver appropriately respond to Laura's needs with labor and delivery?
2. What factors in Laura's database would support the use of the fetal heart monitor? What factors would not support use of the monitor?
3. What political, legal, ethical, and other factors might be relevant to the wide use of monitors in American maternity units today?
4. How does the use of fetal heart rate monitoring fit into a health-promotion approach to labor and delivery?

The process of **conception**, pregnancy, and birth involves a complex interaction of many factors, including the physiological and psychological changes in the woman and family and the development of a **fetus** into a viable newborn. The focus of this chapter is on the pregnant woman, her family, and the developing fetus; discussing one without the others is impossible. The nurse must consider all three entities when seeking to promote a healthy pregnancy and healthy family system after birth.

PHYSICAL CHANGES IN MATERNAL AND FETAL SYSTEMS

The physical changes during pregnancy include natural processes involving fertilization of the egg by the sperm, implantation of the fertilized egg into the uterus, embryonic or fetal growth and development, placental development and function, and maternal changes related to the pregnancy process.

Duration of Pregnancy

Pregnancy begins with the union of a sperm and egg, a process called **fertilization**. Under normal healthy circumstances, a full-term pregnancy lasts approximately 9 solar months, 10 lunar months, or 40 weeks. An accurate estimated date of delivery is determined by using Nägele's rule. This is done by adding 7 days to the date of the first day of the last normal menstrual period and subtracting 3 months. A usual pregnancy consists of 9 months, divided into three equal periods called **trimesters**. Oftentimes these trimesters form the basis for discussion of expected fetal and maternal changes during pregnancy.

Fertilization

The union of sperm and egg requires several crucial factors, many of which are not fully understood. When a sperm cell penetrates an egg in the fallopian tube, the beginning of a human being (called a *zygote*) results. Additional division of **zygotic cells** results in more differentiated structures that eventually produce an embryo and subsequently a fetus.

An absence of one or more critical factors may cause **infertility** (failure of the couple to become pregnant despite usual sexual activity over a year's time). For example, both a sperm cell and an egg cell must be mature and in the fallopian tube for approximately 5 hours for union of sperm and egg to occur (the process of conception). The sperm must be of uniform size, be normally formed, possess high motility, and have an ability to secrete enzymes that dissolve the membrane surrounding the egg (Thornton, 2008). The woman attempting pregnancy must have a certain basal body temperature and fallopian tubes free of adhesions or obstructions. A woman will likely conceive within 24 hours after ovulation.

Implantation

Transplantation of the fertilized egg in the uterine cavity after its trip through the fallopian tube requires approximately 6 days (Wingerd, 2007). Once the zygote reaches the uterus, it stays there for up to 5 days, receiving nutrition from the **endometrium**, the inner lining of the uterus (Tortora & Derrickson, 2007). The process of fertilization and implantation triggers the production of large amounts of the hormone **progesterone**, which stimulates the formation of endometrial cells known as the decidua. The decidua provides nutrition for the **embryo**, a term that defines the growing conceptus up to 8 weeks of age.

Fetal Growth and Development

Much is known about the stages of physical development in each structural system of the embryo. However, metabolic functions, particularly those relevant to the endocrine and neurological systems, are less well defined. Appropriate fetal development depends on these events occurring in a specified period and order during each trimester of pregnancy. If this does not occur, an abnormality in structure or function (a **congenital defect**) may result. This defect may be noted at birth, did not occur at conception (called a genetic defect), but most likely resulted from some disruption that occurred after conception and during fetal development. **Website Resource 16A** presents a summary of fetal growth and development.

Placental Development and Function

After implantation of the zygote, the **placenta** develops through an integration of embryonic and decidual cells. The **chorionic membranes** and **amniotic membranes**, which surround the fetus throughout **gestation**, also begin to form. The amniotic fluid, manufactured by the amniotic membrane, supports the developing fetus and protects it from injury.

The basic structure of the placenta (**Website Resource 16B**) allows maternal–fetal blood exchange to nourish the fetus and allow excretion of fetal waste. Throughout most of gestation, increasing placental development allows maternal blood to flow through the intervillous spaces and fetal circulation to flow through the **chorionic villi** (Cunningham et al., 2005a). The unique structure of the placenta permits the exchange of certain molecules but prevents fetal and maternal blood supplies from mixing for most of the pregnancy. Substances with larger and heavier molecules (such as heparin or insulin) normally do not pass through the placenta to the fetus, but lighter molecules (such as anesthetic gases, oxygen, carbon dioxide, and electrolytes) readily cross

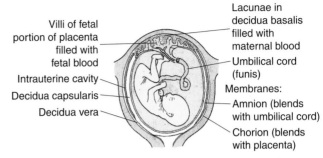

Figure 16-1   Diagrammatic representation of relationship of fetus, placenta, membranes, and uterus during gestation. (From Lowdermilk, D., & Perry, S. [2007]. *Maternity and women's health care* [9th ed.]. St. Louis: Mosby.)

the placenta. Because of the difficulty involved in predicting exactly which substances will cross the placenta, the nurse needs to encourage pregnant women and those contemplating pregnancy to avoid any substance that might cause harm to the fetus.

The fetus, which continues to gain strength and maturity during the later weeks of gestation, generally rests its head in the lower maternal pelvis by the end of pregnancy (Figure 16-1). The membranes protect the fetus from infection and act as a container for the amniotic fluid. As birth begins, the membranes may rupture, causing the loss of amniotic fluid and stronger uterine contractions, reflective of the **labor** process. If the membranes rupture more than 24 hours before birth, uterine infection and potential fetal harm may result.

As gestation nears completion, placental function gradually decreases, which may serve as a stimulus for the onset of labor. When pregnancy continues beyond 42 weeks, or 2 weeks beyond the calculated due date, placental function decreases even more, posing concerns about the well-being of the fetus (Blackburn, 2007).

The discussion of fetal development provides only a brief glimpse about the prenatal period. Maternal changes and culmination of the prenatal period, labor, and birth are also important to address.

Maternal Changes

A woman experiences various physiological effects based on a combination of hormonal and mechanical changes during pregnancy. Hormonal influences tend to increase as the pregnancy progresses. The mechanical (hemodynamic) changes reach a peak in the seventh or eighth month and then gradually decline as the pregnancy nears completion (Cunningham et al., 2005b). Clinical symptoms will manifest during this peak stress time.

Signs of Pregnancy

A woman may assume that she is pregnant because she has skipped her menstrual period or experiences nausea and vomiting, changes in breast sensations and size, or increased urinary frequency (presumptive signs of pregnancy). If she suspects she is pregnant, the woman should undergo a pregnancy test. If performed too early, a home pregnancy test may produce a false-negative result due to a low level of **human chorionic gonadotropin** (HCG). This hormone, produced by the placenta and found in a pregnant woman's urine and blood, triggers a positive pregnancy result. These tests have a high degree of accuracy (97%) if the instructions are followed exactly. As the pregnancy progresses, the woman may have both **probable signs of pregnancy** and **positive signs of pregnancy**, objective changes that increasingly verify that a pregnancy exists (Box 16-1). During the first trimester of pregnancy, using sophisticated testing with **ultrasound**, health care providers can determine fetal presence and placental adequacy early in pregnancy. This technology, using high-frequency sound waves that bounce off the fetus and are interpreted by a computer, allows visualization of the fetus and gestational structures throughout pregnancy (Norwitz and Schorge, 2006).

Adaptive Changes of Other Systems

In addition to pregnancy-related changes in the reproductive system, adaptive changes in other body systems occur. The urinary system undergoes dramatic changes during gestation as follows:

- 50% increase in glomerular filtration rate (GFR) occurs related to the influences of **estrogen** and progesterone.
- Ureters increase in diameter by 25% secondary to progesterone influence.
- Urinary output increases about 80% related to the total body water increase.
- Bladder capacity increases to about 1500 mL to accommodate extra fluids.

Box 16-1 **Signs of Pregnancy**

PROBABLE
- Enlargement of the uterus
- Softening of the uterine isthmus (Hegar sign)
- Bluish or cyanotic color of cervix and upper vagina (Chadwick sign)
- Softening of the cervix (Goodell sign)
- Asymmetrical, softened enlargement of the uterine corner caused by placental development (Piskacek sign)
- Positive test for HCG in the maternal urine or blood serum
- Changes in skin pigmentation (chloasma and linea nigra)

POSITIVE
- Detection of fetal heart tones by auscultation, ultrasonography, or a Doppler
- Palpation of fetal body parts using Leopold maneuvers
- Objective detection of fetal movements
- Radiological or ultrasonographic demonstration of fetal parts

HCG, Human chorionic gonadotropin.

The cardiovascular system changes also beginning early in pregnancy as follows:

- Cardiac output increases up to 50% to meet the demands of pregnancy.
- Total blood volume increases 30% to 45% during pregnancy. Physiological anemia of pregnancy may result because of an increase in the proportion of plasma to red blood cells.
- Heart rate increases by 10 bpm to handle the increase in blood volume.

Respiratory system changes include the following:

- Tidal volume (volume of air inspired) increases by 30% to 40% to increase the effectiveness of air exchange. Total oxygen consumption increases about 20%.
- Diaphragm is displaced upward secondary to the enlarging uterus and causes shortness of breath during the last trimester.

Increased elasticity and softening of connective tissue of the musculoskeletal system cause the following changes during pregnancy:

- The joints relax, especially the pelvic joints that support the pregnancy and create pliability at the time of birth.
- Lumbar and dorsal curves of the spine increase late in pregnancy and contribute to low back pain and the waddle of pregnancy.
- Separation of the symphysis pubis occurs secondary to influence of relaxin hormone.

Changes in the integumentary system occur, which may include:

- Hormones and stretching of the connective tissue of the abdomen due to an enlarging uterus lead to stretch marks (**striae gravidarum**).
- A narrow, brownish line (**linea nigra**) divides the abdomen, running from the umbilicus to the symphysis pubis. The linea nigra fades after the pregnancy ends.
- An increase in pigmentation caused by melanocyte-stimulating hormone causes darkened areas on the face termed the mask of pregnancy (**chloasma**).

The gastrointestinal system undergoes dramatic changes during pregnancy, which include:

- The enlarging and space-occupying uterus cramps the intestinal region causing a slowing of peristalsis and emptying time of the stomach.
- Relaxin causes a decrease in gastric motility leading to constipation.
- Frequent "heartburn" results from reflux of stomach contents into the esophagus secondary to upward displacement of the stomach and a relaxed gastroesophageal sphincter (Blackburn, 2007; Gilbert, 2006; Simpson & Creehan, 2008).

Reproductive System

Effects on the reproductive system include changes in the uterus, breasts, vagina, vulva, and ovaries. The prepregnant uterus is approximately the size of a closed fist. The uterus at

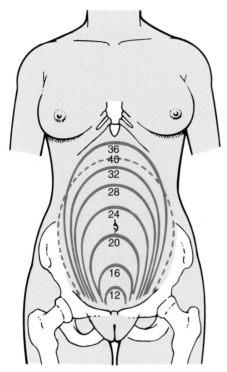

Figure 16-2   Upper level of enlarging uterus by weeks of normal gestation with a single fetus. (From Seidel, H. M., Ball, J. W., Dains, J. E., & Benedict, G. W. [2006]. *Mosby's guide to physical assessment* [6th ed.]. St. Louis: Mosby.)

term has the capacity to contain a 3.2-kg to 4.5-kg (7-lb to 10-lb) infant and the placenta. As the uterus enlarges, the **fundus** (the upper uterine segment) moves higher in the abdomen (Figure 16-2). The breasts begin enlarging early in the pregnancy, and in late pregnancy they may secrete small amounts of **colostrum**, a precursor of mature breast milk. The vagina and vulva receive a greater blood supply and appear darker (cyanotic) as a result. Some women will notice an increase in vaginal secretions (Simpson & Creehan, 2008).

Hormones such as HCG and estrogen, secreted by the placenta and the fetus, create an optimal intrauterine environment for the fetus and stimulate many changes in the pregnant woman's body. The developing fetus contributes to the provision of an adequate environment for its own growth and nourishment, despite the possibility of creating discomforts for the pregnant woman.

Preconception Care of Women

The rates of adverse birth outcomes (preterm and low birth weight, infant deaths and birth defects) and maternal pregnancy complications in the United States are all higher than goals targeted in *Healthy People 2010 Midcourse Review* (2006) and the developing 2020 objectives. Given the adverse trends seen in preterm birth rates and related infant death rates, a comprehensive public health research agenda that investigates the social, genetic, and biomedical

factors contributing to these adverse outcomes was convened by CDC. The National Summit on Preconception Care was charged with developing national recommendations to coordinate services, improve pregnancy outcomes, reduce costs associated with adverse perinatal outcomes, and study the prevention opportunity of preconception care (2006).

Ten recommendations were formulated under the following four goals:

1. Improve the knowledge and attitudes and behaviors of men and women related to preconception health
2. Ensure that all women of childbearing age in the United States receive preconception care services (i.e., evidence-based risk screening, health promotion, and interventions)
3. Reduce risks indicated by a previous adverse pregnancy outcome through interventions during the interconception period, which can prevent or minimize health problems for a mother and her future children
4. Reduce the disparities in adverse pregnancy outcomes (CDC/ATSDR, 2006)

Preconception care offers an effective and efficient means to reduce complications of pregnancy for both the mother and her newborn. Women should be made aware that certain preconception interventions may improve not only the outcomes of pregnancy, but their overall health as well. Such interventions may include:

- Folic acid supplementation to reduce the risk for neural tube defects by two thirds
- **Rubella** vaccination to reduce the risk of severe congenital defects
- Diabetes management to reduce risk of birth defects 3-fold
- Hypothyroidism management to promote healthy neurological development of child
- **Hepatitis B** vaccination for at-risk women to prevent chronic liver disease
- HIV/AIDS screening and treatment to prevent transmission to fetus
- Screening and treatment for STIs to reduce ectopic pregnancy, fetal anomalies
- Oral antiepileptic medication management to minimize birth defect potential
- Cessation of acne treatment with isotretinoin (Accutane) to prevent defects
- Smoking cessation counseling to reduce negative perinatal outcomes
- Screen for and treat depression to reduce the risk of postpartum depression
- Eliminate alcohol use to prevent fetal alcohol disorders and long-term effects (mental retardation; hyperactivity; seizure disorders)
- Obesity control to reduce risks of CVD, diabetes, surgical births (CDC, 2007)

As a group, nurses are challenged to effectively translate the concept of preconception care to all women in their practice setting. By informing women that existing health conditions and medications can affect pregnancy outcomes, nurses can provide a positive environment for the woman's future pregnancy and improve overall health practices.

Normal Discomforts

Changes in the woman's body during pregnancy support a nursing diagnosis of alteration in comfort with relevant interventions for most women. Women may feel a sense of relief that other pregnant women have these concerns and that interventions exist to increase their comfort at various points during gestation. Particularly for those experiencing a first pregnancy, the nurse serves as a valuable support person to help expectant couples adjust to the challenges and discomforts of pregnancy, a goal for the earlier-stated diagnosis.

Teaching Throughout Pregnancy Related to Bodily Changes

In addition to serving as a caregiver, advocate, and support person, the nurse serves as a teacher throughout the pregnancy care process. Active teaching responsive to an individual's concerns about pregnancy may occur in the clinic, physician's office, or other care environments. Nursing interventions should address recommended professional practice guidelines for education during the prenatal period to prevent complications for the family. For example, the nurse may offer textbooks, pamphlets, videotapes, and referrals to websites and other media to increase a couple's knowledge of fetal, maternal, and family changes during gestation and then encourage and answer any questions based on the material. Going beyond one-to-one teaching, the nurse may also refer couples to early pregnancy and **Lamaze** childbirth preparation classes to enlarge their social support network and increase knowledge about labor and delivery. Throughout the care process, the nurse is sensitive to the cultural and ethnic beliefs and behaviors of the individual or family. By incorporating knowledge of these beliefs and behaviors, the nurse protects the pregnant woman and her baby by providing individualized care addressing the childbearing rituals held by various cultural groups (Table 16-1). A summary of perinatal care guidelines is provided in Table 16-2.

Total Weight Gain

Total weight gain during pregnancy reflects not only the growth of the baby and placenta, but that of the uterus, breasts, maternal fat storage, as well as increases in blood and other body fluids. Many practitioners recommend a weight gain of about 25 to 35 lb for a pregnancy involving one fetus (Figure 16-3) (ACOG, 2007; U.S. Department of Health and Human Services [USDHHS], 2000). Additionally, a consistent pattern of gain, with most weight gained during the final two trimesters, has been recommended (ACOG, 2007; USDHHS, 2000).

Labor and Birth

Pregnancy culminates with labor and giving birth. The process of giving birth elicits a significant emotional response from the delivering family. A description of the events of a usual labor and birthing process must occur to establish a background for considering the physiological changes in the mother and the infant.

Several theories offer explanations for the cause of labor. Several factors likely interact, including uterine distention, mechanical irritation, progesterone deprivation, placental aging and hormones, and posterior pituitary activity. Labor usually begins around 40 weeks' gestation, suggesting that hormonal control similar to that regulating the menstrual cycles also contributes to its onset (Cunningham et al., 2005c).

Labor may be divided conveniently into four distinct stages. They are:

1. **Dilation stage**—lasts from the onset of true labor contractions to complete dilation of the cervix. It is divided into three phases: Latent (0 to 3 cm dilation); Active (4 to 7 cm dilation); and Transition (8 to 10 cm dilation)
2. **Pushing stage**—lasts from complete dilation (10 cm) of the cervix to birth
3. **Placental stage**—lasts from the time of birth of the newborn to delivery of the placenta and membranes, which can be from 2 to 15 minutes
4. **Recovery stage**—defined as the first 4 hours after childbirth where physiological and psychological adjustments begin to occur

The first stage of labor starts with regular timing of uterine contractions and ends with complete **dilation** (opening) and **effacement** (thinning) **of the cervix**. Signs of beginning labor include those listed in Box 16-2. The cervix, the lower portion of the uterus, must dilate from a closed position (0 cm) to a totally open position (10 cm, or 4 inches, in diameter). During the first stage, the cervix must also completely efface or shorten from a length of 1 to 2 inches to a barely palpable (paper-thin) thickness. For most women, painless Braxton-Hicks contractions throughout pregnancy cause some cervical dilation and thinning, or at least cervical softening, before the onset of active labor.

During the **first stage of labor**, the presenting part of the fetus begins to press on the cervix, lower uterine segment, and nerve endings around the cervix and vagina. Women's responses to this process vary; pain thresholds and cultural perceptions of and responses to pain differ among laboring women (see Table 16-1). The fundus, the active contractile part of the uterus, becomes thicker as labor progresses, retracts the lower uterine segment and cervix, and helps push the fetus toward the cervix and eventually through the vagina for birth (Ratcliffe et al., 2008). Stage one lasts an average of 12 hours for women experiencing a first birth and somewhat less for women having a second or additional child. Based on a laboring woman's needs, various pain medications, nonpharmacological measures, Lamaze

Table 16-1 Cultural Values Related to Pregnancy and Birth*

Filipino	Structured prenatal care for those who can afford it
	Pregnancy normal event with family focused on pregnant woman's needs
	Pregnant woman encouraged to eat well, sleep often, and not to work out of home
	Sexual intercourse taboo during last 2 weeks of pregnancy
	Pregnant woman encouraged to eat fresh eggs close to delivery to help baby "slide out" with birth
	Woman very modest about body needs and care during pregnancy
	Father passive with birth process; pregnant woman active participant with birth
	Breast-feeding encouraged until child is a toddler
American Indian	In many tribes women are expected to seek prenatal care with pregnancy; some tribes accept late care
	Dialogue with women in tribal community important to maximize pregnancy and birth process
	Meditation, self-control practice, and indigenous plants (herbal teas) used for discomforts of pregnancy and birth
	Pregnant woman stoic about birth process; father present but not active participant
	Female kin present to support woman in labor; breast-feeding and bottle feeding encouraged after birth
	Father may avoid hunting immediately after birth or until infant's cord falls off
Arab American	Pregnancy normal event; may not access prenatal care because of that belief
	Much family support given to pregnant woman to allow maximal rest and minimal work
	Present orientation: little preparation for birth, fears labor pains but responds once they come
	Expressive with labor but not active with control of pain; relies on family members for support; father not active, may feel powerless with birth process
	Very modest about care, especially with opposite gender health care provider
	Prefer bottle feeding; colostrum believed to harm baby
Blacks	Most access prenatal care after first trimester or seek care earlier with problems
	Female kin provide most of support with pregnancy and birth; male support less visible
	Open expression of pregnancy and birth discomfort; active participant in birth process
	May self-medicate with cultural remedies for pregnancy complaints
	May avoid being in photographs due to fear of stillbirth
	May crave certain foods: chicken, greens, clay, starch, or dirt (pica)
	If of Muslim faith, may wish to have head covered during labor and birth process
	Breast-feed if given information on the benefits of this method
Mexican American	Often face barriers to prenatal care due to lack of insurance, fear of health care system, lack of transportation to clinic
	May consider prenatal care not needed due to normal life event
	Education and acculturation influence prenatal care access
	Pregnancy considered to follow marriage; family supports respect and assistance to pregnant woman
	Pregnant woman does not smoke, work, drink alcohol, or use drugs; pregnancy a time to rest, walk, eat well, sleep, drink chamomile tea, and avoid cold air
	Grandmother may move into the home close to delivery time to help and provide folk remedies after birth
	Modest about care and needs; same gender health care provider encouraged
	Generally walks during labor to enhance birth; wants family for support; woman active and father delegates support to female members of family
	Generally breast-feeds for up to 1 year
Vietnamese	Generally early prenatal care unless immigrant status, then depend on family for care
	Encouraged to eat healthy foods, get rest, avoid strenuous activity during last trimester
	Focus on keeping pregnant woman warm, encouraging salt water for oral care, and maintaining good hygiene
	Sexual intercourse taboo with pregnancy
	Father present but not active with pregnancy
	Birth a time of hot and cold imbalance; mother "suffers in silence," may moan or grunt; mother depends on female relatives for support and guidance
	Mother breast-feeds for up to 1 year; avoids cold foods for this period

*General ideas about beliefs and behaviors of each of these cultural groups have been given with no intent to stereotype all persons who represent these groups' beliefs or behaviors. It is hoped that this information will provide direction to the nurse who will continue to assess each individual to render care that meets that person's traditional values in a biomedical model of health care in the United States today.
Compiled from Spector, R. E. (2004). *Cultural diversity in health & illness* (6th ed., pp. 101-137). Upper Saddle River, NJ: Pearson/Prentice Hall; Purnell, L. D., & Paulanka, B. J. (2004). *Guide to culturally competent health care*. Philadelphia: F.A. Davis; Wood, M. J. (2006). Immersion in another culture: One strategy for increasing cultural competency. *Journal of Cultural Diversity, 13*(1), 50-54; Green, M. J. (2007). Strategies for incorporating cultural competence into childbirth education curriculum. *Journal of Perinatal Education, 16*(2), 33-37; Hackley, B., Kriebs, J. M., & Rousseau, M. E. (2007). *Primary care of women: A guide for women's health providers*. Sudbury, MA: Jones and Bartlett; Bowers, P. (2007). Cultural perspectives in childbearing. *Nursing Spectrum* [Online] Retrieved from *www.nurse.com/ce/course.html?CCID=3245*.

Table 16-2 Perinatal Care Guidelines

First Trimester	Second Trimester	Third Trimester	Labor Stages	Postpartum
Complete assessment to identify risk factors	Assess adaptation to pregnancy and fetal well-being	Review physiological changes	Admission to birthing facility	Complete a head-to-toe physical assessment: Breasts Uterus Bladder Bowels Lochia Emotional status Circulatory status Episiotomy
Awareness of subtle or overt physical, sexual, or emotional abuse	Update health history	Monitor changes related to pregnancy	1st stage: Complete maternal/fetal assessments Determine labor progress Assist with comfort measures Monitor FHR Support family in their efforts Praise efforts	Assess for postpartum blues/depression
Assess physical and psychosocial progress in adaptation to pregnancy	Continue to recognize cultural influences	Assess expectant family's readiness for labor, birth, and parenting role	2nd stage: Offer encouragement Assist with pushing efforts Document activities	Encourage bonding and attachment
Inquire about physical changes and discomforts; explain the causes and identify appropriate relief measures	Encourage informed decision-making and positive health care practices	Review finalized birth plan	3rd stage: Provide care as needed Document time of placental delivery Administer meds as ordered	Demonstrate breast-feeding techniques
Provide anticipatory guidance appropriate for her individual needs	Review potential risk factors and when to report	Identify community resources available to family	4th stage: Monitor vital signs; fundus, assess bladder status	Provide anticipatory guidance needed for this family
Educational needs: Hazards during pregnancy Use of drugs, alcohol and smoking Seat belts, high-risk behaviors Warning/danger signs to report Nutrition and weight management Sexuality	Ensure community referrals/resources as needed Educational needs: Oral hygiene Nutritional needs Safety issues in workplace Discomforts of pregnancy Relief of common discomforts of pregnancy Prepared childbirth classes	Explain any diagnostic tests ordered Meet educational needs: Needs for newborn care Monitoring fetal movements Strategies to cope with discomforts Promote family safety Including partner in process Childbirth preparation	Encourage parental-infant interaction Monitor newborn's well-being Provide perineal care, food, fluids Provide family support	Educational needs: Nutrition Fatigue Childcare Immunizations Sexuality Family planning Breast engorgement Family adaptation Follow-up care needed Danger signs to report Sibling readiness for new member Self-care activities

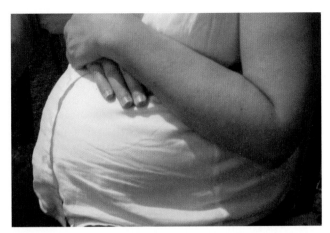

Figure 16-3   Many practitioners recommend a weight gain of 25 to 30 pounds.

> **Box 16-2**   **Signs of Beginning Labor**
>
> - Bloody show or loss of the mucous plug that seals cervical canal during pregnancy
> - Regular uterine contractions
> - Contractions increasing in intensity, duration, and frequency
> - Palpable hardening of the uterus during contractions
> - Pain in the lower back and front of abdomen

---

breathing, and other distractive techniques may alleviate the discomfort associated with first-stage labor. Periodic vaginal examinations by the nurse or other health care provider indicate a laboring woman's cervical dilation and effacement and descent of the fetus into the birth canal (a concept called **station**). In a full-term pregnancy, loss of the amniotic membrane usually increases pressure of the fetal head against the cervix, making dilation and effacement more efficient, and tends to augment the labor process.

During the **second stage of labor**, the fetus descends through the lower birth canal toward the woman's perineum. The upper uterine segment greatly thickens, and the abdominal muscles assist in the fetus' descent and expulsion. Women who have attended childbirth classes often are better prepared to actively push the baby through the pelvis and perineum during contractions. Cultural practices may support pushing from a squatting or upright position, such as that seen with Hmong women (Armstrong & Feldman, 2007). For many women, an overwhelming urge to bear down during uterine contractions occurs at this time. The fetal head accommodates to the mother's pelvis and vaginal structure and, finally, the head becomes flush with the vaginal opening on the woman's perineum. The woman at this point actively pushes to expel the newborn.

The **third stage of labor** begins after the birth of the newborn and lasts until placental expulsion. Placental separation usually takes place within 5 to 30 minutes

after completion of the second stage. After delivery of the placenta the health care provider examines the placenta to determine that all placental tissue is intact and to detect any abnormalities that could affect the infant's condition and adaptation to extrauterine life.

The **fourth stage of labor** generally consists of the first 2 hours after childbirth, during which the mother faces the greatest risk of postpartum hemorrhage. An expected blood loss of 250 to 500 mL may cause the mother to experience a moderate decline in blood pressure (Wylie & Bryce, 2008). She may also experience an increase in pulse rate (**tachycardia**) to compensate for blood loss during the early postpartum period. The Care Plan at the end of this chapter addresses the nurse's role in managing the **stages of labor**.

Overview of Care

Professional members of the health care team play an important role in labor and delivery, but a woman's family or significant other (i.e., husband, partner, friend, family) also inherently contributes to her care during labor and birth, particularly in certain cultures (see Table 16-1). Many practitioners suggest that the expectations and beliefs of a birthing couple have a great effect on how the woman fulfills the mothering role. Therefore the nurse needs to collaborate with the people who care for the pregnant woman to meet that family's needs during pregnancy, labor, and delivery.

The importance of the nurse's knowledge, caregiving, and support cannot be underestimated during the first stage of labor. Active emotional and physical nursing support decreases the length of many women's labors, analgesia and anesthesia use, and number of operative deliveries and may help women reach their birthing goals (Association of Women's Health, Obstetrical, and Neonatal Nursing [AWHONN], 2007). Provided that they are accepted by a woman's culture, independent nursing interventions to increase comfort (e.g., giving backrubs, massages, offering ice or warm fluids by mouth, assisting with ambulation and position changes, and providing a clean and dry environment) may help the laboring woman cope with the challenges of labor. Many women will request medication to diminish the pain of labor and birth, and the nurse may need to review options for medication with each woman or couple. During the first stage the mother must not bear down, because this may cause cervical swelling; often, active nursing support and distractive techniques, such as breathing and visual refocus, can prevent pushing before the second stage of labor. A woman may depend on the nurse to model breathing techniques to relieve labor discomfort. The nurse may need to explain usual interventions during this stage of labor, including the use of a **fetal heart monitor** (a machine that detects and records fetal heart rate and activity during labor), intravenous fluids, digital blood pressure machine, and urinary catheterization. Open and clear communication among the health care providers and laboring woman and her significant others, particularly during frequent and difficult uterine contractions, will improve coping before the pushing stage begins.

During the second stage of labor, the woman needs reassurance and support for her pushing efforts. Constant reinforcement and education by the nurse about labor progress, fetal heart monitor tracings, and other interventions will give the mother and her support system the guidance needed to give birth to the infant. Throughout labor the nurse considers the specific cultural and ethnic needs to support nursing assessment and positive responses to labor by the childbearing family.

Active nursing support during the third and fourth stages of labor includes observing for excessive vaginal bleeding after the placenta is expelled, assisting the woman in breast-feeding her new baby, monitoring vital signs, and implementing uterine massage if the uterus becomes boggy or fails to contract over the placental site. Emotional support during assessments and delivery of information to explain the rationale for assessments are also important nursing roles supported by professional practice standards.

Throughout the entire labor and birth process, the nurse makes careful observations of the laboring woman and fetus so that she can detect early any difficulties with the progress of labor or with maternal or fetal health. Problems may include unusual fetal or uterine activity, presence of **meconium** (fetal stool) in the amniotic fluid, fetal tachycardia (heart rate above 160 beats per minute) or fetal **bradycardia** (heart rate below 110 beats per minute) in a full-term infant, and fetal heart rate decreases with uterine activity during labor (Blackburn, 2007). These events must be reported immediately to the health care provider, with a complete oral and written description of the event. The nurse must be aware that abnormal fetal and maternal signs and patterns may be related to factors such as maternal diabetes or hypertension; type, timing, or dosage of labor medications; uterine contraction pattern; maternal infection; maternal anemia; preeclampsia; presence and character of amniotic fluid; bleeding in the pregnant woman or fetus; or gestational age of the infant (Dangel, 2008).

CHANGES DURING TRANSITION FROM FETUS TO NEWBORN

Most newborns experience a smooth transition from intrauterine to extrauterine life. When difficulty occurs, however, the newborn's viability depends on the nurse's understanding of the fine balance of chemical, physiological, and anatomical changes that occur as it makes the transition to extrauterine life (Blackburn, 2007). **Website Resource 16C** presents details about the adaptation of the fetus to extrauterine life.

Nursing Interventions

Nursing activities during this adaptation process include assessment and interventions aimed at specific protection of the infant and prevention of complications. Cold stress should be avoided by keeping the newborn dry and warmly wrapped and by avoiding environments that cause heat loss. Overall, the nurse should minimally disturb, but maximally observe and document, the newborn's behavior during reactive periods.

Apgar Score

Assessment of the newborn after the first few hours of life is essentially the same as assessment of the young infant (see Chapter 17). One technique, specific to timing after birth, is the **Apgar scoring system**. This scoring historically has been used to provide a simple clinical measure to evaluate the newborn's general condition at birth. The Apgar score, made at 1 minute and 5 minutes of age, may be repeated again at 10 minutes of age until the infant's condition has stabilized. A total score is calculated by adding the values allotted to the categories noted in Table 16-3. The highest possible score is 10. A score of 8 to 10 indicates that the baby is adapting well. The Apgar score does not predict the neurological development of an infant, but may relate to the infant's risk of illness or death during the first year of life, important information for parents of an infant with a low Apgar score to know (Queenan et al., 2007).

Gender

Gender differences occur in fetal growth. Generally boys grow faster than girls in the third trimester, and at birth boys are slightly heavier, longer, and have a larger head circumference than girls (Blackburn, 2007). Although more boys are conceived, they tend to be aborted spontaneously more often than girl embryos; the two X chromosomes possessed by female embryos may protect them from the early hazards of pregnancy. After birth, boys continue to have a lower survival rate than do girls (Coch et al., 2007).

Table 16-3   Apgar Scoring

Sign	Score 0	Score 1	Score 2
Heart rate	Absent	Slow (under 100)	Over 100
Respiratory effort	Absent	Weak cry, hypoventilation	Good strong cry
Muscle tone	Flaccid, limp	Some flexion of extremities	Active motion, extremities well flexed
Reflex irritability	No response	Grimace	Cry
Color	Blue, pale	Body pink, extremities blue	Completely pink

From Arenson, J., & Drake, P. (2007). *Maternal and newborn health.* Sudbury, MA: Jones and Bartlett; Norwitz, E. R. & Schorge, J. O. (2006). *Obstetrics and gynecology at a glance.* 2nd edition. Malen, MA: Blackwell Publishing.

Race and Culture

Race may affect the fetus' health in several ways. For example, in the United States, non-Whites (mainly Blacks) have more fraternal twin pregnancies than Whites (Cunningham et al., 2005d). Because their organs are less mature, twin fetuses face an increased risk for **premature delivery** due to gestational factors in the mother. Currently the United States is 36th in the world ranking for **infant mortality rate** (IMR), with a rate of 6.78 (CDC, 2007). This rate, which reflects the number of infants that die before the end of their first year of life and is the leading indicator of a nation's health, reflects the higher IMRs and low–birth-weight outcomes of Blacks and other ethnic minority populations in the United States. This rate illustrates the complex sociopolitical issues that produce birth outcomes in this country and those needing attention to improve the IMR (CDC, 2007; USDHHS, 2000; USDHHS, 2006).

Race is also a factor in the frequency of certain genetic and congenital malformations. For example, more Native American, Latino, or Asian descent babies have cleft palates (an opening in the oral palate) than do Black babies (Mayo Clinic, 2007). Black babies have higher rates of sickle cell anemia (abnormally shaped red blood cells) than White babies. Interestingly, the total number of malformations tends to be about the same in all races that have been studied (Whites, Blacks, Hispanics, and Asians) (March of Dimes, 2007).

A woman's ethnic background may also influence her fetus' health based on a link to socioeconomic status. For increasing numbers of homeless pregnant women, income may support family survival needs, but not prenatal care. Minority group pregnant women may have fewer economic resources to obtain a nutritious diet or early and consistent high-quality prenatal care. These outcomes may relate to access to health care factors or cultural beliefs that do not support recommended foods or prenatal care (*Healthy People 2010* box).

Healthy People 2010

Selected National Health-Promotion and Disease-Prevention Objectives for the Prenatal Period

- Reduce fetal and infant deaths (28 weeks of gestation to 1 year) to no more than 4.4 per 1000 live births (baseline: 7.3 per 1000 live births in 1998)

Special Population Targets: Infant Mortality	1997 Baseline	2010 Target
Blacks	13.7	4.5
Native Americans–Alaska Natives	7.9	4.5
Asians	4.6	4.5
Hispanics	6.5	4.5

- Reduce the fetal death rate (20 or more weeks of gestation) to no more than 4.1 per 1000 live births plus fetal deaths (baseline: 6.8 per 1000 live births plus fetal deaths in 1997)

Special Population Target: Fetal Deaths	1997 Baseline	2010 Target
Blacks	12.5	6.8

- Reduce low birth weight to an incidence of no more than 5% of live births and very low birth weight to no more than 0.9% of live births (baseline: 7.6% and 1.4%, respectively, in 1998)

Special Population Target	1998 Baseline	2010 Target
Low Birth Weight		
Blacks	13%	5%
Very Low Birth Rate		
Blacks	3%	0.9%

- Reduce the number of unintended pregnancies to no more than 30% (baseline: 51% of pregnancies for females 15 to 44 years of age in 1995 were unwanted or earlier than intended)
- Reduce the number of pregnancies occurring in girls ages 15 to 17 to no more than 46 per 1000 (baseline: 72 pregnancies per 1000 girls of this age in 1995)

- Increase the number of women who breast-feed during the early postpartum period to at least 75% and increase the proportion who breast-feed for 5 to 6 months after birth to at least 50% (baseline: 64% of women chose to breast-feed during the early postpartum period in 1998; 29% chose to breast-feed for 5 to 6 months in 1998)
- Increase abstinence by pregnant women from tobacco to at least 98%, from alcohol to 94%, and from illicit drugs (cocaine and marijuana) to 100% (baseline: 87% of pregnant women abstained from tobacco, 86% abstained from alcohol, 98% abstained from cocaine, and 98% abstained from marijuana from 1996 to 1997)
- Increase the number of women who receive prenatal care during the first trimester of pregnancy to at least 90% (baseline: 83% of live births in 1997)

Special Population Target: Prenatal Care	1997 Baseline	2010 Target
Native Americans–Alaska Natives	68%	90%
Asians	85%	90%
Blacks	72%	90%
Whites	85%	90%

- Increase the proportion of mothers who achieve a recommended weight gain during their pregnancies (baseline: 75% of married women delivering at term gained the recommended weight of 25 to 35 lb with pregnancy in 1988)
- Reduce the cesarean delivery rate to no more than 15 per 100 deliveries (baseline: 17.8 per 100 deliveries in 1997; a rate of 15.5 for primary cesareans and 71 for repeat procedures in 1997)

Continued

Healthy People 2010

Selected National Health-Promotion and Disease-Prevention Objectives for the Prenatal Period—cont'd

- Reduce cesarean births among low-risk (full-term, singleton, vertex presentation) women

Reduction in Cesarean Births	1998 Baseline % of Live Births	2010 Target % of Live Births
Women giving birth for first time	18	15
Prior cesarean birth	72	63

- Reduce the occurrence of fetal alcohol syndrome (FAS)

Reduction in FAS	1995-97 Baseline % of Live Births	2010 Target % of Live Births
	0.4	0.1

- Increase the proportion of pregnancies begun with an optimal folic acid level

	1991-94 Baseline Percent	2010 Target Percent
Consumption of at least 400 micrograms of folic acid daily by nonpregnant women aged 15 to 44 years	21	80

	Concentration in ng/mL	Concentration in ng/mL
Median RBC folate level among nonpregnant women aged 15 to 44 years	160	220

From U.S. Department of Health and Human Services. (2000). *Healthy People 2010*: Vol. 1 (Conference edition). Washington, DC: U.S. Government Printing Office; U.S. Department of Health and Human Services (USDHHS). (2006). *Healthy People 2010 Midcourse Review*. Washington, DC: U.S. Government Printing Office.

Genetics

Genetic influences affect the survival and later well-being of the child through several known mechanisms. **Down syndrome** (trisomy 21) remains the most recognized and most commonly occurring example of an extra chromosome. Extra chromosomes, deleted chromosomes, or translocations usually cause multiple malformations incompatible with life, causing early loss of the fetus via **spontaneous abortion**. Single malformations in an otherwise normal fetus (e.g., clubfoot, cleft palate, or neural tube defect) probably result from a combined effect of many genes (March of Dimes, 2007). These defects, found at birth, may be surgically corrected or managed during the child's life. Modern techniques of **amniocentesis**, chorionic villus sampling, and chromosome analysis have expanded genetic counseling options and interventions for women facing possible fetal genetic defects. The nurse works with other members of the health care team to inform these women and couples of genetic and high-risk screening resources when family history or other factors indicate that a fetal genetic defect may be likely.

GORDON'S FUNCTIONAL HEALTH PATTERNS

Box 16-3 provides an example of a pregnancy assessment using Gordon's functional health patterns (1995).

Health Perception–Health Management Pattern

Based on her culture and life experience, a woman may view pregnancy as an illness, as a completely natural and healthy state, or as a combination of the two. This perception will influence her view of her changing body, attitude toward the usual discomforts of pregnancy such as fatigue or backache, choice of health-oriented or illness-oriented care, and her decision to seek prenatal care. The woman who sees herself as healthy and pregnancy as a normal part of her life most likely will seek a health care provider with a similar outlook. Another woman with the same perception may seek help from a socially approved group, as defined by her culture, and avoid standard Western medicine during pregnancy (e.g., Roma [gypsies]). Generally, women with a positive view of pregnancy will continue active participation in their respective social circles and careers. However, the woman who sees her pregnancy as a time of illness may use this as a reason to withdraw from her work and social obligations.

A woman's acceptance of her pregnancy influences her health management practices and choices. The woman who denies or has strong negative feelings about her pregnancy may fail to eat properly, get enough rest and exercise, breast-feed, or seek prenatal care. A woman may deny a pregnancy because she never intended to become pregnant despite having sexual intercourse without birth control. Approximately 50% of American pregnancies are unintended, particularly among adolescents, women over age 40, women with low income, and women who lack access, cultural acceptance, education, and financial resources to purchase or use contraception (Ahluwalia et al., 2007; USDHHS, 2000). These women, faced with an unplanned or closely spaced pregnancy, may expose a fetus to alcohol, tobacco, and **sexually transmitted infections (STIs)**, abuse a child who was never wanted, or fail to get follow-up care for a high-risk child (i.e., experienced complications from delivery) (USDHHS, 2000; U.S. Preventive Services Task Force, 2006a).

The nurse who works with a pregnant population is sensitive to a wide range of views expressed by these women and work with each to effectively manage their pregnancies. For example, Hispanic women are less likely to get early prenatal care based on a belief that pregnancy is not

Box 16-3 Assessment for Pregnancy According to Gordon's Functional Health Patterns

Health perception–health management pattern: aware of or participates in management of pregnancy, or both; expects an uncomplicated pregnancy based on woman's or significant other's active involvement in her own care; able to state complications of pregnancy that mandate physician notification; engages in health-promotion behaviors specific to pregnancy

Nutritional-metabolic pattern: follows diet changes of pregnancy as recommended by nurse; has appropriate weight for height and has gained adequate weight for gestational age of pregnancy; eats three meals a day and two snacks (afternoon and evening), focusing on increased amounts of vegetables and fruits; drinks healthy fluids including at least 8 glasses of water per day; has elastic skin turgor

Elimination pattern: experiences occasional constipation from iron therapy of pregnancy—usually corrected by increased fluids, nightly walking, and more diet roughage; voids 7 to 10 times a day, depending on amount of fluids consumed; no known hemorrhoids or difficulty in elimination; voiding without excess frequency, urgency, or burning; understands signs of UTI

Activity-exercise pattern: walks 3 times a week for 20 minutes without complaints of unusual fatigue or soreness; active at home with housework and at work teaching primary school; swam 2 times a week before pregnancy and move to current residence

Sleep-rest pattern: generally sleeps 7 to 8 hours a night; has increased total daily sleep somewhat with fatigue of pregnancy—naps for 1 hour on weekends and 30 minutes after work; sleeps on side and with two pillows for comfort; uses no sleep aids; generally able to relax and initiate sleep without difficulty; occasionally has headache at end of workday and takes acetaminophen (Tylenol) for relief or listens to soft music after work to enhance relaxation

Cognitive-perceptual pattern: realizes the need to decrease work activity and increase rest periods as she nears end of pregnancy; answers questions in appropriate tone and words during pregnancy visits; has intact memory (alert and remote); reads about pregnancy and early parenthood to prepare for the birth

Self-perception–self-concept pattern: states she is excited about pregnancy after a year of trying to conceive; well groomed, wears maternity clothes because "I want to"; believes she looks "nice" due to pregnancy

Roles-relationships pattern: lives with husband of 3 years; visits extended family, 60 miles away, every month; shares family roles with husband, accepts this balance; has many friends who support her pregnancy; perceives extensive employee and employer support with pregnancy and time off after delivery

Sexuality-reproductive pattern: states, "I have a satisfying love life and enjoy my husband"; before pregnancy, engaged in sexual intercourse 4 to 5 times a week with desire to become pregnant; with pregnancy and fatigue, has intercourse generally 2 to 3 times a week, with pattern acceptable to both partners; no known STIs in past or present

Coping-stress tolerance pattern: concerned about fatigue affecting performance as primary school teacher; walks 3 times a week for 20 minutes to "center myself and feel good"; smiles often, good sense of humor; supportive family excited about her pregnancy

Values-beliefs pattern: Protestant religion; prays daily and gains strength from religion

Other data:
- Medication history:
  Prenatal vitamin (Materna), 1 tablet each morning
  Ferrous sulfate, 1 tablet each morning
  Acetaminophen (Tylenol) 650 mg for occasional headaches
- Physical examination:
  5 feet, 4 inches tall
  Weight 140 lb (at 14 weeks' pregnancy; weight gain of 5 lb with pregnancy)
  29 years of age
  PERRLA
  TPR 98.2-76-16
  BP 114/78 right arm (sitting, left arm)
  Peripheral pulses equal, strong bilaterally
  Skin warm, dry, elastic turgor; mucous membranes intact, moist; alert, oriented × 3

BP, Blood pressure; *PERRLA,* pupils equally round and reactive to light and accommodation; *STDs,* sexually transmitted diseases; *TPR,* temperature, pulse, respirations; *UTI,* urinary tract infection.
Modified from Peterson, R. (2005). *Clinical companion for fundamentals of nursing* (6th ed). St. Louis: Mosby.

---

an illness. The nurse targets interventions that focus on this group's needs and beliefs while adhering to professional practice standards that will improve their outcomes.

Nutritional-Metabolic Pattern

Massive amounts of literature support the importance of optimal nutrition during pregnancy for maternal and fetal well-being. Maternal malnutrition before and during pregnancy may exert a teratogenic effect on the fetus. A **teratogen** is an agent that causes either a functional or structural disability in the organism based on exposure to that agent (Merriam-Webster, 2007). Teratogens principally affect the central nervous system of the fetus, leading to impaired intelligence and performance later in life. They are discussed more in the Environmental Processes section later in the chapter.

Various factors influence the quality of nutrition needed for positive fetal development and birth outcome. Fetal development suffers in cases of adolescent pregnancy or older women who experience poor nutrition between and during several pregnancies. Maternal nutritional deficiencies during one's own fetal, infant, and childhood periods also contribute to the development of structural and physiological disadvantages to supporting a growing fetus. For example, women who are severely underweight before pregnancy often experience higher rates of low–birth-weight infants and preterm labor than do women of appropriate prepregnant weight (Cunningham et al., 2005e). Inherited maternal stature and pelvic development may influence pregnancy and efficiency of labor and delivery. A lack of income to buy healthy food may also exist, and sometimes cultural values related to food intake influence the quality of nutrition during pregnancy.

To meet increased metabolic, energy, and structural needs for pregnancy, most nutritionists recommend that a pregnant woman increase her intake by approximately 300 calories each day (USDHHS, 2000). This results in a total weight gain of about 25 to 35 pounds. If at the end of 20 weeks of gestation the woman has not gained at least 10 pounds, she risks delivering an ill infant suffering from intrauterine growth restriction (IUGR). These risks also exist when a woman continues to gain insufficient weight throughout the pregnancy or in one who was underweight or overweight before pregnancy. Although the rate of gain and the total gain during pregnancy vary among women, a correlation exists between an erratic pattern of weight gain or a too-rapid weight gain and a lack of fetal well-being (Debruyne et al., 2007). The nurse advises the pregnant woman to eat a well-balanced diet.

A well-balanced diet for a pregnant woman parallels that needed by all human beings, with increases of certain components as recommended by the Food and Nutrition Board of the National Academy of Science (Institute of Medicine, 2007; USDHHS, 2000). The nurse recommends that the entire family eat a healthy diet. The nurse encourages the pregnant woman to drink 8 to 10 glasses of water per day to develop amniotic fluid and prevent urinary tract infections often seen with pregnancy. The nurse may also need to encourage the woman to modify her diet to include more fiber and roughage to avoid constipation during pregnancy (Table 16-4).

Protein requirements during pregnancy increase to about 70 g per day, or a daily increase of 25 grams above normal (Dudek, 2006). This ensures an adequate supply of amino acids for fetal growth and development, blood volume expansion, and maternal tissue growth. Other protein sources, such as cheese, cream soups, puddings, tofu, and yogurt, may be better tolerated by some women and by those from cultures (Hispanic) that do not drink milk. Animal protein and less expensive legume sources provide protein and, if combined with other healthy food sources, provide high-quality meals (e.g., tuna and rice, peanut butter, and whole wheat bread). Protein foods cost more than other foods. Therefore the nurse may need to teach pregnant couples about economical ways to meet protein needs for fetal development.

Mineral intake must also increase during pregnancy. Increased protein intake usually provides the extra needed essential minerals, particularly phosphorus and calcium. The rapid deposit of calcium in fetal bones and teeth during the third trimester of pregnancy requires adequate maternal calcium stores from early pregnancy and continued calcium intake to prevent maternal bone demineralization. Other calcium sources include green leafy vegetables and calcium-fortified foods, sources more acceptable to cultures with a history of lactose intolerance (African, Mexican, and some European groups).

Table **16-4**   Nutritional Needs for Pregnant and Lactating Women

Nutrient	Pregnancy	Lactation	Sources	Comments
Calories	+300	+500	Eat a variety from all food groups	Begin to increase calories in 2nd and 3rd trimesters
Protein	70 g	70 g	Lean meat, fish, eggs, poultry, milk, and dairy products	Supports fetal growth and development; formation of placenta and amniotic fluid; and expanded blood volume
Calcium	1000 mg	1000 mg	Milk, cheese, dark green leafy vegetables, nuts, and dried fruit	Women with low calcium intake require calcium supplements with vitamin D
Iron	27 mg/day	9 mg/day	Lean meats, dark green leafy vegetables, eggs, whole grain, dried fruit, and shellfish	Provides iron for fetal liver storage, which sustains the infant for the first 4 to 6 months of life
Folic acid	400 micrograms	400 micrograms	Fresh green leafy vegetables, liver, peanuts, whole grain breads, and cereals	All women of childbearing age should take 400 micrograms of folic acid daily to prevent neural tube defects in the first trimester
Fats	30% of daily calories	30% of daily calories	Low-fat dairy products and lean cuts of meat	Provides a valuable source of energy for the body during pregnancy
Carbohydrates	7 to 11 servings daily	7 to 11 servings daily	Dairy products, fruits, vegetables, whole grain cereals, and breads	Provides fiber necessary for proper bowel functioning. CHO needs to be sufficient to prevent ketoacidosis from protein use for energy

A woman who eats a well-balanced diet should gain sufficient vitamins and minerals for maternal and fetal needs during pregnancy. However, most health care providers recommend that the pregnant woman include 30 mg of elemental iron daily to benefit both mother and fetus, particularly during the last trimester. Iron deficiency anemia is common among pregnant women, and anemia contributes to hemorrhage, postpartum infection, and preterm birth. Anemia occurs more often among pregnant adolescent, Black, and older White women (Arenson & Drake, 2007). Research supports that women planning pregnancy and those in their first trimester take 0.4 mg (400 micrograms) of folic acid in a daily multivitamin supplement to prevent neural tube defects and anemia. This is particularly important for women with multiple gestations who experience a greater risk of anemia. However, research has shown that only 25% of women of childbearing age consume this amount of folic acid, which is critical for early fetal development (USDHHS, 2000).

Fats and carbohydrates must supply the caloric requirements during pregnancy. Although increased protein intake provides more calories, the body-building requirements of pregnancy and fetal growth demand most of the added protein. Fats and carbohydrates remain the most important sources of energy and essential vitamins and minerals. Supplemental vitamins and minerals, although not known to cause maternal or fetal harm if taken in reasonable dosages, probably cost the pregnant woman more to meet the nutritional needs of pregnancy than does a well-balanced diet.

The practice of **pica**, a psychobehavorial disorder characterized by the ingestion of nonfood substances such as dirt, clay, starch, and ice, may negatively influence the quality of a pregnant woman's nutrition during pregnancy. Pica in humans can be classified by the type of ingested substance. The three main substances consumed by pregnant women are soil or clay (geophagia), ice (pagophagia), and laundry or corn starch (amylophagia). Other pica cravings include burnt matches, stones, charcoal, mothballs, soap, sand, plaster, coffee grounds, baking soda, paint chips, and glue (Mills, 2007). Common in rural pregnant Black women, this practice may contribute to iron deficiency anemia and interfere with nutrient absorption, particularly among women of lower economic status. Other potential complications may include lead poisoning, fecal impaction, parasitic infections, prematurity, perinatal mortality, low–birth-weight infants, and anemia in the infant (Dudek, 2006). The nurse completes a nutritional assessment on any pregnant woman. The nurse identifies instances of pica and suggests a culturally sensitive diet that will better meet the needs of the woman and her developing fetus. It is essential that the nurse remain nonjudgmental but stress the importance of an adequate diet, folic acid, and iron supplements, and the dangers of pica.

The best time to teach a woman about prenatal nutrition is before she becomes pregnant. Most women do not seek prenatal care until they suspect pregnancy. Therefore the nurse often delivers information about optimal nutrition to the pregnant woman after critical fetal development has already begun. If all school children received nutrition information as part of their kindergarten through twelfth grade curriculum (a primary prevention approach), women might have better overall personal nutrition established through lifestyle practices of individuals and families that would support high-quality prenatal nutrition later in their lives. Without such a primary prevention approach, secondary prevention intervention during pregnancy occurs through laboratory monitoring of iron levels, assessment of the woman's feelings of well-being, her actual intake of essential nutrients, and assessment of her pattern and total weight gain during the pregnancy. Many pregnant women work outside the home and may be among the increasing numbers of American families who spend 40% of their food budgets on food eaten outside the home (USDHHS, 2000). The nurse alerts the pregnant woman and her family to the documented high amounts of cholesterol, calories, sodium, and fat and low amounts of iron and calcium that these foods contain so as to improve nutritional intake during pregnancy.

In summary, the pregnant woman needs to follow the USDA MyPyramid as follows:
- Fruits and vegetables—7 or more servings daily (3 servings of fruit and 4 of vegetables)
- Whole-grains or enriched breads/cereals—6 to 9 servings daily
- Dairy products—3 to 4 servings of low-fat or nonfat milk, yogurt, or cheese daily
- Meat and beans—3 servings daily (one serving = 2 ounces) (USDA, 2007).

See Chapter 11 for more information on nutrition including MyPyramid.

Elimination Pattern
Fetus

The fetus accomplishes all essential elimination functions through the placenta. Carbon dioxide, water, urea, and other waste products pass through the placenta, to be eliminated by the mother's body. By the end of the first trimester, the fetus swallows, makes respiratory movements, and urinates. However, these abilities become truly functional only after birth.

Pregnant Woman

The pregnant woman experiences changes in her elimination pattern because of the enlarging uterus and hormonal influences. These changes (urinary frequency during the first and third trimesters, constipation, and hemorrhoids) cause normal, minor discomforts. Anticipatory guidance by the nurse helps the pregnant woman cope with these changes and prevent complications of pregnancy. For example, teaching the pregnant woman commonsense measures (Health Teaching box) may prevent

HEALTH TEACHING   Suggestions for Preventing Urinary Tract Infections and Promoting Genitourinary Health

- Increase fluid intake to approximately 8 to 10 glasses per day; plain water is best to flush the body's systems of potential toxins; drink a glass of water before sexual intercourse to allow urinary output afterward and prevent UTIs.
- Avoid bladder irritants such as caffeine products, alcohol, artificial sweeteners, spicy foods, and carbonated beverages.
- Make urination a regular habit; avoid waiting to urinate until bladder is full.
- Urinate before and after sexual intercourse to cleanse the urethra and empty the bladder.
- Be aware that vigorous or frequent intercourse may contribute to increased risk of UTIs.

- Maintain consistently good perineal hygiene, including wiping from front to back after urination and bowel movements.
- Take all prescription medications given for UTIs, even when the symptoms of the infection have been alleviated.
- Drink cranberry or blueberry juice to acidify the urine or take cranberry pills; these products may relieve some of the symptoms of a UTI.
- Seek health care advice for a vaginal infection, which may contribute to development of a UTI.
- The nurse should assess for increased risk of developing a UTI: congenital or structural abnormalities of the genitourinary system, previous surgery to the genitourinary system; pregnancy; previous UTIs; high intake of carbonated beverages; and poor intake of water.

UTI, Urinary tract infection.

urinary tract infections (UTIs), typically a problem that is more common during pregnancy. With a known correlation between UTIs and premature labor, a focus on preventing and managing these infections must occur during pregnancy.

Activity-Exercise Pattern
Fetus

Early spontaneous movements of the fetus may be reflexive, stimulated by passive uterine movement. Ultrasonographic observation of fetal movement shows repetitive movements early in pregnancy; at about 16 weeks, the pregnant woman feels these movements, termed **quickening**. By the end of the second trimester, fetal movement occurs less frequently because of lack of space in the uterus. The woman and her partner look forward to the regular daily cycle of movements, indicators of fetal well-being. An absence of or dramatic increase in fetal movements for more than 8 hours may indicate fetal distress. The nurse routinely teaches a pregnant woman to count the number of fetal movements each day and report any changes in fetal activity to the health care provider.

Pregnant Woman

The physical changes during pregnancy and the rigors of labor and delivery require that a pregnant woman be in the best physical condition of her life. Fortunately many pregnant women view pregnancy as a normal, natural state, and they often participate actively in physical activities or sports enjoyed before pregnancy. Generally a woman should avoid high-risk sports, such as sky diving and high-altitude climbing, because these could cause trauma to the fetus from low oxygen pressure or a maternal fall. Nurses encourage each woman to choose activities based on her interests, comfort, and good judgment. When a sport or activity causes exhaustion or pain, it should be modified or discontinued. Later in

pregnancy the woman should be encouraged to choose safe physical activities because of changes in her center of gravity due to the enlarging uterus and in the musculoskeletal system.

The woman with a sedentary lifestyle before pregnancy should slowly increase her activity level during pregnancy. A daily swim or 30-minute walk provides a good introduction to a regular exercise program. Regular exercise contributes to joint flexibility, improved cardiovascular and gastrointestinal fitness, uterine tone for an efficient labor, fewer pregnancy discomforts, weight control and a lower risk for diabetes, and overall feelings of well-being in the pregnant woman (USDHHS, 2000). For the self-directed woman, prenatal classes or a consumer-oriented book of prenatal exercises will facilitate an adequate exercise program. For most women, group exercise with other pregnant women is more enjoyable than exercising alone. The nurse encourages women to enter a structured diet and exercise program sponsored by the birthing hospital to help women lose weight after childbirth (Frieden & Chan, 2007).

In an uncomplicated pregnancy, a couple may continue their usual sexual activity. However, threatened abortion or history of abortion in the first trimester, early rupture of membranes, and other complications may call for restrictions on sexual intercourse or orgasm.

Sleep-Rest Pattern
Fetus

Electroencephalographic studies have shown four cyclical states of activity in the fetus: complete wakefulness, drowsy wakefulness, rapid eye movement sleep, and quiet sleep. Evidence suggests that a diurnal (day-night) pattern exists during the fetal period. Sleep is required for somatic and brain growth and development. Sleep-wake patterns change with central nervous system maturation.

Infant development entails increasing amounts of quiet sleep as well as increasing periods of quiet alertness. Both states require remarkable neural organization, thus sleep-wake patterns are an excellent window to the infant's neurological status.

Pregnant Woman

Fatigue reflects the significant physical and emotional changes occurring in the pregnant woman. The nurse counsels a woman that fatigue usually subsides by the fourth month but may return later in pregnancy. Rest breaks during the day and 8 hours of sleep each night help prevent fatigue and increase the pregnant woman's comfort. The nurse encourages each pregnant woman to rest when her body signals it is tired because of the rapidly growing fetus and the woman's needs for physical renewal. This encouragement must be directed particularly toward working women, who may need a doctor's note for their employer that validates the need for rest during the workday.

Many pregnant women do not sleep well because they need to urinate several times a night during the first and third trimesters. In addition, some women experience positional discomfort in late pregnancy that prevents effective sleep and, therefore, increases their fatigue. Fatigue may influence a woman's evaluation of her role as a pregnant woman, her body changes, and her cultural beliefs related to her ability to succeed in pregnancy. The nurse helps the woman express her thoughts and feelings and find ways to support better sleep and rest patterns (e.g., sleeping upright in a chair at night for easier breathing).

Cognitive-Perceptual Pattern
Fetus

During the prenatal period, all fetal sensory systems function or nearly function. These systems include vision, hearing, taste, smell, touch, and proprioceptive and vestibular senses (Blackburn, 2007). The fetus with all senses intact does experience the discomfort of pregnancy and the pain of labor contractions. Although capable of seeing by 30 weeks of age, the fetus has little opportunity to use this ability in utero (Blackburn, 2007). After approximately 25 weeks, pregnant women note that their babies respond to a loud, sudden noise. Some pregnant women and their partners offer sensory stimulation to the fetus by singing or rubbing the woman's abdomen. This parental behavior may assist in the bonding process between parent and baby. Thus the nurse may wish to include this kind of information in prenatal teaching sessions.

Pregnant Woman

Physical and psychological processes remain closely intertwined as pregnancy progresses. Psychological stresses and normal emotional growth affect the physical status of the pregnancy, interactions of the family members, and the eventual relationship between mother and infant. When considering the emotional aspects of pregnancy, the nurse recognizes that the woman's personality, environment, physical state, family, and sociocultural and spiritual background affect the ways in which she handles the psychological changes.

Two major categories of psychological influences are (1) normal psychological growth required of parents to emotionally and physically prepare them for parenthood and (2) internal or external stressors on the pregnant woman that decrease her ability to provide the best environment for the developing fetus. The pregnant woman undergoes many cognitive changes that ultimately result in her psychological readiness for motherhood.

Emotional Changes Hormonal and other physical changes assist the woman in the psychological work of pregnancy. Progesterone level increases affect the woman's general mood, causing her to be more introverted and passive. These mood changes help her to focus her energy on the growing child and her own growth and development. In addition to hormonal changes, the presence, growth, and movements of the fetus become more a part of the woman's experiential self. According to Rubin (1984), the classic researcher on maternal-infant bonding, the pregnant woman receives immediate sensations of touch, motion, and weight from the fetus that she can share only partially with others. These support a maternal feeling of separateness and uniqueness that causes the woman to turn inward. She frequently worries that the shift in energy away from the world toward herself and her child may cause her to lose contact, drift away from valued relationships, and lose feelings of competence in her areas of achievement. She spends time analyzing her experiences and their possible influence on her effectiveness as a future parent. She constantly studies the qualities of human relationships and shows increased sensitivity and perceptiveness to many people. To others, the woman may seem overly sensitive and analytical during pregnancy (Rubin, 1967, 1984).

Although a woman's mood varies based on a variety of factors and at different times during the pregnancy, many women experience wide mood swings, emotional lability, irritability, and changes in sexual desire. Physical discomforts, hormonal changes, feelings about altered body image, cultural considerations, work and relationship adjustments, and demanding cognitive maturational processes may also cause these emotional changes.

Rubin's classic work stimulated nurses to look beyond the physiological and pathological aspects of childbearing to the intricate process of becoming a mother, and to identify areas for providing help. Current research identifies two simultaneous processes in the transition to motherhood: engagement and growth and transformation. Engagement is making a commitment and being engrossed in mothering through active involvement in the child's care. At the same time, the woman's engagement leads to the woman's growth and transition as she becomes a mother (Mercer, 2004).

Current descriptions for the stages in the process of establishing a maternal identity in becoming a mother include the following:

- Commitment, attachment, and preparation for the pregnancy
- Acquaintance, learning, and physical restoration during the first 6 weeks after birth
- Moving toward a new normal from 2 weeks to 4 months
- Achievement of the maternal identity at about 4 months (Nelson, 2003).

The times for achieving the stages are highly variable, and are influenced by maternal and infant variables and the social-environmental context (Mercer, 2004).

Stressors Influencing Development The mother's age, fears related to a previous fetal loss, feelings about the pregnancy, life situation and culture, degree of stress, the presence of other children, loss of control at times, and the influence of loved ones may serve as stressors that influence the ways in which she completes the developmental tasks of motherhood (Richter et al., 2007). A young pregnant woman facing the additional developmental task of adolescence may have difficulty incorporating the pregnant body or the role of mother into her still undefined self-image. Cognitively, she may still be unable to make plans for the baby or even accept the pregnancy until she feels the baby move. Anticipatory guidance is critical when an adolescent faces overlapping developmental challenges of age and pregnancy.

On the other hand, a pregnant woman older than 35 years may feel more isolated by her situation than does the pregnant woman in her 20s. Frequently established in career and family, the older pregnant woman needs to learn to balance her growth and development in these valued areas with her new sense of self. Fears related to being considered at high risk because of age may increase her anxiety and ambivalence about the pregnancy, even if she was previously infertile. As a first-time mother, she may worry about managing the physical demands of labor and delivery, sleeplessness of motherhood, chances of having an abnormal child, and the need to juggle conflicting life responsibilities and relationships.

A woman with other children moves through the developmental tasks differently than does a woman who is pregnant for the first time. Even with a desired pregnancy, the woman may worry about incorporating the new infant into her relationships and managing the time needed for a new baby. She may have fears and anxieties about labor and delivery because of a previous negative experience. She may be much more aware of the problems involved with caring for a new infant and may not be excited about another pregnancy experience that demands a redefinition of motherhood or additional child-rearing expenses.

Developmental Tasks

Rubin (1967, 1977, 1984) describes four major developmental tasks that a woman seeks to accomplish as she learns to become a mother. These include ensuring safe passage through pregnancy and childbirth, ensuring acceptance of the child by significant people in her family, binding into her unknown child, and learning to give of self. According to Rubin, all four tasks must be confronted simultaneously, but each task assumes greater priority at certain times than do other tasks. Each woman works through these tasks based on her unique style, cultural values, and life priorities. At the end of pregnancy, however, all tasks must be integrated to create a presentation, similar to a tapestry (Rubin, 1984).

1. Ensuring Safe Passage

- Engages in a variety of prenatal care options appropriate to her culture and life experience. For example, pregnant Cambodian women rely on older same-culture women to give prenatal care and advice and rely little on prenatal classes or visits. Some Hispanic American women, based on their view that pregnancy is a healthy, natural experience, may not seek prenatal care but seek a strong matriarchal support system for a positive outcome.
- Woman becomes more protective of herself and the fetus by avoiding crowds, revolving doors, small spaces, and people believed to place the mother at risk. She tires of being pregnant but fears the effect of delivery on her safety and that of her child (Rubin, 1972, 1984). Although sharing fears and desires with her partner, family, or health care provider helps, only the safe delivery of a normal child can fully free a pregnant woman from her fears to meet this developmental task (Rubin, 1972, 1977).

2. Ensuring Acceptance of the Child

- The woman must believe that her child will be accepted into her family based on her definition of family. According to Rubin (1984), the partner's receptivity to the child is particularly important, and many women fantasize about the gender of their child based on a partner's preference.
- The woman frequently judges her partner's degree of receptivity to the infant by the amount of love and attention that she, herself, receives from him during her pregnancy.
- She may desire support from other women, rather than her partner, based on her life experience, values, and cultural background.

3. Binding into Her Unknown Child

- This task is the most complex cognitive process for the pregnant woman (Rubin, 1984). To accomplish this task, she must integrate the fetus as an integral part of her but also as a separate being. Completion of this task occurs with birth of the baby.
- Initially, the woman fantasizes about the baby through associative images: when she eats an egg, she thinks of the baby. Fantasies in the second and third trimesters relate more specifically to what the child will be like; the woman may imagine the baby in little girl or little boy clothes.
- During the eighth month, the woman begins nesting activity by preparing the nursery and thinking increasingly of the baby as an external reality in her home.

4. Learning to Give of Herself

- Although the actual mothering activity occurs after birth, the learning process to become a mother begins during pregnancy.
- The woman begins the task by examining what she will gain and lose by becoming a mother.
- She then explores the meaning of giving by examining how others give to her and to others and how she has given to others in the past (Rubin, 1984).
- Gifts for herself and the baby represent meaningful manifestations of her own and others' acceptance of her motherhood and her ability to give to her child and develop her identity as mother (Rubin, 1967, 1972).

Self-Perception–Self-Concept Pattern

To develop a maternal identity, the woman must first accept the pregnant body image. Initially she may show ambivalence based on her need to "fit" the pregnancy with her perception of self. She may dislike the physical changes of pregnancy or gladly "show off" her pregnant body to others. During the second trimester, however, the woman frequently begins to feel more positive about her changing womanly image as she feels the baby move, and increased estrogen and progesterone increase her sense of vitality, inner peace, and acceptance. Her body begins to look pregnant, and generally others respond positively to this change (Rubin, 1972).

By the third trimester, however, the woman frequently tires of the pregnancy. Her sense of awkward moments supersedes feelings of well-being. She may experience uncomfortable, sleepless nights, the constant need to urinate, Braxton-Hicks contractions, and other discomforts. Some women experience infant movement or mild contractions as pleasurable, sensual sensations, whereas others find them extremely uncomfortable. By pregnancy's end, these women yearn to have their former body boundaries back, to hold the baby in their arms, or to have someone else carry the baby.

After birth, the woman gradually sees the infant more and more as a separate individual, dependent on her care. The mother starts to bond with her baby based on her self-perception. If she feels good about herself, she will show love toward the infant; when she feels ugly or unlovable, she may make uncomplimentary remarks about the infant's appearance (Rubin, 1984).

Maternal Role

The pregnant woman's personality, maturity level, and psychological development influence her readiness to assume the role of mother. The way in which society in general and her culture in particular perceive motherhood and the role of women, as well as the way in which her own views mesh with these perceptions, will affect the ease of the transition. The family situation, the availability of peer role models, and the relationship with her mother are also significant. Internalization of the mother role occurs only after the birth, when the woman interacts with the infant in a reciprocal relationship (Rubin, 1977).

Nursing Interventions

The woman may feel overwhelmed by her feelings and thoughts during pregnancy. Although others acknowledge her physical changes, only she experiences the psychological changes of excitement, ambivalence, or confusion associated with being pregnant. During prenatal assessment, the nurse should address expected cognitive changes and self-image issues with each pregnant woman and respond nonjudgmentally to concerns expressed in this area. In one-to-one sessions or group prenatal classes, women and their partners should be encouraged to discuss their ideas and feelings related to the emotional and relationship changes expected during pregnancy, because these changes influence the future intimate relationship.

Roles-Relationships Pattern

The pregnant family changes throughout the pregnancy and postpartum period as each family member explores and responds to new roles and relationships. A pregnant woman without a partner may feel isolated during pregnancy and depend on family or friends as she adjusts to her situation. Cultural beliefs and traditions may produce stresses during pregnancy, change roles and relationships, or provide emotional and physical support to the pregnant family as it prepares for the baby.

The partner of the pregnant woman faces many new situations that influence that person's parental development. The pregnant woman may seem to be a different person to others because of her emotional response to the pregnancy, introspection, fantasies, need for more rest, and changes in sexual drive. The partner may feel a rivalry with the fetus and baby, because the mother is increasing amounts of time with the baby. He may resent the attention that she receives during the pregnancy and the additional demands that she may make on his time. He may experience more financial pressure because of baby expenses and his partner's need to stop working on a short-term or long-term basis. These perceptions may lead him to batter or otherwise abuse his partner, possibly causing a poor pregnancy and newborn outcomes (Hot Topics box). The nurse assesses each pregnant woman for abuse and intervene appropriately to protect the safety and health of the family during gestation.

The male partner may be concerned about his ability to fulfill the father role and support his wife or significant other. His fathering role models may be limited because of a lack of contact with his own father or because he spends time with men who are not actively parenting. He may never have held a baby before and may worry that he might drop or harm his own child. If his partner experiences pregnancy complications, he may feel guilty about causing the

BIRTH OUTCOMES IN ABUSED PREGNANT WOMEN

HOTtopics

Nurses and other providers who deliver health care to women must address the issue of abuse of the pregnant woman by an intimate partner. Intimate partner violence is a significant public health problem with negative physical and psychological outcomes. It has been associated with increased sexually transmitted infections, preterm labor, low–birth-weight infants, and postpartum depression (Kendall-Tackett, 2007). Consider the following research studies and the questions that follow to understand the issue further.

These studies examined the prevalence of different types of intimate partner violence (IPV) during pregnancy, as well as the association between both physical and psychological IPV and negative health behaviors, including smoking, other substance use, inadequate prenatal care utilization, nutrition, physical and psychological adaptations, and birthing outcomes. *Methods:* 104 southern Appalachian women, primarily Caucasian and lower SES, completed a pregnancy interview focused on IPV (CTS2) and health behaviors. Medical records were also reviewed. *Results:* 81% of participants reported some type of IPV during the current pregnancy, with 28% reporting physical IPV, and 20% reporting sexual violence. More than half were current smokers. Physical IPV during pregnancy was associated with significantly increased rates of pregnancy smoking (including decreased rates of quitting and reducing), increased rates of alcohol, marijuana, and harder illicit drug use around the time of conception, increase in sexually transmitted infections, and later entry into prenatal care. The experience of psychological IPV during pregnancy was associated with a significantly decreased likelihood of quitting or reducing smoking during pregnancy, an increased rate of alcohol use around the time of conception, and an increased rate of prepregnancy obesity. *Conclusions:* In this sample, pregnancy IPV and smoking occurred at rates well above national averages. Additionally, while physical IPV during pregnancy was associated with several negative pregnancy health behaviors, the experience of psychological IPV, even in the absence of physical IPV, also placed women at increased risk for negative health behaviors, all of which have been linked to poor pregnancy and newborn outcomes.

Overall, study results indicate a need to tailor nursing interventions supportive of pregnant women facing abuse and mandating that nurses conduct sensitive abuse screening for all pregnant women.

Questions

1. How do the current health care system and the sociopolitical context of care in this country contribute to the high numbers of pregnant women facing abuse from their intimate partners?
2. What kind of interventions do you believe would be effective for these abused women?
3. How should U.S. health care policy ethically and legislatively address the problem of intimate partner abuse during pregnancy?

Compiled from Bailey, B. A. & and Daugherty, R. A. (2007). Intimate partner violence during pregnancy: incidence and associated health behaviors and outcomes in a rural population. *Maternal & Child Health Journal*, 11(5), 495-503; Records, K. (2007). A critical review of maternal abuse and infant outcomes: Implications for newborn nurses. *Newborn & Infant Nursing Reviews*, 7(1), 7-13; Kendall-Tackett, K. A. (2007). Violence against women and the perinatal period. *Trauma, Violence & Abuse*, 8(3), 344-353; Sharps, P. W., Laughon, K., & Giangrande, S. K. (2007). Intimate partner violence and childbearing year: Maternal and infant health implications. *Trauma, Violence & Abuse*, 8(2), 105-116.

pregnancy. Table 16-5 gives a more complete list of both the father's and the mother's emotional responses to a first pregnancy. The nurse must work with the pregnant family to help them adapt to a first pregnancy, because this one affects how they will cope with subsequent pregnancies.

Children in the family also experience role changes during and after the pregnancy. The very young child, unaware of the concept of a new baby before the infant arrives, may experience a changed relationship with his pregnant mother. She may have less time to play, be more irritable from fatigue, or limit or stop active play late in pregnancy because of increased awkwardness and concern about her safety. After the baby arrives, the child may be kept away from both baby and mother by well-meaning friends and relatives, have to share parents with others, or may want to breast-feed from the mother as the baby does. When permitted to see the newborn, the child may be admonished to "be careful" or "don't touch the baby." Thus a young child may not accept the baby with open arms.

The older child understands the newborn's significance more clearly but still experiences apprehensions about the effects of the baby on the family. Older children may have been told that they will become a big brother or sister, but does this mean they will lose toys, time with parents, and have to give up a private bedroom? Older children may worry about their mother, who seems more tired, less available, and perhaps even sick at times. Her enlarging abdomen may appear frightening. With help from the nurse, parents can make pregnancy an exciting time of learning and growing for the family (Box 16-4). Chapter 18 also discusses the sibling relationship in greater detail.

In extended families, expectant grandparents also experience changes during the pregnancy of their daughter or daughter-in-law. The maternal grandmother, seeing her daughter assume the mother role, may now view her daughter as a rival, because they are both mothers. The grandparents may be reminded of their own aging, resenting when their advice about pregnancy and parenting goes unheeded. A positive outcome of a pregnancy may be a new closeness between woman and mother if the daughter turns to her mother to seek advice and share feelings. The nurse may encourage expectant parents to use pregnancy as a transition time for their own parents, which can enhance extended family cohesion in the future.

Table **16-5** Possible Responses to First Pregnancy

Phase of Pregnancy	Father's Response	Mother's Response
First trimester	Fear of losing wife or child Self-doubt as a future father May develop new hobby outside of partner as way of distancing self	Loss of interest in coitus Possible less sexual effectiveness Sleepiness and chronic fatigue Nausea Increased dependence Feels ambivalent toward reality of pregnancy Anxious about process of labor and prospect of caring for a child Worries about miscarriage Becomes aware of physical changes in body May develop a closer relationship with her mother with a common experience of motherhood
Second trimester	Increased respect Awe as quickening comes Names for fetus coined May give partner extra attention she desires	Solemnity, hilarity, and playfulness about fetal movements Talks about and with fetus Increased eroticism Expects partner to demonstrate interest in caring for her and baby Feels movement and thinks of child as an individual
Third trimester	Fear of coitus hurting fetus Abstinence difficult Envy or pride or both at wife's creativity Worry about birth Keen awareness of male-female differences May show a greater level of tenderness and protectiveness	Abstinence (often recommended by physician) Sleepiness Backache Abdominal discomfort Sexual isolation Heightened sense of femininity Assembles the items needed for the care of the infant and selects possible names
Postpartum	Eagerness to resume marital relations Concern over endangering wife's recovery Sense of triumph in becoming a father Tenderness toward wife and baby	Pain and fear of harm from too early coitus Low eroticism Concern about effect on husband of continued abstinence Sense of completion as a mother
Pregnancy as a whole	Increased romanticism Increased nurturance Increased family life participation Anxiety about costs Concern about lack of skills in baby care	Increased romanticism Increased optimism Family roles replacing marital emphases Fear of miscarriage or problems with baby Pride of accomplishment

From Ramer, L., & Frank, B. (2001). *Pregnancy: Psychosocial perspectives* (3rd ed). White Plains, NY: March of Dimes; Hilling, H. and Rutherford, JJ. (2007). *Modern mom's guide to dads: Ten secrets your husband won't tell you.* Nashville: Cumberland House.

Box **16-4** Nursing Strategies to Help Parents Prepare Siblings for the Neonate

- Explain the pregnancy and birth appropriate to the child's age.
- Answer all the child's questions.
- Use relevant literature to educate the child about the coming baby.
- Encourage discussion and questions by talking about the new baby during relaxed family times rather than during busy, rushed times.
- Have the child participate in decisions, such as choosing a name, clothes, and toys for baby.

- When sibling classes are available as part of the childbirth education process, encourage parents and child to attend.
- Suggest that the child go with the mother during clinic or office visits.
- Allow and discuss negative comments about the pregnancy or baby.
- Encourage child to make drawings or give small gifts to the baby when it is born.

During pregnancy and after birth, each family member begins to establish an emotional attachment to the imagined or real new baby. Research shows that when the mother has a strong support system to develop deep feelings of attachment to the fetus, she will most likely attach to the baby after birth. Therefore the nurse assesses the support system of each pregnant woman and implements primary and secondary interventions to increase family bonding with a new baby.

Sexuality-Reproductive Pattern

The pregnant woman's body image and merging of this body image with her definition of femininity greatly influence her feelings about her sexuality. For a previously infertile couple, achieving pregnancy may be a blessed event, despite the need for technology that affects a woman's concept of self and femininity and a man's concept of self and masculinity. The reflections of others, particularly those of a pregnant woman's husband, partner, or friend, help a woman to accept changes in her body, leading to better adjustment in their sexual relations.

On the other hand, women may experience different sexual feelings during pregnancy. Some women experience an increase in desire, but most worry about intercourse during pregnancy, fearing that it will cause **miscarriage**, infection, early delivery, or harm to the baby. Sexual dissatisfaction of the couple may result from restrictions in sexual positions, pain on penetration, increased vaginal discharge, breast tenderness, or the other physical discomforts of pregnancy such as fatigue or heartburn. In some cases the enlarging uterus will require the couple to modify positions for intercourse, particularly during the latter part of pregnancy. The couple's feelings about the woman's changing body may alter their sexual relationship. The nurse's first step in primary prevention intervention in this area is to support the couple's needs and relate, in a sensitive fashion, accurate information that facilitates couple intimacy during pregnancy.

Some women experience a decreased desire for sexual intercourse but an increased desire for holding, touching, and other signs of physical affection from their husbands or partners. The nurse encourages the couple to explore other activities for mutual sexual satisfaction.

Coping–Stress Tolerance Pattern

Physical and psychological adaptations of the woman to pregnancy affect her perception of stressors and her ability to cope with all aspects of her life. Even normal discomforts of pregnancy may be stressful for a woman, mandating her to modify her usual routine to cope more effectively. Anxiety tends to be high during the first trimester as the woman adapts to pregnancy and anticipated life changes. During the second trimester, the woman feels less anxious, but anxiety returns during the third trimester with impending labor and delivery. Throughout pregnancy women may demonstrate their anxieties through psychosomatic complaints and behaviors, such as nausea and vomiting after the first trimester, excessive eating, food cravings, sleeplessness,

and fainting. Realistically, every pregnant woman probably experiences some degree of stress. However, many women have considerable stress or ongoing stress, such as poverty, marital difficulties, or unsatisfactory living or working conditions, that influences their coping abilities.

A pregnant woman's anxieties may be reflected in her dreams and fantasies. Many pregnant women report dreams about their babies being deformed or dead, themselves dying, or a family member being injured. Many women at the end of their pregnancies express fears about body mutilation with delivery. Other women may manifest their anxiety by smoking, drinking, or using drugs (legal or illegal), all of which can harm the fetus. Maternal anxiety may cause increased fetal activity and heart rate, as well as decreased blood flow to the uterus, thus influencing adequate oxygen and food to the fetus (Alder et al., 2007). The nurse must direct a pregnant woman who is not coping well to relevant resources for assistance. The nurse must also assess each woman's progress in taking on the mothering role as the pregnancy nears term. This information can be shared with the postpartum nursing staff to encourage discussion in this important area.

The nurse encourages the pregnant woman to use tension-relieving strategies such as listening to soft music, using humor, crying, sleeping, talking to a friend, meditating, exercising, and fantasizing during times of stress. These strategies are safe for the fetus and provide relief from many normal tensions and anxieties during pregnancy and afterward. Overall, the nurse plays a key role by responding nonjudgmentally and promoting the coping of women during pregnancy.

Values-Beliefs Pattern

Although pregnancy has been described as the fulfillment of the deepest and most powerful wish of a woman, this fulfillment often coincides with a woman's fear of losing part of herself. She gives up some relationships and pleasures to take on other anticipated satisfactions. She may find that she values friendships with other mothers now, whereas before pregnancy her friendships focused on work or school colleagues. She may discover, much to her husband's confusion, that she values different qualities in him than she did before anticipating birth. Her husband may also experience a shift in his values.

Pregnant women and their partners may experience changes in their spiritual values. For women with strong spiritual needs related to their cultural backgrounds, spiritual interventions will help them integrate various dimensions of their lives, develop the ability to parent successfully, and find meaning in the changes and goals of pregnancy. Seen as a mystical event or miracle, conception may lead to an increased faith in God or a favorite saint. Nonreligious couples may start to attend church after the baby's birth, because they want religion to be part of their child's life. Religious beliefs may influence a woman's decision to undergo certain tests or procedures, such as amniocentesis or abortion. Some women may feel forced to reproduce because their religious or cultural mores forbids contraception or encourages large families. In these groups, each pregnancy may be seen as another unwanted, but unavoidable, burden or may be valued because more children signify a stronger family.

ENVIRONMENTAL PROCESSES

A healthy infant is the outcome of most pregnancies. However, genetic abnormalities and environmental hazards may cause fetal harm, spontaneous abortion (natural loss of conceptive products), or minor or serious congenital defects. Diagnostic methods that identify an early pregnancy or a fetal loss may assist couples in practicing healthy decisions to prevent loss or congenital abnormalities. Cunningham and colleagues (2005f) note that congenital defects affect 3% to 4% of all live births and contribute to infant mortality rates by causing structural or functional disability incompatible with life. Real-time ultrasonography identifies approximately 85% of fetal anomalies by 36 weeks of gestation (Gilbert, 2006). This knowledge, gained before giving birth, permits expectant couples and the health care delivery team to access resources for improving the baby's life or support family grieving if the baby is not expected to live. With progress made in diagnostic tools and the Human Genome Project, some couples may be able to prevent fetal defects or manage them during pregnancy to improve the quality of their baby's life after birth (see the Case Study at the end of this chapter). Unfortunately, even when no genetic or congenital defects exist, the fetus may still be injured during the process of labor and delivery and face a lesser quality of life.

Teratogens are environmental agents that cause spontaneous abortions or congenital defects. Unlike genetic abnormalities, which occur only at conception, environmental agents may affect the developing infant at any point during gestation. Fetal organs have critical periods of development and, if affected at that time by a teratogen, the infant may have a defect in that organ system. **Website Resource 16D** depicts the effects of teratogens on the embryo and fetus. Teratogens normally do not cause a congenital defect during the first 14 days after conception. However, the embryo may be lost later during early gestation (a spontaneous abortion). Therefore, as a primary prevention strategy, any woman contemplating or attempting pregnancy should be counseled to avoid teratogens that might cause fetal loss or damage.

Physical Factors and Diagnostic Tools

Modern diagnostic tools, such as ultrasonography, amniocentesis, chorionic villus sampling, and alpha-fetoprotein screening, have been used to identify a number of fetal problems. Many of these tools are presented in **Website Resource 16E**. Certain risk factors, such as family history, maternal and paternal age, maternal illness, or previous fetal abnormalities, may indicate the need for these diagnostic tools during a woman's pregnancy. These tools commonly identify problems related to abnormal size or rate of fetal growth, chromosomal abnormalities, neural tube defects, and fetal lung immaturity. The nurse, in consultation with the health care team, must participate in providing informed consent to women before these diagnostic tools are utilized.

Biological Agents

Biological processes in the fetal environment, which include infections and other health problems of the mother, may affect fetal growth and development. A pregnant woman who acquires an asymptomatic viral infection may not seek health care because she believes that the fetus will not be harmed. However, viral agents may cause fetal damage early in pregnancy. The woman with a health problem, such as diabetes, may also cause fetal damage if she fails to adhere to her health care provider's directives.

When the nurse discusses with pregnant couples the effects of biological processes on the fetus, she must emphasize that the timing of the maternal infection or illness is critical to predicting fetal defects. Maternal infections during the first trimester of pregnancy may cause severe fetal defects or death, depending on the organism. Infections later in pregnancy may also seriously affect the fetus, but less often. Unfortunately, pregnancy renders many women more susceptible to viral illness, supporting an argument for all women of childbearing age to be fully immunized. Many vaccines (measles, mumps, rubella, and polio) cannot be given during pregnancy due to potential risk to the fetus, but others present no risk (tetanus and diphtheria). A TORCH screen may be done to detect the presence of five teratogenic perinatal infections: toxoplasmosis, hepatitis B, rubella, cytomegalovirus, and herpes simplex (Table 16-6).

Toxoplasmosis

Toxoplasmosis is caused by a protozoan that infects people through undercooked meat, handling of cat feces, and exposure to infected soil in countries outside the United States (Friars, 2007). An infected pregnant woman may have flu-like symptoms or mild to severe upper respiratory symptoms believed to be unrelated to an infection. About 60% of maternal infections acquired during the third trimester will result in fetal infection, which might manifest as skin rashes, enlarged lymph nodes and liver, inflammation of the heart, pneumonia, jaundice, or severe central nervous system damage (Ward, 2007) after birth or years later. Pregnant women should use good hand-washing technique, avoid eating raw meat, and avoid handling cats or cleaning cat litter boxes to avoid exposure to Toxoplasma.

Syphilis

An infected mother transfers **syphilis**, an STI that is caused by a protozoan, to her fetus. Although preventable and treatable, the number of congenital and neonatal syphilis cases has increased over the last several years (CDC, 2007). Maternal risk factors for acquiring syphilis

Table **16-6** TORCH Perinatal Infections

Infection	Agent	Source	Fetal-Neonatal Risks	Comments
Toxoplasmosis	Protozoan *Toxoplasma gondii*	Raw or undercooked meat; unpasteurized goat's milk; feces of infected cats	Intrauterine growth restriction (IUGR), microcephaly, hydrocephaly; seizures, neurological and cognitive effects	Instruct mother to not eat undercooked or raw meat; avoid exposure to cat litter
Other/Hepatitis B	Hepadnavirus	Blood or blood products; sexually transmitted via body fluids	Generally asymptomatic, but majority become chronically infected	Newborn should receive HBIG within 12 hours after birth and Hep B vaccine postpartum
Rubella	Rubella virus	Direct or indirect contact with droplets of infected person	CNS defects— developmental delay, deafness, cataracts, IUGR, microcephaly, cardiac defects	Screen all pregnant women with rubella antibody titers
Cytomegalovirus	Herpes virus	Transmitted by droplet infection from person to person	Microcephaly, IUGR, CNS abnormalities, deafness, blindness, jaundice, GI defects	Prevention of maternal primary infection in early pregnancy; stress good personal hygiene
Herpes simplex	HSV 1 and 2	Sexually transmitted infection to mother; fetus contacts it during birth from genital lesions	Intense herpetic lesions on eyes, mouth, and skin	Practice safer sex; careful handwashing; surgical birth if active lesions

Compiled from Blackburn, S.T. (2007) *Maternal, fetal, & neonatal physiology: A clinical perspective.* 3rd edition. St. Louis: Saunders; Arenson, J. & Drake, P. (2007). *Maternal and newborn health.* Sudbury, MA: Jones and Bartlett; Cunningham, F. G., Gant, N. F., Leveno, K. J., Gilstrap, L. C., Hauth, J. C., & Wenstrom, K. D. (2005g). Sexually transmitted diseases. *Williams obstetrics* (22nd ed. pp. 1301-1325). New York: McGraw-Hill.

include homelessness, **human immunodeficiency virus (HIV)**-positive status, single marital status, and a history of STIs. Maternal syphilis has been associated with complications such as **polyhydramnios**, spontaneous abortion, and preterm births. Fetal complications such as fetal syphilis, fetal hydrops, prematurity, fetal distress, and **stillbirth** also occur. Neonatal complications can include congenital syphilis, neonatal death, and late sequelae (Majeroni & Ukkadam, 2007). The infant may be born with localized mucocutaneous lesions, nasal congestion, anemia, and generalized septicemia, but may appear healthy at birth only to have symptoms appear later. Routine testing of high-risk women for syphilis at the first prenatal visit and during the third trimester, as well as antibiotic treatment (benzathine penicillin G) for affected women and their partners, have reduced the number of infants with congenital syphilis (Goh & Thornton, 2007). Treating the infected mother during the first 16 weeks of pregnancy usually protects the fetus (Queenan et al., 2007).

Rubella

Despite the broad use of the measles, mumps, and rubella vaccine, or MMR, and the resulting immunity to rubella, approximately 20% of women reach their childbearing period without immunity to this disease (USDHHS, 2000).

Rubella is associated with an 80% risk of congenital abnormalities if acquired in the first 12 weeks of pregnancy (Best, 2007). The symptoms of rubella may cause the mother to think she has a minor viral infection, but rubella during the first trimester may cause improper fetal development of the ears, eyes, and heart and deafness. No treatment exists for an infected fetus; however, a pregnant woman may receive the vaccine to protect future pregnancies if she has no history of rubella infection. After giving birth, new mothers often receive the vaccine before being discharged with a recommendation to avoid pregnancy for at least 3 months to prevent fetal harm from the vaccine.

Cytomegalovirus

Cytomegalovirus (CMV) is responsible for the most common infection that may cause serious fetal complications. CMV infects an estimated 1% to 2% of all infants born in the United States. Most mothers infected with CMV have mild, often nonspecific symptoms, but their infants may experience hearing loss, blindness, enlarged liver and spleen, and neurodevelopmental disabilities (Malm & Engman, 2007). Unfortunately, no means exist to prevent or manage this viral infection. Perhaps an immunization similar to that for rubella will be developed in the future. Until vaccines and nontoxic antiviral agents are available, hygienic measures are important as prophylaxis.

Herpes Simplex Virus

Herpes simplex virus infections remain extremely common today, with many people unaware that they have the disease. Herpes simplex may cause spontaneous abortion or fetal neurological damage. Infants infected at birth may show localized or generalized disease with symptoms of vesicular skin lesions, conjunctivitis, seizures, respiratory distress, or gastrointestinal bleeding. These symptoms may cause newborn death. An infant from a vaginal birth by a woman with active genital herpes has a 40% to 60% chance of being infected (CDC, 2007), supporting a decision for a cesarean birth for any women with active vaginal or perineal herpes lesions. Risk factors for the transmission of herpes from mother to newborn have been detailed. The pregnant woman who acquires genital herpes as a primary infection in the latter half of pregnancy, rather than prior to pregnancy, is at greatest risk of transmitting this virus to her newborn. This is true for both herpes simplex virus type-1 and type-2 (Baker, 2007). Generally acyclovir (Zovirax) is not recommended during pregnancy for treatment of viral lesions. The nurse educates the infected woman about comfort measures at this time, including ways to keep the lesions dry and application of comfort measures to reduce the pain of the lesions (Hackley et al., 2007).

Chlamydia, Gonococcus, Group B Streptococcus, Bacterial Vaginosis, and Candida albicans

Infections caused by these bacteria and yeast (**Candida albicans**) may occur in the woman's vagina or cervix, infecting the infant during a vaginal delivery. **Chlamydia**, the most common bacterial STI, appears most often among poor women with little access to care. Although few symptoms are seen, infection may cause preterm labor or newborn conjunctivitis or pneumonia. Routine treatment of the newborn's eyes after birth with erythromycin destroys the organisms. Maternal **gonococcus** (GC) infection can be transmitted to the newborn from the mother's genital tract at the time of birth and can cause ophthalmia neonatorum, systemic neonatal infection, maternal endometritis, or pelvic infection. The risk of transmission from an infected mother to her infant is between 30% and 47% (Majeroni & Ukkadam, 2007). Newborn infants often receive erythromycin ointment in the eyes to prevent GC infection. Screening at 36 to 37 weeks of pregnancy for **group B Streptococcus** infection has been recommended, because this infection causes preterm rupture of the amniotic membranes, premature labor, fetal respiratory distress syndrome, fetal septicemia, and meningitis (Gilbert, 2006). **Bacterial vaginosis** may also cause premature labor (U.S. Preventive Services Task Force, 2006b). *Candida albicans*, cause of a common vaginal fungal infection, may also cause an oral infection called thrush in the newborn. Routine assessment of pregnant women, and occasionally their sexual partners (GC), for these bacterial and yeast infections must occur during pregnancy so that treatment can occur and prevent fetal infection at the time of birth.

Human Immune Deficiency Virus (HIV)

Acquired Immunodeficiency Syndrome The U.S. Public Health Service and the U.S. Prevention Services Task Force recommend that all pregnant women in the United States be tested for HIV infection, ideally at the first prenatal visit (USPSTF, 2006f). Any woman in a high-risk group (e.g., an intravenous drug user, one who has bisexual partners, one who has multiple sexual contacts, history of STIs, one who exchanges sex for money or drugs, or Black or Hispanic women living in poverty) should be tested for antibodies to HIV. For the HIV-positive woman or one who engages in high-risk sexual practices, counseling must occur before conception. Counseling should include both the effect of the virus on pregnancy and the effect of pregnancy on HIV disease progression. Although unclear, it appears that HIV infection becomes worse during pregnancy because of a woman's altered immune status. Some early pregnancy discomforts, such as fatigue, anorexia, and weight loss, may mask the early symptoms of HIV infection and thus postpone a definitive diagnosis.

Infants born to HIV-positive women have an infection rate of 15% to 25% (CDC, 2006). Affected infants may not be seropositive for HIV for many months after birth and then later develop the disease. Recent use of zidovudine (AZT) protocol treatments throughout pregnancy has improved the prognosis of an HIV-positive woman and has decreased viral transmission to the fetus, although the drug remains expensive and may be inaccessible for women who do not receive prenatal care.

The pregnant woman who has **acquired immunodeficiency syndrome (AIDS)** or who is HIV positive should be carefully monitored by a health care team for opportunistic infections that occur frequently. The nurse can be instrumental in helping this woman coordinate her contacts with care providers, answering her questions, and working as a member of the team to provide optimal care for her and her child. Frequently the pregnant woman with AIDS does not seek care, based on fears of being reported for her disease. Involving the woman in continuous prenatal care decreases her risk of preterm rupture of membranes, problems with fetal growth, postpartum infection, drug and alcohol abuse, and difficulty in addressing sociocultural barriers to a better life (Dangal, 2008).

Although important in decreasing the transmission of any disease, astute preventive measures are mandatory for nurses who come in contact with HIV-infected body fluids, such as blood, amniotic fluid, and vaginal secretions (universal precautions). All health care providers must follow hospital and birth center policies regarding the use of gloves, gowns, and the disposal of needles and other potentially contaminated equipment to prevent the transmission of this disease in particular.

Hepatitis B

Hepatitis B virus (HBV) infection remains a significant concern during pregnancy, because it affects the maternal liver and has a high fetal transmission rate (60%) if present during the third trimester. High-risk groups for HBV include women from Asia, Pacific Islands, and sub-Saharan Africa, as well as health care workers, intravenous drug users, and women with multiple sex partners (CDC, 2007). Based on the large number of infected women who fail to show symptoms until liver damage has occurred, all pregnant women early in pregnancy and those at risk should be screened routinely for this virus (U.S. Preventive Services Task Force, 2006c). HBV immunization (three injections over a period of 6 months) may be given before or during pregnancy to a mother who is seronegative (CDC, 2007). According to Gilbert (2006), most women harboring the virus transmit it through the placenta to the fetus or through contaminated urine, feces, saliva, or vaginal fluids during birth. Many women carrying the virus deliver prematurely, and some infants may have acute hepatitis or later develop liver cancer.

Other Health Concerns

Pregnant women may also develop any of the infections of nonpregnant women. For example, pregnant women frequently experience upper respiratory and gastrointestinal infections, adding to the discomforts of pregnancy. However, there is no evidence the viruses causing these infections have a teratogenic effect on the fetus.

Fever frequently occurs with illness. A high, prolonged fever (hyperthermia) in a pregnant woman may harm the fetus, especially during the first trimester. Some literature indicates that high fever is associated with miscarriages, stillbirths, and premature deliveries. Whether the high fever or an underlying illness causing the fever has created the problem must be determined. Some reports have also correlated prolonged use of a sauna or hot tub, causing hyperthermia, with birth defects such as microcephaly, anencephaly, and hypotonia. Until health care providers understand this issue better, the nurse should advise pregnant women to avoid prolonged sauna or hot tub use and people who are ill or carrying disease. When a pregnant woman develops a high fever, she should be advised to contact her health care provider immediately.

Pregnant mothers may have other health problems that influence their physiological processes and thus harm the developing fetus. Black women experience twice the rate of hypertension and diabetes mellitus as do White women. These higher rates may account for the three to four times higher maternal mortality rate seen among pregnant Black women as compared with White women (CDC Office of Women's Health, 2007).

Diabetes Diabetes may exist before or during pregnancy, affecting both mother and fetus. Pregnancy increases the need for maternal insulin to balance the woman's blood sugar. Currently the American College of Obstetricians and Gynecologists recommends that all pregnant women complete a glucose tolerance test at 28 weeks' gestation to identify abnormal blood glucose utilization and need for additional monitoring. Complications from diabetes during pregnancy include polyhydramnios (excessive amniotic fluid volume), acidosis, increased rate of infection, vascular complications, and increased risk of pregnancy-induced hypertension. Because of an increased incidence of intrauterine

death after 36 weeks of gestation due to an aging placenta, close monitoring in the last month is essential. Neonatal complications from diabetes include hypoglycemia, respiratory distress syndrome, hyperbilirubinemia, and hypocalcemia. Infants of mothers with diabetes also have a higher incidence of congenital anomalies, such as a heart lesion or meningocele (Gilbert, 2006). The diabetic pregnant woman needs close health care team supervision and ongoing health teaching, including diet and exercise management, in order to control her disease effectively.

Heart Disease and Hypertension Heart disease and hypertension are the two serious maternal cardiovascular problems during pregnancy. Rheumatic heart disease, a common problem, contributes to congestive heart failure, threatening both the mother's and fetus' life. The fetus may be premature because of the need for an early birth. Chronic hypertension, seen more frequently in first-time mothers over age 35, increases the chance of stillbirths, premature delivery, and the development of **gestational hypertension**, which increase both maternal and infant mortality rates. Mothers with these problems must be monitored closely throughout pregnancy to prevent complications (Blackburn, 2007).

Rh Blood Group Incompatibility Rh blood group incompatibility sometimes affects fetal development. This problem usually occurs when the mother has Rh-negative red blood cells and the fetus has Rh-positive red blood cells, inherited from a father who has Rh positive blood. Rh incompatibility affects 10% to 15% of White women, 5% of Black women, but few Asian women (Dangel, 2008). In this disorder, maternal antibodies develop, cross the placental membranes, and destroy the Rh-positive red blood cells of the fetus. Based on the severity of the response, the infant may develop varying levels of hyperbilirubinemia after birth or may die in utero from the anemia of erythroblastosis fetalis (hemolytic disease of the newborn).

All women should be assessed for blood type, Rh factor, and antibody development to Rh-positive cells at their first prenatal care visit and again at 24 to 28 weeks of pregnancy unless the father of the baby is Rh negative (U.S. Preventive Services Task Force, 2006d). Rh incompatibility between a mother and future fetus may be prevented by administering Rho (D) immune globulin (RhoGAM) to an Rh-negative mother at 28 weeks of gestation and within 72 hours after birth. The immunization prevents the mother's sensitization to fetal Rh-negative cells by inactivating fetal red blood cells in the mother before she can develop an antibody response. The ideal injection time is after the mother's first delivery of an Rh-positive infant, miscarriage, or therapeutic abortion. The incompatibility generally does not occur during the first pregnancy, and the immunization prevents problems with later pregnancies.

Chemical Agents

Drugs ingested by the mother may be teratogens to the fetus. The tragic experience with the tranquilizer drug thalidomide, which caused limb deformities during the early

1960s, led to a recommendation that medications should be avoided during pregnancy unless absolutely necessary. The fact remains, however, that during the most critical early weeks of fetal development and growth, when many women do not know they are pregnant, ingested drugs may seriously affect the fetus. Based on fetal gestational age and drug metabolism, drugs may alter the placenta itself or directly affect development and growth of the fetus. The drugs that most commonly cause congenital defects are prescription medications, over-the-counter (OTC) drugs, street drugs, nicotine (cigarettes), caffeine, and alcohol. The U.S. Food and Drug Administration has labeled some of these drugs with an "X"; this means that scientific studies have shown negative fetal effects when pregnant women take them.

Prescription Medications

Women frequently become pregnant while on medications for illnesses diagnosed before pregnancy, such as hypertension, or they may receive medication to treat an illness acquired during pregnancy, such as a UTI. Some of the more common drugs that have been studied for fetal effects include antibiotics and anticonvulsants.

Most short-term and usual-dose antibiotics do not cause fetal harm. The tetracyclines are categorized as pregnancy category D (positive evidence of human fetal risk) because they combine with calcium ions and are deposited in deciduous teeth (causing discoloration) and bones (inhibiting bone growth and causing deformities) (Roe, 2007). Primary teeth seem most affected, but when the antibiotic is given near the time of delivery the permanent teeth may be damaged also.

The effects of anticonvulsants on the fetus have been documented thoroughly. Women with seizure disorders have carried infants to term while being treated with hydantoin, barbiturates, and other antiseizure medications. Infants born to mothers taking hydantoin (Dilantin) may have fetal hydantoin syndrome, reflected in microcephaly, retardation, cleft lip and palate, and congenital heart disease. Barbiturates, such as phenobarbital, may cause newborn addiction. Women with seizure disorders should discuss their medication requirements with their physicians before becoming pregnant and have close health care team monitoring throughout pregnancy.

Over-the-Counter Drugs

Pregnant women frequently choose to treat minor illnesses with OTC drugs. Research on acetylsalicylic acid (aspirin) and acetaminophen (Tylenol) indicates that both medications are safe in recommended dosages. However, aspirin alters platelet function and may cause maternal and newborn bleeding if taken close to delivery. Acetaminophen can be toxic to the liver. Certain ingredients in common cold remedies have been associated with fetal irritability (Rubin & Ramsay, 2007). Ibuprofen has been known to prolong labor based on its antiprostaglandin effect. Any drug may harm a fetus, so all drugs should be avoided during pregnancy unless prescribed by their health care provider.

The nurse includes information on the known and probable effects of medications on the fetus in prenatal teaching of couples. Discussion of herbal treatments is included, because little research exists on their effects and interactions with over-the-counter and prescribed medications. The nurse recognizes that many cultural groups use these nontraditional agents, because they believe that they will effectively manage pregnancy-related concerns. The nurse may need to encourage an individual to reconsider the use of herbs when evidence exists that these may harm the fetus or mother.

Drug Abuse

Given the prevalence of drug use and abuse in our society, it is imperative that nurses be able to recognize, manage, and refer as appropriate substance abuse problems for the women they care for. Substance abuse during pregnancy poses significant risk because all substances consumed by the mother pass freely through the placenta, and thus the fetus as well as the mother experiences substance use, abuse, and addiction.

Maternal use of narcotics, tranquilizers, cocaine, amphetamines, marijuana, and other drugs may cause serious health problems to both the mother and unborn child. These drugs represent an enormous cost to society by causing increased risks of low birth weight, preterm birth, and deficits in child development if the mother ingests them during pregnancy (Chasnoff, 2007).

Narcotics The narcotics heroin and methadone cause infant prematurity, IUGR, respiratory distress at birth, low birth weight and small for gestational age, possible congenital anomalies, fetal addiction in utero, neonatal withdrawal after birth, and long-term cognitive and behavioral problems (Kidder & Hackley, 2007). Signs of narcotic withdrawal in the newborn include tremors, irritability, hyperactivity, vomiting, diarrhea, sweating, poor feeding, and possibly convulsions. No evidence suggests withdrawal in infants whose mothers used cocaine or amphetamines, although there is an increased risk for preterm births, neonatal irritability, placenta abruption, premature rupture of membranes, and fetal distress (Chasnoff, 2007). Frequent maternal marijuana use during pregnancy may cause fetal immunological problems, but evidence conflicts with an unclear impact. To avoid these problems, nurses must recognize women who abuse drugs and assist them in seeking appropriate help. This task may be difficult because drug abusers often try to hide their habit, fear being reported to the police, and may be unable to change their lifestyle without extensive intervention.

Alcohol Many women in today's society drink alcohol regularly. However, alcohol crosses the placenta and may cause fetal death early in pregnancy. Fetal exposure to alcohol throughout pregnancy may cause **fetal alcohol syndrome** (FAS) or fetal alcohol spectrum disorder (FASD), a collection of symptoms including IUGR, increased risk of facial anomalies, structural brain abnormalities, mental health problems, attention deficit hyperactivity disorder, and retardation (Kidder & Hackley, 2007). Recent studies report symptoms of fetal alcohol disorder in children whose mothers may have consumed just a couple of drinks a day at certain stages of pregnancy. A second study confirmed that fetal alcohol syndrome is the not the only problem connected with drinking during pregnancy: It is also a risk factor for early alcohol abuse and dependence in the child (May et al., 2006; Alati et al., 2006). Numerous studies have shown that no safe level of alcohol use exists during pregnancy; therefore, alcohol should be avoided during this time and when attempting conception. Nurses need to stress this alcohol avoidance to all women.

Nicotine Since the 1940s, evidence has existed that cigarette smoking by pregnant mothers causes fetal problems, yet 20% to 30% of women continue to smoke during pregnancy (Norwitz & Schorge, 2006). The U.S. Preventive Services Task Force (2006e) recommends screening of all pregnant women for tobacco use and pregnancy-tailored counseling for those who smoke as proposed by the Association of Women's Health and Obstetric,

innovative practice

Development of Protocol for Smoking Cessation During Pregnancy

Based on a concern about the numbers of pregnant women who smoke and lack of a consistent approach to stopping this habit, AWHONN has proposed testing an evidence-based clinical practice guideline called SUCCESS. This research project will focus on nurses and other health care providers delivering a multifaceted intervention that is expected to increase the success of smoking cessation among childbearing women.

Thirteen clinical sites in the United States and Canada that meet study criteria will participate in the research study involving an expected 6000 women, 1000 of whom currently smoke or face the risk of returning to this habit once they give birth. Using research-based practice guidelines, researchers will investigate whether changed smoking practices decrease health-related risks to women and newborns involved in the study.

The study will incorporate previously tested programs from a variety of agencies focused on smoking cessation. Culturally sensitive tools will be used to screen participants. Trained nurses will deliver standard smoking cessation counseling approaches from previously tested programs. Materials such as the U.S. Department of Health and Human Services, Public Health Service's publication, *Treating Tobacco Use and Dependence: A Clinical Practice Guideline, Healthy People 2010,* and patient education materials developed by Smoke Free Families will structure and evaluate the SUCCESS program.

AWHONN, Association of Women's Health, Obstetrical, and Neonatal Nursing; SUCCESS, Setting Universal Cessation Counseling, Education, and Screening Standards.
From Association of Women's Health, Obstetrical, and Neonatal Nursing. (2004). SUCCESS: Nursing care for pregnant women who smoke. Retrieved September 23, 2007 from *www.awhonn.org/ awhonn/?pg=874-2190-6070-6080.*

Neonatal Nurses (AWHONN, 2004) (Innovative Practice box). The USPSTF recommends using the 5-A behavioral counseling framework for engaging women in smoking cessation discussions:

1. **A**sk about tobacco use
2. **A**dvise to quit through clear, personalized messages
3. **A**ssess willingness to quit
4. **A**ssist to quit
5. **A**rrange follow-up and support

Evidence indicates that maternal smoking causes increased rates of spontaneous abortion, decreased fertility, low birth weight, preterm birth, placental abnormalities, vaginal bleeding, congenital anomalies, perinatal mortality, and premature rupture of the membranes. Neonatal exposure (secondhand smoke) is associated with sudden infant death syndrome, asthma, respiratory infections, and attention deficit disorder (Chasnoff, 2007). The best advice for pregnant mothers or women considering pregnancy is not to smoke at all, decrease smoking if one is a heavy smoker, and avoid places where smoking occurs. The nurse needs to understand the context of a smoking woman's life and the complexity of her choice to quit smoking in order to propose solutions to decrease fetal exposure to nicotine (Research Highlights box).

Caffeine Coffee, cocoa, tea, cola, and chocolate contain caffeine, another addictive drug. Gene mutations have been found in laboratory animals exposed to moderate amounts of caffeine; however, these defects have not been found in human beings. One study found a weak association between excess caffeine intake (more than 300 mg or more than three cups of coffee per day) during pregnancy with spontaneous abortions, but caffeine has no known teratogenic effect (Hey, 2007). Until additional research clarifies the relationship between caffeine intake and fetal effects, nurses should teach pregnant women to avoid excess caffeine intake.

Chemical Agents

The influence of chemicals on human development remains unclear. Some natural substances found to be teratogenic in animals, but not necessarily in human beings, include insect and bacterial toxins, insecticides, herbicides, and fungicides, including dichlorodiphenyltrichloroethane, or DDT. Recent studies involving pregnant women who eat fish with high mercury levels (shark, swordfish, king mackerel, or tilefish) support evidence that mercury negatively affects fetal development, particularly brain development, and may be associated with preterm labor (Xue et al., 2007). Women can safely eat 12 ounces of cooked fish weekly. Some studies report stillbirths, abortions, preterm births, and mental retardation in fetuses exposed to lead. This area needs more study, particularly with more women working in traditional male workplaces where there are environmental contaminants. Nurses assess and provide women in their first trimester with information on environmental agents that are potentially damaging throughout gestation and counsel them on ways to avoid exposure.

Medications Given During Childbirth

The final time that the fetus encounters drugs through the mother is during the birthing process. Many women desire medications for labor discomforts, and usually only medications deemed safe and monitored closely during labor and birth have been used (e.g., epidural anesthesia, opiate agonists in small doses). Some analgesic drugs administered during labor can cause neonatal sedation and respiratory depression and can influence the rate and quality of the infant's adaptation to extrauterine life. Studies of visual attentiveness and sucking behavior, as well as neurological tests and electroencephalography, suggest that fetal depressant effects may last as long as days after birth.

Mechanical Forces

The amniotic fluid reservoir protects the fetus during pregnancy and during mild to moderate trauma to the mother's abdomen. However, major trauma to the mother's abdomen, such as that sustained in a severe car accident, may cause maternal bleeding, preterm labor, and other concerns. The nurse instructs the pregnant woman in the proper way to wear both a lap belt and shoulder harness to protect her and her fetus while driving. All women in the second and third trimester should be encouraged to seek medical care following an accident believed to influence the health of mother or fetus.

The uterus, another mechanical force, also influences the fetus. Near the end of pregnancy, the fetus outgrows the uterus and becomes molded by it, particularly in cases of multiple pregnancy. Some children have congenitally dislocated hips from uterine pressure and fetal position in utero. Most deformities return to normal either naturally or with repositioning after birth. Fetal malposition cannot be prevented; therefore, the neonate is assessed for problems and support provided to the parents about the newborn's appearance.

The actual labor and birth process represents the final mechanical force. Few newborns experience injury during this process, and those who do usually recover with limited effect. Some of the more common injuries that occur during this time are discussed in **Website Resource 16F**. It is difficult to predict and prevent traumas during birth, such as when delivery of an infant who is larger than expected requires vacuum extraction, which may injure the child. In these cases, based on health care team assessment, the mother may undergo cesarean section to protect her and the baby.

Radiation

Scientific evidence indicates that exposure to x-rays, especially early in pregnancy, may cause chromosomal changes, spontaneous abortion, mental retardation, microcephaly, fetal loss, or malignancy later in life (Norwitz & Schorge, 2006). Literature supports a greater incidence of leukemia

---

research highlights

Interventions for Promoting Smoking Cessation During Pregnancy

Smoking remains one of the few potentially preventable factors associated with low birth-weight, preterm birth, and perinatal death. The purpose of this study was to assess the effects of smoking cessation programs implemented during pregnancy on the health of the fetus, infant, mother, and family.

This review included 64 trials. Fifty-one randomized controlled trials (20,931 women) and six cluster-randomized trials (over 7500 women) provided data on smoking cessation and/or perinatal outcomes. Despite substantial variation in the intensity of the intervention and the extent of reminders and reinforcement through pregnancy, there was an increase in the median intensity of both "usual care" and interventions over time.

There was a significant reduction in smoking in the intervention groups of the 48 trials included: (relative risk [RR] 0.94, 95% confidence interval [CI] 0.93 to 0.95), an absolute difference of 6 in 100 women continuing to smoke. The 36 trials with validated smoking cessation had a similar reduction (RR 0.94, 95% CI 0.92 to 0.95). Smoking cessation interventions reduced low birthweight (RR 0.81, 95% CI 0.70 to 0.94) and preterm birth (RR 0.84, 95% CI 0.72 to 0.98), and there was a 33 g (95% CI 11 g to 55 g) increase in mean birthweight. There were no statistically significant differences in very low birthweight, stillbirths, or perinatal or neonatal mortality but these analyses had very limited power. One intervention strategy, rewards plus social support (two trials), resulted in a significantly greater smoking reduction than other strategies (RR 0.77, 95% CI 0.72 to 0.82). Five trials of smoking relapse prevention (over 800 women) showed no statistically significant reduction in relapse. There was a significant reduction in smoking in the intervention groups of the 48 trials included: (relative risk [RR] 0.94, 95% confidence interval [CI] 0.93 to 0.95), an absolute difference of six in 100 women continuing to smoke. The 36 trials with validated smoking cessation had a similar reduction (RR 0.94, 95% CI 0.92 to 0.95). Smoking cessation interventions reduced low birthweight (RR 0.81, 95% CI 0.70 to 0.94) and preterm birth (RR 0.84, 95% CI 0.72 to 0.98), and there was a 33 g (95% CI 11 g to 55 g) increase in mean birthweight.

Cigarette smoking in pregnancy is common, particularly where there is low income and social disadvantage. Smoking in pregnancy increases the risk of infants having low birth weight and being born too early. Infants often struggle to cope with life outside utero and can suffer ill health later in life. Many mothers find it hard to stop, or to reduce, smoking during pregnancy even knowing the benefits this may have, because smoking can help them cope with stress. There are effective strategies to help and support women to stop smoking that lead to fewer premature babies and better birth weights for infants.

From Lumley, J., Oliver, S. S., Chamberlain, C., & Oakley, L. (2006). Interventions for promoting smoking cessation during pregnancy. *Cochrane Database of Systematic Reviews* 2006, Issue 1. Art. No.: CD001055. DOI: Chichester, UK: John Wiley & Sons.

in children of women exposed to x-rays during pregnancy compared with children whose mothers were not exposed. Unless the benefits of radiographic information clearly outweigh the risks of exposing the fetus to x-rays, these examinations should not be performed during gestation. If radiography is deemed necessary, a lead apron, as low a radiation dose as possible, and other recommendations made by the National Council on Radiation Protection and Measurements should be used to protect the developing fetus.

SOCIAL PROCESSES
Community and Work

Many more women now work outside the home, either in careers or in jobs needed for family economic survival. As each woman considers or experiences pregnancy, she will need to ask herself questions that will optimize her pregnancy outcome. These questions include the following: Is my work strenuous or possibly dangerous to my baby because of exposure to toxic substances? Do I need to work for long periods, influencing my need for rest? Will workplace stressors influence my coping with pregnancy and my family needs?

A safe workplace environment (one that does not involve exposure to hazardous substances or organisms and provides adequate breaks for worker rest and body movement), will allow a pregnant woman to work until her baby is due, unless her health becomes impaired. The nurse helps each woman assess the safety of her workplace and suggest ways to decrease hazards in that setting. These hazards include exposure to viruses, fungi, industrial products (hydrocarbons or pesticides), smoke, radiation emitted by medical diagnostic equipment, air pollutants, asbestos, possibility for workplace violence, mental and physical stress, and even noise pollution. The nurse encourages the pregnant worker to consider workplace ergonomics, addressing how the current work space will meet her changing physical needs.

Some employers in this country have been designated creators of "family friendly" work environments, because they have willingly made accommodations to support breast-feeding and pregnant workers and families. These accommodations allow women to prioritize their pregnancy and family needs. Evidence indicates that such approaches reduce pregnancy complications and increase work productivity. Although few in number, family friendly employers offer health-promotion programs focusing on healthy nutrition, stress management, and exercise for employees, who experience better health outcomes.

As a rule, however, too few employers support flexible work schedules for prenatal care visits, rest periods for pregnant workers, or removal of vending machines to support optimal nutrition for pregnant working class women. Some working women, regardless of status, believe that once they announce their pregnancy, they will face workplace pressure to stop working or change positions in the company based on their gestational needs. Based on experience, some employers fear that their pregnant employees will overuse sick time or seek a reduced workload. The pregnant woman must deal with these situations by being factual and assertive about her ability to continue working. National law dictates that it is illegal to discriminate against a woman because she is pregnant. If a woman believes that she has been treated unfairly because of her pregnancy, she may pursue the issue legally or become active in local women's rights organizations to gain support. However, when a woman leaves a job that did not support her pregnancy, she often gives up accrued leave time or takes a lower salary at another job. These outcomes influence her choices during pregnancy and early parenting.

Workplaces vary greatly in allowing leave time during and after pregnancy. Federal legislation, the Family and Medical Leave Act, obligates employers of at least 50 people to provide up to 12 weeks' paid leave for new parents or women who have medical problems during pregnancy. Ideally a woman who desires children should explore the issue of leave during a job interview, but many women fail to do this until they are already pregnant. A woman often requires written verification from her physician if she needs a leave of absence from her job due to pregnancy complications. Although she may wish to return to work shortly after giving birth, the woman is counseled to allow sufficient time to regain her strength and adapt to parenting. The nurse may help the couple make reasonable decisions related to locating resources for child care, exploring "shared-time" with other new mothers or part-time employees (for example middle-age adults caring for their older parents) in the woman's workplace, or for balancing work and family needs.

Culture and Ethnicity

Cultural groups have unique ideas and beliefs related to pregnancy, childbirth, and childbearing that must be understood by the nurse in order to render individualized care to each pregnant woman. **Website Resource 16G** presents a list of questions to ask the person to gain this understanding. As part of the assessment, the nurse determines the cultural attachment of a woman by asking the following question: Does she think that some or most of the childbearing ideas of her culture are old fashioned, but does she feel obligated to follow these ideas, at least superficially, because of family pressure? In this situation, the nurse may need to be a confidant for the woman who needs to vent her frustrations about cultural restrictions. Nursing support may assist the individual in adjusting both her needs and those of the culture she represents to experience a satisfactory pregnancy.

The nurse has an obligation to read about and seek information on cultures encountered in practice and to become

MULTICULTURAL AWARENESS

Nursing Roles in Providing Culturally Competent Care

Delivery of culturally competent care implies that a nurse acknowledges and acts on the unique history that a pregnant woman and family bring to a health care interaction. The nurse supports culturally competent care by:

- Recognizing that cultural diversity exists and affects the process and outcome of health care
- Respecting people as unique individuals who, by their differences from the majority, bring a broadened definition of appropriate health care
- Using data gained from a cultural assessment for completion of a care plan
- Encouraging cultural behavior that protects the biopsychosocial, spiritual, and safety needs of the individual
- Gaining insight into the nurse's own beliefs and values about people who may be different or have different needs than the majority or those of the nurse's own culture; understanding how these beliefs and values influence the outcomes of health care delivery with childbearing families
- Recognizing the values of the health care system reflected in the customs and practices of birthing facilities and responding to these facilities based on one's value system
- Providing interpreters to improve communication between the individual and health care providers
- Becoming literate in languages, customs, and cultural practices of people commonly seen in the health care environment

active in community organizations that represent cultures whose members get prenatal care from the nurse. Above all, the nurse must be open to a variety of viewpoints, judging them not against personal beliefs, but rather in relation to the general concept of health promotion and today's goal to provide culturally competent care to a variety of cultural groups (Multicultural Awareness box).

Legislation

Both legislative actions and social movements influence childbearing. In some countries, such as China, the government decrees the number of children a couple may have and imposes economic or social sanctions to enforce these restrictions. Although Americans may have as many children as they desire, various coalitions lobby strongly for families. The recent Family and Medical Leave Act validates the federal government's commitment to prioritizing family issues by giving new parents time off from work during the early months of parenthood, while supporting these individuals' professional work goals and needs.

The U.S. government remains concerned about the health of pregnant women and ways to decrease fetal and infant morbidity and mortality. Historically states have used federal monies from Medicaid and Title V maternal and child health block programs to provide services for pregnant women and children. Many countries provide universal access to prenatal care, but in the United States low-income women rely on Medicaid, a joint federal-state program, to cover most of the cost of prenatal care. With constraints on state and federal budgets, many of which fund community prenatal clinics, concerns have been expressed about whether sufficient money will exist for funding women and children's care programs. Local health departments may offer free or low-cost prenatal care for women who are pregnant, but again, the extent of services depends on state government or local allocation of funds. Despite this free or low-cost care, over 47 million Americans overall lack health insurance and, therefore, face barriers that affect their easy access to prenatal care (Park et al., 2007; USDHHS, 2000). Many ethnically diverse populations and, in particular, Hispanic groups, lack insurance and a level of education that increases their understanding of health-related information for family health promotion. Educating women during the childbearing cycle is particularly important to increase the chances of families obtaining and understanding health-promotion information for healthier behaviors (USDHHS, 2000).

With the nurse's help in data collection, consumers should be encouraged to express their views and opinions on pregnancy and parenting topics to their elected governmental representatives. This expression indeed works; many states recently legislated hospital stays of at least 48 hours for women with vaginal deliveries and even longer stays for women with cesarean deliveries. These laws evolved from public concern over premature discharges of new mothers as part of managed care insurance directives. Longer stays help health care providers identify potential problems in the mother or the baby before discharge, such as difficulty breast-feeding. Continued legislative work on insurance reform may improve family planning services so that couples can plan pregnancies to better meet their sociocultural and financial goals and needs (USDHHS, 2000). Insurance reform, driven by legislative change, may also improve health care coverage for underinsured individuals who lack a consistent source of prenatal care or report difficulties in receiving care because of communication, structural, or personal barriers within their insurance system (Johnson, 2006).

Economics

When the pregnant woman begins prenatal care, personal financial resources influence the kind of care she receives, whether she works during or after a pregnancy, her acceptance of a pregnancy, her nutritional status, and other choices. The expenses of planning and experiencing a pregnancy may determine whether the woman or her family faces a financial crisis. The nurse needs to understand the financial history and priorities of the couple, because this information will affect access to and use of prenatal care.

The nurse inquires in a sensitive fashion about a woman's or couple's finances to make appropriate referral to resources for care (e.g., Title V or Medicaid programs). Until recently, Medicaid provided no adolescent family planning services, a situation that may have influenced high rates of pregnancy in some sectors of this country (USDHHS, 2000). Many low-income women qualify for the U.S. Department of Agriculture's supplemental feeding program for women, infants, and children (WIC). This program provides essential foods such as milk, cheese, and eggs to pregnant and lactating women. During prenatal visits, the nurse may help a woman or family plan a budget for food and other essential requirements based on individual family needs, cultural values, need for a healthy diet during pregnancy, and income. Local food banks and secondhand clothing and baby supply stores may provide needed items for these families. Occasionally women may access free transportation and child care at the prenatal clinic if the nurse provides information about this program.

Health Care Delivery System

Options for care during pregnancy range from medical-based care by an obstetrician or general practitioner to more health-promotion–focused care by a nurse practitioner or midwife. Geographical availability of options, finances, previous experience, partner's preference, cultural or social acceptability of certain options, and preexisting or newly recognized risk factors will influence a woman's choice of care. Based on her culture and the belief that pregnancy is not an illness, a woman may not seek Western medical prenatal care, but rather may rely on individuals of her culture to provide care until the actual labor, when she will go to a hospital.

Unless complications arise a woman generally chooses where she will labor and give birth and the extent of labor and birthing process intervention. The movement toward home birth that began during the early 1970s continues to meet some consumer needs for a more family-oriented, natural, health-focused experience. However, most couples choose a hospital birth setting because of availability of emergency equipment and personnel in case of complications. Some insurance companies will cover only births done in hospitals and in birth centers or birthing rooms attached to a hospital. The nurse helps expectant couples become aware of the care and birthing alternatives to make an informed choice for a positive labor and birth experience. Women who lack resources to access the health care delivery system and teaching by the nurse during regular prenatal visits generally are less able to make informed decisions that affect their childbearing experiences.

Many expectant couples also make an informed choice about the actual process of labor and birth by developing a birth plan, those components of care and intervention that the couple desires for the birth experience. A pregnant woman and her partner may choose natural childbirth or a method of analgesia or anesthesia. The nurse helps the pregnant woman and her partner choose the most appropriate method by providing information about options and encouraging questions about each one. Collaboration between the nurse and woman or couple in meeting their birth plan goals is important, because research shows that women remember their labor and birthing experiences for a long time. A positively viewed birth experience may support a couple's involvement as active health care consumers, thus facilitating their future health of their family.

The nurse may encourage the pregnant couple or woman to attend prenatal classes. These provide valuable information and preparation for birth for many couples. The International Childbirth Education Association, the American Society for Psychoprophylaxis in Obstetrics (ASPO), and many local groups offer a variety of classes for the expectant couple. These classes may include information on early pregnancy, Lamaze-ASPO or Bradley methods, cesarean birth, breast-feeding, infant cardiopulmonary resuscitation, and parenting. Sibling classes for the newborn and involvement of children in the birth experience may also increase sibling bonding.

NURSING INTERVENTIONS

Teaching the pregnant woman and her partner during the prenatal period is the most important role of the nurse. Even the woman who has previously given birth or who has a high degree of education may need or want information from the health care team that will assist her family to adapt effectively to changes of pregnancy to support a healthy birth outcome.

To provide appropriate teaching, the nurse performs a comprehensive assessment that involves the entire family, such as that presented in **Website Resource 16H**. Assessment, the first step in the nursing process, allows the nurse to determine maternal and fetal physical and psychological risks, the woman's informational base for pregnancy and birth, and cultural and family needs. Assessment should also include physical, spiritual, emotional, and sociocultural inspection and recognition of abuse. Battering increases during pregnancy and may be detected by physical, emotional, and history assessment of the woman (see Hot Topics box). Pregnant women at high risk for abuse include adolescents, those with low incomes, and those with a history of alcohol or drug abuse, as well as a partner with a similar history (American College of Obstetricians and Gynecologists, 2007; U.S. Preventive Services Task Force, 2006a). In cases of suspected abuse, the nurse, in consultation with other members of the health care team, provides support and resources for the woman to make an informed decision about protecting herself and her fetus during pregnancy. The nurse may also want to refer the person to a professional counselor for a brief counseling outreach intervention demonstrated to decrease the incidence of family violence (Paluzzi, 2007).

As discussed in this chapter, assessment may also be made by using Gordon's functional health patterns, a common conceptual framework for clinical assessment (see Box 16-3). Data used in the assessment process will likely be collected during the prenatal visit and may change based on life occurrences of the pregnant woman. A woman may be defined as high risk during her pregnancy if she experiences heavy bleeding, premature labor, elevated blood pressure, extreme anxiety, if there is fetal distress, or if she shows unexpected behavior or symptoms. After noting these high-risk conditions, the nurse should refer the pregnant woman to an obstetrical specialist or other resources for pregnant women and their families (see the Case Study at the end of this chapter).

After a complete assessment during each prenatal visit, the nurse develops a teaching plan for the individual. Throughout the prenatal course, the nurse collaborates with the woman and her partner to assess their learning and support needs. For example, literature on bottle feeding or breast-feeding may be provided to help a woman decide on a method, and books, videos, and websites may help couples understand more about birth and, therefore, feel that they have more control during labor and in meeting their birthing goals. If the woman plans to attend group prenatal classes, the nurse should coordinate her teaching content and process with those expected in the classes, thereby preventing undue repetition. The nurse teaching prenatal classes should provide a list of topics to participants in the class to share with their health care providers. A woman may be knowledgeable in some areas, and the nurse can use this knowledge as a foundation for further individualized teaching. Box 16-5 covers relevant topics to be covered by the nurse during prenatal care interactions with pregnant women. These topical areas relate to nursing interventions covered earlier in this chapter. Basic handouts detailing information such as danger signs will provide information that a woman can post at home should she experience unexpected complications of her pregnancy.

Box 16-5 Topics for Prenatal Care Teaching

1. Rationale for and interpretation of physical findings and laboratory results
2. Value of keeping appointments
3. Danger signs that should be reported
4. Breast care to prepare for lactation
5. Breast-feeding versus bottle feeding
6. Exercise and rest
7. Fetal growth and development
8. Physical and psychological changes during pregnancy and relief measures
9. Effects of smoking, drinking, and drugs on the fetus
10. Nutrition
11. Work and play
12. Body mechanics
13. Personal hygiene
14. Sex during pregnancy
15. Preparation for labor and birth
16. Superstitions and old wives' tales
17. Signs of impending labor
18. Supplies and preparations for the baby
19. Partner's and siblings' responses

SUMMARY

Dramatic changes occur during pregnancy; a new life forms and develops and the expectant family members (mother, father, siblings, and other close members) experience major changes in their roles and relationships with each other. Although all fetal development processes, changes in pregnant women's bodies, and role transitions among family members share common elements, each family uniquely experiences pregnancy because of life experience and personal values. The focus is the entire family, although the nurse most often deals directly with the pregnant woman. The nurse provides valuable resources and information that the family may use to meet its specific needs. The overall nursing goal involves assisting each family to have a healthy pregnancy and birth outcome, to lay the foundation for satisfactory parenting and family life.

CASE STUDY

Active Labor: Susan Wong

Mrs. Wong, a first-time mother, is admitted to the birthing suite in early labor after SROM at home. She is 38 weeks gestation with a history of abnormal α-fetoprotein levels at 16 weeks of pregnancy. She was scheduled for ultrasonography to visualize the fetus to rule out an open spinal defect or Down syndrome, but never followed through. Mrs. Wong and her husband disagreed about what to do (keep or terminate the pregnancy) if the ultrasonography indicated a spinal problem, so they felt they didn't wish to find out.

Reflective Questions:

1. As the nurse, what priority data would you collect from this couple to help define relevant interventions to meet their needs?
2. How can you help this couple if they experience a negative outcome in the birthing suite? What are your personal views on terminating or continuing a pregnancy with a risk for a potential anomaly? What factors may influence your views?

Continued

CASE STUDY

Active Labor: Susan Wong—cont'd

Reflective Questions—cont'd

3. with the influence of the recent Human Genome Project and the possibility of predicting open spinal defects earlier in pregnancy, how will maternity care change in the future?

Prediction of Human Disease

Starting in 1990, the federal government and a private agency engaged in genetic research as part of the International Genome Project, a coordinated effort to map the genetic instructions found on human DNA and within the DNA of several model organisms. Initial sequencing of the human genome has been accomplished, so the ability to predict and manage hereditary diseases is on the horizon. Although this knowledge holds much hope for predicting fetal defects and disease in humans, ethicists have expressed concerns about how this information might be used. Will this material be used to discriminate against individuals with predisposition to genetically related diseases? Will couples wanting the perfect baby seek genome technology to decide whether to maintain a pregnancy or to abort a fetus if a child has a disease perceived as causing a lesser quality of life? Will this information be made available to employers and health care insurers, who might then decide to deny insurance to people with existing or future disease that may increase health care costs? Many have heralded such advances for their effectiveness in detecting certain genetic conditions, while others have argued that they perpetuate discrimination by preventing the birth of children with disabilities. Although the Human Genome Project will provide information intended to help individuals have a better quality of life, many ethical questions remain for society to address concerning the use of this information.

From Munger, K. M., Gill, C. J., Ormond, K. E., & Kirschner, K. L. (2007). The next exclusion debate: Assessing technology, ethics, and intellectual disability after the human genome project. *Mental Retardation & Developmental Disabilities Research Reviews*, 13(2), 121-128. Reprinted with permission of John Wiley & Sons, Inc.

CARE PLAN

Nursing Management for Stages of Labor: Susan Wong

Nursing Diagnosis: Ineffective Individual Coping Related to Active Labor Status

DEFINING CHARACTERISTICS

- Initiation of labor at 2:00 AM with SROM
- First-time mother who did not attend childbirth classes
- Supportive spouse
- Current gestational age of 38 weeks
- Contraction pattern defined as moderate intensity, frequency every 2 minutes, 60 seconds in duration
- After 6 hours of labor, 4 cm dilated, 100% effaced, and stage: active phase
- Moaning, moving around in bed, and stating, "I can't take this much longer; it hurts too much!"

RELATED FACTORS

- Prenatal history of abnormal alpha-fetoprotein levels at 16 weeks
- Prenatal care since 12 weeks pregnant
- History of depression in college
- Works as engineer with large manufacturing firm
- Gravida 1, para 0
- Recent resident of city, moved from East Coast approximately 4 months ago
- 25 years of age, Asian family history, married 1 year

EXPECTED OUTCOMES

- Mother will state level of pain to be less than 4 on a scale of 1 to 10 during labor.
- Mother will successfully use visual imagery techniques, massage, and slow deep breathing for relaxation during labor.
- Mother will state early in labor at least three ways to cope effectively with pain and will implement these strategies as relevant.
- Fetus will demonstrate an expected FHR pattern and will experience no compromise during labor.
- Mother and family will verbalize needs during labor and delivery to health care team.

INTERVENTIONS (BY NURSE)

- Assess level of labor discomfort every 20 to 30 minutes and as needed according to pain scale rating of 1 to 10.
- Implement and document nursing interventions (backrubs, heat and cold, position changes, back pressure and massage, and Jacuzzi therapy, among others) to relieve labor discomforts.
- Assess cultural beliefs with labor and delivery management and implement interventions as needed to meet practice standards.
- Provide teaching about labor and delivery progress and breathing, visual imagery, and massage techniques that may decrease labor discomfort.
- Provide verbal and nonverbal reassurance during labor.
- Teach about fetal response during labor and rationale for nursing interventions to support fetal health, such as left side position to increase placental blood flow.
- Throughout labor, answer any questions from mother and family members about needs and responses to labor process.
- Involve family members as much as possible during labor and as requested by mother to improve her ability to cope.

FHR, Fetal heart rate; *SROM*, spontaneous rupture of membranes.

REFERENCES

Ahluwalia, I. B., Whitehead, N., & Bensyl, D. (2007). Pregnancy intention and contraceptive use among adult women. *Maternal & Child Health Journal, 11*(4), 347–351.

Alati, R., et al. (2006). In utero alcohol exposure and prediction of alcohol disorders in early adulthood: A birth cohort study. *Archives of General Psychiatry, 63*(9), 1009–1016.

Alder, J., Fink, N., Bitzer, J., Hosli, I., & Holzgreve, W. (2007). Depression and anxiety during pregnancy: A risk factor for obstetric, fetal and neonatal outcomes? *Journal of Maternal-Fetal & Neonatal Medicine, 20*(3), 189–209.

American College of Obstetricians and Gynecologists (ACOG). (2007). *Nutrition during pregnancy.* [Online] Retrieved from *www.acog.org/publications/patient_education/bp001.cfm.*

American College of Obstetricians and Gynecologists (ACOG). (2007). *Women's Health: Domestic Violence.* [Online] Retrieved from *www.acog.org/publications/patient_education/bp083.cfm.*

Arenson, J., & Drake, P. (2007). *Maternal and newborn health.* Sudbury, MA: Jones and Bartlett Publishers.

Armstrong, P., & Feldman, S. (2007). *A wise birth: Bringing together the best natural childbirth with modern medicine.* London, England: Pinter & Martin Limited.

Association of Women's Health, Obstetrical, and Neonatal Nursing. (2004). *SUCCESS: Nursing care for pregnant women who smoke.* Retrieved September 23, 2007, from *www.awhonn.org/awhonn/?pg=874-2190-6070-6080.*

Association of Women's Health, Obstetrical, and Neonatal Nursing (AWHONN). (2007). *Evidence-based clinical practice guidelines: Professional nursing support of laboring women.* Washington, DC: Author.

Baker, D. A. (2007). Consequences of herpes simplex virus in pregnancy and their prevention. *Current Opinion in Infectious Diseases, 20*(1), 73–76.

Best, J. M. (2007). Rubella. *Seminars in Fetal & Neonatal Medicine, 12*(3), 182–192.

Blackburn, S. T. (2007). *Maternal, fetal, & neonatal physiology: A clinical perspective* (3rd ed.). St. Louis, MO: Saunders Elsevier.

Centers for Disease Control and Prevention (CDC). (2006). *Guidelines for treatment of sexually transmitted diseases.* [Online] Retrieved from *www.cdc.gov/std/treatment/2006/hiv.htm.*

Centers for Disease Control and Prevention (CDC). (2007). Overall infant mortality rate in United States largely unchanged: Rates among black women more than twice that of white women. *CDC National Center for Health Statistics.* [Online] Retrieved from *www.cdc.gov/od/oc/media/pressrel/2007/r070502.htm.*

Centers for Disease Control and Prevention (CDC). (2007). *Syphilis - CDC fact sheet.* [Online] Retrieved from *www.cdc.gov/std/syphilis/STDFact-Syphilis.htm.*

Centers for Disease Control and Prevention (CDC). (2007). *Hepatitis B fact sheet.* [Online] Retrieved from *www.cdc.gov/ncidod/diseases/hepatitis/b/fact.htm.*

Centers for Disease Control and Prevention (CDC). (2007). *Guidelines for preconception care of women.* [Online] Retrieved from *www.medscape.com/viewarticle/553457.*

Centers for Disease Control and Prevention (CDC) and ATSDR Preconception Care Work Group. (2006). Recommendations to improve preconception health and health care–United States. *MMWR, 55*(RR-6), 1–23.

Centers for Disease Control and Prevention Office of Women's Health. (2007). *Heart disease and stroke fact sheet.* [Online] Retrieved from *www.cdc.gov/women/natstat/hrtstrk.htm.*

Chasnoff, I. J. (2007). *Drugs, alcohol, pregnancy and parenting.* New York: Springer-Verlag LLC.

Coch, D., Dawson, G., & Fischer, K. W. (2007). *Human behavior, learning, and developing the brain.* New York: Guilford Publications, Inc.

Cunningham, F. G., Gant, N. F., Leveno, K. J., Gilstrap, L. C., Hauth, J. C., & Wenstrom, K. D. (2005a). Implantation, embryogenesis, and placental development. In *Williams obstetrics* (22nd ed., Chapter 3, pp. 39–90). New York: McGraw-Hill.

Cunningham, F. G., Gant, N. F., Leveno, K. J., Gilstrap, L. C., Hauth, J. C., & Wenstrom, K. D. (2005b). Maternal physiology. In *Williams obstetrics* (22nd ed., Chapter 5, pp. 121–150). New York: McGraw-Hill.

Cunningham, F. G., Gant, N. F., Leveno, K. J., Gilstrap, L. C., Hauth, J. C., & Wenstrom, K. D. (2005c). Prenatal care. In *Williams obstetrics* (22nd ed., Chapter 8, pp. 201–230). New York: McGraw-Hill.

Cunningham, F. G., Gant, N. F., Leveno, K. J., Gilstrap, L. C., Hauth, J. C., & Wenstrom, K. D. (2005d). Prenatal diagnosis and fetal therapy. In *Williams obstetrics* (22nd ed., Chapter 13, pp. 313–340). New York: McGraw-Hill.

Cunningham, F. G., Gant, N. F., Leveno, K. J., Gilstrap, L. C., Hauth, J. C., & Wenstrom, K. D. (2005e). Antepartum assessment. In *Williams obstetrics* (22nd ed., Chapter 15, pp. 373–388). New York: McGraw-Hill.

Cunningham, F. G., Gant, N. F., Leveno, K. J., Gilstrap, L. C., Hauth, J. C., & Wenstrom, K. D. (2005f). Genetics. In *Williams obstetrics* (22nd ed., Chapter 12, pp. 285–312). New York: McGraw-Hill.

Cunningham, F. G., Gant, N. F., Leveno, K. J., Gilstrap, L. C., Hauth, J. C., & Wenstrom, K. D. (2005g). Sexually transmitted diseases. In *Williams obstetrics* (22nd ed., Chapter 59, pp. 1301–1325). New York: McGraw-Hill.

Dangel, G. (2008). High-risk pregnancy. *Internet Journal of Gynecology & Obstetrics, 7*(1), 2–9.

Debruyne, L., Whitney, E. N., & Pinna, K. (2007). *Nutrition and diet therapy* (7th ed.). Boston: Wadsworth.

Dudek, S. G. (2006). *Nutritional essentials for nursing practice* (5th ed.). Philadelphia: Lippincott Williams & Wilkins.

Friars, C. (2007). Toxoplasmosis and pregnancy. *Practicing Midwife, 10*(4), 20–21.

Frieden, F. J., & Chan, Y. (2007). Antepartum care. In R. E. Rakel & E. T. Bope's (Eds.), *Conn's Current Therapy 2007* (Section 16; pp. 1168–1175). Philadelphia: Saunders.

Gilbert, E. S. (2006). *Manual of high risk pregnancy and delivery* (4th ed.). St. Louis: Mosby.

Goh, B. T., & Thornton, A. C. (2007). Antenatal screening for syphilis. *Sexually Transmitted Infections, 83*(5), 345–346.

Hackley, B., Kriebs, J. M., & Rousseau, M. E. (2007). *Primary care of women: A guide for midwives and women's health providers.* Sudbury, MA: Jones and Bartlett Publishers.

Hey, E. (2007). Coffee and pregnancy. *British Medical Journal, 334*(7590), 377.

Institute of Medicine. (2007). Influence of pregnancy weight on maternal and child health: A workshop report. *Institute of Medicine, National Academy of Sciences.* [Online] Retrieved from *www.iom.edu/CMS/12552/31379/41424.aspx.*

Johnson, K. A. (2006). Public finance policy strategies to increase awareness to preconception care. *Maternal & Child Health Nursing, 10*(Supplement), 85–91.

Kidder, T. J., & Hackley, B. (2007). Substance abuse. In B. Hackley, J. M. Kriebs, & M. E. Rousseau's (Eds.), *Primary care of women: A guide for midwives and women's health providers* (Chapter 8; pp. 213–247). Sudbury, MA: Jones and Bartlett Publishers.

Majeroni, B. A., & Ukkadam, S. (2007). Screening and treatment for sexually transmitted infections in pregnancy. *American Family Physician, 76*(2), 265–270.

Malm, G., & Engman, M. L. (2007). Congenital cytomegalovirus infections. *Seminars in Fetal & Neonatal Medicine, 12*(3), 154–159.

March of Dimes. (2007). Genetic birth defects. *March of Dimes fact sheets.* [Online] Retrieved from *www.marchofdimes.com/pnhec/4439_1206.asp.*

May, P. A., et al (2006). Epidemiology of FASD in a province in Italy: Prevalence and characteristics of children in a random sample of schools. *Alcoholism: Clinical and Experimental Research, I*(9), 1562–1575.

Mayo Clinic. (2007). Cleft lip and cleft palate. *Mayo Clinic Health Library.* [Online] Retrieved from *www.cnn.com/HEALTH/library/DS/00738.html.*

Mercer, R. T. (2004). Becoming a mother versus maternal role attainment. *Journal of Nursing Scholarship, 36*(3), 226–232.

Merriam-Webster. (2007). *Merriam-Webster's Medical Dictionary.* Springfield, MA: Merriam-Webster, Incorporated.

Mills, M. E. (2007). More than food: The implications of pica in pregnancy. *Nursing for Women's Health, 11*(3), 267–273.

Nelson, A. (2003). Transition to motherhood. *JOGNN, 32*(4), 465–477.

Norwitz, E. R., & Schorge, J. O. (2006). *Obstetrics and gynecology at a glance* (2nd ed.). Malden, MA: Blackwell Publishing.

Paluzzi, P. A. (2007). Violence against women and children. In B. Hackley, J. M. Kriebs, & M. E. Rousseau's (Eds.), *Primary care of women: A guide for midwives and women's health providers* (Chapter 7; pp. 193–212). Sudbury, MA: Jones & Bartlett Publishers.

Park, J. H., Vincent, D., & Hastings-Tolsma, M. (2007). Disparity in prenatal care among women of colour in the USA. *Midwifery, 23*(1), 28–37.

Queenan, J. T., Spong, C., & Lockwood, C. (2007). *Management of high-risk pregnancy: An evidence-based approach* (5th ed.). Malden, MA: Blackwell Publishers.

Ratcliffe, S. D., Baxley, E. G., & Cline, M. K. (2008). *Family medical obstetrics.* Philadelphia: Elsevier Health Sciences.

Richter, M. S., Parkes, C., & Chaw-Kant, J. (2007). Listening to the voices of hospitalized high-risk antepartum patients. *JOGNN, 36*(4), 313–318.

Roe, V. A. (2007). Antibiotics. In B. Hackley, J. M. Kriebs, & M. E. Rousseau's (Eds.), *Primary care of women: A guide for midwives and women's health providers* (Chapter 5; pp. 115–137). Sudbury, MA: Jones & Bartlett Publishers.

Rubin, P., & Ramsay, M. (2007). *Prescribing in pregnancy* (4th ed.). Malden, MA: Blackwell Publishers.

Rubin, R. (1967). Attainment of the maternal role. Part I. Processes. *Nursing Research, 16,* 237–245.

Rubin, R. (1972). Fantasy and object constancy in maternal relationships. *Maternal and Child Nursing Journal, 1*(2), 101–111.

Rubin, R. (1977). Binding in the postpartum period. *Maternal and Child Nursing Journal, 6,* 67–75.

Rubin, R. (1984). *Maternal identity and the maternal experience.* New York: Springer.

Simpson, K. R., & Creehan, P. A. (2008). *Perinatal nursing* (3rd ed.). Philadelphia: Lippincott Williams & Wilkins.

Thornton, S. (2008). *Understanding human development.* London: Palgrave Macmillan.

Tortora, G. J., & Derrickson, B. H. (2007). *Introduction to the human body: The essentials of anatomy & physiology* (7th ed.). Indianapolis: John Wiley & Sons Inc.

United States Department of Agriculture (USDA). (2007). *What to eat while pregnant.* [Online] Retrieved from *www.womenshealth. gov/pregnancy/pregnancy/eat.cfm.*

U.S. Department of Health and Human Services. (2000). *Healthy people 2010* (Vol. 1, Conference ed.). Washington, DC: U.S. Government Printing Office.

U.S. Department of Health and Human Services (USDHHS). (2006). *Healthy people 2010 Midcourse review.* Washington, DC: U.S. Government Printing Office.

U.S. Preventive Services Task Force (USPSTF). (2006a). *Screening for family and intimate partner violence.* U.S. Department of Health and Human Services. AHRQ Pub. No. 06-0588; pp. 101–103.

U.S. Preventive Services Task Force (USPSTF). (2006b). *Screening for bacterial vaginosis in pregnancy. I.* AHRQ Pub. No. 06-0588; pp. 157–158.

U.S. Preventive Services Task Force (USPSTF). (2006c). *Screening for hepatitis B virus infection.* U.S. Department of Health and Human Services. AHRQ Pub. No. 06-0588; pp. 90–91.

U.S. Preventive Services Task Force (USPSTF). (2006d). *Screening for Rh (D) incompatibility.* U.S. Department of Health and Human Services. AHRQ Pub. No. 06-0588; pp. 164–165.

U.S. Preventive Services Task Force (USPSTF). (2006e). *Counseling to prevent tobacco use and tobacco-caused disease.* U.S. Department of Health and Human Services. AHRQ Pub. No. 06-0588; pp. 120–123.

U.S. Preventive Services Task Force (USPSTF). (2006f). *Screening for HIV.* U.S. Department of Health and Human Services. AHRQ Pub. No. 06-0588; pp. 94–97.

Ward, T. T. (2007). Toxoplasmosis. In R. E. Rakel & E. T. Bope's (Eds.), *Conn's current therapy 2007* (Section 2; pp. 193–196). Philadelphia: Saunders.

Wingerd, B. (2007). *Human body: Essentials of anatomy and physiology.* San Diego: University Readers.

Wylie, L., & Bryce, H. (2008). *The midwives' guide to key medical conditions: Pregnancy and childbirth.* Oxford: Churchill Livingstone.

Xue, F., Holzman, C., Rahbar, M. H., Trosko, K., & Fischer, L. (2007). Maternal fish consumption, mercury levels, and risk of preterm birth. *Environmental Health Perspectives, 115*(1), 42–47.

Infant

objectives

After completing this chapter, the reader will be able to:

- Evaluate the infant's health status and give examples of basic growth and developmental principles.
- Analyze the developmental tasks for the infant and the behavior indicating that these tasks are being met.
- Explain the immunization schedule and other safety and health-promotion measures to a parent.
- Identify common parental concerns about infants and describe a model for parent education to allay these concerns.
- Describe accidents that occur during infancy and recommend appropriate counseling for accident prevention and safety.
- Indicate ways in which nurses can be active in promoting major policies and influencing legislation concerning health.
- Outline governmental strategies to meet the goals of improving infant health.

key terms

Active immunization

Birth defects

Body mass index (BMI)

Denver Developmental
  Screening Test II

Down syndrome

Failure-to-thrive syndrome

Growth index

Oral stage of development

Passive immunization

Paternal engrossment

Reflexes

Sensorimotor period

Sickle cell anemia

Sudden infant death
  syndrome (SIDS)

Tay-Sachs disease

Trust versus mistrust

Weaning

website materials

ℰvolve

These materials are located on the book's website at *http://evolve.elsevier.com/Edelman/*.

- WebLinks
- Study Questions
- Glossary
- Website Resources

  17A: Denver Developmental Screening Test II and Directions for Administration
  17B: Growth Chart for Girls, Birth to 36 Months
  17C: Growth Chart for Boys, Birth to 36 Months
  17D: Height and Weight Measurements for Girls and Boys
  17E: Detailed Immunization Schedules
  17F: Nursing Interventions to Prevent Cancer in Infants
  17G: Nursing Interventions to Help Economically Deprived Families and Infants
  17H: Infant Health Care Programs

THINK About It

Car Safety Seats

Infants are at particular risk from automobile accidents. The proper use of occupant protection systems (infant car safety seats with seat belts) can reduce the risk of death and injury significantly. Although many public service campaigns encourage parents to restrain their infants while riding in automobiles (and all states have laws requiring some type of passenger safety restraint for infants), some parents neglect or remain unaware of the importance of providing safety for their vulnerable infants.

Nurses must have up-to-date knowledge about car occupant protection systems and their proper use to help parents find new products and obtain the most current information available. Parents often rely on the salesperson of the infant car seat for their information about protection systems and the proper use of car seats. However,

informational brochures and media campaigns fall short because they usually fail to provide explanations or demonstrations. As a result, parents may misinterpret the information that they receive.

1. What type of program might you develop to reach and inform parents about the importance of car seat safety?
2. In what settings might such a program be implemented?
3. How would you modify your teaching plan to meet the needs of illiterate parents?
4. How would you modify your program to ensure that parents who come from cultural backgrounds different than your own would respond well to the information?

Providing a safe and sound source of attachment and interaction is paramount to healthy infant development. Caregiving and mothering activities are the primary ingredients of an infant's preparation for life and ultimate independence. Nurses play a vital role in influencing this positive interaction through health promotion and education.

This chapter focuses on the infant and family during the infant's developmental period of 1 to 18 months. Because the infant is completely dependent, this chapter addresses the infant's parents and significant others as sources of health-promotion activities. The relationship initiated at birth between parents and infant is the basis for the interdependence that is required for proper psychological and physical infant development. Health care professionals must focus on parent education as a means of fostering healthy, satisfying relationships within the family unit and promoting the development of healthy future generations.

The principles of normal growth and development are used as a structural framework for this chapter. Understanding these principles helps the nurse identify deviations from the norm and institute appropriate health promoting interventions.

To promote and maintain health during infancy, a balance between the infant's internal and external environmental forces must be established; any disruption places the infant at risk. Several processes that greatly influence this balance are identified, and appropriate interventions are outlined to assist the nurse in promoting a healthy infant population (*Healthy People 2010* box; American Academy of Pediatrics, 2007; Hockenberry & Wilson, 2006).

AGE AND PHYSICAL CHANGES

Human development begins when a single sperm penetrates a mature ovum. The changes that follow are undeniable and wondrous (Box 17-1). During this early period of growth and development the infant depends completely on others, primarily the parents, to meet all personal needs. To assist

the parents in their understanding of their infant's needs and progress, the nurse must know what behaviors to expect at certain age levels. These developmental landmarks serve as a basis for anticipatory guidance (Table 17-1). Parents are aware of age-appropriate behavior to anticipate and facilitate these developmental landmarks. This knowledge, along with the nurse's anticipatory guidance, can also promote closer family relationships. In addition to the growth landmarks, the infant must accomplish developmental tasks to form a healthy personality.

Developmental Tasks

Every infant faces developmental tasks and must accomplish them individually. Different practices in various societies affect the perception and resolution of the tasks, but all must be faced (Pillitteri, 2007).

The infant's first and most basic task is survival, which includes the physical tasks of breathing, sucking, eating, digesting, eliminating, and sleeping. Because many of these tasks involve the infant's mouth, this stage of life often is referred to as the **oral stage of development**, reflecting the primary importance of the mouth as the center of pleasure. More developmental tasks that must be accomplished during infancy are listed in Box 17-2.

To assist the infant's parents in encouraging achievement of these tasks, the nurse discusses the importance of stimulation and environmental interactions. Many neurological structures are far from completely developed at birth (Coch et al., 2007). To continue growing, the brain depends not only on internal, embryological, and maturational forces, but also on external stimulation. This external stimulation appears to influence the internal, anatomical, and maturational processes by means of at least three different mechanisms (Puckett & Black, 2007):

1. Stimulation favors progressive complex arborization of dendrites (the connection between nerve cells).

Healthy People 2010

Selected National Health-Promotion and Disease-Prevention Objectives for Infants

- Reduce iron deficiency to less than 5% among infants age 1 to 2 years. (Baseline is 9% for children age 1 to 2 years. Note: iron deficiency is defined as having abnormal results for two or more of the following tests: serum ferritin concentration, erythrocyte protoporphyrin, or transferrin saturation.)
- Reduce nonfatal poisonings to no more than 292 nonfatal poisonings per 100,000 population. (Baseline is 348.4 nonfatal poisonings per 100,000 population in 1997.)
- Reduce growth restriction among low-income children age 5 and younger to less than 5%. (Baseline is 8% of low-income children under age 5 years were growth restricted in 1997, depending on race and ethnicity. Note: growth restriction is defined as height-for-age below the fifth percentile in the age-gender–appropriate population using the NCHS-CDC growth charts.)
- Reduce infant deaths to no more than 4.5 per 1000 live births by the year 2010. (Baseline is 7.2 per 1000 live births in 1998.) Reduce infant deaths related to birth defects to 0.7% per 1000 live births. (Baseline was 1.4% per 1000 live births in 1998.)
- Reduce deaths from SIDS to less than 0.23 deaths per 1000 live births by the year 2010. (Baseline is 0.67 deaths per 1000 live births were from SIDS in 1999.)
- Increase the percentage of healthy full-term infants who were put down to sleep on their backs to 70% by the year 2010. (Baseline is 35% of healthy full-term infants put down to sleep on their backs in 1996.)
- Reduce or eliminate indigenous cases of vaccine-preventable disease through universal vaccination by the year 2010. (Target: total elimination for congenital rubella syndrome, diphtheria, Haemophilus influenzae type b, measles, mumps, polio, rubella, and tetanus; 41% improvement for pertussis; 99% improvement for hepatitis B; and 99% improvement for varicella.)
- Increase the number of infants age 18 months and younger that have a specific source of ongoing primary care to at least 96%. (Baseline is 93% in 1997.)

- Increase the proportion of mothers who breast-feed their babies. In early postpartum period to at least 75% by 2010 (1998 baseline was 64%); at 6 months still breast-feeding to 50% (baseline was 29% in 1998); at 1 year still breast-feeding to 25% (baseline was 16% in 1998); breast-feeding exclusively through 3 months to 60% by 2010 (baseline was 43% in 2002); breast-feeding exclusively through 6 months to 25% in 2010 (baseline was 13% in 2002).
- Eliminate elevated blood lead levels in children age 1 to 5 years by the year 2010. (Baseline is 4.4% of children age 1 to 5 years with blood lead levels exceeding 10 μg/dL during 1991 to 1994.)
- Increase the use of occupant child restraints by the year 2010 to 100%. (Baseline is 92% of motor vehicle occupants aged 4 years and under used child restraints in 1998.)
- Reduce low birth weight (LBW) and very low birth weight (VLBW). Reduce LBW infants to 5% in 2010 (baseline was 7.6% in 1998); reduce VLBW infants to 0.9% in 2010 (baseline was 1.4% in 1998).
- Reduce preterm births. Reduce the total preterm births to 7.6% in 2010 (baseline was 11.6% of live births in 1998); reduce live births at 32 to 36 weeks of gestation to 6.4% in 2010 (baseline was 9.6% of live births in 1998); reduce live births at less than 32 weeks of gestation to 1.1% in 2010 (baseline was 2.0% of live births in 1998).
- Increase the proportion of VLBW infants born at level III hospitals or subspecialty perinatal centers. Increase to 90% born there (baseline was 73% of VLBW infants born at level III hospitals or subspecialty perinatal centers in 1996-97.)
- Reduce the occurrence of developmental disabilities. Reduce mental retardation to 124.5 per 10,000 by 2010 (baseline was 131 per 10,000 in 1991-94); reduce cerebral palsy to 31.6 per 10,000 by 2010 (baseline was 33.3 per 10,000 in 1991-94); reduction in age of identification of autism spectrum disorder to 48 months by 2010 (baseline was 50 months in 1996.)

SIDS, Sudden infant death syndrome.
NCHS-CDC, National Center for Health Statistics, Centers for Disease Control and Prevention; U.S. Department of Health and Human Services (USDHHS). (2006). *Healthy people 2010 midcourse review*. Washington, DC: U.S. Government Printing Office.
From U.S. Department of Health and Human Services. (2000). *Healthy people 2010*: Vol. 1 and 2 (Conference ed.). Washington, DC: U.S. Government Printing Office.

2. Stimulation increases the degree of vascularization of certain anatomical structures of the brain, such as the centers associated with vision.
3. Stimulation increases the process of myelination, which is closely related to the rate of development of a variety of functions. Myelin coats the brain and nerve tissue, which then becomes activated.

When counseling parents, the nurse stresses the importance of a variety of stimuli within the infant's environment. A variety of auditory and visual stimuli should be available, such as colorful mobiles, radio, spoken voice, and toys, to assist the infant in achieving developmental tasks. The sense of touch is an extremely important stimulus, bringing the infant in tune with caregivers in different environments,

Growth and Development   Box 17-1

During Infancy

ONE MONTH

- Follows and fixes on bright object with eyes when it moves within field of vision
- Still has head lag when pulled to sitting position
- Displays tonic neck, grasp, and Moro reflexes
- Turns head when prone, but unable to support
- Displays sucking and rooting reflexes
- Holds hands in fists
- Makes small, throaty sounds
- Gains 5 to 7 ounces weekly for 6 months
- Grows 1 inch monthly for 6 months
- Cries when hungry or uncomfortable
- Lifts head momentarily when prone

TWO MONTHS

- Has closed posterior fontanel
- Listens actively to sounds
- Lifts head almost 45 degrees off table when prone
- Follows moving object with eyes
- Recognizes familiar faces
- Pays attention to speaking voice
- Assumes less flexed position when prone
- Vocalizes; distinct from crying
- Turns from side to back
- Begins to have social smile

THREE MONTHS

- Visually inspects object and stares at own hand with apparent fascination when either appears in field of vision
- Has longer periods of wakefulness without crying
- Laughs aloud and shows pleasure in vocalization
- Holds head erect and steady; raises chest, usually supported on forearms
- Smiles in response to mother's face
- Begins prelanguage vocalizations (coos, babbles, and chuckles)
- Carries hand or object to mouth at will
- Actively holds rattle, but will not reach for it
- Turns eyes to object placed in field of vision

FOUR MONTHS

- Begins drooling, indicating appearance of saliva; does not know how to swallow it
- Holds head steady when in sitting position
- Recognizes familiar objects
- Shows almost no head lag when pulled to sitting position
- Rolls from back to side and abdomen to back
- Inspects and plays with hands; pulls clothing or blanket over face in play
- Begins eye-hand coordination
- Chews and bites
- Enjoys social interaction
- Demands attention by fussing
- Reaches out to people
- Is aware and interested in new environment
- Grasps object with two hands
- Squeals

FIVE MONTHS

- Reaches persistently; grasps with entire hand
- Plays with toes
- Smiles at mirror image
- Begins to postpone gratification
- Shows signs of tooth eruption
- Sleeps through night without food
- Weighs twice the birth weight
- Sits with slight support
- Vocalizes displeasure when desired object is taken away
- Is able to discriminate strangers from family
- Makes cooing noises
- Squeals with delight
- Looks for object that has fallen
- Rolls from back to stomach or vice versa

SIX MONTHS

- Gains approximately 3 to 5 ounces weekly during the second 6 months
- Grows approximately 1 inch monthly for 6 months
- Is able to lift cup by handle
- Begins to hitch in locomotion
- Sits in high chair with straight back
- Begins to imitate sounds
- Vocalizes to toys and mirror image
- Babbles with one-syllable sounds: "ma, ma, da, da"
- Has definite likes and dislikes
- Likes to be picked up
- Plays peek-a-boo
- Makes "guh" and "bah" sounds

SEVEN MONTHS

- Has eruption of upper central incisors
- Bears weight when held in standing position
- Sits, leaning forward on both hands
- Fixates on one very small object
- Produces vowel sounds: "ba-ba" and "da-da"
- Shows fear of strangers
- Displays emotional instability by easy and quick changes from crying to laughing
- Repeats activities that are enjoyed
- Bangs objects together
- Approaches toy and grasps it with one hand
- Imitates simple acts

EIGHT MONTHS

- Feeds self with finger foods
- Sits well alone
- Stretches out arms to be picked up
- Greets strangers with bashful behavior
- Begins to show regular patterns in bladder and bowel elimination
- Responds to "no"
- Makes consonant sounds: t, d, and w
- Dislikes dressing and diaper change
- Releases object at will
- Shows nervousness with strangers
- Pulls toy toward self

Growth and Development   Box 17-1

During Infancy—cont'd

NINE MONTHS

- Creeps and crawls (backward at first)
- Shows good coordination and sits alone
- Responds to adult anger; cries when scolded
- Explores object by sucking, chewing, and biting it
- Responds to simple verbal requests
- Drinks from cup or glass with assistance
- Pulls self to standing position
- Begins to show fears of going to bed and being left alone
- Imitates waving "bye-bye"
- Releases object with flexed wrist
- Repeats facial expressions of adults
- Uses thumb and index finger in pincer grasp

10 MONTHS

- Sits by falling down
- Says "da-da" and "ma-ma"
- Understands "bye-bye"
- Looks at and follows pictures in book
- Crawls and cruises about well
- Pays attention to own name
- Picks up object fairly well
- Extends toy to another person without releasing
- Pulls self to standing position and stands while holding onto solid object

11 MONTHS

- Is able to push toys and place several objects in container
- Attempts to walk without assistance
- Begins to hold spoon
- Stands erect with help of person's hand
- May have lower lateral incisors erupting
- Holds crayon to mark on paper
- Imitates definite speech sounds
- Reacts to restrictions with frustration

12 MONTHS

- Loses Babinski sign
- Develops evident hand dominance
- Weighs triple the birth weight
- Has equal circumference head and chest
- Walks with help
- Knows own name

- Has slow vocabulary growth because of increased interest in walking
- Develops lumbar curve
- Uses spoon in feeding, but often puts it upside down in mouth
- Drops object deliberately for it to be picked up
- Shakes head for "no"
- Plays pat-a-cake
- Recovers balance when falling over
- Tries to follow when being read to
- Does things to attract attention
- Imitates vocalization lead

15 MONTHS

- Creeps up stairs
- Uses "da-da" and "ma-ma" labels for correct parents
- Tolerates some separation
- Drinks from cup well, but rotates spoon
- Asks for object by pointing
- Plays interactive games such as peek-a-boo and pat-a-cake
- Expresses emotions; has temper tantrums
- Walks without help

18 MONTHS

- Has closed anterior fontanel
- Has long trunk, short and bowed legs, and protruding abdomen
- Walks up stairs with help
- Turns pages of book
- Has short attention span
- Begins to test limits
- Has bowel movements at appropriate time when placed on potty
- Indicates wet pants
- Gets into everything
- Fills and handles spoon without rotating it, but spills frequently
- Runs clumsily and falls often
- Is extremely curious
- Places object in hole or slot
- Becomes communicative, social being
- Imitates behavior of parents, such as mimicking household chores

making it a reality. Ensuring that appropriate sensory stimuli are available is vital to the infant's growth and developmental progression (Pillitteri, 2007).

Concepts of Infant Development

The study of how a helpless infant grows and develops into a fully functioning, independent adult has fascinated many researchers. Their theories describe the development of human behavior as overlapping stages that occur in somewhat predictable patterns in an individual's life (Burge, 2007). Because these developmental theories are presented in Chapter 15, only their specific application to the infant is discussed here.

Psychosocial Development

Erikson's psychosocial developmental theory is concerned primarily with a series of tasks or crises that each individual must resolve before encountering the next one. The central task during infancy is the development of a sense of **trust versus mistrust**. Establishing this basic trust or mistrust

Table **17-1**	Parenting Tasks for Developmental Landmarks in Infancy	
Age (Months)	**Landmark**	**Parenting Task**
1	Lifts head when prone	Place infant in prone position and dangle colorful object above head
2	Has social smile	Promote by talking to infant and allowing opportunity to smile
4	Squeals	Encourage and praise for doing
5	Rolls from back to front	Place infant in protected area (crib or playpen) and encourage to move by placing toy out of reach
8 to 9	Uses pincer grasp to feed self	Make finger foods available
10	Pulls self to standing position	Provide safe environment; place chair or object of appropriate height within reach
11 to 12	Initiates vocalization	Talk to infant frequently and include in family gatherings
12 to 15	Walks	Encourage and provide clutter-free, safe walkway; praise for attempts
15	Drinks from cup	Supply cup with appropriate drink; do not scold for clumsiness in handling cups or spills
18	Mimics household chores	Give rags to help with chores, dusting, allow to fold clothes, and so on

Growth and Development   Box 17-2

Developmental Tasks Accomplished in Infancy

1. Achieves physiological equilibrium after birth
2. Establishes self as a dependent person, but separate from others
3. Becomes aware of animate versus inanimate and familiar versus unfamiliar and develops rudimentary social interaction
4. Develops a feeling of affection for others and the desire for affection from others
5. Manages the changing body and learns new motor skills, develops equilibrium, begins eye-hand coordination, and establishes rest-activity rhythm
6. Learns to understand and control the physical world through exploration
7. Develops a beginning symbol system, conceptual abilities, and preverbal communication
8. Directs emotional expression to indicate needs and wishes

From Ingoldsby, B. B., Smith, S. R., & Miller, J. E. (2007). *Exploring family theories.* New York: Oxford University Press.

determines the manner in which the infant approaches all future stages of growth. The infant first develops a sense of trust in the mother (or other caretaker) and then in other significant people. Trust influences the infant's future relationships, allowing for deeper commitment and intimacy. To develop trust the infant requires maximal gratification and minimal frustration to experience a healthy balance between inner needs and outer satisfaction. If the mother or caretaker is consistently responsive to the infant, meeting physical and psychological needs, the infant will likely learn to trust his or her caretaker; view the world as a safe place; and grow up to be secure, self-reliant, trusting, cooperative, and helpful towards others.

Prompt, skillful, and consistent response to the infant's needs helps foster security and trust because it enables the infant to predict what will happen within the environment. When unpredictability and disorganized routines exist, the infant will develop fear, anger, and insecurity, which eventually lead to mistrust. The infant can demonstrate desire by crying but depends on the sensitivity and willingness of others to provide relief. If the most important people fail to do this, the infant has little foundation on which to build faith in others or self in adulthood.

Cognitive Development

Piaget's cognitive developmental theory focuses on intellectual changes that occur in a sequential manner as a result of continual interaction between the infant and the environment (Berk, 2007). Piaget's **sensorimotor period** (up to age 18 months) describes the time during which infants develop the coordination to master activities that allow them to interact with the environment. During this period the infant solves problems using sensory systems and motor activity rather than symbolic processes, which develop later.

Research has shown that fetuses are able to distinguish light from dark and that sight is present at birth. Rod cells in the retina of the eyes, which are responsible for light perception, are functional at birth although the retina (the organ of visual perception) is not fully developed until approximately 4 months of age. However, the infant can perceive color and shape. Infants are startled by loud noises and are soothed by soft voices, which indicates that their sense of hearing is functioning. Their hearing can also be tested with audio equipment at birth. Babies cry when pricked with a diaper pin and fuss when too hot or too cold; therefore, the senses of pain and temperature are operative also. Touching, stroking, and rocking typically soothe a fussing infant. Infants will also react to odors and tastes.

In addition to perceiving stimulation, the newborn is capable of reflexive behavior. **Reflexes** are responses that normally are exhibited after particular types of new stimulation (Pillitteri, 2007). Because the response occurs after the stimulus, reflexes are unlearned. Some infant reflexes, such as rooting and sucking, have survival value. The rooting reflex, activated by lightly stroking the angle of the lips or cheek, helps the infant locate the food source.

The infant will turn toward the side that is being stroked and will open the lips to suck. The sucking reflex is initiated when an object is placed in the infant's mouth. Together, these reflexes ensure that the infant can obtain food. Infants also have reflexes that result in grasping, yawning, hiccoughing, coughing, and sneezing.

Armed with these reflexes and sensory capabilities, the infant is ready to begin interacting with the environment (seeing, hearing, touching, tasting, and smelling) to acquire valuable information.

The infant progresses in various ways between birth and age 18 months, with early capabilities changing and becoming intentional. Piaget outlines five stages within the sensorimotor period that describe the infant's development, from the early reflexive behavior to differentiation between self and environment (Table 17-2).

The infant in the sensorimotor period uses behavioral strategies to manipulate objects, to learn some of their properties, and to reach goals by combining several behaviors. The infant's behavior is tied to the concrete and the immediate; schemes can be applied only to objects that can be perceived directly.

Knowledge of child developmental theories is extremely valuable to the nurse during interactions with infants. Understanding the infant's level of cognitive thought and emotional and social development helps the nurse decipher a child's communications more meaningfully and interpret behaviors and the processes that motivate the child more accurately. This knowledge can be incorporated in the anticipatory guidance offered to the parents. The nurse stresses that a variety of sensory and motor stimuli fosters learning within the infant's environment.

Denver Developmental Screening Test II

The Denver Developmental Screening Test (DDST) is a standardized tool that screens for developmental problems in children from birth to 6 years of age. Three purposes have been identified for administering the Denver II: (1) screening apparently healthy infants for developmental problems, (2) validating intuitive concerns about an infant's development with an objective test, and (3) monitoring high-risk children for developmental problems. The **Denver Developmental Screening Test II** and directions for administration are presented in **Website Resource 17A**.

Four areas of development are screened: (1) personal-social, (2) fine motor–adaptive, (3) language, and (4) gross motor. Unique features of the Denver II are its recent and sophisticated standardization and its inclusion of norms for various subgroups based on place of residence, ethnicity, and mother's level of education. The Denver II includes four test behavior descriptors to rate the infant's behavior, reflecting the administrator's subjective impression of the infant's overall behavior. Behavioral ratings are established for compliance with the examiner's requests for alertness and interest in the surroundings, fearfulness, and attention span.

The nurse tells the parents before the test that the DDST is not an intelligence test but, rather, a test of the child's developmental level. By adding the number of accomplished and unaccomplished items on the test form, the screener estimates the child's developmental level. By referring to guidelines on the instruction sheet, the child is scored P (passed) or F (failed) on each item. The DDST can be administered with minimal materials and time and, ideally, should be administered to an infant at approximately 3 or 4 months of age, again at 10 months, and again at 3 years (Coch et al., 2007).

The infant's growth index—height and weight measurements plotted on a standard growth chart to assess for normal progression—is also important. Physical growth (height and weight) is a valid health status indicator that should be measured during each routine office or clinic visit. During the first year of life, growth is rapid. An infant who is growing properly is at low risk for developing a chronic disease (Puckett & Black, 2007).

The nurse plots the infant's length and weight measurements against exact chronological age on growth grids. In 2000 the National Center for Health Statistics published growth grids that have been standardized to the present growth charts for female and male infants from birth to age 36 months. These growth charts are presented in **Website Resources 17B and 17C. Body mass index (BMI)** is a feature of the new pediatric growth charts recently released by the Centers for Disease Control and Prevention (CDC). The charts are used by most pediatricians and were

Growth and Development	Table 17-2

Piaget's Five Stages of Infant Development

Stage	Description
Stage 1: birth to 1 month	Modification of reflexes Practices and perfects reflexes present at birth Sucking reflex becomes more refined and voluntary
Stage 2: 1 to 4 months	Primary circular reactions Repeats behavior that previously led to an interesting event Only the infant's own body involved in activities
Stage 3: 4 to 10 months	Secondary circular reactions begins Repetitions involve events or objects in the external world Appears to perform actions with a purpose Hand-eye coordination
Stage 4: 10 to 12 months	Coordination of secondary reactions Combines two or more previously acquired strategies to obtain a goal
Stage 5: 12 to 18 months	Tertiary circular reactions Uses active experimentation to achieve previously unattainable goals Infant purposely varies movements to observe results

developed by the National Center for Health Statistics in collaboration with the National Center for Chronic Disease Prevention and Health Promotion (2007). With the addition of body mass index to the charts, the CDC significantly increased the usefulness of this tool as a warning signal for potential obesity as early as 2 years of age. Parents have an opportunity to change their children's eating habits before a weight problem develops. The revised pediatric growth charts more accurately reflect the United States' cultural and racial diversity and can track children and young people through age 20. The growth charts indicate data that children are heavier today than in the past, but height has remained virtually unchanged.

An infant's **growth index**, as determined by length and weight, is only one factor in assessing health status. The nurse has an overall understanding of growth and development principles to counsel parents regarding their infant's progress. **Website Resource 17D** presents height and weight measurements for girls and boys.

Gender

The infant's gender is determined at the moment of fertilization. Immediately after delivery, the parents usually ask, "Is it a girl or a boy?" The answer has far-reaching implications for many family units. Gender is one of the many important factors that influence parents' way of relating to the infant.

Studies have revealed many biological and behavioral differences between male and female infants. Boys are, on average, larger and have proportionately more muscle mass at birth. Girls are generally smaller but physiologically more mature at birth and are less vulnerable to stress. Boys show more motor activity, whereas girls display a greater response to tactile stimulation and pain (Polan & Taylor, 2007). As the infant develops, further differences are noted. By 6 months, girls respond to visual stimulation with longer attention spans and are more socially responsive than are boys; girls also tend to sit up, walk, and crawl earlier than do boys. Girls also learn to communicate with language at an earlier age, whereas male infants use their whole bodies in communicating (Coch et al., 2007).

The gender of the infant, a major concern of many expectant parents, may well influence parental relationships and expectations. The infant's gender can evoke disappointment; in some cases, a woman may feel disappointed in a girl because she knows that her husband wanted a boy. Today, the trend is to want one child of each gender. Because of the availability in America of better forms of contraception and economic factors such as the expense of raising children, most couples are having fewer children today when compared with the 1950s. The importance and stress of producing the right-sex infant is evident. Being the "wrong sex" can, combined with other factors, place an infant at risk for child abuse. The parents may find fault with and place blame on the infant for not meeting this expectation (Olson et al., 2007).

Health intervention focuses on the identification of high-risk families and the promotion of positive relationships between infants and parents. The nurse promotes the good health, appearance, and developmental potential of the infant. Increasing the parents' feelings of adequacy and self-esteem will promote their acceptance and care of the infant. Most importantly, follow-up care for these families is a high priority to ensure that adequate support and help are available.

Race

Race refers to the classification of human beings into groups based on particular physical characteristics, such as skin pigmentation, head form, and stature owing to a common inheritance. Caucasoid, mongoloid, and negroid are the three racial types generally recognized (Dorland, 2007). A range of physical variation exists among people of different races with regard to growth rate, dentition, body structure, blood groups, susceptibility to certain diseases, as well as a great many other variables.

In assessing an infant, the nurse not only collects data, but also compares the data with established norms, such as a standardized growth chart. When the norms chosen are not appropriate for the individual (for example, an Asian infant's growth is assessed based on norms for White children), the assessment will not be accurate. The nurse who works with families from a variety of racial groups has an understanding of each background and how it relates to health and health care. To facilitate nursing care for a family from a racial group different from that of the health care provider, effective communication must be established. This communication will help foster an understanding of the other's point of view and frame of reference. Each family member is viewed as an individual, as well as a family unit. There is no stereotyping of families within a racial or ethnic group. Despite common language, color, or historical background, not all members of a particular racial group are alike. This diversity presents, without doubt, considerable challenges for nurses who work with families with infants (Schwartz & Scott, 2006). Universal norms by which to measure one's growth and skill capacity do not exist. The nurse recognizes the differences and intervenes appropriately. The orientation of health maintenance and disease prevention is basic to good health practices, regardless of racial makeup. This concept is the main focus of all health care. (Refer to Chapter 2 for further details.)

Genetics

The desired and expected outcome of any pregnancy is the birth of a healthy, perfect baby. Parents experience disappointment when they discover that their baby has been born with a defect. A **birth defect** is an abnormality of structure, function, or metabolism as a result of a genetic or environmental influence on the fetus, often a combination of both. Couples may refrain from having another child because they have had one with a serious birth defect and do not want to risk another. In these situations, genetic counseling provides information that is needed to understand a hereditary disorder and its associated risks. The main goal of counseling is to explain **birth defects** to affected families and to allow prospective parents to make informed decisions about childbearing.

Using the basic laws governing heredity and knowing the frequency of specific birth defects in the population, the genetic counselor can often predict the probability of recurrence of a given abnormality in the same family. An important aspect of primary prevention is identifying families at increased risk and referring them for counseling (Lashley, 2007). Aspects to be reviewed in the initial interview include:

1. *Maternal age.* The risk of having a child with **Down syndrome** increases significantly for the woman older than 35 years of age. In this syndrome, three chromosomes appear in the 21 chromosome group (trisomy 21). Characteristic features include upward-slanting eyes; small, malformed ears; large, protruding tongue; broad hands and feet; and some degree of mental retardation.

2. *Ethnic background.* Several genetic disorders occur with higher frequency in certain groups. Eastern European Jews have a 10 times greater chance of carrying the Tay-Sachs gene than does the general U.S. population. Abnormal deposits of lipids (fats) in the cells of the cerebral cortex, spleen, liver, and lymph nodes are characteristics of **Tay-Sachs disease.** An autosomal recessive gene transmits it. Blacks have a much greater chance of carrying the sickle cell trait than does the general population. **Sickle cell anemia** is an autosomal recessive condition that occurs in 1 out of every 500 Black births and causes severe hemolytic anemia crises. One in 12 African Americans has the sickle cell trait (CDC, 2007).

3. *Family history.* Certain diseases, such as Huntington's chorea, hemophilia, or mental retardation, are often hereditary. Huntington's chorea (an autosomal dominant disease involving the brain) is characterized by deterioration of intellectual functions and involuntary movements of the limbs, face, and trunk. Once manifested, a steady deterioration leads to death after some years. Hemophilia is a sex-linked recessive coagulation disorder caused by a functional deficiency of a clotting factor; that leads to prolonged bleeding. Hemophilia passes from an unaffected carrier mother to her male offspring and affects 18,000 people in the United States (CDC, 2007).

4. *Reproductive history.* Spontaneous abortions, stillbirths, and previous live-born children with birth defects or slow development may indicate an increased risk.

5. *Maternal disease.* Several maternal disorders are associated with a higher frequency of birth defects, including diabetes mellitus, seizure disorder, mental retardation, and phenylketonuria. Prenatal diagnosis offers the couple the option of aborting a fetus that is affected with certain genetic disorders. For

many people, however, this option is unacceptable. Chapter 16 discusses the various tests used for prenatal diagnosis.

The nurse's role throughout the genetic counseling process is to provide the vital link between the counseling team and the high-risk couple. The nurse is involved in case finding, referral, and family education. The nurse has a sound background in the principles of genetics to provide families with appropriate information as part of preventive guidance (Lashley, 2007).

GORDON'S FUNCTIONAL HEALTH PATTERNS
Health Perception–Health Management Pattern

Health promotion is aimed at assisting the infant and family to change behavior to produce better physical and emotional health in adulthood. To reach this goal, the nurse encourages child-rearing practices that promote normal growth and development, fosters attitudes and values compatible with health, and teaches appropriate use of health services (Wilhelmsson & Lindberg, 2007). The nurse promotes the infant's health through the parents, who determine the care practices for the dependent infant.

Health is largely a subjective judgment. Each person's perception of health is related to physical and mental capabilities, self-concept, relationships with others and the environment, and personal goals and values (Jarvis, 2007). With this understanding, the nurse uses every opportunity to convey confidence in the parents' health perception–health management pattern and their ability to act to enhance the infant's health. When parents learn and adopt behaviors that improve their own health, they are more likely to ensure that the health needs of their infant are met. Parental modeling increases the chances that good health practices will be retained throughout the child's life.

The goals of nursing practice with infants and their families are to promote individual motivation for health, to assist the family to identify health needs, and to develop problem-solving skills using the family's own resources. To meet these goals, the nurse identifies the family's perception of good or bad health practices, which greatly influences participation in health-promoting activities. Age, gender, educational level, cultural orientation, financial status, and occupation combine to influence health perception. When parents believe that the infant is more susceptible to a health problem if promotional behavior is not enacted, they become more motivated to adopt the behavior.

The nurse's task helps the parents recognize their infant's susceptibility and the potential consequences when healthy practices are not instituted. The nurse works within the family's health perception framework to become acquainted with the characteristics that influence the infant's health. Unless caregivers meet their own personal needs, they will be unable to meet their infant's developmental needs (Clark, 2008). The nurse supports the parents, strengthening their parental confidence and self-esteem, providing information on meeting their infant's needs, and reinforcing their health perception–health management pattern.

Nutritional-Metabolic Pattern

One of the most important aspects of health promotion in the infant is nutritional status. Many opinions have been expressed about the infant's nutritional needs. As research in this area continues, recommendations and opinions will change; however, some basic facts about nutrition remain fairly consistent. Infant nutritional requirements are based on what is considered necessary to (1) support life, (2) provide for growth, and (3) maintain health.

Essential Nutrients

Water, proteins, fats, carbohydrates, vitamins, and minerals are the essential nutrients in any diet. Because the first year of life is a period of rapid growth, nutritional needs during this period are especially important and always changing. Water is vital to survival. A person can live for several weeks without food but can survive only a few days without water. Because the infant's body weight is approximately 75% water, the baby must consume large amounts of fluid to maintain water balance. Water requirements average between 125 to 150 mL/kg of body weight per day during the first 6 months of life and 120 to 135 mL/kg per day during the second 6 months (DeBruyne et al., 2007). The sources of water are fluids (primarily milk) and food; most strained foods are 75% to 85% water. Most infant diets meet the basic water requirement.

The infant must also consume sufficient high-quality protein to facilitate growth and development. Recommended protein requirements are 2.2 g/kg per day during the first 6 months and 2 g/kg per day during the second 6 months (Shaw & Lawson, 2007).

Carbohydrates should supply 30% to 60% of the energy intake during infancy. Approximately 37% of the calories in human milk and 40% to 50% of the calories in commercial formulas are derived from lactose or other carbohydrates (Dudek, 2006).

A minimum of 3.8 g/kcal and a maximum of 6 g/kcal of fat (30% to 54% of calories) are recommended for infants (Shaw & Lawson, 2007). This quantity is present in human milk and in all formulas prepared for infants. Significantly lower intakes, such as in skim milk feedings, can result in an inadequate energy intake.

Vitamins are essential nutrients in the infant's diet that regulate metabolism and allow more efficient use of carbohydrates, fats, and proteins within the body. Although most infants receive adequate vitamin intake through formula, breast milk, and food, recent research has raised a concern about a vitamin D deficiency in infants who receive only breast milk. According to the Institute of Medicine (2007), nutritional rickets is on the rise in the United States among American children with certain risk factors: dark-skinned infants, breast-fed for long periods without receiving any vitamin supplementation, and decreased exposure to sunlight. They recommend that this population needs vitamin D supplementation of 200 international units/day to be initiated within the first two months of life, and it needs to be continued throughout the time the infant is breast-feeding (Institute of Medicine, 2007).

Minerals are found in relatively small amounts in the infant's body but are vital elements in body structure and control of certain bodily functions. Mineral intake for infants appears to be adequate, except for iron and fluoride.

The full-term infant is born with stores of iron adequate to meet bodily needs for hemoglobin production for approximately 4 to 6 months. After this time, body stores may need to be replenished. Although iron in human milk is bioavailable, both breast-fed and formula-fed infants should receive an additional source of iron by 6 months of age. Iron-fortified formula and cereals are the most commonly used food sources.

Fluoride, concentrated in the bones and teeth, helps reduce dental caries. The Institute of Medicine (2007) has recommended that optimal fluoride intake for an infant is 0.25 mg per day. Supplementation is necessary when the diet contains insufficient fluoridated water.

A review of these requirements shows that milk (breast or formula) meets most of the infant's nutritional needs when consumed in adequate amounts, plus vitamin D supplementation for the high-risk infants. No data support the theory that solid foods are needed to meet these nutritional needs, at least during the first 6 months of life.

Food Additives

In addition to their questionable nutritional value, additives in commercial baby food can negatively influence an infant's health status. The purposes of food additives vary, including (1) adding nutritional value; (2) preserving or extending shelf life; (3) facilitating preparation; (4) improving flavor, color, and texture; and (5) keeping flavors and textures consistent (Fullerton-Smith, 2007).

Commercially prepared baby foods are generally safe, nutritious, and of high quality. In response to consumer demand, baby food manufacturers have removed much of the added salt and sugar that their products once contained and have eliminated most food additives.

Nutrition problems include undernutrition, in which infants do not receive an adequate supply of an essential nutrient, and overnutrition, in which they receive more of a certain nutrient than is needed for healthy growth and development (Dudek, 2006). For infants in the United States, both of these problems are present. A parent who wants the infant to have family foods rather than commercial baby food can blenderize a small portion of the table food at each meal. This choice necessitates cooking without salt or sugar as is the practice of baby food manufacturers. Making baby food is easy and economical. Written resources are available for parents who are interested in more details about home food preparation for infants.

Parents should be encouraged to read baby food labels carefully. Nurses can obtain lists of baby foods and their ingredients from the manufacturers. The best overall recommendation that nurses make to parents is to provide their infants with a well-balanced diet and avoid excesses.

Breast-Feeding

Research throughout the years has demonstrated unequivocally that exclusive breast-feeding is the preferred method of infant feeding for the first 6 months of life and should be continued for at least the first year of life and beyond for as long as mutually desired by mother and child (American Academy of Pediatrics [AAP], 2005). Breast milk is often called the perfect food for the infant and for the mother, because of its composition and it doesn't have to be bought, cooked, or stored. Both the American Dietetic Association and the AAP have released position statements in support of breast-feeding. This has influenced a number of health-promotion strategies in the United States. In the *Healthy People 2010 Midcourse Review* (2006), two new subobjectives were added to breast-feeding (16-19): breast-feeding exclusively through 3 months from 43% in 1998 to 60% of mothers by 2010; and breast-feeding exclusively through 6 months from 13% in 1998 to 25% of mothers by 2010. These two new subobjectives are consistent with recommendations from the AAP and the World Health Organization (WHO). The surgeon general has recommended that by the year 2010, 75% of all postpartum women should be breast-feeding when they leave the hospital, and 50% should still be breast-feeding 6 months later (Research Highlights box). If the nation is to meet the surgeon general's goal by the year 2010, efforts to promote breast-feeding must be strengthened in hospitals, health maintenance organizations, private health care offices, and public health clinics.

WHO, the United Nations Children's Fund (UNICEF), and the *Healthy People 2010 Midcourse Review* (2006) have adopted the Baby-Friendly Hospital Initiative in an attempt to establish a global effort to increase breast-feeding. To become a baby-friendly health care facility, the 10 steps to successful breast-feeding must be implemented, as shown in Box 17-3.

Box **17-3**	**Baby-Friendly Hospital Initiative Breast-Feeding Guidelines**

1. Have a written breast-feeding policy that is communicated routinely to all health care staff.
2. Train all health care staff in the skills necessary to implement this policy.
3. Inform all pregnant women about the benefits and management of breast-feeding.
4. Help the mother initiate breast-feeding within 30 minutes after birth.
5. Show mothers how to breast-feed and how to maintain lactation even when they are separated from their infants.
6. Give newborn infants no food or drink other than breast milk unless medically indicated.
7. Practice rooming-in; allow mothers and infants to remain together 24 hours a day.
8. Encourage breast-feeding on demand.
9. Give no pacifiers to breast-feeding infants.
10. Foster the establishment of breast-feeding support groups and refer mothers to these groups when discharged from the hospital or clinic.

From World Health Organization and United Nations Children's Fund. (2006). *Global strategy for infant and young child feeding: Baby-friendly hospital initiative.* (Section 2) [Online] Retrieved from *www.who.int/nutrition/topics/bfhi/en/index.html*; *Healthy People 2010 Midcourse Review* (2006).

research highlights

Pacifiers and Breast-Feeding

Improving nutrition is a key area in the government's *Healthy People 2010* initiative, and breast milk is widely acknowledged to be the most complete form of nutrition for infants. There is strong evidence for both short-term and long-term benefits of breast-feeding, including reduced mortality in preterm infants and reduced infant morbidity. Breast-feeding has also been associated with reduced risk of type 1 diabetes, lower blood pressure, and lowered risks of urinary tract and middle ear infections. The benefits appear to increase with longer duration of breast-feeding.

The UNICEF Baby-Friendly Initiative statement recommends that pacifiers should not be given to breast-feeding infants. Shorter breast-feeding duration has been associated with pacifier use by a number of researchers. This research review aimed to answer the question: Does the use of pacifiers shorten breast-feeding duration in infants?

The Cochrane Library, Medline, CINAHL, and Embase databases were searched for systematic reviews, random-

ized controlled trials, and cohort studies examining the effect of pacifier use on breast-feeding duration. This review found evidence to suggest that there is a relationship between pacifier use and shortened breast-feeding duration. Several of the research studies reviewed a classic "dose-response" relationship, with greater pacifier use being associated with earlier cessation of breast-feeding. Most studies confirmed this association between frequency and duration.

The weight of evidence suggests that pacifier use may cause a reduction in long-term breast-feeding (beyond 3 months), although there is little evidence of harm associated with occasional pacifier use (e.g., restricted to the period when the infant settles). The recommendation is that nurses should inform breast-feeding mothers of this association and advise them according to the "ten steps to successful breast-feeding" recommended by the Baby-Friendly Initiative.

From Santo, L. C., de Oliveira, L. D., & Giugliani, E. R. (2007). Factors associated with low incidence of exclusive breastfeeding for the first 6 months. *Birth: Issues in Perinatal Care, 34*(3), 212-219.

Box **17-4** Advantages of Breast-Feeding

BREAST MILK

- Has the correct balance of all essential nutrients for infants
- Is full of immunological agents to protect against disease
- Is easier to digest than is formula
- Contains anti-inflammatory properties
- Promotes growth of Lactobacillus bifidus

BREAST-FEEDING

- Is cheaper and more convenient than formula
- Provides a unique bonding experience for both infant and mother
- Assists in process of uterine involution for mother
- Decreases postpartum vaginal bleeding
- Decreased costs for public health programs (e.g., WIC)
- Decreased SIDS rate, overweight, and obesity in adulthood
- Decreased environmental burden for disposal of formula cans and bottles
- Promotes weight reduction for new mother

Research shows that women's decisions of whether to breast-feed are influenced by information they receive from their health care providers (Miller et al., 2007). Given that important role in the mother's choice of infant feeding, nurses can be instrumental in working toward the national goal to increase breast-feeding by educating all women about the advantages of the practice (Box 17-4). Community nurses who are caring for breast-feeding mothers stress the following tips to increase the duration of this activity:

- Drink up to eight glasses of fluids daily to produce sufficient quantity of breast milk.
- Consume 2300 to 2700 cal/day to avoid excessive weight loss (Farrell & Nicoteri, 2007).
- Learn the appropriate interventions for engorged breasts, sore nipples, plugged ducts, infection, and leaking (Health Teaching box).
- Learn about the use of breast pumps and milk storage.
- Join breast-feeding support groups for continued help within the community.
- Learn about the effects of drugs, environmental pollutants, alcohol, and nicotine on breast milk.

Introduction of Solid Foods

No scientific evidence is available on the best time to introduce solid foods during infancy. At approximately 4 to 6 months of age, the infant is usually physiologically and developmentally ready to have solid foods, either commercial or home prepared. AAP (2007) recommends that waiting until the child is 6 months of age to introduce solid food decreases the tendency to develop food allergies. The introduction of various foods was recommended to (1) supply a more appealing, diversified diet for the infant; (2) supply energy, iron,

and vitamins; and (3) provide needed trace elements (AAP, 2005). The decision to start solid foods at 4 to 6 months of age is based more on neuromuscular and developmental readiness of the infant than on any hard scientific data, but research does validate the lowered risk of developing food allergies if solid foods are not introduced until 6 months of age (Maloney et al., 2006).

All infants develop according to their own schedules, and some are ready to start eating solid foods before others are. The addition of foods should be governed by an infant's nutritional needs and readiness to handle different forms of foods (Jacknowitz et al., 2007). The order of food introduction and specific amounts to be given is based on tradition rather than on scientific fact. No scientific studies have been performed to determine whether there is a specific order of infant food introduction necessary or amounts needed for optimal development. The sequence of solids typically recommended by the AAP is cereal, fruits, vegetables, and meats. The typical sequence in which foods are introduced is shown in Box 17-5. A few tips to assist the parents in making the introduction of solid foods to their infant's diet a smooth process are listed in Box 17-6.

Recommendations for food introduction by age and sequence are shown in Table 17-3.

Weaning

Weaning is a gradual, caring process that introduces the infant to a cup, which replaces the bottle or breast. Weaning should be started when the infant is ready. Developmentally, the infant can usually learn to use a cup by age 5 to 6 months; however, many children continue to nurse after they start using a cup. The infantile extrusion reflex needs to be absent. This reflex is present in very young infants and involves the tongue pushing out any material in the mouth not associated with sucking. The safety advantages of this are obvious, but weaning cannot be commenced until the infant has matured sufficiently for the reflex to be absent. In addition, weaning should not be started until the infant can sit only slightly supported and turn away his/her head to indicate food refusal. The AAP recommends breast-feeding for at least the first year of life. WHO and UNICEF suggest that the health benefits of breast milk are important throughout the second and third years of life. Weaning should be started at this age by periodically offering sips of water or juice. Initially the infant may not be eager to accept these offers but should become accustomed to this new experience fairly quickly.

Box **17-5** Solid Food Introduction Sequence

1. Cereals, particularly rice because of nonallergenic property
2. Fruits such as peaches, pears, and applesauce
3. Vegetables, with yellow vegetables (squash and carrots) given before green vegetables (peas or beans)
4. Strained meats, such as nonallergenic lamb or veal

HEALTH TEACHING   Breast-Feeding

How to Hold Your Baby for Feedings

- Sit or lie down comfortably with your back supported.
- Make sure your baby has one arm on either side of your breast as you pull the baby close.
- Use firm pillows or folded blankets under the baby as a means of support during the feeding. As your baby gets older, the extra support will likely be unnecessary.
- Support the baby's back and shoulders firmly. Do not push on the back of the baby's head.
- After the baby's mouth is open wide, pull your baby quickly to your breast.

Four Common Breast-Feeding Positions

Football

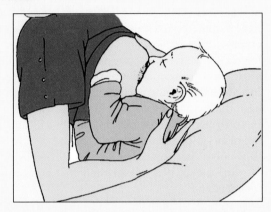

- Hold the baby's back and shoulders in the palm of your hand.
- Tuck the baby up under your arm, keeping the baby's ear, shoulder, and hip in a straight line.
- Support the breast. After the baby's mouth is open wide, pull the baby quickly to you.
- Continue to hold your breast until the baby feeds easily.

Lying Down

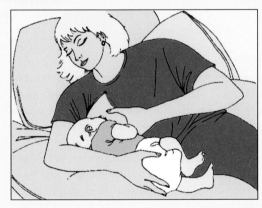

- Lie on your side with a pillow at your back and lay the baby such that you are facing each other.
- To begin, prop yourself up on your elbow and support your breast with that hand.
- Pull the baby close to you, lining up the baby's mouth with your nipple.
- After the baby is feeding well, lie back down. Hold your breast with the opposite hand.

Cradling

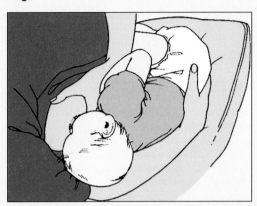

- Cradle the baby in the arm closest to the breast with the baby's head in the crook of your arm.
- Have the baby's body facing you, tummy to tummy.
- Use your opposite hand to support the breast.

Across the Lap

- Lay your baby on firm pillows across your lap.

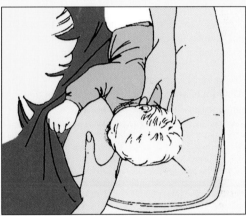

- Turn the baby, facing you.
- Reach across your lap to support the baby's back and shoulders with the palm of your hand.
- Support your breast from underneath to guide it into the baby's mouth.

Breast-Feeding is Going Well When ...

- Your newborn is feeding approximately 8 times in 24 hours for 30 to 40 minutes at each feeding. Some newborns need to eat more frequently until they learn to breast-feed efficiently. Other babies gain weight although they feed less often.
- At least one breast softens well at each feeding.
- You feel a tug, but not pain, when the baby sucks.
- The baby's arms and shoulders are relaxed during the feeding.
- The baby has bursts of 10 or more sucks and swallows at the beginning of each feeding.
- As your breast softens, the baby slows down to two to three sucks and swallows at a time.
- Your baby is content when you finish breast-feeding.
- By the time the baby is 4 days old, you should see at least six wet diapers and two bowel movements every 24 hours.

Used with permission of Lactation Consultants of North Carolina. Illustrations from a handset accompanying the video, *Breastfeeding: A special relationship.* Courtesy of Eagle Video Productions.

Box **17-6** Tips for Introducing Solid Foods

1. The infant's first solid foods should be smooth and runny. Gradually, the infant will be ready to accept a slightly rougher texture.
2. Puréed foods are used until the infant has teeth; chopped foods are used when the infant can chew.
3. Introduce only one new food at a time and in small amounts for a period of 5 to 7 days. When the new food is not tolerated or the infant is allergic to it, the new food can be identified quickly and discontinued.
4. The infant must learn how to handle solid foods. Because infants use sucking movements, part of the food is ejected from the mouth. With time and practice, the infant learns how to take solid food from a spoon.
5. Do not mix solid foods together; the infant should learn to appreciate different tastes and textures.
6. Always feed the infant in an upright position; do not feed the infant solids from the bottle.
7. Do not start to reduce the milk supply until the infant is taking food successfully from the spoon.
8. Until 1 year of age, feed the baby milk before solid foods.
9. Look at, smile at, and talk to the infant during feeding.
10. Do not give honey to infants less than 12 months of age because of the risk of infant botulism.*
11. Respect the infant's likes and dislikes; rejected foods may be reintroduced later.
12. Avoid peanuts and peanut butter because of the potential for severe allergic reactions.

* Honey has been credited throughout the centuries with therapeutic and medicinal uses. However, honey should not be given to infants under 1 year of age. Honey is a known source of bacterial spores that produce a toxin that can cause infant botulism. This rare, but serious, form of food poisoning affects the nervous system of infants and can result in death. Researchers also suspect a link between infant botulism and some cases of SIDS, because breathing is affected in the most severe stages of food poisoning. Botulism spores are quite common, found in dust, soil, and uncooked food. Honey is the only food implicated in infant botulism. Because honey is not essential for the nutrition of infants, parents and caregivers should be reminded not to feed it to infants younger than 1 year. Honey should never be added to baby food or placed on the nipple of a pacifier.

Table **17-3** First Foods for the Infant

Age (Months)	Addition
4 to 6	Iron-fortified rice cereal, followed by other cereals
5 to 7	Strained vegetables and fruits and their juices
6 to 8	Protein foods (cheese, meat, fish, chicken, and yogurt)
9	Finely chopped meat, toast, teething crackers
10 to 12	Whole egg, whole milk (allergies less likely now)

Some infants accept the cup readily; other infants are extremely reluctant to give up the bottle, especially the bedtime bottle. Allowing infants to sleep with propped bottles can lead to aspiration if the milk flows too rapidly or the infant becomes too sleepy to coordinate sucking and swallowing. Another potential problem is baby bottle tooth decay, of all upper teeth and some of the lower posterior teeth, from direct contact with sugar, syrup, honey-sweetened water, or fruit juice. When the infant falls asleep and stops sucking on the bottle, the sugary solution pools around the infant's teeth and remains there for long periods. The carbohydrate in the solution is fermented into organic acids that demineralize the teeth until they decay. By not using the bottle as a pacifier, parents can prevent this condition.

Some additional tips for counseling parents are as follows:
1. Keep a calm, relaxed attitude throughout the weaning process.
2. Do not force an infant to use a cup; it is more detrimental to wean sooner than later.
3. Introduce the cup for one feeding per day and progress until the breast or bottle is surrendered.
4. Put only purified tap water into the bottle, and give the infant juice and milk from a cup.
5. Remember that infants enjoy the accomplishment of using a cup; it is one of their first steps toward independence.

Anticipatory Guidance

The infant progresses from a diet of milk alone to a diet of milk and solid foods within a short period. Understanding the infant's nutritional needs and developmental capabilities, the nurse can guide the parents in meeting them and in the process foster healthy family-infant relationships. The health-promotion activity used in meeting proper infant nutrition focuses on parent education and positive reinforcement of parenting abilities.

Elimination Pattern

The infant develops an elimination pattern by the second week of life, usually associated with the frequency and amount of feedings. Both breast-fed and bottle-fed infants progress to a pattern of fewer stools per day after the first few months of life.

A breast-fed infant's stools have an orange-yellow color and a soft, even consistency, with a slightly sour but clean smell, dissimilar to stools passed later in life. A bottle-fed infant's stools are harder, smellier, and resemble those of an infant eating solid food. The breast-fed infant has many daily stools during the first and second months of life, progressing to one stool per day or even every one stool every 4 to 5 days in the later months before solid foods are introduced. The bottle-fed infant has two to four stools per day during the first month, tapering to one a day or even fewer at the end of infancy (Polan & Taylor, 2007).

For the first year of life, an infant cannot control the bowels. Bowel evacuation remains under involuntary, reflexive control until myelination of the spinal cord is complete, usually by 14 to 18 months of age (Pillitteri, 2007). Nurses advise overanxious parents to delay toilet training until the infant is developmentally ready. The stress in American culture on daily bowel movements makes many mothers concerned about their infant's elimination patterns. The breast-fed infant may go for several days without having a bowel movement, which usually is not a problem. When the infant's behavior and feeding and sleeping patterns are normal, no elimination problem exists. A breast-fed infant rarely becomes constipated when consuming adequate amounts of breast milk. Usually the nurse only has to reassure the parents and discuss normal elimination patterns. Urination increases as fluid intake increases. An infant who voids 6 to 12 times a day during the first few months of life is usually healthy and well hydrated. Voiding is involuntary until some time during the second year of life, when bladder sensation develops. Irregular patterns of voiding characterize the remaining period of infancy.

Anticipatory Guidance

Anticipatory guidance and health promotion concerning elimination patterns of the infant consists of parental teaching and reassurance, with special emphasis on good hygienic practices. Reassuring the parents about the infant's inability to control elimination is important so that their expectations are realistic.

Activity-Exercise Pattern

Physical activity and exercise contribute to development and coordination throughout the life span; infants receive their exercise through play. Initially infants engage in play with themselves with their hands or feet, with sounds, and by rolling and getting into various positions. By manipulating objects and achieving pleasurable sensations, infants learn about themselves and the objects in the environment.

Activity Through Play

Although the word *play* suggests physical activity, the infant's first play is actually an exercise of the senses. The infant's first toys are visual. Through play, infants learn to hone their senses, to exercise their physical abilities, and to relate to other people. Most of the infant's play is solitary and repetitious. As each discovery is made, self-confidence and pride in the achievement are reinforced (as is the skill) through repetition.

As the infant enters the second half of the first year and becomes mobile, the family should provide the infant with increasing opportunities for spontaneous play and exploration. A planned play period in a safe environment should be established. The infant should have unrestrictive clothing so that movement can be free and unhampered. The caregiver should not interfere directly with the play but should be attentive to the infant's needs.

An important nursing role is assisting parents to promote play, stressing the importance of providing opportunities that are appropriate for the infant's age. Buying expensive toys is unnecessary; common household items, such as pots, pans, lids, and spoons, provide excellent objects for play purposes.

Activity Through Stimulation

Parental stimulation of the infant is an important developmental technique; the infant needs stimulation to learn about the world. This activity does not require expensive objects, but rather involves experiences in sight, sound, and touch that are free and can be provided by any parent (Figure 17-1). Examples of stimulating experiences for infants include the following:
- Having lullabies sung to them
- Listening to tape recordings of a heartbeat
- Seeing colorful mobiles in crib
- Being rocked in a rocking chair
- Having a familiar face smiling close by
- Having space to wander when developmentally ready
- Looking at themselves in mirrors
- Listening to music

Anticipatory Guidance

Knowledge of developmental landmarks allows the nurse to guide parents in proper play and stimulation for infants. Handing a 15-month-old child a ball and placing the child in a fenced-in back yard to play is not enough. These activities must provide interpersonal contact, activity, and exercise. Activity and exercise through stimulation and play are extremely important for adequate and healthy development (Berk, 2007).

Sleep-Rest Pattern

The amount of sleep that infants need is closely related to their rate of growth. Initially infants sleep approximately 80% of the time, as demanded by their rapid growth.

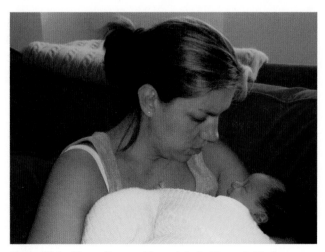

Figure 17-1   The mother provides an infant with comfort by her closeness.

As growth begins to slow toward the middle of the first year of life, less sleep is needed. The 12-month-old infant sleeps only 12 of 24 hours, a pattern that remains essentially unchanged through the second year (Waldburger & Spivak, 2007). To assist parents in understanding normal sleep and rest patterns, the nurse stresses that no set schedule exists (Table 17-4).

Anticipatory Guidance

Health-promotion activities can also help the parents determine the individual needs of their infant. The nurse stresses that longer sleep patterns are signs of maturation and that sleep and rest are recognized as having a significant influence on the infant's growth and development. The nurse

Growth and Development — Table 17-4

Normal Sleep Patterns for Infants

Age (Months)	Hours In 24-Hour Period
2 to 3	Low: 10 Average: 16½ High: 23
3 to 4	Low: 8 to 10 nightly High: 11 to 12 nightly (2 or 3 naps daily)
6 to 12	11 to 12 nightly (2 or 3 naps daily)
12 to 18	8 to 12 nightly (1 or 2 naps daily)

may offer the parents helpful comments for promoting infant sleep patterns, such as the following:

1. Provide a quiet room for the infant that is separate from the parents' room.
2. Learn behavioral clues that signal that the infant is going to sleep and is not interacting socially.
3. Learn to become sensitive to sleep cycles and rest periods that the infant is establishing and base care accordingly.
4. Attempt to schedule feeding times during wakeful rather than drowsy periods.
5. Learn that certain cycles are intrinsic to infants and that each infant is unique.
6. Perform rituals for the infant, such as rocking or reading a bedtime story, to provide comfort and security and let the infant know the expected behavior.

If parents express a sleep concern, the nurse assesses their reactions, considers their definition of the concern, assesses the sleep environment, and observes the infant's own unique sleep patterns. Only then can the nurse's health-promotion approach be individualized to assist the family in caring for the infant.

Sudden Infant Death Syndrome

Sudden infant death syndrome (SIDS) is the sudden, unexplained death of an infant younger than 1 year of age that remains unexplained after review of the clinical history, examination of the scene of death, and postmortem examination (Damato, 2007) (Hot Topics box). The incidence

HOT topics — INFANT SLEEP POSITION AND SUDDEN INFANT DEATH SYNDROME

SIDS is the third leading cause of infant mortality between 1 month and 1 year of age in the United States, occurring in approximately 4 per 1000 live births. SIDS, defined as the sudden death of an infant less than 1 year of age, remains unexplained after a thorough investigation. SIDS tends to occur at a higher-than-usual rate in the infants of adolescent mothers, infants of closely spaced pregnancies, and underweight male infants. However, even these profiles are inconsistent.

A variety of population characteristics have been explored, such as families with smokers, breast-feeding versus bottle-feeding practices, or side or back sleeping positions for the infant. The primary contributor to a 50% decline in SIDS deaths in seven countries, including the United States, over a 12-year period was a decline in the facedown sleeping position of infants. Studies indicate that infants being put down to sleep should be positioned on their sides or backs.

In 1992 the American Academy of Pediatrics published a recommendation that "healthy infants, when being put down to sleep, be positioned on their side or back" in an attempt to decrease the incidence of SIDS. Since that time, the frequency of prone sleeping has decreased from greater than 70% to less than 20% of U.S. infants, and the SIDS rate has decreased by more than 50%. APP also recommends pacifier use for infants for sleep through the first year of life (AAP Task Force on SIDS 2005). Nurses need to educate parents regarding both recommendations as well as the risk factors of SIDS.

SIDS Facts

1. Incidence is highest between 1 and 8 months of age, with peak incidence at 2 to 3 months.
2. Infants of families of low socioeconomic status with a history of heavy smoking or drug abuse are at greater risk.
3. Low–birth-weight infants are at greater risk of dying from SIDS than are term infants of normal weight.
4. SIDS occurs most often during the infant's sleep cycle.
5. Peak incidence is during the fall and winter seasons.
6. SIDS affects more male infants than it does female infants.
7. SIDS is a specific disease entity.
8. No evidence to date suggests hereditary or contagious causes.
9. SIDS is unexpected and unexplained.
10. No sign of distress, crying, or coughing is apparent at the time of death.
11. A mild upper respiratory infection may be present in some infants, but not all.
12. Autopsy findings are remarkably similar, including pulmonary congestion, intrathoracic petechiae, edema, and inflammatory infiltrates in the upper airway.

SIDS, Sudden infant death syndrome.
From American Academy of Pediatrics Task Force on Sudden Infant Death Syndrome. (2005). The changing concept of sudden infant death syndrome: Diagnostic coding shifts, controversies regarding the sleeping environment, and new variables to consider in reducing risk. Pediatrics, 116(5), 1245-1255; Damato, E.G. (2007). Safe sleep: Can pacifiers reduce the SIDS risk? Nursing for Women's Health, 11(1), 72-76.

of SIDS has varied over time and among nations. It is the third leading cause of infant death in both the United States and Canada (congenital anomalies and prematurity/low birth weight are first and second) (Minino et al., 2006). By definition, the cause of SIDS is not known. Observational studies have found an association between SIDS and several risk factors, including prone (on abdomen) sleeping positions, prenatal or postnatal exposure to tobacco smoke, soft sleeping surfaces, hyperthermia or over wrapping, bed sharing, face covered by bedding, and lack of breast-feeding (Moon & Fy, 2007).

Research focuses on sleep pathophysiology, particularly in relation to apneic spells that last longer than 10 seconds (Moon & Fy, 2007). The carotid body network and brainstem reflexes normally control physiological variations in heart and respiratory rates during sleep. For unexplained reasons, in SIDS cases these mechanisms likely fail to work during sleep and respiration ceases. The mechanism of the relationship between apnea and SIDS is unsubstantiated. It has been proposed that a sleeping infant can become hypoxic with positional narrowing of the airway and respiratory inflammation. Research is ongoing.

The AAP Task Force on SIDS (2005) recommends the following: (1) healthy infants should be placed to sleep in the supine position (on back) with the teaching aid "back to sleep" in a crib that meets Consumer Product Safety Commission and American Society for Testing and Material standards; (2) avoid allowing infants to sleep on soft bedding (including waterbeds, sofas, and soft mattresses) or with pillows, soft comforters and coverings, loose bedding, or stuffed toys; (3) avoid overheating that occurs, for example, by placing excessive clothing or blankets on infants or by keeping the room temperature too high; (4) stop maternal smoking in the infant's environment; (5) avoid bed sharing; and (6) offer a pacifier when placing the infant down for sleep through the first year of life (AAP, 2005).

Objective 16-1 of the *Healthy People Midcourse Review* (2006), reduce deaths from SIDS from 0.67 deaths per 1000 live births in 1999 to .23 deaths per 1000 live births in 2010, was revised after data was collected after November 2000.

Infants considered at high risk for SIDS include survivors of near-SIDS, subsequent siblings of SIDS victims, and premature infants with recurrent apneic episodes during sleep. From a preventive perspective, apnea monitors have been used in certain cases. However, controversy remains over this type of respiratory monitoring at home; parents face a heavy psychological responsibility when left in charge of their extraordinarily vulnerable young infant's life and monitoring may increase their anxiety and protectiveness of the infant.

When an infant dies suddenly, unexpectedly, and for no apparent reason, a family crisis occurs. The parents are devastated and completely unprepared for the shock, reacting with intense guilt, blaming themselves and each other, and agonizing over the part they may have played in the infant's death. Because many unanswered questions remain, these feelings are universal. Parents think there is something they could have done to prevent the tragedy. In most cases, nothing could have been done. Too frequently, the first sign that something was wrong is death. The nurse is in an excellent position to help the family through this crisis. Dealing with the family's grief is very difficult. Many families find strength in their faith to help them through this difficult time. Other family members and close friends can assist the family in their grieving process. Many receive solace and support from talking to other parents who have lost an infant to SIDS. Several parent groups are available from local chapters of the SIDS Foundation; the nurse can refer them to their local chapter.

The nurse's main supportive role with families coping with SIDS is listening and offering compassionate guidance through the weeks and months that follow. The nurse encourages parents to talk about their infant. Too soon, family and friends expect the surviving family to "get over it." A parent, however, is never able to "get over it"; it is only put in perspective and not so near the surface (Moon & Fy, 2007).

Nursing assessment of the infant at risk for SIDS includes observing the infant for apneic episodes. Usually, however, nursing assessment occurs after death and consists of support and providing appropriate resources for the family. Nursing diagnoses for sudden infant death might include the following:

- Spiritual distress related to coping with death
- Ineffective family coping related to the loss of an infant
- Dysfunctional grieving related to the parents' inability to cope

Nurses also discuss with the family feelings about caring for future children. Life can appear out of control and parents may believe that they cannot care for another infant. These feelings must be resolved before another pregnancy is contemplated. When dealing with the families of SIDS victims, nurses can feel uncomfortable and helpless. As health professionals, they might speak in terms of easing the pain or alleviating the guilt of these families, but many times simple nonverbal human contact is sufficient to express concern and understanding.

Cognitive-Perceptual Pattern

Cognition is the process by which an individual recognizes, accumulates, and organizes the knowledge of the environment, beginning with the perception or recognition of an event within that environment. Cognitive development is concurrent with biological, adaptive, and psychosocial achievement. The infant's biological and cognitive developmental patterns (Piaget's sensorimotor period) are discussed earlier in this chapter. The focus of this section is on the infant's sensory and language development and the importance of stimulation to both developmental areas. From birth, infants possess sensory capabilities; all sensory organs are well developed and functioning. As the infant is cared for and handled, the special senses become organized neurologically into a pattern of behavior that will greatly influence subsequent development.

Vision

The infant's initial visual impressions are unfocused, bizarre, unfamiliar, and without meaning. Because everything is new and only somewhat significant, visual stimuli must be moving, bright, or flashing to capture the infant's attention. The infant's eyes are well developed at birth, but the muscles that attach the eyes to their sockets are weak. This weakness may be stressful to parents, because the infant's eyes do not appear to function together. Parents can be assured that most infants coordinate their eye movements by the age of 3 months; by 6 months this function is mature. Table 17-5 summarizes visual developmental milestones.

Hearing

After the amniotic fluid drains from the middle ear several days after birth, the infant's hearing becomes acute. Hearing is one of the better-developed senses in the infant; the fetus can even hear in utero and responds to loud sounds (Figure 17-2). The newborn can distinguish sound frequencies and turns toward a voice or another sound. The infant may be familiar with the mother's voice early in life. Sounds gradually gain significance and meaning when they are associated with caregivers, food, and pleasure.

The ability to listen and discriminate among sounds is an important task during infancy. The closer the infant is to the sound, the more easily the sound can be discriminated. The groundwork for verbal ability begins to develop long before words appear, and many believe that infants whose mothers talk to them tend to speak earlier than infants who are not exposed to these sounds (Dacey & Travers, 2006). Table 17-6 summarizes the infant's auditory development.

Smell

The ability to smell is fully developed at birth. The infant has many receptors in the nose, but it lacks the cilia that line the inside of the adult's nose. As a result, the infant has a keen sense of smell, because odors reach the receptor cells easily. Within 2 weeks after birth, an infant can differentiate the odor of the mother's milk from others', an ability developed when the infant is held close (Puckett & Black, 2007). At this time the infant begins associating the parents with their body odors, a perception that is important to infant-parent bonding.

Taste

The sense of taste is present at birth and salivation begins at approximately 3 months of age. The four primary sensations are sour, salty, sweet, and bitter. The taste buds for sweet tastes are more abundant during early life than they are in later life, which may account for the preference for sweets that is characteristic of infants and children.

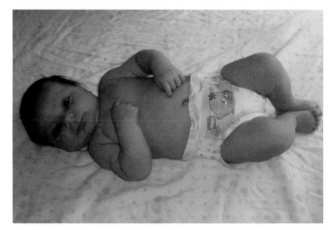

Figure 17-2   Babies respond to startling, loud noises, confirming their sense of hearing.

Growth and Development	Table 17-5

Visual Development During Infancy

Age	Behavior that Indicates Vision
1 to 3 months	Fixes gaze on object 12 to 24 inches away
	Takes interest in bright colors and faces
	Follows objects in field of vision
3 to 6 months	Begins to show interest in hands
	Follows in range of 90 degrees
	Recognizes familiar objects
	Able to see full color by now
6 to 9 months	Visual scanning becomes more integrated
	Capable of organized depth perception
	Begins to perceive distances accurately
	Both eyes should focus equally now
9 to 12 months	Able to look for concealed items
	Converges on objects in close proximity
	Peripheral vision is well developed
	Judges distance well
12 to 18 months	Eye-hand coordination develops
	Depth perception more refined
	Ability to identify forms and shapes

Growth and Development	Table 17-6

Normal Development of Hearing

Age	Behavior that Indicates Hearing
1 to 3 months	Is startled by loud noises
	Stops activity when spoken to
3 to 6 months	Turns eyes and head toward sound
	Responds to mother's voice
	Imitates own noises: "ooh" and "ba-ba"
6 to 9 months	Responds to own name
	Looks toward sounds
	Recognizes familiar sounds
9 to 12 months	Points to familiar objects or people
	Imitates simple words and sounds
	Locates a sound in any direction
12 to 18 months	Follows simple spoken directions
	Distinguishes between sounds
	Spoken words are well on their way

Touch and Motion

Tactile sensation is well developed at birth, particularly on the lips and tongue. Perceptions of motion and touch are perhaps the most important of all senses. Rocking and other motions are sensations of equilibrium picked up by the middle ear. Skin-to-skin touching should be performed regularly; evidence shows that touch helps relieve the unspent tensions that infants develop and accelerates neuromuscular development (Puckett & Black, 2007). Infants respond with pleasure to rocking and other motion and to tactile sensations of warmth, closeness, and cuddling.

Language Development

Language development, an important aspect of the infant's cognitive and perceptual pattern, is affected by intellectual development, maturation of the central nervous system, development of the organs of speech, and exposure to human verbalization.

As in other areas of development, language acquisition follows a definite sequence. During the first 2 months, most of the infant's sounds are vowels and are made primarily in the front part of the mouth (Coch et al., 2007). Crying is the major means of communication during this period. Cooing sounds are heard at approximately 2 to 3 months, usually in response to an adult's voice. By 6 months, babbling sounds are heard, and by 9 to 10 months, the infant forms two-syllable sounds. By 12 months, words such as "ma-ma," "bye-bye," and "dada" are emerging. From 15 to 18 months, an expressive jargon with rhythmic intonations develops, but words are recognized only rarely. The infant uses jargon along with pointing to express wishes.

Anticipatory Guidance

The nurse's knowledge and understanding of an infant's cognitive and perceptual behavior facilitates interaction with infants and serves as a guide in parental counseling. The main focus centers on stimulation, because each of the infant's senses is receptive to environmental stimulation. This activity helps the infant learn from the environment. When an infant is exposed to appropriate sensory stimulation, greater curiosity, improved mental capabilities, accelerated neuromuscular growth, enhanced gastrointestinal functioning; quicker weight gain, more rapid language development, and pleasing mother-infant interactions are likely to occur (Burge, 2007; Stamm & Spencer, 2007).

Parents are the primary providers of pleasurable and stimulating experiences for the infant. The nurse assists them by offering suggestions about suitable stimuli for each sensory modality.

Self-Perception–Self-Concept Pattern

Self-perception has a pervasive influence on all aspects of life. Self-concept consists of a set of attitudes regarding what each person thinks, believes, and feels about the self. These attitudes form a personal self-belief that is an abstraction referred as "me." Many researchers believe that the infant determines self-existence by first noting that actions such as crying or smiling have an effect on others, which depends on receiving feedback (Berk, 2007). Studies confirm that infants can identify themselves and therefore form a self-concept. Infants at 4 months of age were found to be particularly fascinated with their images in mirrors and smiled more at themselves than they did at pictures of other infants (Puckett & Black, 2007).

As the infant continues to grow and mature, many circumstances combine to influence self-concept. How others relate to the infant's body and the messages that the infant receives from the body lead to knowledge of a physical self. The ability to use the body to influence others can lead the psychological self to conclude that someone cares about the infant (Coch et al., 2007).

The infant's development of body image is gradual. At birth the infant has diffuse feelings of hunger, pain, anger, and comfort, but no body image. Initially, the infant knows only the self and regards the external world as an extension of the self. Only when infants begin to experience the environment through sensory modalities are they able to distinguish their bodies from animate and inanimate objects.

Nursing Suggestions

The nurse plays a vital role in assisting parents to foster the development of a positive self-concept and a good body image in their infant. The nurse first identifies personal self-concept and how it influences individuals (Stamm & Spencer, 2007). The nurse stresses that the way in which parents treat the infant influences the infant's self-concept. Basically, infants and young children incorporate their parents' interactions with them (good or bad) into their own view of self. Parents must understand that their infant's self-concept is an important, continuing event. What the infant knows and later believes about the self will affect all interactions with others, and by influencing what the infant will later attempt, the self-concept may have broad effects on the development of new skills (Stamm & Spencer, 2007).

Roles-Relationships Pattern

Researchers have explored extensively the effect of early bonding between parents and their infants, emphasizing that this initial attraction sets the stage for the later development of love and affiliation. The bonding process has many other implications for the infant's future development as well (Oppenheim & Goldsmith, 2007).

Attachment and Bonding

The parent-infant relationship does not begin with the birth of the infant; many aspects have been molded by the life experiences of the parents long before they reached parenthood. The kind of mothering that a woman received as an infant and the concept of mother that she developed as she grew represent early effects that can influence the mother-infant relationship. The mother's overall self-concept will affect her ability to relate to her infant, as will her relationship with the infant's father.

The establishment of this emotional bond between the mother and her infant is known as attachment. This emotional bond is considered crucial for the optimal physical and emotional development of the infant. Maternal behaviors such as how the mother holds, feeds, and looks at the infant demonstrate the process of attachment (Figueiredo et al., 2007).

Various theories have attempted to explain the basis for attachment behavior. Freudian psychoanalytical theory emphasizes that the bond between child and mother develops as a result of the mother's satisfying the infant's innate desire to socialize and the physical requirements for survival. Social learning theory contributes the principles of reinforcement to the attachment process; as the mother meets the infant's needs, discomfort is reduced or removed. The infant associates the pleasurable feeling of being satisfied with the mother, who becomes a significant other in the infant's life. The bonding process is the basis for the mother-infant relationship, which, in turn, forms the basis for the interdependence that is necessary for the infant's psychological and physical development (Carter et al., 2006).

In their early studies on attachment, Klaus et al. (2000) formulated the following seven crucial principles:

1. A sensitive period appears to exist during the first minutes and hours after birth, when it seems necessary for the mother and father to have close contact with their infant for later development to be optimal.

2. Species-specific responses to the infant appear to exist in the human mother and father when the infant is first given to them.

3. The attachment process seems to be structured such that the parents become attached to one infant at a time or in the case of a multiple birth to each infant simultaneously.

4. For attachment to occur appropriately, the infant must respond to the mother and father by some signal, such as body or eye movements. This principle has been called the "you can't love a dishrag" phenomenon.

5. Individuals who witness the birth process become strongly attached to the infant.

6. Some adults find it difficult to go through the processes of attachment and detachment simultaneously. Becoming attached to an infant while mourning the loss or threatened loss of another person is difficult for parents.

7. Some early events may have long-lasting effects. For example, anxiety over an infant with a transient disorder in the child's early days may result in long-term concerns or behavior that will have implications for future development.

Just as the infant's behavior influences attachment, it also continues to influence the evolving maternal-paternal-infant relationship as the infant develops. Studies have shown that if the process of attachment is encumbered, later problems are more likely to occur, such as child abuse, **failure-to-thrive syndrome**, and behavior problems (Schwerdtfeger, 2007).

Many factors are present when a relationship is being established and maintained. Most people enter a relationship with unrealistic expectations. Parents are no exception—they are going to be wise, patient, and devoted, and they will nurture their infant. Because the parents' self-esteem is associated closely with their infant's interactions and accomplishments, when parents' self-esteem is low, disappointment, anger, and a disturbance in the relationship with their infant can occur. In some instances this disturbed parent-infant relationship is short-lived and nothing harmful develops. When a disturbed parent-infant relationship continues, however, the infant is at risk for abuse and behavior problems (Innovative Practice box).

The process of bonding is also important for fathers. Recently, a process called **paternal engrossment** has been

---

innovative practice

The Touchpoints Model

The birth of a baby is a life-changing event for a couple and family. Although most infants develop through predictable yet individual patterns of development, parents, especially first-time parents, are usually unaware of these patterns or have difficulty assessing their infant's progress and problems. All of these processes can be stressful for the parents, the entire family, and the infant.

The Touchpoints Model Program at Children's Hospital in Boston, Massachusetts, delivers a training model for practitioners, emphasizing the building of supportive alliances between parents and professionals around key points in the development of young children. The model is an outgrowth of Dr. T. Berry Brazelton's book *Touchpoints* (2006) and research at Children's Hospital in Boston. The Touchpoints model provides a form of outreach through which multidisciplinary practitioners can engage parents around important, predictable phases of their baby's development. The Touchpoints model stresses preventive health through development of relationships between parents and providers; acknowledges that developing and maintaining relationships is critical to appreciating cultural, religious, and societal family dynamics; and encourages the practitioner to focus on strengths in individuals and families. Touchpoints is not a stand-alone model; it is intended to be integrated into ongoing pediatric, early childhood, and family intervention programs.

Contact Information:
The Touchpoints Project
Child Development Unit
Children's Hospital
1295 Boylston Street, Boston, MA 02215
Touchpoints has gone on-line. Parents and professionals can get advice and information from Dr. Brazelton at: Brazelton, T. B. (2007). Brazelton Touch Points Center (online). Available at *www.touchpoints.org*.

used to describe the behavior pattern of fathers when they interact with their infants. The major characteristics of engrossment include: (1) visual awareness of the infant; (2) tactile awareness, often expressed in a desire to hold the infant; (3) awareness of distinct characteristics, with emphasis on the features that resemble the father; (4) perception of the infant as perfect; (5) development of a strong feeling of attraction to the infant that leads to intense focusing of attention; (6) a feeling of extreme elation; and (7) a sense of deep self-esteem and satisfaction (Berk, 2007).

Child Abuse

Family traditionally has been considered a safe place for its members, but many infants are at risk for maltreatment. Infant and child abuse has always been a part of human history. Acceptable behavior toward infants is largely a learned phenomenon; the art of parenting is not instinctively acquired, as many people believe. Abusing parents are seldom "monsters"; they are merely individuals ineffectively coping with the demands of parenthood, for which there is little or no preparation, as well as other life stressors.

The scope of child abuse is extensive: estimates indicate that more than 3 million infants and children in the United States are victims of abuse annually, which means 1 in 20 children are physically abused each year (AAP, 2007). Children under 3 years of age are the most frequent victims. Women are more frequent abusers than are men, because they are the primary caregivers. Men abuse more severely and commit sexual abuse more frequently. Child abuse does not discriminate; it occurs in families of every race, creed, and socioeconomic class.

The child-abuse syndrome is a clinical condition in infants who have suffered serious active or passive abuse at the hands of their parents or other caregivers. Physical trauma is not the only facet, but it is the most overt indicator of a dysfunctional family unit and a disturbed parent-infant relationship (AAP, 2007).

Active manifestations of abuse include the following:
1. Brain injuries, subdural hematomas, and skull fractures
2. Soft-tissue injuries, such as bruises, lacerations, or burns
3. Fractures of the long bones and ribs; multiple fractures in varying stages of healing
4. Sexual abuse manifested by genital tissue injury; sexually transmitted infections

Passive manifestations of abuse include the following:
1. Poor nutrition, failure to thrive, and severe malnutrition
2. Poor physical condition: neglected safeguards against disease, poor skin condition, and lack of medical attention
3. Emotional neglect: rejection, indifference, and deprivation of love
4. Moral neglect: allowing the infant or child to remain in an immoral atmosphere

Abusing parents often have common patterns of behavior. As children, their own parents may have abused them. In this way, child abuse is cycled from generation to generation.

The development of the maternal role on which the infant depends for health, progress, and survival begins during the mother's early childhood. Unless she received love and proper mothering, she will have difficulty with a relationship that entails the complete dependency of another person. She may find the relationship with her own infant to be unrewarding, threatening, and frustrating. Feelings of inadequacy and guilt in the mother and father roles compound the problems.

Abusing parents are often socially isolated and have few people to whom they can turn during times of crisis; they also cannot support one another emotionally. These parents may view the infant as the person who can provide the love, support, and nurturing that is lacking in their own lives. When the infant does not fulfill their expectations, the risk of abuse becomes acute (St James-Roberts, 2007).

The abused infant or child is frequently singled out as someone who is different. This infant may be chronically ill, may have been premature, may be hyperactive, may have been the product of a difficult and complicated pregnancy, or may have an obvious anomaly. Early bonding disturbances (inadequacies in feeding, holding, and caring for the infant) are characteristic signals.

The long-term effects of child abuse are profound. The victims lack basic trust (a major task of infancy) and confidence and self-worth. These deficits follow the victims into adulthood and parenthood, and the vicious cycle continues. One of the discouraging findings is that infants and children who were abused frequently grow up to be abusing parents (AAP, 2007).

Across the United States great interest has been generated in attempts to identify parents in the prenatal and perinatal periods who have significant potential for child abuse. Nurses play a critical role in recognizing infants who have been intentionally harmed, because they are often the first to begin taking a history on the infant. Nurses work collaboratively with community agencies to provide follow-up care for the infant in danger of continued abuse. Nurses take appropriate action if they suspect an infant is at risk. Doing nothing is not an option. The following measures have been undertaken to help prevent child abuse:
1. Predictive questionnaires to be given to parents on postpartum units
2. Recognition of parents who have difficulty relating to their infants through body language clues or verbalizations
3. Closer follow-up during the postpartum period by the public health nurse
4. Crisis hot lines made available to parents in distress

Before focusing on nursing interventions (Box 17-7), the nurse makes several observations to assist in identifying a high-risk infant by answering the following questions:
- Does the mother hold the infant close and establish eye contact?
- Does the mother speak negatively about the infant?
- Does the mother intensely dislike the duties of motherhood, such as diapering, feeding, and so on?

Box 17-7	Nursing Interventions to Prevent Abuse of Infants

- Promote and facilitate early parent-infant bonding.
- Promote a trusting relationship.
- Provide more frequent office visits and be available by phone.
- Provide infant care instructions to enhance mothering ability.
- Provide for community health person to make home visits.

- Does the mother expect too much of the infant at a particular stage of development?
- Does the mother focus her attention on the infant rather than on her husband?
- Does the mother have a good support system available?
- Does the mother act overly concerned about the infant's gender?

Most communities are seeking ways in which child abuse can be prevented through educational efforts, improved agency coordination, and development of new collaborative efforts and services for parents and infants. Laws for reporting abuse have been enacted in every state. Reporting all cases of suspected abuse and neglect is mandatory. Everyone must assist in this endeavor to prevent continued abuse. It takes a community effort to address the problem.

Homelessness

Along with food, health, and personal safety, probably no greater basic need for human beings exists than shelter. The loss of shelter is detrimental to the health and well-being of all people. Homelessness in the United States is a national disgrace. Most estimates place the number of homeless people at 3 million. One of every four homeless people is a child (NHCHC, 2007).

To say that the well-being of the next generation is being jeopardized by homelessness is not an exaggeration. Homelessness devastates every aspect of a child's life, doing damage with long-term implications that remain unknown. Homelessness endangers a child's health throughout childhood. Homeless infants are often exposed to unsafe and unsanitary conditions in shelters in which infectious diseases thrive. These dangers are combined with a lack of access to regular health care; common childhood ailments such as ear infections become extremely serious and sometimes life-threatening illnesses before they are treated.

Ear infections are among the most common health problems encountered in children. For a bacterial infection, a course of antibiotics usually relieves the condition. Rarely are long-term complications encountered. For the homeless infant, however, the story is different. Families are cut off from their regular clinics and providers. The struggle for basic life needs is intense. The poverty, isolation, and disorientation of prolonged homelessness can be complicated by drug or alcohol abuse, provoked, at least in part, by situational despair.

The fundamental ability of a family to function is hampered or paralyzed.

For the homeless family, the fever caused by an infant's acute ear infection may not have the highest priority. Availability, accessibility, and affordability of health care are serious concerns. As a result, the infection may never be treated, and the problem becomes prolonged (the infection evolves to a chronic state). Hearing and language development can be impaired.

These children simply do not receive routine, reliable health care. They remain at high risk for many health problems. Their health problems remain undiagnosed and undertreated, if they receive attention at all. Complications and secondary problems abound. Infants are born onto the streets without cribs and are rarely held. They may find refuge in an overcrowded shelter one night, and the next night their shelter is a doorway hidden in an alley; the following night home is an abandoned car. From the beginning of life these infants encounter an unbeatable cycle of nowhere to go, no place to call home, no safe sanctuary, only the feeling of aloneness and unpredictability (Gerson, 2007).

The pioneering work of Erik Erikson has defined the necessary stages of human development. Each level of maturation must be mastered sequentially, but to do so takes a secure environment, opportunities to succeed, and emotional support. The hidden tragedy for homeless children is the stifling development of their personal growth. Homelessness can be eliminated. The key factors are increased affordable housing, increased income for low-income families, and strengthened service and support for families at risk of homelessness. Families at risk of homelessness for solely economic reasons can often be helped with short-term loans and grants. Community-based programs can help identify these families before they lose their homes, which increases including more families.

Efforts are increasingly made to link the homeless with all available programs and services, such as the Special Supplemental Nutrition Program for Women, Infants, and Children (WIC), food stamps, Head Start, and housing subsidies. These programs should continue to provide assistance after the family is resettled in permanent housing. These families will need more comprehensive services with special problems such as domestic violence, mental illness, and substance abuse.

Because there is a multitude of needs, a partnership that provides a multitude of resources must be developed. Nurses can take a leadership position in helping the homeless achieve a sense of security and adequate health care. Nursing involvement in community health care for the homeless and providing compassionate care gives the homeless a clear signal of hope and concern about their plight. Bringing attention to this social problem by speaking to community groups to obtain their support is another way that nurses can help. Volunteering time in community shelters and organizing health care days through the local health department is another way to address the problem.

Nurses can become active in raising the nation's conscience and helping to call attention to this national disgrace. Housing and support services must be provided to assist the homeless in regaining a foothold in society. With the right support services and health care, many homeless people can be stabilized and reintegrated into the community. These families with infants are not "throwaways", but people who have fallen on hard times need to be offered a variety of helping hands. Through this help, the nation's health can improve (see the Case Study and Care Plan at the end of this chapter).

Sexuality-Reproductive Pattern

An infant's identity begins at birth, when the gendered child is identified and caretakers behave a certain way toward the infant because of its gender. The infant's sexuality gives direction to its physical, emotional, social, and intellectual responses throughout life. Infants have a great oral sensitivity, enjoy skin-to-skin contact, and explore their own bodies for pleasure during the first year of life. A healthy, accepting attitude by caretakers is important in an infant's evolving sexual development.

Coping–Stress Tolerance Pattern

The term *stress* implies intense reaction to an experience and changes in usual behavior. Stress is a normal phenomenon that occurs throughout the life span, as, for example, when an individual experiences a developmental or situational crisis.

Developmental Crisis

Developmental crises are turning points or periods of great change. Most stressors that the infant experiences are a necessary part of growth and development. For example, learning new skills creates stress. The infant who is unable to move forward while learning to crawl experiences stress. The infant expresses this stress by crying for help. Other stressors are more psychosocial in nature, such as being left with a babysitter or in an unfamiliar place.

Situational Crisis

Situational crises are not anticipated easily and do not occur necessarily as part of the normal growth and development process. One major situational crisis during infancy is separation from the significant other. The following three distinct phases are evident in the reaction to separation (Puckett & Black, 2007):

1. Protest. Infant cries loudly, screams for the mother, and refuses attention of the substitute caregiver.
2. Despair. Infant stops crying and becomes less active, withdraws, and becomes apathetic.
3. Withdrawal. Infant takes an interest in surroundings but tends to ignore or reject the mother when she returns, because she failed to meet the infant's needs.

Initially, with no time framework and no understanding of waiting, the infant has little ability to cope with stress.

As maturity and a sense of security provided by the caregiver increases, the infant begins to wait a short time to have needs met without protest. An infant who experiences stress reacts by crying, the main tool of communication. The infant gradually learns to tolerate greater stress with time.

Nursing Interventions

Nursing interventions that assist the infant and family in stressful situations are listed in Box 17-8. By allaying anxiety in the infant's caregiver, the nurse facilitates coping behaviors in the infant. The stressful situation and the problem-solving activities can be turned into growth-producing experiences for the family, with coping capacities strengthened for the future.

Values-Beliefs Pattern

A value is a standard or principle that reflects a person's judgment on what is important in life. When people communicate, they send both the content message of the spoken words and the unspoken message of who they are and what they believe. Values are pervasive and important and give a focus to both individuals and groups within a particular culture. Because values are attitudes learned especially from significant others within the environment, the parents' values-beliefs pattern greatly influence the care and development of the infant.

Nursing Interventions

By understanding and respecting the parents' value system, the nurse works within their framework of values in the counseling situation. The nurse communicates personal values to the family. To work successfully within a different value system, the nurse incorporates the following attitudes concerning the values-beliefs pattern into the nursing process (Clark, 2008):

Box 17-8 Nursing Interventions to Assist in Stressful Situations During Infancy

- Attempt to meet the infant's needs promptly.
- Allow favorite toy or item of security to be present during stressful experiences.
- Allow familiar caregiver to be present to calm the infant.
- Attempt to keep the number of strangers interacting with the infant to a minimum.
- Attempt to provide a warm and accepting environment for the infant.
- Allow freedom of expression (crying) to reduce tension in the infant.
- Identify the infant's established daily routine and try to follow through with it.
- Reinforce the infant's need for expression.
- Establish a trusting relationship with the infant.
- Provide opportunity for play so the infant can vent fears.
- Provide emotional support for the parents so they can, in turn, give support to their infant.

1. Believe in the ultimate worth of the infant and the family, regardless of their behavior or situation.
2. Grant families the freedom to make their own informed choices and to experience the responsibilities and consequences of their decisions.
3. Use knowledge of the family's value system in specific ways to reward and reinforce positive health practices.
4. Value the growth potential inherent in developmental and situational crisis situations.
5. Recognize your own value system and its influence on your behavior.
6. Work with families without applying your personal value system in judging their behavior.
7. Broaden your value system by accepting lifestyles different from your own.

The nurse influences the behavior of the parents, who have the greatest influence on their infant's values-beliefs pattern. The nurse accomplishes this task by modeling (living congruently with professed values), acting as a consultant by sharing pertinent information with parents, and modifying one's own values (Kenner & Lott, 2007).

Modeling can be a potent influence on another individual's behavior. In the counseling situation, the family looks to the nurse for guidance and assistance in promoting healthy child-rearing practices. The methods by which the nurse interacts with the infant, listens to the parents' concerns, and demonstrates respect for the family unit are influencing factors in changing behavior.

Second, the nurse acts as a consultant to influence values. Advice on child-rearing practices is overwhelming to parents; everyone has opinions. The nurse listens before giving advice to determine whether parents will accept the advice and to allow them to decide whether the advice can be useful. Repeated attempts to convert parents to the nurse's value system can make them defensive and resistant to the advice.

Third, by expressing values and attitudes, but remaining open to other approaches, the nurse influences the values-beliefs pattern. Parents can realize that they are free to change and are not bound to values that others outside their value system express (Kenner & Lott, 2007). Communication skills can more effectively promote the health of the infant and family.

ENVIRONMENTAL PROCESSES

This section discusses various factors within the environment that can affect the infant's health status. The entire realm of accident prevention and safety promotion is applicable here.

Accidents are always unexpected and, in retrospect, usually could have been prevented. Unintentional injuries are the leading cause of death for children in the United States and globally. Research shows that every minute and a half an infant is seen in the emergency department for an unintentional injury (APHA, 2006). Adults take for granted that they are living in a world designed by adults for adults. They must remind themselves constantly that infants also live in this complex world and that they learn at a remarkable rate, primarily by exploring and playing in the environment. These experiences render them extremely vulnerable to accidents, a major problem and a challenging field for preventive measures.

Accidents occur in many situations: in the home, outside, on the playground, and in automobiles. The use of safety belts prevents infant injury (Figure 17-3). Most accidents, however, occur in the home. Their number and seriousness are closely linked to the infant's developmental stage. Accidents tend to increase with the mobility of the infant, but even a 2 month old can wiggle or fall from a high place. Keeping the environment free from hazards and caregiver supervision are crucial at this time.

Nurses have the opportunity to help parents and caregivers anticipate and understand the common hazards of early life and provide specific guidance for accident prevention.

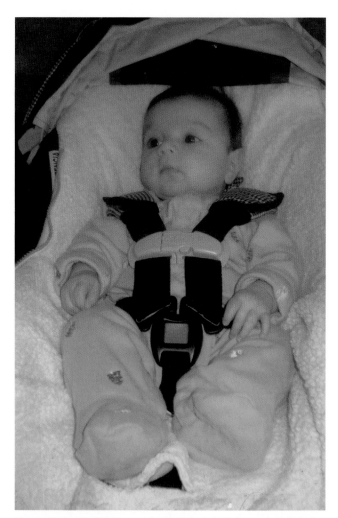

Figure 17-3 Accident prevention for infants in their car seats includes the use of safety belts.

Unintentional Injuries

Falls

Falls are most common after 4 months of age, when the infant has learned to roll over, but they can occur at any age. Falls involving infants happen more often in the home environment, on stairs, from furniture, and out of windows. The best advice is never to place an infant unattended on a raised surface that has no type of guardrails. When in doubt, the safest place is the floor (Gardner, 2007). Safety tips to assist parents in preventing falls are listed in Box 17-9.

Burns

Burns are the most frequent and frightening of all accidents during infancy. The majority of fire deaths occur in the home and most victims die from smoke or toxic gases and not from the burns (Gardner, 2007). Because nearly all burns are preventable, the attendant caregiver can experience severe guilt.

Fire from matches or other sources, hot liquids, ultraviolet light from the sun, electricity or electrical outlets, and heating elements such as radiators, registers, and floor heaters can all cause burns. Box 17-10 lists safety tips to assist parents in preventing burns.

Swallowing/Choking on Foreign Objects

Any small object that an infant puts in the mouth has the potential to be swallowed and choked on. More than 65% of deaths from foreign body aspiration occur in infants. Liquids are the most common cause of choking in infants, whereas balloons, small objects, and foods are the most common causes of foreign-body airway obstruction in children (AHA, 2006). Parents should be advised that objects such as safety pins, peanuts, beads, coins, hot dogs, paper clips, nuts, corn, buttons, popcorn, chips, apple with peel, and parts of broken toys are frequently swallowed. Many objects can fit into this category and into the infant's mouth. The carelessness of a caregiver, relative, friend, or babysitter in leaving small objects available and within reach, or giving toys unsuited to the infant's stage of development, frequently cause these accidents.

When choking occurs, the adult should place the infant across the adult's knees and deliver 5 back blows (slaps) followed by 5 chest thrusts repeatedly until the object is expelled or the infant becomes unresponsive. Abdominal thrusts are not recommended for infants because they damage the relatively large and unprotected liver (American Heart Association, 2006). CPR should be performed if the infant becomes unresponsive. The American Heart Association does not recommend using the Heimlich maneuver (series of under-the-diaphragm abdominal thrusts) for choking infants under the age of one.

Box 17-9 Safety Tips to Prevent Falls

1. Whenever the infant is in the crib, keep sides up and securely fastened.
2. Place the infant seat in the playpen or on the floor; always strap the infant in securely.
3. Check high chairs, strollers, and carriages for safety, and restrain the infant who is active.
4. Lock windows if the infant is capable of climbing on the windowsill.
5. Clean up food or liquid spills immediately from the floor.
6. Remember that polished floors are hazardous, especially when throw rugs are present.
7. Close off stairways with doors, gates, or some other safety device as the infant becomes mobile.
8. Do not leave items that the infant might use to climb out of the crib.
9. To prevent falls, set the crib mattress at the lowest adjustment level after the infant can pull up and stand.
10. Strap the infant into a shopping cart to prevent falls.
11. Keep chairs, cribs, and other furniture away from windows
12. Avoid the use of baby walkers.

From Reich, J. B. (2007) *Babyproofing bible: The exceedingly thorough guide to keeping your child safe from crib to kitchen to car to yard.* Beverly, MA: Fair Winds Press.

Box 17-10 Burn Prevention Guidelines

1. Keep the infant out of the sun when ultraviolet rays are strongest, generally from 10 AM to 3 PM.
2. Sunscreen, clothing with long sleeves, pant legs, and a brimmed hat are essential to prevent sun overexposure.
3. Remember that fireplaces can be a serious hazard. Fine-mesh screens attached to a frame are safer than freestanding screens. Never leave an infant alone in a room where a fire is burning; make sure the fire is out before going to bed.
4. Avoid bathing the infant in a sink or adult tub near hot water faucets. Test the bath water temperatures before placing the infant in it; keep one hand on the infant at all times during the bath.
5. Be sure that all infant's clothing is made of nonflammable materials.
6. Avoid handling hot liquids near the infant.
7. Turn the handles of cooking utensils toward the back of the stove.
8. Keep all electrical cords taut, especially those for coffee pots; keep cords out of the infant's sight.
9. Cover electrical outlets with protective plastic caps.
10. Place a barrier in front of any heat-producing element, especially floor heaters.
11. Keep all matches and lighters out of the infant's reach.
12. Teach the older infant the meaning of hot.
13. Close oven doors when the oven is in use or when cooling.
14. If you must smoke, keep the heat of cigarettes or cigars away from the infant.
15. Install smoke detectors on every level of the home and in every sleeping area.

Box **17-11** Nursing Interventions to Reduce Choking Hazards for Infants

- Keep small objects out of an infant's reach.
- Avoid propping bottles and making large holes in nipples to prevent aspiration of formula into the infant's lungs.
- Discourage the use of powder on infants to reduce the risk of pneumonia from inhaling zinc stearate.
- Burp the infant thoroughly before placing in the crib; place infant in side-lying position.
- Older children should not give food to the infant, who may choke on it. An adult should be near to supervise children around infants.
- Adults should not set a bad example by putting pins or other objects in their mouths; older infants like to mimic adults.
- Inspect toys for loose, removable parts that could end up in the infant's mouth.

Box **17-12** Home Childproofing Tips

1. Remove any heavy, sharp, or breakable objects from tables and low shelves.
2. Bolt bookcases to the wall and remove heavy books to prevent falls.
3. Test floor and table lamps to make sure they cannot be pulled over.
4. Disconnect unused appliances and wrap up cords.
5. Secure all other cords to prevent appliances from being pulled down.
6. Safely discard unused and unneeded medicines.
7. Avoid referring to medicines as candy.
8. Store potentially toxic substances out of sight and reach.
9. Close reachable outlets with safety covers.
10. Tie drapery and blind cords out of the infant's reach.
11. Choose stair gates with openings too small for an infant's head and child-resistant fasteners such as pressure bars.
12. Avoid accordion or expandable gates with openings that can trap an infant's head.
13. Install smoke detectors and check the batteries at least once a month.
14. Use sturdy screens in front of fireplaces.
15. Place crib, playpen, and high chair well away from heaters, fans, and electrical outlets.
16. Install childproof latches on drawers and cupboards. Store all cleaning compounds and detergents in a high, locked cupboard.
17. Buy all medicines in bottles with childproof lids and keep them in their original labeled containers for identification in case of accidental ingestion.
18. Install lids on garbage pails and never leave any harmful materials in them, such as sharp can lids or spoiled food.
19. Check the floor regularly for objects small enough to be swallowed.
20. Cut blind cords into two pieces.

Prevention of swallowing foreign objects is the best treatment. Some safety measures for parents and caregivers of infants are listed in Box 17-11.

The entire balance of safety for infants rests on allowing them plenty of opportunity to explore and play within the environment while protecting them from harmful agents. According to the AAP, the greatest threat to the health of infants is not illness but injuries, many of which can be prevented. The nurse informs the infant's parents, babysitters, family friends, and day care workers about the need to childproof their environments when an infant is present. The nurse can explain ways to promote the safety of these varied environments (Box 17-12).

Biological Agents

The fetus is partially protected from some biological agents in the environment by the placental barrier and the mother's defense system. After birth, however, the infant is thrust into an environment that is filled with infectious, disease-causing agents. These bacterial or viral organisms can be found in food, cribs, the air, pets, the parents, and the siblings—literally everywhere. Even the healthiest environment harbors disease-causing agents. Although the infant cannot escape exposure to these pathogens without being completely isolated, immunizations are given to assist the infant's defense against some communicable diseases.

Acquired Immunodeficiency Syndrome

Acquired immunodeficiency syndrome (AIDS) is spread by contact with the human immunodeficiency virus (HIV) through blood and bodily secretions. The virus attacks the T cell lymphocytes, affecting formation of TH4 (T helper or T inducer) cells, which direct the immune response. The infant with HIV infection is unable to resist normal infections. Transmission of HIV from mother to infant is the most likely cause of childhood HIV. Transmission can occur during pregnancy, at delivery, or during breast-feeding

(Walsh, 2007) (see Chapter 16). There is no immunization against HIV infections currently, but frequently preventative options are offered to mothers, and babies are frequently delivered by C-Section.

Because infants can retain maternal antibodies for HIV infection for as long as 18 months, the diagnosis of HIV infection in an at-risk infant (one whose mother is infected) is extremely difficult. In the last few years, investigators have demonstrated the utility of highly accurate blood tests in diagnosing HIV infection in infants 6 months of age and younger (Peragallo & Gonzalez, 2007). Although signs and symptoms of illness can occur at any time, they usually begin during the first year of life. In infants the symptoms of the disease include failure to thrive, oral candidiasis, recurrent bacterial infections, persistent pulmonary infiltrates, delays in reaching important milestones in motor skills and mental development such as crawling, walking and speaking, and chronic diarrhea (Sarnquist et al., 2007). Early diagnosis is essential for effective treatment.

In response to the urgent need to reduce the number of new HIV infections globally, WHO and the UNAIDS (Joint United Nations Program on HIV/AIDS) convened in 2007 to determine whether male circumcision should be recommended for the prevention of HIV infection. Based on the evidence presented, which was considered to be compelling, experts recommended that male circumcision be recognized as an important intervention to reduce the risk of heterosexually acquired HIV infection in men (WHO & UNAIDS, 2007). Research brought forth strong evidence that male circumcision reduces the risk of heterosexually acquired HIV infection in men by approximately 60% (WHO & UNAIDS, 2007). Parents must weigh their decision to circumcise their male infant based on their own values, religious backgrounds, and culture in light of this new information.

Nursing assessment focuses on a careful and complete history of the infant and mother, signs and symptoms of the disease, growth and development history, and psychosocial concerns. Parents are assessed carefully to determine their level of anxiety; knowledge of the disease process, including prognosis, treatment, and transmission; and awareness of resources, support systems, coping strategies, and the infant's needs.

No other disease causes as much public awareness and panic as does AIDS. Part of this behavior is ignorance. Nurses play a major role in educating the public about the disease process, its mode of transmission, and most of all, preventive measures. Preventive education should begin with young children. Most school health programs include information on AIDS. School nurses can contribute to the success of these programs, as can nurses working in prenatal clinics, to spread the prevention word. Nurses in all settings can engage in research related to AIDS to gather further clarification of this fatal disease.

Although the infant is not an active participant in the spread of HIV, parents should understand the means by which the virus is transmitted and not allow their infant to become a passive participant because of their own high-risk behaviors.

Immunization

Disease prevention by immunization is a public health priority in the *Healthy People 2010* and the following *Healthy People 2020* initiative and society as a whole. Progress continues toward the goal of protecting children from serious disease through immunizations. The most recent schedule recommends the new rotavirus vaccine (Rota) in a 3-dose schedule at ages 2, 4, and 6 months. The influenza vaccine is now recommended for all children aged 6 to 59 months annually. In addition, varicella vaccines should be administered at age 12 to 15 months, and a newly recommended second dose should be administered at age 4 to 6 years (CDC, 2007).

The two types of immunization are active and passive. In **active immunization,** all or part of a disease-causing

Table 17-7 Recommended Immunization Schedule for Infants

Age (Month)	Immunization
Birth	HepB-1
1 month	HepB-2
2 months	DTaP-1, Hib-1, IPV-1, PCV-1, Rota-1
4 months	DTaP-2, Hib-2, IPV-2, PCV-2, Rota-2
6 months	HepB-3, DTaP-3, Hib-3, IPV-3, PVC-3, Rota-3 Influenza (yearly)
12 to 15 months	Hib-4, MMR, PCV, IPV, Varicella
15 to 18 months	DTaP-4, Influenza yearly

DTaP, Diphtheria, tetanus, acellular pertussis vaccine; *HepB*, hepatitis B vaccine; *Hib*, Haemophilus influenza type b conjugate vaccine; *IPV*, inactivated polio vaccine; *PCV*, pneumococcal vaccine; *MMR*, measles, mumps, rubella vaccine, Rotavirus vaccine (Rota).
Modified from the Centers for Disease Control and Prevention. (2007). Recommended immunization schedules for persons aged 0-18 years—United States, 2007. MMWR, 55(51-52): Q1-Q4.

microorganism or a modified product of that microorganism is injected into the body to make the immune system react defensively. This substance is generally a toxin of the disease organism; depending on the virulence and certain other characteristics of the organism, it is used in the vaccine in a live, killed, or attenuated form (Clark, 2008). The attenuated form is alive, but its virulence has been reduced significantly by treatment with laboratory procedures that use, for example, heat or chemicals, which reduces potency of microorganisms. Examples of active immunization include diphtheria, tetanus, and acellular pertussis (DTaP); inactivated polio vaccine (IPV); and measles, mumps, and rubella (MMR). Active immunity is relatively long lasting, waning over several years if at all.

Passive immunization is accomplished by injecting blood from an actively immunized person or animal. After an individual has been exposed to a disease, a passive immunization is given to prevent the disease from developing. Passive immunizations provide a short immunity, usually 1 to 6 weeks, which will protect the person until the danger of contracting the disease is passed. Passive immunization also helps reduce the severity of the disease when it is contracted. Because of the short duration, active immunization is still needed to remain permanently immune. Passive immunity occurs naturally in newborns when maternal antibodies are passed through the placenta or in breast milk.

The Committee on Infectious Diseases of the AAP and the CDC (2007) recommends immunization schedules that are revised periodically as new information arises. Table 17-7 lists the current recommendations for healthy infants. More detailed immunization information is provided in **Website Resource 17E.**

Immunization provides one of the most cost-effective means of preventing infection in infants. Immunizations not only help protect those receiving the vaccinations from developing potentially serious diseases, they also help protect entire communities by preventing and reducing the spread of infectious agents. Immunization is additionally important because currently available antibiotics cannot destroy viruses; therefore, immunization offers the only means of control. Nurses have a special responsibility to keep informed of the recommendations and document all vaccinations given. Emphasis must be placed on educating parents about the importance of immunization. Children need a series of vaccinations, starting at birth, to be fully protected against 12 potentially serious diseases. To motivate parents to have their infants immunized, the nurse can work toward increasing health education to achieve greater health maintenance knowledge, send reminders for upcoming visits and needed immunizations, vigorously advocate for all infants to receive comprehensive health care, including immunizations, provide health services that make immunizations feasible and available, develop a close relationship with the family, and continue the surveillance of the immunization status of every infant in the health care system.

Chemical Agents

Drugs

Aspirin is the medicine most commonly ingested, with acetaminophen and vitamins close behind. Ibuprofen and other aspirin substitutes are becoming increasingly popular with parents as antipyretics. Vitamins can be harmful; however, many vitamins contain iron, making them potentially lethal. Infants are frequently attracted to vitamins because of their appealing colors, scents, and flavors, especially children's vitamins.

Recent changes in packaging and limits on the number of tablets contained in each bottle have reduced deaths resulting from overdose. Drug manufacturers are using childproof caps increasingly as a safety measure. Despite a concerted effort by manufacturers, childproof bottle caps vary in effectiveness (Clark, 2008). Frequently the safety caps are adult-proof, although children can readily open them.

This points to the dangers of medications, regardless of the bottle. All medications still must be locked away when infants are in the home or visiting other homes. Some additional guidelines to help prevent accidents involving drugs include the following:

1. Use a prescription drug only for the purpose and the person for whom it is intended. Do not use medication prescribed for someone else for a similar condition in the infant.
2. Discard unused drugs by taking them to dump into trash on toxic dump days; many infants have been poisoned by eating tablets found in the trash at home.
3. Request safety caps on all prescription drugs.
4. Keep all medicines under lock and key.
5. Have the telephone number of the nearest poison control center readily available.

The main points to be emphasized in giving parents guidance in accident prevention are (1) to eliminate specific environmental hazards, such as drugs, from exploring infants and (2) to supervise infants while they play, gradually replacing supervision with safety training (Reich, 2007).

Plants

Houseplants are another source of poison. Most people fail to think of houseplants as potentially poisonous, because people do not consider eating them. However, infants test almost everything by putting it in their mouths, and a number of plants can be deadly when eaten. As a result, plants are one of the leading sources of poisoning of infants, and amateur foragers frequently learn the hard way that not everything that looks good can be eaten.

Household plants are frequently placed on the floor, where the leaves or flowers are easy to pull off and taste. The best interventions for plant poisoning is prevention which, in this case, means previous knowledge. Table 17-8 identifies several common household and garden plants that are poisonous. The nurse must know which plants are harmful when ingested and must inform parents of the potential dangers to infants.

The National Clearinghouse for Poison Control Centers lists plants as the third most commonly ingested poison, after aspirin and household cleaning agents. Safety education is stressed at all well-baby visits beginning in the first 6 months of life. Prevention of plant poisoning and other accidents depends on a reciprocal relationship between protection and education that must be related to age. Keep all poisonous substances, medicines, cleaning agents, health and beauty aids, paints, and plants locked in a safe place out of an infant's sight and reach. Never store poisonous substances in container other than original ones, for example, empty jars or soda bottles. Safe behavior is a learned behavior, gradually acquired in a progressive process with increasing age. Box 17-13 lists specific safety measures for parents to prevent plant poisoning for infants (Leikin & McFee, 2007; Nelson et al., 2007; Hagan et al., 2007).

Toxins

Infants are at particular risk from toxic factors in the environment; as dependent, developing organisms, they are inherently vulnerable. Generally the exposure of infants to potential toxins is quite different from that of adults because of differences in physical environment, activities, and diet. Daily activities of infants, such as proximity to the floor or carpet inside the home and the lawn or soil outside, hand-to-mouth behaviors, and smaller body size and composition, place them at great risk for environmental toxins. Infants are exposed to a host of environmental pollutants on a regular basis. These exposures occur through all possible environmental media: air, water, soil, and food. Infants have a unique exposure pattern and unique vulnerabilities. For example, some studies identify that the infant's

Table **17-8** Poisonous Parts of Common House and Garden Plants

Plant	Toxic Part	Symptoms
Apple	Seeds	Release cyanide when ingested in large quantities; can be fatal
Azalea	All parts	Nausea, vomiting, dyspnea, paralysis; can be fatal
Buttercup	All parts	Inflammation around mouth, stomach pains, vomiting, diarrhea, and convulsions
Castor bean	Seeds	Burning of mouth and throat, excessive thirst, and convulsions; one or two seeds are near the lethal dose for adults
Croton species	Plant juice	Gastroenteritis
Daffodil	Bulb	Nausea, vomiting, and diarrhea; can be fatal
Dieffenbachia	All parts	Intensive burning and irritation of the mouth and tongue; death can occur when base of tongue swells enough to occlude air passages
English holly	Berries	Nausea, vomiting, diarrhea, central nervous system depression; can be fatal
English ivy	Leaves and berries	Dyspnea, vomiting, diarrhea, coma, and death
Hyacinth	Bulb	Nausea, vomiting, and diarrhea; can be fatal
Iris	Underground stems	Digestive upset
Jasmine	All parts	Hallucinations, elevated temperature, tachycardia, and paralysis
Lily of the valley	All parts	Arrhythmia, mental confusion, weakness, shock, and death
Mistletoe	Berries	Acute stomach and intestinal irritations with diarrhea; can be fatal
Oak tree	Acorns	Kidney failure, gastritis
Oleander	All parts	Digestive upset, bloody diarrhea, respiratory depression, cardiac arrhythmia, blurred vision, coma, and death
Philodendron	All parts	Burning of lips, mouth, and tongue; swelling of tongue; dyspnea, kidney failure; death
Poinsettia	Leaves	Severe irritation to mouth, throat, and stomach; can be fatal
Potato	All green parts	Cardiac depression; can be fatal
Tomato	Green parts	Cardiac depression; can be fatal
Violet	Seeds	Taken in quantity, cathartic effects can be serious to infant
Yew	Foliage, seeds, bark	Nausea, vomiting, diarrhea, dyspnea, and dilated pupils; death is sudden

Box **17-13** Nursing Interventions to Prevent Plant Poisoning in Infants

- Keep plants out of reach of infants and young children.
- Never eat any part of a plant except the parts that are grown or sold as food.
- Keep jewelry made from unknown seeds or beans away from exploring infants.
- Learn to identify poisonous plants around your house and garden.
- Do not use unknown plants as medicines or teas.
- Pay close attention to infants at play inside and outside.
- Seek help whenever anyone chews or swallows a poisonous plant.
- Be aware that infants are more susceptible than are adults to the effects of poisonous plants.
- Keep the poison control center telephone number handy (800-222-1222).

oral habits and unique diet (ingesting more fruits, vegetables, and water than do adults) magnify their exposure to certain agents. Finally, because infants have a longer life span, toxins that have a long latency or cumulative toxicity (such as certain carcinogens) pose a greater risk to them than to adults (Leikin & McFee, 2007).

Some pesticides that are used to control insects that feed on cereal grains, fruits, and vegetables are notorious for their slow accumulation in human tissue. Produce washes are available now to rid vegetables and fruits of these potential toxins. Over sufficient time, exposure to relatively small amounts of pesticides can result in the buildup of toxic quantities and lead to chronic disease in humans.

Lead is another environmental toxin, which has no known physiological role in the human body. Although lead is essentially a contaminant, most people absorb a certain amount through exposure to lead-based paint in older homes, contaminated soil, household dust, drinking water, lead crystal, and lead-glazed pottery. Numerous toys made in China have been recalled and deemed unsafe because they contain lead-based paint. Studies have revealed a high lead content in dust, dirt, and soil. Lead in the air comes primarily from automobile emissions (NIEHS, 2007). Absorption of lead is closely related to particle size. Airborne lead of small particle size is readily absorbed through the lungs, whereas larger particles fall to the ground. Lead affects practically all systems within the body. At high levels, lead can cause convulsions, coma, and even death. Lower levels of lead can adversely affect the brain, central nervous system, blood cells, and kidneys.

Infants are vulnerable to lead exposure for several reasons. In proportion to their weight, infants breathe in more air and more lead than do adults. Additionally, infants breathe closer to the ground, where a higher concentration of lead is located. Their dust-raising play and habit of putting their hands in their mouths add to their lead consumption; they also have a greater rate of gastrointestinal absorption of lead and other chemicals than do adults. Both exercise and blockage of the nasal passages increase mouth breathing, and the mouth is a far less capable filter than the nose. Mouth breathing, coupled with their greater frequency of respiratory tract infections, exposes infants to a greater amount of environmental toxins. The growing prevalence of asthma is also evidence of environmental exposure to lead and other pollutants. Approximately 5 million children have asthma. Statistics show that asthma rates have doubled in the last decade and death rates from asthma have increased in recent years. The reality is that we do not know why asthma is becoming more prevalent, but air pollution is a contributing factor (NIEHS, 2007).

Human potential and development are clearly important natural resources, and a growing body of evidence now links increased lead exposure to impaired intellectual performance and potential. Clinical lead poisoning affects many children, but it is preventable; excess lead in the infant's environment is made by, and should be eliminated by, human beings. Progress has been made in reducing blood lead levels in infants and young children. The following factors have contributed to these improvements (U.S. Department of Health and Human Services [USDHHS], 2000):

- Decline in lead used in gasoline
- Decline in manufactured food and soft drink cans containing lead solder
- Ban on leaded paint for residential (indoor) use
- Established standard for lead exposure in industry
- Ban on lead-containing solder in household plumbing
- Implementation of lead poisoning prevention programs
- Ban of toys manufactured in China containing lead-based paint.

Parents need to be educated to take steps to reduce their infant's exposure to lead:

- Keep areas in which infant plays as dust free and clean as possible.
- Do not remove lead paint yourself.
- Do not bring dust into the home.
- If work or a hobby involves lead, change clothes, and bathe before entering the environment of infants, for example, day care.
- Do not burn painted wood in fireplace.
- Eat a balanced diet, rich in calcium, iron, and vitamin C.

Infants do not necessarily escape noxious chemicals when they are indoors. The contaminants that cause air pollution are approximately the same indoors as they are outdoors, with perhaps more indoors from carbon monoxide, nitrogen dioxide, and various hydrocarbons from tobacco smoke, poorly ventilated heating and cooking equipment, and aerosol sprays. There are radon checks and carbon dioxide detectors that can be used to assess the presence of these contaminants. Many air pollution aftereffects may not be observed during infancy, but can surface in problems that affect both physical and mental well-being over a lifetime.

Among the acute illnesses of infancy, respiratory disease is ranked number one, representing between 50% and 75% of all childhood diseases (NIEHS, 2007). In addition to the inconvenience and incapacity induced by respiratory diseases, medical costs are high. Dirty air aggravates, and in some cases, causes nearly all respiratory problems. Infants with chronic respiratory disease can become adults with respiratory problems.

Water pollution can cause gastrointestinal disturbances in the infant. Parents and health care providers are quick to blame food, teething, or a virus for simple diarrhea, when the underlying cause may come from the kitchen tap. Numerous strong chemicals are used today to purify drinking water. These chemicals can irritate the delicate lining and cause disturbances in the infant's gastrointestinal tract. Nurses encourage parents to boil all water for 20 minutes before they give it to their infant to help eliminate any potential problem.

Table 17-9 lists major pollutants and their health effects.

Table **17-9**	Major Pollutants and Their Health Effects	
Pollutants	**Major Sources**	**Effects**
Carbon monoxide	Vehicle exhaust	Replaces oxygen in red blood cells; causes dizziness, coma, or death
Lead	Antiknock agents in some gasoline, old paint chips, metal pieces, pottery, and soil	Accumulates in the bones and soft tissues; affects blood-forming organs, kidneys, and central nervous system
Nitrogen dioxide	Industrial wastes, vehicle exhaust	Causes structural and chemical changes in lungs; lowers resistance against URI
Radon	Earth and rock beneath homes, well water, and building materials	Lung cancer
Ozone	Formed when hydrocarbons and nitrogen dioxide react	Produces smog; irritates mucous membranes, causing coughing, choking, and impaired lung function; contributes to asthma and bronchitis
Sulfur dioxide	Burning coal and oil, industrial processes	Increases colds, coughs, and asthma; contributes to acid rain
Passive smoking	Tobacco products	Causes high incidence of URI, pneumonia, bronchitis, and asthma; linked to cancer

URI, Upper respiratory infection.
From the Environmental Protection Agency. (2007). *Air quality* (On-line). Retrieved October 20, 2007, from *www.epa.gov/iaq*.

Motor Vehicles

This section refers to the effects of motion or action of forces on the infant; the focus here is on motor vehicle accidents.

Automobiles present a danger to people of all ages, but especially to infants. Usually an infant is injured because of improper restraint inside the automobile. Many parents have been misled by thinking that it is better to be thrown clear of an accident than it is to be restrained. Many also think that it is safer to hold an infant on the lap in the front seat rather than to have the infant restrained in the back seat. On the contrary, these practices increase the probability of a fatality. A free-moving child not only distracts the driver, but is in a more vulnerable position for being thrown.

Adult seat belts are unsuitable for infants or children under 4 years of age, because their pelvic structure is small; the AAP recommends that safety seats for infants be used (USDHHS, 2000). A variety of car seats is available: for infants up to 20 pounds, the recommended type is the rear-facing, molded plastic shell seat, which includes a shoulder restraint and employs the adult seat belt (AAP, 2007). The shield-type or infant only car seat offers maximal protection for the child weighing up to 30 pounds. All children should be in the back seat because of the potential danger posed by air bags. Infant safety in motor vehicles depends entirely on the responsible adults.

Each year infants die from heat stroke after being left unattended in motor vehicles. Research has found that on days when ambient temperatures exceeded 86° F, the internal temperatures of a vehicle quickly reaches 134° F to 154° F (McLaren et al., 2005). Even at relatively cool ambient temperatures, the temperature rise inside vehicles is significant and places the infant at risk for hyperthermia. Vehicles heat up rapidly, with the majority of the temperature rise occurring within the first 15 to 30 minutes. Leaving the windows opened slightly does not significantly slow the heating process or decrease the maximum temperature attained (Researchers, 2007).

Nurses can take the lead in increasing public awareness and improving parental education regarding heat rise in motor vehicles. The take home message here is to never leave an infant alone in a motor vehicle.

The nurse can also suggest the automobile safety precautions listed in Box 17-14.

Much of automobile safety is common sense, but the nurse must cover all areas in anticipatory preventive teaching. The importance of automobile safety cannot be overemphasized.

Radiation

In its broadest sense, radiation means the transfer of electromagnetic waves or energy through space (Leikin & McFee, 2007). Radiation of all types presents a potential hazard in the infant's environment. The risk level depends on the amount of radiation and the length of exposure and on the particular tissues involved. The infant's rapidly growing and immature cells are especially vulnerable.

The infant is exposed to two basic categories of radiation: (1) natural background radiation, which comes from cosmic rays and radioactive material existing naturally in the soil, water, and air; and (2) human-made radiation, which includes x-rays and radiation from nuclear power plants, microwave ovens, and other electronic devices found in the home (USDHHS, 2000).

Cancer

Most people think of cancer as a disease of adults. Cancer, however, is the leading cause of death from disease in children more than 1 year of age. The most common cancers found from infancy to age 5 years are Wilms tumor, retinoblastoma, acute lymphocytic leukemia, neuroblastoma, and rhabdomyosarcoma (NCI, 2007). Nursing interventions to prevent cancer in infants are listed in **Website Resource 17F**.

Nursing intervention to identify risk factors includes taking a careful history, which usually reveals a slow progression of symptoms (e.g., cat's eye reflex, strabismus, painful red eye, and blindness). For example, the nurse who suspects retinoblastoma should ask questions such as the following to identify risk factors:

- Are tumors of the eyes common in your family?
- If so, can you identify which relatives had this and what was done for these tumors?
- Have you noticed your child having any eye problems, such as crossed or lazy eyes, or difficulty seeing?
- Have you noticed any changes in your child's eyes?

Nurses with physical assessment skills can perform screening and ophthalmoscopic examinations on high-risk infants and children. These eye tests include checking for the following:

1. Visual acuity, which can be determined by the fixation test, used to screen vision in infants and children 6 months to 5 years of age

---

Box 17-14 **Automobile Safety Precautions**

1. Be a good role model. Make sure you always wear your seat belt.
2. Never leave a child unattended in a parked car or around cars.
3. Never hold a child in the lap in the front seat.
4. Always use an infant car seat that is properly installed by following the manufacturer's instructions.
5. Keep car doors and windows locked.
6. Use safety restraints for passengers and driver.
7. Do not be distracted by an infant while driving.
8. Continue to use car seats as directed by the manufacturer, then use seat belts.
9. Never place an infant in a rear-facing car safety seat in the front seat of a vehicle that has a passenger air bag.
10. Make sure the seat belt is routed through the correct belt path for adult seat belts.

2. Red reflex, which appears whitish in the infant with retinoblastoma (the cat's eye reflex, the most common presenting sign of this cancer)
3. Lid lag, which is found in exophthalmos

Nurses play a big role in cancer detection, treatment, and prevention through their astute assessment skills, interview techniques, and community education to increase awareness of this disease to parents.

SOCIAL PROCESSES
Community and Work

As infants grow and develop, their boundaries extend beyond the home environment. Many mothers and fathers of infants return to the work force, placing them in community day care centers.

Today few young families can escape financial burdens. The two-income and single mother families are ways of life and the trend will continue. With more than one half of all American mothers working outside the home, the need for child care service is growing. This situation is usually an emotional issue for families; the separation process can be traumatic for both infant and parent.

Findings from social science research regarding the effects of day care on an infant's development and health can be summarized as: (1) little evidence suggests that day care permanently enhances or slows intellectual development, (2) day care can be used, even from earliest infancy, without damaging the mother-infant relationship, and (3) day care can lead to a slight increase in minor illnesses, but excluding ill infants from the center is not an effective means of reducing the spread of illness (Clark, 2008).

The question of how old an infant should be before being placed in day care is frequently asked of health professionals. Many experts believe that a mother and infant should have 4 to 6 months together before the mother goes to or returns to work. Brazelton and Sparrow (2006) make a good case for the mother and infant going through four stages of attachment together before the mother goes to work.

- In the first stage, which takes 10 to 14 days, the infant learns to be attentive to the mother, and the mother learns cues from the infant about being both ready for and tired of attentiveness.
- The second stage, which lasts 8 weeks, is a stage of playful interaction, when the mother learns how to recognize the infant's nonverbal cues and helps the infant maintain the alert state.
- The third stage, from the tenth week to the fourth month, is when the mother and infant learn to play games together.
- During the fourth stage, which occurs in the fourth month, infants rapidly learn about themselves and their world. Brazelton suggests that a mother, when possible, should spend the first 4 months with her new infant.

A nationwide survey of family day care found that nearly 50% of all infants in day care centers in the United States are cared for in one of three types of arrangements (Clark, 2008):

1. Private homes that provide informal day care to infants of relatives, friends, and neighbors
2. Regulated independent care licensed by state agencies
3. Regulated, sponsored care provided by licensed workers operating as part of home networks under umbrella agencies

The nurse has a vital role in assisting families with infants who need day care. Many factors are reviewed when a family is looking for an appropriate day care program; the nurse can counsel and guide the family in its search. The means by which the nurse counsels and guides the family in selecting a day care center are as follows:

1. Promote awareness of the three types of day care available in their local communities.
2. Counsel parents on what to ask employees of a prospective day care facility (Box 17-15); (American Academy of Pediatrics, 2003).
3. Help parents to deal with the separation behaviors manifested by their infant:
   - Remain calm in the situation.
   - Attempt to reduce the number of adults who interact with the infant and always introduce them.
   - Encourage the parents to bring an infant's special cuddly toy from home to the day-care facility to promote security.
   - Discuss the parent's understanding of the separation and expected behaviors.
   - Reassure parents that it takes time for the infant to make the transition from parent to another caregiver and vice versa.
   - Emphasize that at certain developmental levels stranger anxiety may be heightened (8 months), and separation behaviors of crying and clinging may be repeated.
   - Work toward promoting a good relationship among parents, infant, and caregiver by providing opportunities for open discussions of concerns.

Box 17-15 **Prospective Day Care Facility Questions**

- Licensed by the state?
- Open all year?
- Number of children present?
- Age range of children?
- Teacher-to-child ratio? (For infants, 1:3 is recommended.)
- Describe day care program.
- What meals are served?
- What is the cost?
- Are there openings?
- What are the qualifications of caregivers?
- Are the caregivers happy and interacting with the infant?
- Are infants content?
- Are parents welcome to drop in?

Culture and Ethnicity

The developing infant is subject to the influences of culture from the moment of conception. Partly because of the long dependency period, the family environment is the setting within which the infant experiences overall cultural attitudes. The lives of infants tend to be more under the direct control of parents or other caregivers than the lives of older children, who often are actively involved in selecting their own environments through contacts with peers, teachers, and other adults. The special demands of infancy require extensive and specific caregiving routines across cultures. The parents' perceptions of illness, wellness, roles, child-rearing practices, religious values, language, and health practices are all modeled for the infant. In short, culture helps form the infant's view of the world (Giger & Davidhizar, 2007).

The family's ethnicity includes ideas about health, illness, food preferences, moral codes, and family life that persist across generations and survive even the upheaval of coming to a new country. All cultural groups confront repeated challenges as they transfer their families from familiar to unfamiliar surroundings. Infants are exposed to an appropriate mode of behavior that is in accordance with their families' cultural standards. By observing and imitating family members, infants take cues for behavior. These perceptions are then incorporated into their own self-concepts (Puckett & Black, 2007).

To assess and plan appropriate interventions for different ethnic groups, nurses must be aware of their own cultural backgrounds. An important consideration is to examine all customs and values in relative terms, seeing none as altogether good or bad. Change is inevitable in family life, whether it is resisted or welcomed. An important function of the nurse is to help families monitor the rate of change that is acceptable to various members and reach a consensus (Box 17-16).

Box **17-16**	Factors that Facilitate Multicultural Health Care by Nurses

- Self-exploration of values and beliefs concerning other cultures and their beliefs
- Knowledge of the historical experience, recent and long-term, of ethnic groups that live in the community
- Demographic data that include family size, socioeconomic status, and future expectations that are characteristic of diverse ethnic groups
- Understanding and sensitivity to cultural health care practices different from own
- Recognition of folk beliefs and cultural attitudes toward health and illness
- Awareness of the nature of problems encountered by ethnic group members when they enter the health care system, including fear and distrust of health care professionals, language barriers, and discrimination by caregivers

From Giger, J. N., & Davidhizar, R. E. (2007). *Transcultural nursing: Assessment and intervention.* Philadelphia: Elsevier; Andrews, M.M., & Boyle, J. S. (2007). *Transcultural concepts in nursing care.* 5th edition. Philadelphia: Lippincott Williams & Wilkins.

The nurse identifies the power structure within a given cultural group. This knowledge may help dictate which family member to approach with the health teaching. Although the nurse might assume it would be the infant's mother, this may not necessarily be the case. Among some Native American tribes, the grandmother, not the parents, has the authority over the grandchildren. In many Latin cultural groups, the infant's father, not the mother, makes decisions about the infant's welfare (Andrews & Boyle, 2007). The nurse assesses the cultural groups' practices and beliefs before planning interventions. Approaches to infant care practices vary among cultural groups (Multicultural Awareness box).

MULTICULTURAL AWARENESS

Quick Guide for Cross-Cultural Nursing Care

The dominant American attitudes about infants and approaches to infant care have undergone many changes in the past several years. With the increased numbers of women in the work force, fathers are becoming more involved in infant care and day care for infants is increasing. Although children are valued, and raising children within the nuclear family remains a priority, an increasing number of American women are focusing on careers, delaying childbirth, and limiting family size.

Members of some cultures view childbearing and child-rearing differently. The birth of a child is crucial for many Hispanic, Navajo, Black, Middle Eastern, and Mormon women, whose social role and status are attained through reproduction within the marital relationship. Preference for a male child exists among families of many cultures, particularly Middle Eastern and Asian (Giger & Davidhizar, 2007).

In the dominant American culture, an infant frequently is wrapped warmly in blankets, placed in an infant seat or stroller, and put to sleep in a crib in a room separate from the parents. Mothers of other cultures may choose to carry or wrap their infants differently; women from some cultures carry their infants with them at all times and sleep with them. Southeast Asian infants may be carried in a hip sling or a blanket carrier. Native American infants often are carried in a cradleboard (a wooden frame into which an infant is bundled and tied). The cradleboard is properly blessed before it is used and can be carried, attached to the mother's back, hung from a tree, or propped up to keep the infant comfortable, safe, and secure (Andrews & Boyle, 2007).

Cultural beliefs and practices are continually evolving and changing. Nurses acknowledge and explore their meanings with all the families with which they meet. Nurses work actively to reduce the experience of culture shock for ethnic minority families, remembering that American medical beliefs and practices may appear strange to others. All behavior must be evaluated from within the context of the family and their cultural background and experience.

Nurses must facilitate health-promoting attitudes and practices and show empathic concern and respect for individuals of all cultural backgrounds. By incorporating the assessment of cultural beliefs and practices into the individual's plan of care, nurses can demonstrate respect and take a step forward in developing culturally appropriate patterns of caring.

In American culture the number of women choosing to breast-feed has steadily increased in recent years. Many factors are involved in the decision-making process. Nurses who care for families of newborns are aware of the multiplicity of factors influencing feeding choice and encourage and support parents in their decisions to promote health of newborns.

The family is the primary health care provider for the infant. The family determines health promotion of the family including when an infant is ill. Many cultural groups choose between the traditional or folk beliefs that they believe to be appropriate to them and Western medical treatment. The Vietnamese use both. For example, to decrease an infant's fever, a basil leaf is tied to the wrist with a piece of cheesecloth. For colic, a silver coin is dipped in wine and rubbed or scratched on the infant's back. Nurses are cautious in imposing their own values, beliefs, and attitudes on others. Rather than judging people by the nurse's ascertains how each family influences his practice's health outcomes.

The nurse remembers that all behaviors must be evaluated from within the context of the family's cultural background and experiences. Nurses who strive to foster health-promoting attitudes and behaviors begin at the most basic level: empathic concern and respect for the individual. By incorporating the assessment of cultural beliefs and practices into the infant's plan of care, nurses demonstrate respect, reduce alienation, and take a step toward developing culturally appropriate patterns of health promotion. Respecting another's language and religion is extremely important.

Language

Language is an important medium for understanding and working together. The nurse may avoid or tend to mumble a person's name when it is foreign; people hesitate to express themselves when the material is unfamiliar. The nurse must consider how the individual who speaks a different language feels about being unable to express thoughts and feelings or to understand what is being said. Both parties may play the avoidance game.

The nurse takes steps to remove communication barriers, including the following:

1. Using a professional interpreter to help in the communication process
2. Using pictorial flash cards in the individual's native language to assist in explaining instructions
3. Sending a health care worker to school to learn the basics of the language to help in the interpreting process in the health care facility

Even a person who speaks the nurse's language may not understand and comprehend instructions the nurse gives them.

Religion

In this pluralistic and democratic society, Americans are confronting the ethical and religious values that impinge on health care services. Interestingly, some providers believe that religion plays no role in individuals' health care practices; therefore, they eschew people's religious or ethical concerns and deal mainly with the physical or psychological problems at hand. However, the individual's religious and ethical concerns are generally the major source for human values when evaluating health care services.

Religious beliefs can become risk factors when they affect decisions concerning treatment. An example may be the parents who refuse a blood transfusion, surgery, or other medically indicated treatment required to save their infant's life. A court order is needed in many instances to treat these infants. The decision is the parents' responsibility, based on their customs and beliefs, and should be respected. Deciding not to offer an opinion may be extremely difficult, but usually the opinion is unwanted. Religion is often a powerful force, and when the nurse causes conflict and interferes, a gap can be formed. This gap may force the parents to seek nonprofessional health care to help them with their health-related and religious ideas about birth, death, stress, birth control, and other matters. To work successfully with an individual, the person's religious background should be investigated and understood thoroughly.

Legislation

Health and well-being have become generally accepted rights of everyone, without regard to color, gender, age, economic or social status, or creed. The federal government has pledged to promote the general welfare of the United States in the belief that it belongs to everyone.

To fulfill this pledge, several goals were established. One of these concerns is infant health. The goal, as described by the U.S. Department of Health and Human Services, is to "Improve the health and well-being of women, infants, children and families." (USDHHS, 2000, p. 16-10; *Healthy People Midcourse Review,* 2006 and the upcoming *Healthy People 2020*).

The infant mortality rate has been on a steady decline since the turn of the century, a result of better infant nutrition; improved technology; improved housing; and improved prenatal, obstetrical, and pediatric care (USDHHS, 2000). To meet the goal of improving infant health, major health problems in this age group must be reduced. A major hazard for infants is low birth weight. To address this problem, factors that increase the risk of low birth weight in infants must be identified (Box 17-17).

Many of these factors can be prevented, or risks can be identified early and managed to prevent low birth weight in infants. The major focus for prevention is prenatal care for all women.

Another major threat to infant survival is congenital disorders, such as malformations of the brain and spine (e.g., microcephaly and myelomeningocele), congenital heart defects (e.g., ventricular septal defects), and combinations of malformations, such as Down syndrome or Tay-Sachs disease. Some congenital abnormalities cannot be prevented, but many can be through prenatal screening and research to discover the "why" in the development of these birth defects.

| Box 17-17 | Low–Birth-Weight Risk Factors |

MATERNAL FACTORS
- Low socioeconomic status
- No prenatal care
- Preeclampsia and eclampsia
- Hypertension
- Chronic renal disease
- Advanced diabetes
- Malnutrition
- Cigarette smoking (10 per day or more)
- Drug addiction
- Maternal age (under 15 or over 35)
- Alcohol abuse
- Marital status

FETAL FACTORS
- Multiple gestation (twins)
- Congenital malformation
- Chromosomal abnormality
- Chronic intrauterine infection
- Placental insufficiency

Other factors identified by the U.S. Department of Health and Human Services (2000) and the *Healthy People Midcourse Review* (2006) and developing 2020 that contribute to the high infant mortality rate are (1) injuries at birth, (2) SIDS, (3) accidents, (4) respiratory distress syndrome, and (5) inadequate parenting.

The federal government's plans to attain the goal of healthy infants are the following:

1. Promote family planning services such that all pregnancies are planned and all infants are wanted.
2. Provide pregnancy and infant care services through Maternity and Infant Care (MIC) projects to high-risk populations. The WIC program improves the nutritional status of both mother and infant.
3. Encourage educational efforts by schools, health providers, and the media to promote prenatal care.
4. Promote massive immunization efforts such that each infant is protected from communicable disease.

Nursing's Role

Nurses have important roles in bringing about change in response to a continually expanding knowledge base, consumer health care needs, and governmental legislation. By actively participating in groups involved with health planning, the nurse helps make governmental policy more responsive to infants' health care needs.

The nurse's role in the development of health care policies has three stages: (1) identifying resources for the community to meet its specific need, (2) planning for resources not available to the community, and (3) coordinating the resources available to the community to promote better use of them.

The nurse can become a member of a health planning council, a concerned citizen's group, or an advisory group to a local legislator or to a state health department grant task force. In this capacity, the nurse's responsibility is to inform the other committee members. Because nurses have first-hand experience with many community needs, they are in a good position to speak out and inform others.

The nurse within the community also has several resources available to assist when a need is identified to promote the infant's health, including resources on the federal level (U.S. Department of Health and Human Services), state level (public health department), local level (MIC clinics and well baby clinics), and community groups (Parents Anonymous, hot lines, La Leche League, March of Dimes, and SIDS groups).

Coordinating for resources, the nurse actively participates in assessing the availability of services within the community and makes recommendations to consolidate or expand existing services. Making the public aware of community resources, their services, and existing needs is the basis of the nurse's role in developing policy.

Economics

Even in this society of considerable affluence, many people live below the poverty level. Poor families tend to be characterized as lacking education, having high unemployment rates, being large in size with female heads of household, residing in crowded living areas, and lacking adequate bathroom facilities (U.S. Census Bureau, 2000a). Virtually every major health problem is found more frequently in segments of the population with low income than in high-income groups. The infant mortality rates in low-income families remain significantly higher than do rates in high-income families, despite an overall decrease in infant mortality rate nationally (Guyer, 2008; *Healthy People 2010 Midcourse Review*, 2006 and the developing *Healthy People 2020*).

Studies have demonstrated that parents with low incomes are often unaware of their infant's developmental needs; they frequently are faced with many environmental and social stresses that demand their time, energy, and other resources (Hutchings, 2007). Many parents have so many unfulfilled needs of their own that they cannot meet their infants' needs.

In many cases, infants from families in poverty have delayed language development. With limited educational and life experiences, their parents are often unable to be ideal models for language development. Infants learn early language sounds from their parents, but their attempts at language must be reinforced.

Armed with the knowledge of how economics can affect the infant's growth, development, and health status, the nurse, before deciding interventions (see **Website Resource 17G**), assesses the family situation by performing the following tasks:

1. Establish a relationship with the family to obtain pertinent information.
2. Evaluate the home environment in which the infant interacts.
3. Elicit the parents' health perceptions about their own health and that of the infant.

4. Complete a thorough physical examination of the infant to identify any problem areas.
5. Identify community resources that are available to the low-income family.

Health Care Delivery System

The U.S. health care delivery system is diverse and large; many different sectors merge to provide infant care. Within this enormous, multidisciplinary system, the nurse is an advocate who facilitates the family's passage through the many facets of care. **Website Resource 17H** lists health care programs that have been established for the infant and the family for the purpose of disease prevention and health promotion and maintenance. Table 17-10 lists a suggested schedule for health-promotion infant care.

The value of health promotion and preventive health care has been validated; it is cost-effective and is here to stay. As nurses' roles continue to expand within the various parts of the health care system, their duty is to keep pace with the needs, concerns, and available strategies (Clark, 2008; Stanhope & Lancaster, 2008). Because many conditions that cause morbidity or mortality in infants are preventable when

Table 17-10 Suggested Schedule for Health-Promotion Infant Care

Age (Months)	Promotional Activity	Age (Months)	Promotional Activity
1	Complete physical assessment PKU test Immunizations: HepB-2 **Parent discussion includes:** Basic infant needs: to be touched, held, fondled, rocked, and talked to Appropriate toy: colorful mobile Nutrition: formula or breast milk		Use of finger foods Playing games with infant: pat-a-cake, peek-a-boo, waving bye-bye, and shaking hands Appropriate toys: blocks, stack toys, and jack-in-the-box Fear of strangers
2	Complete physical assessment Immunizations: DTaP-1, Hib-1, IPV-1, and PCV-1, Rota-1 **Parent discussion includes:** Placing infant in prone position to allow lifting of head Need of infant to be exposed to a variety of stimuli within environment Need of infant for change of scenery Colic and other common problems	12	Complete physical assessment Immunizations: TB test Laboratory work: CBC **Parent discussion includes:** Accident prevention Getting into things Infant's need to touch and investigate environment, with supervision Parent's need to read, show pictures, and repeat body parts to infant Infant's need for limited independence Sleeping patterns Appropriate toys: sets of measuring cups, nesting toys, pots and pans, and wooden spoons
4	Complete physical assessment Immunizations: DTaP-2, Hib-2, IPV-2, PCV-2, Rota-2 **Parent discussion includes:** Stimulation of infant Providing a mirror in which the infant can see reflection Being talked to and played with Appropriate toy: rattle	15	Complete physical assessment Immunizations: MMR, Hib-4, Varicella **Parent discussion includes:** Negativism as normal aspect of development Age of curiosity in infant Toys appropriate for age: push-pull toys and ball Accident prevention Elimination patterns Discipline: stress positive aspects of behavior, when possible
6	Complete physical assessment Immunizations: DTaP-3, Hib-3, HepB-3, IPV-3, PCV-3, Rota-3, and flu vaccine Laboratory work: hematocrit level **Parent discussion includes:** Accident prevention Teething and use of cool rings Allowing infant to crawl to explore environment Stranger anxiety	18	Complete physical assessment Immunizations: DTaP-4 **Parent discussion includes:** Accident prevention Begin toilet training, if child is ready Encourage vocalization Socialization with other small children Importance of reading to child Setting limits on behavior Coping mechanisms of parents
9	Complete physical assessment **Parent discussion includes:** Accident prevention Dental caries prevention: cleaning teeth with gauze daily Infant's need for space to crawl about Use cup if weaning		

CBC, Complete blood count; *DTaP*, diphtheria, tetanus, acellular pertussis vaccine; *HepB*, hepatitis B vaccine; *Hib*, Haemophilus influenza type B conjugate vaccine; *IPV*, inactivated polio vaccine; *MMR*, measles, mumps, rubella vaccine; *PCV*, pneumococcal vaccine; *Rota*, Rotavirus; *PKU*, phenylketonuria; *TB*, tuberculin.

health-promotion practices are employed, nurses have the mission of working within the health care system to promote infant health (*Healthy People 2010 Midcourse Review*, 2006).

SUMMARY

Society is changing, as are people's needs and ideas. Families today want more information and knowledge, and they demand that health care professionals be more responsive to their needs. Their demand has been a catalyst for the nurse's expanded health care role and responsibility for health promotion.

Health-promotion and disease prevention practices that are applicable during infancy can be used in the nurse's expanded role. A four-pronged approach is stressed:

1. Giving anticipatory guidance to the family unit as the infant grows and develops
2. Teaching and counseling to ensure the infant's optimal development
3. Being a family advocate to ensure the safety and development of the family unit
4. Screening to identify infants at risk of developing a condition via history gathering, physical exam, observation of parent-child interaction, and laboratory testing

Anticipating potential health problems during infancy and effectively intervening to avert these problems are nursing processes that promote health. Early detection and reduction of risk factors avoid many health problems, such as abuse. By anticipating problems and helping families to avoid them, the nurse promotes health maintenance.

Using the infant's normal growth and development, psychosocial tasks, common health problems, and health maintenance strategies, the nurse makes an assessment of the infant, the family, and the infant's developmental status to provide anticipatory guidance.

By teaching, an essential component of the nursing process, the nurse transmits knowledge to families to ensure continuity of care and long-term health maintenance. By counseling, the nurse listens to the identified problem, helps the family to recognize the real issues, and allows the family to make its own decisions regarding health care.

Because the infant is in no position to advocate effectively, the nurse assumes this role. The ultimate goal of nursing intervention in maintaining the infant's health is future self-care. As the infant grows and matures, well-established family health maintenance habits can only enhance the lives of healthy future generations. The nurse is challenged to join this effort of investment in the future.

CASE STUDY

Homelessness: Homeless Infants

As a community health nurse in an inner-city health center, you are increasingly aware that the homeless population in your city appears to be the forgotten aggregate. Your community health center provides primary care to a culturally diverse and indigent population. As a nurse, you believe that the homeless population within your city has numerous health needs. Beyond the basic requirements, many homeless people have mental and substance abuse problems, lack of life skills, poor family support, and most of all no child health access.

The homeless population has all of the usual health problems you would expect in the general population in addition to other problems resulting from their homeless lifestyle. Although there are several glaring concerns, you plan to focus your attention first on securing immunizations for the homeless infants and, secondly, to obtain formula for them.

Reflective Questions:

1. In planning health services for this special population, what facts do you need to know?
2. What barriers to accessing health care for infants confront the homeless family?
3. How can you overcome some of the barriers in developing your plan for health care?

Discussion

1. In planning health services for this special population, what facts do you need to know? Some of the first questions that should be asked are:
   - How many homeless infants are in this aggregate?
   - Where are they?
   - How can they access health care in the city?

To answer these questions, it might be prudent to collaborate and partner with other health and social service agencies, local hospitals, and the state health and human services agency. Collaboration and partnering can bring in additional resources and reduce duplication and gaps in services.

2. What barriers to accessing health care for infants confront the homeless family?
   - Lack of transportation
   - Lack of trust in the medical establishment
   - Judgmental care on the part of health care providers
   - No health insurance to cover medical visits
   - Preventive care, such as immunizations, not a priority when you are hungry
   - No money to get prescriptions filled
   - Waiting until condition is serious before seeking treatment

3. How can you overcome some of the barriers in developing your plan for health care?
   - Provide health care in the city shelters for use by homeless families.
   - Set up a mobile health care team and visit the shelters to provide care.
   - Offer free immunizations for all family members.
   - Set up educational sessions within the shelters to provide information.
   - Stress importance of preventive measures to reduce illness in infants.
   - Obtain free formula from company or hospitals to give to homeless infants.
   - Work closely with other health care interests within the community.

CARE PLAN

Homelessness: Homeless Infants

Homelessness is a community dilemma and an example of an economic problem that places infants at risk. Families are the fastest growing group of homeless people. Homeless families do not have health insurance; infants within these families are more likely to lack immunizations, proper nutrition, safe environment, and a stable family situation. The community health nurse in this chapter's Case Study wants to address two aspects of homeless infants: (1) immunizations and (2) nutrition.

Nursing Diagnosis: Altered Health Maintenance Related to Nonadherence to Appropriate Immunization Schedule as Manifested by Increased Incidence of Communicable Diseases

DEFINING CHARACTERISTICS

History of lack of health-seeking behavior by caregiver; lack of financial or other resources; reported or observed impairment of personal support systems; lack of knowledge regarding health-promotion practices; inability to access health care; limited basic personal resources

RELATED FACTORS

Ineffective family coping; perceptual-cognitive impairment; lack of material resources; ineffective individual coping

EXPECTED OUTCOMES

Caretaker of infant will:
- Begin health-seeking behavior on behalf of infant
- Increase health-promotion and health-maintenance knowledge
- Gain access to available health care resources
- Participate in life change to improve health status; meet goals for health care maintenance

NURSING INTERVENTIONS

- Assess caretaker's feelings, values, and personal situation.
- Assess for family patterns, economic issues, and cultural patterns that influence compliance.
- Assist caretaker and family to access health care resources available to them.
- Refer caretaker and family to community agencies to address social and economic issues.

- Educate caretaker and family on the importance of immunizations and disease prevention.
- Provide for follow-up to increase chance of health status change taking place.

Nursing Diagnosis: High Risk for Altered Nutrition—Less than Body Requirements; related factors and socioeconomic factors as manifested by low height and weight measurements for chronological age on growth chart

DEFINING CHARACTERISTICS

Pale conjunctival and mucus membranes; poor muscle development; inadequate food intake to maintain body weight; weight loss, fatigue, frequent irritable, fussy, crying behavior; growth and development milestones not met; frequent illnesses suggesting depressed immunity

RELATED FACTORS

Inability to obtain adequate food or fluid or both to nourish body because of socioeconomic factors

EXPECTED OUTCOMES

Infant will demonstrate the following:
- Progressive weight gains toward desired goal
- Weight within normal range for height and weight
- Infant consuming adequate nourishment
- Infant free of signs of malnutrition

NURSING INTERVENTIONS

- Assess healthy body weight for age and height.
- Observe infant's ability to consume food and fluids.
- Monitor food and fluid intake weekly.
- Access nutritional resources for the caretaker or family.
- Refer to appropriate community agencies to meet needs.
- Assist the caretaker or family to identify area needing change that will make the greatest contribution to improve nutrition.
- Implement instructional dialogue that is appropriate for their level.
- Provide for follow-up care to assist them in changing their health status.

For further information on developing care plans, see: Carpenito-Moyet, L. J. (2008). *Nursing diagnosis: Application to clinical practice* (12th ed.). Philadelphia: Lippincott, Williams & Wilkins.

REFERENCES

American Academy of Pediatrics (AAP). (2005). Breastfeeding the use of human milk. *Pediatrics, 115*(2), 496–506.

American Academy of Pediatrics Task Force on Sudden Infant Death Syndrome. (2005). The changing concept of sudden infant death syndrome: Diagnostic coding shifts, controversies regarding the sleeping environment, and new variables to consider in reducing risk. *Pediatrics, 116*(5), 1245–1255.

American Academy of Pediatrics (AAP). (2007). *Child Abuse.* [Online] Retrieved from *www.aap.org/publiced/BK0_ChildAbuse.htm.*

American Academy of Pediatrics (AAP). (2007). *Car safety seats: A guide for families 2007.* [Online] Retrieved from *www.aap.org/family/carseatguide.htm.*

American Academy of Pediatrics. (2003). *Campaign launched to avoid sudden death in childcare settings.* Retrieved October 27, 2007, from *www.aap.org/advocacy/archieves/jansids.htm.*

American Academy of Pediatrics. (2007). *Bright futures: Guidelines for health supervision of infants, children, and adolescents* (3rd ed.). Elk Park, IL: American Academy of Pediatrics.

American Heart Association (AHA). (2006). American Heart Association guidelines for cardiopulmonary resuscitation and emergency cardiovascular care of pediatric and neonatal patients: Pediatric basic life support. *Pediatrics, 117*(5), 989–1004.

American Public Health Association (APHA). (2006). *Unintentional injuries in children. APHA 134th Annual Meeting and Exposition.* [Online] Available at *www.cmemedscape.com/viewarticle/553273*

Andrews, M. M., & Boyle, J. S. (2007). *Transcultural concepts in nursing care* (5th ed.). Philadelphia, PA: Lippincott Williams Wilkins.

Brazelton, T. B., & Sparrow, J. A. (2006). *Touchpoints: Your child's emotional and behavioral development* (2nd ed.). Cambridge, MA: Perseus/Da Capo Press.

Burge, T. (2007). *Foundations of mind.* New York: Oxford University Press.

Berk, L. E. (2007). *Infants and children: Prenatal through middle childhood* (6th ed.). Boston: Allyn & Bacon/Longman Publishers.

Carter, C. S., Lamb, M. E., Hardy, S. B., Porges, S. W., & Ahnert, L. (2006). *Attachment and bonding: A new synthesis.* Cambridge, MA: MIT Press.

Centers for Disease Control and Prevention (CDC). (2007). *Hemophilia* [Online] Retrieved from *www.cdc.gov/ncbddd/hbd/hemophilia.htm.*

Centers for Disease Control and Prevention (CDC). (2007). Recommended immunization schedules for persons aged 0-18 years—United States, 2007. *MMWR, 55*(51-52), Q1–Q4.

Centers for Disease Control and Prevention (CDC). (2007). *Sickle cell disease: Data and statistics.* [Online] Retrieved from *www.cdc.gov.mill1.sjlibrary.org/ncbddd/sicklecell/hcp_data.htm.*

Clark, M. J. (2008). *Community health nursing: Advocacy for population health* (5th ed.). Upper Saddle River, NJ: Pearson Prentice Hall.

Coch, D., Dawson, G., & Fischer, K. W. (2007). *Human behavior, learning, and the developing brain: Typical development.* New York: Guilford Publications.

Dacey, J., & Travers, J. (2006). *Human development across the lifespan* (6th ed.). Boston: McGraw-Hill.

Damato, E. G. (2007). Safe sleep: Can pacifiers reduce SIDS risk? *Nursing for Women's Health, 11*(1), 72–76.

DeBruyne, L., Whitney, E. N., & Pinna, K. (2007). *Nutrition and diet therapy* (7th ed.). Belmont, CA: Wadsworth Publishers.

Dorland, N. W. (2007). *Dorland's illustrated medical dictionary* (31st ed.). Philadelphia, PA: Elsevier Health Sciences.

Dudek, S. G. (2007). *Nutritional essentials for nursing practice* (5th ed.). Philadelphia, PA: Lippincott Williams & Wilkins.

Farrell, M. L., & Nicoteri, J. L. (2007). *Nutrition* (2nd ed.). Sudbury, MA: Jones & Bartlett.

Figueiredo, B., Costa, R., Pacheco, A., & Pais, A. (2007). Mother-to-infant and father-to-infant initial emotional involvement. *Early Child Development & Care, 177*(5), 521–532.

Fullerton-Smith, J. (2007). *The truth about food: What you eat can change your life.* New York: Bloomsbury USA.

Gardner, H. G. (2007). Office-based counseling for unintentional injury prevention. *Pediatrics, 119*(1), 202–206.

Gerson, J. (2007). *Hope springs maternal* (2nd ed.). New York: Altschuler & Associates.

Giger, J. N., & Davidhizar, R. E. (2007). *Transcultural nursing: Assessment and intervention* (5th ed.). St. Louis: Mosby.

Guyer, R. L. (2008). *Baby at risk.* Sterling, VA: Capital Books, Incorporated.

Hagan, J. F., Shaw, J. S., & Duncan, P. (2008). *Bright futures guidelines for health supervision of infants, children, and adolescents* (3rd ed.). Elk Grove Village, IL: American Academy of Pediatrics.

Hockenberry, M. J., & Wilson, D. (2006). *Wong's nursing care of infants and children* (8th ed.). St. Louis: Mosby.

Hutchings, J. (2007). *Enhancing parenting skills.* Oxford: Routledge.

Institute of Medicine (IOM). (2007). *Dietary supplement fact sheet: Vitamin D.* [Online] Retrieved from *http://ods.od.nih.gov/factsheets/vitamind.asp.*

Institute of Medicine (IOM). (2007). *Dietary reference intakes: The essential guide to nutrient requirements.* [Online] Retrieved from *www.iom.edu/CMS/3788/29985/37065.aspx.*

Jacknowitz, A., Novillo, D., & Tiehen, L. (2007). Special supplemental nutrition program for women, infants, and children and infant feeding practices. *Pediatrics, 119*(2), 281–289.

Jarvis, C. (2007). *Physical examination and Health assessment* (5th ed.). St. Louis: Elsevier.

Kenner, C., & Lott, J. W. (2007). *Comprehensive neonatal care: An interdisciplinary approach* (4th ed.). St. Louis: Elsevier.

Klaus, M. H., Kennell, J. H., & Klaus, P. H. (2000). *Bonding: Building the foundations of secure attachment and independence.* New York: Perseus Book Group.

Lashley, F. R. (2007). *Essentials of clinical genetics in nursing practice.* New York, NY: Springer.

Leikin, J. B., & McFee, R. B. (2007). *Handbook of nuclear, biological, and chemical agent exposures.* Baca Raton, FL: CRC Press.

Maloney, J. M., Sampson, H. A., Sicherer, S. H., & Burks, W. A. (2006). Food allergy and the introduction of solid foods to infants: A consensus document. *Annals of Allergy, Asthma & Immunology, 97*(4), 559–560.

McLaren, C., Null, J., & Quinn, J. (2005). Heat stress from enclosed vehicles: moderate ambient temperatures cause significant temperature rise in enclosed vehicles. *Pediatrics, 116*(1), 109–112.

Miller, L. C., Cook, J. T., Brooks, C. W., Heine, A. G., & Curtis, T. K. (2007). Breastfeeding education: Empowering future health care providers. *Nursing for Women's Health, 11*(4), 374–380.

Miniño, A. M., Heron, M. P., & Smith, B. (2006). Deaths: Preliminary data for 2004. *National Vital; Statistics Reports, 54*(19), 1–49.

Moon, R. Y., & Fu, L. Y. (2007). Sudden infant death syndrome. *Pediatrics in Review, 28*(6), 209–214.

National Cancer Institute (NCI). (2007). *Childhood cancers.* [Online] Retrieved from *www.cancer.gov/cancerinfo/types/childhoodcancers.*

National Center for Health Statistics, Health Resources and Services Administration, U.S. Department of Health and Human Services. (2007). *Height and weight measurement for girls.* Hyattsville, MD: National Center for Health Statistics.

National Health Care for the Homeless Council (NHCHC). (2007). *Homeless children: What every health care provider should know.* [Online] Retrieved from *www.nhchc.org/Children/.*

National Institute of Environmental Health Sciences (NIEHS). (2007). *Lead.* [Online] Retrieved from *www.niehs.nih.gov/health/topics/agents/lead/index.cfm.*

National Institute of Environmental Health Sciences (NIEHS). (2007). *Asthma.* [Online] Retrieved from *www.niehs.nih.gov/health/topics/agents/asthma/index.cfm.*

Nelson, L. S., Shih, R. D., & Balick, M. J. (2007). *Handbook of poisonous and injurious plants* (2nd ed.). New York: Springer-Verlag LLC.

Olson, D. H., DeFrain, J. D., & Skogrand, L. (2007). *Marriages and families: Intimacy, diversity and strengths* (6th ed.). Boston: McGraw-Hill Higher Education.

Oppenheim, D., & Goldsmith, D. F. (2007). *Attachment theory in clinical work with children: Bridging the gap between research and practice.* New York: Guilford Publications.

Peragallo, N., & Gonzalez, R. M. (2007). Nursing research and the prevention of infectious diseases among vulnerable populations. *Annual Review of Nursing Research, 25,* 83–117.

Pillitteri, A. (2007). *Maternal and child health nursing: Care of the childbearing and childrearing family* (5th ed.). Philadelphia, PA: Lippincott Williams & Wilkins.

Polan, E., & Taylor, D. (2007). *Journey across the lifespan: Human development and health promotion* (3rd ed.). Philadelphia: F.A. Davis.

Puckett, M. B., & Black, J. K. (2007). *Understanding infant development.* St. Paul, MN: Redleaf Press.

Reich, J. B. (2007). *Babyproofing bible: The exceedingly thorough guide to keeping your child safe from crib to kitchen to car to yard.* Beverly, MA: Fair Winds Press.

Researchers: Don't let infants sleep unattended in car seats. (2007). *Family Safety & Health, 66*(1), 4.

Sarnquist, C. C., Cunningham, S. D., Sullivan, B., & Maldonado, Y. (2007). The effectiveness of state and national policy on the implementation of perinatal HIV prevention interventions. *American Journal of Public Health, 97*(6), 1041–1046.

Schwartz, M. A., & Scott, B. M. (2007). *Marriages and families: Diversity and change* (5th ed.). Paramus, NJ: Prentice Hall.

Schwerdtfeger, K. L. & Goff, B. S. (2007). Intergenerational transmission of trauma: Exploring mother-infant prenatal attachment. *Journal of Traumatic Stress, 20*(1), 39–51.

Shaw, V., & Lawson, M. (2007). *Clinical paediatric dietetics* (3rd ed.). Boston: Blackwell Publishing Professional.

Stamm, J., & Spencer, P. (2007). *Bright from the start: The simple, science-backed way to nurture your child's developing mind from birth to age 3.* New York: Penguin Group (USA).

Stanhope, M., & Lancaster, J. (2008). *Public health nursing: Population-centered health care in the community* (7th ed.). St. Louis: Mosby.

St James-Roberts, I. (2007). Helping parents to manage infant crying and sleeping: A review of the evidence and its implications for services. *Child Abuse Review, 16*(1), 47–69.

U.S. Census Bureau. (2000a). *Characteristics of the population below the poverty level.* Washington, DC: U.S. Government Printing Office.

U.S. Census Bureau. (2000b). *Statistical abstract of the United States: 2000. Child abuse* (120th ed.). Washington, DC: U.S. Government Printing Office.

U.S. Department of Health and Human Services. (2000). *Healthy People 2010* (Vol. 1 and 2, Conference ed.). Washington, DC: U.S. Government Printing Office.

U.S. Department of Health and Human Services (USDHHS). (2006). *Healthy People 2010 Midcourse Review.* Washington, DC: U.S. Government Printing Office.

Waldburger, J., & Spivak, J. (2007). *The sleepeasy solution: The exhausted parent's guide to getting your child to sleep—from birth to age 5.* Deerfield Beach, FL: Health Communications.

Walsh, C. (2007). Treatment and follow-up for infants born to HIV-positive women. *Clinical Nurse Specialist, 7*(2), 8–10.

Wilhelmsson, S., & Lindberg, M. (2007). Prevention and health promotion and evidence-based fields of nursing—A literature review. *International Journal of Nursing Practice, 13*(4), 254–265.

World Health Organization (WHO) and Joint United Nations Program on HIV/AIDS (UNAIDS). (2007). *New data on male circumcision and HIV prevention: Policy and programme implications.* Retrieved from *http://data.unaids.org/pub/Report/2007/mc_recommendations_en.pdf.*

Chapter 18

Martha Driessnack*

Toddler

*The author acknowledges the work of Marinda Allender as the author of this chapter in a previous edition.

objectives

After completing this chapter, the reader will be able to:

- Describe the physical growth, developmental, and maturational changes that occur during the toddler period.
- Outline the recommended health promotion and disease prevention visits for the toddler and the appropriate topics for anticipatory guidance for their parents.
- Discuss developmentally appropriate approaches to toddlers.
- Analyze the factors that contribute to the heightened vulnerability of toddlers to injury and abuse.

key terms

Amblyopia
Autism spectrum disorders
Autonomy
Child abuse
Conditioned-play audiometry
Doubt
Egocentrism

Lumbar lordosis
Masturbation
Night terrors
Object permanence
Otitis media
Parallel play
Preoperational stage
Rituals

Sensorimotor stage
Shame
Strabismus
Styes
Temperament
Toilet training
Visual-reinforcement audiometry

website materials

evolve These materials are located on the book's website at *http://evolve.elsevier.com/Edelman/*.
- WebLinks
- Study Questions
- Glossary

455

THINK About It

Reframing the Terrible Twos

A young mother tells the nurse that she is convinced that her 22 month old, who used to be the sweetest child around, has entered what must be the terrible twos. She reports that her child's favorite words include "mine" and "no," with "no" being the response to every request the mother makes. In addition, the child is getting increasingly stubborn and just threw her first public temper tantrum. The mother says that she is tired of saying and hearing "no" and turns to the nurse for help.

1. How does the nurse explain the relationship between the child's stage of psychosocial development and meaning behind the child's behaviors?
2. What suggestions can the nurse give to the mother to respond sensitively to her child's evolving need for independence while balancing her own need to provide for and protect her child?

Having spent their first year of life getting to know and trust their parents and other child care providers and their immediate environments, toddlers' increasing mobility now allows them to begin to expand their worlds, bringing excitement and challenges to both themselves and their parents. Toddlers are ready to develop a sense of self and separate from their parents, and understanding and respecting this evolving independence is a common parental challenge. Their behaviors can be frustrating, but the toddlers' delight in their own emerging competence and achievements can bring a sense of joy and accomplishment to everyone around them (Figure 18-1; Warren et al., 2008).

Nurses explain to parents and other primary care providers the many physical and developmental changes that occur in toddlers and how these changes contribute to their vulnerability to injury, their overall health, and that of the family unit. Unfortunately, the recommended schedule for health-promotion and disease-prevention visits for this age group provides for fewer contacts than during infancy. Parents may begin to fall into a pattern of illness care, missing the continued opportunity to receive anticipatory guidance and health-promotion information until preschool or school requirements bring them back in. The nurse plays an integral role in encouraging health-promotion efforts and behaviors (American Academy of Pediatrics, 2008; Hockenberry & Wilson, 2006).

AGE AND PHYSICAL CHANGES

The toddler period extends from 12 to 18 months to 3 years of age. The overall growth rate slows significantly, and the increasingly active toddlers begin the process of shedding baby fat and straightening their posture. Toddlers have a protuberant abdomen, accentuated by a **lumbar lordosis**, and a characteristic gait, in which their feet are planted wide apart and appear flat because of an extra fat pad in the instep for stability.

A slow, steady growth in height of 2 to 4 inches per year and in weight of 4 to 6 pounds per year occurs during toddlerhood and remains steady until puberty. Birth weight usually quadruples by 2½ years of age, and the toddler's height at age 2 years is approximately 50% of final adult height (Hockenberry & Wilson, 2007). The toddler's stature may be measured in a recumbent position for length, as in infancy, or in a standing position for height. Depending on the position, the nurse selects the appropriate Centers for Disease Control and Prevention (CDC) growth chart. The nurse continues to measure head circumference throughout the toddler period. The anterior fontanel usually closes by 18 months, the skull begins to thicken, and by 24 months it is 80% of its adult size (Hockenberry & Wilson, 2007).

The kidneys are well differentiated by the toddler years, and specific gravity and other urine findings are similar to those of adults. The daily excretion of urine for the 2-year-old child is 500 to 600 mL, increasing to 750 mL for the 3 year old. Toddlers empty their bladders less frequently than infants and begin to develop voluntary control of urination. However, full control comes later.

The toddler's gastrointestinal tract also reaches functional maturity, although it continues to grow into adulthood. The toddler tends to need meals and snacks more frequently than an older child or adult. Most toddlers develop sufficient voluntary control of internal and external anal sphincters to accomplish successful bowel training.

Bowel control typically precedes urinary control. Lung capacity continues to increase as the toddler grows, and the respiratory rate decreases from a mean of 30 breaths per minute at 1 year of age to 25 breaths per minute at 3 years. The diameter of the toddler's upper respiratory tract is small when compared with that of an older child or adult. This small diameter, coupled with toddler's exploratory nature and lack of judgment in deciding what to place in the mouth, can result in accidental airway obstruction, which demands emergency action.

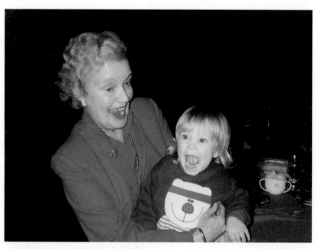

Figure 18-1 A toddler and her grandmother share a happy moment.

The anatomy of the ear, eustachian tube, and nasal pharynx continue to resemble those of the infant more closely than those of the adult, continuing the risk for otitis media. The tonsils and adenoids remain proportionately large during the toddler years (Seidel et al., 2006).

With the exception of reproductive functions, most endocrine organs become functionally mature during the toddler and preschool years, although function continues at a minimum. The production of glucagon and insulin can be limited or labile, producing variations in blood glucose levels throughout early childhood. The production of cortisol, aldosterone, and deoxycorticosterone by the adrenal cortex remains somewhat limited, but they appear to function effectively in protecting the young child from the hazards of fluid and electrolyte imbalance well known in infancy. Secretion of epinephrine and norepinephrine from the adrenal medulla increases sufficiently to perform homeostatic functions of the autonomic nervous system and to mediate certain aspects of increased emotional components of behavior. Regulation of growth during early childhood remains one of the most important functions of the endocrine system.

Changes in the circulatory system include a decrease in heart rate, increase in blood pressure, and changing vascular resistance in response to growth in the size of various vessel lumens. The toddler's heart rate ranges from 80 to 120 beats per minute and the mean blood pressure is 90/56 mm Hg. Getting the toddler to sit still for a blood pressure reading can be difficult, but it is worth the effort to obtain several baseline readings for future reference.

The capillary beds gradually increase their capacity to respond to heat and cold in the environment, providing the toddler with more effective thermoregulation. Toddlers can also begin to take voluntary measures to relieve the discomfort of heat or cold. For example, the older toddler can put on clothing or move to warmer or cooler areas, assisting physiological efforts to maintain a constant internal thermal environment.

The immune response continues to mature. As toddlers expand their worlds through playgrounds and day care centers, exposure to new and different organisms is greatly increased. They may experience a period during which they appear to succumb to many minor respiratory and gastrointestinal infections. As immunity begins to develop against the organisms in their new environments, their resistance similarly increases.

Passive immunity to communicable disease acquired through transfer of maternal antibodies during fetal life has disappeared, and active immunity through the initial immunization series is usually completed by the age of 18 months. The next scheduled immunizations do not occur until age 4 to 6 years, prior to entering kindergarten. If a toddler is behind in the initial immunization series, a separate schedule is available that gives catch-up schedules and minimum intervals between doses. See **Website Resource 17E** for detailed immunization schedules.

All 20 primary or deciduous teeth erupt by the end of toddlerhood (Figure 18-2). Timing of these eruptions can vary widely, but a variation in the sequence alerts the nurse to inquire about early trauma to the mouth or familial traits for out-of-sequence tooth eruption. Other important aspects of dental care at this age that are included in health teaching are listed in Box 18-1.

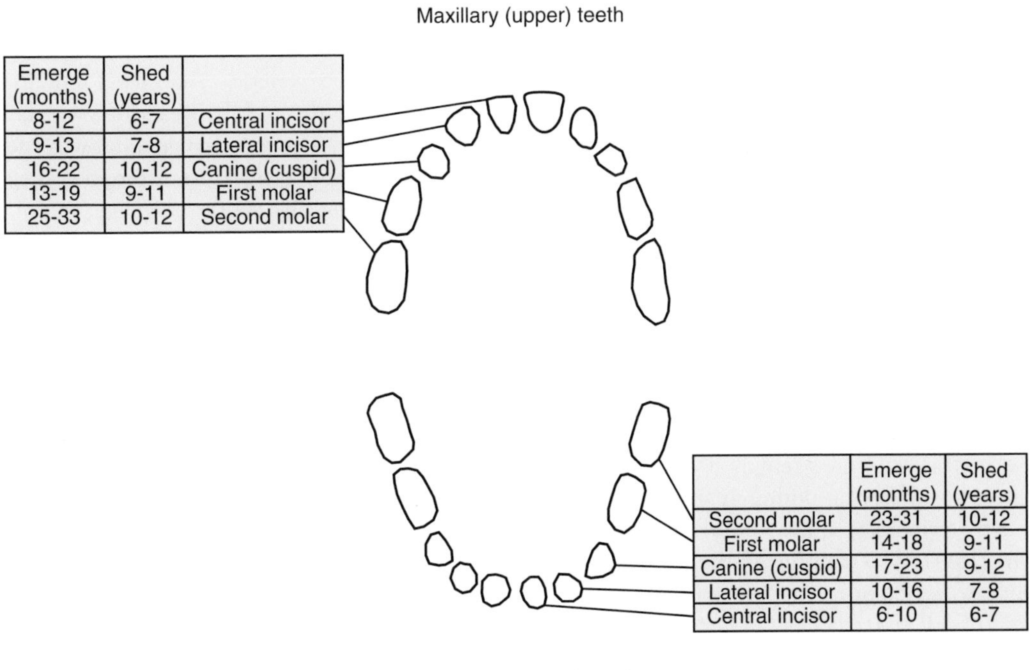

Maxillary (upper) teeth

Emerge (months)	Shed (years)	
8-12	6-7	Central incisor
9-13	7-8	Lateral incisor
16-22	10-12	Canine (cuspid)
13-19	9-11	First molar
25-33	10-12	Second molar

	Emerge (months)	Shed (years)
Second molar	23-31	10-12
First molar	14-18	9-11
Canine (cuspid)	17-23	9-12
Lateral incisor	10-16	7-8
Central incisor	6-10	6-7

Mandibular (lower) teeth

Figure 18-2 Eruption (and shedding) of primary teeth.

Box **18-1** | **Nursing Interventions to Promote Dental Health Care for Toddlers**

BRUSHING

- Use a soft-bristled brush. The gauze method used during infancy is no longer adequate because the teeth are too close together to allow a finger wrapped in gauze to reach all surfaces.
- Introduce only a moist toothbrush at first. After the toddler has accepted the toothbrush, begin using toothpaste. A pea-size amount is adequate. If the child does not like the taste of the toothpaste, use plain water.
- Toothpaste should contain fluoride.
- Toddlers do not have the motor coordination to brush their own teeth. They may enjoy imitating parents and put the toothbrush in their mouths, but an adult should be responsible for the actual brushing.
- Brush daily; for many toddlers, this practice becomes part of the bedtime routine. When the child appears too tired to cooperate in the evening, the parent should choose some other time of day when this important task will not be so difficult.

FOODS

- Limit foods high in sugar.
- When the young toddler still drinks from a bottle, only plain water should be given. Milk and juices should be offered by cup. If milk or juice is given in a bottle, it should never be done at naptime or bedtime.

VISITS TO THE DENTIST

- The first visit to the dentist should occur during the toddler years. Many dentists suggest an introduction-orientation, inspection-consultation type of visit when the child is approximately 18 months of age. This type of visit provides an early, enjoyable introduction to professional dental health promotion and care.

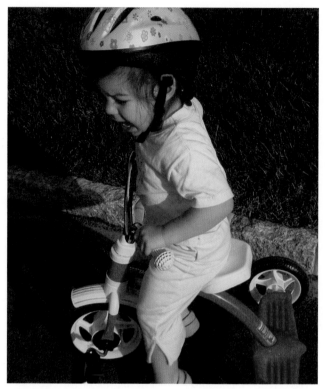

Figure 18-3 Toddlers enjoy learning coordination of large muscle groups.

A mature swallowing pattern, using the tongue rather than the cheeks, has not yet developed, and toddlers continue to be at risk for choking. Toddlers who are mouth, rather than nose, breathers because of ongoing respiratory illness or allergies may have an underdeveloped palatal arch. With normal breathing, the tongue rests on and naturally widens the palate; however, when the child is forced to breathe through the mouth, the tongue rests in the lower jaw, not on the palate. This resultant narrowing of the palatal arch sets these toddlers up for dental crowding when the permanent teeth erupt.

An increase in the size and strength of muscle fibers continues. During this period, as during infancy, the use of muscle tissues is the primary stimulus for increased size and strength (Figure 18-3). Myelination of the corticospinal tract is functionally sufficient to support most movement, but achievement of full control does not occur until much later in life. Throughout early childhood, voluntary motor movement is often accompanied by involuntary movements on the other side of the body. This mirroring of action is more pronounced in children who suffer some damage of the central nervous system, but the mechanisms by which this occurs are unknown. The toddler generally does not show complete dominance of one-sided body function and may still switch hands when eating, throwing a ball, or engaging in other-handed activities.

Most genetic syndromes and disease entities are diagnosed either during the prenatal period or during infancy. However, some genetic syndromes and diseases are not detected until the toddler years or even later. The most common initial sign is a change in growth pattern or developmental delays. Delays are often not diagnosed during infancy because the subtle language, motor, or cognitive deficiencies do not interfere with the expected performance and behavior.

GORDON'S FUNCTIONAL HEALTH PATTERNS
Health Perception–Health Management Pattern

Toddlers may come to know that being sick means feeling bad or having to stay in bed, but they have little, if any, understanding of the meaning of health. They may perform or request some health-promotion activities, such as brushing teeth, but they do it as part of their bedtime ritual and not because they know this activity will prevent caries. Toddlers depend on their parents for health management, and their overall health will be greatly influenced by their parents' health perceptions and health management priorities (*Healthy People 2010* box).

Healthy People 2010 (Midcourse Review)

Selected Health-Promotion and Disease-Prevention Objectives for Toddlers

- Reduce iron deficiency to less than 5% among children between ages 1 and 2 (baseline is 9% among children between ages 1 and 2 in 1994).
- Reduce drowning deaths among children ages 4 and younger to no more than 0.7 per 100,000 (adjusted baseline is 1.6 per 100,000 in 1998; 0.9 per 100,000 in 2000).
- Increase use of child restraints to 100% of children ages 4 and younger (baseline is 92% in 1998).
- Reduce nonfatal poisoning among children ages 4 and younger to no more than 292 per 100,000 (baseline is 348.4 per 100,000 in 1997).
- Achieve total elimination of blood lead levels exceeding 10 mg/dL among children ages 1 to 5 years (baseline is 4.4% of children ages 1 to 5 years had blood level exceeding 10 mg/dL in 1994).

From *Healthy People 2010*: Midcourse Review. (2007). Office of Disease Prevention and Health Promotion (ODPHP) of the Office of Public Health, U.S. Department of Health and Human Services. *http://odphp. osophs.dhhs.gov/pubs/*.

Toddlers identify with parents, caregivers, and other important role models, internalizing a wide range of lifestyle attributes. Parents' and caregivers' health perceptions and health behaviors should model the perceptions and behaviors desired for health promotion. Toddlers whose parents eat a variety of foods are more likely to try new foods. Such modeling increases the chances that good practices will be retained throughout the toddler's life. The nurse's task is to help parents strengthen their confidence and self-esteem as parents and provide them with the information needed to anticipate and meet the developmental needs of their toddler as they develop as a family.

Nutritional-Metabolic Pattern

Weaning from the breast (Gubala, 2007) or bottle usually occurs before or during toddlerhood. Adequate iron intake must be ensured as the toddler changes from breast milk or iron-fortified formula and cereal to whole cow's milk, which is low in iron. Milk also interferes with the absorption of iron from other food sources. A toddler who continues to ingest whole milk from a bottle tends to drink up to 32 ounces per day. This practice blunts the child's appetite at meal-times including foods that contain iron (Wright et al., 2007). The use of a bottle with milk or juice, especially at bedtime, has also been associated with dental caries (baby bottle tooth decay). If parents want to give a bottle at bedtime, it should contain only water.

Fruit juice and drinks are often overconsumed because they taste good, are conveniently packaged and carried around by the toddler, and because they are viewed as nutritious. The American Academy of Pediatrics (AAP) Committee on

research highlights

NEAT: Nutrition Education Aimed at Toddlers

Healthful eating behavior, developed early in life, has the potential to persist into adulthood. And the toddler years appear to be a critical period for influencing children's eating habits. While toddlers are learning to feed themselves, they are also being introduced to new foods and experiencing fluctuation in rates of growth and appetite. The Nutrition Education Aimed at Toddlers (NEAT) curriculum, developed at Michigan State University, was part of an interventional study designed to help parents gain the knowledge and skills needed to help their toddlers acquire healthful eating habits. It is based on Social Cognitive Theory (SCT), in which personal factors, environmental influences, and behavior interact.

The NEAT curricular intervention contained a series of 4 lessons and 18 reinforcing activities. The lessons and reinforcing activities included strategies for introducing new foods to toddlers, dealing with "picky" eaters, developing parenting skills related to feeding toddlers, dealing with toddlers' behaviors, and involving toddlers in food preparation. Different tools were provided to parents, including a development wheel and a child-sized utensil.

The results indicate that parents in the intervention group significantly increased their knowledge, allowed their children more independence when eating, and had the television on less frequently than parents in the control group. The lessons and reinforcing activities could be delivered by nurses working with families on a one-to-one basis or incorporated into parenting classes.

Coleman, G., Horodynski, M. A., Contres, D., & Hoerr, S. M. (2005). Nutritional Education Aimed at Toddlers (NEAT) Curriculum. *Journal of Nutrition Education and Behavior, 37*(2), 96-97.

Nutrition (2001) cautions parents to use only 100% juice that is pasteurized. The AAP also recommends children 1 to 4 years of age have 2 fruit servings each day and only one should be juice. They further state that 4 to 6 oz of fruit juice equals 1 fruit serving. Fruit juice has no nutritional advantage over whole fruit and in fact lacks the fiber in whole fruit.

A decrease in the growth rate during toddlerhood results in a decrease in appetite. Parents need to be reminded of this if they begin to worry about their toddler's nutritional intake. Keeping a record (Figure 18-4) over 3 to 5 days, rather than daily, presents a better picture of a child's intake and is a useful teaching tool for this age group.

Toddlers often use mealtime as an occasion to assert individuality and control as well as exploration. Families will vary in their expectations of feeding behavior and mealtime routines. The nurse's best guide for parents of toddlers is to remind them that parents are in charge of what food is offered, when it is offered, and where (Research Highlights box). Box 18-2 lists some nursing interventions to promote healthy eating in toddlers. However, it is up to the toddler to decide how much to actually eat. Periodically, a toddler may even refuse a meal altogether. Parents need to be encouraged to offer healthy, age-appropriate food choices. Toddlers will eat them, as long as they do not fill up on empty calories

PLAN FOR YOUR YOUNG CHILD...The Pyramid Way

Use this chart to get an idea of the foods your child eats over a week. Pencil in the foods eaten each day and pencil in the corresponding triangular shape. (For example, if a slice of toast is eaten at breakfast, write in "toast" and fill in one Grain group pyramid.) The number of pyramids shown for each food group is the number of servings to be eaten each day. At the end of the week, if you see only a few blank pyramids...keep up the good work. If you notice several blank pyramids, offer foods from the missing food groups in the days to come.

	SUNDAY	MONDAY	TUESDAY	WEDNESDAY	THURSDAY	FRIDAY	SATURDAY
Milk Meat Vegetable Fruit Grain	▲▲ ▲▲ ▲▲▲ ▲▲ ▲▲▲ ▲▲▲	▲▲ ▲▲ ▲▲▲ ▲▲ ▲▲▲ ▲▲▲	▲▲ ▲▲ ▲▲▲ ▲▲ ▲▲▲ ▲▲▲	▲▲ ▲▲ ▲▲▲ ▲▲ ▲▲▲ ▲▲▲	▲▲ ▲▲ ▲▲▲ ▲▲ ▲▲▲ ▲▲▲	▲▲ ▲▲ ▲▲▲ ▲▲ ▲▲▲ ▲▲▲	▲▲ ▲▲ ▲▲▲ ▲▲ ▲▲▲ ▲▲▲
Breakfast							
Snack							
Lunch							
Snack							
Dinner							

Figure 18-4   Plan for Your Young Child…the Pyramid Way. An easy teaching system to log the food a child eats. (From U.S. Department of Agriculture.)

Box 18-2   **Nursing Interventions to Promote Healthy Eating in Toddlers**

1. Offer simple, single foods, because mixtures of foods are often rejected.
2. Serve your toddler's favorite foods along with new ones. Several introductions may be necessary before the toddler accepts a new food. Make sure you eat it, too.
3. Encourage the use of utensils, but accept that toddlers still often need to use their fingers.
4. Routines are important to toddlers. Serve scheduled meals and snacks. Parents are responsible for what, when, and where the toddler eats. The toddler decides whether to eat and how much.
5. Turn off the TV. Mealtime should be a relaxed and pleasant time, free of distractions.
6. Do not use food to bribe, reward, or punish your toddler.
7. Schedule meals and sleep periods such that the child is awake and alert during mealtime.
8. Serve small portions and let your toddler ask for more.
9. Avoid foods that may cause choking, such as hard candy, mini-marshmallows, popcorn, pretzels, chips, spoonfuls of peanut butter, nuts, seeds, large chunks of meat, hot dogs, raw carrots, dried fruits, and whole grapes.
10. Drinking more than 24 ounces of milk per day can reduce your child's appetite for other healthy foods. For those under age 2 years, do not use reduced-fat, low-fat, or fat-free (skim) milk because children less than 2 years old need the extra fat for their developing nervous systems.

from juice and high carbohydrate snacks that are often nervously given to children "so they eat something." Further, parents should not put too much attention on food intake or punish children for refusing food. Toddlers may learn how easily the parents can be controlled by their behavior around food intake and may continue the behavior for the attention alone. Using a record of food intake over time (see Figure 18-4), the nurse can demonstrate the adequacy of the nutrients that the toddler is already receiving during other meals and help parents work out a plan to offer more of the essential foods during these meals (Story et al., 2002). Children with inadequate nutrition are predisposed to impaired immune systems leading to infections and delayed healing and recovery. They are also predisposed to depletion of muscle mass leading to diminished functional capacity. In addition, although inadequately understood, nutrients and neurotropic factors interact with one another in brain development and function (More, 2008; Rosales & Zeisel, 2008).

The family who has a vegetarian or vegan diet may need some assistance from the nurse or a dietician. Vegetarian and vegan diets vary widely, so it is important to assess precisely what foods are eaten, what foods have been eliminated from the diet, and what supplements are used.

Elimination Pattern

Toilet training is often a major parental concern during toddlerhood. The nurse anticipates this developmental stressor and initiates discussion with the parents to determine their understanding of the child's signs of developmental readiness and their attitude and commitment to establishing a toileting pattern for their toddler. Emotional and physical readiness for toilet training rarely develops before 18 months of age. Parents who begin before their child is ready usually experience frustration.

Nursing Interventions

By suggesting the sequence in the Health Teaching box, Initiating a Toileting Program for Toddlers, the nurse assists parents with toilet training. The parent who can approach toilet training with a relaxed attitude, accepting some delays and frustrations, will have a better chance of success and a more positive outcome for the toddler.

Activity-Exercise Pattern

Toddlers are always busy—emptying wastebaskets and drawers, building and destroying towers, throwing, kicking, chasing after balls, or dressing and undressing. Many of their activities are repeated over and over, providing practice opportunities for their newly realized skills.

During the toddler period, children will advance from taking their first step to running, climbing stairs, and even pedaling a tricycle. They enjoy pushing and pulling, whether it is an unsuspecting laundry basket or a push-pull toy made for the job. They scribble spontaneously, usually with vigor, and will emerge from toddlerhood capable of copying a circle and creating tadpole-like figures (Figure 18-5). They learn to use a spoon and a fork with fairly good success and to wash their hands (Figure 18-6). They also advance from being dressed by others to dressing themselves with assistance, although at times they resist it.

Toddlers spend most of their waking hours at play—exploring their expanding environment, imitating others' actions, and creating a safety net of **rituals** around eating, sleeping, and everything in between. In their enthusiasm to try many activities, toddlers invariably take on tasks that are beyond their abilities, which can result in frustration and an occasional well-known temper tantrum. Their exploratory nature and limited, but advancing, skills also make them vulnerable to injury.

Most toddlers are interested in other children. However, this interest is limited because toddlers, although ready to be with other children, are not ready to share. Successful social encounters with toddlers are best described as **parallel play**, where children play side by side, doing similar things with similar toys, but each working independently (Berger, 2004). Sharing and cooperative play will not develop until well into the preschool age.

HEALTH TEACHING   Initiating a Toileting Program for Toddlers

- Interest in and awareness of bowel and urinary elimination usually begins by 18 months of age.
- Before beginning toilet training, parents should begin to check their toddlers for the prerequisite skills, which include being able to walk well, stoop and recover, stay dry for at least 2 hours during the day, and communicate sensation before elimination, as well as the discomfort of wet or messy pants and the need for assistance.
- When these prerequisites are present, introduce the child to a potty seat or chair. The potty chair should provide secure seating with the child's feet touching the floor. The potty seat should be used with a small step stool to create the same effect.
- Because of the gastrocolic reflex, bowel elimination is more likely after a meal, so this is a good time to place the

toddler on the potty. When a pattern of bowel or urinary elimination is noticed, use this pattern as a guide for placing the child on the potty.
- Encourage the toddler to stay on the chair for 2 to 3 minutes and always explain what to do ("Go potty") rather than what not to do ("Don't wet your pants"). Do not refer to elimination as dirty or yucky. Remember this is your child's first creation.
- Praise the child for desired behavior. Introduce underwear as a badge of success. Ignore undesired behavior and never punish the child by scolding, spanking, or other punitive measures.
- Anticipate that your toddler may want to touch his or her genitals.
- Remember that daytime dryness usually is achieved by 3 years of age and ahead of nighttime dryness.

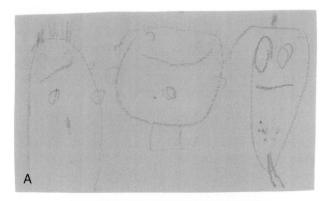

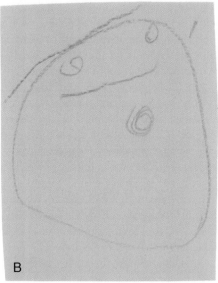

Figure 18-5 Tadpole-like drawings created by a toddler. **A,** Family portrait. Everyone looks the same but there are a few distinguishing details. The dad is on the right, with the scratchy face. The toddler is in the center, and the mom is on the left. Both the mom and the toddler (a girl) have bellybuttons. Mom was 8 months pregnant at the time. **B,** The same toddler drawing herself. Note the bellybutton.

Nursing Interventions

When parents inquire about what toys and activities to provide for their toddler, the following are suggested:

1. Provide toys that challenge the child to develop new skills: toys that require skills slightly above the child's present level, but not advanced such that the child cannot achieve some success.
2. Provide opportunities for new learning. This may be as basic as a book with pictures of new animals or a walk through the produce section of the grocery store to point out fruits and vegetables.
3. Provide opportunities for social encounters with other children, but do not force playing together. Creating separate, yet parallel space, with the use of small mats or hoola hoops is recommended.
4. Follow the child's lead. Let the toddler choose and explore new toys or objects, within safe limits.

The desire of some parents to raise the smartest, most coordinated, or most musically talented super kids often begins in the toddler period. The American Academy of Pediatrics (AAP) (2007) recommends no screen time, including television and videos, for children under age 2. For older toddlers, the AAP recommends no more than 1 to 2 hours daily of high-quality television and videotapes. Instead, children should be allowed to explore what they are interested in, with parents responding to their cues. It is interaction with parents and others in their environment that provides the advantage. Recent research demonstrates that for every hour daily that infants or toddlers watch *educational* television or video, they know 6 to 8 fewer words than those infants or toddlers who do not. For more information on helping parents support their toddler's activity and exploration in a safe and educational way go to *Zero to Three, www.zerotothree.org.*

Sleep-Rest Pattern

Toddlers' need for sleep has decreased to 12 hours a day, including 1 or 2 naps of shorter duration (Figure 18-7). One of the naps usually is replaced by quiet time, a brief period to unwind

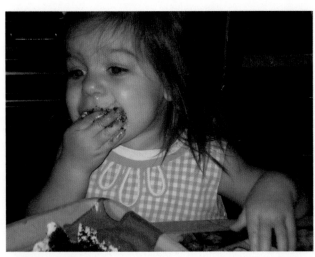

Figure 18-6 Toddlers can slip back to entry with their fingers.

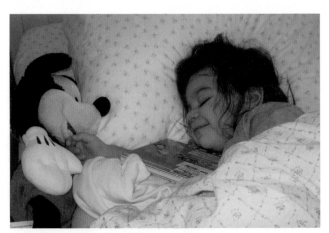

Figure 18-7 Toddlers' need for sleep declines to 12 hours a day, including 1 or 2 naps of shorter duration.

from a busy or noisy activity. Occasionally the parents or caregivers need these rest breaks as much or more. Sitting together in a rocking chair for a soothing song or quiet music or reading side by side or together can be suggested by the nurse.

The toddler may be highly involved in an activity and not be aware of fatigue, especially when visitors are in the home or some interesting new toys have been discovered. All parents are familiar with the child who is overtired but unable to relax enough to sleep. Parents can potentially avoid this dilemma by scheduling nap and quiet time even when there are houseguests or holidays that preempt the toddler's routine.

Rituals are characteristic of this age, and most toddlers have a nap and bedtime ritual. A typical pattern might be: a snack, followed by bathing, brushing teeth, a story, a kiss, and overhead lights out and night light on. Following this ritual is important, because the toddler gets a sense of security when ending the day. Changing this ritual can be upsetting. The nurse encourages parents to establish and follow the sleep time ritual as closely as possible, even when visitors, family illness, or travel makes the routine more difficult.

Many toddlers will try to delay sleep by calling for water, another story, another kiss, or by making other requests. Parents should be certain that the toddler has ample opportunity for interaction with them during the day, follow the usual bedtime ritual, and be firm and consistent in resisting any requests for attention after the final good nights have been said. Encouraging toddlers to use transition or security objects, such as stuffed animals or blankets, helps them to self-quiet and console themselves both at bedtime and in new situations.

Night terrors may begin in toddlerhood. Night terrors are different from nightmares, which generally begin at a later age and result in the child awakening and being able to recall the frightening dream. The child who experiences night terrors does not waken completely, but cries out, looks terrified, and cannot be aroused for several minutes. Eventually, usually after 5 to 10 minutes, the child falls back into quiet sleep. Parents need to be reassured that these episodes will become less frequent as the child develops. The parents should talk in a soothing voice but should not try to awaken the child. If the child does waken, the parents should then provide comfort and tuck the child back in bed.

Cognitive-Perceptual Pattern

Toddlers who experienced the security of a nurturing and reliable source of protection and attachment during infancy have a strong base from which to begin to explore and learn about their expanding world. They begin toddlerhood in Piaget's **sensorimotor stage** of cognitive development and begin moving to the **preoperational stage**. Their advancing thought-processing skills and abilities to use the language are heralded by the development of **egocentrism**, an inability to put oneself in another's shoes. Toddlers who come running into a room asking their parents "Where is it?" are confused when parents respond "Where is what?" They assume their parents and all others share their same thoughts and cannot understand why they don't.

Toddlers interpret and learn about objects and events, not in terms of general properties, but in terms of their relationship with them or their use to them. Their thoughts are dominated by what they see, hear, or otherwise experience, and they want to experience everything. Their two- to three-word phrases are most often related to present events, describing an action, a desire, or possession (example: "Mommy, me up!").

Both receptive and expressive language skills are developing rapidly in toddlers; however, their receptive language skills far outweigh their expressive language ability, and toddlers often use gestures until words are found to represent the meanings already acquired. Toddlers also learn the use of inflection. "Mommy" may mean "pick me up," on one occasion and "I'm scared" or "Where are you?" on another. Often frustrated by their limited repertoire of expressive language, which usually includes about 400 words, young toddlers default to using "NO" as a method of gaining control over a situation or expressing themselves (see Think About It).

By age 3, children have mastered the basics of language function, form, and content, and these fundamentals will continue to be refined throughout childhood and adolescence. Table 18-1 outlines the landmarks of speech, language, and hearing ability in this age group.

Toddlers have a solid understanding of **object permanence** and are no longer easily distracted when a desired toy, blanket, or parent is not to be found. Many toddlers will sit patiently in front of the washing machine while a favorite blanket is laundered or stare out a front window awaiting a parent's return. They often inadvertently put themselves in harm's way as they pursue an object or person they sense is just out of view.

The toddler period is dominated by play, but often referred to as "child's work", which is repetitive and ritualistic. When toddlers bounce a ball over and over and over again they are not trying to drive their parents crazy. They are trying to learn about balls, and repetition is the best teacher. Toddlers' ritualistic behaviors help them master skills and decrease anxiety, and the addition of a seemingly endless string of questions to these behaviors can test the limits of the most patient parents. These queries, however, must be acknowledged and responded to in a manner that not only provides answers but also validates and reinforces the toddler's burgeoning curiosity. The nurse explains the "terrible twos" by teaching parents and caregivers that toddlers might better be viewed as "young scientists" in need of a safe "laboratory" in which to conduct their trial and error research. Better now and in parents' close proximity than in adolescence, a developmental period that mirrors and repeats many of the parent-child challenges of toddlerhood. The American Academy of Pediatrics (2008) has recommended administering autistic screening at the 18th month preventive care visit. At present, Autism Spectrum Disorders are defined as pervasive developmental disorders with onset in infancy or childhood characterized by impaired social interactions, impaired communications, and significantly restricted activities and interests. There is no known cause. The current prevalence is one in every 150 American children and almost one in 94 boys (Robins, 2008; Wetherby et al., 2008). See *www.autism.society.org* for more information.

Hearing

The ability to hear and listen to others is critical for speech and language development. Listening includes attending to what is heard, discriminating among the various qualities of sound, cognitively associating what is heard with previously learned experiences, and remembering what is heard. The quantity and quality of language that the toddler is exposed to is thought to be more important for the development of listening ability and therefore receptive language skills than it is for the development of expressive language skills

Growth and Development Table 18-1

Landmarks of Speech, Language, and Hearing Ability During the Toddler Period

Age (Months)	Receptive Language	Expressive Language	Related Hearing Ability
18	Up to 50 words; recognizes between 6 and 12 objects by name, such as *dog, cat, bottle, ball;* identifies three body parts, such as *eyes, nose, mouth;* understands simple, one-step commands such as *give me the doll, open your mouth, stick out your tongue*	Up to 20 words; jargon and echolalia are present; uses names of familiar objects and one-word sentences, such as *go* or *eat;* uses gestures; uses words such as *no, mine, eat, good, bad, hot, cold,* and expressions such as *oh-oh, what's that, all gone;* use of words can be quite inconsistent, 25% of speech intelligible	Has begun to develop gross discrimination by learning to distinguish between highly dissimilar noises, such as doorbell and train, barking dog and auto horn, or mother's and father's voices
24	Up to 1200 words; knows *in, on, under;* identifies *dog, ball, engine, bed, doll, scissors, hair, mouth, feet, nose, cup, spoon, car, key;* distinguishes between one and many and formulates a negative judgment (a knife is not a fork); understands simple stories; follows simple, two-step directions; is beginning to make distinctions between *you* and *me*	Up to 270 words; jargon and echolalia almost gone; average 75 words per hour during free play; talks in words, phrases, and two-word to three-word sentences; averages two words per response; first pronouns appear, such as *I, me, mine, it, who, that;* adjectives and adverbs are only beginning to appear; names objects and common pictures; refers to self by name, such as *Katrina go bye-bye;* uses phrases such as *I want, go bye-bye, want cookie, ball all gone,* 60% of speech intelligible	Refinement of gross discriminative skills
30	Up to 2400 words; identifies action in pictures and objects by use; carries out one-part and two-part commands, such as *pick up your shoe and give it to mommy;* knows what is used to drink liquids, what goes on the feet, what is used to buy candy; understands plurals, questions, difference between boy and girl, the concepts *one, up, down, run, walk, throw, fast, more, my*	Use up to 425 words; jargon and echolalia no longer exist; averages 140 words per hour; names words such as *chair, can, box, key, door;* repeats two digits from memory; average sentence length is approximately two and one-half words; uses more adjectives and adverbs; demands repetition from others, such as *do it again,* nearly always announces intentions before actions; begins to ask questions of adults; 75% of speech intelligible	—
36	Up to 3600 words; understands *both, two, not today,* what to do when thirsty (hungry, sleepy), why people have stoves, understands *wait, later, big, new, different, strong, today, another,* and taking turns at play; carries out two-item and some three-item commands, such as *give me the ball, pick up the doll,* and *sit down;* identifies several colors; is aware of past and future	Up to 900 words in simple sentences, averaging three to four words per sentence; averages 170 words per hour; uses words such as *when, time, today, not today, new, different, big, strong, surprise, secret;* can repeat three digits, name one color, say name, give simple account of experiences, and tell stories that can be understood; begins to use more pronouns, adjectives, and adverbs; describes at least one element of a picture; is aware of past and future; uses commands such as *you make it* and expressions such as *I can't, I don't want to;* verbalizes toilet needs; expresses desire to take turns; communication includes criticisms, commands, requests, threats, questions, answers; 85% of speech intelligible	Starts to distinguish dissimilar speech sounds, such as the difference between ee and er, although there may be some difficulty with the concepts of *same* and *different*

Modified from Chinn, P. L. (1976). *Child health maintenance: Concepts in family-centered care* (2nd ed.). St. Louis: Mosby; Ports, N. L., & Mandleco, B. L. (2007). *Pediatric nursing: Caring for children and their families* (2nd ed.). Clifton Park, NY: Thomson Delmar Learning; Pan, B. A., Rowe, M. L., Singer, J. D., & Snow, C. E. (2005). Maternal correlates of growth in toddler vocabulary production in low-income families. *Child Development, 76*(4), 763–782.

(Genesee, 2008; Pan et al., 2005). Toddlers often seek repetition of auditory input, as observed in their seemingly endless repetition of sounds, words, and combinations of words. This repetition is their way of practicing and organizing new language (Gillam et al., 2001; see Table 18-1).

Hearing loss is one of the most common conditions present at birth. If undetected, even mild hearing loss can impede speech, language, cognitive, and emotional development (Green & Palfrey, 2002). Health care providers need to continue to monitor, screen, and refer children for formal audiological evaluation if they develop signs of identified risk factors for hearing loss. The timing and number of hearing re-evaluations for children with risk factors should be individualized. Infants who pass the neonatal screening but have a risk factor should have at least one diagnostic audiology assessment by 24 to 30 months of age (AAP, 2007). Early and more frequent assessment may be indicated for children with cytomegalovirus (CMV) infection, syndromes associated with progressive hearing loss, neurodegenerative disorders, head trauma, or culture-positive postnatal infections associated with sensorineural hearing loss (e.g. herpes viruses); toddlers who spent more than 5 days in an NICU; children who have received extracorporeal membrane oxygenation (ECMO), exchange transfusions, or chemotherapy; and when there is caregiver concern or a family history of hearing loss (AAP, 2007).

Younger toddlers are screened using **visual-reinforcement audiometry**, in which stimulus tones and visually animated reinforcers (e.g., a lighted toy) are paired and presented together. After the toddler has been conditioned to expect this relationship, the visual reinforcer is withheld and the sound is presented alone. The toddler looks for the visual reinforcer in response to the sound, and the visual reinforcer is then presented as a reward. **Conditioned-play audiometry** is used for older toddlers and preschool children. The child is first taught to play listening games, using blocks or rings. The child learns to wait and listen for a sound and then perform a motor task (e.g., places a block, a bucket, or a ring on a stacking stick) in response. The motor task is followed by social reinforcement. Noncalibrated toys or noisemakers and signals that lack frequency specificity are inappropriate screening methods and should be used only as gross indicators for monitoring.

Otitis media, or inner ear infection, is one of the leading causes of visits to health care providers during the toddler years and the number one reason for which antibiotics are prescribed for these children. Discussing the current literature and evidence-based reports and recommendations often helps parents understand the proper use of antibiotics, which is also imperative in preventing antibiotic resistance. When it is deemed necessary to use an antibiotic, nurses teach how to administer the medication safely and stress the importance of taking the medication at the prescribed time and for the full duration of the course.

Vision

Toddlers' visual acuity is usually around 20/40, although gaining their cooperation for screening is often difficult and not recommended unless parents, caregivers, or health care providers identify a concern. Depth perception is still immature, although more developed than in infancy.

Amblyopia is one of the major health care concerns of this age group and occurs in 2% to 5% of children. It is defined as diminished, or loss of, vision in an eye that has not received adequate use. The eye looks normal, but it is not being used normally. Because the brain favors the other eye, the term "lazy eye" is often used. The most common cause of amblyopia is strabismus, but it may also occur when one eye is more nearsighted, farsighted, or astigmatic than the other. Occasionally amblyopia is caused by other eye conditions such as a cataract.

Strabismus is a deviation of the line of vision from the midline resulting from extraocular muscle weakness or imbalance and is commonly referred to as crossed eye. One or both eyes may turn in, out, up, or down and can be constant or intermittent. Marked or continuous strabismus usually is noticed early by the parents and health care providers and is therefore treated early; the more subtle deviations are often unnoticed until older toddlerhood or the preschool years. Every toddler should be screened for strabismus as part of the routine eye examination that is performed by the physician or nurse practitioner during well-child visits. Best results are obtained when the condition is diagnosed and treated early.

Management of amblyopia depends on the cause and may include surgery or paralytic, autonomic, and centrally acting pharmacological agents. However, no matter what the cause, management will involve making the child use the lazy eye, the eye with reduced vision. There are two ways to do this: (1) atropine eye drops or (2) patching the stronger eye. Researchers have found that atropine eye drops, when placed in the stronger eye once a day, work as well as eye patching and may result in better compliance (The Pediatric Eye Disease Investigator Group, 2002). In addition, 2 hours of patching may produce an improvement in visual acuity that is of similar magnitude to the improvement produced by 6 hours of daily patching (The Pediatric Eye Disease Investigator Group, 2002). Shorter patching time should lead to better compliance and improved quality of life (Innovative Practice box).

innovative practice

The Eye Patch Club

It is estimated that 2% to 5% of all children suffer from amblyopia. Prevent Blindness America is creating a support group called the Eye Patch Club for families coping with a child's amblyopia treatment. The Eye Patch Club News is a newsletter featuring tips and techniques for promoting compliance, stories from and about children whose eyes are patched, and professional advice from optometrists, ophthalmologists, and orthoptists. Each issue also includes a Kid's Page, and there is a classroom guide for teachers with explanations for the classroom, as well as activities for everyone to learn more about their eyes. An Eye Patch Club calendar and stickers that allow children to track their patch-wearing activity, a refrigerator magnet with helpful hints, and pen pal opportunities are also available. To learn more about Prevent Blindness America and The Eye Patch Club, visit their Web site at: *www.preventblindness.org/children/EyePatchClub.html*.

Other signs of vision problems that the nurse observes or parents report in their toddlers include the following red flags:

1. Rubs eyes excessively
2. Shuts or covers one eye, tilts head, or looks sideways to view an object
3. Has difficulty or is irritable when doing close work
4. Blinks, squints, or frowns when viewing objects
5. Holds books close to eyes
6. Has red, encrusted, or swollen eyelids
7. Has red, inflamed, or watery eyes
8. Develops recurring **styes** (swelling at the edge of the eyelid)

Taste and Smell

Toddlers are beginning to take control of their world and have the capacity to taste and smell, new skills that are rapidly put to use. Toddlers often refuse to even taste something that looks or smells displeasing to them or eat something that they recall as tasting terrible. They are able to react accurately to a sensation that a taste or smell arouses in them, and they begin to learn conditioned association between certain smells and culturally acceptable values. Foods and smells found in one family or culture become palatable and accepted, and those that are unacceptable become displeasing. Many of our adult eating habits, food likes and dislikes, and visceral responses to odors have their roots in this period.

Self-Perception–Self-Concept Pattern

According to Erikson (1995, 1998), the developmental task of toddlers is to acquire a sense of **autonomy** while overcoming a sense of **doubt** and **shame**. To exert autonomy, toddlers must relinquish the dependence on others that was enjoyed during infancy. Continued dependency has the potential to create a sense of doubt in toddlers about their ability to take control of, and ultimately take responsibility for, their own actions. Toddlers seem to thrive when parents can accommodate their increasing autonomy yet maintain a strong parenting presence that includes a full measure of patience, enough parental self-confidence to set appropriate limits, and the ability to realize that their toddler's negative behavior is not directed at them and that their egocentrism is not a reflection on them.

The toddler must explore the world, not only the physical aspects but also the interpersonal aspects of relationships, to develop a true sense of autonomy. Exploring the physical world involves poking into, climbing onto, crawling under, tasting, smelling, and taking apart the objects encountered. The child explores relationships with others by searching for the limits of the child's power: if a "no" or a temper tantrum means control of another person's behavior, the child learns that one's own self is more powerful than the other person's self. The toddler continually practices separateness to develop a sense of autonomy.

This process can be trying and confusing for parents. The toddler may say a vehement "no" when offered a drink and then scream and cry when the drink is put away; the parents may wonder if the toddler wants the drink or not. Likely the answer is "yes," but the toddler may also need to express

autonomy by refusing it. Occasionally the same toddler who displays a strong need for autonomy spontaneously cuddles or even clings to a parent. These conflicting desires can be confusing to both the parent and the toddler.

The toddler's need for more autonomy may conflict with parental expectations, safety limits, or the rights of other children or adults. Any of these conflicts results in feelings of frustration. A typical toddler response to frustration is the well-known temper tantrum.

In one study, parent-reported socioemotional/behavioral problems at 12–36 months of age significantly predicted teacher- and parent-reported sub-clinical and clinical emotional-behavioral problems (Briggs-Gowan & Carter, 2004).

Nursing Interventions

The nurse assesses the toddler-parent relationship to determine the following:

1. How is the toddler expressing the need for autonomy?
2. How do the parents perceive these actions?
3. How does the toddler respond to frustration in exploring the environment or controlling personal and others' actions?
4. How do the parents respond to the toddler's display of frustration?
5. What provisions are the parents making to allow safe choices for the toddler?

The nurse's teaching focuses on the aspects that are troublesome for the toddler-parent relationship. Some general concepts to include are:

1. Match the environment to the child's needs and abilities. Childproof the home such that the child can explore safely. Provide toys that the child can master. Give opportunities to play with more challenging toys, but do not make these toys the rule.
2. Give advance notice of a change in activity, such as lunch or nap time. Utilize transition rituals and objects.
3. Do not offer a choice if there isn't one. For example, rather than ask if the toddler wants to take a bath, say it is time to take a bath, do you want to take it upstairs or downstairs, or do you want to start at the face and move down to the toes or start with the toes and wash the face last? This allows for the toddler to be in charge and the task of bathing achieved.
4. Set and enforce consistent limits such that the toddler will come to develop control within these limits.
5. To prevent temper tantrums, keep routines simple and consistent, set reasonable limits and give rationales, avoid "head-on clashes," and provide choices.
6. If temper tantrums occur, provide a safe environment for the toddler, identify the tantrum's cause, and help the toddler regain control. Do not reason, threaten, promise, hit, or give in. Respond consistently and follow through on discipline free of anger. Overcriticizing and restricting the toddler may dampen enthusiasm and increase feelings of shame and doubt.

7. Praise the toddler's skills and abilities. Never miss an opportunity to catch your toddler being good. Be positive. Remember to say "yes" once in a while.

Roles-Relationships Pattern

By toddlerhood, children typically know their mother, father, and older siblings and have established some form of reciprocal relationship with them (Treyvaud et al., 2009). Toddlers' capability for relationships is limited and usually reflects their egocentric approach to everything else. Parents' and siblings' roles are understood, just like everything else in their lives, in terms of how those roles relate to the toddler. One family member may be the fixer of toys or the comforter of bruises, another the troublemaker who takes away toys.

Toddlers are interested in everything, and their parents' and siblings' activities and possessions are often imitated and preferred. Frequently the desire to be like or have something that belongs to a sibling creates sibling rivalry. This happens between toddlers and their older siblings, but even more when a new younger sibling is introduced (Figure 18-8). A new baby who is often loud, unable to play, not to be touched or explored too vigorously, and demands and gets too much parental attention quickly becomes a nuisance to toddlers who have been known to inform their parents that they can "Take the new baby back where it came from now." Realizing the new sibling is here to stay, toddlers often regress, reverting to earlier, previously abandoned infantile behavior such as losing toileting skills, wanting to be fed or dressed, or even talking baby talk. They are usually trying to retain or regain a sense of mastery and, once reassured, will move on. This process is not the end of sibling rivalry, but only the beginning of what will take on many forms and require ongoing negotiation from all family members. Parents cannot stop sibling fighting by forbidding it, but reasonable limits can be established. One way to tone down fighting is to remove the gain. Generally the desired outcome in the toddler's mind is to see the self rewarded and the sibling punished. When parents do not reward or punish, or when they do not take sides, the gain is missing and fight-

ing becomes less satisfactory. This approach does not mean that all fighting will stop, but the child will look for other ways of getting approval.

Sibling relationships and parent-child relationships can be difficult subjects for parents to discuss. Parents may think that any hint of discord indicates an unhealthy family (Bergman & Harpaz-Rotem, 2004). The nurse should include normal family development and role relationships as part of the anticipatory guidance given during the toddler years (Warren et al., 2008). Toddler behaviors are trying for all parents, and discipline can often be influenced as much by parental emotions as by parenting knowledge and skill (Caughy et al., 2009). When parental anger, depression (Del Vecchio & O'Leary, 2008; Eshbaugh, 2006; Gartstein & Bateman, 2008; Treyvaud et al., 2009; Weinfield et al., 2009), criticism, and restrictions go unchecked, physical and emotional abuse can occur.

Child Abuse

Child abuse and maltreatment is not limited to a particular age or particular families (Siebel et al., 2008). However, it is more likely to occur with a major change or turmoil (Mann & Kretchmar, 2006; Norris, 2008) in the family and when parental role models were abusive. Toddlerhood is a trying time for the most patient of parents, and nurses need to be alert to family changes and stresses as well as to warning signs of abuse (Box 18-3). Many injuries are difficult to differentiate from accidental injury and, at times, may even be confused with culturally appropriate healing practices (Multicultural Awareness box).

Typically parental responses to childhood injuries include a spontaneous reporting of the details of the illness or injury accompanied by concern, questions about progress and discharge, difficulty in leaving the child, and an attempt to identify with the child's feelings. These parents may also experience guilt for not protecting the child from the accident and may offer gifts to compensate for these feelings of guilt. In contrast, neglectful or abusive parents are often hesitant to provide information about the illness or injury; they

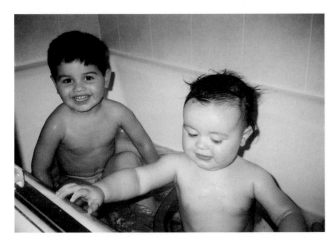

Figure 18-8 Toddlers often have to learn to deal with a new family member.

Box **18-3** Warning Signs of Child Abuse
• Parental delay in seeking help • Inconsistencies in the history of how the injury occurred • Injury inconsistent with the history or child's developmental capability • Old, unexplained fractures evident on radiographs • Bruises confined to back surface of the body—neck to knees • Bare spots and broken hair • Pattern of injury or bruising descriptive of object used to inflict injury (belt or belt buckle, hand, cigarette, hot water) • Burns with sharply demarcated edges or circumferential patterns • Perineal injuries of any kind

From Butchar, A., Harvey, A. P., Mian, M., & Furniss, T. (2006). *Preventing child maltreatment: A guide to taking action & generating evidence.* WHO Press.

MULTICULTURAL AWARENESS

Evaluating for Child Abuse with Cultural Sensitivity

Nurses are required by law to report cases of suspected child abuse to Child Protective Services. The nurse who takes a careful health history may discover that what might appear to be characteristic burns or bruises associated with child abuse may instead be the product of a traditional culturally appropriate healing practice. The following are two examples of healing practices found in the Pacific Islander and Asian populations that might create such confusion.

COINING (CAO GIO)

Coining is a common healing practice used among Pacific Island and Asian families within the United States. Traditionally, coining is used for conditions associated with "wind" illnesses, as well as a wide variety of febrile illnesses. The lesions seen from coining are produced by rubbing a warm oil or balm on the skin and firmly abrading the skin with a coin or special instrument. The practice produces linear petechiae and ecchymosis on the chest and back that often resemble strap or belt marks. The appearance of the deep red-purple skin color is confirmation that the person had bad wind in the body.

CUPPING (VENTOUSE)

Cupping involves creating a vacuum inside a special cup or glass by burning the oxygen out of it and then promptly placing it on a person's skin surface. Cupping draws blood and lymph to the body surface that is under the cup or glass, increasing local circulation. The purpose for doing this is to remove cold and damp "evils" from the body or to assist blood circulation or both. The procedure frequently is used to treat lung congestion. The resulting circular ecchymotic marks are approximately 2 inches in diameter and resemble nonaccidental trauma.

---

may be evasive or even contradict themselves, irritated by the inconvenience of being asked questions. Abusive parents may not exhibit guilt feelings and often contend that the toddler was solely responsible for the injury.

Although these signs of potential abuse are certainly not present in all abusive parents, their presence alerts the nurse to assess and observe further. The nurse also remembers that some of these signs may be found in nonabusive parents, and their presence serves only as a cue for further assessment. All nurses are required by law to report suspected child abuse to the local child protective services agency.

Sexuality-Reproductive Pattern

The toileting process, during which attention is focused on the genital area, may precipitate curiosity about the genital organs. The nurse includes this aspect in early teaching about toilet training, giving parents time to consider their feelings and decide on their approach to genital exploratory behavior and **masturbation**. Some parents accept the child's curiosity, whereas others see this as an opportunity to introduce their own sexual values and taboos.

The nurse helps parents approach this curiosity and exploration, as well as masturbation, as a normal developmental process. These behaviors provide toddlers with an opportunity to become better acquainted with their bodies. Many parents are uncertain about the vocabulary they should use and often create cute, unrelated words rather than provide the correct anatomical terms. The use of cute alternative words often is a reflection of parental discomfort or embarrassment. Using correct terms will help toddlers develop accurate knowledge about sexuality and communicate more effectively if inappropriate touching by others occurs. For example, a young boy was initially ignored by day care providers because he said an older boy ate his "pickle." After repeated episodes, the parents were contacted because the child seemed so upset (even though day care gave him a new pickle to eat). The parents shared that "pickle" was their name for penis.

Coping-Stress Tolerance Pattern

Perceptions of events and reactions to them are filtered through children's developing cognitive, emotional, and social capacities. The relevance of life events and the child's vulnerability to their impact depend on the given developmental period (see the Case Study and Care Plan at the end of this chapter). A child's **temperament**, which is defined as an individual's style of emotional and behavioral response across situations, especially those involving change or stress, serves as a foundation for coping (Burns et al., 2008). Although temperament generally has been accepted as inborn, it is influenced by environmental characteristics and exerts an influence on psychosocial adjustment by way of its effect on parent-child interactions. Nurses assist parents in recognizing their toddler's innate behavioral qualities as expressions of temperament and in developing management strategies (Hot Topics box).

Toddlers are developing new ways to cope with the myriad new stresses that come with being a toddler. As is typical of their stage of development, coping is egocentric and reflective of their need for autonomy. Typical stressors include new siblings, babysitters, day care, toilet training, parental limit setting, and an endless string of tasks involving skills they have yet to develop.

Toddlers often imitate their parents' behavior and this includes their methods of dealing with stress. They also regress, at times, to earlier infantile behavior when overwhelmed, until they regain some sense of mastery. Parents can help to anticipate and prepare toddlers for stressful experiences before they happen. However, they need to remember that toddlers' sense of time and ability to recall are limited. Preparations should be honest, simple, and focused on what the toddler will experience. Enough time should be allowed for the toddler to rehearse the coping behavior with the parent, but not so far off from the event that the toddler forgets.

The nurse helps the parents anticipate developmental stressors and suggests age and temperament-appropriate coping

HOTtopics

COPING WITH A CHILD'S TEMPERAMENT

Temperament is defined as the style of behaviors that a child habitually uses to cope with demands and expectations of the environment. Chess and Thomas (1986) originally described three common temperament patterns that they believe are innate: (1) the easy child, (2) the difficult child, and (3) the slow-to-warm-up child.

The easy child is cuddly, affectionate, and easy to manage. The way in which a child with an easy temperament elicits positive reactions from adults is obvious.

Children with a difficult temperament, however, are less adaptable, are more intense and active, and have more negative moods. These behaviors can be distressing to parents and caregivers and may cause them to feel ineffective in their roles.

Temperament affects development throughout the life span but is especially significant for toddlers when placed in the context of development. Toddlers are increasingly mobile and are striving for independence at a time when parents become more demanding. Various approaches to parenting, teaching, and providing health care, including the adults' own temperament styles, culture, and gender-related biases, can influence the way in which the child's behavior is viewed.

According to the goodness-of-fit interactive model of temperament, adults can accommodate their demands and expectations in ways that match the child's behaviors, including learning strategies to help toddlers adapt positively to social expectations.

Questions

1. What are some of the consequences of labeling a toddler as difficult, easy, or slow to warm up?
2. What are common reactions to girls who are extremely active and highly distractible? Boys who are clingy, cry often, and prefer to play with dolls? What influences these reactions in adults? What influence do they have on children?

From Burns, C. E., Dunn, A. M., Brady, M. A., Starr, N. B., & Blosser, C. (2008). *Pediatric primary care* (4th ed.). St. Louis: W. B. Saunders; Chess, S., & Thomas, A. (1986). *Temperament in clinical practice.* New York: Guildford Press.

behaviors for toddlers. Early efforts at dealing with stress are an essential step to more mature coping responses as the child grows (DeVos et al., 2006; Kolak & Vernon-Feagans, 2008).

Values-Beliefs Pattern

Healthy behaviors are expressions of positive values and beliefs. These values and beliefs are learned, and their recognition and acceptance are fundamental to the integrity of every child. Toddlers believe rules are absolute and behave, according to Kohlberg, out of a fear of punishment. However, toddlers' environments should not only help them become aware of right and wrong but also contribute to their sense of security, belonging, and autonomy. Development of moral integrity is enhanced if toddlers believe they are valued.

Because most of toddlers' developing values and beliefs depend on their interactions with parents, the nurse's assessment questions are often directed to or focused on the parent or caregiver. Examples are:

- What are the family's values and beliefs about what is right and wrong?
- How does the parental approach to limit setting reflect these values and beliefs?
- What religious, spiritual, or cultural traditions and activities does the family have?
- How is the toddler included in these traditions and activities?

Children are exposed to and begin to participate in and imitate their family's religious rituals and practices during toddlerhood. They are often taught prayers and songs with a religious theme that are tied into what the family believes is right and wrong. Toddlers may be able to learn the words to these simple prayers and songs, but parents should be cautioned that knowing the words does not mean that toddlers understand the full meaning of what is said. This early introduction into the family's religious beliefs is important as a socialization factor but should not be assumed to produce a good child.

The creation of values and beliefs in young children is related to their developmental stage and reflected in their behaviors. An important aspect of teaching young children what is right and wrong involves stating what acceptable behavior is and then reinforcing the behavior when it occurs. Parents often attend to toddlers only when they are misbehaving, leaving them alone when they are being good. In this scenario, toddlers receive no attention for acceptable behavior but gain their parents' attention when they misbehave. The nurse can remind parents to catch their toddlers being good and give them the same or more attention.

ENVIRONMENT
Accidents

"If a disease were killing our young children in the proportions that injuries are, people would be outraged and demand that this killer be stopped"
C. Everett Koop, M.D., Former Surgeon General

Toddlers are at high risk for accidental injury, because they lack judgment and experience and have only rudimentary problem-solving skills, limited physical coordination, and a heightened level of curiosity about their environment (Garzon et al., 2007). Most parents think that it is natural for children to get hurt and that childhood injuries are just a part of growing up. However, most injuries are predictable and preventable and can cause disabilities requiring long-term care. Furthermore, they cause more deaths than all childhood disease combined.

One out of every 10 toddlers who comes to the emergency room is treated for accidental injury. Male toddlers tend to have more injuries than their female counterparts, but the overall numbers of accidental injuries peak during toddlerhood for both males and females. A second peak occurs for males during adolescence. Major causes of accidental injury in toddlers involve structural hazards, sports, drowning, burns, motor vehicles, and poisoning.

Recent research indicates that although overall injury rates for young children have decreased over the past 20 years, mortality rates from injury remain higher in Black and American Indian/Alaskan Native children. The young children in both of these groups had higher injury risk for residential fires, suffocation, and poisoning. These findings suggest new strategies and approaches are needed to narrow the disparities that continue to exist.

Structural Hazards

Houses and other buildings can be hazardous for toddlers. Their desire to explore lures them to locations to which older children or adults would not consider going. The toddler will climb onto furniture or fixtures, out of windows, or into small spaces. Injuries that result from these explorations can range from minor scrapes and bruises to fatal head injuries. Ideally homes are "baby-proofed" before the infant begins scooting and crawling and toddler-proofed before the toddler becomes increasingly mobile. Parents should reassess the safety of their home as their child acquires new skills. Injuries to toddlers occur most often when they fall from furniture, high chairs, changing tables, stairs, windows, and playground equipment. When the child or family visits the home of a friend or relative, it must be inspected for hazards, or the toddler must be confined to one safe room. Many injuries occur in unfamiliar environments.

Preventive measures for structural hazards include the following:

- Don't leave a toddler unattended.
- Use gates at the top and bottom of stairways and at doors.
- Keep chairs away from countertops and tables to prevent toddlers from climbing.
- Lock doors to dangerous areas and use gates and window guards.

Toys

Toys commonly found in homes are another source of injury. Parents should inspect not only the toys that are in their own homes, but also the toys given to the toddler outside the home by relatives, friends, babysitters, or day care personnel (see the Case Study and Care Plan at the end of this chapter). Many toys that are likely to be safe for older children are extremely hazardous for the toddler. Of concern are small, removable parts and batteries, toxic paint or stuffing, sharp edges, and flammable material.

Sports

Although sporting and recreational equipment is recognized as a major source of accidents in older children and adolescents, parents and health care personnel occasionally forget that these items can also be dangerous to toddlers. Improper storage of this equipment is a primary danger. Firearms that are left loaded and unlocked are deadly hazards, and bodybuilding weights and other heavy equipment

easily overwhelm toddlers who may pull these objects down on themselves. Toddlers should always be supervised closely, especially in new environments or on playground equipment.

As toddlers become more mobile, they are introduced to riding toys, tricycles, and bicycles. Nurses remind parents about the need for, and in most states the requirement of, bicycle helmets that are fitted properly and worn every time the toddler rides or is a passenger on a bicycle.

Drowning

Children between the ages of 1 and 3 years are at highest risk of drowning, because most do not know how to swim and do not have the skills to keep their heads above water or to get out of the water. Toddlers can drown in water just deep enough to cover their noses and mouths. Although swimming pools and other natural bodies of water are a big part of the problem, even pails of water, toilets, bathtubs, and wading pools are dangerous. When toddlers fall into a pail of water or toilet it is hard for them to straighten up because all of their weight is forward. Toddlers should never be left unattended—even for a few seconds—near a bathtub, hot tub, wading or swimming pool, toilet, or pail of water. All swimming pools should be fenced and have self-closing gates and latches. Toddlers must be supervised constantly and competently whenever they are near any body of water and fitted properly with personal flotation devices whenever they are on a boat.

Burns

Each year more than 100,000 children between the ages of 0 and 4 years require emergency room treatment for scalds from hot liquids. Hot tap water, boiling water, coffee, tea, and food are the most common sources of injury. These very painful and often debilitating injuries often happen as toddlers begin to gain mobility and explore their environments, inadvertently touching hot surfaces or spilling hot liquids on themselves. They may also put their mouths on live electrical cords or their fingers into electrical sockets and get serious burns, as well as tip their walkers or themselves into fireplaces or woodstoves.

Nurses give parents reminders including:

- Never eat, drink, or carry anything hot while holding a child.
- Lower water heater temperature to 120° to 125° Fahrenheit.
- Never leave hot beverages or foods within a child's reach.
- Put children in a playpen while cooking.
- Never leave a toddler unattended in the bathtub. It takes only a moment to turn on the hot water.
- Put screens around fireplaces or woodstoves.
- Do not let children handle food directly from the microwave oven.
- Use burners at the back of the stove and turn pot handles in toward the stove.
- Install and maintain smoke detectors, replacing batteries annually.

Motor Vehicles

Motor vehicle–related injuries, which include both passenger and pedestrian injuries, are leading in children from 1 to 4 years of age. For the toddler, passenger injury is more frequent and often involves the lack of use or misuse of child safety seats. Child safety seats, when properly installed and used, have reduced the risk of death and serious injury to children. Unfortunately, improper installation and use of child safety seats are widespread problems, with some experts reporting that more than 80% of them are misused in some way. Certified Child Passenger Safety Technicians are trained in installing car safety seats properly and can help parents make sure their children are as safe as possible on the road. To find the closest inspection station, the nurse can visit or direct parents to visit *www.seatcheck.org* or call toll-free 866-SEATCHECK (866-732-8243).

As children reach 20 pounds, the nurse confirms with parents that they are switched to forward-facing child safety seats. Rear seat position is preferred and safer than the front seat, and a special warning has been issued that no child should be seated in the front passenger seat if the car has airbags. During the toddler years, children may progress in size and weight to a transition or booster seat. The nurse can provide a list of approved car seats and local retail outlets or agencies that sell, lend, or rent car seats. The AAP has published a comprehensive pamphlet on choosing a car seat (AAP, 2005).

Toddlers are also injured or killed when they are hit by driver backing up in their own driveways and often by members of their family or nearby neighbors. They are too small to be seen by a driver backing up and quick to run out after a departing parent or relative who thinks they are still safely inside.

Biological Agents

Recent events have heightened concern about bioterrorism, and concerns about agents such as anthrax are becoming more common questions for health care providers. Nurses provide information that can assist parents in dealing with their toddler's and their own fears. Nurses encourage parents to:

- Talk about their fears and worries
- Stick to family routines that help toddlers feel comfortable and secure
- Supervise toddlers' television viewing
- Educate themselves, the best protection against unnecessary fear. Toddlers will be less fearful if they see that parents are not afraid.

Many parents feel that toddlers, because of their exploratory nature and limited cognitive competence and understanding, are especially vulnerable to certain agents such as anthrax. This is accentuated by knowing that no anthrax vaccine exists for this age group. Fearful parents might request antibiotics that they can keep on hand, just in case. The nurse teaches parents that giving children antibiotics when they are not needed can do more harm than good. Many antibiotics, especially those identified for anthrax

management, have serious side effects and using them when they are not needed can lead to the development of drug-resistant forms of bacteria. If this happens, the antibiotics will not be able to kill the resistant bacteria the next time the child needs the same antibiotic to treat common ear, sinus, or other infections.

The AAP website addresses numerous issues related to bioterrorism and children (*www.aap.org*), including the development of a teaching toolkit for parents to use with their children.

Poisoning

Studies have shown that poisoning happens 10 times more often among young children between the ages of 1 and 4 years than in their older counterparts. Toddlers between the ages of 1 and 2 years are at the greatest risk. They are becoming more mobile, enabling them to explore and discover poisonous substances in the home. These include prescription and over-the-counter medications, alcohol, household products, plants, cosmetics, lead-based paint, and cigarettes (Box 18-4). They are also at risk because they still use their mouths as a way of exploring. Although many parents take precautions against poisoning in their own homes, some forget that toddlers can be poisoned away from home, while visiting grandparents or other relatives, for example (see the Case Study and Care Plan at the end of this chapter).

The toddler, because of limited experience and cognitive level, is unaware that these items are harmful. Many emergency room calls and visits are precipitated by a toddler's ingestion of a potentially or actually harmful substance. These incidents are likely to occur in the kitchen, bathroom, bedroom, or work area and usually are discovered by the parent or caretaker who finds an open or empty container or a half-eaten leaf or other substance.

When parents or caregivers suspect that a toddler has ingested a poisonous substance, they should call the poison control center, even if the child appears perfectly healthy.

Box 18-4   Interventions to Prevent Poisoning in Toddlers

- All household, garden, and car products should be kept out of reach.
- Keep medications out of reach in locked cabinets.
- Use childproof caps on medication.
- Keep all products and medication in their original containers for easy identification.
- No poisonous plants should be kept in the house. A list, which includes poinsettia, amaryllis, aloe vera, English ivy, mistletoe, mums, and spider plants, is available from local poison control centers.
- Avoid outdoor plants and shrubs that are poisonous, including azaleas and mums.
- Supervise toddler's activity at all times.
- Post the poison control center number (800-222-1222) next to every telephone, including your cell phone.

For more information on prevention poisoning and locating the closest poison control center, visit the American Association of Poison Control Centers at *www.aapcc.org*.

Each center is part of a nationwide effort to provide immediate information about poisonings. Parents should not attempt to induce vomiting without specific instructions from the center. Vomiting can cause further harm if the child is drowsy, unconscious, or convulsing, or if the substance ingested is corrosive, such as lye or a strong acid. When vomiting is recommended by the poison control center, instructions often are given to use ipecac syrup to stimulate the vomiting rapidly. This medication should be stored as carefully as any other medication or hazardous household product and replaced often because of its short shelf life.

Chronic poisonings, such as lead poisoning, are often undetected until irreversible damage has occurred. Primary prevention involves teaching parents about risk factors and dangers of lead poisoning and the importance of a diet that encourages decreasing fat intake, because lead is retained in fat. Vitamin C, calcium, and iron intake reduce lead levels in the body. Secondary prevention involves doing periodic screening of blood lead levels on all young children identified at risk. See the Multicultural Awareness box in Chapter 15 about childhood lead poisoning.

Consumer protection laws in the United States require that all toys and furniture manufactured for small children be free of lead-based paint products. However, imported toys and furniture or antique and older family furniture may have been painted with a lead-based product.

SOCIAL PROCESSES
Day Care

During the toddler years many parents return to work or decide that an experience in a group setting would be beneficial for their child. The nurse can provide counseling about the decision to place a child in day care and the resulting emotions, as well as guidelines for selecting a child care or day care provider (Siebel et al., 2008).

The U.S. Department of Health and Human Services Administration for Children and Families recommends a four-step approach as a guideline for selecting a child care provider or day care center (*www.acf.hhs.gov/programs/ccb/parents/index.htm*):

Step 1: Interview potential child-care providers and observe the program or setting.
- Ask about cost; enrollment; ages served; daily activities; accreditation and licensing regulations; caretaker credentials and experience; and policies about visiting, illness, and nutrition.
- Look at provider-child interactions, safety, and the quality of the learning material and toys.

Step 2: Check references.
- Talk to parents with children in the center or being cared for by the provider about discipline and responsiveness to parents, and talk to local child care resource or referral agencies and licensing offices.

Step 3: Make a decision based on specific criteria.
- Think about safety, values, fit for you and your toddler, and affordability.

Step 4: Get and stay involved.
- Talk to the provider regularly about how your child is doing, to your child about what the children are doing each day, and to other parents.
- Visit often, announced and unannounced, and at various times of the day.

Many organizations have developed guidelines and checklists on choosing child care. Child Care Aware (*www.childcareaware.org* or 800-424-2246) is a national initiative designed to improve the quality of care and increase the availability of high-quality child care in local communities. Services include helping to find child care and connecting parents with local child care resource and referral agencies. Their brochure, *Give Your Child Something That Will Last A Lifetime—Quality Child Care,* outlines the steps to finding child care and includes an observation checklist.

Regardless of the reasons for the parents wanting or needing day care for their child, the traditional expectation of caring for the young child at home continues to influence the parents' concept of what they should do for their child. Parents must be reassured that a day care environment congruent with the family environment is not detrimental to the child. If a child has been placed in a setting that is detrimental to physical or emotional development, the parent may need assistance in selecting an alternative setting. Changes in caregivers are difficult for toddlers, and regressive behaviors may surface during transition periods.

Culture and Ethnicity

Culture influences everything we do, know, and believe in. Each culture possesses its own values, attitudes, and practices with regard to family and child-rearing. Toddlers continue to be shaped by the cultural values and beliefs of their parents and families, the first of many socializing forces they will encounter. As their world expands, other forces and subcultures, including peers, the media, and their schools, will also be encountered.

Unlike older children, toddlers do not question the cultural practices of the family. The toddler who refuses to do certain expected things usually does so out of a need for autonomy and control rather than a questioning of beliefs. However, nurses remind parents of this, because parents may be feeling the pressure of cultural norms and expectations. This is especially true for families that have emigrated recently.

Nurses are prepared to provide culturally sensitive and competent care. Knowledge and respect for various cultural world views, customs, values, and traditions are needed to negotiate different approaches in developing a health-promotion plan with families. Health care practices are culturally influenced. For example, if a culture views immunizations as dangerous or unnecessary, the toddler may go unprotected from certain communicable diseases. Incorporation of knowledge, respect, and negotiation facilitates the development of a therapeutic relationship grounded in trust, as well as effective, high-quality health care outcomes (Burns et al., 2008).

Legislation

Local and state legislation specific to the toddler is directed primarily toward safety and injury prevention. Many states have passed laws requiring use of child safety seats, bicycle helmets, and temperature limits for household hot water heaters.

Each state has passed laws that provide protection for a child or developmentally disabled adult, define abuse and neglect, require that a report be made to a designated agency in the case of actual or suspected abuse or neglect, and define the responsibility of the protecting agency. These laws also provide for a central registry of reported cases of abuse. Nurses are aware that they are required by law to report suspected child abuse and should familiarize themselves with the child abuse and neglect laws in their states.

Based on current neuroscience and developmental research, as well as "data from a recent 50 state study of current health, child care, and family support policies," Knitzer (2008, p. 18) proposes 5 care policy challenges: 1) enacting a national family leave; 2) expanding access to child and family programs like Early Head Start; 3) providing policy incentives and resources for high quality infant and toddler child care; 4) strengthening the early identification and treatment for infants and toddlers at risk for poor development; and 5) building a policy framework to support, in every state, an infant and early childhood mental health infrastructure (Knitzer, 2008).

Another legislative issue for the toddler is the Education of the Handicapped Act amendment of 1986 (Public Law 99-457). This law creates programs that assist states in planning, developing, and implementing systems within states for handicapped children from birth to 3 years of age. Nurses who work with young children with disabilities need to investigate and familiarize themselves with the programs in their states.

Economics

Toddlers are completely incapable of contributing to the economic resources of the family; however, a lack or paucity of economic resources is capable of affecting the toddler's health and well-being. Toddlers who live in poverty have higher mortality rates, poorer health, poorer growth, and more physical morbidity from respiratory infections, gastrointestinal infections, anemia, asthma, dental caries, otitis media, and visual loss, as well as higher rates of accidental injury and psychological and developmental disorders (Burns et al., 2008).

About 25% of all children in the United States are enrolled in Medicaid programs and another 10 million are uninsured. In 1997 the State Children's Health Insurance Program (S-CHIP) was developed to address this need. The S-CHIP program expired on September 30, 2007. After much discussion by Congress and two presidential vetoes of revised S-CHIP proposals, President Bush signed legislation that would extend the S-CHIP program through March 2009. Other services that are available to low-income families with toddlers include Temporary Assistance for Needy Families and the Special Supplemental Nutrition Program for Women, Infants, and Children. The nurse can play a critical role in mobilizing these resources for families.

Health Care Delivery System

The health of toddlers is significantly affected by the health care delivery system in the place where they live (Burns et al., 2008). Private physicians or nurse practitioners and public well-child clinics are the most frequently used resources for ongoing health maintenance or illness care for toddlers. Some public clinics sponsor special immunization days for young children who do not receive routine health care.

Each health care visit includes an interval history, assessment of growth and development, physical assessment, a discussion of age-appropriate developmental concerns, and anticipatory guidance. Immunizations are given according to the current Recommended Childhood and Adolescent Immunization Schedule, which is published at least once a year in January by the CDC (*www.cdc.gov/vaccines*) (see **Website Resource 17E**). The nurse informs parents that they can anticipate and keep track of their toddler's immunizations with the CDC Childhood Immunization Scheduler available at *www2a.cdc.gov/nip/kidstuff/newscheduler.le*.

Toddlers need to explore their environment to master it, and this is also valid for their health care encounters. They may need to observe and listen as their parents interact with the health care providers, be introduced to and allowed to manipulate examination equipment, and be given simple explanations and choices so that they can maintain some degree of control. Taking the time to enlist the cooperation of a toddler will make the health care visit more productive and conducive to information exchange and health care teaching.

SUMMARY

This period can be an exciting and challenging time for both toddlers and their parents. Parents who have encouraged their toddlers' desire to explore can now delight in their developing sense of adventure as they enter their preschool years. The world is a wonderful place for the toddler who has known and experienced support, affection, and protection.

CASE STUDY

Grandparents Provide Care: Jeremy

Mary and John are the parents of 18-month-old Jeremy. They plan to take a week-long vacation while leaving Jeremy with his grandparents at their house. Because Jeremy is the first grandchild, the older couple is eager to spend time with him, but they have expressed concern about caring for a toddler.

Reflective Questions:
1. What do the parents need to discuss with the grandparents concerning safety issues?
2. What psychosocial issues of a toddler are important for both the parents and the grandparents to consider?
3. What resources are available for today's grandparents?

CARE PLAN

Grandparents Provide Care: Jeremy

Nursing Diagnosis: At risk of injury related to change in environment and change in primary caregiver(s)

Definition: At risk of injury as a result of the interaction of environmental conditions interacting with the individual's adaptive and defensive resources.

SELECTED RISK FACTORS

- Change in living environment to grandparents' home
- Grandparents home not "child-proofed"
- Change in primary caregiver(s) from parents to grandparents
- Grandparents not up-to-date with caregiver/safety knowledge for toddlers

SUGGESTED INTERVENTIONS

- Surveillance: Safety
  - *Conduct a safety check in grandparents' home/community*

- *Provide a safety checklist for grandparents*
  - *Assist grandparents in identifying resources/support*
- Risk Identification
  - *Identify potential risk factors in grandparents' home/community*
- Teaching: Toddler Care/Safety
  - *Teach grandparents about toddler care/safety issues*

EXPECTED OUTCOMES

- Grandparents will receive instruction re: toddler care/safety.
- Grandparents will take necessary precautions to childproof their home.
- Grandparents will identify available resources to assist in toddler care/safety.
- Toddler will remain free of injury while in grandparents' care.

Based on Johnson, M., Bulechek, G. M., Dochterman, J. M., Maas, M. L., Moorhead, S., Swanson, E., & Butcher, H. K. (2006). *NANDA, NOC, and NIC Linkages: Nursing Diagnosis, Outcomes & Interventions* (2nd ed.). St. Louis: Mosby; NANDA-International (2008). *Nursing Diagnosis: Definitions & Classifications 2009-2011* (2nd ed.). Philadelphia: Wiley-Blackwell. For further information in developing care plans, see: Carpenito-Moyet, L. S. (2008). *Nursing diagnosis: Application to clinical practice* (12th ed.). Philadelphia: Lippincott, Williams & Wilkins.

REFERENCES

American Academy of Pediatrics. (2008). *Bright futures: Guidelines for health supervision of infants, children, and adolescents* (3rd ed.). Elk Grove Village, IL: American Academy of Pediatrics.

American Academy of Pediatrics. (2005). *Car safety seats: A guide for families*. Elk Grove, IL: The Academy. Available from: AAP, 141 Northwest Point Blvd., P.O. Box 927, Elk Grove Village, IL 60007-0927. Retrieved April 5, 2005, from *www.aap.org*.

American Academy of Pediatrics Committee on Nutrition. (2001). The use and misuse of fruit juice in pediatrics. *Pediatrics, 107*(5), 1210–1213.

American Academy of Pediatrics. (2007). *Television and the family*. Elk Grove Village, IL.

American Academy of Pediatrics. (2007). Year 2007 position statement: Principles and guidelines for early hearing detection and intervention programs. Joint Committee on Infant Hearing. *Pediatrics, 120*, 898–921.

Berger, K. S. (2004). *The Developing Person Through the Life Span* (6th ed.). New York: Worth.

Bergman, A., & Harpaz-Rotem, I. (2004). Revisiting reapproachement in the light of contemporary developmental theories. *Journal of the American Psychoanalytic Association, 52*(2), 555–570.

Briggs-Gowan, M. J., & Carter, A. S. (2004). Social-emotional screening status in early childhood predicts elementary school outcomes. *Pediatrics, 121*(5), 957–962.

Burns, C. E., Dunn, A. M., Brady, M. A., Starr, N. B. & Blosser, C. (2008). *Pediatric primary care* (4th ed.). St. Louis: W. B. Saunders.

Caughy, M., Huang, K., & Lima, J. (2009). Patterns of conflict interaction in mother-toddler dyads: Differences between depressed and non-depressed mothers. *Journal of Child and Family Studies, 18*(1), 10–20.

Del Vecchio, T., & O'Leary, S. G. (2008). Predicting maternal discipline responses to early childhood aggression: The role of cognitions and affect. *Parenting: Science & Practice, 8*(3), 240–256.

DeVos, E., Spivak, H., Hatmaker-Flanigan, H., & Sege, R. D. (2006). A Delphi approach to reach consensus on primary care guidelines regarding youth violence prevention. *Pediatrics, 118*(4), 1109–1115.

Erikson, E. H. (1995). *Childhood & society* (35th anniversary ed.). New York: Norton.

Erikson, E. H. (1998). *The life cycle completed*. New York: Norton.

Eshbaugh, E. M. (2006). Adolescent mothers and depression: Predictors of resilience and risk through the toddler years. *Journal of Family Social Work, 10*(3), 13–29.

Garfunkel, L. C., Kaczorowski, J., & Christy, C. (2002). *Pediatric clinical advisor*. St. Louis: Mosby.

Gartstein, M. A., & Bateman, A. E. (2008). Early manifestations of childhood depression: Influences of infant temperament and

parental depressive symptoms. *Infants and Child Development, 17*(3), 223–248.

Garzon, D. L., Lee, R. K., & Homan, S. M. (2007). There's no place like home: A preliminary study of toddler unintentional injury. *Journal of Pediatrics Nursing, 22*(5), 368–375.

Genesee, F. (2008). Early dual language learning. *Zero to Three, 29*(1), 17–23.

Gillam, R. B., Marquardt, T. P., & Martin, F. N. (2000). *Communication sciences and disorders: From science to clinical practice*. San Diego: Singular Publishers.

Green, M., & Palfrey, J. S. (Eds.). (2002). *Bright futures: Guidelines for health supervision of infants, children, and adolescents* (2nd ed., Rev.). Arlington, VA: National Center for Education in Maternal and Child Health.

Grodner, M., Anderson, S. L., & DeYoung, S. (2003). *Foundations and clinical applications of nutrition: A nursing approach* (3rd ed.). St. Louis: Mosby.

Gubala, J. A. (2007). Merits of breastfeeding children through the toddler years. *American Family Physician, 76*(6), 765, 769.

Guyton, A. C., & Hall, J. E. (2006). *Textbook of medical physiology* (11th ed.). Philadelphia: W. B. Saunders.

Hockenberry, M. J., & Wilson, D. (2006). *Wong's nursing care of infants and children* (8th ed.). St. Louis: Mosby.

Knitzer, J. (2008). Giving infants and toddlers a head start: Getting policies in sync with knowledge. *Infants and Young Children, 21*(1), 18–29.

Kolak, A. M., & Vernon-Feagans, L. (2008). Family-level coparenting processes and child gender as moderators of family stress and toddler adjustment. *Infant and Child Development, 17*(6), 617–638.

Mann, J., & Kretchmar, M. D. (2006). A disorganized toddler in foster care: Healing and change from an attachment theory. *Zero to Three, 26*(5), 29–36.

More, J. (2008). Don't forget the undernourished children in our midst. *Journal of Family Health Care, 18*(5), 159–160.

Norris, F. W. (2008). Decision-making criteria in child custody disputes that involve requests for overnight visits with infants and toddlers: Derived from a review of the literature. *Journal of Child Custody, 4*(3-4), 33–43.

Pan, B. A., Rowe, M. L., Singer, J. D., & Snow, C. E. (2005). Maternal correlates of growth in toddler vocabulary production in low-income families. *Child Development, 76*(4), 763–782.

Pediatric Eye Disease Investigator Group. (2002). A randomized trial of atropine vs. patching for treatment of moderate amblyopia in children. *Archives of Ophthalmology, 120*(3), 268–278.

Repka, M. X., Beck, R. W., Holmes, J. M., Birch, E. E., Chandler, D. L., Cotter, S. A. et al. (2003). A randomized trial of patching regimens for treatment of moderate amblyopia in children. *Archives of Ophthalmology, 121*(5), 603–611.

Robins, D. L. (2008). Screening for autism spectrum disorders in primary care settings. *Autism: The International Journal of Research and Practice, 12*(5), 537–556.

Rosales, F. J., & Zeisel, S. H. (2008). Perspectives from the symposium: The role of nutrition in infant and toddler brain and behavioral development. *Nutritional Neuroscience, 11*(3), 135–143.

Siebel, N. L., Gillespie, L. G., & Temple, T. (2008). The role of child care providers in child abuse prevention. *Zero to Three, 28*(6), 33–40.

Seidel, H. M., Ball, J. W., Dains, J. E., & Benedict, G. W. (2006). *Mosby's guide to physical examination* (6th ed.). St. Louis: Mosby.

Story, M., Holt, K., & Sofka, D. (2002). *Bright futures in practice: Nutrition.* Arlington, VA: National Center for Education in Maternal and Child Health.

Treyvaud, K., Anderson, V. A., Howard, K., Bear, M., Hunt, R. W., Doyle, L. W., et al. (2009). Parenting behavior is associated with the early neurobehavioral development of very preterm children. *Pediatrics, 123*(2), 555–561.

Warren, H. K., Denham, S. A., & Bassert, H. H. (2008). The emotional foundations of social understanding. *Zero to Three, 28*(5), 32–39.

Weinfield, N., Ingerski, L., & Moreau, S. (2009). Maternal and paternal depressive symptoms as predictors of toddler adjustment. *Journal of Child and Family Studies, 18*(1), 39–47.

Wetherby, A. M., Brosnan-Maddox, S., Peace, V., & Newton, L. (2008). Validation of the Infant-Toddler Checklist as broadband screener fo autism spectrum disorders from 9 to 24 months of age. *Autism, 12*(5), 487–511.

Wilson, A. L. (2007). The state of South Dakota's child: 2006. *South Dakota Medicine, 60*(1), 7–9, 11.

Wright, C. M., Parkinson, K. N., Shipton, D., Drewett, R. F. (2007). How do toddler eating problems relate to their eating behavior, food preferences, and growth? *Pediatrics, 120*(4), e1069–1075.

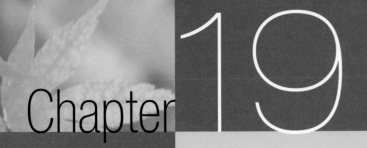

Chapter 19

Anne Rath Rentfro

Preschool Child

objectives

After completing this chapter, the reader will be able to:

- Explain physical and psychosocial changes occurring during the preschool years that influence child and family health needs.
- Discuss the concepts of cognitive development of preschoolers using Piaget's theory.
- Review *Healthy People 2010* concepts that pertain to preschool children and their families.
- Describe family teaching and nursing support for the typical sleep disturbances of the preschooler years.
- Differentiate the nursing roles regarding vision and hearing screening for preschoolers.
- Compare coping skills of preschoolers with those of younger children.
- Outline primary prevention immunization requirements for preschoolers.
- Identify warning signs of cancer in preschoolers.
- List risk factors for asthma in preschoolers.
- Identify major causes of injuries during the preschool years.

key terms

Acquired lactase deficiency
Acute lymphocytic leukemia
Amblyopia
Asthma
Centering
Chloroma
Classroom Assessment Scoring System
Deduction
Doll or puppet play
Draw-a-Person and Draw-a-Family tests
Early and Periodic Screening, Diagnosis, and Treatment (EPSDT)
Eccrine sweat gland function

Egocentrism
Expressive language
Heterophoria
Heterotropia
Homeostasis
Induction explanation
Initiative
Irreversibility
Ishihara's test
Mnemonic techniques
Mutual storytelling
Myopic vision
Neuroblastoma
Nightmares
Night terrors
Otitis media

Parental divorce
Peabody Picture Vocabulary Test
Preoperational stage
Preschool Readiness Experimental Screening Scale (PRESS)
Quiet
Receptive language
Refractive errors
Retinoblastoma
Snellen E chart
Strabismus
Transductive reasoning
Vineland Social Maturity Scale
Wilms tumor

website materials

THINK About It | Aggressive Behavior

Phillip, age 4, started preschool 2 weeks ago after spending his early years at home with his mother and his 18-month-old sister. His mother recently returned to her job as an accountant, works 9 hours a day, and is fatigued when she picks up Phillip at 5:00 pm. Phillip's father travels for his job but is home on weekends to spend time with his family. Although Phillip's mother always believed that he was shy because he was quiet, during the last week at child care he started hitting his peers and becoming loudly vocal at story time. His mother, believing that Phillip's behavior is related to her return to work, feels embarrassed and frustrated by his behavior, especially because she enjoys her new job and the extra income.

1. What factors might be contributing to Phillip's changed behavior?
2. How might you define Phillip's temperament? Why?
3. What discussions might you have with Phillip's parents to help them understand, respond to, and change their son's behavior for the better?

The preschool child (ages 3 to 6 years) has a more developed body structure, an ability to control and use the body, and a facility with language that more closely resembles that of the adult than that of the toddler. The major psychological thrust of this period of development is mastery of self as an independent human being, with a willingness to extend experiences beyond those of the family. Although historically the end of early childhood in the Western world was marked by entrance into the formalized educational system, increasing numbers of children are starting formalized schooling during their preschool years. The *Healthy People 2010* box presents objectives related to this developmental stage (American Academy of Pediatrics, 2007; Hockenberry & Wilson, 2006).

AGE AND PHYSICAL CHANGES

The protuberant abdomen of the toddler disappears during the preschool years as the pelvis begins to straighten and the abdominal muscles develop. Hips gradually rotate inward, replacing out-toeing with straight or slight in-toeing. Mild in-toeing (metatarsus adductus) may remain during the preschool years, but anything beyond a mild level should be investigated and treated.

Growth rates remain steady from ages 3 to 6 years. Average preschoolers gain approximately 2 kilograms (4 pounds) of body weight and 7 centimeters (2 inches) of height each year, whereas head circumference increases less than 2 centimeters during the entire preschool period. During early childhood, skin matures in its ability to protect the child from outer invasion and loss of fluids. The skin's capacity to localize infection increases but remains less than mature. Negligible secretion of sebum makes the skin fairly dry. Changes occur both in color and texture of the hair. Hair usually turns darker and becomes straighter. **Eccrine sweat gland function**, which is the body heat–regulation mechanism, gradually matures, but the quantity of eccrine sweat produced in response to heat or emotion remains minimal. Apocrine sweat glands, located primarily in the axillae, areolas of the breast, and the anal area, remain nonsecretory during this period.

Kidneys reach full maturity by the end of infancy and early toddlerhood with only their size changing during the preschool years. By the end of the preschool years, urine excretion totals from 650 to 1000 milliliters (19 to 30 ounces). Under normal homeostatic conditions, the preschooler's renal system conserves water and concentrates urine on a level that approximates adult abilities. Under conditions of stress, however, their kidneys lack the ability to respond fully and to maintain **homeostasis** when compared with the more rapid response of the adult system.

Healthy People 2010
Selected National Health-Promotion and Disease-Prevention Objectives for Preschool Children

- 01-04a—Increase the proportion of people who have a specific source of ongoing care to 96% (baseline is 93% for children and youth in 1997; 86% in 2006).
- 01-06—Reduce the proportion of families that experience difficulties or delays in obtaining care or do not receive needed care to 7% (baseline is 12% in 1997; 12% in 2001).
- 01-12—Establish a single toll-free telephone number for access to poison control centers on a 24-hour basis throughout the United States to 100% (baseline is 15% of poison control centers shared a single toll-free number in 1999; 100% in 2006).
- 01-13i—Increase the number of tribes, states, and the District of Columbia with trauma care systems that maximize the prevention, survival, and functional outcomes of trauma patients to 100 (baseline = 5 states in 1998; 47 in 2005).
- 01-14a—Increase the number of states and the District of Columbia that have statewide pediatric protocols for on-line medical direction to 100% (baseline is 17 states in 1997; 44 in 2002).
- 08-11—Eliminate elevated blood lead levels in children (baseline is 4.4% of children age 1 to 5 years had blood lead levels exceeding 10 mcg/dL in 1994; 1.1 in 2004).
- 08-16a—Reduce indoor allergen levels to 29 million homes with dust mite allergens exceeding 2 mcg of dust in the bed (baseline is 36.3 million homes in 1999; new data unavailable).
- 18-8—Increase the proportion of people visiting primary health care who receive mental health screening and assessment (baseline 50%; 53% in 2002).
- 21-01a—Reduce the proportion of children and adolescents who have dental caries to 11% (baseline is 18% of children age 2 to 4 years from 1988 to 1994; 24% in 2004).
- 22-11—Increase the proportion of children and adolescents who view television two or fewer hours per day (baseline 57%; 63% in 2005).
- 28-02—Increase the proportion of preschool children age 5 years and under who receive vision screening (baseline 36%; no new data available).
- 28-12—Reduce otitis media in children and adolescents to 294 per 1000 (baseline is 344.7 per 1000 in 1997; 243.2 in 2006).
- 16-2a—Reduce the rate of death for children age 1 to 4 years to 25.0 per 100,000 (baseline is 34.2 per 100,000 in 1998; 29.9 in 2004).
- 24-1a—Reduce deaths from asthma to 1 per million children under age 5 (baseline is 1.7 per million in 1998; 1.8 in 2004).
- 01-09a—Reduce hospitalization rates for pediatric asthma to 17.3 per 10,000 (baseline is 23 per 10,000 in 1996; 22.6 in 2003).

From U.S. Department of Health and Human Services. (2007). *Healthy people 2010: Midcourse review*. Washington, DC: U.S. Government Printing Office. Accessed January 22, 2008, from *http://wonder.cdc.gov/data2010/objsearc.htm*.

Growth of gastrointestinal organs continues through the preschool years without functional changes. Children achieve full voluntary control of elimination. **Acquired lactase deficiency**, intolerance to milk products manifested by diarrhea, often appears during the preschool years. This condition, more common in Black, Asian American, and Native American children, can be managed successfully by eliminating lactose from the diet.

Lung capacity continues to increase, with a gradual decrease in respiratory rate. Preschoolers make better decisions than toddlers about what to put in their mouths resulting in fewer instances of choking and obstruction. Gradual increase in size and shape of ears coincides with decreases in incidence of **otitis media** (inner ear infection). Tonsils and adenoids are large compared to their throat, which may contribute to noisy breathing and upper respiratory infection in preschoolers.

The cardiovascular system enlarges in proportion to general body growth. Heart rate for preschoolers ranges from 40 to 70 beats per minute with a mean blood pressure of 100/60 mm Hg. Early hypertension develops in some children during the preschool years; therefore, measuring blood pressure routinely is indicated, particularly in children with a strong family history of hypertension (see Chapter 20). Preschool children maintain adequate hemoglobin levels when dietary intake is sufficient. Bone marrow of the ribs, sternum, and vertebrae become fully established as primary sites for red blood cell formation. Liver and spleen continue to form erythrocytes and granulocytes.

The immune system continues to develop. Preschoolers boost their immune response to common pathogens as exposure occurs. Group activities, such as joining preschool or play groups, increase exposure and subsequently escalate incidence of common contagious illnesses during the time of exposure, regardless of the child's age. Initial encounters with such group activities usually results in increases in illness. Later these children may be less prone to common contagious diseases because of their early exposure to infectious illnesses and their consequent immunity.

Primary teeth finish erupting by late toddler or early preschool years. Initial permanent teeth generally erupt toward the end of the preschool period. Permanent teeth tend to erupt approximately 6 months earlier in girls than in boys. Older preschoolers usually take responsibility for dental hygiene, although all children need gentle guidance about proper brushing and appropriate nutritional intake for healthy teeth. Parents should continue to assist with and supervise flossing. Because the preschool period is an age of caries formation, regular dental checkups are essential. Nurses assess whether the child is receiving preventive dental care. Parents should be encouraged to begin or maintain this care. Suggestions for promoting good oral hygiene as part of general health-promotion teaching can be found in Chapter 20.

Musculoskeletal and neurological development reaches a level that allows for seemingly effortless walking, running, and climbing. Older preschoolers' ability to copy figures and draw recognizable pictures indicates their advancing fine motor abilities, and they are eager to demonstrate these skills to others. Practice, increases in muscle size, continuing associations among existing neural pathways, and the establishment of new pathways for already accomplished tasks are a few of the many complex factors that contribute to the advances in function observed during early childhood. These advances in fine motor and gross motor skills are outlined in Table 19-1.

Gender

Boys tend to experience more childhood illnesses than do girls during ages 3 to 6 (see Chapter 18). Preschoolers are more aware of their sexual identity than are toddlers and may imitate societal stereotypes more closely. Traditionally boys have been encouraged to take more risks than girls have been and they have more accidents than do preschool girls, who may have been encouraged to choose more sedentary activities. In today's society, boys and girls have opportunities to choose the same activities. Whether this change will reflect accident statistics in the future will be interesting to observe.

Race

Race, with its related economic and cultural issues, can influence health care practices at this age, as is the case during all ages. Cultural preferences and economic issues, therefore, influence the environments and other health-promoting behaviors, such as nutrition and recreation (Brotanek et al., 2005; Harrison, 2006).

Genetics

Signs and symptoms of most genetic problems appear during infancy or the toddler years, whereas other genetic problems will be noted during adolescence. Those most likely to appear during the preschool years are cystic fibrosis, Duchenne muscular dystrophy, fragile X syndrome, and Williams's syndrome (Hockenberry & Wilson, 2006). Genetic conditions diagnosed early in life affect the child's health, and nursing strategies focus on continuing parent education, assessing the development, including complications, and interventions to support family coping (Hockenberry & Wilson, 2006).

GORDON'S FUNCTIONAL HEALTH PATTERNS
Health Perception–Health Management Pattern

Preschoolers have a fairly accurate perception of the external parts of their own bodies based on what they can see and do; they may be extremely curious about the body of a member of the opposite sex. Their concept of what is inside the body and how its internal functions operate are vague and inaccurate. Preschoolers view the internal part of the body as hollow. Most preschoolers can name one or two items inside the body (blood, bones). Many of their questions involve body functions. Anxiety surrounding the body and fear of mutilation and death pervade the children's concerns. Their size as compared with that of adults produces a sense of vulnerability and fear of loss of control (Vagnoli et al., 2005).

Growth and Development	Table 19-1

Developmental and Behavioral Milestones for Preschool Children

Age	Expectations
3 years	At this age, the typical child: Opens doors Kicks a ball; jumps in place; rides on a tricycle Builds a tower of nine cubes; imitates bridge made from three cubes Demonstrates speech that is mostly intelligible. (The child who fails to speak in sentences or whose speech is unintelligible to strangers should be referred for speech, language, and hearing evaluation.) Knows own name, age, and gender May comprehend cold, tired, hungry; may understand the prepositions over and under; differentiates bigger and smaller; can convey the use of scissors, key, and pencil Copies a circle, may imitate a cross, and begins to visually discriminate colors Describes action in picture books and shows some early imaginative behavior Puts on some clothing and shoes Eats without assistance

Growth and Development   Table 19-1

Developmental and Behavioral Milestones for Preschool Children—cont'd

Age	Expectations
4 years	At this age, the typical child:
	Alternates feet when descending stairs; jumps forward; hops on one foot, and can stand on 1 foot for up to 5 seconds
	Climbs a ladder
	Rides a tricycle or a bicycle with training wheels
	Can walk on tiptoes
	Throws a ball overhand
	Holds and uses a pencil with good control
	Builds a tower of 10 or more cubes
	Is able to cut and paste
	Gives first and last name
	Engages in conversational give-and-take
	Asks, why, when, how, and inquires about meanings of words
	Talks about daily experiences and things that are used at home (food, appliances)
	Can name three or four primary colors
	Can count from 1 to 5
	Enjoys jokes
	Can sing a song
	Knows about things used at home (e.g., food, appliances)
	Washes and dries hands and brushes teeth
	Dresses and undresses with supervision, except for handling laces and buttons, when allowed sufficient time to dress; begins to be selective about clothes
	Initiates dramatic make-believe and dress-up play during which the child assumes a specific role
	Is imaginative and intensely curious
	Distinguishes between fantasy and reality
	Has formed gender identification
	Copies a cross and circle
	Draws a person with two to three parts
	Enjoys the companionship of other children, plays cooperatively, and shows interest in other children's bodies
	Meets the challenges of kindergarten class
	Rides with training wheels
	Is aware of gender of others
5 years	At this age, the typical child:
	May be able to skip; can walk on tiptoes; broad jumps
	Can cut and paste
	Names four or five colors and can identify coins
	Tells a simple story and knows several nursery rhymes
	Defines at least one word (ball, shoe, chair, table, dog)
	Dresses and undresses without supervision
	Knows address and telephone number
	Can count on fingers
	Copies a triangle from an illustration
	Recognizes many letters of the alphabet
	Prints some letters
	Draws a person with a head, body, arms, and legs
	Begins to understand right and wrong, fair and unfair
	Engages in dramatic make-believe and dress-up play during which the child assumes a specific role; engages in domestic role playing and dressing up
	Enjoys the companionship of other children; plays cooperatively
	Has formed gender identification ("Are you a boy or girl?")
6 years	At this age, the typical child:
	Bounces a ball 4 to 6 times; throws and catches
	Skates
	Rides a bicycle
	Ties shoelaces
	Counts up to 10; prints own first name; prints numbers up to 10
	Understands right from left
	Draws a person with six body parts, with the figure depicted wearing clothing

Modified from American Academy of Pediatrics. (2007). *Bright futures: Guidelines for health supervision of infants, children, and adolescents* (3rd ed.). Elk Park, IL: American Academy of Pediatrics.

By age 4 or 5, children have amassed their beliefs about health from the family. They begin to understand that they play a role in their own health. The preschooler often becomes upset over minor injuries. Pain or illness may be viewed as a punishment. The preschooler's declaration, "If you don't put your seat belt on you will get in an accident" is a statement that reflects the idea of expected immediate and absolute cause and effect. The preschooler cannot conceive that the purpose of the seat belt is to prevent injury in the event of an accident, not prevention of the accident itself.

Although preschoolers are not completely responsible for their own health management, they certainly contribute by brushing their teeth, taking medication, wearing appropriate clothing for inclement weather, and performing other actions. Preschoolers' memory for these activities can be sporadic, but they are at least beginning to be health care agents for themselves (Hockenberry & Wilson, 2006).

Reinforcement of health-promotion activities, which occurs in the home and the child-care environment, helps to instill behaviors that affect self-esteem, safety, and an individual's overall balance with life. For example, family support for active lifestyles provides one way for parents to assume a positive role to model for children (Floriani & Kennedy, 2007). The National Association of Pediatric Nurse Practitioners has designed resources to use with families and children to promote Healthy Eating and Activity Together (HEAT) (Gottesman, 2007). Many community bookstores carry health-promotion–focused books appropriate to the preschool population; these references provide information for discussion among parents, caregivers, and children on the importance of healthy behaviors for success in life. See **Website Resource 19A** for a detailed list of recommended books.

Nutritional-Metabolic Pattern

Establishing healthful nutritional and physical activity behaviors begins during childhood. Children should eat a variety of foods with at least five servings of fruits and vegetables per day. Preschool children should consume approximately half of their diet in carbohydrates, with the other half consisting of protein (5% to 20%) and fat (30% to 40%) (Burrowes, 2007). With over half of the preschool diet consisting of carbohydrates, whole grains and other complex carbohydrates should be plentiful to attain a total fiber of 20 to 25 grams per day. Fat consumption in preschool children is higher than in older children, but should include primarily unsaturated fat, with saturated fat, transfatty acids, and cholesterol intake as low as possible (Burrowes, 2007). Although iron-deficiency anemia is decreasing generally, it is more prevalent in vulnerable populations (McCann & Ames, 2007). Studies that have been conducted, although small in number, demonstrate support for the idea that iron deficiency results in behavioral and cognitive deficits (McCann & Ames, 2007). Salt and sugar intake should be moderate. Marshall's study group (2007) provides support for limiting nonmilk sugar intake in order to limit carcinogenicity. Their findings suggest that sugar delivery agents along with

their mode of exposure (rather than the type of sugar) present more of a risk for caries than the type of sugar. Guidance for the types and amounts of foods are depicted in the system called MyPyramid (U.S. Department of Agriculture, 2005). MyPyramid, which replaces the Food Guide Pyramid, was developed as a personalized approach to healthy eating and physical activity (Marshall, 2006; Peregrin, 2006; U.S. Department of Agriculture, 2005). A child-friendly version of MyPyramid addresses the special needs of children 6 to 11 years old (U.S. Department of Agriculture, 2005).

The Fitness Pyramid depicts typical situations intended to encourage physical activity among children (Haven & Britten, 2006). The pyramid website uses interactive strategies to produce more personalized recommendations. A figure climbing up the left side of the pyramid links to recommendations for physical activity (Coleman, 2005).

Bone growth needs in 1- to 4-year-old children following American diets are met by a daily calcium intake of 470 mg/d, which suggests that the current Adequate Intake of 500 mg/d is close to the actual Estimated Average Requirement. The benefits and risks of higher calcium intakes consistent with threshold values should be evaluated in a controlled trial before those intakes could be used as a basis for dietary recommendations.

Preschooler dietary patterns are unique to their age group, making estimates for consumption of nutrients difficult. Generally, estimates for preschoolers are adapted from food intake patterns of other age groups (Lynch et al., 2007). Adequate calcium intake for this age group has been set at approximately 500 mg/dL. Preschoolers need approximately 90 kcal/kg of body weight per day for health maintenance, activity, and growth. **Website Resource 19B** lists a typical daily distribution of foods that provides the essential calories and nutrients. As early childhood progresses, intense food preferences emerge. This behavior is a natural outgrowth of the increased physical capacity to react to the taste and textures of foods and the realization that expressing an opinion about food is a way to control the environment. Older preschoolers frequently refuse to try new foods. Favorite foods for this age are meat, cereal grains, baked products, fruits, and sweets. Parents should provide nutritious foods, avoiding salty and sweet foods. Parents should encourage good nutritional habits to help establish healthy eating behaviors (Hockenberry & Wilson, 2006). Increased consumption of fats and processed foods along with diminished physical activity have contributed to a significant increase in obesity and type 2 diabetes in children and adolescents (Kumanyika, 2007; U.S. Department of Health and Human Services, 2007).

Family tolerance for individual food preferences varies, and children vary in their tendency to develop strong likes and dislikes. When families reach extreme differences over food preferences, major conflicts may arise requiring insightful counseling to achieve a mutually satisfying solution. Nurses collaborate with families to discover comfortable approaches to maintain nutritional adequacy of foods that children prefer. Community nurses use a variety of approaches and recognize the wide range of possibilities that exist for families of varying cultures (Donohue et al., 2006; Leininger & McFarland, 2006).

Preschoolers frequently eat meals away from home. Minimal standards require licensed child-care centers and preschools to serve foods using recommended dietary allowances of basic nutrients. Parents should communicate regularly with agency personnel about foods eaten at home and away to provide healthy food variety. Preschoolers in group settings learn both positive and negative eating habits and food preferences from care providers and other children. Communication about these habits reinforces positive behaviors and discourages negative habits at home (Innovative Practice box).

Nutrition and dentition impact health at all ages. Pain from dental caries, infection, and poorly cared-for teeth affects appetite and chewing ability with a subsequent impact on future nutritional status. Dental caries in children have declined dramatically in recent years because of preventive measures such as tooth brushing with fluoride toothpaste, community water fluoridation, sound dietary

practices, and dental sealants. Children from low-income families carry the bulk of the burden of these dental caries (Fisher-Owens et al., 2007; Gilbert, 2005). Oral health promotion involves self-care and population-based initiatives, along with professional care. Adequacy of professional dental care varies significantly by age, race, educational level, family income, and dental status (Fisher-Owens et al., 2007; Gilbert, 2005).

Preschoolers struggle with the intricacies of using utensils. In the later years of the preschool period, children attain skill with spoons, demonstrate fair proficiency with forks, and manage knives for spreading soft foods on bread or crackers. Most preschool children, however, need help cutting meat and pouring from large, heavy containers. Preschoolers enjoy helping to prepare family meals and may be capable of simple tasks, such as washing fruits and vegetables. Involving young children in meal preparation teaches them about healthy nutrition. Sharing important family functions nurtures self-esteem and a sense of value.

Prevalence of food allergy in children in the United States continues to increase (Collier et al., 2004). Most allergies develop before the age of 2. Foods most likely to cause allergic reactions include: milk and milk products; eggs and egg products; peanuts and peanut products; tree nuts and tree nut products; soybeans and soybean products; fish and fish products; shellfish and shellfish products; cereals containing glutens; and seeds. Reactions to peanuts tend to decrease over time; however, children who experience peanut allergy should keep epinephrine available until tolerance can be ensured (Collier et al., 2004). Clear food labeling and education are essential for preventing allergic reactions. A food labeling law passed in 2006, the Food Allergen Labeling and Consumer Protection Act (FALCPA), requires manufacturers to use specific terminology and to state clearly when ingredients include one of eight major food allergens or any protein derived from these allergens: milk; eggs; peanuts; tree nuts such as almonds, walnuts, and pecans; wheat; soybeans; fish such as bass, flounder, and cod; and crustacean shellfish such as crab, lobster, and shrimp (Bren, 2006). Many preschools have banned foods such as peanut products as a precautionary measure. Parents may need help identifying potential hazardous situations and communicating their child's needs to agency personnel. A Food Allergy Action Plan should be developed for parents to use to facilitate communication regarding the child's allergies (Collier et al., 2004).

innovative practice

Healthy Start

Risk factors for cardiovascular diseases are prevalent by 3 years of age, the most common of which are hypercholesterolemia and obesity. Healthy Start, a project located in Valhalla, New York, sponsored by the Child Health Foundation and the American Health Foundation, is a 3-year demonstration and research program to evaluate the effectiveness of interventions for reducing cardiovascular risk factors in preschool centers. Two interventions are recommended. The first is the preschool food service, which is designed to reduce the total fat in the preschooler's meals and snacks to less than 30% of calories and to reduce saturated fat to less than 10% of calories. The second intervention is a comprehensive preschool health education curriculum, which focuses on nutrition and exercise.

The effectiveness of this program is evaluated using many components. Changes in the nutritional behaviors (including dietary intake of school snacks and meals of the preschoolers) are being recorded, as are those in snacks and meals consumed at home. Special attention is being given to the intake of total and saturated fat. Additionally, changes in the health knowledge of preschoolers are being assessed to evaluate the education component. Physical examination data include semiannual assessments of growth and body weight and blood lipid levels.

The specific details of rationale and methods of the randomized controlled trial studies within the Healthy Start project are described at the website: *www.healthy-start.com*.

Healthy-Start, LLC
PO Box 115
Huntington, NY 11743

Telephone: (631) 549-0010
Fax: (631) 824-9182 (TIN# 010533895)
Email: info@healthy-start.com

Elimination Pattern

Older preschool children are capable of and responsible for independent toileting. They may forget to flush the toilet or wash their hands when they are rushed, but they have the physical ability to perform the skills. Preschoolers should not be teased or punished when they are unable to perform independently. If their clothing becomes soiled, they should be responsible for changing their clothes and reminded gently and encouragingly of ways to avoid problems in the future. (Enuresis and encopresis are discussed in Chapter 20.)

Activity-Exercise Pattern

Play continues to be the primary activity for preschoolers as well as for toddlers. Preschoolers explore intently and demonstrate increased coordination and confidence with motor activities. They venture farther from home than toddlers do. Many activities involve other children (Figure 19-1) and involve modeling behavior. Particularly in group care settings, children should be monitored for safe activities that enhance gross and fine motor skills while creating fun in movement.

Most 4-year-old children separate easily from their parents, play simple interactive games, dress themselves, copy a number of basic geometric figures well, and draw recognizable people. Preschoolers enjoy using language skills to tell stories and ask questions. Their physical abilities include balancing on one foot, jumping, and running (Hockenberry & Wilson, 2006). Generally, preschoolers appreciate an audience, enjoy practicing new skills, and demonstrate mastered skills to others.

Play constitutes an important role in preschoolers' social and psychological development. Play offers a vehicle that allows them to explore while experimenting with who they are, who they might become, and how they relate to others socially. The drama of play allows preschoolers to view themselves from another perspective. Play often reveals the child's reality and perception of the world.

Children mimic the behavior of people familiar to them, rehearsing what has been demonstrated to them as appro-

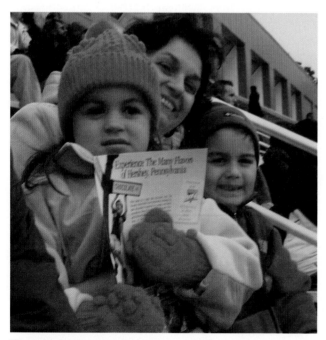

Figure 19-1   Preschool children enjoy a sporting event with their grandmother.

priate behavior. Young children seldom assume the role of a younger child or infant while playing. They usually assume adult roles and use a doll for the younger child. Through play preschoolers learn to exert control over their own behavior. Assuming an adult role in play allows children to consciously adopt more mature behaviors.

Patterns of behavior used in play can be transferred to actual situations. For example, children who express their anger in a play situation aggressively by vocalizing their distress, scolding the offending party, or using withdrawal of attention are likely to respond with aggression or tantrum behavior when facing frustration or anger in real life situations. Observing children at play reveals their natural physical capacities better than observing them in an examination or testing environment and provides further evidence of the child's social and inner development.

Observing imitation play in peer groups helps nurses assess social competency. At first the new child in a peer group may be expected to stand back and observe other children before manipulating a toy (Hockenberry & Wilson, 2006). Preschool children engage in more interactive play, particularly dramatic play, than at any other age. Two or more children may become involved in an imaginary plot, especially when toys and equipment support a particular scenario, such as toy kitchen equipment. Much of the preschooler's play involves fantasy. The young child frequently invents an imaginary companion who plays, eats, and sleeps with the child. (The section about cognition and perception addresses more fully the aspects of fantasy during the preschool stage.)

Most preschoolers spend some time in a group setting each week. Ground rules at these facilities govern sharing, quiet times, and group activities. The preschooler regulates bodily activity and copes with limit setting better than the toddler.

Although time orientation remains incompletely developed in preschoolers, they have an idea about past and future. They enjoy planning activities with their parents for the future. Visiting the library to review books about wild animals, packing lunches, and choosing what clothes to wear may preface a trip to the zoo.

Many preschoolers spend long periods each day watching television. Occasionally parents use the television inappropriately to entertain the child. Although some excellent television shows are available for preschoolers, a significant amount of airtime focuses on adult themes and violence. Many experts agree that television disengages the child's mind and supports less learning (see Chapter 20). Parents should remember that preschoolers who watch television (1) do not have enough life experiences to interpret many of the issues presented in adult shows (violence, interpersonal relationships, moral decisions), (2) might be missing opportunities for interacting with other children or adults and other opportunities for active learning, and (3) cannot judge which shows are appropriate for them. In addition, television, a sedentary activity, inhibits children from developing an active healthy lifestyle.

Parents should choose which shows are appropriate for their child and, when possible, watch these shows with the child, which provides an opportunity for discussion and for the child to ask questions (Bryant et al., 2007; Gable et al., 2007; Shivers & Barr, 2007). Nurses explain to parents and preschoolers the relationship between watching television and lack of physical activity that leads to health problems such as obesity (Atherson & Metcalf, 2005; Nelson & Gordon-Larsen, 2006; Zabinski et al., 2007).

Sleep-Rest Pattern

Most preschoolers sleep from 8 to 12 hours during the night, with wide variation from child to child. For many older preschoolers, a nap is not necessary (Jenni & LeBourgeois, 2006). The preschooler who still naps usually requires only 30 to 60 minutes a day (Hockenberry & Wilson, 2006). Quiet time provides a welcome respite for the parent, along with a chance for the active preschooler to relax before afternoon activities. Many child-care environments routinely provide these rest periods, enhancing rest and relaxation with soft music and a story. An afternoon rest also gives the young child energy for the evening routine when family members have other duties beyond work and school.

Bedtime Ritual

Preschoolers usually require a ritual of activities at bedtime to move from playing and being with others to being alone and falling asleep. These children prolong bedtime routines more often than the toddler. They insist on sleeping with the light on, take a treasured object to bed, request parental attention after being told good night, and experience delays falling asleep. The bedtime ritual generally lasts 30 minutes or longer. Parents should honor reasonable rituals, but repeated requests for attention afterward should generally be handled firmly and consistently. Vigorous resistance to bedtime challenges parents more during the preschool period than at any other developmental stage. Preschoolers learn to use the behaviors that meet their needs and control the family regardless of the disruption created.

Nursing Interventions

When a demanding bedtime behavior extends beyond one year or an episode persists longer than 1 hour, the nurse explores the family situation. A comprehensive assessment in this case includes the following elements:

1. Description of early episodes
2. The manner in which these early episodes were managed and the progression of events since then
3. Current bedtime behaviors of the child and siblings
4. Identification of parental temperament and the resulting responses of parent and family members
5. Feelings of the parents and child about each other and about the bedtime situation
6. Stressful events and changes that have occurred over the past several years
7. Behavior of the child at other times of the day
8. Parents' thoughts about reasons why these episodes continue
9. Parents' ideas about strategies to use now

The nurse observes interactions within the family. A home visit at mealtime provides an excellent method to observe active interaction. In the office or clinic setting the nurse can ask a parent to teach the child a task or give directions. The nurse remains as unobtrusive as possible while observing the interaction. The first-hand observation of parent-child interaction, along with the detailed history, usually provides the nurse with adequate baseline information to decide whether to manage the situation in the primary care setting or refer the family to a child behavior specialist. Sharing recent literature about management techniques for children with differing temperaments helps families understand more about the behaviors. Research-based strategies should be used to help parents reach their goals related to managing bedtime concerns.

Sleep Disturbances

Night terrors and **nightmares** characterize the nighttime wakening problems that generally occur during the preschool years. Night terrors manifest as frightening dreams that cause the child to sit up in bed, scream, stare at an imaginary object, breathe heavily, perspire, and appear in obvious distress (see Chapter 18). The child, not fully awake, may be inconsolable for 10 minutes or more, before he or she relaxes and returns to a deep sleep. In most cases the child does not recall the dream and in the morning does not remember the incident. These night terrors can start at approximately age 2 but are more common during the preschool years. Night terrors rarely occur in older children and adults, and only approximately 6% of preschool children have them. Night terrors and *nightmares* trigger apprehension for the parents (Mason & Pack, 2005).

Nightmares (anxiety dreams) are a more common cause of night wakening. Although infants and toddlers likely have nightmares, their limited verbal skills hinder relating details of the incidents. After age 3, nightmares occur frequently. Approximately 20% of the night is spent dreaming. Dreams frighten preschoolers as they connect to the larger world with their active imaginations and fantastic ideas. These children usually waken fully and feel fearful and helpless. Usually they provide vivid descriptions at the time, and they frequently remember the event the following morning. Consolation can be given by a parent who sits with the child, listens to descriptions and fears about the dream, and reminds the child that dreaming is natural and sleep will soon return.

Helping children appreciate the meaning of the words *pretend* and *real* facilitates growth during this phase of childhood. When the parent reads a story to the child or the child tells a make-believe tale, the parents can specify that these are "pretend" and did not really happen. The parent relating a true event can say, "This is real." Children differentiate between the two concepts as they develop cognitively.

Recommendations

Parents of a preschooler can benefit from knowing the following facts:

1. Bedtime rituals of 30 to 45 minutes are common for preschoolers. These rituals, because of their importance to children, should be respected within reasonable limits.
2. Night-wakening events are common during the preschool years. Children who waken at night should be reassured and encouraged to remain in their own beds.
3. Parents should have clear rules about children sleeping with them if the children will not stay in their own beds.
4. Restricting frightening television shows and stories and discussing "real" versus "pretend" ideas and stories can help lessen the incidence of nightmares.

Cognitive-Perceptual Pattern

During the preschool years, children cultivate their conceptual and cognitive capacities. The quality of the child's care environment enhances these gains. The child gradually differentiates today from yesterday and defines tomorrow and future more clearly as concepts of time emerge. The child becomes more oriented in space and develops an awareness of the location of the home within the neighborhood. The child also begins to structure daily activities and to value certain activities, objects, and people above others.

Piaget's Theory

The older toddler enters the first substage of the **preoperational stage** described by Jean Piaget (see Chapter 18). The hallmark of this preconceptual substage includes the ability to function symbolically using language. The preschool child demonstrates increased symbolic functioning during the intuitive substage, from age 4 to 7 years. The predominant feature of this and the following period is the concrete thought process, as compared with adult thinking. As they experience symbolic mental representations, preschoolers process mental symbols as though they were actually participating in the event. An adult analyzes and synthesizes symbolic information without concrete connections between the mental process and the actual event. At this stage, mental abstraction, such as skipping from one part of an operation to another, reversing the operation mentally, or thinking of the whole in relation to the parts is not feasible.

The **egocentrism** that is characteristic of the preschool years exemplifies this concept of concrete thinking. At this stage, children concentrate solely on their own perspective. They consider only their own personal meanings for symbols. The preschooler wonders why another person fails to follow these idiosyncratic communications.

Furthermore, attention focuses solely on one part of an object without shifting. This behavior, termed **centering** by Piaget, illustrates the child's inability to consider more than one factor at a time when solving simple problems. For example, a child can be given two identical cups containing equal amounts of water and asked which cup contains the greater amount of water. During the preoperational stage, the child responds that they contain the same amount of water. The child is then asked to pour the water from each cup into two different containers (one flat and wide, the other tall and narrow). When asked which container has more water, the child always identifies one, usually the taller, narrower container in which the water reaches a higher level. When the water is again transferred to the identical cups and the experiment repeated, the child returns to the original conclusion that the amounts are equal.

This experiment also illustrates the trait of **irreversibility**. The child is unable to connect the reversible operation, the transfer of the water back into the original cup, to reach the logical conclusion that the differently shaped containers may hold the same amount of water. The child cannot mentally associate that the transformation from one state to another relates to the shape of the container, not the amount of the water.

Finally, Piaget describes the preoperative stage of thinking as **transductive reasoning**. The child cannot proceed from general to particular (**deduction**) or from particular to general (induction); rather, the child moves only from particular to particular in making associations and solving problems. For example, Piaget relates an association made by one of his children between being hunchbacked and being ill. When a hunchbacked neighbor was unable to visit one day because he had a communicable illness, the child understood that the neighbor was ill. However, when the child was told later that the neighbor was better and that she could go see him, her conclusion was that now his hunched back was straight and well. She thought in terms of the man being well or ill, but she placed the man in one or the other category and assumed that he possessed all the attributes and meanings that she linked symbolically with either trait.

The cognitive development of preschoolers is reflected in their symbolic games, which becomes significantly more orderly and representative of reality (Box 19-1). They begin to incorporate the reality of the world, as it exists outside the self. They increasingly seek play objects that represent models of authentic objects in their environment. Preschoolers progressively imitate more social rules in their play. Social interactive play predominates as the young child develops a more secure sense of self.

The preschooler may have one or more imaginary companions who exist for varying periods. These fantasy companions assume the form of another child, an animal, or some other friendly or fearsome creature. The preschooler may save special chairs, insist that an extra place be set at the table, and talk at length to this companion. Imaginary companions serve an important function; they are controlled totally by the

Box 19-1 Play as a Method of Learning: Preschool-Age Child

Throughout life, play develops cognitive, affective, and psychomotor skills that are important to the effective performance of life skills. For the preschool-age child, the following play activities provide the foundation for later competency and socialization-skill refinement:
- Arts and crafts (jewelry making, painting, drawing, ceramics, printmaking)
- Group sports (softball, volleyball, soccer, swimming)
- Skating, skateboarding
- Bicycling
- Puzzles
- Gymnastics
- Games (board, card, knock-knock jokes, computer)
- Secret clubs
- Imaginary play (being in playhouse productions)
- Horseback riding

child and are not a threat. The preschooler practices social interactions, controls a fearsome beast, or blames someone for naughty behavior without fear of scolding, shame, or attack. Imaginary companions do and say only what the child wills.

Vision

Vision capabilities, which are well developed by 2 years of age, continue to undergo refinement during the early childhood period. By approximately age 6, the child should approach a 20/20 visual acuity level. The possibility of developing **amblyopia** decreases; it appears most frequently during infancy through approximately the fourth year (see Chapter 18). Depth perception and color vision become fully established, and the child recognizes subtle differences in color shading by the sixth year. Maximal visual capability usually is achieved by the end of the preschool years.

Visual capacity throughout the rest of life deteriorates rather than improves. This phenomenon relates partly to changes in the refractive power of the lens and developmental changes that occur in the shape of the eyeball. In the normal sequence of growth, the eyeball becomes increasingly spherical, losing the short shape typical of infancy and progressing to the point at which light converges accurately on the surface of the retina. This change occurs at approximately 6 years of age. When this change occurs before the sixth year, growth continues past the point of ideal light conversion, the eyeball lengthens, and the child may develop early **myopic vision**, which will progress with age. Glasses are always indicated for the child who develops myopia before approximately age 8.

Early detection requires regular screening with standardized tests such as the Denver Eye Screening Test or the Snellen Screening Test. The Denver Eye Screening Test was designed for preschool children and includes detection of the commonly occurring visual problems, such as **refractive errors**, **strabismus** (crossing of the eyes), and amblyopia.

The Snellen Screening Test, when administered under standardized procedures, has the advantage of rendering a reliable estimate of actual visual acuity. The child must be able to understand the test requirements of either pointing in the direction of the Es or naming the letters.

The **Snellen E chart** is designed for preschool children; a version for home testing is available from the National Society for Prevention of Blindness. Home testing has been demonstrated to be reliable and offers the advantage of obtaining an estimate for younger children who might not cooperate with this type of testing in a strange environment.

The pupillary light reflex provides a screening approach for **heterotropia**, a condition in which the child's eyes do not focus together to transmit effective, coordinated binocular vision. When the child has heterotropia, the light from a penlight held approximately 20 inches from the eyes reflects off the pupil slightly off center. Consistent and observable *strabismus* may be noted. The cover test provides further evidence of a tendency for the child's eyes to cross, known as **heterophoria**. The child focuses on a spot 14 inches away, then 20 feet away. As the child gazes at the designated spot, one eye is covered completely for several seconds (the eye and eyelashes must not be touched), and then the cover is removed abruptly. If the covered eye moves from the line of vision of the uncovered eye, that eye has a tendency toward muscle imbalance and must be evaluated further (Bickley & Szilagyi, 2007; Hockenberry & Wilson, 2006).

Color blindness presents a particular problem for younger children, because many cues encountered at school depend on the child's ability to distinguish colors. With early detection, the child is able to receive assistance to interpret visual cues, thus minimizing the disadvantage of being color blind. The nurse screens for certain types of color discrimination difficulties by asking the child to respond to various colors in the environment; however, accurate testing for all types of color blindness requires a specialized tool, such as **Ishihara's test**, which uses a series of cards with color-tinted letters and figures.

The preschooler may be aware of some discomfort or limitations with vision. The nurse gathers history from the parents, including the questions listed in the Vision section in Chapter 18, about signs of eye problems. The preschooler is asked questions to elicit information about the following symptoms:

1. Itching, burning, or "scratchy" eyes
2. Poor vision
3. Dizziness, headaches, or nausea after close eye work
4. Blurred or double vision

Hearing

During the preschool years, hearing develops to the level of an adult's, when the ability to attend to and interpret what is heard becomes more refined. The 4-year-old preschooler begins to discriminate among remarkably similar speech sounds, such as the difference between sounds made with "f" and "th" or "f" and "s." It is generally accepted that hearing ability of the preschooler can be hindered by repeated middle ear infections (otitis media). Otitis media with effusion occasionally can result in temporary hearing loss. Parents who notice language delays because of ear infections should be referred to their health care provider for appropriate follow-up (Hockenberry & Wilson, 2006). Parental reports of difficulty should be taken seriously. Not all cases of hearing impairment are identified with newborn screening. One study reported nine cases where hearing loss was identified subsequent to a normal newborn hearing test (Norris et al., 2006).

Audiometric methods most accurately measure the child's ability to hear. Preschool children possess the developmental capability to perform the standard audiometric test. The child can follow directions by this age, and most preschoolers enjoy demonstrating their abilities and cooperate easily during vision and hearing screening (Hockenberry & Wilson, 2006). Refractive error can be significant in the preschool child. The prevalence of refractive errors (5% to 7%) and amblyopia (2% to 4%) in preschool children places vision loss as an important pubic health concern (Ramsey & Bradford, 2006). Children under 7 years of age demonstrate significant improvement in amblyopia when treated, providing a rationale for screening and early recognition programs (Ramsey & Bradford, 2006). The American Academy of Pediatrics on-line resources supply a wealth of information for nurses and families at *www.aap.org/healthtopics/vision-hearing.cfm*.

To ensure success, the nurse encourages a positive experience by adhering to the following points:

- Use equipment skillfully.
- Use age-appropriate language. Avoid the word test to limit anxiety or fear of failure.
- Encourage the child to ask questions and scrutinize the equipment.
- Perform screening before other intrusive or painful procedures.
- Perform screening in a quiet, private area without distractions.
- Praise the child for cooperating.
- Allow rest periods when the child becomes distracted or tired.
- Discuss results with the child in age-appropriate language.

Sensory Perception

Sensory abilities contribute to preschoolers' skill to perceive and interact with the world. Both sensory acuity and sensory perceptual abilities mature during the preschool years. The nature of the visual stimulus determines the response. Preschoolers respond powerfully to visual illusions and have difficulty discriminating right and left mirror images.

Confusion commonly occurs with the letters "b," "d," "p," and "q."

Language

Cognitive and sensory abilities contribute to preschool language development. Toward the end of the preschool period, **expressive language** rivals that of an adult except for minor deficiencies in refinement, vocabulary, and structure. Language ability depends on aptitude, opportunities to use language, quality and quantity of language used at home, and range of experiences. Regardless of expressive capacity, the child develops **receptive language** during the preschool years that provides a vital foundation for later communication (Hockenberry & Wilson, 2006). Throughout early childhood, receptive capacity exceeds expressive capacity. Children comprehend meanings of words and phrases not contained in their expressive vocabulary. Associations between concepts materialize, although the child lacks the ability to explain these concepts. Table 19-2 outlines the receptive and expressive language skills of the preschooler.

During the early childhood years, rhythm develops as an important dimension in speech capacity. Between ages 3 and 5 years, children practice speaking by mimicking adult language patterns. Practice expands neuromotor capacities, and verbal interaction develops vocabulary and sense of grammatical structure. Hesitations, repetitions, and frequent revisions in speech reflect attempts to expand language capacity. Adults may label such preparation as stuttering, but these inaccuracies actually represent normal speech maturation. Many authorities believe that stuttering originates during this developmental period, arising not from inadequacy of the child, but rather from adult response to this normal broken speech pattern. Adult reactions of impatience while waiting for the child to express thoughts decrease the child's opportunities to use language. Insisting children use correct speech before capacity for fluent speech develops may hinder normal speech development. As many as 60% of expressive language delays resolve during the preschool years (Glogowska et al., 2006). In their study of 196 children, however, Glogowska et al. (2006) determined that approximately 30% continued to struggle with language literacy and social difficulties after treatment. These researchers concluded that although language impairment resolves in most children, a substantial number require ongoing support (Glogowska et al., 2006). As nurses help parents provide anticipatory guidance for language development, they should maintain vigilance to identify those children who are not outgrowing their language difficulties. These children encounter lifelong obstacles with learning and socialization. Suggestions for nurses to assist parents and to facilitate preschoolers' language development are listed in Box 19-2.

Growth and Development   Table 19-2

Landmarks of Speech, Language, and Hearing Ability During the Preschool Period

Age (Months)	Receptive Language	Expressive Language	Related Hearing Ability
42	Up to 4200 words; knows words such as *what, where, how, funny, we, surprise, secret*; knows number concepts to 2; knows how to answer some questions accurately, such as, Do you have a dog? Which is the girl? What toys do you have?	Up to 1200 words in mostly complete sentences averaging 4 to 5 words per sentence; uses all 50 phonemes; 7% of sentences are compound or complex; averages 203 words per hour; rate of speech is accelerating; relates experiences and tells about activities in sequential order; such as what, where, how, see, little, funny, they, we, he, she, several; can recite a nursery rhyme; asks permission; 95% of speech is intelligible	Begins to make fine discriminations among similar speech sounds, such as the difference between *f* and *th* or *f* and *s*. Child has matured enough to be tested with an audiometer. At this age, formal hearing testing usually can be carried out. Not only has hearing developed to its optimal level, but listening has also become considerably refined.
48	Up to 5600 words; carries out 3-item commands consistently; knows why people have houses, books, umbrella, key; knows nearly all colors; knows words such as *somebody, anybody, even, almost, now, something, like, bigger, too*, full name, one or two songs, number concepts to 4; understands most preschool stories; can complete opposite analogies such as brother is a boy, sister is a girl and in daytime it is light, at night it is dark	Up to 1500 words in sentences averaging 5 to 6 words per sentence; averages 400 words per hour; counts up to 3, repeats 4 digits, names 3 objects, repeats 9-word sentences from memory; names the primary colors, some coins; relates fanciful tales; enjoys rhyming nonsense words and using exaggerations; demands reasons why and how; questioning is at a peak, up to 500 a day; passes judgment on own activity; can recite a poem from memory or sing a song; uses words such as *even, almost, something, like, but*; typical expressions might include "I'm so tired," "You almost hit me," "Now I'll make something else"	
54	Up to 6500 words; knows what materials a house, window, chair, and dress are made of and what people do with eyes and ears; understands differences in texture and composition, such as hard, soft, rough, smooth; begins to name or point to penny, nickel, dime; understands *if, because, why, when*	Up to 1800 words in sentences averaging 5 to 6 words; now averages only 230 words per hour—is satisfied with less verbalization; does little commanding or demanding; likes surprises; about 1 in 10 sentences is compound or complex, and only 8% of sentences are incomplete; can define 10 common words and counts up to 20; common expressions are "I don't know," "I said," "tiny," "funny," "because"; asks questions for information and learns to manipulate and control people and situations with language	
60	Up to 9600 words; knows number concepts to 5; knows and names colors; defines words in terms of use, such as a bike is to ride; defines wind, ball, hat, stove; understands qualifiers such as *if, because, when*; knows purpose of horse, fork, and legs; begins to understand *left* and *right*	Up to 2200 words in sentences averaging six words; can define ball, hat, stove, policeman, wind, horse, fork; can count five objects and repeat four or five digits; definitions are in terms of use; can single out a word and ask its meaning; makes serious inquiries—"What is this for?" "How does this work?" "Who made those?" "What does it mean?"; language is now essentially complete in structure and form; uses all types of sentences, clauses, and parts of speech; reads by way of pictures, and prints simple words	

Modified from Hockenberry M. J., & Wilson, D. (2006) *Wong's nursing care of infants and children*. (8th ed.). St. Louis: Mosby.

Box **19-2** Nursing Suggestions to Encourage Language Development in Preschoolers

- Read to the child. Encourage the child to be an active listener. Pause during the story to ask questions, such as "What do you think will happen next?" and "Why do you think the boy said that?" and "What would you do now?" See **Website Resource 19A** for a list of suggested books to read aloud to a child.
- Praise the child's storytelling and creativity with stories.
- Always respond to the child's questions. Occasionally a response must be delayed; for example, when the parent is driving in heavy traffic and the child asks a question that requires a complex answer, the parent might say, "That's a very good question; let's talk about that as soon as we get home." The parent should remind the child of the question later and respond if the child still expresses interest.
- Never tease or criticize a child about speaking style. If the child speaks so fast as to be fumbling over words, then the parent might say, "I can't listen that fast. Slow down a little for me." This is much more encouraging than is the statement, "You talk too fast. No one can understand you."
- Play language-focused games, such as naming the colors of houses or kinds of flowers as parent and child walk to the store.

Memory

Memory plays an important role in language development and learning in general (Girbau & Schwartz, 2007; Montgomery, 2003; Rescorla, 2005). In her study of 28 adolescents who had been late to talk, Rescorla (2005) found that these late talkers tended to display limitation with verbal memory ability. At the preschool level children label pictures, group objects, and mimic others as ways to aid memory, performing these tasks with less precision than the older child. Younger children benefit from suggestions about how to group items using characteristics to remember. Preschoolers remember pictures better by saying names of pictures rather than simply hearing the name of a picture when it is first shown. Preschoolers do not spontaneously use rehearsal or other **mnemonic techniques** for remembering, but they do use and benefit from rehearsal when it is suggested (McGuigan & Nunez, 2006). The nurse tests memory by asking the child to repeat an arbitrary sequence of numbers. By approximately age 5, children should be able to repeat four consecutively named numbers easily (Hockenberry & Wilson, 2006).

Testing of Developmental Level

Parents of preschool children determine their child's readiness for school programs. The child's skill level, the child and family's psychosocial status, and the characteristics of the school program under consideration each contribute to readiness determination. Questions about readiness should be answered considering all three of these components. Developmental testing modalities used during the toddler

years appear less accurate as the child approaches school age. Tools designed for this purpose can help identify the child's skill level.

Historically, tools to evaluate readiness skills have been used. The **Preschool Readiness Experimental Screening Scale (PRESS)** has been used in the past. This tool screens easily for developmental lags or abnormalities that might interfere with academic and social success in school. Constructed for use with 5-year-old children, it may also estimate readiness of slightly older or younger children. The test measures school readiness and addresses specific skills, not intellectual level.

Other components of readiness, family dynamics and school environment, have concerned experts. Children develop the ability to cope with a school setting through a complex interaction of social relationships with peers, parents, teachers, and other caregivers (Mashburn & Pianta, 2006). La Paro et al. (2004) have developed and tested a 9-point assessment of the environment called the **Classroom Assessment Scoring System**. The scales assess global classroom quality: positive climate, negative climate, teacher sensitivity, overcontrol, behavior management, productivity, learning formats, concept development, and quality of feedback (La Paro et al., 2004). Evaluating the environment holistically using a comprehensive approach contributes important information about readiness. Children who are ready for school demonstrate competencies in areas other than measurable skill performance. Complex home environments with stable caring adults or safe, predictable physical environments with regular, stimulating activities, peers, and materials contribute to readiness. Social norms define expectations; therefore, home values that align with school values are more likely to result in children characterized as ready for school. Conversely, when school expectations differ from those at home, children are less likely to be considered ready for school (Allor & McCathren, 2003; Ionescu & Benga, 2007; Mashburn & Pianta, 2006).

To obtain a more specific measure of developmental age, the nurse uses one of several screening tools designed for use with the preschool child (Ionescu & Benga, 2007; Snow, 2006). These validated instruments provide rough estimates of ability for school and help determine whether a child needs referral for further evaluation. The **Peabody Picture Vocabulary Test** examines verbal intelligence but also estimates verbal ability. When used with predominantly middle class children who have acquired standard English-speaking ability, accuracy is reliable (Rock & Stenner, 2005). Insufficient language stimulation or cultural differences may influence scores negatively. Children from bilingual backgrounds, nevertheless, acquire letter recognition readily once they encounter an environment that emphasizes these abilities (Hammer & Miccio, 2006; Hammer et al., 2007). Also children sometimes become disinterested with the process randomly pointing to options to finish more quickly. Examiners must remain alert to eye movement to identify changes in children's response behaviors (Bracken &

HEALTH TEACHING   Health Promotion with Preschoolers: Environmental Accountability

Rationale for Teaching Preschoolers about Environmental Protection

- Environmental education at an early age will produce environmental practitioners of the future.
- Preschoolers can learn basic concepts of environmental accountability and gain a sense of empowerment when they perceive that they make a difference to the future world.
- Health care providers, in consultation with child care providers, can promote environmental education that is based on their knowledge of child growth and development and concerns about overall health.

Basic Ways for Preschoolers to Help the Environment and Promote Overall Societal Health

- Use water wisely.
- Use electricity only when necessary.

- Recycle.
- Avoid using balloons.
- Plant trees, protect plants, and grow a garden.
- Create a compost pile.
- Care for birds.
- Clean up the neighborhood.
- Decrease the amount of trash; say "no" to Styrofoam and plastic garbage bags, and use paper cups and reusable cloth bags for groceries.
- Recycle old toys by giving them to less fortunate people.
- Buy and use only earth-friendly school supplies.
- Walk rather than ride in the car.
- Use live Christmas trees and replant.

Shaughnessy, 2003). Readiness tests continue to improve in their ability to predict performance. The Early Childhood Longitudinal Study, for example, predicts about 60 percent of third grade performance (Rock & Stenner, 2005).

Draw-a-Person and Draw-a-Family tests approximate intelligence and emotional development; however, scoring figure drawings requires standardized test conditions and analysis of findings by a psychometric specialist. Nurses, however, use these methods in conjunction with other information to help establish rapport and to provide a starting point to guide assessment (Flanagan & Motta, 2007).

Drawings may indicate general developmental level, fine motor control, and evidence of concept formation. Perceptions of family relationships can also be assessed. Preschool children will draw a person with at least six body parts in the appropriate locations. Normally children name the parts correctly. The representation may be an approximation, but it should resemble the actual body parts and be drawn with strong, evenly flowing lines. The family drawing may be less sophisticated than a drawing of a single person and may lack some family members. The normal child names the family members readily and describes unique characteristics of each member from a child's perspective (Hockenberry & Wilson, 2006). The nurse provides a pencil and plain sheet of paper and asks the child to draw the best picture possible. The nurse explains that the picture will remain with the nurse but that another sketch may be drawn to take home (Vygotsky, 2004).

Self-Perception–Self-Concept Pattern

During the preschool years, basic self-concept emerges from the child's personal struggle for autonomy. As children develop beyond the toddler years, they refine their sense of self through both task-oriented and socially oriented experiences. By reinforcing skills and successfully accomplishing tasks, the preschooler builds self-esteem,

enhancing overall health. Social acceptance helps children feel successful in their role as child, sibling, and friend. Preschoolers investigate roles through rich imagination. Pretending to be the parent or baby allows the preschooler to imagine experiences and feelings of others and safely experiment with new ideas (Hockenberry & Wilson, 2006; Vygotsky, 2004).

Preschool children learn about their roles in their child care environments and learn that being dependable within their world is important. When children perceive their value in improving the world in which they live, they experience good feelings about themselves and, ultimately, demonstrate improved mental and physical health. Many simple ways to improve the environment are available, and when children learn ways to contribute to environmental health, they often reinforce these behaviors in their parents (Health Teaching box).

Erikson's Theory

Preschoolers develop a sense of **initiative** through their vigorous motor activity and active imagination. Erikson views this growth as the most central developmental task in the emerging self-concept of the preschool years. By praising preschoolers' efforts and providing opportunities for new experiences, parents promote development of initiative. Rather than requiring a particular behavior, parents should provide avenues for experimentation. The preschooler then feels mastery, thus encouraging repetition. With mastery, preschoolers become more confident about trying new actions.

Preschoolers remain sensitive to criticism by others. When ridiculed for ideas or behaviors, they may develop feelings of guilt and inadequacy. Parents, caregivers, and health care professionals should nurture their ideas, while encouraging behaviors to support a positive self-concept.

Roles-Relationships Pattern

Family members continue to play a vital role in the preschooler's life, but peers become increasingly significant as development progresses. Preschoolers receive ideas and information from peers. They may subsequently question rules or expectations at home comparing them to their friends'. Discussion about family values and behaviors that are acceptable one place but not another help them understand differences.

Preschoolers understand gender expectations regarding jobs, activities, and competencies of people in their lives. Ideas about gender differences in work roles or activities are based on models in the home, at child care or preschool centers, and on television. Parents and caregivers should be aware of the powerful influence that environment has on role perceptions (Box 19-3). When inaccurate portrayals of male and female roles are depicted, parents and caregivers should discuss more accurate ones with children. Preschoolers experiment through play, including adopting family roles. As the mother or father in a play situation, preschoolers set limits, punish, praise, and make outlandish demands on the invented child. Play represents an important strategy for preschoolers to use for stress reduction and experimentation with new roles. By playing different roles, children safely experience effects of their behavior and understand others' roles more clearly. Parents also better understand effects of their own actions when they observe the behaviors of their child. Nurses help parents use their observations to improve interactions with their child.

Preschoolers relate to older children in the family on a more equal basis than toddlers do. Although their cognitive, motor, and language skills are less refined, preschoolers participate in some activities with their older siblings. Younger children may admire and imitate an older sibling.

This behavior flatters the older child initially, but with continued persistence develops into a source of frustration for the sibling.

Social interaction during this period prepares preschoolers for school. Through experience within the family, with peers, and with other adults, the child acquires readiness to interact in group situations, follow directions, take turns, recognize others' rights, channel energy toward an assigned activity, and demonstrate increasing independence. School readiness can be assessed by using several relevant tests, as discussed in this chapter. The nurse who sees the child repeatedly in an office, clinic, or group care or preschool setting assesses progress as the child develops social competencies. Comparing the child's current, more mature behavior with previous behavior provides insight into the preschooler's readiness for school. This method of evaluation, however, prevents comparison with other children of the same age. For example, school personnel may view a child who reflects a **quiet** temperament and is introverted or subdued as overly attached to the mother in comparison with other children the same age. However, if the child's earlier social behavior is known, the behavior may be interpreted as a progression toward independence. When the mother is not available, the child may make sufficient adaptations to remain comfortable and secure.

Evidence of social competency can be obtained by discussion and evaluation of the child's family drawings. The nurse observes the drawing and responds to any comments or questions volunteered by the child. When asked for advice or assistance, the nurse encourages the child to proceed with drawing. Positive encouragement for the child's efforts may be used, particularly with reluctant children. After the drawing is finished, the nurse discusses the sketch with the child to identify the people and describe individual characteristics.

Box **19-3** Evaluating a Child Care Setting

Child care that meets the needs and expectations of parents will most likely ensure a happy preschooler as well. Questions that parents should consider in evaluating and choosing a child care setting include the following:

- Will my needs and those of my child be best met with a caregiver in a family home, commercial center, or preschool, or by having a person come to my home to care for my child?
- What kinds of backup plans will I need or will be available if the provider becomes ill?
- What are my standards for nutrition, safety, sanitation, and health, and can these standards be met at the chosen child care facility?
- How important is it to my child to be with other children? How many children would be ideal for my child's socialization needs?
- What personality attributes and educational preparation do I desire in my child's caregivers? What attributes do I dislike and how will I deal with these attributes to maximize the care given to my child? How important is caregiver stability

to me? Can I comfortably communicate with the staff to collaborate with my child's learning?
- What educational philosophy do I want in the setting? What involvement do I wish to have in the educational mission of the facility?
- Do the hours of the facility meet my personal and professional needs? Is close access to my job or home important to me?
- How are the children grouped, and what is the caregiver-to-child ratio?
- Does the cost of the service meet my financial needs? Can I pay part-time fees during vacation or when my child is ill for a lengthy period?
- Is accreditation of the facility mandatory for me to use it?
- What is my internal response or my general feelings about the setting when I visit it before my child's enrollment? Are the caregivers interacting with and responsive to the children? Are the children happy and interactive? Are the children's individual needs addressed appropriately? Is the environment supportive of my child's care? Is discipline appropriate?

The nurse writes the names of each family member on the picture and documents the perceptions the child describes. Open-ended questions such as "What do you like best about your brother?" or "When do you get angry with your sister?" can be posed to encourage the child to describe the family interaction patterns. When an adult family member is present, the nurse explains the purpose of the drawing and interview and requests that the adult withhold comments or questions until the activity is completed. Any areas of concern or questions should be discussed, assuring the parent that confidentiality will be maintained. The child's perceptions can be verified with the adult at the conclusion of the interview, or further information can be sought to clarify them.

The **Vineland Social Maturity Scale** provides an objective, standardized estimate of social functioning and social maturity. This tool profiles the child's self-help skills, self-direction, locomotion, communication, and social relations. The scoring system seems to be culturally and socioeconomically neutral. The investigator collects data by observing the child's behavior and interviewing the mother or primary caregiver. Designed to measure progression toward independence, this instrument uses direct observation of the child's behavior whenever possible, using the interview data only if needed to complete the assessment (Hockenberry & Wilson, 2006).

These kinds of tools elicit cues indicative of family stress and strain. **Parental divorce** commonly creates disruption in family relationships. Discussion of results of the assessment offers the opportunity to discuss family situations that otherwise might have gone unmentioned. Children's responses to changes in family circumstances depend on their developmental stages and their relationships before the change. Divorce represents a final decision, usually culminating from a period of conflict, stress, and changing relationships that the child has had only a limited relationship to. Although preschoolers definitely sense stress in the home, they cannot articulate their feelings or determine their origin. Children react to changes in various ways, including regression, confusion, or irritability. Asking the same questions repeatedly, such as, "Is Daddy coming home for supper tonight?" or "Why doesn't Daddy stay here anymore?" can be a child's way of expressing difficulty in coping with or comprehending the situation.

Parents in the midst of marital problems or divorce frequently lack the psychological energy or patience to deal with questions and altered behavior. Nonetheless, these children desperately need closeness, patience, and consistent responses from their parents. Nurses advocate for children by helping parents explore ways to address regression and irritability. As parents develop skills to explain situations, they realize children are deeply affected during times of family disruption, regardless of their behavior (McGuinness, 2006). Parents need to connect emotionally with their children to demonstrate that love will continue for the child despite dissolution of the marriage. Books appropriate to the preschooler's cognitive and emotional level can help parents address children's feelings and needs during divorce.

Child Abuse

Social processes within families and communities that create child abuse are multifaceted and complex. Research focuses on the complexity of the abuse cycle and the challenges involved in resolution. In some communities, hitting children as a form of discipline remains socially acceptable. Parents and caregivers who experience workplace stressors, financial worries, and other frustrations may project their anger and abuse their children physically, emotionally, or sexually. Effective primary and secondary prevention interventions involve promoting awareness of violence as a social problem, opposing violence to women, and offering community or school programs to teach nonviolent conflict resolution skills to people of all ages. Apparent child abuse, however, must be reported.

Sexuality-Reproductive Pattern

Preschoolers recognize there are two genders and identify with their own gender. Appropriate and positive representations of both genders on television and in role models, such as working mothers, allow preschoolers to interpret gender roles broadly and define their own roles more realistically (Bowie, 2007). Body image, a part of gender identity, also includes perception of sex organs. Preschoolers develop curiosity at this age, including inquisitiveness about bodies and sexual functions of others. Questions should be answered simply and factually. Teasing preschoolers about this interest or implying that sexual information is unacceptable or naughty promotes negativity. Positive feelings about all aspects of the self (including gender role) create positive self-esteem. Many children's books address self-esteem in young children and provide interesting and informative approaches to nurturing overall health promotion in this age group. See **Website Resource 19A** for a list of recommended books for preschool children.

Coping-Stress Tolerance Pattern
Play Approaches

Assessing self-concept in preschool children who struggle to articulate their feelings presents a challenge for the nurse. Play can elicit behaviors that indicate sense of self and self-esteem, future success or failure, sense of acceptance, and competence. **Doll or puppet play** provides valuable insight into a child's sense of self. Dolls or puppets, including those representing a young child of the same gender, race, and cultural background as the preschooler, should be available (Hockenberry & Wilson, 2006; Rudisill & Wall, 2004). If the child spontaneously begins to engage the dolls or puppets in imaginary activity, no further guidance should be given. With a reluctant child, the nurse begins to pretend, using examples for the child, such as going to the store, moving the dolls through the related activities, and then involving the child. Frequently preschoolers continue the scenario to tell their personal stories.

A related technique is **mutual storytelling**. The nurse begins a story for the child to finish. The nurse might begin with a standard line, such as, "Once upon a time there lived a [girl, boy, cow, monkey, etc.] who..." The nurse then pauses for the child to continue. If the child hesitates, the nurse resumes the story for another sentence or two and asks what the figure in the story is doing. As the child supplies details, the nurse offers encouragement to continue, asking questions such as "And then what happened?" or "How did the child feel?"

The child's inner nature can be explored along several dimensions. The emotional theme of the story is noted and should be congruent with the child's tone and expression. For example, a child who centers on a theme of aggression and destruction but describes the character's anger in a monotone is demonstrating incongruence between content and expression. The child's emotionless response suggests difficulty with expressing feelings. At the conclusion of the story, possible meanings can be revealed by asking whether the child feels similar to any of the characters or would like to be any of the characters.

Although these dimensions may be explored for meaning, interpretation of a child's behavior in these play situations remains highly speculative. To determine possible themes or estimate the child's self-esteem requires several encounters. Additionally, the nurse's personality and approach influence the child's spontaneity and ability to tell a story. Observed behavior and responses without associated interpretation should be recorded for future reference. Interpretations are avoided until validated by a specialist.

Coping Mechanisms

Preschoolers use coping mechanisms similar to those of the toddler (separation anxiety, regression, denial, repression, and projection). Protest behavior in the form of temper tantrums normally disappears as a stress response in the older preschooler. Temper tantrums that persist through the fifth year indicate a lack of matured coping responses. The child uses tantrums and continues to gain the desired result.

Preschoolers lack the cognitive awareness, social abilities, and motives for communication of adults and older children. They display temperaments and tantrums that appear oppositional to older individuals. Through positive interactions with parents and caregivers, preschoolers frequently learn how to organize their bodies, abilities, and environment to move successfully to the next stage of development (Hockenberry & Wilson, 2006; Kalpidou et al., 2004). A positive relationship between the child's temperament and the demands of the environment (also known as goodness of fit) can be attained by social interaction which, in turn, prevents the development of problem behaviors later (Hot Topics box).

Preschoolers possess a considerable range of experiences and memories; therefore, they respond more maturely to stress than do toddlers. Positive coping resources are determined by some of the following variables:

1. Availability of emotional comfort and the child's inner resilience;
2. Ability to work on task;

HOTtopics

THE CHALLENGE OF TEMPERAMENT AND PRESCHOOLERS

Temperament describes the way in which an individual behaves or responds to new situations and to life occurrences. Most children can be defined as *easy, difficult,* or *hard to warm up to* based on how they react to their surroundings and to people. For many adults the challenge in parenting is to learn how to work with a child's temperament, which can vary from the parents' or other children's temperaments, in efforts to attain family happiness.

3. Availability of play materials and toys; and
4. Opportunity to engage in activities (Kalpidou et al., 2004).

Preschoolers use many of the coping mechanisms developed during their toddler years, but they generally show greater ability to verbalize frustration, fewer temper tantrums, and more patience in experimentation to resolve difficulty than the typical toddler. Preschoolers refine their problem-solving skills. Through fantasy play, they investigate solutions or responses to stressful events and find inner control for challenging situations.

Occasionally projection and fantasy lead parents to consider their child dishonest. When faced with the question, "Did you break this dish?" the preschooler might respond, "No, Teddy did it." The child might even relate a detailed story of the toy bear's mishap. Preschoolers tend to project blame. Active fantasies help tell the story. Parents should not accuse preschoolers of lying, but rather the adult should help the child decide whether the story is pretend or real. The concepts of pretend and real help encourage children to discuss nightmares, television shows, stories, and their own active imaginations (Hockenberry & Wilson, 2006; Vygotsky, 2004).

Preschoolers perceive their ability to control and manage situations better than does the toddler. Strict adherence to rituals or game rules controls situations. As discussed, the preschooler has a longer and more rigid bedtime ritual than the toddler. The preschooler also dislikes losing games and may structure the rules to ensure winning. Older children and adults may be able to accept these structures, but these controlling behaviors frustrate other preschoolers, because they also need to win. Gentle, consistent direction by parents and caregivers about how to play games fairly and how to move toward positive group outcomes helps the preschooler to develop a sense of morality, which is important for later life success and happiness. See the Case Study and Care Plan at the end of this chapter for an example of ineffective coping in a preschool child.

Values-Beliefs Pattern

Preschoolers, like toddlers, lack fully developed consciences; however, at age 4 to 5 years these children do demonstrate some internal controls on their actions. Immaturity limits the consistency and effectiveness of these internal controls. With the child's concrete perspective, the internal controls may be rigid; therefore, a preschooler may feel overwhelming guilt when behavior and internal controls conflict. Cognitive developmental level determines, for the most part, preschoolers' maturity and their feelings about their behavior fluctuations. Cognitive development continues with dramatic transformation during these years, explaining the differences from child to child and from time to time in the same child. Modeling and **induction explanation**, moving from specific to general, influences moral behaviors appreciably. Modeling stems from many sources, not all of which leave positive impressions. Parents affect the availability of models by screening television shows, carefully selecting child-care situations, and monitoring play sessions. Responsible parents verify suitability of the models. More detailed inductive explanations, based on the child's cognitive level, generally are comprehended by the preschool population.

Preschoolers control their behavior to retain parental love and approval. From their perspective, parental disapproval represents a decrease in a child's importance from the parent's viewpoint. The child therefore suffers a decline in self-esteem, which motivates a change in behavior. Guilt results from perceived reduction of self-esteem, a critical step in the development of conscience. Moral actions are demonstrated in simple activities, such as taking turns and sharing. These actions stem from the assumption that other people have rights and desires that are as important as the rights and desires of the preschooler.

Preschoolers frequently express their values by stating who or what they like or what they want to be when they become adults. These values change frequently, even within a few minutes. Preschoolers occasionally use statements of value as punishment for playmates or family members and display insensitivity to the effect of their remarks on others. Preschoolers ask endless questions. When they ask these questions about moral actions or feelings, they may simply be asking, "How does this work?" and not questioning the underlying parental value. The same intent exists when the child asks about the spiritual values that the parent may be teaching. Parents may enroll their child in Sunday school or other faith-oriented classes or activities. The preschool child generally enjoys the social aspects of these activities and receives some important modeling of values from the involved adults and from working with peers as they struggle to develop morality.

Life beginnings and death concepts fascinate preschoolers. Because of their limited emotional experiences with death, some ask about dead insects and the process of death with great interest, occasionally with insensitivity. Others become upset with the idea of dying, assuming that when someone becomes angry and wishes them dead, they will cease to exist. Many children worry about who will care for them if their caregivers die, whether pain comes with death, what causes death, and what happens after

someone dies. Children who actually lose a loved one to death can experience sleep disturbances and other behavioral changes as part of the grieving process. Parents, based on their own religious and cultural values, should respond to children in a supportive and open manner to provide an accurate interpretation of death. In some cases, counseling may be needed if the parents are unable to cope with their duties or if the child has significant behavioral problems as a result of the family disruption. Increasingly, books appropriate to the preschooler's level of understanding are available to help deal with this delicate issue (Elkins & Cavendish, 2004).

PATHOLOGICAL PROCESSES

For many children physiological, psychosocial, and environmental factors create health problems that interfere with physical, social, and educational activities of normal development (Hockenberry & Wilson, 2006). Major disruptions limit fulfillment of the child's potential in adulthood. Environmental processes that affect toddlers also affect preschoolers. Occurrence rates and outcomes of health problems differ in this age group, likely because of developmental differences (U.S. Department of Health and Human Services, 2007). Preschoolers have more refined problem-solving skills, are more coordinated, and have more experience with a variety of situations than do toddlers. Although preschoolers recognize and avoid some environmental hazards, they remain impulsive and immature. Population-based programs ensure that screening takes place at the most developmentally appropriate time (Research Highlights box and Box 19-4).

research highlights

Screening Preschoolers

The goal of this study was to measure the effectiveness of vision screening carried out in two different settings using the protocol recommended by Maternal and Child Health Bureau and National Eye Institute for vision screening in the preschool child that was developed by a task force. The protocol was designed to screen preschool children using monocular visual acuity and stereopsis testing. The protocol was implemented in four sites with 3- and 4-year-old children (n = 47). Each site recorded the testing and the documented referral and follow-up. Two sites were primary care sites where staff members conducted the testing. The other two sites were community-based programs where volunteers conducted the testing.

Successful screening ranged from 70% to 98%; referral rates ranged from 2% to 41%; and follow-up rates ranged from 29% to 100%. Significant differences were demonstrated in all three measures between the primary care sites and the community-based sites. These data that vary across pilot sites indicate that preschool vision screening depends on thorough training and detailed protocols.

From Hartmann, et al. (2006). Project Universal Preschool Vision Screening: a demonstration project. *Pediatrics, 117*(2 Supp), e226.

Box **19-4** Environmental Safety for Preschoolers

A safe and developmentally stimulating environment allows children of all ages to explore without negative consequences. When teaching parents how to modify their homes for preschoolers, the following requirements for child safety should be considered.

SAFE SLEEP ENVIRONMENT

Provide beds with guardrails (as needed), soft corners, and appropriate bedding to prevent suffocation.

WELL-VENTILATED BUT OPTIMAL TEMPERATURE ENVIRONMENT FOR PLAY

Provide safe play areas by using electrical outlet covers, handrails in stairwells, toy boxes with lids that lock securely, nonslip floor materials, well-anchored furniture, and appropriate soft ground coverings and padding for outdoor play equipment.

BURN PREVENTION

Use only cool mist humidifier for management of upper respiratory infections; dress child only in flame-retardant clothing, particularly at bedtime.

APPROPRIATE INSTALLATION AND USE OF EMERGENCY HOME EQUIPMENT

Discuss the importance of properly operating smoke detectors, fire extinguishers, and practicing an escape plan from the home in case of emergency.

CONNECTION TO EMERGENCY SERVICES

Post 911 on all phones; teach the child how to use 911 and how to report the child's name and address over the phone; parents should be trained in cardiopulmonary resuscitation and the Heimlich maneuver.

PREVENTION OF ASPIRATION

Monitor use of balloons and eating habits of the preschooler.

SAFE DAILY HOME ENVIRONMENT

Close doors of dishwasher, oven, washer, and dryer; mark all glass doors with decals to delineate doors; use gates at the top and bottom of stairs for the younger child; set water heater temperature at a maximum of 120° F to avoid burns; store all poisonous substances out of the reach of children; discourage running in the house; avoid throw rugs on bare floors.

PREVENTION, RECOGNITION, AND MANAGEMENT OF POISON INGESTION OR EXPOSURE

Know how to use syrup of ipecac and have the nearest poison control center phone number within easy access; learn how to evaluate burns or blisters around the mouth, odor of poisons, empty containers around the child, stomach distress, or changes in normal activity level that might indicate poison ingestion.

WATER SAFETY

Monitor bathtub and pool activity; teach preschooler swimming skills (usually by age 4); ensure that all pools are fenced.

BICYCLE SAFETY

Ensure that the child is riding a developmentally appropriate bicycle with a federally approved safety helmet and is schooled in the rules of riding in the street and interacting with strangers.

LEAD CONCERNS

Avoid items with a high lead content in home (paint, wrapping paper, earthenware, colored newspaper); ensure that children are monitored when lead exposure is a concern.

ENVIRONMENTAL CONTAMINANTS HAZARDOUS TO THE CHILD'S HEALTH

Avoid exposure to tobacco smoke, nitrous oxide from wood-burning stoves, asbestos, pesticides, radiation, and factory-produced irritants.

Adapted from Hockenberry, M. J., & Wilson, D. (2006). *Wong's nursing care of infants and children* (8th ed.). St. Louis: Mosby.

Because many preschoolers attend child care programs, many have been trained to use 911 and can access help in emergencies when this phone code exists. At this age, children need to know their name, address, and how to say "no" to strangers.

Injuries

Approximately 55 American children die every day from injuries; 43% of the deaths of children age 1 through 4 years are a result of injuries, "4 times the number of deaths due to birth defects, the second leading cause of death for this age group" (U.S. Department of Health and Human Services, 2007).

Accidents and injuries are often predictable and preventable (Hockenberry & Wilson, 2006; U.S. Department of Health and Human Services, 2007). As preschoolers become more independent, causes of injury change; they may chase a ball into a busy street or suffer from sports-related injuries. Preschoolers continue to need supervision to prevent injury related to their developmental age.

Of all injuries, two thirds occur in children and adolescents. The rate of death from injuries is decreasing in the United States. On the other hand, death rates continue to be higher than in countries with long-term comprehensive preventive approaches that focus on widespread community change (e.g., Great Britain and Scandinavian countries) (Hockenberry & Wilson, 2006).

Although preschoolers have fewer accidents than toddlers, motor vehicle accidents continue to be a major cause of fatalities in this age group (Fallat et al., 2006; U.S. Department of Health and Human Services, 2007). Although many state laws mandate federally approved car seats for children who are less than

4 feet tall or weigh less than 40 pounds and booster seats for children up to the age of 6, many parents fail to place their children in appropriate restraint systems, or they use them incorrectly. Although parents may know that infants should be placed in the back seat, they do not always know that children in the front seat of a motor vehicle face danger, even if they are using restraint systems. Federal investigations concluded that children under age 13 should ride in the back seat of a motor vehicle, particularly because of potential injury or death from a passenger seat air bag that could inflate in a severe car accident (Hockenberry & Wilson, 2006).

Household furniture and fixtures also remain a hazard for preschoolers, as do structural features such as stairs and windows. Nursery and toy injuries decrease during the preschool years. Sports and recreational injuries increase markedly. This elevated incidence likely reflects a change in the preschoolers' involvement in group sports, riding bicycles, and using playground equipment. Preschoolers need a broad range of play areas and experiences. Conscientious parents supply age-appropriate limits and supervision (Hockenberry & Wilson, 2006).

Preschoolers lack the skill or judgment to ride bicycles in the street. They need instruction about safe use of playground equipment. Adult supervision of most preschooler activities, group sports in particular, is required to prevent injury.

Preschoolers begin to safely handle basic tools, kitchen equipment, and cleaning supplies. Children at this age take pride in participating in household projects with a supervising parent. They spend much of their time in the home and in the preschool or child care center. The facilities pose the same potentially harmful environmental conditions as the home, as well as some additional threats to safety (Hockenberry & Wilson, 2006; U.S. Department of Health and Human Services, 2007).

In response to concern about firearm safety in homes with small children, most states have passed Child Access Protection (CAP) legislation to encourage safe storage of firearms (Hepburn et al., 2006). For young children, CAP means a decline in the rate of deaths due to firearms. Greater effect has been demonstrated in states that permit felony prosecution of offenders (Hepburn et al., 2006). Most deaths from firearms are preventable (Emergency Nurses Association, 2005). Geographical areas with more firearms are likely to produce more deaths (Miller et al., 2007). Over one third of U.S. homes contain firearms, with most stored inappropriately (Emergency Nurses Association, 2005). Children are physically capable of pulling a trigger before they are able to cognitively depict cause and effect of their actions. Even if gun safety training occurs, most curious children will handle firearms given the opportunity. Firearms remain the second leading cause of overall injury-related deaths in the United States (Emergency Nurses Association, 2005).

Burns

Scalds and direct flame burns are major hazards for the preschooler. For young children the number of burn injuries is second only to the number sustained in motor vehicle accidents (Hockenberry & Wilson, 2006). The highest death rates from residential injuries in the United States result from fires (Nagaraja et al., 2005). In preschool children the number of deaths in house fires is nearly double that of other ages. Children of this age experiment with matches and fire, and they may be unable to escape from a fire once it starts. Home fire deaths occur more often in the African American, Hispanic, and Native American preschool population than in the non-Hispanic White population (Nagaraja et al., 2005). Measures discussed in Chapter 18 to reduce scald burns in the home apply to this age group as well. Preschoolers should be taught about the dangers of matches, open flames, and hot objects. Parents and caregivers should model appropriate use of active and potentially dangerous burning devices.

Drowning

Children over age 3 years are at lower risk for drowning in the bathtub, but at greater risk for drowning in a swimming pool, than the toddler. Children aged 1 to 4 years are at highest risk for drowning with two near-drowning episodes for every fatality (Burford et al., 2005). Most children are close to safety when drowning occurs (Burford et al., 2005). With this in mind, it is important to supervise young children when they are near a body of water, install fencing to isolate a residential pool from the house, use personal floatation devices while bathing or playing near a natural body of water, and to teach children how to swim and that swimming alone is unsafe. Preschoolers should receive instruction in water safety and swimming and should always be supervised by a trained adult or older person. Because a good outcome depends on early resuscitation, it is reasonable to encourage parents and pool owners to learn cardiopulmonary resuscitation (Burford et al., 2005).

Preschoolers have the cognitive ability to learn water survival. They should always wear a personal flotation device (i.e., life jacket) when they are on boats, even when they know how to swim, and they must be supervised when near water, even shallow water. Safety campaigns provide one effective measure to prevent unnecessary injury and death (Burford et al., 2005).

Mechanical Forces

Bicycle accidents become a greater source of injury during the preschool years. Many bicycle accidents involve automobiles, and most of these accidents result from the child's errors. Parents should set reasonable and age-appropriate limits on bicycle use. The transition from tricycle to bicycle provides an excellent time to begin using a helmet. Federally approved bicycle helmets are effective in reducing head trauma, a major cause of death among young children (Pardi et al., 2007).

Preschoolers, as passengers or pedestrians, present with great risk for an auto-related accident. At this age, pedestrian injury is more likely to occur than is passenger injury. Preschoolers should be taught proper street-crossing techniques and, generally, should be supervised when crossing streets. Approved car seat restraint systems should be used by young children at all times during car travel. Many accidents occur as a result of improper use of restraint devices. It is important for nurses to be informed and to instruct families about how to restrain the child in the car (Hockenberry & Wilson, 2006; Taft et al., 1999). The back seat is safer than the front seat, and all car doors should be locked. If the preschooler refuses to use the seat belt or appropriate restraint, parents must insist that the outing be postponed. Parents who provide a good example by using their seat belts directly influence the child's acceptance, and it meets the child's desire at this age to imitate the parent. The child who uses a car seat from infancy on will generally accept the seat belt quite well.

Biological and Bacterial Agents

Preschoolers seem healthier than toddlers, with fewer respiratory and gastrointestinal illnesses. They have developed antibodies to many common organisms through exposure. Children usually become ill more often when they enter their first group situation, where they are exposed to organisms new to them. This concerns parents and should be discussed by the nurse before the child begins attending a group setting. Increasingly, child-care settings provide instruction to children about appropriate hand-washing techniques to decrease disease transmission and provide relevant health-promotion teaching (Hockenberry & Wilson, 2006).

The child with a full course of immunizations as an infant receives a booster dose of the diphtheria, tetanus, and pertussis vaccine in the fourth year (Hockenberry & Wilson, 2006; Paulson & Hammer, 2002). A second injection to protect against measles, mumps, and rubella is recommended between ages 4 and 6 years. Many states require that all children in a school setting be fully immunized. The American Academy of Pediatrics (AAP) publishes their most current recommendations annually. The 2008 recommendations can be found at: *www.cispimmunize.org/IZSchedule_Childhood.pdf.*

Parents who choose not to immunize their children usually make this choice for religious reasons, but some parents worry about the risk of the immunization itself. Although vaccines provide an extremely safe way to combat communicable disease, issues about safety do arise. Because autism is often diagnosed around the same time a child is vaccinated, some parents have connected the onset of their child's autism with the vaccine (Paulson & Hammer, 2002; Woo et al., 2004). The American Academy of Pediatrics position statement refutes this association as coincidental (see *www.cispimmunize.org/aap/aap_main.html?* and *www.cispimmunize.*

org/fam/autism/autism.html for more information). The risk of consequences of the disease itself far outweighs any vaccine risk. However, nurses must remain informed about the risks in order to provide accurate information to parents.

Nurses who remain informed about reasons for avoiding immunization will be better able to increase parents' understanding of the possible consequences of omitting a dose. Incomplete immunization may also occur as a result of parental forgetfulness or procrastination. Mandatory immunization for school entry provides an effective incentive for these parents. In addition, community immunization initiatives make administration less expensive and more accessible in many communities (Kempe et al., 2004).

One of the newer developments in childhood immunizations is the introduction of a conjugate vaccine to prevent pediatric pneumococcal disease, which was added to the recommended schedule in the United States in 2001. Other advances on the horizon are more combination vaccines to decrease cost of administration. Noninjectable vaccines that could be inhaled or eaten would greatly enhance pediatric immunization programs with ease of administration and simplified storage.

Continued efforts to vaccinate all children are needed, especially children living in poverty, particularly in large cities, where they are traditionally undervaccinated (Tung et al., 2003). Nurses use immunization registry programs to consolidate records, to remind parents, to evaluate the client's scheduled program, and to analyze issues for a particular population. With registry programs duplication may be avoided in the preschooler whose immunizations are not up to date. The Centers for Disease Control and Prevention (CDC) publishes recommendations for scheduled immunizations and for individuals who have omitted doses for some reason. These schedules are updated regularly and are available on-line in a variety of formats, in both Spanish and English, at the CDC website (*www.cdc.gov/nip/recs/child-schedule.htm*). When immunizations have been omitted or delayed, the immunization schedule continues from the dose of the last vaccine (Centers for Disease Control and Prevention, 2007; Rennels et al., 2004). Parents should be fully informed about the potential side effects of immunizations. In most office and clinic settings, parents sign state-developed informed consent documents that describe potential side effects.

Occasionally parents of children with disabilities do not allow them to attend preschool in an effort to protect them from inadvertent harm or scorn from other children. Financially and socially disadvantaged children remain at home because of economic constraints or ignorance about advantages of preschool preparation. Nurses facilitate the exploration of advantages and disadvantages of preschool for these children, helping their families obtain information about local opportunities and sources for assistance with cost.

Chemical Agents

Preschoolers face exposure to environmental pollutants. The young child's skin area relative to body mass is twice that of an adult's, which increases the risk of toxicity. Environmental exposure has been implicated in the increased prevalence of learning disabilities, because of the unique vulnerability of a child's brain to chemicals (Rehfuess et al., 2006). Disparities exist among populations with regard to their risk. Ethnicity, socioeconomic status, and geographical location all have an impact on the risk of exposure.

In particular, lead is found in products used in folk remedies for many reasons. In the preschool group, lead may be found in products used to treat upset stomach (*empacho*), constipation, diarrhea, and vomiting. In Hispanic traditional medicine, these products, known as *greta, azarcon, alarcón, coral, luiga, maría luisa,* or *rueda,* may contain extremely high lead contents. Lead has also been found in traditional remedies from cultures other than the Hispanic group. For example, *ghasard,* an Indian traditional tonic, and *ba-baw-san,* a Chinese herbal remedy for colic, have also been found to contain lead.

Sources of lead other than those found in traditional medicine include pottery, cosmetics, and food additives. Common sources of environmental lead are listed at the CDC website for Managing Elevated Blood Lead Levels among Young Children: Recommendations from the Advisory Committee on Childhood Lead Poisoning Prevention: *www.cdc.gov/nceh/lead/CaseManagement/ caseManage_appendixes.htm#Appendix%20I.* Chemical agents of concern for toddlers, such as pesticides, lead, and passive smoke, continue to merit consideration in the preschool population (Lu et al., 2006). Preschoolers, however, become more independent and understand the concepts of safe and poisonous.

More than one half of all poisonings occur in children under the age of 6. Each year poison control centers receive more than 2 million calls about accidental poisonings among children ages 5 and under (Criddle, 2007). Calls to poison control centers peak between 4 PM and 10 PM, which is known by poison centers as the arsenic hour. Most poisonings occur in the home (Nagaraja et al., 2005; University of Pittsburgh, 2004). Even though companies enclose many children's medications in childproof packaging, the product may be administered incorrectly by the caregiver, or the child may experiment with another family member's colorful pills. For example, the medication used to treat attention-deficit/hyperactivity disorder, methylphenidate, poisons many children. Klein-Schwartz's analysis (2003) of data from a 7-year period indicates that more than 40% of these methylphenidate poisonings were in children under the age of 6 years. About 60% of all poisonings in children, however, involve products other than medicines, such as plants, cleaning products, cosmetics, pesticides, paints, and solvents, with the remaining 40% attributed to medications

(University of Pittsburgh, 2004). **Website Resource 19C** presents recommendations on how to childproof a home from poisons.

Many household products, drugs, carbon monoxide, pesticides, lead, mercury, polychlorinated biphenyls, ethers, and poisonous plants pose hazards to the preschooler. Secondary smoke and lead exposure represent negative chemical influences on the growing child.

Preschoolers should receive verbal explanations about poisonous or dangerous substances, but parents cannot rely on the preschooler to remember instructions. A poison control program from the University of Pittsburgh introduced a character called Mr. Yuk in 1971. The ability to identify warning symbols such as Mr. Yuk helps preschoolers remain safe. Preschools and child care facilities often incorporate topics about environmental pollutants and dangerous substances into their curricula to promote the health of the preschooler. Information about poison control is widely available on-line (*www.aapcc. org/*) (American Association of Poison Control Centers, 2002; Criddle, 2007; University of Pittsburgh, 2004). The national, toll-free poison control center number is 800-222-1212. From that number the caller is directed to the nearest poison control center.

Parents should teach children about the four forms of poison, which are (1) solids: air fresheners, pills, vitamins, aspirin, lipstick; (2) liquids: cleaning products, fuel, alcohol; (3) sprays: furniture polish, oven cleaner, room deodorizer; and (4) invisibles: carbon monoxide, space heater fumes. Communication with parents about environmental dangers remains a major role of the child care provider.

Cancer

Cancer mortality in preschool children has declined over the past 20 years (Ries et al., 2007). Almost 600 cancer deaths annually in children aged 0 to 4 are a result primarily of leukemia, brain/CNS, endocrine (primarily neuroblastomas), and soft tissue malignancies (Ries et al., 2007). However, with an average of 1 to 2 children (per 10,000) developing some kind of cancer each year, the diseases are considered rare (Ries et al., 2007). Even though incidence of brain and other CNS tumors has increased, mortality has decreased (Ries et al., 2007). **Acute lymphocytic leukemia** (ALL), the most common childhood cancer, accounts for over one third of the cases of cancer in preschool children (Ries et al., 2007). Although less common than other solid tumors, **retinoblastoma** merits attention because of the possible loss of vision (Hockenberry & Wilson, 2006). Remarkable advances in long-term survival of children with cancer have occurred. Early detection remains the key to successful treatment; therefore, early, aggressive efforts have been put into detection programs. Some of the increases in rates of diagnosis may be attributed to improved imaging techniques and early detection (Hockenberry & Wilson, 2006).

Leukemia

ALL accounts for one third of the mortality from childhood cancer. The incidence of ALL rises from age 2, peaks at age 5, and diminishes through later childhood and adolescence. The dominant signs and symptoms of ALL appear suddenly, but often the child demonstrates a prodromal period of weakness, malaise, anorexia, fever, and tachycardia. Bone pain, petechiae, and hemorrhages after minor procedures such as dental extractions are encountered frequently. When an unexplained infection does not respond to management, suspicion should arise. Early detection and treatment of ALL has resulted in a marked increase in 5-year survival rates. Survival depends on age at diagnosis, with the best survival rates occurring when diagnosis occurs during the preschool years (Hockenberry & Wilson, 2006).

With suspected leukemia, the nurse institutes secondary prevention strategies with an assessment that includes the following parameters:

1. Examination of the cervical and peripheral lymph nodes
2. Palpation and percussion of the liver and spleen
3. Inspection of the skin for systemic signs of leukemia, such as pallor, purpura, petechiae, and **chloroma**, a localized tumor mass that has a greenish appearance and may be found in the skin, orbits, or other tissues in granulocytic forms of leukemia
4. Inspection of the mouth for enlarged tonsils; hyperplasia of the gums; and red, friable gingivae
5. Palpation of the sternum, bones, and joints for tenderness and pain

The rate of leukemia is higher in children with Down syndrome; therefore, school nurses and public health nurses should monitor these children for early signs of the disease.

Wilms Tumor

Most cases of **Wilms tumor** occur in children under 5 years of age. A strong correlation exists between Wilms tumor and several congenital malformations. Genetic links may contribute to its occurrence in children with bilateral tumors and those who have family members with the disorder. When Wilms tumor, aniridia (a congenital malformation of the iris of the eye), genitourinary malformations, and mental retardation occur together, the genetic association strengthens. However, survivors of Wilms tumor that is unilateral at diagnosis possess a low risk for producing a child who will develop the disease. Information about the risk factors for Wilms tumor is not definitive. The 5-year survival rates for children with this disease are excellent (Hockenberry & Wilson, 2006).

Retinoblastoma

Even as the most common intraocular tumor in younger children, retinoblastoma affects only 300 children younger than 20 years of age each year. Most of these children are less than 5 years old. Genetic mutations contribute to the incidence of retinoblastoma, usually causing the bilateral form

of the disease. Even though the tumor is uncommon, the scientific work surrounding its diagnosis and management has resulted in many of the methods used for other cancers. Survival rates are excellent (Wilson et al., 2006).

The history usually reveals a slow symptom progression. To reveal risk factors, the following questions should be asked:
Do tumors of the eye run in your family?
If tumors of the eye run in your family, which relatives were affected and how were they treated?
Have you noticed that your child has eye problems (crossed or lazy eyes or difficulty seeing)?
Have you noticed any changes in your child's eyes?
Screening eye examinations for high-risk children include:

1. Visual acuity
2. Red reflex, which appears whitish with retinoblastoma (cat's eye reflex)
3. Ophthalmoscopic findings
4. Lid lag, which is found with exophthalmos
5. Strabismus, by doing the cover-uncover test

The cat's eye reflex and strabismus are the most common signs of retinoblastoma. Any suspicious findings indicate referral for further evaluation.

Neuroblastoma

Neuroblastoma, a cancer of the sympathetic nervous system, begins in the abdomen, primarily in the adrenal gland, approximately 70% of the time. The remaining 30% of cases originate in cervical, thoracic, or pelvic areas. Approximately one half of these cancers occur in individuals younger than 2 years, suggesting the contribution of prenatal or perinatal factors (Urayama et al., 2007). More than 90% of diagnoses occur by age 5. Unfortunately, many of the children have metastases when the cancer is identified. Frequently symptoms of secondary spread bring the child to the health professional. The survival rate for children diagnosed during the preschool years is improving, but in other age groups it has remained static. There is little convincing evidence of specific risk factors. Prenatal exposure to pesticides, hormones, and use of certain medications suggest an increased risk (Urayama et al., 2007).

Cancer in a child can be frightening to parents, particularly if there is a strong family history of cancers of any kind. Early detection continues to be associated with increased survival rates. Secondary prevention programs should include the warning signs of cancer in children. Routine procedures, such as a bath, provide opportunities for parents to examine the child for physical symptoms of disease that are outlined in Box 19-5.

Asthma

The incidence of **asthma**, a chronic inflammatory disorder of the airways, is rising more rapidly in preschool-age children than in any other group (Danov & Guilbert, 2007).

Box 19-5 Warning Signs That May Indicate Childhood Cancer

Cancer remains a leading cause of death in children under 15 years of age, second only to injuries.

GENERAL

- Documented weight loss without explanation, failure to thrive
- Persistent poor appetite
- Tires easily or lack of energy

LEUKEMIA OR LYMPHOMAS: "LIQUID TUMORS" (CANCER OF THE BLOOD, BLOOD-MAKING SYSTEM, LYMPH NODES)

- Persistent fever (more than 2 weeks)
- Bruising without injury and purple or red patches appearing on the skin
- Swollen glands (lymph nodes) unrelated to infection
- Persistent bone pain or limping
- Paleness of the lips, skin, nails, or lining of the eyes

BRAIN TUMOR

- Recurrent headaches, especially accompanied by vomiting, particularly in the morning

- Reflection in the pupil of the eye (eye tumor)
- Unexplained, persistent changes in behavior

KIDNEY TUMORS

- Lump in the abdomen or abdominal enlargement
- Blood in the urine
- Bulging of the eyes
- Unexplained, persistent cough or chest pain
- A firm mass in the muscles

MAKE BATH TIME EXAMINATION TIME

- These complaints or physical findings should be interpreted only as warnings of possible serious disease. When these warnings are present, you should consult your physician at once.
- Do not forget that your children must be examined by a physician every year. The earlier cancer is detected, the better the chances are for a cure. With current treatment methods of surgery, radiation therapy, and chemotherapy (administration of anticancer drugs), the survival rate of children with certain forms of cancer has improved dramatically.

Modified from the Children's Cancer Research Fund website; Main Headquarters 7801 East Bush Lake Road, Suite 130; Minneapolis, Minnesota 55439-3152. Telephone Numbers: 1-888-4CCRF48; 952-893-9355; Fax: 952-893-9366; Email: webmaster@childrenscancer.org; Website: *www.ccrf. org/learning-center/kids-and-cancer/recognizing-the-symptoms-of-childhood-cancer.html.*

The inflammation in this disorder contributes to a hyperresponsive airway, limited airflow, and respiratory symptoms that include breathlessness, wheezing, cough, and chest tightness. Causes include genetic predisposition, allergens such as animal dander or dust mites, and nonspecific precipitants such as infections, exercise, weather, or stress. Rates for boys exceed those for girls, and rates in the Black and Hispanic population exceed those in the non-Hispanic White population. Poverty contributes significantly to asthmatic illness, disability, and death (Smith et al., 2005). Multiple factors contribute to exacerbation of asthma symptoms. High levels of exposure to tobacco smoke, pollutants, and allergens contribute. In addition to the generally known allergens of house mite dust and pet and rodent dander, cockroach particles have been implicated. Access to quality medical care, financial resources, and social support to manage the disease on a long-term basis exist in significantly different proportions from one population to another in the United States (U.S. Department of Health and Human Services, 2007).

SOCIAL PROCESSES
Community and Work

Some preschoolers become involved with groups outside their families, such as group child care settings, church groups, or family involvement in other activities, by age 3. Other children of the same age experience little outside contact. A preschool setting introduces the child to a wider social arena. Parents learn to release their child to encourage independent activity in a safe, supervised setting. Preschoolers test their independence, interactive skills, and self-discipline as they learn to function in a group. Preschool provides a transition to kindergarten and first grade, where group interaction skills are expected. Parents often select a preschool based on geographical closeness to their home or a friend's recommendation, using the most practical approach. With many child care facilities and options now available, parents frequently visit and evaluate a number of settings to determine the most appropriate for their needs (Hockenberry & Wilson, 2006).

Culture and Ethnicity

Family cultural heritage continues to shape preschoolers. Unlike toddlers, preschoolers frequently ask why the family follows certain practices. These young children notice differences from one family to another. Their playmates may celebrate different holidays or practice family rituals different from their own. As preschoolers experience more activities outside their home, differences become more apparent. Discussion about the strength of cultural differences provides an excellent learning opportunity (Multicultural Awareness box) (Andrews & Boyle, 2008).

MULTICULTURAL AWARENESS
Preschool

Three groups of 36 Chinese children (each with a mean age of 61 months) were studied to identify cognitive abilities that might distinguish children at risk for dyslexia: (1) teacher- or parent-reported (and health care professional–confirmed) language delay; (2) family history of dyslexia; and (3) not at risk.

The cognitive skills studied included syllable awareness, tone detection, rapid automated naming, visual skill, and morphological awareness. Compared to the control, the language-delayed group of children scored significantly lower on all measures. Children in the familial risk group performed significantly worse only on tone detection, morphological awareness, and word recognition.

Testing these skills may be important assessment tools for diagnosing risks for reading problems and may be associated with broader cognitive impairment as found previously in various Indo-European languages.

From McBride-Chang C., Lam F., Doo S., Wong S. W., & Chow Y. Y. (2008). Word recognition and cognitive profiles of Chinese pre-school children at risk for dyslexia through language delay or familial history of dyslexia. *Journal of Child Psychology and Psychiatry, 49*(2), 211-218.

Preschoolers also notice ethnic differences in appearance and pronounce skin colors, eyes, and hairstyles as "pretty" or "ugly." The socialization process forms presumptions similar to those of their family or playmates. Parents and caregivers who teach and role model positive behaviors allow children to see differences in others as being positive rather than negative. Mass media influences on physical attractiveness also contribute and become more significant to the adolescent.

Certain cultures apply more pressure for children to assume responsibility for younger siblings or household tasks. Confusion develops in the preschooler when the family's culture varies from that of most playmates. Disciplinary approaches vary from culture to culture. Uncertainty also results when parents integrate their cultural background into the community standards, but the grandparents adhere to traditional cultural practices, rituals, and child-rearing ideas.

Legislation

Many safety-focused legislative bills have affected the preschooler (see Chapter 18). School issues, as discussed in Chapter 20, also affect this age group. With current concern about health care costs, financial programs that focus on children may lose when competing with the whole of health care. If overall funding for vulnerable populations such as the homeless and the poor decrease, child health care in general in this country suffers. In the United States, one in every four children under the age of 6 lives in poverty. More than 50% of the occupants of urban homeless shelters at a given time will be children under the age of 6 years (Nilsen, 2007; U.S. Census Bureau, 2003).

Economics

Poverty influences the preschooler as it does any child. Unlike toddlers, preschoolers become more aware of family economic status. A preschooler may know that the family lacks money for toys but recognizes less the comprehensive limits to resources that influence the family lifestyle. In some cases the family's financial history prevents attendance at preschool or influences exposure to expanded learning activities. Preschoolers realize money acquires food, toys, and clothes, but they do not yet have a concept of economic values. The child might trade an expensive item for a trinket that looks more interesting. A child who uses the earnings to buy something realizes that more must be earned to buy more things. The child thus begins to learn the concepts of earning and spending.

Health Care Delivery System

Access to health care resources remains the same for preschoolers as toddlers. When preschoolers enter a school setting, admission may require that a health care worker screen them physically and developmentally. For indigent children **Early and Periodic Screening, Diagnosis, and Treatment (EPSDT)**, a Medicaid program, may fund the visit. Screening for children under age 21 who meet the economic criteria for Medicaid occurs in private offices, local health departments, and community clinics. Medicaid provides one screening examination per year, which includes the following elements:

1. Medical history
2. Assessment of physical growth, nutritional status, and mental development
3. Inspection of ears, eyes, nose, mouth, teeth, and throat
4. Vision screening
5. Auditory screening
6. Screening for cardiac abnormalities
7. Screening for anemia
8. Screening for the sickle cell trait
9. Urine sampling
10. Blood pressure reading
11. Assessment and updating of immunizations
12. Tuberculosis screening, when indicated
13. Referral to a dentist for diagnosis and treatment for children 3 years of age and older

Referral for a complete physical examination addresses any health or developmental concerns identified during this screening. Eligible children receive EPSDT as a comprehensive service administered by Medicaid.

NURSING INTERVENTIONS

Preschoolers show much interest in the tools and procedures of a health screening examination (Hockenberry & Wilson, 2006) (Box 19-6). These inquisitive children may play with the stethoscope, otoscope, and other diagnostic instruments. The nurse explains the tests in age-appropriate terminology and expects the child to cooperate for most of the visit. The preschooler may show self-control during injections but definitely needs a parent close by to offer support and encouragement. The nurse includes the preschooler in the history by directing questions about dietary intake and health practices, such as tooth brushing, favorite activities, and friends. At this age children begin taking some interest in health, developing the cognitive maturity to learn many health-promotion skills that they will use for the rest of their lives.

SUMMARY

Schedules for preventive health care during the preschool years include visits at 4 and 5 years of age. Each visit includes an ongoing history; growth, physical, and developmental assessment; and discussion of age-appropriate developmental concerns.

In addition to the office or clinic contact, the nurse may consult with a preschool nurse or a nurse for a primary school and preschool. Early exposure to and reinforcement of health care information as part of preschool education lays a foundation for later healthy lifestyle habits, which influence overall societal health. Health as a curricular subject during the school-age years continues this focus. The school nurse's role in health promotion and prevention of illness is discussed in Chapter 20.

Box 19-6 | Health-Promotion Interventions for Preschool Children

ANNUALLY
- Health history
- Height and weight
- Blood pressure
- Vision screening (age 3 to 4 years)
- Developmental and behavioral assessment
- Physical examination

PERIODICALLY
- Immunizations based on recommended schedule
  - Ensure currency
  - Diphtheria, tetanus, pertussis
  - Oral poliovirus
  - Pneumococcal
  - Measles, mumps, rubella
  - Haemophilus influenzae type b
  - Hepatitis B
  - Varicella
- Hematocrit or hemoglobin level at least once after age 9 months
- Urinalysis at 5 years old

SCREENINGS FOR HIGH-RISK CHILDREN
- Lead
- Tuberculosis
- Cholesterol

ANTICIPATORY GUIDANCE
- Injury Prevention
  - Child safety car seat (age less than 5 years) or seat belt
  - Lap and shoulder belt (age 5 years and older)
  - Use helmet and avoid traffic when bicycling
  - Smoke detectors, flame-retardant sleepwear
  - Hot water temperature less than 125° F
  - Window and stair guards, pool fence
  - Safe storage of drugs, toxic substances, firearms, matches
  - Close availability of syrup of ipecac, poison control phone number
  - Parents and caretakers trained in cardiopulmonary resuscitation
- Violence prevention
- Nutrition and exercise
  - Limit saturated fats; maintain caloric balance; and emphasize grain, fruit, vegetable intake
  - Regular fun physical activity
- Tobacco
  - Effects of passive smoking
  - Antitobacco messages
- Dental health
  - Floss, brush with fluoridated toothpaste at least daily
  - Regular visits to dentist

CASE STUDY

Preschool Child: Ricky

Ricky, age 4, arrives in the clinic with his mother. Ricky lives with his mother and father, who both work full time, and his infant sister. Their extended family lives in a different state more than 100 miles away. Both parents are of average height and in good health. Ricky's mother mentions that Ricky often expresses frustration, particularly in regard to food. Conflict over food occurs every day. Mealtime is a battle to get him to eat, unless his mother feeds him. Ricky's baby sister eats no table food and seems to be able to tolerate any food given. Ricky's mother is quite frustrated and concerned that he will become malnourished.

Reflective Questions:
1. What additional assessment information would you collect?
2. What questions would you ask and how would you further explore this issue with the mother?
3. In what ways does the distance of the extended family influence this family's approach to health promotion?
4. What factors would you consider to determine whether malnourishment is a factor in this family?

CARE PLAN

Ineffective Coping in Preschool Child: Ricky

Nursing Diagnosis: Ineffective Coping Related to Parental Feedback for Regressive Behaviors and Lack of Consistent Limits and Fulfillment of Appropriate Responsibilities

DEFINING CHARACTERISTICS

- Parent verbalization of need for help
- Changes in the usual behavior patterns of the child

RELATED FACTORS

- Inconsistent methods of parental discipline
- Inadequate impulse control
- Lack of social skills

EXPECTED OUTCOMES

- The child will separate from his parents without incident (tantrum, crying).
- The child will join a community or church peer group activity.
- The child will perform one household task (picking up his toys) before bedtime every evening.
- The child will demonstrate independent self-care behaviors (feed himself).
- The parents will have clear, consistent, and age-appropriate expectations for behavior.
- The parents will explain the rationale for limiting a socially unacceptable or unsafe behavior as soon as it is displayed.

INTERVENTIONS

- Discuss with parents the process of growth and development and the child's need to learn how to compromise, take turns, and channel energy appropriately.
- Use a prescreening developmental questionnaire to validate general assessment data.
- Encourage the parents to leave the child in someone else's care while they go shopping or to see a movie.
- Encourage the mother to formulate a bedtime ritual with the child that does not include her sitting in his room until he falls asleep.
- Discuss with the parents and the child what "jobs" he can do at home and the expectation that they be performed daily.
- Suggest laying out the child's clothes so that he can dress himself. Set a time to be dressed, such as before or after a certain television program.
- Explore with the parents the availability of playgroups or community activities for the child.
- Encourage the parents to take the child to the neighborhood playground so that he can meet and play with other children.
- Have the child help around the house alongside his parents. Specify "work" and "play" times.
- Encourage the parents to praise the child for age-appropriate behaviors, being careful not to bribe him to perform.
- Discuss the principles of discipline consistency, immediacy, realistic expectations, and clear explanations.
- Recognize the parents' frustration and encourage them to try different approaches, such as limited choices, diversion, and incentives ("when you finish your meat, we'll play a game").
- Suggest that the parents keep a diary of how long an approach was tried and how consistently the child responded.
- Discuss the decrease in appetite and reliance of food fads that typify the child's age. Review the principles of nutrition, timing of snacks, and ways of making food attractive to children.
- Refer the parents and the child to a nutritionist for nutrition counseling.

EVALUATION

- Parents make appropriate verbal, nonverbal, and eye contact.
- Parents demonstrate correct caregiver techniques.
- Parents verbalize intent to maintain relationships.
- Parents attend to routine well child care appointments.
- Parents provide developmentally appropriate play activities.
- Parents describe healthy ways to express frustration.

For further information on developing care plans, see: Carpenito-Moyet, L. J. (2008) *Nursing diagnosis: Application to clinical practice* (12th ed.). Philadelphia: Lippincott, Williams & Wilkins; and Sparks, S. M., & Taylor, C. M. (2007). *Sparks and Taylor's nursing diagnostic reference manual* (7th ed.). Philadelphia: Lippincott Williams & Wilkins.

REFERENCES

Allor, J. H., & McCathren, R. B. (2003). Developing emergent literacy skills through storybook reading. *Intervention in School & Clinic, 39*(2), 72–79.

American Academy of Pediatrics. (2008). *Bright futures: Guidelines for health supervision of infants, children, and adolescents* (3rd ed.). Elk Park, IL: American Academy of Pediatrics.

American Association of Poison Control Centers. (2002). *Toxic Exposure Surveillance System (TESS)*. Retrieved January 22, 2008, from *www.aapcc.org/poison1.htm.*

Andrews, M. M., & Boyle, J. S. (2008). *Transcultural concepts in nursing care* (5th ed.). New York: Lippincott Williams & Wilkins.

Atherson, M. J., & Metcalf, J. (2005). Television watching and risk of obesity in American adolescents. *American Journal of Health Education, 36*(1), 2–7, 14.

Bickley, L., & Szilagyi, P. G. (2007). *Bates' guide to physical examination and history taking.* (9th ed.). Philadelphia: Lippincott Williams & Wilkins.

Bowie, B. H. (2007). Relational aggression, gender, and the developmental process. *Journal of Child and Adolescent Psychiatric Nursing, 20*(2), 107–115.

Bracken, B., & Shaughnessy, M. F. (2003). An interview with Bruce Bracken about the measurement of basic concepts in children. *North American Journal of Psychology, 5*(3), 351–363.

Bren, L. (2006). Food labels identify allergens more clearly. *FDA Consumer, 40*(2; 2), 37–38.

Brotanek, J. M., Halterman, J. S., Auinger, P., Flores, G., & Weitzman, M. (2005). Iron deficiency, prolonged bottle-feeding, and racial/ethnic disparities in young children. *Archives of Pediatrics & Adolescent Medicine, 159*(11), 1038–1042.

Bryant, M. J., Lucove, J. C., Evenson, K. R., & Marshall, S. (2007). Measurement of television viewing in children and adolescents: A systematic review. *Obesity Reviews, 8*(3), 197–209.

Burford, A. E., Ryan, L. M., Stone, B. J., Hirshon, J. M., & Klein, B. L. (2005). Drowning and near-drowning in children and adolescents: A succinct review for emergency physicians and nurses. *Pediatric Emergency Care, 21*(9), 610–619.

Burrowes, J. D. (2007). Nutrition for a lifetime: Childhood nutrition. *Nutrition Today, 42*(4), 160–167.

Carpenito-Moyet, L. J. (2008). *Nursing diagnosis: Application to clinical practice* (12th ed.). Philadelphia: Lippincott Williams & Wilkins.

Centers for Disease Control and Prevention. (2007). Recommended immunization schedules for persons aged 0-18 years—United States, 2007. *Morbidity and Mortality Weekly Report, 55*(51), Q-1-Q-4.

Centers for Disease Control and Prevention, National Center for Environmental Health & Childhood Lead Poisoning Prevention Program. (2007). *Folk Medicine and Childhood Lead Exposure.* Retrieved June 14, 2008, from *www.cdc.gov/nceh/lead/faq/folk%20meds.htm.*

Coleman, E. (2005). Physical activity and the new pyramid. *Nutrition & the M.D., 31*(6), 1–4.

Collier, S., Fulhan, J., & Duggan, C. (2004). Nutrition for the pediatric office: Update on vitamins, infant feeding and food allergies. *Current Opinion in Pediatrics, 16*(3), 314–320.

Criddle, L. M. (2007). An overview of pediatric poisonings. *AACN Advanced Critical Care, 18*(2), 109–118.

Danov, Z., & Guilbert, T. W. (2007). Prevention of asthma in childhood. *Current Opinion in Allergy and Clinical Immunology, 7*(2), 174–179.

Donohue, B., Strada, M. J., Rosales, R., Taylor-Caldwell, A., Hise, D., Ahman, S., et al. (2006). The semistructured interview for consideration of ethnic culture in therapy scale: Initial psychometric and outcome support. *Behavior Modification, 30*(6), 867–891.

Elkins, M., & Cavendish, R. (2004). Developing a plan for pediatric spiritual care. *Holistic Nursing Practice, 18*(4), 179–184.

Emergency Nurses Association. (2005). Position statement: Firearm safety. *Topics in emergency medicine, 27*(3), 233–236.

Fallat, M. E., Costich, J., & Pollack, S. (2006). The impact of disparities in pediatric trauma on injury-prevention initiatives. *Journal of Trauma, 60*(2), 452–454.

Fisher-Owens, S. A., Gansky, S. A., Platt, L. J., Weintraub, J. A., Soobader, M., Bramlett, M. D., et al. (2007). Influences on children's oral health: A conceptual model. *Pediatrics, 120*(3), e510–e520.

Flanagan, R., & Motta, R. W. (2007). Figure drawings: A popular method. *Psychology in the Schools, 44*(3), 257–270.

Floriani, V., & Kennedy, C. (2007). Promotion of physical activity in primary care for obesity treatment/prevention in children. *Current Opinion in Pediatrics, 19*(1), 99–103.

Gable, S., Chang, Y., & Krull, J. L. (2007). Television watching and frequency of family meals are predictive of overweight onset and persistence in a national sample of school-aged children. *Journal of the American Dietetic Association, 107*(1), 53–61.

Gilbert, G. H. (2005). Racial and socioeconomic disparities in health from population-based research to practice-based research: The example of oral health. *Journal of Dental Education, 69*(9), 1003–1014.

Girbau, D., & Schwartz, R. G. (2007). Nonword repetition in Spanish-speaking children with specific language impairment (SLI). *International Journal of Language & Communication Disorders, 42*(1), 59–75.

Glogowska, M., Roulstone, S., Peters, T. J., & Enderby, P. (2006). Early speech- and language-impaired children: Linguistic, literacy, and social outcomes. *Developmental Medicine & Child Neurology, 48*(6), 489–494.

Gottesman, M. M. (2007). HEAT: Healthy eating and activity together. *American Journal of Nursing, 107*(2), 49–50.

Hammer, C. S., Lawrence, F. R., & Miccio, A. W. (2007). Bilingual children's language abilities and early reading outcomes in Head Start and kindergarten. *Language, Speech, and Hearing Services in Schools, 38*(3), 237–248.

Hammer, C. S., & Miccio, A. W. (2006). Early language and reading development of bilingual preschoolers from low-income families. *Topics in Language Disorders, 26*(4), 322–337, 385-390.

Harrison, K. (2006). Fast and sweet: Nutritional attributes of television food advertisements with and without black characters. *Howard Journal of Communications, 17*(4), 249–264.

Hartmann, E. E., Bradford, G. E., Chaplin, P. K., Johnson, T., Kemper, A. R., Kim, S., et al. (2006). Project universal preschool vision screening: A demonstration project. *Pediatrics, 117*(2), (Supplement), e226–e237.

Haven, J., & Britten, P. (2006). My pyramid—the complete guide. *Nutrition Today, 41*(6), 253–259.

Hepburn, L., Azrael, D., Miller, M., & Hemenway, D. (2006). The effect of child access prevention laws on unintentional child firearm fatalities, 1979-2000. *Journal of Trauma, 61*(2), 423–428.

Hockenberry, M. J., & Wilson, D. (2006). *Wong's nursing care of infants and children* (8th ed.). St. Louis: Mosby.

Ionescu, T., & Benga, O. (2007). Reconceptualizing early education on scientific grounds: School readiness in focus. *Cognitie, Creier, Comportament/Cognition, Brain, Behavior, 11*(1), 49–65.

Jenni, O. G., & LeBourgeois, M. K. (2006). Understanding sleep-wake behavior and sleep disorders in children: The value of a model. *Current Opinion in Psychiatry, 19*(3), 282–287.

Kalpidou, M. D., Power, T. G., Cherry, K. E., & Gottfried, N. W. (2004). Regulation of emotion and behavior among 3- and 5-year-olds. *Journal of General Psychology, 131*(2), 159–178.

Kempe, A., Beaty, B. L., Steiner, J. F., Pearson, K. A., Lowery, N. E., Daley, M. F., et al. (2004). The regional immunization registry as a public health tool for improving clinical practice and guiding immunization delivery policy. *American Journal of Public Health, 94*(6), 967–972.

Klein-Schwartz, W. (2003). Pediatric methylphenidate exposures: 7-year experience of poison centers in the United States. *Clinical Pediatrics, 42*(2), 159–164.

Kumanyika, S. K. (2007). The obesity epidemic: Looking in the mirror. *American Journal of Epidemiology, 166*(3), 243–245.

La Paro, K. M., Pianta, R. C., & Stuhlman, M. (2004). The classroom assessment scoring system. *Elementary School Journal, 104*(5), 409–426.

Leininger, M., & McFarland, M. R. (2006). *Culture care diversity and universality: A worldwide nursing theory* (2nd ed.). Sudbury, MA: Jones and Bartlett.

Lu, C., Barr, D. B., Pearson, M., Bartell, S., & Bravo, R. (2006). A longitudinal approach to assessing urban and suburban children's exposure to pyrethroid pesticides. *Environmental Health Perspectives, 114*(9), 1419–1423.

Lynch, M. F., Griffin, I. J., Hawthorne, K. M., Chen, Z., Hamzo, M., & Abrams, S. A. (2007). Calcium balance in 1-4-y-old children. *American Journal of Clinical Nutrition, 85*(3), 750–754.

Marshall, T. A. (2006). Dietary guidelines for Americans and MyPyramid. *The Journal of the American Dental Association, 137*(9), 1344.

Marshall, T. A., Eichenberger-Gilmore, J. M., Larson, M. A., & Levy, S. M. (2007). Comparison of the intakes of sugars by young children with and without dental caries experience. *Journal of the American Dental Association: JADA, 138*(1), 39–46.

Mashburn, A. J., & Pianta, R. C. (2006). Social relationships and school readiness. *Early Education and Development, 17*(1), 151–176.

Mason, T. B., 2nd, & Pack, A. I. (2005). Sleep terrors in childhood. *Journal of Pediatrics, 147*(3), 388–392.

McCann, J. C., & Ames, B. N. (2007). An overview of evidence for a causal relation between iron deficiency during development and deficits in cognitive or behavioral function. *American Journal of Clinical Nutrition, 85*(4), 931–945.

McGuigan, N., & Nunez, M. (2006). Executive functioning by 18–24-month-old children: Effects of inhibition, working memory demands and narrative in a novel detour-reaching task. *Infant and Child Development, 15*(5), 519–542.

McGuinness, T. M. (2006). Marriage, divorce, and children. *Journal of Psychosocial Nursing and Mental Health Services, 44*(2), 17–20.

Miller, M., Lippmann, S. J., Azrael, D., & Hemenway, D. (2007). Household firearm ownership and rates of suicide across the 50 United States. *Journal of Trauma, 62*(4), 1029–1035.

Montgomery, J. W. (2003). Working memory and comprehension in children with specific language impairment: What we know so far. *Journal of Communication Disorders*, 36(3), 221-231.

Nagaraja, J., Menkedick, J., Phelan, K. J., Ashley, P., Zhang, X., & Lanphear, B. P. (2005). Deaths from residential injuries in US children and adolescents, 1985-1997. *Pediatrics*, 116(2), 454–461.

Nelson, M. C., & Gordon-Larsen, P. (2006). Physical activity and sedentary behavior patterns are associated with selected adolescent health risk behaviors. *Pediatrics*, 117(4), 1281–1290.

Nilsen, S. (2007). *Poverty in America: Economic research shows adverse impacts on health status and other social conditions as well as the economic growth rate.* (Government No. GAO-07-344). Washington, DC: United States Government Accountability Office, (poverty). Retrieved January 22, 2008, from *www.gao.gov/new.items/d07344.pdf.*

Norris, V. W., Arnos, K. S., Hanks, W. D., Xia, X., Nance, W. E., & Pandya, A. (2006). Does universal newborn hearing screening identify all children with GJB2 (Connexin 26) deafness? Penetrance of GJB2 deafness. *Ear and Hearing*, 27(6), 732–741.

Pardi, L. A., King, B. P., Salemi, G., & Salvator, A. E. (2007). The effect of bicycle helmet legislation on pediatric injury. *Journal of Trauma Nursing*, 14(2), 84–87.

Paulson, P. R., & Hammer, A. L. (2002). Pediatric immunization update 2002. *Pediatric Nursing*, 28(2), 173–181.

Peregrin, T. (2006). Making MyPyramid for kids a successful tool in nutrition education. *Journal of the American Dietetic Association*, 106(5), 656–658.

Ramsey, J. E., & Bradford, G. E. (2006). Legislative issues facing pediatric ophthalmology in 2006. *Current Opinion in Ophthalmology*, 17(5), 441–446.

Rehfuess, E., Mehta, S., & Prüss-Ustün, A. (2006). Assessing household solid fuel use: Multiple implications for the millennium development goals. *Environmental Health Perspectives*, 114(3), 373–378.

Rennels, M. B., Baker, C. J., Baltimore, R. S., Bocchini, J. A., Dennehy, P. H., Frenck, R. W., et al. (2004). Recommended childhood and adolescent immunization schedule—United States. *Pediatrics*, 113(5), 1448.

Rescorla, L. (2005). Age 13 language and reading outcomes in late-talking toddlers. *JSLHR: Journal of Speech, Language, and Hearing Research*, 48(2), 459–472.

Ries, L. A. G., et al. (2007). *SEER cancer statistics review, 1975-2004.* Retrieved January 22, 2008, from *http://seer.cancer.gov/csr/1975_2004/.*

Rock, D. A., & Stenner, A. J. (2005). Closing racial and ethnic gaps: Assessment issues in testing of children at school entry. *The Future of Children*, 15(1), 15–34.

Rudisill, M. E., & Wall, S. J. (2004). Meeting active start guidelines in the ADC-motion program: Preschool. *Teaching Elementary Physical Education*, 15(2), 25–29.

Shivers, E. M., & Barr, R. (2007). Exploring cultural differences in children's exposure to television in home-based child care settings. *Zero to Three*, 27(5), 39–45.

Smith, L. A., Hatcher-Ross, J. L., Wertheimer, R., & Kahn, R. S. (2005). Rethinking race/ethnicity, income, and childhood asthma: Racial/ethnic disparities concentrated among the very poor. *Public Health Reports*, 120(2), 109–116.

Snow, K. L. (2006). Measuring school readiness: Conceptual and practical considerations. *Early Education and Development*, 17(1), 7–41.

Sparks, S. M., & Taylor, C. M. (2007). *Sparks and Taylor's nursing diagnostic reference manual* (7th ed.). Philadelphia: Lippincott, Williams & Wilkins.

Taft, C. H., Mickalide, A. D., & Taft, A. R. (1999). Child passengers at risk in America: A national study of car seat misuse. Retrieved July 27, 2004, from *www.safekids.org/tier3_ed.cfm?falders_id=680&content_item_id=2530.*

Tung, Y., Duffy, L. C., Gyamfi, J. O., Wojtaszczyk, F., Dozier, A., Tempfer, T., et al. (2003). Improvements in immunization compliance using a computerized tracking system for inner city clinics. *Clinical Pediatrics*, 42(7), 603–611.

U.S. Department of Health and Human Services. (2007). *Healthy people 2010 midcourse review.* Retrieved January 22, 2008, from *www.healthypeople.gov/Data/midcourse/.*

U.S. Census Bureau. (2003). *Current population survey: Poverty: 2002 highlights.* Retrieved January 16, 2008, from *www.census.gov/prod/2003pubs/p60–222.pdf.*

U.S. Department of Health and Human Services. (2007). *The Surgeon General's call to action to prevent and decrease overweight and obesity.* Retrieved January 22, 2008, from *www.surgeongeneral.gov/topics/obesity/calltoaction/fact_glance.htm.*

University of Pittsburgh. (2004). *Child health library: Common childhood injuries and poisonings.* Retrieved January 22, 2008, from *www.chp.edu/besafe/index.php.*

Urayama, K. Y., Von Behren, J., & Reynolds, P. (2007). Birth characteristics and risk of neuroblastoma in young children. *American Journal of Epidemiology*, 165(5), 486–495.

U.S. Department of Agriculture. (2005). *My-pyramid for kids web site.* Retrieved January 22, 2008, from *www.mypyramid.gov.*

Vagnoli, L., Caprilli, S., Robiglio, A., & Messeri, A. (2005). Clown doctors as a treatment for preoperative anxiety in children: A randomized, prospective study. *Pediatrics*, 116(4), (Supplement), e563–e567.

Vygotsky, L. S. (2004). Imagination and creativity in childhood. *Journal of Russian & East European Psychology*, 42(1), 7–97.

Wilson, M. W., Haik, B. G., & Rodriguez-Galindo, C. (2006). Socioeconomic impact of modern multidisciplinary management of retinoblastoma. *Pediatrics*, 118(2), e331–e336.

Woo, E. J., Ball, R., Bostrom, A., Shadomy, S. V., Ball, L. K., Evans, G., et al. (2004). Vaccine risk perception among reporters of autism after vaccination: Vaccine adverse event reporting system 1990-2001. *American Journal of Public Health*, 94(6), 990–995.

Zabinski, M. F., Norman, G. J., Sallis, J. F., Calfas, K. J., & Patrick, K. (2007). Patterns of sedentary behavior among adolescents. *Health Psychology*, 26(1), 113–120.

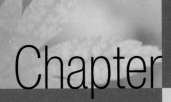

Chapter 20

Leslie Kennard Scott*

School-Age Child

objectives

After completing this chapter, the reader will be able to:

- Identify expected physical and developmental changes occurring in the school-age child.
- Explore stages of cognitive development of the school-age child, particularly its relation to academic skills and performance.
- Distinguish relevant health promotion needs and common health risk factors found in the school-age child.
- Analyze cultural, societal, peer influence, and stress on development in the school-age child.
- Propose common developmental problems that occur in the school-age child including ways to assist parents in the management of these common problems.
- Describe strategies for family (parents) to improve child's self-concept, socialization abilities, and stress reduction in the school-age child.

key terms

Astigmatism
Attention-deficit/hyperactivity disorder (ADHD)
Auditory acuity
Auditory learners
Child abuse
Chronic serous otitis media
Classifying and ordering
Concrete operation
Conservation
Coping strategies
Dental caries
Depression
Discipline
Disorders of arousal
Dyslexia
Encopresis
Enuresis
Gastroenteritis
Healthy People 2010
Human papilloma virus (HPV)
Hyperopic (farsighted)
Hypertension
Individualized Educational Plan (IEP)

Individuals with Disabilities Education Act (IDEA)
Industry versus inferiority
Intelligence
Intelligence quotient (IQ)
Kinesthetic learners
"Latchkey children"
Learning disability
Lice (pediculosis)
Limit setting
Malocclusion
Menarche
Meningococcal vaccination
Moral development
Myopia (nearsightedness)
No Child Left Behind Act of 2001
Obesity
Orthodontic care
Ossification
Overweight
Peer groups
Phonics
Preconventional
Puberty

Public Law 94-142 (Education for All Handicapped Children Act)
Punishment
Scabies
Section 504 of the Rehabilitation Act of 1973
Self-concept
Self-discovery
Self-esteem
Sexual abuse
Sleep talking
Sleepwalking
Snellen 'E' Chart
Socialization
Somatization
Standardized growth charts
State Children's Health Insurance Program (SCHIP)
Talismans
Tooth eruption
Tympanograms
Visual acuity
Visual learners
Vision screening programs

*The author acknowledges the work of Carolyn Spence Cagle in a previous edition of the chapter.

website materials

evolve

These materials are located on the book's Website at *http://evolve.elsevier.com/Edelman/*
- WebLinks
- Study Questions
- Glossary
- Website Resources

  20A: Blood Pressure Levels for Girls and Boys by Age and Height Percentiles
  20B: Development of Deciduous and Permanent Teeth
  20C: Dental Health Education
  20D: Helpful Information for Parents About Nocturnal Enuresis
  20E: Common Developmental and Cognitive Tests

THINK About It

School-Age Shyness

Rebecca Sims, 7 years of age, has demonstrated withdrawn behavior. Her mother reports she has "always been a quiet and reserved child." She performs well in school; however, her teacher has reported that Rebecca is very quiet, withdrawn, and speaks in a hesitant fashion when called on. Rebecca's step-father has voiced frustration with her withdrawn behavior and has enrolled her in a cheerleading group and an after-school soccer team to combat her shyness. Rebecca will frequently not speak during cheerleading ("she'll just go through the motions") and her soccer coach reports she does not engage with the other players. This pressure has created an intense home environment that has Rebecca's parents feeling frustrated about her behavior. Her step-father will frequently mention what others are saying about her shyness to Rebecca. "I don't know how else to get her involved with her classmates and get over this shyness."

Rebecca says that she prefers to be alone and is afraid to speak up in school. She has poor eye contact, speaks hesitantly, and shrugs her shoulders in initial response to assessment questions. "I'm afraid they'll laugh at what I say." She reports she "has no friends."

Her parents are divorced and both are remarried. She visits her father every other weekend and on various holidays. Her mother and step-father are both employed full-time outside the home. They often try to engage her in conversation and include her in activities, but "she seems like she would rather be alone."

1. Is Rebecca's behavior typical for a 7-year-old child?
2. Discuss the values inherent in Rebecca's and her parents' behavior and how these might be related to the scenario as described.
3. How might you, as the health care professional, guide this family in finding ways to encourage Rebecca and thus decrease family stress?
4. Are there any further underlying issues that may be contributing to Rebecca's behavior?

"The school-age years" is a span of time between a child's entrance into kindergarten and the beginning of adolescence, a range from 5 to 12 years of age. During this time period observable differences in growth, development, and cognitive ability are prominent. Consider how different the child entering kindergarten is from the preadolescent, particularly the differences in size as well as mental ability. Children grow (physically) much more slowly during this time period as compared with growth during infancy and adolescence. Fine and gross motor skills are being perfected and mental abilities grow tremendously as the child learns to read, write, and compute mathematics in addition to other topics of interest. Relationships outside the family including **peer groups** are also developing during this phase of growth and development.

Most children are relatively healthy during this time period. Health-promotion and health-maintenance strategies are important. During this period of development children learn to accept personal responsibility and participate in the management of self-care tasks in the areas of personal hygiene, nutrition, physical activity, sleep, and safety. Nurses fill a significant role in the facilitation of parental roles and child roles in meeting growth, developmental, and self-care aspects of the school-age child (American Academy of Pediatrics, 2007; Hockenberry & Wilson, 2006).

PHYSICAL CHANGES

A child's growth and development is influenced by genetic inheritance, nutrition, and the physical sociocultural environments in which they live. The school-age child has an overall slimmer appearance as compared with the preschool-age child. Their legs are longer as compared to the rest of the body allowing greater strength, balance, coordination, and fluidity of motion in running, jumping, climbing, throwing, and riding a bicycle (Hockenberry & Wilson, 2007).

Most bodily systems reach adult level of function during the school-age years. Before 6 years of age, children use the diaphragm as the primary breathing muscle. After 6 years of age, thoracic muscles develop and the respiratory rate slows to 16 to 22 breaths per minute (Ball & Bindler,

2008). The school-age child's head circumference continues to grow. However, after age 5 years head growth slows until puberty, at which time the head and brain reach adult circumference (53 to 54 cm; 21 inches) (Hockenberry & Wilson, 2007). The heart slowly grows in size and the heart rate slows to an average rate of 70 to 100 beats per minute, approaching that of an adult. Mean blood pressure is lower in this age group than in adults and ranges from 104 to 106 mm Hg systolic and from 58 to 62 mm Hg diastolic (U.S. Department of Health and Human Services [USDHHS], 2004). The gastrointestinal system is maturing with increased stomach capacity, resulting in less need for snacks and decreased calorie needs as compared to the preschooler. Bladder capacity improves. The immune system is better able to produce an antibody-antigen response (Hockenberry, 2005). By puberty, the endocrine system (with the exception of reproductive function) approaches adult capacity and function.

Elevated Blood Pressure

The long term effects of elevated blood pressure, **hypertension**, in adults are well known and documented. The realization that adult hypertension often begins in childhood has encouraged efforts to screen young children for elevated blood pressure. The American Academy of Pediatrics and the American Heart Association recommend that children have their blood pressure measured annually, beginning at age 3 years of age (Flynn, 2004; American Heart Association [AHA], 2007). This recommendation has come about due to concerns of higher blood pressure values in children over the past two decades, demonstrating risk of cardiovascular disease (Urrutia-Rojas et al., 2006). In 1980, 11% of American children had high blood pressure. By 2002, the incidence increased to 15% (AHA, 2007). Blood pressure values among school-age children may vary greatly. See **Website Resource 20A** for detailed tables of blood pressure levels for boys and girls according to height and weight.

Black children and Mexican-American children should be followed closely due to earlier onset and end-stage organ damage in those with hypertension as compared to Caucasian children (AHA, 2007; Hansen et al., 2007; Hayman et al., 2007; Lane & Gill, 2004). A family history of hypertension or identification of an elevated blood pressure in a child mandates close monitoring and assessment of cardiovascular risk factors during well-child check-ups during the school-age years (Chiolero et al., 2007; Din-Dzietham et al., 2007; Podoll et al., 2007). Differentiation between primary and secondary hypertension should be determined in any school-age child with elevated blood pressure (Flynn, 2002, 2004).

Physical Growth

Although many children have "spurts" of growth alternating with periods of minimal growth, height and weight growth velocities assume a slower and steadier pace as compared with earlier years of growth. The school-age child gains approximately 5 cm (2 inches) per year in height and 2-3 kg (4.4 to 6.6 lb) per year in weight (Hockenberry & Wilson,

2007). Black children tend to be slightly larger and Asian-American children somewhat smaller than their Caucasian counterparts, as plotted on growth charts that are believed to be standardized for various ethnic groups (World Health Organization [WHO], 2007; Butte et al., 2007). Before the onset of **puberty**, there is little difference in size between boys and girls. However, towards the latter part of this developmental stage, girls tend to grow more rapidly in height and weight (Gavin, 2007). A preadolescent increase in height and weight tends to occur around 10 years of age in girls, 12 years of age in boys. However, maturation rates vary resulting in a wide range of sizes in both boys and girls, particularly among 10 to 12 year olds (Hockenberry & Wilson, 2007; Gavin, 2007).

Black and Asian-American children mature earlier than do Caucasian children (National Institute of Child Health & Human Development, 2007). Black children are often taller and heavier than their Caucasian counterparts. They also tend to have longer and denser bones, slimmer hips, more muscle, and less fat on their limbs than on their central body as compared to Caucasian children (Hockenberry, 2005). Girls tend to mature, enter puberty, and stop growing earlier than boys. From birth, girls tend to have more fat than boys, and after puberty girls have a greater percentage of body weight devoted to fat. In fact, adiposity has a direct correlation to puberty onset in girls (Herman-Giddens et al., 2004).

School-age children tend to be concerned about their rate of growth, weight, time of menarche, and final height. These children need to understand that the timing and extent of their physical changes usually reflect their genetic inheritance. When assessing a child's height and weight and before referring to **standardized growth charts**, the height of the child's family must be taken into consideration (Centers for Disease Control [CDC], National Center for Health Statistics, 2009). For more information, see *www.cdc.gov/ nchs/nhanes/growthcharts/clinical_chart.htm*. For example, the child whose height is in the third percentile may have parents who are shorter than average. Shorter height can be expected because of the family's genetic make-up. Likewise, although the average age of **menarche** is around 12.8 years in Caucasian girls and 12.2 years in Black girls, most girls experience their menarche at about the same age their mothers did (Nield et al., 2007). With sufficient body fat to stimulate hormones needed for menses, girls can have their first menstrual period between ages 11 and 15 and still be considered normal (Herman-Giddens et al., 2004). Due to better nutrition and differences in lifestyle, girls appear to experience menarche earlier than did girls of 30 years ago (Lee et al., 2007). Although the school-age child experiences numerous physical changes before adolescence, changes in three physical areas are of particular interest: oral development, lymphoid tissue, and motor skills development.

Oral Development

Teeth enable a person to speak, chew, and smile. They also help give the face shape and form. The school-age child appears to be constantly losing or gaining a tooth.

Deciduous or baby teeth are usually lost in the same order in which they initially erupted. School-age children begin shedding their first teeth when they are around 6 to 7 years of age, and the process is complete with the loss of the second molars at 11 to 13 years of age. The first permanent teeth, the 6-year molars, erupt at 6 to 7 years of age and continue to erupt until the third molars (wisdom teeth) appear at about 17 to 22 years of age. **Website Resource 20B** shows deciduous teeth and the 32 adult teeth and their average time of appearance. The child between ages 6 and 13 loses and gains approximately four teeth per year. A 13-year-old child should have 28 teeth, having lost 20 deciduous teeth (Hockenberry & Wilson, 2007). When deciduous teeth come out, only the crown is lost; the root has been reabsorbed in the developing permanent tooth. As the child's mouth becomes filled with the larger, permanent teeth, the shape of the jaw and the facial appearance normally change. Girls tend to experience earlier permanent **tooth eruption** than do boys (American Dental Association, 2007).

Dental problems, primarily **dental caries** (cavities), periodontal disease, and **malocclusion**, are among the most common health problems in school-age children today (Fisher-Owens et al., 2007). In fact, it remains the most common chronic disease of children 5 to 17 years of age, 5 times more prevalent than asthma (Centers for Disease Control and Prevention [CDC], 2005). Present in up to 42% of children 6 to 17 years of age, caries occur more frequently in poor and ethnically diverse children and those who lack insurance or access to preventive dental care (Bethram-Aguilar et al., 2005). School dental programs are necessary to educate school-age children on proper care and maintenance of their teeth. School-based oral health education programs are in line with the *Healthy People 2010* and the 2020 initiatives and objectives for reducing dental caries among children (American Dental Association, 2005; USDHHS, 2000). At the midcourse review of progress towards the *Healthy People 2010* initiatives, small gains were made in the proportion of children receiving overall dental care and the application of dental sealants on their molar teeth (USDHHS, 2005b). In fact, community-based and school-based sealant programs have reduced new decay by up to 60% for 2 to 5 years after a single application in high-risk children (CDC, 2005).

The rapid change in the number and type of teeth and the uneven growth in the child's jaw may cause malocclusion, an unacceptable relationship of the teeth in one jaw to those in the other. Dentists evaluate children with overbites, gaps between teeth, and other alignment problems that may influence speech and eating (American Association of Orthodontics, 2006). Some children will grow out of these problems, but others may need **orthodontic care** and appliances (braces) to correct problems or improve their appearance. Peer reaction to braces is addressed as part of the teaching about body changes; this teaching may decrease problems with the child's self-concept or body image as a result of looking different. School dental programs include education about conscientious tooth care for the child who wears braces, because these frequently make brushing and flossing more difficult, especially for the school-age child who lacks manual dexterity (see **Website Resource 20C**).

Lymph Tissue

Lymph tissue grows rapidly throughout childhood, reaching maximum size before puberty, after which it begins to decrease in size, most likely due to sex hormones. The amount of lymphoid tissue of a child up to 10 years of age often exceeds that of an adult (McClain & Fletcher, 2007). This is most often reflected in the size of the tonsils. As a result what appears pathologically enlarged to a parent can be normal for the child's age. Additional lymphoid tissue during the school-age period generally helps this group to have a stronger immune response than do younger and older children. This is a result of the immune system being activated by environmental antigens and exposure to common organisms (McClain & Fletcher, 2007).

Motor Skills Development

Neurological, skeletal, and muscular changes combine to increase the child's overall motor abilities. With maturation of the nervous system by age 7 or 8 years, the brain's two hemispheres articulate to allow the child more control over and coordination with motor tasks (Hockenberry & Wilson, 2007).

The child grows taller because of lengthening of the long bones that continues into adolescence. **Ossification**, replacement of cartilage with bone, occurs throughout childhood but is not complete until adulthood (Rauch, 2007). Therefore special attention must be paid to well-fitting shoes, appropriately sized chairs and desks, and backpack loads to avoid strain on an evolving musculoskeletal system (Hockenberry & Wilson, 2007; Moore et al., 2007). Children at this age also need protective sports equipment and conditioning exercises before sports to prevent sports fractures (Spinks & McClure, 2007). However, the child builds new bony tissue during the entire period of childhood, which generally allows for rapid healing of fractures (Rauch, 2007). Overweight children typically have greater bone density as compared to their normal weight peers. Although they have greater bone density, this does not translate into reduced risk of fractures and joint pain. In fact, overweight children are more likely to suffer bone fractures, have joint pain, and more muscle pain than their normal weight counterparts (USDHHS, 2005a). The etiology of this finding is not clearly understood at this time.

Muscle mass also increases with muscle strength. During the school-age years, physically active boys are slightly stronger than girls, but this difference is not significant until adolescence (Faigenbaum, 2007). With these changes, the child has the potential to perform more complex fine motor and gross motor functions but must practice to perfect these skills (Kaufman & Schilling, 2007). Children willingly exercise their newfound skills and feel pride when others see their improved skill level when bike riding, tying shoes, and engaging in team sports.

GORDON'S FUNCTIONAL HEALTH PATTERNS

Health Perception–Health Management Pattern

The school-age child understands an abstract definition of health and sometimes the factors causing illness, but this understanding differs from that of an adult. Most school-age children perceive symptoms and show an ability to participate in health-promoting behaviors. Health-promoting behaviors taught at school and home must meet the school-age child's cognitive level (concrete operation) and moral level (external rules and forces) to be effective. Teaching strategies using cognitive, psychomotor, and affective senses can help children learn responsibility for their own health (Hagan et al., 2007). This knowledge provides an excellent foundation for health-promotion behaviors during the school years.

School-age children's understanding of illness is directly correlated with their cognitive development and follows a direct sequence of developmental stages. It is important for nurses to integrate the child's developmental views on illness as this has direct implications for plans related to health education (Koopman et al., 2004). When specifically asked about their ideas on causes of illness, school-age children usually state the germ theory, the punishment theory, or the external forces theory. Although many younger school-age children know that germs play a role in illness, they have limited understanding of how germs work (Siegal & Peterson, 2005). They may believe that a misdeed or misbehavior caused their illnesses.

Various cultural influences may also contribute to a child's understanding of illness. Hinduism ascribes to the theory of karma (law of cause and effect). Persons create their own destiny by thoughts, words, or deeds (University of Virginia Health System, 2006). Illness, accident, or injury result from the karma one creates and are often seen as a means of purification. Belief in the "evil eye," another cultural influence, occurs in many cultures and manifests itself in slightly different ways depending on where it arises. Most cultures believe that the victims are primarily babies or young children because they are so often praised and commented upon by strangers. The evil eye is thought to be based on jealousy and can have significant implications for the health of the victim (Stevens, 2005). This belief is strongest in Middle-Eastern countries, Asia, Latin America, and Europe. Attempts to ward off the curse have led to the use of a number of **talismans** within the various cultures. It is important to be aware of such cultural and developmental beliefs of the school-age child in defining strategies for teaching health promotion.

School-age children face challenges in meeting health-promotion goals as defined by *Healthy People 2010* (USDHHS, 2000). The *Healthy People 2010* and coming 2020 initiatives present selected objectives related to this age group (*Healthy People 2010* box). However, people in the school-age child's life can facilitate societal attainment

---

Healthy People 2010
Selected National Health-Promotion and Disease Prevention Objectives for School-Age Children

- Reduce proportion of children and adolescents who experience dental caries in their primary or permanent teeth to 42% for all children in 2010 (baseline is 52% of children ages 6 to 8 from 1988 to 1994).

Special Population Targets

Dental Caries Prevalence	1999 Baseline
Native American–Alaska Native	90%
Asian American–Pacific Islander*	90%
Black	50%
White	51%
Mexican American	68%

*1993 to 1994 baseline.

- Reduce untreated dental caries such that the proportion of children who have them (in permanent or primary teeth) is no more than 21% among all children ages 6 through 8 and no more than 15% among adolescents age 15 (baseline is 29% of children ages 6 to 8 from 1988 to 1994; 20% of adolescents age 15 from 1988 to 1994).

Special Population Targets

Untreated Dental Caries	1988 to 1994
Children ages 6 to 8 whose parents have less than a high school education	44%
Native American–Alaska Native (ages 6 to 8)	69%
Black (ages 6 to 8)	36%
Mexican American (ages 6 to 8)	43%

- Increase the proportion of children who have received protective sealants on surfaces of molar teeth to at least 50% (baseline is 23% of children age 8 and 15% of adolescents age 14 from 1988 to 1994).
- Reduce physician visits for otitis media among children and adolescents to 294 in 1000 visits (baseline is 344.7 in 1000 visits in 1997).
- Reduce the proportion of children and adolescents regularly exposed to tobacco smoke at home to 10% (baseline is 27% of children 6 years and younger in 1994).

Continued

Healthy People 2010

Selected National Health-Promotion and Disease Prevention Objectives for School-Age Children—cont'd

- Increase the proportion of people age 2 and older who consume less than 10% of their calories from saturated fat to 75% (baseline is 36% of all children from 1994 to 1996).

Special Population Targets

Saturated Fat Consumption	1994 to 1996
Hispanic-Latino	39%
Mexican American	37%
Black	31%
White	35%

- Reduce the number of asthma deaths among children ages 5 to 14 years to 1% (baseline is 3.3% in 1998) (rate per million).

Special Population Targets

Asthma	In 1998
Black	9.7
White	2.0

- Increase the proportion of the nation's public and private schools that require daily physical education for all middle and junior high students to 25% (baseline is 17% in 1994).

- Reduce the proportion of children and adolescents ages 6 to 11 years who are overweight or obese (defined as at or above gender-specific and age-specific 95th percentile) to 5% (baseline is 11% from 1988 to 1994).
- Decrease the incidence of maltreatment of children under age 18 to less than 11.1 per 1000 (baseline is 13.9 per 1000 in 1997).
- Increase the proportion of children and adolescents who view television 2 or fewer hours a day to 75% (baseline is 60% of children ages 8 to 16 years from 1988 to 1994).
- Increase the use of helmets by motorcyclists and passengers to at least 79% (baseline is 67% of motorcyclists and passengers in 1997).
- Reduce deaths caused by motor vehicle crashes to no more than 9.2 per 100,000 people (baseline is 15.6 per 100,000 people (age adjusted) to the year 2000 standard population).

Special Population Targets

Deaths from Motor Vehicle Crashes	1998
Children 14 years and younger	4.4

From U.S. Department of Health and Human Services. (2000). *Healthy people 2010*: Vols. 1 and 2 (Conference ed.). Washington, DC: U.S. Government Printing Office.

of these goals. Parents, caregivers, and teachers teach health-promotion concepts when they spend time monitoring and reinforcing preventive health practices, such as personal hygiene, dental care, and good nutrition. Role playing, reading an age-appropriate book, and modeling of health-promotion behaviors (e.g., washing hands) also may help children make the link between behavior and improved health. Unfortunately, by imitating some caregivers, children can become passive health care consumers, asking few questions, doing as they are told, and perpetuating poor choices. These responses may also be caused by children's developmental and cultural obligation to obey authority figures. Parents, caregivers, and teachers need to make commitments to demonstrate and teach healthy behaviors at home and in school; this helps children develop health values as part of their educational process toward reaching a healthy adulthood (Hagan et al., 2007; Lozano, 2004).

Counseling the child and family on a broad definition of health, one that includes personal and environmental health and safety, requires an awareness of the school-age child's normal perceptions of health (Seigal & Peterson, 2005). The nurse, in consultation with teachers, is in a prime position to use such information in order to present content in a manner beneficial to the school-age child's level of understanding. Topics may include some of the following content areas: cultural difference of causes and management of illnesses, causes of personal and environmental health

problems, and critical issues affecting the school-age child's general health (e.g., backpack safety) (Moore et al., 2007). All of these issues may be integrated into general academic studies to establish a foundation for teaching prevention as well as help the school-age child develop advocacy skills to become an assertive health care consumer.

Nutritional-Metabolic Pattern

School-age children, like all people, need a well-balanced diet. An average of 1200 to 1800 calories per day is recommended to meet growth requirements (based on sedentary behavior) (U.S. Department of Agriculture, 2005). Usually these calories are consumed in three daily meals and one or two snacks. School-age children often eat foods low in iron, calcium, and vitamin C, and foods that have a higher fat and sodium content than foods their parents ate when they were this age. There is a disjuncture between current dietary practices and recommended dietary intake of children. These behaviors place children at risk for poor nutritional habits, iron deficiency anemia, and chronic illnesses such as diabetes and hypertension (CDC, 2007a).

Factors Influencing Food Intake

Access to food, mass media, and contemporary busy lifestyles play a role in poor food choices. At the midcourse review of the *Healthy People 2010* initiatives, 89% of American households were food secure throughout the year, approaching initiative target rate of 94% (USDHHS, 2005c). Federal food assistance programs are in existence to assist in the achievement of these initiative targets.

A multitude of television and billboard messages pressure children to eat certain foods, many of which contain large amounts of salt, sugar, and calories. In 2004, 36.4% of nonprogram content time was for food-related advertisements (Powell et al., 2007). Frequent and lengthy watching of television has been linked to childhood obesity (Proctor et al., 2003). In 2005, American children watched an average of 3 hours, 19 minutes of television daily (Powell et al., 2007). Working parents spend 40% of their budget on dining outside the home, a behavior that contributes to more "fast food" consumption and food of poor nutritional quality (Gerberding, 2003). On a typical day, 30.3% of children consume fast food (Bowman et al., 2004). Healthy food costs more and may be less accessible than unhealthy food (Lee, 2006). Some cultures value food that has high salt and fat content.

Cultural factors as well as food access influence poor nutrition among the homeless and children in child care centers and contribute to the high level of obesity, especially among Hispanic, Black, and Native American children (Lee et al., 2007). These groups often lack access to safe and nutritious food. Thus, successful interventions for school-age overweight and nutrition must focus on economic, social, and cultural factors that influence access to and use of food.

Although some school-age children willingly try new foods, many continue to dislike vegetables, fruits, casseroles, spicy foods, and iron-rich foods and prefer a small range of foods. Some children may eat only raw vegetables and fruits and go through a phase of eating only one food at lunch, such as a peanut butter sandwich. These practices seldom hurt the child nutritionally (Haines, 2007). Unfortunately, at the midcourse review of the *Healthy People 2010,* initiatives with a focus on the reduction of dietary fat intake and the increased consumption of fruits and vegetables in children, no progress has been made in initiatives focused on reducing dietary fat intake and increasing consumption of fruits and vegetables in children (USDHHS, 2005c).

Children frequently make their own after-school snacks and need supervision regarding the content. Foods high in vitamins A and C, fruits, and vegetables should be encouraged daily. With parental, caregiver, or teacher help and positive reinforcement, school-age children can learn to calculate nutrition needs, plan family meals, and eat better for their overall health (Ball & Bindler, 2008). These activities also assist school-age children in developing wise decision-making practices, feelings of empowerment about health, and healthy food habits for the rest of their lives.

American families have such busy lives that they eat few meals together. A positive environment for nutrition and socialization during a shared meal time is important. Parents encourage positive food habits for each family member, and pressure to eat certain foods are avoided to prevent power struggles between parent or caregiver and child (Van Voorhees, 2006). A child's nutritional pattern usually reflects family patterns. For example, parents who skip breakfast tend to have trouble convincing their children to eat breakfast. Educating children as a group to eat healthy foods can be successful because of the powerful influence of a peer group (people of the same age, experience, and usually gender) (Stock et al., 2007). The child whose friend is eating a candy bar usually prefers the same rather than an apple for a snack.

Nutrition Education

Nutrition education incorporates into the general curriculum of school-age children throughout their education experience is important (Box 20-1). Despite evidence that the school can serve as an environment for nutritional health-promotion education, not all schools require nutrition education from kindergarten through 12th grade (Hockenberry & Wilson, 2007). School nurses and teachers, as part of core concepts usually taught in school, teach students about choices related to weight control and health and help them understand the role of media and culture in nutritional choices (School Nutrition Association, 2006). Teachers and school personnel also serve as role models for optimal eating and exercise habits for children in their charge. Lunch and breakfast programs exist in most schools and meet guidelines established by the U.S. Department of Agriculture [USDA] (2008). Many of these programs continue in after-school programs and during the summer when school is out of session to support needs for quality food intake in 30 million U.S. children (Martin & Oakley, 2008; USDA, 2007).

The American Academy of Pediatrics and the American Heart Association have established dietary guidelines for children and adolescents (Gidding et al., 2006). Daily nutritional needs of a child who is 9 to 13 years old include the following (Figure 20-1; U. S. Department of Agriculture, Center for Nutrition Policy and Promotion, 2005):

1. Milk group: 3 cups (24 oz total) of fat-free milk
2. Meat group: 5 oz of lean meat or beans; or equivalent combinations of these foods
3. Vegetable group: 2 to 2½ cups vegetables daily

Box 20-1   Child Nutrition and Activity Websites

Below is a list of child-focused websites promoting nutrition and increased activity behaviors.

- *www.kidshealth.org*
- *www.mypyramid.gov*
- *www.kidnetic.org*
- *www.Bam.gov/sub_physicalactivity/index.html*
- *www.smallstep.gov/kids/html/index.html*
- *www.nutritionExplorations.org*
- *www.healthfinder.gov/kids/*
- *www.LearnToBeHealthy.org*

From American Dental Association. *Smile Smarts! An Oral Health Curriculum for Preschool – Grade 8.* Chicago: American Dental Association, 2005.

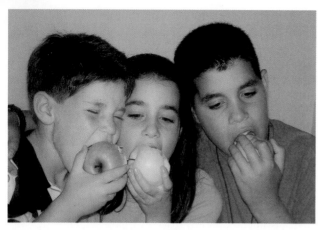

Figure 20-1 Children 9 to 13 years old should eat two or more portions of vegetables and fruit totaling 3 to 4 cups daily.

4. Fruit group: 1½ cups of fruit
5. Grains group: 5 to 6 oz daily. Half should be whole grain items (Gidding et al., 2006).

Overweight and Obesity

Overweight and **obesity** are major nutritional problems that have reached alarming proportions among adults and children in the United States. The Expert Committee on the Assessment, Prevention, and Treatment of Child & Adolescent Overweight and Obesity list the following definitions for use in children and adolescents (American Medical Association, 2007):

- Individuals 2 to18 years of age with BMI >95th percentile for age and gender or BMI exceeds 30 (whichever is smaller) should be considered obese.
- Individuals with a BMI >85th percentile, but <95th percentile, should be considered overweight.

The problem of overweight and obesity in children and adolescents has increased significantly over the last 40 years, with 17% of children ages 6 to 19 years estimated as obese (BMI above the 95th percentile for age and gender) (American Medical Association, 2007; Ogden et al., 2006). Unfortunately, this demonstrates movement away from the *Healthy People 2010* initiative target of 5% (USDHHS, 2005a). Of similar concern is the finding that as many as 36% of children 6 to 19 years of age are overweight (BMI between 85th and 95th percentile for age and gender) (American Medical Association, 2007; Ogden et al., 2006). Evidence suggests that adult obesity begins in infancy or childhood and results from both genetic and environmental factors. For example, a child whose overweight parents constantly use food as a reward faces a greater risk for obesity than does a child of thin parents who do not reward with food (Lumeng et al., 2007). Excessive food intake and lack of physical activity also leads to obesity, and once overweight these children tend to exercise even less. A recent study showed that in an ethnically diverse population, 22% of fourth graders in Texas were overweight (Hoelscher et al., 2004). Overweight occurs more in Black and Hispanic children than in Caucasian children (28.8%, 26.2%, and 15.7%, respectively) (Hoelscher et al., 2004). These higher overweight and obesity rates may reflect less physical activity of Black and Hispanic children due to living conditions and an inability to purchase higher-cost healthy food choices (USDHHS, 2000; Freedman et al., 2007).

Overweight increases the risk of hypertension, diabetes, sleep apnea, orthopedic problems, and heart disease. In fact, experts believe that overweight and sedentary behaviors are the primary risk factors for the development of insulin resistance, hyperlipidemia, hypertension, type 2 diabetes, and heart disease (Lau et al., 2007). There is also evidence that postprandial hyperinsulinemia may result in excessive weight gain (Slyper, 2004). Also, hormones released during the pubertal years make the situation worse in that these hormones make the body use insulin less effectively, leading to insulin resistance—thus increasing risk for the development of type 2 diabetes (Lau et al., 2007).

Current evidence suggests that overweight is associated with obstructive sleep apnea. Whether each disease state increases the expression of the other is unclear at this time (Redline et al., 2007). The potential association between short sleep duration and childhood overweight has been described in the literature (Research Highlights box). Longer sleep durations are associated with higher degrees of activity, which may assist with weight loss. Recent findings support the preventive approach of ensuring adequate sleep in the prevention of overweight in children (Lumeng et al., 2007).

The overweight and obese child faces ridicule by peers and discrimination later in life. These responses reinforce an already low self-esteem and poor body image and cause a cycle of personal isolation that influences a child's success, current and future (Hayden-Wade et al., 2005). Helping the overweight and obese child change lifestyle patterns requires intensive intervention, including support of parents (Stein et al., 2005). Even with such work, few overweight children achieve or maintain significant weight loss because of the complexity of factors (environmental, cultural, economic, and psychological) involved (Hockenberry & Wilson, 2007). In addition, there are reports that failure of maintained weight loss may be associated with impulsivity behaviors (Nederkoorn et al., 2007). Some success has been achieved by programs that include reasonable caloric restriction, eating a variety of low-fat and low-cholesterol foods, diet support groups, physical exercise, peer counseling groups, and habit changes (American Medical Association, 2007). However, intervention sometimes fails because some school-age children do not show concern about being overweight (Braet, 2006). Nursing suggestions for parents who are interested in preventing obesity in their school-age children appear in Box 20-2.

research highlights

Sleep Duration Relation to Overweight in Children

The purpose of this study was to better describe the association between short sleep duration or sleep problems with childhood overweight. Emerging research has introduced the association between sleep and regulation of many physiological functions including energy balance, appetite, and weight maintenance. The researchers sought to determine if the association of short sleep duration and overweight in children existed while controlling for measures such as quality of the home environment, parenting, and child behavior problems.

A longitudinal study of 785 children and their parents who were enrolled in the National Institute of Child Health and Human Development Study of Early Childcare and Youth Development was conducted. Data was collected on BMI, gender, socioeconomic status, and race in 3rd and 6th grades. Questionnaires regarding sleep and home environment were completed by the participant's mother at the same time intervals.

Findings reported an association between short sleep duration in the 6th grade and overweight in 6th grade. Shorter sleep duration in 3rd grade was independently associated with overweight in the 6th grade regardless of the child's weight in 3rd grade. For every additional hour of sleep received in the 6th grade, the child was 20% less likely to be overweight in 6th grade. For every additional hour of sleep in the 3rd grade, the child was 40% less likely to be overweight in the 6th grade. Interestingly, sleep problems were not associated with overweight in children.

Adequate sleep duration in childhood may offer a protective effect on weight maintenance and overweight risk in children. One preventive approach to overweight in children may simply be to ensure adequate sleep in childhood.

Lumeng, J., Somashekar, D., Appugliese, D., Kaciroti, N., Corwyn, R. and Bradley, R. (2007). Shorter sleep duration is associated with increased risk for being overweight at ages 9 to 12 years. *Pediatrics, 120,* 1020-1029.

Box 20-2 Nursing Interventions to Prevent Overweight/Obesity During the School-Age Years

- Incorporate discussion of healthy food intake and daily activity into daily school life.
- Encourage parents to be a role model for their child—be active, plan physically active family outings.
- Make activity FUN!
- Limit the amount of TV, videogames, time on computer/internet use.
- Discourage eating while watching TV.
- Encourage parent(s) to consider cultural influences on dietary intake. Evaluate snacking habits and food choices. Balance healthy foods with ethnic food choices.
- Encourage family to assess "fast food" consumption and explore/develop eating habits that support a healthier diet as defined by the food-guide pyramid.
- Encourage child to participate in food/meal selection and preparation.
- Support lunch choices that meet overall healthy nutrition intake.

Compiled from Hagan, J., Shaw, J., and Duncan, P. (2007). *Bright Futures Guidelines for health supervision of infants, children, and adolescents.* (3rd ed.) American Academy of Pediatrics; Bruss, M., Applegate, B., Quitugua, J., Placios, R., & Morris, J. (2007). Ethnicity and diet of children: Development of culturally sensitive measures. *Health Education Behavior, 34*(5):735-747.

Elimination Pattern

Most children have full bowel and bladder control by 5 years of age. Control involves the ability to undress and dress and to wipe, flush, and clean hands. The child's elimination patterns are similar to the adult's, with urination occurring 6 to 8 times a day and bowel movements averaging 1 or 2 times a day (Ball & Bindler, 2006; Hockenberry & Wilson, 2007). For some school-age children, however, elimination continues to be a problem.

Enuresis

Involuntary urination at an age when control should be present is called **enuresis** (Ball & Bindler, 2006). Children with primary enuresis have never achieved bladder control, and those with secondary enuresis have periods of dryness and recurrent enuresis. Involuntary nocturnal urination (bedwetting) that occurs at least once a month

is defined as nocturnal enuresis, and wetting during the day has been termed diurnal enuresis (Ball & Bindler, 2008). Enuresis should not be considered a disease but a variation of normal development. Enuresis affects 5-7 million U.S. children >6 years of age (Landgraf et al., 2004; Ball & Bindler, 2008).

Nocturnal enuresis causes disruption for both child and family. The child may frequently experience teasing from classmates and siblings. It can have profound effects on life socially, emotionally, and behaviorally (Landgraf et al., 2004). Although many forms of enuresis do not pose any significant health risk, there are social stressors. A night away from home appears impossible because of fear of wetting. Parents may be angry about the frequent bed changes and washes and may try punishments, thinking that the child should be able to control the problem. Parental stress places additional pressure on the child, who may already have low self-esteem and lack self-confidence due to perceived inability to control the problem (Hjalmas et al., 2004).

Often because they lack information, frustrated families seek help. Many therapies exist yet require a high degree of motivation from the child and parents. Their views must be taken into consideration when considering various treatment options (Landgraf et al., 2004). In addition to providing information, the nurse provides active support to facilitate coping. **Website Resource 20D** presents helpful information for parents about nocturnal enuresis. If a child does not have a urinary tract infection, various forms of management may be considered. These include wet alarm systems, bladder training and retention control, waking schedules, drug therapy, and hormone therapy. Each method has advantages, disadvantages, and cost considerations, but all require consistency and time from the child and parents, as well as positive reinforcement by the parents, to reach a successful outcome (Ball & Bindler, 2008).

Diurnal enuresis is often called daytime dribbling. This term describes a urinary pattern most often seen in school-age girls. These children demonstrate "holding on" behaviors, including not voiding first thing in the morning, voiding only 2 or 3 times a day, and voiding exceptionally quickly (Ball & Bindler, 2008). It is not clear why children delay urination or empty their bladders only partially, thus promoting overflow incontinence. Evaluation of these children begins with a urine culture to rule out urinary tract infection. If no infection exists or symptoms persist after treatment, then the intervention is focused on increasing fluid intake to prevent "holding" and establishing a voiding routine of every 2 hours, with a conscious effort to empty the bladder completely. The nurse can be instrumental in helping the child and parents understand the problem and its management.

Encopresis

Another elimination problem that may occur in children is **encopresis**, defined as the persistent voluntary or involuntary passing of stool into the child's underpants after age 4 (Hockenberry & Wilson, 2007). In most cases, the problem has no discernable physiological cause and is not related to laxative use. There may be a history of inconsistent toilet training or early life stress in affected children. Encopresis is a common complication of chronic constipation. In fact, over 80% of children with encopresis have a history of recent constipation and/or painful bowel movements (Borowitz, 2006). Once the child becomes constipated or has hard and painful stools; they begin to hold their bowel movements to prevent further pain. This creates a cycle that leads to fecal impaction and rectal distension. Stool then begins to leak around the impaction and leaks through the child's rectum; often times without the child's knowledge. In most cases, soiling occurs during the day when the child is awake and active. Soiling at night is uncommon (Borowitz, 2006).

Encopresis is often associated with complaints of recurrent abdominal pain and, for many, enuresis as well. Often these children have emotional difficulties that began before or resulted from encopresis. They experience poor peer relationships and self-esteem, perhaps due to their offensive odor. Awareness of this childhood problem is necessary to appropriately identify the affected child, refer the child for treatment, and support the child and family during a bowel management program and counseling.

Activity-Exercise Pattern

Physical activity in children is an important aspect of health and an integral component of health promotion. Childhood is considered to be a critical time in which

Growth and Development	Table 20-1	
Motor Development of the School-Age Child		
Age (Years)	**Gross Motor**	**Fine Motor**
5 years	Independent in dressing Runs well, jumps	Prints letters Ties shoes, buttons Draws triangle, square
6 to 8	Balances on one foot for 10 seconds Can perform tandem gait Pedals a bicycle Skilled physical activities, running, skipping	Spreads with knife Holds pencil with fingertip Draws a person with 3 to 6 parts Cuts and pastes Aligns letters horizontally Knows right from left
8 to 10	Has good body balance Enjoys vigorous activities Increased coordination	Spaces words and letters with writing Draws a diamond Has good eye-hand coordination Bathes self Sews and builds models
10 to 12	Balances on one foot for 15 seconds Catches a fly ball May experience clumsiness due to prepubertal growth spurt Possesses all basic motor skills similar to adult	Writes well Has skills similar to those of an adult

From Ball, J. & Bindler, R. (2006). Child health nursing: Partnering with children & families. Pearson-Upper Saddle River, New Jersey: Prentice Hall.

regular physical activity behaviors are acquired and fostered. Generally, the school-age child is naturally active, although Hispanic-American and Black children may be less active than Caucasian children (USDHHS, 2005c). Also, those who perceive their neighborhood as unsafe or do not have at least one parent who exercises are less likely to exercise themselves (Kellert, 2005). Physical activity and participation in sport activities tends to decrease with age; 78% of 10-11 year olds compared with 63% of 15-17 year olds. Boys are typically more active than girls; this is particularly so in the older child (USDHHS, 2005c).

As previously discussed, impressive changes in motor skills occur between the ages of 6 and 12 years, allowing the child to engage in many activities that develop strength, balance, and coordination (Table 20-1). Exercise typically occurs through group activities and organized sports such as Little League baseball and soccer, through individual activities such as gymnastics and ballet, and through unorganized play such as bike riding,

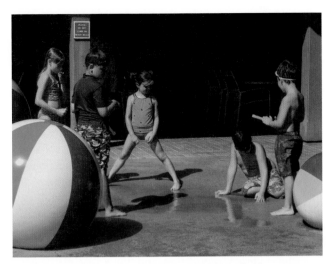

Figure 20-2   Peer play is important during the school-age years.

sledding, rollerblading, and imaginary play (Reid, 2003). Typically play provides important learning and health promotion and for this reason should be encouraged consistently during the school-age years. For many children, involvement in physical activities is fun and connects them to their peers, family members, and other important people in their lives (Allgier, 2007).

Play activities also promote social, personal, and cognitive development. School-age children frequently prefer interacting with peers rather than with family. This desire for peer interaction, usually with one of the same gender, extends beyond school and carries over to play and outside activities (Hockenberry & Wilson, 2007). A child's skill in motor tasks wins the respect of other children and provides a feeling of self-accomplishment (Allgier, 2007). Organized sports such as baseball teach team cooperation, competition, and other social skills. Concerns exist that young children have experienced too much physical and psychological pressure to perform in sports. This has generated a renewed commitment by many parents to focus more on the fun of sports than on the winning of games (Robinson, 2006). In addition, organized activities such as Scouts and 4-H clubs teach children about group functioning, processes involved in carrying out a task, and the power of social relationships to create change. These lessons can prepare them for discipline needed for a job later in life (McKinney et al., 2005). Overall, children who perform well in these activities, evidenced by prizes or trophies, feel good about themselves, their competence, and their sense of industry (Hockenberry & Wilson, 2007). Parents and teachers who compliment children when they perform well enhance self-esteem, as well.

As part of play, school-age children incorporate new cognitive skills, including the ability to count and sort objects. Children of this age express pleasure in their collections of stamps, rocks, or other objects. Understanding the concepts

of fair and consistent rules found in games requires cognitive skills of memory, logical reasoning, and the desire to work with others (Hockenberry & Wilson, 2007). Many children like to read, which provides ideas about life and cultures that differ from their own, thereby enhancing their acceptance of human diversity. The nurse helps parents promote healthy play activities for children by encouraging the following (Fackler, 2005):

- Family activities that focus on physical activity and togetherness between parents or caregivers and children, such as daily reading (out loud or silently)
- Use of a library card to encourage reading on a variety of topics and to teach responsibilities involved with borrowing
- Purchase of personal magazines for children's learning and ownership
- Monitoring of daily television and computer use that detract from physical activity and more active mental activities
- Encouragement of both group and solitary activities to support the child's overall development

Sleep-Rest Pattern
Sleep Patterns

Most school-age children have no difficulties with sleep. Generally their sleep requirements and patterns are more similar to those of an adult than those of a younger child. Individual needs vary based on activity, age, and state of health, but most school-age children sleep between 8 and 12 hours a night without naps during the day (Homeier, 2004). Unlike younger children, school-age children experience few difficulties with going to bed. Most children and parents can agree on a bedtime with some flexibility on non-school nights and adhere to that agreement. When problems arise regarding bedtime, children may be testing parents who have not been clear and firm about their expectations for going to bed or have not been willing to discuss the arrangement with their children (American Academy of Sleep Medicine, 2006). Although most Americans accept the idea that school-age children should sleep in their own beds, some Black, Hispanic, or Japanese families may encourage the family or siblings to sleep together (Owens, 2004). Studies have shown that in the school-age child, bed-sharing does not have any impact on sleep patterns, nor does it show any long term effects towards health, positive or negative (Jenni et al., 2005).

Sleep Disturbances

The most common sleep problems that occur during the preschool and school-age years are night terrors (see Chapter 19), **sleepwalking**, **sleep talking**, and enuresis. As a group, these disturbances have been called **disorders of arousal** (Harvard Health Publications, 2007) and share the following characteristics:

- They occur immediately before a REM, or rapid eye movement, state of sleep.

- Most occur 1 to 2 hours after going to sleep.
- There is a family history of sleep problems, and more boys experience sleep problems than girls.
- Problems reflect normal central nervous system (CNS) immaturity of the child.
- Problems may be influenced by fatigue and stress within the child.
- Problems do not involve the respiratory system (Moore et al., 2006).

Approximately one out of six children (15%) between ages 5 and 12 has sleepwalked at least once, but far fewer children walk in their sleep persistently. Sleepwalking is most likely due to the brain's inability to regulate sleep/wake cycles due to immaturity of the nervous system. It occurs more often in boys and often occurs with enuresis (Harvard Health Publications, 2007). Shortly after going to sleep, the child may suddenly sit up in bed, make repetitive finger and hand movements, or walk, usually for a short time. In most cases, however, the child stays in bed. The child may mumble when talking to a parent or other person (sleep talking). The words tend to be simple but unclear to the listener. Often the child falls back to sleep quickly after talking or walking (Hockenberry & Wilson, 2007).

Parents who are concerned about sleepwalking or sleep talking need to know that most children outgrow these episodes with CNS maturation. However, parents protect their child from injury by placing gates at the top of stairs and removing sharp objects from the child's path. Most parents find that the easiest solution is to direct the sleepwalker back to bed, where the child returns to a normal sleep (Hockenberry & Wilson, 2007). Occasionally parents can intervene effectively by implementing relaxation techniques for their child before bedtime, avoiding stressful and fatiguing situations, and providing consistency with sleep preparation patterns (American Academy of Sleep Medicine, 2006). If a child has many episodes of sleepwalking or sleep talking or if parents express particular concern, he or she may need further evaluation and treatment by health care professionals (Gaylor et al., 2005; Guilleminault et al., 2003; Harvard Health Publications, 2007).

Cognitive-Perceptual Pattern

The school-age child spends extensive time in settings that require mastery of new ideas and concepts. The child's basic intelligence, heredity, and environment encourage or discourage learning. Mastery of ideas and learning requires intact senses, such as vision, hearing, language, and memory capabilities that allow for cognitive development and acquisition of skills needed for later life success (Better Brains for Babies, 2007). Unfortunately, many children in society lack these capabilities and will have learning problems if not identified early through parental awareness, school observations, or routine health care

assessments. For further information about school-age tests or procedural preparations, see *www.nlm.nih.gov/medlineplus/ency/article/002058.htm.*

Piaget's Theory

Piaget (2001) refers to the age span of 7 to 11 years as the period of **concrete operation**, a stage when children learn by manipulating concrete objects and lack the ability to perform thinking operations that require abstraction. During this time, the child moves from egocentric interactions to more cooperative interactions and increased understanding of many concepts gained through environmental connections (Harkreader et al., 2007). Children increasingly change their reasoning from intuitive to logical or rational operations (rule-governed actions) and engage in serial ordering, addition, subtraction, and other basic mathematical skills. The operations of this period are termed concrete because the child's mental operations or actions still depend on the ability to perceive specific examples of what has happened. Older school-age children use both concrete and recently acquired abstract operations, which add flexibility and control to their thinking and meet developmental needs of adolescence. Unlike the egocentric preschooler, a school-age child begins to take the other person's point of view into account. This trait does not emerge suddenly and completely (Hockenberry & Wilson, 2007). The new skill appears occasionally and then more frequently as the child's mental capacity and experience grow (Piaget, 2001).

During the school-age period, the child understands a number of expanding concepts regarding objects, including the concept of **conservation** of substance (Harkreader et al., 2007). When asked if a difference exists in the amount of liquid poured into two glasses of different shapes, the preschool, preoperational child focuses on the different shapes and says "yes." The concrete operational school-age child realizes that no change has occurred in the substance despite the change in shape (Hockenberry & Wilson, 2007). Conservation of numbers, weight, volume, and quantity, required to understand basic mathematics, sequentially develops as the school-age child gains chronological age and experience (Ball & Bindler, 2008; Hockenberry & Wilson, 2007).

The concept of time also develops during this period. Children begin to learn to tell time and understand the passage of time (Lucile Packard's Children's Hospital, 2007). By age 8, most children understand the difference between past and present, and history becomes meaningful (Hockenberry & Wilson, 2007). The concept of human aging becomes increasingly understandable, and the child can comprehend the difference between an 18-year-old and an 80-year-old person.

Two major operations of the school-age period are **classifying and ordering**. The child classifies or groups objects by their common elements and understands the relationship between groups or classes (Hockenberry & Wilson, 2007). For example, when given 12 wooden beads, some brown and some white, the child understands that the beads may be grouped by their color and by their material. Conversely, the preschool child focuses only on one property of the beads, such as color. The newfound ability to classify shows in the school-age child's interest in collections, such as stamps or coins (McKinney et al., 2005). Children in school frequently "order" their world; they line up in school according to height, they repeat numbers and letters in their classic order, and they receive numbers in school to reflect an alphabetized surname. These two operations (classifying and ordering) must exist to learn to read, understand the concepts of numbers, and learn subjects based on relations, such as history (the relation of events in time) and geography (the relation of places in space) (Hockenberry & Wilson, 2007).

Vision

The child's sensory abilities continue to develop during the school-age years. Visual capacity should reach optimal function by the sixth or seventh year (Ball & Bindler, 2006). Peripheral vision and the ability to discriminate fine color distinctions should be fully developed as well. Although many 4 year olds have 20/20 vision, a school-age child should have a **visual acuity** of at least 20/30 in each eye, as measured by the **Snellen 'E' Chart**, an assessment tool for children who can read some letters (Ball & Bindler, 2006).

Physiological changes occur in the eye during the school-age years. Eyes in the preschool years are normally **hyperopic (farsighted)**, a condition in which the visual image of an object falls behind the retina (Hockenberry & Wilson, 2007). However, unlike older individuals, preschool children do not need glasses because their eyes normally accommodate by adjusting their lenses. For most children, vision becomes normal as the shape of the eye changes and lengthens with maturation. However, many school-age children need visual correction to prevent academic difficulties and headaches and dizziness when reading or doing close work.

Only about one third of all children have had an eye examination or vision screening prior to entering school (American Optometric Association, 2007). **Vision screening programs** for school children are intended to help identify those children who have or may potentially have a vision problem that may affect physiological or perceptual processes of vision or that could interfere with school performance. At the midcourse review of the *Healthy People 2010* initiatives there was sufficient evidence to assess progress towards objective targets related to vision screening in school-age children (USDHHS, 2005d). Vision screenings are not diagnostic nor do they lead to treatment, but rather only indicate a potential need for further care. The school nurse is in an optimal position to ensure eye screenings are performed and the nurse encourages parents of children with deficits to seek further optometric care to correct these defects so that these children can learn more effectively.

It is estimated that nearly 25% of school-age children have vision problems (American Optometric Association, 2007). Two other visual problems are common in the school-age child group. Many school-age children inherit **myopia (nearsightedness)**, a condition in which the visual image of an object falls in front of the retina, causing the child to have difficulty seeing distant objects (Hockenberry & Wilson, 2007). The other condition, **astigmatism**, causes blurred vision because the image is focused poorly on the retina due to changes in the surface of the cornea or lens (Hockenberry, 2005). Eyeglasses correct the defects, but the problem must be identified before it can be solved (American Optometric Association, 2007). For example, a child with myopia may not realize that his visual images are impaired. Children with corrective lenses often express delight and surprise when they first see the fully focused and rich detail of the world after experiencing less refined visual acuity for some time.

Hearing

The child's hearing ability (**auditory acuity**) is nearly complete by 7 years of age, although some maturation continues into adolescence. Hearing deficits occur less frequently than visual deficits, but hearing loss affects more than 1 million children from birth to age 21 years in the United States. This deficit compromises learning in school and important socialization with peers. **Chronic serous otitis media**, or long-term fluid in the middle ear, remains a common cause of hearing deficit in both the preschool and the early school-age years (Hockenberry, 2005). Fortunately, reduction in rates of otitis media in children has met the *Healthy People 2010* initiative targets. The success of meeting this initiative has been attributed to the introduction of heptavalent pneumococcal conjugate vaccine in 2000 (USDHHS, 2005d). Additionally, concerns about the potential for long-term hearing loss in children who listen to loud music have been raised (Hockenberry & Wilson, 2007).

All school-age children, especially those with a history of recurrent ear infections or fluid behind the eardrum, should have periodic hearing evaluations performed as part of a health-promotion program in school and as required by many states (Allen et al., 2004). Various treatments exist for acute otitis media, including antibiotics and the recent discovery that Xylitol gum may be of some preventive benefit (Fuller, 2007). Additionally, work continues on a vaccination for otitis media. **Tympanograms**, used to measure the sensitivity of the tympanic membrane to vibrations induced by pressure and sound waves, help detect and monitor this problem as part of well-child and ill-child care (Ball & Bindler, 2008). The nurse considers education on hearing protection for school-age children in order to maintain this important sense for the future.

Sensory Perception

Children learn simultaneously through many senses, and most teaching approaches incorporate this concept. For example, young school-age children see a letter, hear its sound, and feel its shape. With this approach, children learn in a number of ways to interpret an event. For example, some children learn best by listening (**auditory learners**), others by doing (**kinesthetic learners**), and others by engaging all sensory modalities (auditory, kinesthetic, and **visual learners**). Because no two children have exactly the same sensory acuity, sensitivity, or discrimination, all children build slightly different perceptions and conceptions of the world around them and do not follow the same timetable to grasp concepts (Kramer, 2007). Therefore, teaching approaches must be individualized to meet the learning needs of most children.

Of all the senses, visual perception has been studied the most, primarily because of its role in helping children learn to read. Studies have examined children's abilities to discriminate parts of a picture (to see a figure within a picture). Children usually progress from the preschool stage, during which they perceive visual stimuli more as a whole, to the school-age stage, during which they perceive more details, and finally to the point at which they perceive and integrate both. This process helps children recognize letters, the first step needed for reading. Children may first be able to differentiate between obviously different letters, such as "h" and "o," but may have difficulty with letters similar in appearance, such as "b" and "d," until they can distinguish details more effectively (Hockenberry & Wilson, 2007).

Language

Language develops rapidly during the school years. Most school-age children enter this period with an ability to understand and speak a language, but with only a basic knowledge of reading and writing. By the end of the school-age period, most children have acquired at least a functional ability in both areas. Language development mandates that a child have visual perception for reading, auditory acuity and perception for understanding spoken language, and fine motor skills for both articulation and handwriting.

The full capacity to imitate sounds develops during the childhood years. Between 6 and 7 years of age, the child shows the ability to produce proper articulation for most vowel and consonant sounds. However, some have difficulty expressing sounds for "s," "l," "z," "sh," "ch," and "r" (Hockenberry & Wilson, 2007). By 7 years of age the child should be able to articulate all sounds for speaking and by age 12 years has a vocabulary of around 4000 words. Understanding of the syntax (grammar) and semantics (meaning) of language continues to develop. The child uses more complex sentences and understands multiple meanings for the same word and metaphors (Golanka, 2005). The child should be able to recognize and correct spelling and grammatical errors by 8 or 9 years of age. The capacity to learn foreign languages is at an optimal level at this stage

and provides rationale for foreign language instruction during the school-age years. Foreign language instruction also provides children with information about other cultures and an opportunity to understand people who are different from themselves.

Much of the child's time in school focuses on learning to read and write. Learning to read is a complex process, beginning with letter and sound recognition (Needlman, 2004). Letters combine to form words that the child must learn to decode. Words combine to form sentences, and so on. Most children need help from teachers, peers, parents, or older children to learn to read effectively (National Institute for Family Literacy, 2006). Some researchers believe that children learn best by sounding out the individual letters of a word (**phonics**), whereas others think that learning the word as a whole unit is better. Both processes have value, and likely a combination of both is most effective (National Institute of Family Literacy 2006). Considering the wide range of processes that support development of reading skills (conceptual, perceptual, verbal, and motor), it's not surprising that most children experience some difficulty in learning to read (National Institute for Family Literacy, 2006).

Handwriting requires eye-hand coordination, motor control, and perceptual abilities (American Occupational Therapy Association, 2007). Primarily a motor skill, handwriting does not reflect mental capacity. Many bright children and adults have poor handwriting, and vice versa. Boys tend to have more problems with legible handwriting than do girls. Writing style does not approach adult-level maturity until the end of late childhood, but the handwriting should reflect the child's handedness. No reversal of letter outlines should occur by age 7 or 8, and the relative size of letters should be uniform. By age 8 or 9, letter strokes should be firm, even, and flow with ease (Hockenberry, 2005). The individual who has difficulty with handwriting may use a typewriter, computer, or graphics to produce a satisfactory written product. Tutoring by a handwriting specialist can help children with **dyslexia**, a term defining the tendency to reverse the normal appearance of letters and numbers in writing.

Memory

Memory abilities, both short term and long term, improve for school-age children. Strategies such as organizing, classifying, and labeling information help them retain information. Rehearsal, repeating an item to be learned, is also a helpful memorization strategy (Ball & Bindler, 2008). At age 5 children use rehearsal when someone suggests or models it; at age 10 they rehearse spontaneously. Memory abilities improve with practice and through various strategies, such as placing the words that need to be remembered in a song or by rhyming words (Kramer, 2007).

Intelligence

Intelligence tests assess a person's mental abilities and compare them with the abilities of other people through the use of numerical scores. Although the term **intelligence** is used as if there is agreement on what it means, in reality there is much debate as to how this term should be and has been defined. For example, debate has surrounded whether intelligence should be considered an inherent cognitive capacity, an achieved level of performance, or a qualitative construct that cannot be measured. Psychologists have debated whether intelligence is learned or inherited, culturally specific or universal, one ability or several abilities (Warwick, 2001). While these debates are ongoing, evidence is increasing that traditional intelligence tests measure specific forms of cognitive ability that are predictive of school functioning, but do not measure the many forms of intelligence that are beyond these more specific skills, such as music, art, and interpersonal and intrapersonal abilities. **Website Resource 20E** contains a list of common developmental and cognitive tests.

The concept of intelligence usually conveys an ability to think and process information learned earlier in life. Scores on an intelligence test should measure the child's basic abilities as compared with others of the same age and experience level and, ideally, should predict performance in school or society. However, this is not always the case. Intelligence test scores tend to differ because each test, or each form of the same test, measures slightly different samples of abilities and reflects the test author's philosophy on intelligence. It is important to note that some intelligence tests may be culturally insensitive (Benson, 2003). For example, the protectionism of the Asian culture may cause lower test scores on self-help skills and socialization among Asian children who demonstrate in other ways that they are good students. Furthermore, words on the test may not be part of an ethnic group's usual vocabulary, causing children to miss these items on an intelligence test.

Children also take achievement tests that measure the amount of information learned in a specific area and offer insight into a child's overall intelligence. Although intelligence and achievement tests should measure different issues (basic ability versus learned achievement), their results correlate well. Some researchers believe this correlation exists because both tests actually measure the same thing (achievement, not ability).

Reports from intelligence and achievement testing differ. Intelligence tests usually provide a number that represents **intelligence quotient (IQ)**. An IQ of 90 to 110 is considered average (Logsdon, 2009). Achievement tests compare the child's performance with that of other children and report scores as percentiles. For example, a score in the 20th percentile of a test means the child scored better than only 20% of other children of the same age in that skill. Current beliefs accept that people inherit some of their intelligence but that environmental factors also influence opportunities for learning and overall intelligence. Most likely the greatest environmental influence is socioeconomic, reflected in the correlation in scores: children from low-income families tend to score lower on intelligence tests than do children from middle-income or high-income families. The reason

for this probably relates to many subfactors, such as nutrition, language, parental reinforcement and encouragement, and sociocultural environmental stimuli. Social programs such as the federal nutrition program for women, infants, and children (WIC) and preschool stimulation programs such as Head Start have attempted to address these subfactors to improve the potential of young children from diverse populations. Many people have suggested less focus on IQ tests, primarily because they label children early in life and influence, often negatively, their self-perception and their performance.

Learning Disabilities

Educators estimate that 5% to 10% of children 6 to 17 years of age have a **learning disability** (Boyse, 2008). Many terms and definitions have been used to describe the impairments of children who have normal or above-normal intelligence and usually do not have visual, hearing, or motor handicaps or emotional problems yet have difficulties in school learning. Some children have minor, almost unnoticeable difficulties, whereas other children are so impaired that they appear to be mentally retarded until diagnosed and helped. An individual child may have more than one developmental disorder. Some children will develop behavior and self-esteem problems as a response to their inability to function satisfactorily (Boyse, 2007).

One well-known condition that causes difficulty in the child's adjustment to the school setting is **attention-deficit/hyperactivity disorder (ADHD)**, a behavior that reflects developmentally inappropriate degrees of inattention, impulsiveness, and hyperactivity (National Institute of Mental Health, 2007). ADHD is the most common neurobehavioral disorder of childhood and among the most prevalent chronic health conditions affecting school-age children. Frequently these children have high energy, intuitiveness, and creativity, personal characteristics that help them succeed in some facets of their lives. Despite diagnostic criteria for ADHD developed by the American Psychiatric Association (2000), the problem has been difficult to assess, primarily because the child manifests symptoms in varying degrees in different settings and with different people (Box 20-3). Treatment of children with ADHD has been controversial but includes behavior management, family counseling, classroom management, nutrition therapy, and medication (National Institute of Mental Health, 2007). These interventions may also be successful in management for ADHD-affected adults.

The nurse's role with the child who has a learning disability varies. The nurse may participate in detection of the problem, consultation during evaluations, collaboration with school administration on implementation of a treatment plan, referral to resources, serving as a liaison between school and home environments, and counseling the child and family to improve overall development and the family's adaptation to meet the needs of this unique child (National Institute of Mental Health, 2007).

Box **20-3** Diagnostic Criteria for Attention-Deficit/
Hyperactivity Disorder

Note: Consider a criterion met only if the behavior occurs
more frequently than that noted in most people of the same
mental age as the child.
1. A disturbance of at least 6 months exists during which
   at least six of the criteria for either inattentive behavior
   or hyperactivity-impulsivity behavior are met.*
2. Some inattentive or hyperactive-impulsive symptoms
   that caused impairment existed before age 7 years.
3. Some impairment for the symptoms exists in two or
   more settings (at school or at home).
4. Clear evidence of clinically significant impairment
   exists in social or academic functioning.
5. The symptoms do not occur only with a pervasive
   developmental disorder, schizophrenia, or other
   psychotic disorder and do not support another mental
   disorder (mood disorder, anxiety disorder, dissociative
   disorder, and personality disorder).

*For specific criteria, refer to American Psychiatric Association. (1994).
Diagnostic and statistical manual of mental disorders. DSM-IV (4th ed.).
Washington D.C.: Author.
From American Academy of Pediatrics, Committee on Quality
Improvement, Subcommittee on Attention-Deficit/Hyperactivity
Disorder. (2000). Clinical practice guideline: Diagnosis and evaluation of
the child with attention-deficit/hyperactivity disorders. *Pediatrics, 105,*
1158-1170.; Leslie, L., Weckerley, J., Plemmons, D., Landsverk, T, and
Eastmen, S. (2004). Implementing the American academy of pediatrics
attention deficit/hyperactivity disorder guidelines in the primary care
setting. *Pediatrics, 114,* 129-140. National Institute of Mental Health
(2007). ADHD. [on-line] Retrieved from *www.nimh.nih.gov/health/
publications/adhd/complete-publication.shtml*

There are two laws protecting children with disabilities, including those with ADHD: (1) the **Individuals with Disabilities Education Act (IDEA)** of 1997 and (2) **Section 504 of the Rehabilitation Act of 1973** (U.S. Department of Justice, 2005). The IDEA is a special education law, whereas Section 504 is a civil rights statute. Both guarantee qualified students a free and appropriate public education and instruction in the least restrictive environment. This means that students are to be instructed among those who are not disabled and to the maximum extent appropriate for the student's needs (American Academy of Pediatrics, 2002).

The nurse plays a vital role in promoting the school-age child's overall cognitive and perceptual health, helping to prevent problems in these areas. The nurse must talk to parents and school administration personnel about any child who has language articulation problems beyond 6 or 7 years, because this child should be evaluated by a professional. The nurse helps parents understand their child's level of cognitive and sensory abilities so that learning expectations are realistic. Through educational materials sent home or provided during school meetings, the nurse may address the **socialization** needs and development of school-age children. The nurse also needs to help parents understand common tests used for child intelligence and achievement screening (National Institute of Mental Health, 2009). In addition, the nurse helps evaluate a child believed to have a learning

disability when the child may actually suffer from a health problem, general immaturity, or an environmental deficit (poverty or divorce).

Self-Perception–Self-Concept Pattern

Through each of the developmental processes of physiological growth, cognitive development, and social development, children progressively engage in an important process of **self-discovery**. Through these processes, children actively build and create their own personalities, develop relationships with others, and expose themselves to a wide range of experiences that influence their behavior, attitudes, and values.

Erikson's Theory

The stage of personality development described by Erikson for the school-age child is **industry versus inferiority** (Ball & Bindler, 2008). The major task to be accomplished is full mastery of whatever the child is doing (sense of industry). The child focuses on success in personal and social tasks and avoidance of a sense of inferiority. Inferiority occurs with repeated failures at attempted tasks and with little encouragement or trust from people important to the child (Hockenberry & Wilson, 2007). With mastery of the tools of the culture in relation to those of the peer group, a sense of worth and understanding of the self develops (Erikson, 1993, 1994).

Self-Concept

Self-concept develops over time and through a variety of experiences and relationships. For example, by being responsible for a pet's care and by showing love to this animal, the older school-age child nurtures a positive self-concept. The way in which others, especially peers, view the child influences the sense of self (Hockenberry, 2005). Increasing cognitive abilities facilitate better understanding of the identifying factors of others (race, ethnicity, disability, or gender) and how those others compare with the child. Self-concept includes self-esteem, sense of control, body concept, and gender role.

Self-Esteem **Self-esteem** has been defined as the extent to which an individual believes oneself to be capable, significant, successful, and worthy (Sheslow, 2008). The younger school-age child has a limited self-concept, but one that develops with successful completion of the tasks of this period (Erikson's sense of industry). Although engaged in more activities outside of the home, the child still depends on family, as defined by one's culture, to develop high self-esteem. In school, teachers or group leaders frequently reward those who have succeeded in a task with badges, stars, or privileges (tangible objects that validate success).

The peer group's influence on the school-age child's self-esteem is unquestionable. Acceptance by a peer group contributes to feelings of self-worth and sense of belonging to a desired group. Competition or collaboration with peers in school, clubs, and activities also influences feelings of adequacy and feelings of success (Harkreader et al., 2007). In one study, Black children ages 9 to 14 years voiced higher self-esteem than did Asian, Hispanic, or White children because they believed they could make others laugh and others wanted to be like them (Jordan et al., 2003). Parents must be encouraged to expose their school-age children to interesting activities of their choice, involving peers, to nurture their self-esteem and sense of uniqueness.

Concern has been voiced about school-age girls suffering a decline in self-esteem that affects their school achievements. Some research indicates that boys receive more praise in school than do girls, that girls receive criticism on the content of their work but that boys receive more criticism on the appearance of their work (Myers, 2009). Girls experience greater competition now than in earlier times, and they face pressures about personal appearance, particularly if they are White (Jordan et al., 2003). Various authors report that girls need strong adults to support their ways of thinking and behaving in a world often built on "male values". Girls tend to have high self-esteem if they perceive parental harmony that supports perceptions of balance within themselves and promotes their emotional health (Myers, 2009).

In encouraging development of self-esteem in all school-age children, the nurse remembers that a child needs to experience success with tasks, and completely structured activities may not provide this opportunity for some children. A child who succeeds in some things and receives acceptance by peers gains a sense of competence and worth, is self-confident, and has high self-esteem, which are important qualities for life survival.

Sense of Control As the school-age child matures and makes choices, a sense of control develops about the self and the environment. Children with an internal locus of control believe they are responsible for their behavior and accomplishments and tend to have higher levels of achievement than do children who believe in an external locus of control. The latter think that fewer reasons exist for them to try hard at a task, because others or fate determines life results. Hispanic and Black cultures may more often support an external locus of control based on a strong belief that God determines one's outcome (Tynan, 2008). Older children and girls tend to have a more internalized locus of control than do younger children and boys.

Body Concept The school-age child's concept of the body and its functioning also changes from the preschool period and adds to overall self-concept. By ages 8 to 11, children know that parts of the body constitute a related whole (Hockenberry, 2005). The 11-year-old child can name twice the number and functions of internal body structures that a 6-year-old child can and frequently understands the functions of the cardiovascular, musculoskeletal, and nervous systems. For example, the 7-year-old child knows that the heart is important and that it beats, whereas the 13-year-old child knows that the heart pumps blood. Changes or differences in the body may frighten the school-age child

until one understands normal developmental processes such as losing deciduous teeth. Physical differences, such as freckles, can provoke ridicule and isolation. Children in this age group frequently feel threatened by others with deformities (Hockenberry & Wilson, 2007). Children with chronic illness worry that their peer relationships will be negatively influenced if others know about their illness. Children who learn about body differences, meeting people with chronic health problems, as well as through reading and discussion of anxiety about differences, increase their knowledge about the body and ways to maintain health. They also gain an understanding of the value of each person, despite their differences (Ball & Bindler, 2006). Ways in which the nurse can help children develop positive self-concepts are listed in Box 20-2.

Roles-Relationships Pattern

The family environment provides a sense of security that allows the school-age child to cope with uncertainties in the external environment (Hockenberry, 2005). Although many live in single, divorced, mixed-race, or same-gender parenting households, the family structure generally encourages a child's cognitive growth through exposure to a variety of experiences that bolster the desire to achieve and develop positive self-esteem.

Parents, caregivers, and children interact in a variety of ways to show love and companionship for each other. Caregivers, such as grandparents or extended family members, protect the dependent child and teach the learning child. The caregiver-child relationship is not equal, primarily because caregivers and parents serve as authority figures that establish the rules needed for the functioning of the family and safe growth of the child. During the school-age years, the child's increasing maturity, independence, and responsibility begin to reduce the amount of parental authority and structure needed. In one study, Black parents set higher standards for child independence than did parents of other diverse populations (Jordan et al., 2003). With increasing independence, the child prioritizes school and peer group relationships to develop socialization skills and understand group social mores (Elliot, 2007). These connections will help prepare the child for future heterosexual relationships.

School-age children also begin to broaden their interests outside the home, often encouraged by parents (Ball & Bindler, 2006). Unfortunately, some older ones may become involved in gangs, behavior that causes much stress for both children and their parents. The child's changing world frequently alters family schedules and patterns, supporting studies that have found that parents express the least amount of parental satisfaction when their oldest one is between the ages of 6 and 13. The relationships between siblings vary, depending on birth order, culture, gender, and age differences and perceived power of siblings (Hockenberry & Wilson, 2007). Siblings interact with one another in a number of roles, such as playmates, teacher-learner, protector-dependent, and adversaries, based on feelings of jealousy and rivalry that often occur in families. School-age children cope with these feelings better than do preschool children because they have outlets outside the family, including school and friends. Parents can minimize conflicts by recognizing each child's needs and level of maturity and by providing guidance and support.

As children mature, they take on more responsibilities within the family and the community. School-age children learn responsibility for allowance, household chores, self-care, and pets and acquire a sense of empowerment as an integral part of the family (Hockenberry & Wilson, 2007). This is the period during which families often give allowances or children earn money through chores or small jobs, such as paper routes. The amount of an allowance may relate to cultural values. In one study Asian children earned higher allowances than did other children from diverse population groups for completing fewer chores and for meeting higher standards of academic performance (Jordan et al., 2003). School-age children learn valuable life lessons by earning and spending their allowances.

Children learn socially accepted behaviors when their parents engage in **limit setting** (defining expected behavior and consequences when limits are not honored). Some cultures enforce consequences when a child engages in behavior that does not foster the good of the community, a strong cultural value (Maiter, 2004). Violent behavior must be discouraged, and nonviolent methods to reach resolutions for personal problems should be encouraged. Parents who express their feelings, explain why things happen, and listen to their children while setting limits encourage the development of self-control and positive self-esteem. Some families with school-age children find it helpful to have periodic family meetings during which everyone discusses family issues, rules, and responsibilities. Behavior contracts between parent and child provide direction and may also encourage improved behavior by delineating favorable consequences when the terms of the contract are followed.

Children frequently model their behavior after that of people they love or admire (parents, friends, and other adults). Positive reinforcement (rewards for good behavior) is an effective form of limit setting, i.e., **discipline**, used often by upper class parents. **Punishment**, a negative reinforcement as reflected in shaming a child in front of his community or family (seen with some Asian cultures [Hockenberry, 2005]), may stop an undesired behavior, but often only until the child repeats the action and is not caught. Lower-class parents tend to use more punishment directed toward misbehavior or failure to adhere to parental values and requirements (Hockenberry, 2005).

Child Abuse

Child abuse (physical, sexual, or emotional exploitation of children) and neglect (lack of adequate food, shelter, or emotional support) continue to be significant societal problems. According to the American Academy of Pediatrics

(2007), 2.5 million cases of abuse or neglect in children are reported annually. Abused children have an increased likelihood of becoming violent adults and of abusing their own children. Factors that increase the risk of abuse include family poverty, culture, limited maternal education, needy child syndrome, presence of a stepfather, single-parent status, parental drug addiction, and teenage parenthood (American Academy of Pediatrics, 2007). However, child abuse occurs in families that do not have these risk factors. Cultural factors must be considered in detecting abuse. For example, coin rubbing of the chest (used in the Asian ethnic group for treatment of respiratory infections) leaves abrasions that may be perceived as abuse by a nurse assessing an ill child (Hockenberry & Wilson, 2007). Both national governmental agencies and professional organizations recommend that health care providers report suspected abuse and participate in preventing, assessing, and treating victims. Many state nurse practice acts require nurses to report suspected cases of abuse. Ultimately nurses help interrupt the vicious cycle of abuse by becoming involved in community coalitions and innovative evidence-based programs that prevent and intervene with child and family abuse (Box 20-4).

Unfortunately, relationships between children and adults are not always positive. **Sexual abuse**, use of a child for sexual exploitative purposes, has become a more common but often hidden problem for a variety of reasons (American

---

| Box **20-4** | Warning Signs of Child Abuse |

- Physical evidence of abuse or neglect, including previous injuries
- Conflicting stories about the "accident" or injury from the parents or others
- Injury or complaint inconsistent with the child's history or developmental level (e.g., the child received a concussion and broken arm from falling off a bed)
- Signs and symptoms consistent with signs of abuse and inconsistent with history, vague recall of event (e.g., chief complaint is a cold when there is evidence of first-degree and second-degree burns)
- Inappropriate response of caregiver, such as an exaggerated or absent emotional response, refusal to sign for additional tests or agree to necessary treatment, excessive delay in seeking treatment, or absence of the parents
- Inappropriate response of child, such as little or no response to pain, fear of being touched, excessive or lack of separation anxiety, or indiscriminate friendliness to strangers
- Child's report of physical or sexual abuse
- Previous reports of abuse in the family
- Repeated visits to emergency facilities with injuries

Compiled from Kellogg, (2007). Clinical report: Evaluation of suspected child physical abuse. *Pediatrics, 119*(6), 1232-1241; Hockenberry, M. J., & Wilson, D. (2006). *Wong's Nursing Care of Infants and Children* (8th Ed.). St. Louis: Mosby.

Academy of Pediatrics, 2007). The child may be too frightened to talk about the situation, families and society do not want to admit its existence, Internet traffic has supported pornography and pedophilia, and fewer agencies exist to respond to these cases. Many victims know their abusers (many are parents), and people in positions of authority (e.g., doctors or clergy) may be abusers. The child may comply for a variety of reasons, such as a need to be good or a need to keep the family together. Emotions are complex and change as the child grows, but they often lead to adult anxiety, depression, and physical symptoms and illnesses. Males less often report sexual abuse but are more likely than girls to suffer negative emotional effects from incest, a form of sexual abuse (Hockenberry, 2005).

As in any type of suspected abuse, nurses assist these children by recognizing those at risk and those experiencing abuse and referring them to relevant resources. All people who work with young children must acknowledge the warning signs of abuse (see Box 20-4). When sexual abuse is suspected, an in-depth interview and examination must be conducted by a multidisciplinary team that is sensitive to the needs of the child and can validate the abuse. Most authorities believe that children who describe sexual abuse are telling the truth, because the details are usually specific and trauma is evident. Therefore a child's story should be believed unless it is disproved.

Sexuality-Reproductive Pattern

The preschool child learns about gender and begins to model the general societal behaviors expected of a female or male child (Ball & Bindler, 2006). The child enters the school-age years with a strong identification with the parent of the same gender. The child continues to learn the concepts and behavior of the gender role and incorporate these into the self-concept. This challenge is significant for all children, but more so for homosexual children. Societal stereotypes related to gender roles continue to influence the school-age child's ideas of male and female roles (Hockenberry & Wilson, 2007). Fortunately, most children receive early teaching about gender roles that emphasizes that gender does not determine one's choices, personality, or behavior. Due to this teaching, children increasingly choose occupations based on their skills and interests, rather than on what appears appropriate because of their gender.

The school-age child's increasing awareness of the body, its functioning, and a need for sexual identity combine to foster a desire for knowledge about the biological aspects of sexual function. Late in the school-age period, when the physical changes of puberty have begun, concern and curiosity about sexual issues frequently grow. A child may become extremely attached to another of the same gender, and they may explore one another's sexual organs. This is common exploratory behavior and does not reflect true homosexuality, even though parents and children may express concerns about it. With the advent of physical changes of puberty,

the school-age child desires more privacy in a bedroom shared with no one. As noted earlier, the physical changes of puberty appear gradually over several years.

Children frequently share questions about sexual matters with their peer group. Parents are frequently uncomfortable or unsure of what sexual information to give to their children and when to give it. Many health care agencies sponsor short programs to educate parents and older school-age children, in a supportive environment, about bodily and mental changes during preadolescence and puberty. An increasing number of age-appropriate books that focus on emotional and body changes can be used at home and in school to increase children's understanding. Particularly because menstrual cycles start earlier now than they did 50 years ago, education about bodily changes and puberty appears appropriate as part of later school-age education.

The nurse plays an important role in sex education in health care and education settings. This professional should be receptive to answering questions in this area and at each health care visit (Hockenberry & Wilson, 2007). The nurse employed in the school is in an ideal position to teach group sex education programs using literature and games. Children at this age appear to respond most favorably with gender-segregated classes, based on their general discomfort with sexual topics and unique needs and questions (Hockenberry & Wilson, 2007). Some schools appropriately incorporate these classes into school curricula as part of a health-promotion curriculum. Other schools have special programs focused only on sex education based on parental desires or school board policies. Most school-age children have the cognitive skills to respond to programs on responsible sexuality, including discussions on abstinence and condom use, pregnancy, sexually transmitted diseases, and the human immunodeficiency virus (Schmitt, 2006). The nurse also wants to include program content specific to disabled children who face unique body changes and concerns and need to understand ways others can express affection to them without causing accusations of abuse.

Coping-Stress Tolerance Pattern

The school-age child must learn to cope with stress as part of the developmental process. Through a health-promotion program, children can learn to identify symptoms of stress (pounding heart, stomach "butterflies," and sweaty hands) and ways to cope with these perceived stresses (e.g., deep breathing and walking) before they cause illness. The child actually faces many stressful experiences in life, including competition, homework deadlines, failure at home or school, and decisions whether to cheat, steal, or even join an unpopular peer group. The young school-age child may never have shared his life with other children his age, and cultural values learned earlier in life may not be reflected in school or in peer relationships. Threats to the child's security (e.g., bullying) cause feelings of helplessness and anxiety that may affect the ability to function successfully. Grief over the death of a loved one, parental divorce, loss of a favorite activity because of misbehavior, or expulsion from a favorite peer group may cause negative behavior. Parents need to provide appropriate discipline in responding to this behavior but should also listen and analyze factors related to the problem in order to increase the child's feelings of control and decrease stress for the family (Health Teaching box).

Children use a variety of **coping strategies**, healthy behaviors intended to buffer perceived stressful events. However, in a very stressful situation or many stressful situations, a child may be unable to move beyond the coping behaviors. In conversations with teachers and parents, the nurse may offer a variety of strategies for coping with a school-age child's problems, enabling the child to cope and learn from others (Table 20-2). These strategies may

---

HEALTH TEACHING   The School-Age Child: Points for Effective Discipline

Effective discipline is essential to family harmony and individual child growth and reflects cultural beliefs. The goal of discipline is to encourage and reinforce positive child behaviors, eliminate inappropriate child behaviors, improve parent-child communication, and meet parental needs. Effective discipline requires these essential components: a positive, supportive, loving relationship between parent/child, use of positive reinforcement strategies to increase desired behavior, and removal of reinforcements or application of punishment to reduce/eliminate undesired behaviors.

Specifics of discipline strategies include
- Ignoring the misbehavior and acknowledging the appropriate behavior
- Using distraction or substitution to avoid a problem situation
- Offering choices to prevent inappropriate behavior such as whining or emotional outbursts

- Using humor to decrease the intensity of a situation
- Modeling the appropriate behavior
- Setting age-relevant limits
- Giving specific and clear commands for behavior appropriate to the child's age
- Talking calmly, being a good listener, and encouraging negotiation, perhaps in a family meeting, to promote problem resolution
- Limiting a child's environment (distractions such as music and television)
- Setting clear and consistent consequences for misbehavior (withholding privileges, using contracts)
- Providing one-to-one time, focusing on positive attention
- Taking time for oneself to replenish one's energies as a parent and as an individual

Compiled from Hockenberry, M. J. (2005). *Wong's essentials of pediatric nursing* (7th Ed.). St. Louis: Mosby; Hockenberry, M. J., & Wilson, D. (2007). *Wong's nursing care of infants and children* (8th Ed.). St. Louis: Mosby; American Academy of Pediatrics (2004). AAP guidelines of effective discipline. (Re-affirmation of 1998 recommendation; Pediatrics (1998) *Pediatrics 114*(4), 1126.

Table **20-2**   The School-Age Child's Coping Strategies and Nursing Interventions to Promote Coping

Coping Strategies	Nursing Interventions
Use of defense mechanisms (regression, denial, repression, projection, displacement, sublimation)	Accept child's use of defense mechanisms as temporary, healthy coping responses; provide child options for moving to more age-appropriate ways of responding to stressors
Cognitive mastery (problem solving, communication)	Ask children what they know of situation and how they might handle it; encourage questions; use diagrams and models to help explain; encourage child to verbalize feelings and use past successful strategies that might help deal with present stressors; try personalized approaches such as books, puppets, manipulation of equipment, to increase feelings of control when faced with stressful situation; encourage praying and other communications to a chosen deity as appropriate
Controlling, holding behaviors	Encourage child to participate and to make decisions; accept child's need to direct as appropriate; set consistent age-appropriate limits; respond to signals for help; let child be responsible for self-care
Use of repetition	Use books, games, and other communication media to work through feelings; emphasize "ok" for child to continue to ask questions and to receive answers that assist in coping
Use of humor	Be a good listener and participate in riddles and jokes used by child; be a good sport with school-age children's desire to play jokes on each other; share stories and cartoons with child
Motor activity, aggression, protest behavior	Encourage physical activity to deal with stress; accept appropriate behavior; establish limits on behavior for group safety
Withdrawal (resurgence of separation anxiety)	When child is separated from family, may have separation anxiety; encourage close emotional contacts between child and significant others (friends, family, church members); allow favorite objects from home to be brought to hospital or new environment for child

involve role playing or referral to literature on the problem topic to interrupt the child's negative behavior cycle to improve family health. The nurse may also refer a child to relevant religious and spiritual leaders, based on school-age children's belief that prayer will help them cope with an otherwise uncontrollable situation (Hockenberry, 2005).

Parental Divorce

More than one half of all marriages end in divorce, leaving many school-age children to face stress related to their parents' separation. Often children experience a feeling of loss, although they may hope that their parents will reunite at some point. Box 20-5 discusses the effects of divorce on a school-age child. Children's responses vary with their level of development. Factors such as economic security, availability of both of their parents, other family, church, and school supports, and quality of interactions with their parents can influence the child's ability to cope with divorce. Unfortunately, many parents become so immersed in their own feelings that they fail to support their children. Conflicts over custody, child support, and visitation rights add to the child's difficulty in coping. Sometimes the school

---

Box 20-5 Effects of Divorce on the School-Age Child

School-age children tend to view life in black and white, and are likely to blame one parent for the break-up. Boys, especially, mourn the loss of their fathers and frequently express anger at their mothers. Both boys and girls have great difficulty accepting their parents' new dates. Crying, daydreaming, and problems with friends and school are common divorce-related behaviors in children this age.

Here are some suggestions that might help the school-age child cope with divorce of parents.

1. *Discourage reconciliation fantasies.*

   Have parents avoid dinners, outings, or holiday celebrations with ex-spouse. This only fuels the child's fantasies. Instead, emphasize the finality of divorce.

2. *Make sure the child has the phone number of the absent parent.*

   Both parents should encourage easy access and frequent conversations with the noncustodial parent.

3. *Do not allow the child to manipulate parents into buying more possessions.*

   School-age children are likely to feel deprived. Although they may intensify requests for playthings or other possessions, do not try to retain child's affection through material objects. Even children of divorce need to be told "No!"

4. *Talk to child's teachers or school counselors about the divorce.*

   School personnel may better understand possible learning or behavioral problems and will likely offer extra support.

From University of Michigan Health System, 2006. Divorce: The effects on children. *Pediatric Advisor 2006.* [on-line]. Retrieved from *www.med. umich.edu/1libr/pa/pa_divorce_pep.htm.*

---

system becomes the child's advocate to encourage the parents to provide a supportive environment during divorce proceedings. Despite this intervention, some children do not cope well with the divorce and have emotional aftereffects that result in juvenile behavior problems or require long-term counseling (see the Case Study and Care Plan at the end of this chapter).

Somatization and Depression

Children, like adults, use defense mechanisms to cope, with varying degrees of success. Two strategies used by the school-age child to respond to uncontrollable situations are **somatization** and **depression**.

Some children respond to a stressful situation by transferring their feelings to a physical problem (somatization). In this phenomenon, school-age children, unable to discuss their concerns, complain of stomachaches or headaches, symptoms reflective of functional or psychogenic pain. These children may also develop discrete, repetitive movement habits called tics. In many cases the child with these problems must be evaluated to determine whether an underlying physiological cause exists. The child and the family will then need assistance in understanding the child's concerns to define successful ways to cope with the behavior.

Depression occurs in 0.8% to 2% of children (National Institute of Mental Health, 2009) and more often in boys than girls during the school-age period. Depression reflects a disturbance of mood, when a child displays sadness, guilt, or worthlessness, and other unusual behaviors that disengage the child from peers and family. In defining depression in children, most authors point out that they refer to a more long-term syndrome in which the child's normal development and functioning become impaired, not a periodic sadness that all children occasionally experience. Factors that place a child at risk for depression include homelessness, death of a parent or significant other, divorce, long-term hospitalization, chronic illness, learning problems, or emotional turmoil at home. Parents and teachers look for symptoms of depression, including anorexia, sleeplessness, lethargy, changed affect, aggressive behavior, frequent crying, or withdrawal from previously enjoyed activities.

Although it has been concluded that there is insufficient evidence to routinely screen all school-age children for depression, the nurse can serve an important role in identifying any child who appears to be depressed and in notifying parents about the need for further assessment (National Institute of Mental Health, 2009). Depending on the child and the situation, varying amounts of counseling and individual child guidance may be required. Antidepressant medication may also be prescribed (National Institute of Mental Health, 2009). Nurses in schools and outpatient settings are often the ideal helpers, because they have the skills and time needed to help a child cope with a helpless feeling and its cause.

Values-Beliefs Pattern

Children make decisions related to moral and ethical issues every day. Should they tell the teacher which classmate broke the rule? Should they share their candy with a younger sibling? For these situations, the child makes a decision based on the level of moral development. **Moral development** involves choosing the most appropriate behavior based on one's values and feelings related to the situation. Environmental factors and culture strongly influence a child's moral development, as do the type of family discipline, role models, people with whom the child identifies, and the child's rehearsal and practice of moral behavior (Hockenberry & Wilson, 2007).

Kohlberg's Theory

Most researchers agree that the younger school-age child is at the **preconventional** level, a level of moral development characterized by self-interest only. The child continues to do many things simply to avoid getting in trouble, does not understand the reason for rules, but also performs actions that will benefit the self (Kohlberg, 1981; Ball & Bindler, 2006). During later childhood (10 to 13 years) most children progress to the conventional level, a stage of moral development defined by concern about group interests and values. The conventional level of moral judgment involves the child looking to others for approval and to societal authority for a definition of rules. Children 10 to 12 years old judge a behavior in terms of the intention of the offender, understand the "golden rule" concept, and engage in behavior that maintains a valued relationship. The conventional level coincides with Piaget's cognitive level of concrete operations and the child's increased social involvement with people outside the home (Kohlberg, 1981; Hockenberry & Wilson, 2007).

Moral Behavior Problems

Some moral behavior problems, such as lying, stealing, or cheating, are common during the school-age years. Cultural, religious, and parental values influence a child's moral development, concept of right and wrong, and consequences of not demonstrating moral behavior. Preschool and younger school-age children frequently lie due to fantasy, exaggerations, or inaccurate understanding. As children grow, they may use the defense mechanism of denial to block upsetting situations and maintain self-esteem. The lie then becomes an unconscious act. Older children often lie because they fear punishment or ridicule. Children may cheat because of a desire to win, do well in competitive society, or "look good" for their peers. Children usually steal when they think they will not be caught and they think that there is no other way to get what they want. Although these actions can be quite upsetting for parents, they are common developmental behaviors. Parents frequently need reassurance that the child is normal and probably will outgrow the behavior with parental assistance. They may need help in developing fair rules for behavior and communicating their expectations for a child's behavior to meet parental and cultural values. Therefore the nurse encourages the parents to warn the child clearly not to steal, lie, or cheat, offer other, more socially acceptable, ways to cope with the stressor causing the behavior, and then apply appropriate punishment congruent with an understanding of the event (Hockenberry & Wilson, 2007).

ENVIRONMENTAL PROCESSES

School-age children, similar to those of all other age groups, face daily exposure to environmental agents and factors that may cause injury, illness, or death. Many of these agents and factors are harmless if appropriately used or when exposure is minimal. Examples include physical agents such as fires; mechanical agents such as bicycles, skateboards, and cars; biological agents such as bacteria; chemical agents such as asbestos; and radiological agents such as x-rays. Death rates from these agents vary among ethnic groups because of access to health care and environmental issues (Hockenberry & Wilson, 2007). For example, Native Americans and Alaska Natives experience higher death rates from motor vehicle accidents, residential fires, and drowning than do other groups. Blacks experience higher death rates for unintentional injury than do other ethnic group members (National Safety Council, 2007).

Accidents

Accidents are the leading cause of death in children over age 1 year in the United States (USDHHS, 2000). Most accidents do not result in death, but many serious ones cause significant morbidity and disability. Because of this effect, the nurse has a significant role in educating parents and school personnel on ways to prevent dangers to school-age children and to become involved in public initiatives to create a safer society for them.

The agent, host, and environment must be considered in developing solutions to decrease the number of accidents. The type of agent varies with the child's age. Most fatal accidents during the school-age period derive from motor vehicle accidents when the child (host) is a passenger or pedestrian (walking or riding a bike). Other fatal accidents occur from fires and burns, bicycles, drowning, and firearm accidents. Most common nonfatal accidents tend to be caused by simple agents that produce simple injuries. Despite helmet laws in several states, many school-age children continue to experience head injuries related to recreational equipment, such as bicycles, swings, skateboards, and trampolines (Hockenberry & Wilson, 2007; SafeKids, 2007). Slightly older children have an increased number of accidents from contact sports and cuts, falls, burns, and injuries from firearms.

Specific accident factors relate to the host, the school-age child (Hot Topics box). Children in this age group tend to become hurt because of their happy-go-lucky attitude,

HOTtopics

SAFETY CONCERNS SPECIFIC TO SCHOOL-AGE CHILDREN

Because of increased independence, school-age children face significant exposure to situations threatening their health. Consequently, parents of these children must be involved in community and legislative activities that provide safe play environments. Additionally, at appropriate health visits, health care workers should provide anticipatory guidance to parents in the following areas:

Bicycle Safety

Each child should have a well-maintained bicycle, ride only in safe areas approved by parents, observe rules for vehicle traffic, ride on the side of road with traffic, "bike defensively," and use a federally approved riding helmet

Street Safety

Children should look right, left, then right again to check safety of crossing a street; cross only at safe and well-monitored intersections, preferably with an adult present; ensure parental supervision when children play close to streets and heavy traffic areas

Motor Vehicle Safety

Children should wear a seat belt or be in age-appropriate booster seat as needed; older children should ride with restraint system and in back seat until age 12

Pool Safety

All children should have swimming lessons and swim with a buddy or adult who swims well; all pools should have drain covers; children should avoid swimming after a heavy meal and avoid "roughhousing" behavior around the pool; children should be monitored by parents during swimming

Firearm Safety

Adults need to lock away guns and ensure gun safety locks are intact; parents need to educate children NEVER to touch guns

Playground Safety

All playground equipment should meet federally approved standards; children should be trained on how to use equipment safely; equipment should be evaluated for safety and repaired before children use it

Fire Safety

Working smoke detectors should be in place in home and school; family needs to have a fire evacuation plan and practice it; children need to wear fire-retardant clothing at night; children should not play with matches, open fires, fireworks, or open wires that can cause injury and fire

Toxin Safety

Children should avoid insecticides, radiation sources, inappropriate use of medications, and pollution sources; parents need to store all known toxins, chemicals, and household cleaning agents in an adequately ventilated location that is inaccessible to children

Stranger Safety

Children should play with friends, have a plan for returning home, know home phone number and address, play in safe and known area, and report any suspicious activity threatening their safety to an appropriate adult; children should know how to say "no" and how to locate assistance when in an unsafe situation

Sports Safety

Children need to engage in age-appropriate activities and wear protective equipment relevant to the sport; parents need to ensure safety and maintenance of all sports equipment; parents need to caution children against hazardous sports, such as trampolines

Animal Safety

Parents should teach children to avoid strange animals, especially sick or injured ones, and ensure that personal pets receive vaccinations; need to teach children not to mistreat pets and not to place their faces close to any animal

---

curiosity, love of mimicking older people, and their intense oral tendencies. Typically school-age boys have more accidents than girls, perhaps due to differences in personalities, societal expectations, child-rearing practices, and more risk-taking behaviors. The mechanism varies with the gender of the host. For school-age boys, drowning is the most common fatal accident; for girls, automobile accidents are the most common (Centers for Disease Control and Prevention, 2008b).

The physical environment of the child dictates the type or frequency of accidents, which occur in the home, neighborhood, and school. Most accidents happen outdoors, which means that school-age children face greater risk for automobile or bicycle accidents than for poisoning or falls, indoor accidents that occur predominately in the younger set. More

accidents (drowning and pedestrian-vehicle accidents) occur in the summer than in the winter because of children's outside play. Socioeconomic level affects children's physical environments and access to dangers. For example, space heaters place children of low-income families at risk for burns, whereas skiing places wealthier children at risk for injury.

The social environment, which includes the family, school, and playmates, also plays a role in accidents. Although little research has focused on the physical trauma caused by heavy backpacks that many school-age children use, appliances such as these exert significant pressure against functionally immature muscles of the back and torso. Daily carrying of bulging backpacks causes muscle strain, headaches, improper posture, shoulder slouch, and other physical problems. Also to be considered are teachers' expectations all textbooks being used for learning, both in the classroom and at home. At least one study has shown that children will change their backpack carrying behaviors if involved in a school-based program focused on this topic (Goodgold & Nielsen, 2003).

As part of the social environment, the family may influence the rate of accidents in the school-age child. Chronic familial stress (parental unemployment) or a sudden acute stress (parental illness) may contribute to homicide as the third-leading cause of death among children ages 5 to 14 years (USDHHS, 2000). Homicide is a more common cause of death among Black and Hispanic children than White children (Finkelhor & Ormod, 2001). Children also face increased risk of accidents when parental supervision is limited, such as during holidays or a move to a new home.

Drowning

Fewer school-age children than infants and adolescents die from drowning. More Black children of this age drown than do White children (USDHHS, 2000). According to the midcourse review of the *Healthy People 2010* initiatives, movement toward meeting initiative targets had been found (USDHHS, 2005e). Water safety measures can help reduce drowning, along with the many other injuries that occur around water, such as falls in slippery areas. Environment and safety teaching can influence the number of school-age children dying as a result of drowning.

Burns

Each year many children become victims of house fires, many of which occur during the winter months from Christmas trees, space heaters, and fireplace malfunctions. At the midcourse review of the *Healthy People 2010* initiatives, a 10% movement toward the initiative target of 1:100,000 population was found (USDHHS, 2005e). Many homes lack working smoke detectors because of incorrect installation or inadequate testing. If a fire occurs in a home with a smoke detector, the risk of death is decreased by 40% to 50% (Ahrens, 2004). Most burned children survive, frequently with varying degrees of physical and psychological scars. Children need to learn about fire safety, including the need to avoid situations involving fire and to practice fire drills routinely at school and home. The nurse encourages parents to understand other practices to prevent fire-related problems, including parental purchase of flame-retardant sleepwear for children.

Firearms

People in the United States who use firearms frequently cause fatal injury through homicide, suicide, or accidents. Every 3 hours someone's child dies due to a gun accident (American Academy of Child & Adolescent Psychiatry, 2008). With many U.S. homes containing a handgun and because of recent shootings by adolescents, concern about children's safety remains well founded.

Possibly the best means of preventing accidents with firearms is to ban them from private ownership as seen in England. However, because handgun ownership is an important individual right in this country, several states have passed legislation that allows handguns for individual protection. Families with firearms in the home should store guns in a locked area apart from ammunition and consider using nonlethal (wax) bullets. All family members should practice about gun safety.

Sports and Recreation

Accidents from sports and other recreational activities increase during the school-age years and include lacerations, contusions, hematomas, concussions, sprains, and fractures. Some evidence exists that adolescents now have more musculoskeletal injuries due to involvement in repetitive team sports earlier in their lives. This suggests that society needs to examine the current emphasis on initiating young children with musculoskeletal immaturity into team sports such as football, hockey, soccer, and basketball. Intense social pressure for children to participate in these sports means that parents and school systems must ensure that each child has protective body devices to prevent injuries, as well as psychological support to allow a child to benefit from the team sport. There is a further need to increase safety by ensuring that each child fits the sport, has adequate hydration during the game, and engages in conditioning exercises before and after the game for prevention of injuries. There is not enough evidence of any change towards *Healthy People 2010* initiative targets related to sports equipment use and safety in children (USDHHS, 2005e). Furthermore, literature supports societal need to focus more on the collaborative skills children learn by being part of a team, rather than the winning-despite-the-costs philosophy found in many school-age team sports.

Recreation area injuries may be prevented by several measures. The National Bureau of Standards set guidelines in 1976 for home playground equipment, regulating things such as sharp edges, moving parts, and equipment design. Nurses help prevent accidents by participating in decisions about school playground equipment and counseling families on a variety of issues. Playground safety has become an important issue because 200,000 children need emergency room assessment each year for related injuries. Many of these occur in low-income neighborhoods where playgrounds fail to meet safety standards (USDHHS, 2000).

Nursing Interventions

Although nurses offer suggestions to parents to improve their children's play safety, studies have shown that few parents follow these suggestions. Reasons for this behavior include parental difficulty in assessing the safety of and age appropriateness of play equipment, the amount of effort involved, and a lack of money to create a safe play area.

The nurse helps parents respond to these perceived barriers. With more children using skateboards and rollerblades, the nurse also encourages the use of child safety helmets and knee, elbow, and wrist guards to prevent muscle sprains and bone fractures. The school offers an on-site opportunity for teaching children, teachers, and parents about accident prevention. In addition to providing this guidance, nurses can participate in legislative and educational actions to increase community consciousness about child safety (Box 20-6).

Mechanical Forces

Motor vehicles and bicycles represent the two most common mechanical agents that cause injury to school-age children.

Motor Vehicles

The leading cause of death in the United States in all individuals from age 1 to 34 years of age is motor vehicle accidents (Daly et al., 2006). Children die as passengers in cars, as pedestrians, and as bicycle riders. In this country, more children die from pedestrian-related accidents than passenger-related accidents (Centers for Disease Control and Prevention, 2008b). More than 37% of the people

killed in bicycle accidents are children, many of whom did not wear helmets to prevent head injury (National Highway Traffic Safety Administration, 2008). Although not all accidents result in death, children may also sustain injury that causes permanent disability as a result of motor-vehicle accidents.

Automobile passenger injuries can be prevented, or the severity reduced, by altering some aspects of the child's environment. Lower speed limits, alcohol-related laws, better automobile and highway designs, door lock mechanisms, and effective restraint system requirements in all states have reduced the severity and number of accidents and injuries (USDHHS, 2007b). However, more injuries have been correlated to higher speed limits instituted in the United States several years ago. Furthermore, many children remain at risk for injury because various school districts and states do not require seat belts in buses used to transport students, despite a recommendation by the American Academy of Pediatrics to do so.

Studies indicate that proper and consistent use of federally approved belt-positioned booster seats for children ages 4 to 7 years decreases the likelihood of child death and serious injury significantly (American Academy of Pediatrics, 2007). However, one study showed that only 19% of such children used these seats (National Highway Traffic Safety Administration, 2008). Less than 10% of children needing the protection of a booster seat ride in one, and younger, smaller school-age children (under 4 feet, 9 inches) often fail to use them correctly (National Highway Traffic Safety Administration, 2008). Reasons given by parents and children for not using seat belts or booster seats include forgetting to use, difficulty reaching and fastening belts, seat belt or seat discomfort, and misinformation about the need for the belt or seat for short trips. Clearly, consistent use of booster seats by young children and seat belts by older children and adults, who model seat belt behavior to their children, will occur only when legal enforcement occurs. Federal government and national professional groups recommend that all children under the age of 12 years ride in the automobile's back seat in an appropriate restraint due to the potential for death from an air bag activated in a motor vehicle accident (Hockenberry, 2005). Many families have difficulty meeting this recommendation because of long-term acceptance of older children riding in the front seat after they have outgrown booster seats.

Urban children under the age of 15 years experience more than one half of all pedestrian-automobile accidents (Hockenberry & Wilson, 2007). These occur when using rollerblades, skateboards, and skate scooters and tend to be more severe (head injuries) than passenger injuries. Many factors cause pedestrian accidents: children often have difficulty interpreting traffic signs and judging the speed of cars, and they forget to look carefully before crossing the street. Although overcrowding, poverty, high volume of traffic, stress, and unsafe play areas influence children's street safety, various principles can direct interventions to decrease the number of street dangers.

Bicycles and Motorized Vehicles

Many accidents occur each year with young children on bicycles, motorized skateboards, and all terrain vehicles (ATVs). Most of these are not serious, but deaths occur among young children who have suffered head trauma or significant bodily injury from inappropriate use of this equipment. The American Academy of Pediatrics (2000) recommends that only people at least age 16 years ride ATVs and then only in rural areas with adult supervision. Bicycle accidents occur most frequently near the child's home and during the day and commonly involve injuries from the spokes when children ride behind the bike seat. More boys than girls experience these injuries from bicycles, motorized skateboards, and ATVs, perhaps based on their greater risk-taking behavior.

In response to children's developmental behavior related to bicycles, motorized skateboards, and ATVs, the nurse addresses safety issues. Additionally, nurses encourage parents to teach and reinforce safe bicycling habits to their children and should sponsor helmet and bike programs within the school.

Biological Agents

School-age children face constant exposure to bacterial, viral, and other biological agents that pose threats to or improve their overall health (e.g., immunizations). Compared with the preschool child, the school-age child has fewer illnesses. The most frequent illness continues to be upper respiratory infections (URIs), illnesses shared among school children who fail to practice good hand washing and avoidance of ill peers. These illnesses cause children to lose school days and learning opportunities. Most URIs result from viruses, but bacteria can play either a primary or a secondary role. Two problems associated with URIs are streptococcal infection ("strep throat") and otitis media.

Strep throat occurs frequently among school-age children. A child with an infection from Group A streptococcus may have a severe sore throat, fever, and malaise or may have only a minor sore throat. A throat culture confirms the diagnosis, and antibiotic treatment typically cures the infection. Children are noninfectious after 24 hours of treatment and may return to school (AAP, Committee on Infectious Diseases, 2006). If not treated, the affected child may develop rheumatic fever or acute glomerulonephritis as a secondary infection following the sore throat. Greater transmission of streptococcal infection occurs in areas where there is close person-to-person contact during colder weather. The school nurse's preventive efforts focus on teaching the children good hand washing techniques and identifying children who complain of sore throats. Children with throat infections caused by other strains of streptococcus, such as group B, do not usually require treatment, because these infections generally do not cause the same serious complications.

The school-age child may experience other illnesses. The frequency of gastrointestinal infection (**gastroenteritis**) decreases during the school-age years but is still the second most common acute condition of childhood. Usually caused by a virus, gastrointestinal infections cause vomiting and diarrhea. Older and larger school-age children have little chance of rapid dehydration; they basically react to the illness the same as do adults and need to be treated similarly. Gastroenteritis is contagious and, therefore, the nurse should monitor school children for symptoms of illness and encourage hand washing to prevent transmission of the virus from one child to another.

Scabies and **lice** (**pediculosis**) are common skin disorders among school-age children. This problem causes extreme itchiness of either the body (scabies) or the head (lice) and is easily spread to other children. The nurse educates parents to visualize or use a lice comb to check their children for scabies and lice when they complain of itchiness or seem to be constantly scratching their heads (Gavin, 2008). Previously, children diagnosed with lice could not come to school until they were lice free. This isolated students from their peers and influenced state school funding based on student attendance. The American Academy of Pediatrics now recommends that if children are under treatment for the problem, they should be allowed in school (AAP, Committee on Infectious Diseases, 2006).

A biological agent that many children know about is human immunodeficiency virus, or HIV, which causes acquired immunodeficiency syndrome (AIDS). Of all age groups, the young school-age child is at the lowest risk for contracting the disease, because AIDS acquired by the perinatal route emerges in infancy and toddlerhood, and most young school-age children do not use intravenous drugs or engage in high-risk sexual practices. However, the school-age child may know a person with AIDS or may have heard something about the disease from adults, older children, or the news media. The school-age child and school staff should know basic facts about the disease, its transmission and, most importantly, that it cannot be transmitted through casual contact, such as being in the same classroom with a child who has it. Due to widespread misinformation and fear, the United States Surgeon General has called for mandatory, explicit AIDS education beginning with children 8 years of age. The involvement of parents, students, and school personnel in AIDS education programs through age-appropriate materials will increase each group's knowledge and acceptance of people who have the disease. Accepting parents assist their own children in learning to accept others with special needs and in taking better control of their own health.

Children with AIDS may attend school as long as they will not be exposed to illness from other children. Most children with AIDS receive routine immunizations but may need further immunization if exposed to a usual childhood disease (AAP, Committee on Infectious Diseases, 2006). During outbreaks of contagious disease, the chronically ill child may have home tutoring; this approach will need to be evaluated annually to identify the risks versus benefits of school attendance. Certainly, long periods of isolation from peers will contribute to feelings of loneliness in the child with AIDS and may even appear to be a punishment for being ill. The school nurse undoubtedly has an important role in facilitating the multidisciplinary nature of AIDS care while maximizing the learning environment of affected children.

Most states require that the child's immunizations be current before entering kindergarten or the first grade and that additional tetanus immunization be given every 10 years or with an unclean wound. Other immunizations recommended by the American Academy of Pediatrics include a **meningococcal vaccination** at age 11 or 12 years and the series of three injections for hepatitis B and **Human Papilloma Virus (HPV)** during the late school-age and early adolescent years (CDC, 2007b). If the child has no history of chickenpox, a varicella immunization is also recommended (AAP, Committee on Infectious Diseases, 2006; Hockenberry, 2005). In many states the school nurse has a responsibility to ensure that all students' immunizations are current and, if not, the nurse informs the parents that the children may not attend school until their immunizations have been brought up to date (CDC, 2008a). Any child lacking age-appropriate immunizations can "catch up" according to a schedule developed by the American Academy of Pediatrics (AAP, Committee on Infectious Diseases, 2006). Although 95% of American children receive immunizations by school entrance time (USDHHS, 2000), increasing numbers of immigrants and transient workers have deepened concern about exposure of Americans to previously conquered diseases (e.g., tuberculosis). Strides towards meeting the *Healthy People 2010* initiative targets related to immunizations continue to be made according to the midcourse review and the 2020 objectives (USDHHS, 2005f).

Chemical Agents

A number of potentially toxic chemical agents exist in the environment, and the child is exposed to these through inhalation, ingestion, or direct contact. Children are particularly susceptible to chemical hazards. Food and drugs are two sources of chemicals ingested by children on a regular basis, and some older school-age children ingest tobacco as a result of cigarette smoking. Although normally safe, some foods and drugs can be harmful when used inappropriately. Other environmental hazards include pollution, heavy metals (lead and mercury), and pesticides.

The nutritional needs of the school-age child were discussed earlier in this chapter. As stated, children frequently eat foods with large quantities of sugar, salt, and fat and with chemical additives. The effects of some of these additives have been questioned, and concern has been expressed about the effect of biochemically altered food on children and future generations. On a short-term basis, some foods may cause allergic reactions; on a long-term basis, some may contribute to the development of coronary disease, hypertension, and cancer. Nurses are aware that the child's diet may contribute to future health problems and assess intake and counsel the child and parents accordingly about ways to improve it.

The incidence of poisoning decreases during the school-age years as children become more aware of the appropriate uses of drugs and other agents. Childproof containers have decreased exposure of children to dangerous poisons and chemicals in the home. However, children continue to face exposure to drugs (alcohol and glue inhalants) due to less monitoring by working parents, and older school-age children face exposure to recreational drugs, primarily through their peers and older children. In the school environment the nurse and school personnel need to encourage students to engage in wise decision-making about recreational drug use that will affect their future and overall health.

With pressure on older school-age children to smoke cigarettes, attention must be paid to effective strategies to prevent these behaviors. Every day, more than 6000 school students try to smoke a cigarette (Stop Smoking Update, 2009). Most students who smoke initiate their habit around 11 years of age (American Heart Association, 2008). White students start smoking at a younger age than Black students. Males tend to begin smoking earlier than females; however, girls catch up in smoking rates during middle school-age years (Stop Smoking Update, 2009). The Federal Tobacco Settlement Project (1998) provides funds to address the public health problem posed by tobacco smoke in the U.S. Although funding for tobacco prevention and cessation programs has reached its highest level in six years, many states continue to fall short of the minimum recommendations by the CDC (*Tobacco Free Kids*, 2007). Attention to smoking as part of a health-promotion program seems merited, because so many begin so young and, because nicotine is highly addictive, many believe that this habit leads people to experiment with more risky drugs (cocaine and methamphetamines).

School policies have been instrumental in supporting a tobacco-free environment. By 2006, 63.6% of schools prohibited all tobacco use in all locations and those associated with school-sponsored events. To further assist in health-promotion, many institutions require staff development and education programs related to the effects of tobacco use on health. By 2006, 67.6% of elementary schools had implemented required instruction on tobacco use prevention (Centers for Disease Control and Prevention, 2009b). Various governmental efforts to reduce exposure to environmental tobacco have occurred. For example, 22 states and numerous cities nationwide have enacted smoke-free laws.

Pollution has become a fact of life for many Americans and, particularly, for the 25% of urban-dwelling children who must breathe air that exceeds federal government levels for acceptable ozone (USDHHS, 2000). Air pollution irritates the eyes and the respiratory tract, causing URIs, ear infections, and allergies. More children now experience asthma, and many inner city children face higher rates of this disease due to poor air quality including secondary and tertiary smoke. Death rates from this illness escalated 67% from 1980 to 1993, and 40% of all activity restrictions of children result from asthma (USDHHS, 2000). Knowing the negative effects of air pollution and smoking to their health, many school-age children participate in school projects to improve their environmental health.

Children also face exposure to various toxic materials in their environment. Progress has been made over the past decades to reduce children's exposure to chemical hazards (Commission for Environmental Cooperation, 2006). Lead for example, has been removed from gasoline and paint. This in turn has resulted in significant reductions in children's blood lead levels. Lead exposure continues to exist. Children are exposed to lead through parents' clothes, shoes contacting lead-infused soil, lead in older residential water pipes, traditional medications in some cultures, or in school building structures. Children living in poverty receive high exposure from lead-based paint used on older and cheaper homes. The long-term effects of these metals on children remain unclear, but some evidence indicates children suffer neurotoxic effects from this type of exposure. High lead levels in children contribute to dental caries and hearing loss.

Routine use of chemicals to control insects and undesirable weeds in landscaping has led to increasing concerns about children's exposure to these agents. With increased interest in more natural substances to control insects and gardening problems, perhaps less reliance will be placed on biological chemicals for these problems in the future. Knowing the primary source of exposure to the most hazardous materials and avoiding these materials is often sufficient to accomplish real risk reduction and offer substantial protection within the child's environment (Children's Health Environmental Coalition, 2008). Various behaviors can be implemented to create a safe environment and minimize health risks associated with hazardous chemical exposure. Nurses are instrumental in the assistance and support of parents, schools, and community agencies in the implementation of these behaviors such as the use of nonhazardous cleaners, pesticide-free foods, and further monitoring of the environment for hazardous materials.

Radiological Agents
X-ray Exposure

The child receives exposure from both naturally occurring radiation and human-made ionizing radiation. Exposure occurs in varying degrees with radiographic examinations of teeth and bone, from nuclear power plants and explosions, and in the management of many childhood cancers. Children exposed to high levels of radiation risk developing breast or thyroid cancer or leukemia and compromised growth. With little advocacy in this area, nurses and other professionals improve children's health by becoming active in initiatives that focus on prevention of chemical and radiation hazards.

Cancer

Leukemia is the most common form of childhood cancer. Of those affected under 5 years of age, 90% will be cured with current medical treatment (Leukemia & Lymphoma Society, 2007). Among the 12 major types of childhood cancers, leukemia and cancers of the brain and central nervous system (second most common forms of childhood cancers) account for more than 50% of all new cases (National Cancer Institute, 2007). Lymphomas (Hodgkin disease and non-Hodgkin lymphoma) also affect school-age children and adolescents as the third most common group of malignancies. Non-Hodgkin lymphoma is more common during the school-age years, and boys experience this malignancy 3 times more often than do girls. Mortality rates in the United States tend to be greater in densely populated areas, particularly where the more-educated and wealthy live (Hockenberry & Wilson, 2007). The most common symptom is abdominal pain caused by intestinal obstruction and symptoms resulting from organ compression. With effective treatment regimens, children with limited disease may be cured but may experience side effects of treatment later in life (e.g., development of cataracts, dental problems, learning difficulties) (Chustecka, 2006). These children present a challenge to the nurse because they are in various stages of recovery, may be developmentally delayed, and may fear a recurrence of their disease. The nurse provides psychological and emotional support to affected children and their families, to help children develop peer relationships and meet developmental goals important to them during the school-age years.

SOCIAL PROCESSES

The school-age child interacts daily with other children and adults to become more independent by age 12. Mutual problem solving of child and parents or friends frequently occurs at this age related to a higher level of maturity in social relationships and concerns. Exposure to a variety of social roles and expectations of others strengthens the process of socialization so that the child develops social competence, the ability and skills to participate effectively in the social interactions of society. Social competence includes both the obvious social behaviors and an inner understanding of the appropriateness of behaviors.

Several elements play a role in the development of the child's social competence. The child's desire for a sense of industry encourages interactions, positive relationships, and accomplishments within society. Cognitive development supports understanding of relationships and effective problem solving. Moral judgment helps the child understand consequences and fairness in relationships. Understanding and obeying authority helps to maintain order in society. Social sensitivity is a result of social interactions and requires the child's ability to perceive the social cues of others, understand the roles of others, and communicate verbally with them. Social behaviors are also a part of social competence; these are learned most frequently through imitation, role modeling, and reinforcement of others' behaviors. The interaction of all these elements produces a level of social competence and simultaneously plays a role in the child's self-perception. Individuals frequently see themselves as others see them.

Community and Work

Peers

The strongest relationships that school-age children develop outside their families are with their peers (other children encountered in the neighborhood and school). The peer group acts as a new social system, becoming increasingly influential in the child's life. All children continue to be influenced significantly by the family, the culture of the family, and many other environmental factors, but the peer group begins to influence lifestyle, habits, and speech patterns and formulate standards of behavior and performance. The standards of the peer group become vitally important, and children attempt to conform to its rules. Being accepted by the peer group becomes more important than being accepted by anyone else. Conforming to the pressures of peers becomes an issue, especially when it interferes with the parents' expectations. When children realize that their own goals, desires, and aspirations might be quite different from those held by the peer group or the school, they must find ways to cope and perform according to the new standards if they are to succeed. The degree to which children fit in socially, learn to cope, and receive satisfaction from the group is a powerful determinant of healthy socialization.

A child may have one best friend or several important friends and a mutual understanding and willingness to help each other. Friendship groups that form during this age may change and become goal directed, such as groups composing a sports team. These groups frequently have set rules or rituals that connect the members. During the middle school-age years, friendships often revolve around same-gender relationships, videos, songs, books, and media shared by the group. Later in the school-age years, the development of sexual relationships with the opposite gender occurs during dating and mixed parties.

School-age children also become increasingly involved with adults outside the family, including teachers, coaches, and others who become role models, all of whom influence the child's view of the world and self. Although this influence may not be as significant as that of a child's peers, long-term ideas and beliefs frequently develop from these relationships. Children usually perceive some similarity between themselves and their models, those of the same gender with similar physical or behavior traits. During these years children may not maintain a strong identification with the parent of the same gender, but they tend to adopt other adult models with whom they can identify.

Working Parents

Both dual-career couples and single-parent families influence their children's safety when no adult is present to monitor the environment after school. Many **"latchkey children"** who are left alone until their parents return from work follow directions given by their parents. These directions may include beginning dinner in anticipation of their parents' return or completing homework while remaining inside the home with the doors locked.

Parents and school-age children often disagree about how old is "old enough" to be left at home alone or with an older sibling. Although the school-age child might consider being at home alone to be a real mark of maturity, children who look after themselves after school can become more isolated and miss peer relationships important to their development. Nurses give guidance to families who must cope with the issue of after-school care for school-age children to ensure that relevant and safe decisions are made.

Culture and Ethnicity

School-age children focus more on the influences of their culture on their lives than do younger children. Aspects of American culture that the child must confront include poverty and affluence, ethnic and racial differences, acceptance of these differences, and the power of media as a cultural phenomenon in American society.

Ethnic Groups

Preschool children may notice racial and ethnic differences, but school-age children increasingly show evidence of being aware of these differences. This is a time during which attitudes toward race develop based on family and community attitudes. Studies of children 5 to 7 years of age show that most identify with and prefer to play with members of their own race. As children get older, they may continue this behavior. Although prejudice exists among some school-age children, they may be encouraged to view people from different cultures and ethnic backgrounds in a positive light. Many schools appropriately focus on the importance of other cultures by having multicultural awareness weeks. During these times, children dress, eat, and live as other cultures do, allowing them to recognize the uniqueness of individual cultural beliefs and values (Multicultural Awareness box).

Television and Video and Computer Games

Television and video and computer games exert a major influence on ideas and behavior in American culture. Unfortunately, many television programs and games pose harm to children because of their messages and because such activities prevent children from engaging in physical activity. Recent advances in gaming offers an option for increased activity during gaming activities. New video games and gaming systems, such as Wii, have been developed that encourage movement during gaming. Energy expenditure more than doubled when sedentary screen times were converted to active screen time (Lanningham-Foster et al., 2006).

Computers connected to the Internet pose danger unless locking devices have been installed to prevent school-age children from accessing inappropriate websites. Additional concerns have focused on the violent themes of programming, persuasive television commercials, unrealistic depiction of the world, unhealthy food intake, and the passivity of television viewing.

MULTICULTURAL AWARENESS
Expectations for Child Behavior Related to Culture

AMERICAN INDIAN

Expect child to respect elders and take pride in heritage; develop natural talents as child matures; personal independence must balance with accountability to family, community, and tribe; help sought from family members, not outsiders

MEXICAN AMERICAN

Family environment protects child; child expected to be obedient, respectful, and to work hard to reach goals; "next" generation expected to do better than current generation

FILIPINO

Family raises child in protective environment; expect child to conform to values of culture and child shamed if fails to meet expected behaviors; child taught to avoid direct confrontation and hide emotions and to be respectful and shy; strong emphasis on education for personal and financial gain

BLACK

Child expected to complete family chores, complete schooling, and develop talents such as music or sports to improve self for future; discipline and respectful behavior encouraged

CHINESE AMERICANS

Child is highly valued, particularly male child; child expected to honor elders and family needs; high value of education to honor family and child

---

Many times, certain ethnic or racial groups implement the violence in these media sources, leading children to stereotype these groups as the perpetrators of violence. Research has shown that television facilitates negative attitudes and values among children, increases their aggressive behavior, decreases their emotional sensitivity when aggressive acts occur, and leads them to accept aggressive acts (AAP, Committee on School Health, 2004). One positive note is that adults who discuss violence with children by pointing out that these acts are unacceptable and cause pain to others can help inhibit some childhood aggression. Discussion of recent acts of violence committed by young people in such a context also help. Anger control programs, as part of school health-promotion programs, also help decrease societal violence and produce more collaborative workers needed for the future.

The average child views an overwhelming number of television commercials by age 18, and these commercials influence daily and future choices and behaviors. Many television commercials focus on sugary foods that cause damage to teeth, diminish overall healthy habits, and lead to increased rates of obesity. Young children cannot always separate the program from the commercials and believe that they must purchase products the television says to buy. Many

childhood authorities question the ethics of exposing children to any type of advertising. Although concern about the effect of advertising has led to programming changes during children's watching time, more work is needed to send more socially responsible messages.

The world as presented on many television shows does not accurately reflect the real world. Despite an increasingly diverse and aging population, stereotypes of women and minority groups and a predominance of younger actors continue to make money for the media industry. Parents and health care providers should monitor television viewing to ensure the age appropriateness of the material, respond to television stations about inaccuracies in the content, and write letters to their newspaper or television networks to express concerns about the material presented. Parents may also participate with their children in responding to media presentations on learning and moral themes. Parents follow recommendations from the American Academy of Pediatrics, Committee on School Health, (2004) to limit television and media viewing to 2 hours per day, have media-free bedrooms, disallow television viewing while eating, and participate in national Turn Off the Television Week.

Some positive aspects of television viewing exist. A number of children's programs, such as "Sesame Street," "Wishbone" and "Kratt's Creatures" for younger children and "Bill Nye, the Science Guy," "Cyberchase," and "Zoom" for older children, have been deemed developmentally appropriate for children (PBS, 2008). Likewise, there are excellent websites for school-age children that stimulate their learning and promote their health.

Increasingly, parents engage their school-age children in learning and playing on a home computer. Although this technology serves as a good resource for locating information, writing papers, and organizing information, parents must limit the time students spend on computers. Likewise, limitations must be put on computer games that detract from socialization with peers and family and take time away from school work.

Legislation

Throughout this chapter, laws that support the health and well-being of the school-age child have been discussed. These laws include guidelines for the safe use of products, flame-retardant clothes, mandates against tobacco advertisements, and the nutritional guidelines for federally supported school lunch programs. Another important law is mandatory public education for disabled children. **Public Law 94-142 (Education for All Handicapped Children Act)**, established in 1977, states that any child with special needs (disabled) aged 5 to 21 years has the right to free appropriate public education in the least restrictive environment and evaluation by school or health professionals to identify learning needs. Disability includes having a limitation in one or more functional areas (USDHHS, 2000) and affects as many as 10% of children ages 5 to 17 years.

Many states begin educational services for affected children at 3 years of age based on an **individualized educational plan (IEP)** for that child and as mandated by law (Hockenberry & Wilson, 2007). The school nurse is responsible for collaborating with other school personnel and parents in ensuring that the IEP, including the health care needs of the child and connection to resources addressing the unique learning needs, receives attention. However, some parents have expressed concern that their "normal" or "gifted" child receives less attention in school systems because of the cost and time expenditures associated with implementing IEPs for disabled children. To add further concern, with recent school budgetary shortfalls, lesser-trained people than the school nurse often have responsibility for implementing IEPs. Despite these concerns, the value of Public Law 94-142 has been that disabled people have had their problems addressed in the educational arena.

To ensure access to educational opportunities for every individual, the U.S. Department of Education was developed in 1980. Through the U.S. Department of Education, President Bush enacted the **No Child Left Behind Act of 2001**, aimed at improving the academic achievement of the disadvantaged (U.S. Department of Education, 2008). The No Child Left Behind Act of 2001 intended to help ensure that all children have the opportunity to obtain a high-quality education and reach proficiency on challenging state academic standards and assessments. As a result of the No Child Left Behind Act of 2001, more reading progress was made by 9-year-olds in 5 years than the previous 28 years combined. Reading and math scores of 9-year-olds and fourth graders have reached all-time highs, and 46 states improved or held steady in all categories of students tested in reading and math (U.S. Department of Education, 2008).

Economics
Poverty

In the United States more than 22% of children less than 18 years of age live in families whose incomes are below the poverty level (National Center for Children in Poverty, 2009). Among diverse population groups, 50% of Black, 30% of Hispanic, and an unknown percentage of Native American children live in poor economic conditions that negatively influence their health. These conditions include unemployment, inadequate or crowded housing, poor sanitation, poor nutrition, low educational levels, and limited or sporadic access to health and social services perhaps due to lack of health insurance or contextual factors of these persons' lives. The number of uninsured children continues to be high, particularly among Hispanics (30%), and limits the number of children and families receiving primary health care (National Center for Children in Poverty, 2009; USDHHS, 2000). The lack of primary care among Black, Hispanic, and White children in rural areas prevents needed asthma management, dictating an expanded role for health care providers to connect families to resources for more effective disease control.

Many homeless children face poor living conditions and high rates of depression related to few friends and poor health status. Migrant children face more disease (e.g., tuberculosis, scabies, ear infections), injury, and dental caries and pose treatment challenges due to their transient status (Hockenberry & Wilson, 2007). The effects of limited financial resources on children include higher mortality rates at all ages than in those who are not poor or migrant and more lost school days because of illnesses. Numerous problems exist for children in poverty, including developmental delay due to poor nutrition, peer rejection, poor self-concept, increased risk of accidents and drug abuse, abuse or neglect from parents, and overall poor coping.

Nurses interacting with poor families and their children are familiar with federal health resources, such as the **State Children's Health Insurance Program (SCHIP)**. This program, part of the Balanced Budget Act of 1997 and implemented at the state level, supports comprehensive care to children 0 to 18 years who do not meet Medicaid criteria but live in families too poor to afford private insurance. This program has improved children's health by improving access for many groups (USDHHS, 2005h). The nurse improves the overall health of poor children by encouraging relationships with appropriate role models and by reinforcing strong family relationships that help children develop strong and positive self-images.

Affluence

Family wealth may have a negative influence on the school-age child if there is frequent substitute caregiving of varying quality due to parental absence, extremely high or unreasonable parental expectations, availability of material possessions but little child awareness of relevant responsibilities, and easy access to drugs and alcohol and similar dangers. The nurse reinforces the need in wealthy families for consistent demonstration of parental love and support, firm limits on appropriate behavior, and the value of recognizing the child's unique abilities. The nurse also offers ideas that will help decrease risk-taking behavior (e.g., drugs) and increase parent-child connection until a parent is in the home.

When discussing children raised in poverty or affluence, the nurse remembers at least two points. First, many variables affect each child, often in different ways, to influence overall development. Second, although personality and support networks help a child in a socially poor environment to excel later in life, most authorities believe that problems of affluence are easier to overcome than are the all-pervasive problems of poverty.

Health Care Delivery System
Well-Child Care

The American Academy of Pediatrics recommends that children 6 years and older have a well-child examination at least every 2 years by either a physician or a nurse practitioner (Hockenberry, 2005). In the ideal situation, the child has a primary health care provider, one person or practice from which the child receives wellness and illness care coordinated by members of a health care team. Unfortunately, many American children still do not have this quality of care (see the earlier section on economics). With increasing numbers living in poverty because of family violence, single parenthood, and divorce, many lack a primary care provider for their physical and emotional needs often due to a lack of health insurance. In this situation, they often receive emergency care only when they are very ill or injured.

The nurse encourages the school-age child and parents to be active members of any health evaluation. Children may give some of their own history, answer questions, and discuss their health concerns. During the history, the child's privacy should be respected. Some children in this age group want a parent present during the examination; others do not. When possible, the nurse spends at least some time alone with the child to allow discussions that the child may not feel comfortable with when parents are present. The examinations can also be a time for education on how the body works and ways to keep it healthy. Preventive information on diet and exercise can be offered relevant to prevention of obesity, cardiovascular disease, and diabetes. Information also can be obtained on school adjustment and performance, particularly because this is a major portion of the child's life. School performance can reflect the child's cognitive and general development. If there are any concerns, the nurse obtains more information through separate testing or discussion with school officials. Health education is directed to both the child and the parents for the best results. Activities that the child performs alone and with the family can give a picture of relationships and adjustments that relate to the child's health (see the Care Plan at the end of this chapter).

NURSING INTERVENTIONS

A challenge for nurses who work with school-age children is to maintain their normal healthy status and prevent illness. This task is accomplished through a variety of health-promotion mechanisms, such as examination, guidance, education, and legislation. The success of this health-promotion approach has been illustrated in at least one study in which Black children improved lifestyle choices when engaged in an intervention focused on cardiovascular health. Many professionals have noted that school-age children guided by the nurse generally seek health and use various resources to attain, maintain, or regain optimal health for their future productivity. Aspects of the nursing process are implemented when structuring a program to maintain the child's health (such as seen with an assessment of immunization status), promote health habits (seen with teaching bicycle safety), and prevent illness (seen by obtaining throat cultures to detect streptococcal infection).

Nurses have many opportunities and settings to help carry out their interventions as consultants, board members, and active providers of care. For example, nurses and school-age children interact during well-child evaluations and at school. Nurses in other roles, such as in public health and hospitals, also play a role in health promotion, although these nurses must often focus more on helping the child and family respond to an illness or a crisis. Local and national groups influence the health of children through their activities and regulations. These include organizations such as Boy Scouts and Girl Scouts, Big Brothers and Big Sisters, charities such as the Red Cross, and government agencies such as the Consumer Product Safety Commission.

School and the Nurse

As an integral part of the community, the school system has the responsibility to provide a healthy school environment and a comprehensive health education program. In some areas, nurses, physicians, and other health care workers work as a team in the school health program, which includes health care and maintenance and education. The nurse advocates and searches for resources so that each child has a source of health care, or the nurse is a nurse practitioner who delivers care. School health programs range from an occasional mention of body care and the changes of puberty to a full program that integrates physical and mental health principles into all aspects of the educational experience.

Comprehensive school health services require an interdisciplinary, coordinated effort between health care providers and educators. Recommendations state that each school should have an on-site nurse to conduct and mentor students and faculty in health-promotion areas. Nevertheless, many schools share nurses due to budgetary concerns (USDHHS, 2000). However, when available, nurses offer educational and interpersonal skills to initiate health-promotion teaching that improves the overall health of consumers (students, parents, teachers, community). Nurses have a wide scope of practice, including that of referring parents to relevant resources aimed toward activities that improve the school environment and its inhabitants.

The nurse's role in planning health maintenance for children of a school varies, depending on the type of health maintenance program. In one system, the school nurse may refer children to resources available to provide a source of health care, whereas in another system, the school nurse functions as a nurse practitioner. Based on scope of practice and state legal requirements, the school nurse monitors and updates children's immunizations and identifies and intervenes with children who have acute or chronic health care problems, such as scoliosis, strep throat, common cold, or child abuse. Increasingly school nurses provide sophisticated care according to evidence-based protocols for chronically ill school-age children who have been integrated into the regular academic environment. Based on state regulations, the nurse also engages in completing vision, hearing, and scoliosis screening at regular intervals. In most schools the nurse works with the school's physician, community physicians, and parents in meeting children's and community health needs.

For all school-age children, the school nurse plays a role in developing a healthy educational environment through promoting a comprehensive and age-appropriate health education program focused on children becoming responsible for their own health. A program aimed at accident prevention in and around the school is part of the nurse's role. The race includes assessing the school for pedestrian and automobile traffic patterns, broken playground and classroom equipment, ice and snow dangers, poorly maintained toilet facilities, and inappropriately prepared food. Regular practice drills are held to acquaint teachers and students with emergency procedures (i.e., fire, bomb, or intruder threats or actual events) (Hot Topics box). All people in the school are prepared to respond to chemical hazards. The nurse implements existing school-based programs on drug and alcohol abuse.

It is also important to consider the role of the nurse in fostering a healthy social environment in the school. The nurse examines the social interactions of the children and interacts with them to promote positive relationships. However, social problems continue to constitute a major concern for many children during this time. Children may experience difficulty in making the initial transition away from family and gaining satisfaction from a group of peers. Children may

HOTtopics

SCHOOL EMERGENCY PREPAREDNESS

Because children spend a significant portion of their day in school, pediatric emergencies such as exacerbation of a medical condition, behavioral crisis, and accidental /intentional injuries are likely to happen. Due to such risk, the American Academy of Pediatrics and the American Heart Association recommend the implementation of a Medical Emergency Response Plan (MERP; Hazinski, et al., 2004). The purpose of a MERP is to establish procedures within the school for the administration of emergency first aid services, emergency treatments, and administration of emergency medications for students. A plan helps schools prepare to respond to life-threatening medical emergencies in the first minutes before the arrival of EMS personnel. All procedures established in the MERP are to be followed during school hours, at school-sponsored activities, and while on school buses and other school property.

Due to the fact that injuries are the most common life-threatening emergency encountered, teachers, trainers, school nurses, and other school personnel should be trained and know general principals of first aid. Schools now employ fewer nurses, and school nurses often rotate between schools resulting in many schools without medical coverage for several hours/ days each week. As a result, much of the emergency care is the responsibility of teachers and other school personnel.

MERP should put the following core elements in place to provide the ability to save the greatest number of lives with the most efficient use of school equipment and personnel.
1. Establish an efficient and effective campus-wide communication system for each school
2. Develop a coordinated and practiced medical emergency response plan with the school nurses, physicians, athletic trainers, and the EMS system, with appropriate evaluation and quality improvement
3. Reduce the risk of life-threatening emergencies by identifying students at risk and ensuring that each has an individual emergency care plan and by reducing the risk of injury and disease triggers at the school
4. Train and equip teachers, staff, and students to provide CPR and first aid
5. Establish an (automated external defibrillator) AED program in schools

A recent study of school nurses assessing school disaster preparedness found 86% of school nurses surveyed had a Medical Emergency Response Plan in place, although 35% of those schools did not practice the implemented plan. Of the schools without a full-time school nurse, 17% did not have a MERP, and 17% did not identify a key responder for medical decisions in the event of a life-threatening emergency (Olympia et al., 2005).

Although most schools are in compliance with many of the recommendations for emergency preparedness, specific areas for improvement exist such as practicing the MERP and ensuring the identification of authorized personnel in the case of an emergency. Preparedness of schools to manage life-threatening emergencies requires the commitment of the entire community. The nurse is in a prime position to facilitate these community efforts and orchestrate partnerships between school officials, local EMS, school personnel, and local pediatricians to ensure the planning and implementation of a disaster plan.

Compiled from Hazinski, M., Markenson, D., Neish, S., Gerardi, M., Nichol, G. Taras, H. et al. (2004). Response to cardiac arrest and selected life-threatening medical emergencies—The medical emergency response plan for schools. *Circulation 109*(2), 278-291; Olympia, R., Wan, E., and Avner, J. (2005). The preparedness of schools to respond to emergencies in children: A national survey of school nurses. *Pediatrics, 116*, e738-e745.

CASE STUDY

Change in Usual Communication Pattern in School: Joey

Joey is an 8-year-old in elementary school. His teacher has voiced a growing concern regarding his classroom behavior. Over the past two months he has become more withdrawn from his classmates and rarely participates in class discussion. This is a new behavior in that he "used to talk all the time, and raise his hand to answer questions in class." His teacher reports that they were discussing family and family roles in class this week. Joey became very aggressive and yelled, "my dad isn't at home anymore 'cause of my mom,'" "I really miss dad. My mom's new boyfriend isn't nice and won't buy me stuff, like my dad does." His teacher determines Joey's parents are divorced. A parent-teacher conference has been scheduled to discuss Joey's behavior as it is now affecting his grades in school.

Continued

CASE STUDY

Change in Usual Communication Pattern in School: Joey—cont'd

Reflective Questions:

1. Is Joey's behavior appropriate for his age?
2. Joey's parents don't understand his change in behavior. His father yells. "If she would let me spend more time with MY son, Joey wouldn't be having trouble with school. She doesn't care about MY son now that *she* has *her* new boyfriend." How might the nurse respond to this situation?
3. What interventions might be effective for Joey's parents and teacher in improving his classroom behavior and school performance?

CARE PLAN

Change in Usual Communication Pattern in School: Joey

Nursing Diagnosis Ineffective coping related to disruption of home environment

DEFINING CHARACTERISTICS

- Frequent absences from school (1 day per week over the past 2 months)
- Change in quality of schoolwork. Grades have deteriorated over the past month.
- Verbal outbursts in class.

RELATED FACTORS

- Parents separated 9 months ago.
- Lives with mother, her boyfriend moved into home two months ago.
- Mom reports "he frequently complains of headache and stomachaches, but his doctor can't find anything wrong." Results in frequent absence.
- Visits father every other weekend.
- No siblings.

EXPECTED OUTCOMES

- Child will decrease number of absences from school related to "headache/stomachache" complaints.
- Child's grades will improve over the 9-week period.
- Parents will become more involved with the school in order to establish a relationship with the school that addresses the needs of the child related to home and school.

INTERVENTIONS (SCHOOL NURSE)

- Assess level of family problems within the home regarding communication between parents and visitation with child.
- Assess somatic complaints by the child. Have child complete "headache diary"/"stomachache diary" to determine aggravating/alleviating factors. Document frequency of complaints and discuss/review with parents.
- Meet with child to assess academic and emotional needs as they relate to home and school. Discuss findings with child's parents.
- Meet with the parents to develop a plan to help child meet academic goals and address emotional needs of the child. Involve child's teacher in plan development.
- Offer community resources to address emotional needs for the child such as support groups for children of divorced parents, Boy's Club of America, peer play groups. Include information for parent support resources as well.
- Offer after-school tutoring to facilitate meeting academic goals as desired.

For further information on developing care plans, see: Carpenito-Moyet, L. J. (2008). *Nursing diagnosis: Application to clinical practice* (12th ed.). Philadelphia: Lippincott, Williams & Wilkins.

make the initial adjustment but then have difficulties interacting with others (e.g., bullying). When problems such as these arise, the nurse, parents, and school system determine reasons for this behavior and intervene appropriately.

SUMMARY

Many changes occur in children during the exciting period of the school-age years. The child's development progresses from the immaturity of the preschooler to the beginning of adolescence and eventual adulthood. Cognitive abilities increase dramatically, adding to the desire to master tasks and the ability to develop moral judgment. The child's world expands beyond the family unit as school and peers begin to exert a major influence. Opportunities for nurses during this period occur primarily in ambulatory settings, with the school nurse frequently the most effective and influential health care provider for children of this age group and their families.

REFERENCES

Ahrens, M. (2004). *U.S. experience with smoke alarms & other fire detectors/alarm equipment.* Quincy, MA: National Fire Protection Association, Fire Analysis & Research Division.

Allen, R. L., Stuart, A., Everett, D., & Elangovan, S. (2004). Preschool hearing screening: Pass/refer rates for children enrolled in a head start program in eastern North Carolina. *American Journal of Audiology, 13*(1), 29–38.

Allgier, M. (2007). *Boosting sports to boost self-esteem* [on-line]. Retrieved from *www. articleclick.com/Article/Boosting-Sports-to-Boost-Self-Esteem/816.*

American Academy of Child & Adolescent Psychiatry. (2008). *Children and firearms.* Retrieved from *www.aacap.org/cs/root/ facts_for_families/children_and_firearms.*

American Academy of Pediatrics. (2002). *Educational rights for children with ADHD.* San Francisco: Jossey-Bass Publishers.

American Academy of Pediatrics. (2007). *Parenting corner Q&A: Child abuse.* Retrieved from *www.aap.org/healthtopics/childabuse.cfm.*

American Academy of Pediatrics. (2007). *Bright futures: Guidelines for health supervision of infants, children, and adolescents* (3rd ed.). Elk Park, IL: American Academy of Pediatrics.

American Academy of Pediatrics, Committee on Infectious Diseases. (2006). *Red Book: Report of the Committee on Infectious Diseases* (27th ed.). Elk Grove Village, IL: AAP.

American Academy of Pediatrics, American Heart Association. (2006). Policy Statement: Dietary recommendations for children and adolescents: A guide for practitioners. *Pediatrics, 117*(2), 544–559.

American Academy of Pediatrics, Committee on Injury and Poison Prevention. (2000). All-terrain vehicle injury prevention: Two-, three-, four-wheeled unlicensed motor vehicles. *Pediatrics, 105*(6), 1352–1354. Reaffirmation printed May 1, 2007.

American Academy of Pediatrics, Committee on School Health. (2004). *School health: Policy and practice* (6th ed.). Elk Grove Village, IL: AAP.

American Academy of Pediatrics, Committee on Quality Improvement, Subcommittee on Attention-Deficit/Hyperactivity Disorder. (2000). Clinical practice guideline: Diagnosis and evaluation of the child with attention-deficit/hyperactivity disorder. *Pediatrics, 105,* 1158–1170.

American Academy of Sleep Medicine. (2006). *Sleep & children* [on-line]. Retrieved January 30, 2009, from *www.sleepeducation.com/topic.aspx?id=8.*

American Association of Orthodontics. (2006). *Want information about orthodontic treatments for children? (Through age 12 years).* Retrieved October 12, 2007, from *www.braces.org/beautifulsmile/.*

American Dental Association. (2005). *Smile smarts curriculum* [on-line]. Retrieved January 30, 2009, from *www.ada.org/public/education/teachers/smilesmarts/smilesmarts_curriculum.pdf.*

American Dental Association. (2007). *Eruption charts, primary/secondary* [on-line]. Retrieved January 30, 2009, from *www.ada.org/public/topics/tooth-eruption.asp.*

American Heart Association. (2007). *High Blood pressure in children: AHA Recommendations* [on-line]. Retrieved January 30, 2009, from *www.americanheart.org/presenter.jhtml?identifyer=4009.*

American Heart Association. (2008). *Cigarette smoking in children* [on-line]. Retrieved January 30, 2009, from *http://americanheart.org/presenter.jhtml?identifier=4549.*

American Medical Association. (2007). *Appendix: Expert committee recommendations on the assessment, prevention, and treatment of child and adolescent overweight and obesity* [on-line]. Retrieved January 30, 2009, from *www.ama-assn.org/ama1/pub/upload/mm/433/ped_obesity_recs.pdf.*

American Occupational Therapy Association. (2007). *Helping your child to better handwriting.* Retrieved from *www.aota.org/Consumers/Tips/Youth/Handwriting/35181.aspx.*

American Optometric Association. (2007). *School vision: 6–18 years of age.* Retrieved from *http://aoa.org/x9451.xml.*

American Psychiatric Association. (2000). *Diagnostic and statistical manual of mental disorders* (4th ed.). Washington, DC: Author.

Ball, J., & Bindler, R. (2006). *Child Health Nursing: Partnering with Children & Families.* Upper Saddle River, NJ: Pearson-Prentice Hall.

Ball, J., & Bindler, R. (2008). *Pediatric Nursing: Caring for Children* (4th ed.). Upper Saddle River, NJ: Pearson-Prentice Hall.

Benson, E. (2003). Intelligent intelligence testing. *APA Monitor on Psychology, 34*(2), 48.

Bethram-Aguilar, E., Barker, L., Canto, M., Dye, B., Gooch, B., Griffin, S., et al. (2005). Surveillance for dental caries, dental sealants, tooth retention, edentulism, and enamel fluorosis. Retrieved January 30, 2009, from *www.cdc.gov/mmwr/preview/mmwrhtml/ss5403a1.htm.*

Better Brains for Babies. (2007). *Brain basics: Overview.* Retrieved from *www.fcs.uga.edu/ext/bbb/brainBasics.php.*

Borowitz, S. (2006). *Encopresis: Overview.* Retrieved from *http://emedicine.medscape.com/article/928795-overview.*

Bowman, S. A., Gortmaker, S. L., Ebbeling, C. B., Pereira, M. A., & Ludwig, D. S. (2004). Effects on fast-food consumption on energy intake and diet quality among children in a national household survey. *Pediatrics, 113,* 112–118.

Boyse, K. (2008). *Learning disabilities.* Retrieved from *www.childdevelopmentinfo.com/learning/learning_disabilities.shtml.*

Braet, C. (2006). Patient characteristics as predictors of weight loss after an obesity treatment for children. *Obesity, 14,* 148–155.

Butte, N., Garza, C., & de Onis, M. (2007). Evaluation of the feasibility of international growth standards for school-aged children and adolescents. *Journal of Nutrition, 137,* 153–157.

Centers for Disease Control and Prevention (CDC). (2005). *Preventing dental caries with community programs.* Retrieved from *www.cdc.gov/OralHealth/topics/child.htm.*

Centers for Disease Control and Prevention (CDC). (2005). *Preventing dental caries with community programs* [on-line]. Retrieved January 30, 2009, from *www.cdc.gov/OralHealth/factsheets/dental_caries.htm.*

Centers for Disease Control and Prevention (CDC). (2006). Mortality weekly report: General recommendations on immunization. *MMWR, 55*(RR15), 1–48.

Centers for Disease Control and Prevention (CDC). (2007a). *Healthy youth! Health topics nutrition* [on-line]. Retrieved January 30, 2009, from *www.cdc.gov/HealthyYouth/nutrition/index.htm.*

Centers for Disease Control and Prevention (CDC). (2007b). *Department of health and human services: CDC & prevention vaccine information statement—HPV.* Retrieved from *www.cdc.gov/std/Hpv/the-facts/default.htm.*

Centers for Disease Control and Prevention (CDC). (2008a). *Recommended immunization schedule for persons 0–6 years, 7–18 years.* Retrieved from *www.cdc.gov/vaccines/recs/schedules/child-schedule.htm#printable.*

Centers for Disease Control and Prevention (CDC). (2008b). *CDC childhood injury report.* Retrieved from *www.cdc.gov/safechild/Child_Injury_Data.htm.*

Centers for Disease Control and Prevention (CDC). (2009). *National Centers for Health Statistics: Clinical growth charts.* Retrieved from *www.cdc.gov/nchs/nhanes/growthcharts/clinical_charts.htm.*

Centers for Disease Control and Prevention (CDC). (2009b). High school students who tried to quit smoking cigarettes: US-2007. *MMWR, 58*(16), 428–431.

Children's Health Environmental Coalition. (2008). [on-line]. Retrieved January 30, 2009, from www.chenet.org/prodres_sche_overview.asp.

Chiolero, A., Bovet, D., Paradis, G., & Paccaud, F. (2007). Has blood pressure increased in children in response to the obesity epidemic? *Pediatrics, 119*(3), 544–553.

Chustecka, Z. (2006). Childhood cancer often cured, but damage from treatment persists for years. *New England Journal of Medicine, 355,* 1572–1582.

Commission for Environmental Cooperation. (2006). *Toxic chemicals and children's health in North America.* Retrieved from *www.cec.org.*

Daly, L., Kallan, M. J., Abogast, K. B., & Durbin, D. (2006). Risk of injury to child passengers in sport utility vehicles. *Pediatrics, 117*(1), 9–14.

Din-Dzietham, R., Liu, Y., Bielo, M., & Shamsa, F. (2007). High blood pressure trends in children and adolescents in national surveys, 1963-2002. *Circulation, 116,* 1488–1496.

Elliot, R. (2007). *Overcoming shyness.* [on-line]. Retrieved January 30, 2009, from *www.overcoming-shyness.com.*

Erikson, E. H. (1993). *Childhood and society* (2nd ed., reissued). New York: W. W. Norton.

Erikson, E. H. (1994). *Identity, youth and crisis* (35th ed., reissued). New York: W. W. Norton.

Fackler, A. (2005). *Growth and development, ages 6-10 years* [on-line]. Retrieved January 30, 2009, from *http://health.yahoo.com/children-behavior/growth-and-development-ages-6-to-10-years/healthwise_te6244.html.*

Faigenbaum, A. (2007). State of the art reviews: Resistance training for children and adolescence. *American Journal of Lifestyle Medicine, 1*(3), 190–200.

Finkelhor, D., & Ormod, F. (2001). *Homicide of children and youth.* Retrieved from *www.ncjrs.gov/pdffiles1/ojjdp/187239.pdf.*

Fisher-Owens, S., Gansky, S., Platt, L., Weintraub, J., Soobader, M., Bramlett, M., et al. (2007). Influences on children's oral health: A conceptual model. *Pediatrics, 120,* e510–e520.

Flynn, J. T. (2002). Differentiation between primary and secondary hypertension in children using ambulatory blood pressure monitoring. *Pediatrics, 110,* 89–93.

Flynn, J. T. (2004). New blood pressure guidelines call for early intervention. *AAP News, 25,* 290.

Freedman, D. S., Kahn, H. S., Mei, Z., Grummer-Strawn, L. M., Deitz, W. H., Srinivasan, S. R., et al. (2007). Relation of body mass index and waist-to-height ratio to cardiovascular disease risk factors in children and adolescents: The Bogalusa Heart Study. *American Journal of Clinical Nutrition, 86*(1), 33–40.

Fuller, C. (2007). Xylitol and ear infection treatment. *EzineArticles* [on-line]. Retrieved January 30, 2009, from *http://ezinearticles.com/?Xylitol_and_Ear_Infection_Treatment&id=571801.*

Gavin, M. L. (2007). *All about puberty* [on-line]. Retrieved January 30, 2009, from *www.kidshealth.org/kid/grow/body_stuff/puberty.html.*

Gavin, M. L. (2008). *Head lice.* Retrieved from *http://kidshealth.org/parent/infections/parasitic/lice.html#.*

Gaylor, E., Burnham, M., Goodlin-Jones, B., & Anders, T. (2005). A longitudinal follow-up study of young children's sleep patterns using a developmental classification system. *Behavioral Sleep Medicine, 3*(1), 44–61.

Gerberding, J. (2003). *CDC's role in promoting healthy lifestyles before Senate committee on appropriations, subcommittee on labor HHS, education & related agencies* [on-line]. Retrieved January 30, 2009, from *www.hhs.gov/asltestify/t030217.html.*

Gidding, S., Barton, B., Dorgan, J., Kimm, S., Kwiterovich, P., Lasser, N., et al. (2006). Higher self-reported physical activity is associated with lower systolic blood pressure: The Dietary Intervention Study in Childhood (DISC) *Pediatrics, 118*(6), 2388–2393.

Golonka, D. (2005). Reading and language development. *Healthwise.* Retrieved from *www.svcmc.org/18131.cfm.*

Goodgold, S. A., & Nielson, D. (2003). *Effectiveness of school-based backpack health promotion program-backpack intelligence.* Retrieved from *www.biomedexperts.com/Abstract.bme/14501090/Effectiveness_of_a_school-based_backpack_health_promotion_program_Backpack_Intelligence.*

Guilleminault, C., Palombini, L., Pelayo, R., & Chervin, R. D. (2003). Sleepwalking and sleep terrors in prepubertal children: What triggers them? *Pediatrics, 111,* e17–e25.

Hagan, J., Shaw, J., & Duncan, P. (2007). *Bright Futures Guidelines for health supervision of infants, children, and adolescents* (3rd ed.). Elk Grove, IL: American Academy of Pediatrics.

Haines, C. (2007). *Medline Plus: Food jags* [on-line]. Retrieved January 30, 2009, from *www.nlm.nih.gov/medlineplus/ency/article/002425.htm.*

Hansen, M., Gunn, P., & Kaelber, D. (2007). Underdiagnosis of hypertension in children and adolescents JAMA, 298(8), 874–879.

Harkreader, H., Hogan, M., & Thobaben, M. (2007). *Fundamentals of nursing care and clinical judgment.* St. Louis: Saunders.

Harvard Health Publications. (2007). *Sleepwalking and sleep terrors* [on-line]. Retrieved January 30, 2009, from *www.healthcentral.com/sleep-disorders/guide-154811-75.html.*

Hayden-Wade, H., Stein, R., Ghaderi, A., Saelens, B., Zabinski, M., & Wilfley, D. (2005). Prevalence, characteristics, and correlates of teasing experiences among overweight children vs. non-overweight peers. *Obesity Research, 13*(8), 1381–1392.

Hayman, L., Meininger, J., Daniels, S., McCrindle, B., Helden, L., Ross, J., et al. (2007). Primary prevention of cardiovascular disease in nursing practice: Focus on children and youth: A scientific statement from the American Heart Association Committee on Atherosclerosis, Hypertension, and Obesity in Youth of the Council on Cardiovascular disease in the Young, Council on Cardiovascular Nursing, Council on Epidemiology and Prevention, and Council on Nutrition, Physical activity, and Metabolism. *Circulation, 116*(3), 344–357.

Hazinski, M., Markenson, D., Neish, S., Gerardi, M., Hootman, J., Nichol, G., et al. (2004). Response to cardiac arrest and selected life-threatening medical emergencies: The medical emergency response plan for schools: A statement for healthcare providers, policy makers school administrators, and community leaders. *Circulation, 109*(2), 278–291.

Herman-Giddens, M., Kaplowitz, P., & Wasserman, R. (2004). Navigating the recent articles on girls' puberty in pediatrics: What do we know and where do we go from here? *Pediatrics, 113,* 911–917.

Hjalmas, K., Arnold, T., Bower, W., Caione, P., Chiozza, L. M., von Gontard, A., et al. (2004). Nocturnal enuresis: An international evidence based management strat-

egy. *The Journal of Urology, 171*(6 Pt 2), 2545–2561.

Hockenberry, M. J. (2005). *Wong's essentials of pediatric nursing* (7th ed.). St. Louis: Mosby.

Hockenberry, M. J., & Wilson, D. (2006). *Wong's nursing care of infants and children* (8th ed.). St. Louis, MO: Mosby.

Hoelscher, D., Day, R. S., Lee, E., Frankowski, R., Kelder, S., Ward, J., et al. (2004). Measuring the prevalence of overweight in Texas schoolchildren. *American Journal of Public Health, 94*(6), 1002–1008.

Homeier, B. (2004). *All about sleep* [on-line]. Retrieved January 30, 2009, from *www.kidshealth.org/parent/general/sleep/sleep.htm.*

Jenni, O., Fuhrer, H., Iglowstein, I., Molinari, L., & Largo, R. (2005). A longitudinal study of bed sharing and sleep problems among Swiss children in the first 10 years of life. *Pediatrics, 115,* 233–240.

Jordan, C. H., Spencer, S. J., Zanna, M. P., Hoshino-Browne, E., & Correll, J. (2003). Secure and defensive high self-esteem. *Journal of Personality & Social Psychology, 85*(5), 969–978.

Kaufman, L., & Schilling, D. (2007). Implementation of a strength training program for a 5-year-old child with poor body awareness and developmental coordination disorder. *Physical Therapy, 87*(4), 455–467.

Kellert, S. R. (2005). *Nature and childhood development. Building for life: Designing and understanding the human-nature connection.* Washington DC: Island Press.

Kohlberg, L. (1981). *The philosophy of moral development.* San Francisco: Harper & Row.

Koopman, H., Baars, R., Chaplin, J., & Zwinderman, K. (2004). Illness through the eyes of the child: The development of children's understanding of the causes of illness. *Patient Education Counseling, 55*(3), 363–370.

Kramer, S. (2007). *Kinesthetic math and language lessons.* Amsterdam: Susan Kramer.

Landgraf, J. M., Abidari, J., Cilento, B. G., Cooper, C. S., Schulman, S. L., & Ortenberg, J. (2004). Coping, commitment, and attitude: Quantifying the everyday burden of enuresis on children and their families. *Pediatrics, 113*(2), 334–344.

Lane, D., & Gill, P. (2004). Ethnicity and tracking blood pressure in children. *Journal of Human Hypertension, 18,* 223–228.

Lanningham-Foster, L., Jensen, T. B., Foster, R. C., Redmond, A. B., Walker, B. A., Heinz, D., et al. (2006). Energy expenditure of sedentary screen time compared with active screen time for children. *Pediatrics, 118*(6), e1831–e1835.

Lau, D. C., Douketis, J. D., Morrison, K. M., Hramiak, I. M., Sharma, A. M., & Ur, E. (2007). 2006 Canadian clinical practice guidelines on the management and prevention of obesity in adults and children [summary]. *Canadian Medical Association Journal, 176*(8), S1–S13.

Lee, M. (2006). *The neglected link between food marketing and childhood obesity in poor* neighborhoods. *Population Reference Bureau* [on-line]. Retrieved January 30, 2009, from *www.prb.org/Articles/2006/Theneglected linkfoodmarketingandchildhoodobesityinpoor-neighborhoods.aspx*.

Lee, J., Appugliese, D., Kaciroti, N., Corwyn, R., Bradley, R., & Lumeng, J. (2007). Weight status in young girls and onset of puberty. *Pediatrics, 119*, e624–e630.

Leukemia & Lymphoma Society. (2007). *Leukemia facts & statistics* [on-line]. Retrieved January 30, 2009, from *www.leukemia-lymphoma.org/all_page.adp?item_id=9346#_survival*.

Logsdon, A. (2009). *Average tests scores-Average test scores in special education*. Retrieved from *http://learningdisabilities.about.com/od/ac/g/average.htm*.

Lozano, J. A. (2004). Study: Texas kids among the nation's most overweight. *Fort Worth Star Telegram*, 5B, May 28, 2004.

Lucile Packard's Children's Hospital. (2007). *Growth and development 6-12 years* [on-line]. Retrieved January 30, 2009, from *www.pch.org/DiseaseHealthInfo/HealthLibrary/growth/schag612.htm*.

Lumeng, J., Somashekar, D., Appugliese, D., Kaciroti, N., Corwyn, R. & Bradley, R. (2007). Shorter sleep duration is associated with increased risk for being overweight at ages 9 to 12 years. *Pediatrics, 120*(5), 1020–1029.

Maiter, S. (2004). Considering context and culture in child protection services to the ethnically diverse families: An example from research with parents from the Indian sub continent (South Asians). *Social Work Research and Evaluation, 5*(1), 63–80.

McClain, K., & Fletcher, R. (2007). *Causes of peripheral lymphadenopathy in children* [on-line]. Retrieved January 30, 2009, from *http://gslbpatients.uptodate.com/topic.asp?file=gen_pedi/6167#5*.

McKinney, E., James, S., Murray, S., & Ashwill, J. (2005). *Maternal-child nursing* (2nd ed.). St. Louis: Elsevier.

Moore, M., Allison, D., & Rosen, C. L. (2006). A review of pediatric nonrespiratory sleep disorders. *Chest, 130*(4), 1252–1262.

Moore, M., White, G., & Moore, D. (2007). Association of relative backpack weight with reported pain, pain sites, medical utilization, and lost school time in children and adolescents. *Journal of School Health, 77*, 232–239.

Myers, B. (2009). *Helping your child develop self-esteem*. Retrieved from *www.healthyplace.com/adhd/add-focus/helping-your-child-develop-self-esteem/menu-id1580/*.

National Cancer Institute. (2007). *A snapshot of pediatric cancers* [on-line]. Retrieved January 30, 2009, from *http://planning.cancer.gov/disease/Pediatric-Snapshot.pdf*.

National Center for Children in Poverty. (2009). *Ten important questions about child poverty and family economic hardship*. Retrieved from *www.nccp.org/faq.html#question8*.

National Centers for Health Statistics. (2000). *2000 CDC growth charts: United States*. Retrieved from *www.cdc.gov/nchs/nhanes/growthcharts/clinical_charts.htm*.

National Highway Traffic Safety Administration. (2008). *Child passenger safety*. Retrieved from *www.nhtsa.gov/portal/site/nhtsa/template.MAXIMIZE/menuitem.9f8c7d6359e0e9bbbf30811060008a0c/?javax.portlet.tpst=4427b997caacf504a8bdba101891ef9a_ws_MX&javax.portlet.prp_4427b997caacf504a8bdba101891ef9a_viewID=detail_view&itemID=ce45e2542a964110VgnVCM1000002fd17898RCRD&viewType=standard*.

National Institute of Child Health & Human Development. (2007). *What is Puberty?* Retrieved October 7, 2007, from *www.nichd.nih.gov/health/topics/Puberty.cfm*.

National Institute for Family Literacy. (2006). *The effect of family literacy interventions on children's acquisition of reading*. Portsmouth, NH: RMC Research Corporation.

National Institute of Mental Health. (2007). *ADHD* [on-line]. Retrieved January 30, 2009, from *www.nimh.nih.gov/health/publications/adhd/complete-publication.shtml*.

National Institute of Mental Health. (2009). *Depression*. Retrieved from *www.nimh.nih.gov/health/publications/depression/complete-index.shtml*.

National Safety Council. (2007). *Workplace venue alerts*. Retrieved from *www.nsc.org/email/library_alerts/79253_workplace/index.htm*.

Nederkoorn, C., Jansen, E., Mulkens, S., & Jansen, A. (2007). Impulsivity predicts treatment outcome in obese children. *Behavior Research & Therapy, 45*(5), 1071–1075.

Needlman, R. (2004). *Pathways of learning: The quiz*. Retrieved from *www.drspock.com/article/0,1510,6215,00.html?r=hott*.

Nield, L., Cakan, N., & Kamat, D. (2007). A practical approach to precocious puberty. *Clinical Pediatrics, 46*(4), 299–306.

Ogden, C., Carroll, M., Curtin, L., McDowell, M., Tabak, C., & Flegal, K. (2006). Prevalence of overweight and obesity in the United States, 1999-2004, *JAMA, 295*(13), 1549–1555.

Olympia, R., Wan, E., & Avner, J. (2005). The preparedness of schools to respond to emergencies in children: A national survey of school nurses. *Pediatrics, 116*, e738–e745.

Owens, J. (2004). Sleep in children: Cross cultural perspectives. *Sleep & Biological Rhythms, 2*(3), 165–173.

Piaget, J. (2001). *Psychology of intelligence*. Florence, KY: Routledge, Taylor and Francis Group.

Podoll, A., Grenier, M., Croix, B., & Feig, D. (2007). Inaccuracy in pediatric outpatient blood pressure measurement. *Pediatrics, 119*(3), e538–e543.

Powell, L., Szczypka, G., & Chaloupka, F. (2007). Exposure to food advertising on television among US children. *Archives of Pediatric Adolescent Medicine, 161*(6), 553–560.

Proctor, M. H., Moore, L. L., Gao, D., Cupples, L. A., Bradlee, M. L., Hood, M. Y., et al. (2003). Television viewing and changes in body fat from preschool to early adolescence: The Framingham Children's Study. *International Journal of Obesity and Related Metabolic Disorders, 27*(7), 827–833.

Public Broadcast Station. (2008). [on-line]. Retrieved January 30, 2009, from *www.pbs.org*.

Rauch, F. (2007). Bone accrual in children: Adding substance to surfaces. *Pediatrics, 119*(suppl), s137–s140.

Redline, S., Storfer-Isser, A., Rosen, C. L., Johnson, N. L., Kirchner, H. L., Emancipator, J., et al. (2007). Association between metabolic syndrome and sleep-disordered breathing in adolescents. *American Journal of Respiratory and Critical Care Medicine, 176*(4), 401–408.

Reid, P. (2003). More than a game? The role of sports governing bodies in the development of sport education programmes. *European Physical Education Review, 9*(3), 309–317.

Robinson, S. (2006). Victimization of obese adolescents. *The Journal of School Nursing, 22*(4), 201–206.

SafeKids. (2007). *SafeKids: Walk this way*. Retrieved from *www.usa.safekids.org/wtw/tips.html*.

Schmitt, B. D. (2005). *Your child's health: The parent's one-stop reference guide to symptoms, emergencies, common illnesses, behavior problems, and healthy development*. New York: Bantam.

School Nutrition Association. (2006). *Study: Schools offering more nutritious food and beverage items* [on-line]. Retrieved January 30, 2009, from *www.schoolnutrition.org/Index.aspx?id=1970*.

Sheslow, D. (2008). *Developing your child's self-esteem*. Retrieved from *www.kidshealth.org/parent/emotions/feelings/self_esteem.html*.

Siegal, M., & Peterson, C. (Eds.). (2005). *Children's understanding of biology & health*. New York: Cambridge University Press.

Slyper, A. H. (2004). The pediatric obesity epidemic: Causes and controversies. *The Journal of Clinical Endocrinology and Metabolism, 89*(6), 2540–2547.

Spinks, A., & McClure, R. (2007). Quantifying the risk of sports injury: A systematic review of activity—specific rates for children under 16 years of age. *British Journal of Sports Medicine, 41*, 548–557.

Stein, M. T. & Perrin, E. L. (1998). Guidance for effective discipline. American Academy of Pediatrics. Committee on Psychosocial Aspects of Child and Family Health (Abstract). *Pediatrics, 101*(4 Pt 1), 723–728.

Stein, R., Epstein, L., Raynor, H., Kilanowski, C., & Paluch, R. (2005). The influence of parenting change on pediatric weight control. *Obesity Research, 13*, 1749–1755.

Stevens, S. (2005). What is the evil eye? *ezineArticles* [on-line]. Retrieved January 30, 2009, from *http://ezinearticles.com/?what-is-the-evil-eye?&id=20447.*

Stock, S., Miranda, C., Evans, S., Plessis, S., Ridley, J., Yeh, S., et al. (2007). Health buddies: A novel, peer-led health promotion program for the prevention of obesity and eating disorders in children in elementary school. *Pediatrics, 120,* e1059–e1068.

Stop Smoking Update. (2009). *Helping your child to stop smoking.* Retrieved from *www.stop-smoking-updates.com/quitsmoking/family/care/helping-your-child-stop-smoking.htm*

Tobacco Free Kids. (2007). [on-line]. Retrieved January 30, 2009, from *www.tobaccof-reekids.org/script/Display/PressRelease.php3?Display=1049.*

Tynan, W. D. (2008). *Teaching your child self-control.* Retrieved from *http://kidshealth.org/parent/emotions/behavior/self_control.html#.*

University of Virginia Health System. (2006). *Hindu beliefs & practices affecting healthcare* [on-line]. Retrieved January 30, 2009, from *www.healthsystem.virginia.edu/internet/chaplaincy/hindu.cfm#illness.*

Urrutia-Rojas, X., Egbuchunam, C., Bae, S., Menchaca, J., Bayona, M., Rivers, P., et al. (2006). *High blood pressure in school children: Prevalence and risk factors.* [on-line]. Retrieved January 30, 2009, from *www.medscape.com/viewarticle 548588_1 posted 1/8/2007.*

U.S. Department of Agriculture. (2008). *National School Lunch Program* [on-line]. Retrieved January 30, 2009, from *www.fns.usda.gov/cnd/Lunch/AboutLunch/NSLPFactSheet.pdf.*

U.S. Department of Agriculture, Center for Nutrition Policy and Promotion. (2005). *MyPyramid.* Retrieved May 31, 2005, from *www.mypyramid.gov.*

U.S. Department of Education. (2008). *No Child Left Behind update* [on-line]. Retrieved January 30, 2009, from *www.ed.gov/print/about/overview/mission/mission.html.*

U.S. Department of Health and Human Services [USDHHS]. (2000). *Healthy people 2010.* (Vol. 1 and 2) (Conference ed.). Washington, DC: U.S. Government Printing Office.

U.S. Department of Health and Human Services [USDHHS]. (2004). *Average blood pressure levels on the rise among American children/teenagers. NIH News,* [on-line]. Retrieved January 30, 2009, from *www.nih.gov/news/pr/may2004/nhlbi-04.htm.*

U.S. Department of Health and Human Services. (2005a). *Overweight and physical activity among children: A portrait of states and the nation, 2005* [on-line]. Retrieved January 30, 2009, from *http://mchb.hrsa.gov/overweight/portrait/2children.htm.*

U.S. Department of Health and Human Services. (2005b). *Healthy people 2010 midcourse review (oral health)* [on-line]. Retrieved January 30, 2009, from *www.healthypeople.gov/data/midcourse/focusareas/FA21ProgressHP.htm.*

U.S. Department of Health and Human Services. (2005c). *Healthy People 2010 midcourse review (nutrition and overweight)* [on-line]. Retrieved January 30, 2009, from *www.healthypeople.gov/data/midcourse/focusareas/FA19ProgressHP.htm.*

U.S. Department of Health and Human Services. (2005d). *Healthy People 2010 midcourse review (vision and hearing)* [on-line]. Retrieved January 30, 2009, from *www.healthypeople.gov/data/midcourse/focusareas/FA28ProgressHP.htm.*

U.S. Department of Health and Human Services. (2005e). *Healthy People 2010 midcourse review (safety and violence)* [on-line]. Retrieved January 30, 2009, from *www.healthypeople.gov/data/midcourse/focusareas/FA15ProgressHP.htm.*

U.S. Department of Health and Human Services. (2005f). *Healthy People 2010 midcourse review (immunizations and infectious disease)* [on-line]. Retrieved January 30, 2009, from *www.healthypeople.gov/data/midcourse/focusareas/FA14ProgressHP.htm.*

U.S. Department of Health and Human Services. (2005g). *Healthy People 2010 midcourse review (respiratory disease)* [on-line]. Retrieved January 30, 2009, from *www.healthypeople.gov/data/midcourse/focusareas/FA24ProgressHP.htm.*

U.S. Department of Health and Human Services. (2005h). [on-line]. Retrieved January 30, 2009, from *www.cms.hhs.gov/NationalSCHIPPolicy/07_EvaluationsAndReports.asp#TopOfPage.*

U.S. Department of Health and Human Services. (2006). School Health Policies and Programs Study (SHPPS, 2006). *Tobacco-use prevention,* [on-line]. Retrieved January 30, 2009, from *www.cdc.gov/shpps.*

U.S. Department of Health and Human Services. (2006). School Health Policies and Programs Study (SHPPS, 2006). *Violence prevention,* [on-line]. Retrieved January 30, 2009, from *www.cdc.gov/shpps.*

U.S. Department of Health and Human Services. (2006). *Youth overweight increased risk of bone fracture, muscle & joint pain* [on-line]. Retrieved January 30, 2009, from *www.nih.gov/news/pr/Jun2006/nichd.htm.*

U.S. Department of Health and Human Services. (2007a). *National Center for Health Statistics: CDC Growth Charts,* [on-line]. Retrieved January 30, 2009, from *http://cdc.gov/nchs/about/major/nhanes/growthcharts/datafiles.htm.*

U.S. Department of Health and Human Services. (2007b). *Healthy eating and physical activity across your lifespan. Helping your child: Tips for parents* [on-line]. Retrieved January 30, 2009, from *http://win.niddk.nih.gov/publications/child.htm.*

U.S. Department of Justice. (2005). *A guide to disability rights laws* [on-line]. Retrieved January 30, 2009, from *www.usdoj.gov/ada/guide.htm.*

Van Voorhees, B. (2006). *Medline Plus: Weight Problems and Children* [on-line]. Retrieved January 30, 2009, from *www.nlm.nih.gov/medlineplus/ency/article/001999.htm.*

Warwick, K. (2001). *QI: The quest for intelligence.* Loughton, Essex: Piatkus Publishing.

World Health Organization. (2007). [on-line]. Retrieved January 30, 2009, from *www.who.int/growthref/en/.*

Chapter 21

Martha Driessnack*

Adolescent

objectives

After completing this chapter, the reader will be able to:

- Distinguish between the terms *puberty* and *adolescence*.
- Summarize the physical growth, developmental, and maturational changes that occur during adolescence.
- Outline the recommended schedule of health-promotion and preventive health visits and the appropriate topics for discussion with the adolescent during each visit.
- Analyze factors that contribute to risk-taking behaviors and situations during adolescence.
- Develop a health teaching plan addressing some of the physical, emotional, social, and spiritual challenges facing adolescents.

key terms

Acne	Formal operations	Primary sexual characteristics
Adolescence	Gynecomastia	Puberty
Anorexia nervosa	Idealism	Purge
Binge eating disorder	Identity vs. role confusion	Risk-taking behaviors
Body image	Introspection	Scoliosis
Bulimia nervosa	Klinefelter syndrome	Secondary sexual characteristics
Comedones	Menarche	Sexually transmitted diseases (STDs)
Date rape	Menstruation	Tanner staging
Depression	Nocturnal emissions	Turner syndrome
Egocentrism	Obesity	
Ejaculation	Overweight	
Emancipated minors	Peer group	

website materials

evolve These materials are located on the book's website at *http://evolve.elsevier.com/Edelman/*.
- WebLinks
- Study Questions
- Glossary

*The author acknowledges the work of Marinda Allender in a previous edition of the chapter.

Risk Behaviors in Adolescents

The mortality rate for adolescents is 3 times higher than it is for school-age children.

Suicide rates in adolescents are increasing across all ethnic groups.

Increasing numbers of young adolescents are not only becoming sexually active but also are choosing not to use any protection or contraception.

1. What growth and developmental factors make adolescents susceptible to these risky situations?

2. What anticipatory guidance and strategies might be offered to adolescents and their families to prevent this risky behavior?

THINK About It

Healthy People 2010

Selected Health-Promotion and Disease-Prevention Objectives for Adolescents

- Reduce the prevalence of overweight and obesity in adolescents ages 12 through 19.
- Reduce the incidence of suicide and injurious suicide attempts among adolescents ages 15 through 19.
- Reduce deaths caused by motor vehicle accidents among youths ages 15 through 24.
- Increase the proportion of high school seniors who associate risk of physical or psychological harm with heavy use of alcohol, regular use of marijuana, and experimentation with cocaine.
- Increase the proportion of adolescents in grades 9 through 12 who abstain from intercourse or use condoms if sexually active.

From U.S. Department of Health and Human Services. (2000). *Healthy People 2010.* Washington, DC: U.S. Government Printing Office. Centers for Disease Control and Prevention (CDC). (2004). *Improving the Health of Adolescents and Young Adults.* Official companion document to *Healthy People 2010.* For information on the upcoming *Healthy People 2020,* go to *www.healthypeople2020.gov.*

The period of **adolescence** is defined as beginning with the onset of puberty, around age 11 to 13 years, and ending with the achievement of independence from the primary family unit, which occurs around ages 18 to 22 years but varies with prolonged undergraduate and graduate education (e.g., undergrad, grad school). The term adolescence refers to the psychosocial, emotional, cognitive, and moral transition from childhood to young adulthood, while **puberty** refers to the development and maturation of the reproductive, endocrine, and structural processes that lead to fertility.

Rapid change in physical, psychosocial, spiritual, moral, and cognitive growth—the most characteristic trait of adolescence—creates an extremely tenuous sense of balance. A pivotal developmental period, adolescence offers health care providers unique opportunities for health-promotion and preventive services. Providing knowledge about the changes, challenges, and choices adolescents will encounter, as well as the tools with which to approach them, encourages and reinforces developing competencies and sense of responsibility (American Academy of Pediatrics, 2008; Berger, 2004; Seidel et al., 2006). The *Healthy People 2010* box presents selected general objectives related to adolescent health.

AGE AND PHYSICAL CHANGES

In contrast to the slow, steady growth of childhood, adolescents experience accelerated growth that dramatically alters their body size and proportions. The most noticeable changes in adolescence involve physical and sexual growth, including the appearance of **secondary sexual characteristics**. These changes occur in a predictable sequence, but the onset and duration of the sequencing varies from individual to individual. Females usually begin puberty 2 years earlier than males and experience their growth spurt earlier. The appearance and sequence of secondary sexual characteristics and pubertal events are summarized in Table 21-1 and later illustrated in Figure 21-3.

The physical changes experienced during adolescence are mediated primarily by the hormonal regulatory systems in the hypothalamus, pituitary gland, gonads, and adrenal glands (Pinyerd & Zipf, 2005) (Figure 21-1). The hypothalamus releases gonadotropin-releasing hormone, which stimulates the anterior pituitary to release the gonadotropin hormones (GnRF), luteinizing hormone (LH), and follicle-stimulating hormone (Ball & Bindler, 2008). In females, this stimulates ovarian development and estrogen production. Estrogen produces all secondary sex characteristics except axillary and pubic hair, which are controlled by adrenal androgens. In males, luteinizing hormone results in testicular enlargement and the development of Leydig cells in the testes, which produce testosterone. Follicle-stimulating hormone stimulates the development of the seminiferous tubules of the testes, leading to spermatogenesis and fertility. Once sexual maturation is completed, the ongoing release of hormones controls menses, pregnancy, and lactation. **Menarche**, the onset of menses in females, usually occurs late in puberty as the growth spurt is subsiding (Ball & Bindler, 2008). Adolescents who do not follow the normal sequence or who have not begun pubertal development by age 14 years, for males, and age 13 years, for females, should have an endocrine evaluation (Greydanus et al., 2006; Pinyerd & Zipf, 2005).

Before the growth spurt, many adolescents experience a transient increase in body fat or adipose tissue. As puberty progresses, the proportion of total body weight composed of fat usually declines, particularly in boys. Body fat begins to accumulate again in both genders after their growth spurt, but at a slightly higher rate in females.

The heart grows in size and strength. Blood volume and blood pressure increase, and the heart rate decreases to adult levels. These cardiovascular changes occur earlier in females and parallel puberty. Adolescent females also generally have higher pulse rates and slightly lower systolic blood pressure than males. Adolescents are identified as hypertensive when their systolic or diastolic blood pressure is at or above

Growth and Development   Table 21-1

Sexual Maturity Rating, Tanner Stages: Developmental Stages: of Secondary Sexual Characteristics

Stage	Male Genital Development	Pubic Hair Development	Female Breast Development	Other Changes
1	Prepubertal	No distinction between hair over pubic area and hair over abdomen		
2	Initial enlargement of scrotum and testes; reddening and texture changes of scrotum	Sparse growth of long, straight, downy hair at base of penis or along labia	Enlargement of areolar diameter; small area of elevation around papillae (breast bud)	Usual time of peak height velocity for girls
3	Initial enlargement of penis, mainly in length; further growth of testes and scrotum	Hair becomes dark, coarse, and curly; spreads sparsely over entire pubic area	Further elevation and enlargement of breasts and areolas, with no separation of their contours	Usual time of menarche; facial hair begins to grow on upper lip and voice deepens in boys
4	Further enlargement of penile diameter, testes, scrotum, and glans	Further spread of hair distribution, not extending to thighs	Areolas and papillae project from breast to form secondary mound	Usual time of peak height velocity for boys; axillary hair begins to grow
5	Adult in size and contour	Adult in amount and type; spreads to inner surface of thighs	Adult, with projection of papillae only; recession of areolas into general breast contour	

Modified from Hockenberry, M. J., & Wilson, D. (2007). Wong's nursing care of infants and children (8th ed.). St. Louis: Mosby.

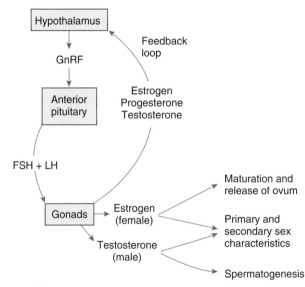

Figure 21-1   Hormonal interaction among hypothalamus, pituitary, and gonads. FSH, follicle-stimulating hormone, GnRF, gonadotropin-releasing hormone; LH, luteinizing hormone. (From Hockenberry, M. J., & Wilson, D. [2007]. *Wong's nursing care of infants and children* [8th ed.]. St. Louis: Mosby.)

the 95th percentile (based on age, gender, and height) on three separate occasions.

Respiratory rate decreases throughout childhood, reaching an average rate of 15 to 20 breaths per minute during adolescence. Respiratory volume and vital capacity increase, particularly in males. The larynx and vocal cords grow, producing the characteristic voice changes of puberty. Both male and female voices become deeper and laryngeal cartilage enlarges, with both effects more pronounced in males.

The gastrointestinal system reached functional maturity during school-age years. However, it continues to grow along with the growth spurt (Ball & Bindler, 2008; Guyton & Hall, 2006).

Permanent teeth begin erupting around 6 years of age, and all 32, except the third molars, or wisdom teeth, are in place by 13 to 14 years of age. Third molars are often pulled during adolescence to make space for the other permanent teeth. However, it is increasingly common for them never to develop (Burns et al., 2008).

Both the sweat and sebaceous glands become more active during adolescence. The sweat glands are located primarily in the axillary, genital, and periumbilical areas and are the primary source of body odor. The sebaceous glands are located primarily on the face, neck, shoulders, upper back, chest, and genitals. They can become clogged and inflamed, leading to the common teenage condition called **acne**. Acne occurs in up to 80% to 85% of all adolescents and young adults (Burns et al., 2008).

Acne

Adolescents typically are concerned about their skin changes. The sebaceous glands increase production of sebum, a primary factor in the pathogenesis of acne. The sebaceous follicles become clogged with sebum and debris, forming open (blackheads) or closed (whiteheads) **comedones**. The incidence of acne within families suggests that hereditary factors are involved.

Thorough examination of the adolescent's skin and a discussion of its impact on the overall body image are necessary to determine appropriate management strategies. Intervention should include teaching the individual about the pathophysiological nature of acne. Knowledge allows the adolescent to become instrumental in its management and helps dispel common myths about acne and its care.

Washing with soap and water 2 or 3 times a day is the best way to remove dirt and oil. Vigorous scrubbing should be discouraged, because the skin can become irritated, leading to follicular rupture. The adolescent should not attempt to remove the pustules and papules that form. Squeezing the lesion can result in further irritation of the gland and permanent injury to the tissue. Many nonprescription topical medications contain benzoyl peroxide, which is bacteriostatic and comedolytic. Unfortunately, these agents cause drying and peeling; therefore, therapy is begun with application of 5% strength once a day. If tolerated, after 2 weeks the application is increased to twice a day.

Adolescent females need to be careful when selecting makeup. Most preparations, when applied extensively over the face, prevent adequate exposure to air and light, especially those that have a fat base. Sunlight can have a beneficial effect on acne; however, prolonged exposure should be avoided. Stress can exacerbate acne in some adolescents. In these cases, stress management techniques should be considered. The effect of diet on acne is a highly controversial issue. Evidence indicates that dietary restrictions specific to acne are unnecessary.

Adolescents with acne need support and understanding. The nurse can help adolescents and their families understand that management does not result in immediate improvement. In fact, topical agents may make acne appear worse initially, with any improvement occurring slowly over several months.

Scoliosis

A common skeletal deformity found in adolescents is **scoliosis**, a lateral S-shaped curvature of the spine (Figure 21-2). The curve is typically convex to the right. Classifications of scoliosis include secondary or functional, congenital, neuromuscular, constitutional, and idiopathic, which has an infantile, juvenile, or adolescent onset. Approximately 10% of all adolescents have a mild truncal asymmetry; however, curves greater than 15 degrees are abnormal and can progress to significant curvature during the growth spurt (Burns et al., 2008). Idiopathic scoliosis is the most common type and is significantly more prevalent in females. Early intervention is important, because untreated scoliosis can result in disfigurement, impaired mobility, and cardiopulmonary complications.

The nurse includes scoliosis screening in the assessment of both prepubertal and pubertal adolescents, paying close attention to the timing of the growth spurt. Most adolescents with scoliosis will require only observation; however, bracing and surgical correction may be necessary and early referral to an orthopedic surgeon is important. Early identification can help avoid more invasive care and prevent the long-term consequences.

Gender

During puberty, **primary sexual characteristics** begin to develop and secondary sexual characteristics emerge. Primary sexual characteristics involve the organs necessary for reproduction, such as the penis and testes in boys and the vagina and uterus in girls. Secondary sexual characteristics are external features that are not essential for reproduction.

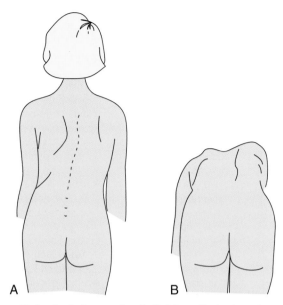

Figure 21-2   Scoliosis screening. So that the entire back can be seen, the adolescent should remove all clothing from the upper body when being assessed for scoliosis. **A,** While the adolescent stands up straight, check for any asymmetry; observe and palpate for differences in shoulder or scapular height, prominence of either scapula or hip, waist asymmetry, and misalignment of the spinous processes. Lateral curvature and thoracic convexity of the spine indicate scoliosis. **B,** With feet together, legs straight, and arms hanging freely, the adolescent bends forward until the back is parallel with the floor. Check for prominence of the ribs, or rib hump, on one side only and hip and leg asymmetry. With scoliosis, the chest wall on the side of convexity is prominent, and the scapula on the side of convexity is elevated.

Breast development, facial and pubic hair growth, and lowering of the voice are examples of secondary sex characteristics (see Table 21-1). Sexual maturity rating, also referred to as **Tanner staging,** is used widely to assess and monitor the degree of maturation of an adolescent's primary and secondary sexual characteristics. Each of the characteristics, breast, pubic hair, and genitals, is staged separately (from 1 to 5) and compared with the expected sequencing (Figure 21-3).

Breast development usually is confined to females; however, some degree of unilateral or bilateral breast enlargement, termed **gynecomastia,** may appear early in male puberty, just before the growth spurt. Gynecomastia is usually temporary and typically disappears. However, occasionally it persists and leads to body image problems and can be surgically reduced if psychological assessment warrants it.

The first sign of puberty in males is a thinning of the scrotal sac and enlargement of the testicles. **Ejaculation** is considered a milestone of male puberty and precedes fertility by several months. **Nocturnal emissions,** or "wet dreams," can concern adolescent males, because the event happens beyond their control.

For females the first sign of puberty is the appearance of breast buds, followed by the growth spurt. The onset of **menstruation,** or menarche, occurs approximately 2 years after the appearance of the breast buds and near the end of the growth spurt.

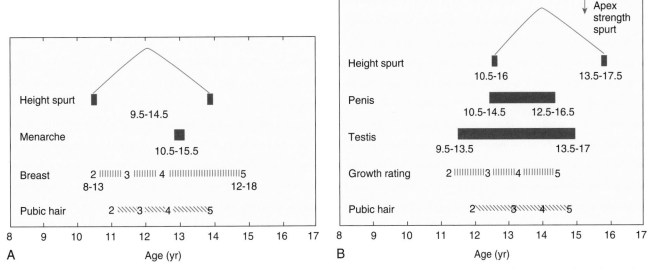

Figure 21-3   Diagram of sequences of events at adolescence in girls **(A)** and boys **(B)**. Single numbers *(2, 3, 4, 5)* indicate stages of development. The average is represented. A range of ages when each event may begin and end is indicated by inclusive numbers listed below each event. (Modified from Marshall, W. A., & Tanner, J. M. [1969]. Variations in pattern of pubertal changes in girls. *Archives of Disease in Childhood, 44,* 291-303; Hockenberry, M. J., & Wilson, D. [2007]. *Wong's nursing care of infants and children* [8th ed.]. St. Louis: Mosby.)

Familiarity with the stages of development of sexual characteristics and their expected sequence helps the nurse monitor the adolescent's progression through puberty and detect any variations that might herald an alteration in normal growth and development.

Genetics

Most genetic problems are discovered during infancy and early childhood. Some syndromes, however, may not be diagnosed until adolescence. These genetic disorders frequently are discovered during the assessment of an adolescent with delayed or irregular pubertal development (Innovative Practice box).

Turner syndrome (XO) is a female disorder in which only one X chromosome is present instead of two. Assessment findings include short stature, a webbed neck, a low posterior hairline, low-set ears, a shield-shaped chest with widely spaced nipples, and gonadal-ovarian dysgenesis, resulting in a lack of sexual development and menses during puberty. Cardiac and renal anomalies are often present. Learning disabilities are common. Management consists primarily of growth hormone, to increase height, and estrogen therapy to help develop secondary sexual characteristics and menses. However, the female with Turner syndrome remains sterile. Ongoing emotional support for the adolescent and her family is important.

Klinefelter syndrome (XXY) is seldom diagnosed before puberty. Males have an extra chromosome and typically are tall, initially thin, and do not develop secondary sexual characteristics. They often have gynecomastia. Klinefelter syndrome is associated with learning or behavior problems during childhood. As with Turner syndrome, management typically involves androgen therapy and counseling; however, the adolescent remains sterile.

innovative practice

My Family Health Portrait

Teens can create a simple pedigree with the Surgeon General's *My Family Health Portrait* at *http://familyhistory.hhs.gov. My Family Health Portrait* is a downloadable, web-based tool for use on a personal computer. It helps individuals create their own family health history and is a part of the National Human Genome Research Institute (NHGRI) and the U.S. Surgeon General's Family History Initiative. Because it is web-based, teens may be the family member best prepared (or most technologically comfortable) to coordinate the input of data. With their family's help, teens gather their family health history, then, using any type of computer, build a drawing of their family tree and a chart of their family health history. Both the chart and the drawing can be printed and shared with other family members and health care providers.

In November, 2004, the U.S. Surgeon General, Richard Carmona, and the Department of Health and Human Services (HHS) launched a national public health campaign to focus attention on the importance of the family health history in predicting the disorders individuals may be at risk for and in helping individuals take action to keep themselves and their families healthy. It was called the Family Health Initiative and Thanksgiving, the time when families gather, was declared National Family History Day. The headline read: "Knowing your family health history may save your life!" 2007 marks the fourth straight year of the U.S. Surgeon General's designation and focus on the importance of the family health history.

In 2006, the Centers for Disease Control and Prevention (CDC) sponsored a meeting on the use of family history in pediatric and adolescent primary care. For access to more information about the CDC meeting, visit *www.cdc.gov/ ncbddd/bd/family_history.htm*. In addition, the National Coalition for Health Professional Education in Genetics (NCHPEG) has published a summary of other family history tools at *www.nchpeg.org/newsletter/inpracticespr05.pdf*.

When the nurse recognizes signs of either of these syndromes during routine screening, the child is referred to specialists who are qualified to diagnose and manage the physical, social, spiritual, and emotional aspects of these problems.

Most adolescents with delayed development do not have a genetic disorder; their pattern of growth merely falls at the far end of the normal curve and is referred to as a constitutional delay. Whatever the cause, delays can have a tremendous effect on psychosocial development, and these adolescents need ongoing assessment and support to promote development of positive self-esteem.

GORDON'S FUNCTIONAL HEALTH PATTERNS
Health Perception–Health Management Pattern

Teens have fewer acute illnesses than do younger children and fewer chronic illnesses than adults. They are seen in health care facilities less frequently than younger children and adults, and they rarely are hospitalized. Yet they need to be monitored, because adolescence is a pivotal developmental period with numerous physical, psychosocial, and spiritual changes. Box 21-1 lists interventions recommended for periodic health examinations for adolescents.

A crucial component for understanding adolescent health is an adolescent's own perceptions of health, illness, and health care services. Too often, their sense of invincibility and "Peter Pan" ideology couples with typical adolescent experimentation and **risk-taking behaviors** to produce deleterious health care choices and outcomes. Caught somewhere between childhood and adulthood, teens may no longer feel as if they are being attended to by pediatricians, pediatric nurse practitioners, and pediatric nurses, yet, at the same time, are often misunderstood by adult health care providers. Health care services for adolescents need to be developed that are available, visible, confidential, and flexible. For information regarding health care services for adolescents, visit the National Adolescent Health Information Center (NAHIC) at *http://nahic.ucsf.edu*.

Adolescents are in the process of developing health habits and patterns of problem solving that are likely to last a lifetime. The cognitive and psychological changes that they experience can affect their adherence to health-promotion and disease-prevention strategies. Teens do not always consider the health risks of their behavior and have an overall sense of insusceptibility to illness or injury. Peer influence is

---

Box 21-1   Interventions Recommended for the Periodic Health Examination: 11 to 21 Years of Age

SCREENING
- Height, weight, and BMI
- Blood pressure
- Scoliosis
- Vision and hearing
- Tanner stage
- Anemia
- Hyperlipidemia
- Urinalysis
- TB
- Eating disorders
- Sports injuries
- Tattoos and piercings
- If sexually active, Pap test and STD screening
- Counseling

Injury and Violence Prevention
- Lap and shoulder belts in car
- Bicycle, motorcycle, all-terrain vehicle helmets
- Protective gear for sports, work, and other physical activities
- Learn first aid and CPR
- Skin cancer, sun exposure, sunscreen SPF 15 or higher
- Safe storage and use of firearms

Substance Use
- Avoid tobacco, alcohol, and drug use
- Avoid alcohol or drug use while driving, swimming, boating, riding a bike or motorcycle, or operating farm equipment or other machinery

Sexual Behavior
- Abstinence, resisting sexual pressures, saying no
- STD prevention and protection
- Unintended pregnancy, contraception
- Date rape

Diet and Exercise
- Choose a variety of healthy foods
- Balance caloric intake and energy expenditure
- Limit fat and cholesterol; emphasize grains, fruits, vegetables
- Adequate calcium, iron, and folic acid

Dental Health
- Regular (every 6 months) visits to dental care provider
- Brush at least twice a day and floss daily
- Avoid tobacco products

IMMUNIZATION
- DT vaccine: booster if at least 5 years since last dose of DTP, DTaP, or DT
- Hepatitis B virus vaccine (if not given previously)
- Hepatitis A virus vaccine (if indicated)
- MMR vaccine
- VAR vaccine (if not given previously or no reliable history of chickenpox; if 13 or older, two doses 4 to 8 weeks apart)
- Meningitis vaccine
- HPV vaccine

BMI, Body mass index; *SMR*, sexual maturity rating; *TB*, tuberculosis; *Pap*, Papanicolaou; *STD*, sexually transmitted disease; *CPR*, cardiopulmonary resuscitation; *SPF*, sun protection factor; *DT*, diphtheria tetanus; *DTP*, diphtheria, tetanus, pertussis; *DTaP*, diphtheria, tetanus, acellular pertussis; *MMR*, measles, mumps, rubella; *VAR*, varicella.

primary, and parental input often is rejected. Nurses need to be sensitive to the changes that occur as adolescents become increasingly capable of more independent decisions about their health behavior (Green & Palfrey, 2002).

Parents, teachers, and health care providers will be more successful in assisting teens to manage their health needs wisely if they treat them as joint partners in planning the care for which the adolescents, themselves, will assume responsibility. Key components of successful health supervision include a respect for individual differences, support for the adolescent's emerging autonomy, a developmental approach, and a focus on the individual's strengths (Green & Palfrey, 2002).

Nutritional-Metabolic Pattern

Many teens have concerns about their body, proper nutrition, and exercise. The media not only portrays the ideal body as thin, lean, or muscular, but at the same time promotes fast food, soda pop, sweets, and alcohol consumption (Dixon & Stein, 2005). Asserting their newfound autonomy, teens may choose dietary intake as a mechanism to gain control over their changing bodies, exert independence, or experiment with a new **identity** or cause, such as becoming a vegetarian. All of this occurs as their bodies' nutrient and energy demands increase in preparation and response to the adolescent growth spurt. Teen activities, including sports and other vigorous extracurricular physical activity, can further increase these demands. Gymnasts, runners, body builders, rowers, wrestlers, dancers, and swimmers are particularly vulnerable to eating disorders because their sports necessitate weight restriction. Complicating matters are teens' overwhelming desire to "fit in" with their peers, which often prevail and can lead to unhealthy dietary practices.

In the United States, up to 10% of adolescent females suffer from an eating disorder (AACAP, 2008) and 62% of female and 20% of male adolescents participate in "fad" dieting (Dixon & Stein, 2005). Adolescents who meet the criteria for eating disorders should be referred to an interdisciplinary team that is experienced and skilled in working with these disorders (Dixon & Stein, 2005). Research shows that early identification and treatment at either end of the spectrum leads to more favorable outcomes (AACAP, 2008).

Eating Disorders

At one end of the eating disorder spectrum is anorexia nervosa and bulimia nervosa. At the other end is **binge eating disorder** and **obesity**. Adolescents with **anorexia nervosa** are typically female, perfectionists, and high achievers with families that tend to be achievement oriented and experiencing marital discord. Symptoms or warning signs include a relentless pursuit of thinness, self-starving with significant weight loss, lack of menstruation (in females) and decreased sexual interests (in males), compulsive physical activity, preoccupation with food, portioning food carefully, eating only small amounts of only certain foods, and a distorted body image.

The adolescent may also have brittle hair and nails; dry, yellowish skin; growth of fine hair over the body; constipation; mild anemia and muscle weakness; and often complains of feeling cold. The onset of anorexia is typically in response to low self-esteem and real or imagined obesity. Needing mastery, the teen with anorexia nervosa experiences a sense of control when able to say no to the body's normal food demands (AACAP, 2008). Eventually, the teen becomes dangerously malnourished and in some cases dies.

Another eating disorder, **bulimia nervosa**, also affects females more than males. The symptoms or warning signs are different from those of anorexia nervosa. Teens with bulimia nervosa typically binge on huge quantities of high-caloric foods and then purge by self-induced vomiting and/or laxatives. Binge episodes may alternate with diets, resulting in dramatic weight fluctuations. These teens often try to hide the signs of vomiting by running water as a sound cover. Purging poses serious threats to the teen's health, including dehydration, sometimes fatal electrolyte imbalances, and erosion of teeth enamel.

At the other end of the eating disorder spectrum is *binge eating disorder* and obesity. Binge eating disorder is a relatively newly recognized disorder that is often referred to as compulsive overeating (AACAP, 2008). Similar to bulimia nervosa, the teen with binge eating disorder frequently consumes large amounts of food while feeling a lack of control over eating. However, this disorder is different from bulimia nervosa because these teens usually do not **purge** their bodies of the excess food they consume during their binge episodes, often leading to obesity.

The obese adolescent consumes too many calories for the amount of energy expended. Studies have shown a strong correlation between inactivity, such as viewing television, playing computer games, and Internet surfing, and the tendency to be **overweight**. Other research has identified depression as one of the strongest predictors of adolescent obesity. Obesity can be detrimental to adolescents' self-esteem and social development, as they often become trapped in a vicious cycle of social rejection, isolation, inactivity, and continued obesity. Adolescent obesity has a poor prognosis, with most obese adolescents becoming obese adults. In addition, obesity increases the risk of and occurrence of Type 2 Diabetes Mellitus.

Obesity, Type 2 Diabetes, and Teens

Soaring obesity rates are making Type 2 Diabetes, a disease that used to be seen mostly in adults over age 45, more common among teens and young people. Diabetes is a group of diseases marked by high levels of glucose in the blood, which left unattended lead to blindness, kidney failure, amputations, heart disease, and stroke. Type 2 Diabetes, formerly called adult onset diabetes, is the most common form. People can develop it at any age. However, being overweight and inactive increases your risk. Teens can access information about weight control with *Take Charge of Your Health! A Teenager's Guide to Better Health* available at *www.win.niddk.nih.gov/publications/take_charge.htm.* Further, the National Diabetes Education Program (NDEP) has now developed a new *Tips for Teens with Diabetes* series that includes a tip sheet on how to *Lower Your Risk for Type 2 Diabetes* that is "teen-friendly." Nurses can

Box **21-2** Adolescent Preparticipation Sports Examination

AREAS FOR SPECIAL CONCERN
- Previous trauma, including concussion
- Cardiovascular disease
- Hypertension
- Asthma
- Seizure disorder
- Splenomegaly, or enlarged spleen, often seen with infectious mononucleosis
- HIV infection
- Absence of paired organs: eye, kidney, testicle, or ovary

HIV, Human immunodeficiency virus.

direct high-risk teens or teens with Type 2 Diabetes to visit their website at: *http://ndep.nih.gov/diabetes/youth/youthtips_lowerrisk.htm*.

More than anything, adolescents need reassurance about their bodies. Parents, teachers, and health care providers will be more successful in helping teens assume responsibility and manage their ongoing health needs if they approach and treat them as partners in planning their care. Nurses need to engage adolescents and help them create an individualized wellness plan that addresses body image, diet, weight concerns, and physical activity.

Elimination Pattern

The renal and gastrointestinal systems are functionally mature by adolescence, and elimination patterns are consistent with those found in adults. Abnormal variation can occur in teens with eating disorders. It is important to remember that an adolescent's need for privacy or self-protection may inhibit normal elimination in public places, such as schools.

Activity-Exercise Pattern

During adolescence, the alterations in body composition and growth of lean muscle mass allow the teen to experience increased physical strength and endurance. All adolescents should be taught that regular exercise can improve their endurance, appearance, and general state of health and that these positive effects can extend into adulthood.

Many teens participate in organized sports, and the preparticipation sports examination is one of the most common reasons to seek primary care. This examination offers an opportunity for nurses to identify adolescents at risk, evaluate their general state of health, and promote healthy lifestyle behaviors (Box 21-2). Frequent injuries, stress fracture, secondary amenorrhea, extreme dietary measures to gain or lose weight, exclusion of other activities, deteriorating school work, and chronic pain are a few of the signs of overuse, overexertion, or overinvestment (Dixon & Stein, 2005). An increase in the incidence of community-acquired–methicillin-resistant *Staphylococcus aureus* (CA-MRSA) infections is also being reported in teens, especially teen athletes (Research Highlights box).

research highlights

New CA-MRSA May Be Harsher on Teens

Recent reports suggest the rate of methicillin-resistant *Staphylococcus aureus* (MRSA) infections in children and teens is on the rise. Researchers note that while the first peak of incidence is in infancy, MRSA infections peak again between 14 and 15 years of age. What is of particular concern is it appears adolescent clients are more likely to die from their infection.

The evidence is growing that current strains of community acquired MRSA (CA-MRSA), rather than hospital acquired MRSA, are more virulent and dangerous to healthy young people. But why? And, why does it appear commonly in teen athletes?

Contaminated equipment and the nature of skin-to-skin contact sports may put teen athletes at an elevated risk for CA-MRSA. To avoid the spread of this infection, experts advise parents and coaches to ensure their teen athletes:
- Receive adequate wound care and cover any skin wounds (If wounds cannot be covered, athletes should be side-lined)
- Practice proper hygiene, including showering with soap and hot water after each practice or competition
- Avoid sharing personal items (e.g., towels, razors, clothing, uniforms)
- Launder uniforms and towels after each use
- Clean and disinfect helmets, pads, and other protective equipment at least once a week with a diluted bleach solution and allow to air dry

In addition, coaches need to establish routine cleaning schedules for shared equipment and mats. School nurses may suggest athletes receive a total body check before any game or match. Nurses, interacting with teens, also need to review basic skin care and hygiene guidelines. They should also discourage the sharing of personal items that is often commonplace among teens and their peers. Particular attention needs to be paid to teen athletes, male and female.

Compiled from AAP News. (2007). Take precautions to keep infections from spreading among teen athletes. Online at: *www.aapnews.org*; Creech, C. B., Johnson, B. G., Bartilson, R.E., Yang, E., & Barr, F. (2007). Increasing use of extracorporeal life support in methicillin-resistant *Staphylococcus aureus* sepsis in teens. *Pediatric Critical Care Medicine* 8(3), 231-235.

Sleep-Rest Pattern

During adolescence, the amount of time needed each night in sleep declines in comparison to earlier childhood needs. Although their sleep patterns vary greatly, adolescents need at least 8 hours of sleep per night. Working adolescents, those involved in after school sports, and those who have "too much on their plate," are at increased risk for sleep deprivation. They stay up late and are then forced to wake up before their sleep cycles have finished because the high school day has such an early start. Some high schools are now considering moving high school start times to later in the day (Wood, 2005). Nurses help adolescents cope with the challenge of balancing their varied responsibilities and prevent exhaustion or burnout by exploring with them various strategies for daily living.

Cognitive-Perceptual Pattern

Piaget's Theory of Cognitive Development

Adolescence is characterized by a shift in cognitive abilities to Piaget's stage of **formal operations**. Piaget's theory used the term *formal* to represent the emergence of ability to focus on the "form" of thoughts, objects, and experiences rather than on the exact content, which in turn lays the groundwork for abstract thinking. These new cognitive abilities are reflected in adolescent behaviors in several ways.

The first change is that, because of their new ability to "think about their thinking," adolescents become highly introspective. As introspection increases, they develop an internalized audience that provides them with a means to evaluate questions such as "Who am I?" "How do others see me?" and "Where am I going?" **Introspection** also combines with a reemergence of **egocentrism**, leading to their sense of being the primary focus—special, unique, and exceptional. Being exceptional to the adolescent means being the exception, giving rise to the risk-taking behaviors for which they are well known:

- I can get drunk on weekends and not develop a drinking problem.
- I won't get pregnant; I've had sex for 6 months and haven't gotten pregnant yet.
- I can take those turns at 60 miles per hour and not lose control.

Another behavioral manifestation of adolescents' formal operations is an intolerance of things as they are. They are able to conceptualize things as they might or could be, rather than how they are, and can think of elaborate means for achieving these changes—now. With this newfound capability, they constantly challenge the ways things are and challenge themselves to consider the way things can or should be. Teens can be vehement in trying to convince others of their viewpoints and untiring in their support of causes that align with them. This **idealism** can lead to a rejection of family beliefs, religion, or social causes, which do not appear to the adolescent to be working fast enough to solve the problems of society. Although this idealism appears to most adults to be a flight from reality, it is a necessary stage in formal thinking. Reality is recognized, but only as a subset of many other possibilities that needs to be brought in line with their own thinking. Eventually, their thinking becomes less egocentric and omnipotent, giving way to an appreciation of differences in judgment between themselves and others. This becomes the basis of an adolescent's ability to think about politics, law, and society in terms of abstract principles and benefits rather than focusing only on the punitive aspects (Burns et al., 2008).

Erikson's Theory of Psychosocial Development

According to Erikson's theory of psychosocial development, the central task of adolescence is the establishment of **identity**, with the primary risk being **role confusion**. Although it may appear that adolescents are involved in a final, rather than a transient or initial, identity formation, adolescence provides a means of moving into and through what might be termed an identity crisis.

This crisis involves a restaging of each of the previous stages of psychosocial development. Development of trust in self and others, as emphasized in infancy, is encountered again as the adolescent searches for people and ideologies in which to have faith. Toddlerhood, and its search for autonomy, is also revisited as adolescents search for autonomy from their primary family units. However, searching for autonomy while avoiding shame and doubt leads to an interesting paradox for adolescents. They would rather behave shamelessly in the eyes of their parents than be forced into behavior that would bring ridicule from their peers. The preschooler's challenge, a sense of initiative rather than guilt, resurfaces as the adolescent searches for direction and purpose. The school-age child's developing sense of industry is carried into the adolescent period also, as teens make choices in social, recreational, volunteer, academic, familial, and occupational activities. The confusion and hesitation in making these choices arise from fears of participating in activities that will not afford them the opportunity to excel or win the approval of their peers.

The extent to which these earlier tasks were accomplished successfully influences an adolescent's resourcefulness and success in experimenting with the new identity. When the threat of identity confusion is exceedingly great, delinquent behavior and alterations in mental health can occur. This threat is enhanced by conditions of poverty, racism, and other social inequities (see the Multicultural Awareness box later in the chapter).

The pursuit for something to which to be devoted and the search for a meaningful ideology frequently create a puzzling combination of shifting devotion and sudden extremes in action (Hot Topics box). Erikson views this behavior as an attempt to try on various roles and to search for some stable principle that might last through the testing of extremes and be carried into adulthood.

Time Orientation

Adolescents look at time differently than they did as younger children. They realize that the response to a problem can, and sometimes should, be delayed to think through the possibilities for approaching the problem. Additionally, teens develop a future orientation and are able to delay immediate gratification to gain more satisfaction in the future.

Language

Advances in cognitive skills are reflected in an increased understanding of language. Formal operations and more abstract thought processes require expression in different words than did the more concrete thoughts of younger children. Adolescents give complex definitions, frequently including all possible meanings or uses. Interpretations of pictures or stories are complex and abstract. Older teens are capable of using and understanding complex sentence

HOTtopics

BODY PIERCING AND TATTOOING

Adolescence is a developmental period full of identity experimentation and risk-taking behavior. Body piercing and tattooing have become popular forms of expression of identity, particularly among adolescents. Each carries health risks and potentially fatal complications.

There are very few sites on adolescent bodies that have not been pierced. Ears, nipples, navels, noses, and eyebrows have all succumbed to metallic rings, rods, studs, and barbells. However, approximately one in three piercings suffers a complication. Most commonly these include localized infection, bleeding, and dermatitis. Intraoral soft tissue piercing of the lips, cheek, uvula, and tongue harbor additional and potentially fatal complications, including a constant risk of aspiration, hemorrhage, and swelling leading to airway compromise, nerve damage, keloid scar formation, abscess, and tetanus. There is also an increased risk of hepatitis and HIV, as well as tooth injury, gingival recession, and difficulty with speech, taste, and swallowing.

Tattooing carries similar risks of infection, with a heightened concern for the transmission of blood-borne diseases including hepatitis and HIV, especially with colorful tattoos. Color ink is expensive and is often reused to cut costs, increasing exposure risks. Tattoos are also permanent markings and do not age well.

Nurses need to provide health education that allows adolescents to make informed decisions about body piercing, tattooing, and other forms of self-expression.

Box 21-3   Deciphering and Conversing in the Latest Text Messaging Lingo

GR8	Great
LOL	Laughing out loud
BRB	Be right back
AFC/AFK	Away from computer/keyboard
POS/MOS/DOS	Parent over shoulder/Mom over shoulder/Dad over shoulder
9	Parent watching
99	Parent no longer watching
CD9	Code 9: Parent watching or in room
RUOK	Are you ok?
XLNT	Excellent
F2F	Face to face
ZZZ	Sleeping, bored, tired
Y	Why
B4N	Bye for now
YYSSW	Yeah yeah sure sure whatever
PCM	Please call me

Assessment, anticipatory guidance, education, and counseling are strategies the nurse can use to guide the adolescent in developing a healthy self-perception that incorporates a healthy body image. It is important for parents, teachers, and health care providers to remember to praise adolescents for who they are rather than for what they do, value each of them as unique, demonstrate belief in their abilities to grow and develop, and delight in their discoveries of themselves and their unique means of expressing it.

Roles-Relationships Pattern

Until adolescence, the younger child is highly dependent on the parents and other adults. Striving for identity and increased independence, the adolescent begins to spend increased time away from the family. Parents sense a narrowing of their influence as their teen not only begins to prefer the company of peers and other adults but also begins to question familial beliefs and values. Parents may respond by setting unreasonably strict limits and asking intrusive questions about their teen's activities, friends, and ideas or decide to drop all rules and limits and assume that the adolescent can now manage alone. Neither of these approaches works well.

While adolescents strive for a sense of identity and independence, their parents try to learn how to let go. Each is temporarily unsure of the relationship with the other, and the family unit may experience more stress than at any previous time. Further, this period is often prolonged as more teens remain financially dependent on their families as they move into young adulthood.

Some families experience better outcomes than do other families. Families in which parents maintain a willingness to listen, demonstrate an ongoing affection for and acceptance of their adolescent, yet still maintain some consistent limits experience more constructive, positive outcomes during this

structure, although they, like adults, may not use these complex sentences routinely in their speech.

Both receptive and expressive vocabularies increase during adolescence. As with all ages, receptive far exceeds expressive vocabulary. The adolescent's vocabulary frequently includes slang. Slang may be centered on topics such as drug use, popular dress, music, and certain peer activities, or it may be more pervasive, in which case adults or "outsiders" may have difficulty following a conversation between two teens. The surge in cell phone use, instant and text messaging, and online chat rooms has given rise to an entirely new set of communications to decipher (Box 21-3).

Self-Perception–Self-Concept Pattern

The term *self-perception*, which often is used interchangeably with the terms *self-concept* and *self-esteem*, refers to both the description of the self and the evaluation of that description. **Body image**, on the other hand, specifically refers to the picture of and feelings about one's body. Tied together and brought to the forefront in adolescence, both self-perception and body image dominate, influence, and are influenced by individual, peer, and societal norms and expectations.

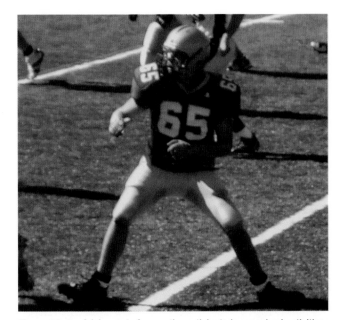

Figure 21-4 Adolescents frequently participate in organized activities, especially sports.

period. This situation does not mean that parents necessarily agree with their teen's ideas or actions, but rather that they are willing to hear what the adolescent has to say and to negotiate some limits. Parents may need assistance in determining negotiable versus nonnegotiable rules and in developing ways to voice their concerns in an honest, open way. Even when teens do not want to "discuss" a topic, they need to know why their parents are concerned. This is the message in many TV ads referring to parents as the Anti-Drug (see Innovative Practice box).

Peers

Faced with the need to become autonomous, achieve identity, and become productive, the adolescent often turns from family to peer group to find a safe psychosocial shelter in which to develop. Belonging to an informally organized clique, crowd, gang, or group is the primary means with which to make the transition from primary allegiance as a young child in the family to a member of a group. Identification with a group is proclaimed through conformity to standards of clothing, behavior, language, and values. This feature of the adolescent subculture persists despite the strong inclination in society as a whole toward greater levels of individuality.

The **peer group** is a vehicle for movement out of and away from the family unit and, as such, provides a means of achieving the goals of independence and individualization (Figure 21-4). It provides a sounding board against which young teens can test ideas, as well as a barometer for their own growth and development (Dixon & Stein, 2005).

Adolescents talk a great deal with their peers. Whether on the phone, online, or in person, they can discuss a 10-minute situation for hours on end. This sharing of thoughts and impressions is important. The telephone or computer can

provide a "safe" mechanism for the teen to interact with members of the opposite sex as they share intimate ideas and concerns and begin to experience the closeness and caring that develops into the capacity to form a future intimate relationship.

Sexuality-Reproductive Pattern

The emergence of secondary sexual characteristics increases adolescents' awareness of themselves as sexual human beings. They fantasize about relationships and sex and gradually experiment with dating and a myriad of noncoital physical contacts, as well as coital contacts. Adolescents become sexually active for a variety of reasons. They have sex for affection, peer pressure, as a symbol of maturity, as spontaneous experimentation, to feel close, because it feels good or right, and at times without their consent (see the Case Study and Care Plan at the end of this chapter). In the process of establishing a sexual sense of themselves, it is not uncommon for them to question if they are homosexual. Same-sex arousal or experimentation with same-sex physical activity does not necessarily indicate homosexuality or future sexual orientation (Dixon & Stein, 2005).

Knowing adolescents are heavily invested in these and other sexual issues, nurses are capable and willing to discuss them. Nurses need to be comfortable with their own sexuality; able to discuss the subject of sex and sexual orientation, contraception, protection against STDs; and aware of their own limitations, beliefs, and biases. Anticipatory guidance about the decision to become sexually active, contraception, and protection from **sexually transmitted diseases (STDs)** needs to be provided before adolescents encounter a situation in which they need the information (see Tables 22-2 and 22-3). This is also a good time to introduce the adolescent to breast and testicular self-examinations (Health Teaching Box).

Adolescent Pregnancy

For health care providers adolescent pregnancy is viewed as a high-risk situation, due to the serious health risks and potential complications for both the mother and the infant. For politicians and governmental agencies it is a social problem that makes overwhelming demands on social and economic resources. For adolescents and their families it may be seen as positive and normal or the worst disaster imaginable. No matter what the perspective, adolescent pregnancy represents a myriad of concerns with far-reaching effects.

Until 2005, adolescent pregnancy and birthrates in the United States had been declining steadily, down 34% since their peak in 1990 (Gruttmacher Institute, 2006; Santelli et al., 2007). However, according to the National Vital Statistics Reports, the preliminary estimates of teens giving birth in 2006 was 4,265,996, an increase in 3% from 2005 (Hamilton et al., 2007). This represents the largest single-year increase in teens giving birth since 1991. The birthrates for teenagers 15 to 17 years of age

HEALTH TEACHING   Performing Breast and Testicular Self-Examination

BSE or TSE should be performed once a month, so that teens become familiar with the usual appearance and feel of their breasts or testicles. This routine makes noticing any changes from one month to another easier. Finding a change from "normal" is the main idea behind regular self-examination. The best time for females to perform a BSE is 2 or 3 days after their period ends, when breasts are least likely to be tender or swollen. For males, the best time for a TSE is during or right after a warm shower.

Breast Self-Examination

1. Stand in front of a mirror. Inspect both breasts for anything unusual, such as any discharge from the nipples, puckering or dimpling of the skin, or marked asymmetry.
2. While watching closely in the mirror, clasp your hands behind your head and press your hands forward, and inspect again.
3. Next, press your hands firmly on your hips and bow slightly toward the mirror as you pull your shoulders and elbows forward, and inspect again.
4. Next, raise one arm (HT Figure 1). Use three or four fingers to explore the breast firmly, carefully, and thoroughly. Beginning at the outer edge, press the flat part of your fingers in small circles, moving the circles slowly around the breast. Gradually work toward the nipple. Be sure to cover the entire breast. Pay special attention to the area between the breast and the armpit, including the armpit itself. Feel for any unusual lump or mass under the skin.

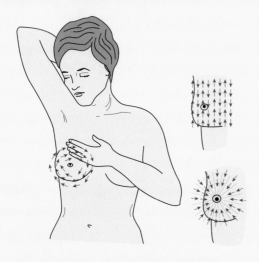

5. Gently squeeze the nipple and look for a discharge. Repeat the examination on the other breast.

Steps 4 and 5 should be repeated lying down (HT Figure 2). This position flattens the breast and makes examination easier. Some women perform BSE in the shower. Fingers gliding over soapy skin make concentrating on the texture underneath easier (HT Figure 3).

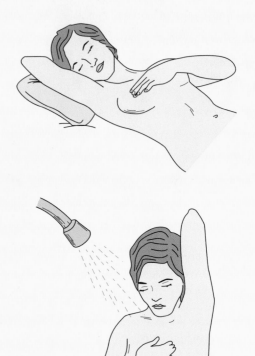

Testicular Self-Examination

1. Cup or support the testicles with one hand and feel with the other.
2. Gently roll each testicle between the thumb and fingers. There should not be any pain. Feel for any swelling or hard lumps on the surface of the testicle. Testicles are normally oval, firm, smooth, and rubbery. One may be slightly larger than the other.
3. A natural tubelike structure, the epididymis, is along the back of the testicle. Learn what it feels like.

BSE, Breast self-examination; *TSE*, testicular self-examination.
Compiled from Lowdermilk, D. L., & Perry, S. E. (2006). *Maternity nursing* (7th ed.). St. Louis: Mosby; and Neinstein, L. S., Gordau, C. M., Katzman, D. K., Rosen, D. S., & Woods, E. R. (2007). *Adolescent health care: A practical guide* (5th ed.). Lippincott Williams and Wilkins.

rose 3% whereas the birthrate for teenagers 18 to 19 rose 4%. The youngest teenagers, ages 10 to 14 years, were the only age group under 20 years whose birthrate did not increase in 2006. The largest single-year increase was reported in non-Hispanic Black teenagers, whose overall rate rose 5%. A 2% increase was noted for Hispanic

teenagers, 3% for non-Hispanic White teenagers, and 4% for American Indian or Alaska Native teenagers. The birthrate for Asian or Pacific Islander teenagers was essentially unchanged.

A review of recent studies identified more than 100 precursors to adolescent pregnancy, including economic disadvantage; family structure; family, peer, and partner attitudes and behavior; early menarche and other biophysical changes; detachment from school; and adolescent risk-taking attitudes and behaviors (Perrin & Dorman, 2003). Many of these factors are used to identify at-risk youth and design education and prevention programs.

The National Campaign to Prevent Teen and Unplanned Pregnancy emphasizes the likely negative outcomes of adolescent pregnancy in outreach efforts. For the mother these include a significant decline in her future prospects, especially educational and economic; serious health risks, including an increased risk of obesity and hypertension; single parenthood; and poverty. For the child born to adolescent mothers there is a higher risk of low birth weight. Low birth weight is associated with infant mortality and other health problems, including cerebral palsy, mental retardation, dyslexia, and hyperactivity. Further, these children often fall victim to abuse and neglect and suffer from poor school performance.

While research has primarily focused on the negative outcome of teen pregnancy, teen mothering has also been identified as a potential anchor for some teens that fosters a sense of purpose and meaning, an ability to reweave connection, and provide a sense of the future, although this is often the exception (Smith Battle, 2000).

When pregnancy occurs, adolescents and their families deserve honest and sensitive counseling about all of the options available to them, as well as the support systems available for them throughout the pregnancy, birth, and subsequent parenting. Nurses not only need to reinforce reproductive health education efforts, they also need to encourage adolescents to build on the strengths in their lives and opportunities available to them.

Coping–Stress Tolerance Pattern

When all of the changes that occur in adolescents are aligned with their need to separate from their parents and gain a sense of their own independence, their ability to cope is put to the test over and over again. Common coping mechanisms, and the strategies the nurse can use to encourage teens to use them in adaptive ways, are listed in Box 21-4.

However, too often adolescents are unable to balance the stresses, lacking the appropriate skills and outlets, adequate support systems, or available mental health intervention. Depression, suicide, and substance abuse emerge as life becomes overwhelming and the future unimaginable.

Depression

As with many other diseases, the rate of depression increases with age and the incidence continues to increase during adolescence. The term **depression** includes both major depressive and dysthymic disorders. A depressive disorder is defined as a depressed or irritable mood or a diminished interest and pleasure in usual activities, while dysthymia is a depressed or irritable mood that extends over a year-long period with symptom relief for no more than 2 months (Burns et al., 2008).

| Box **21-4** | Coping Mechanisms of Adolescents |

COGNITIVE MASTERY

The adolescent attempts to learn as much as possible about the situation or stressor. This strategy is common for the adolescent with a chronic illness. The nurse can assist by clarifying any misinformation, sharing research findings, and encouraging a discussion of feelings.

CONFORMITY

The adolescent attempts to be a mirror image of peers, which includes dress, language, attitudes, and actions. The nurse must respect this need for sameness and can also encourage discussion of feelings about differences among teens.

CONTROLLING BEHAVIOR

Adolescents must be in charge of some aspects of life and can no longer accept family and school rules without question as they did in the past. This need to control extends to health care. The nurse cannot simply give directions or instructions, but rather should present the options and allow the adolescent to partner with the nurse to work out an acceptable plan.

FANTASY

The adolescent may use fantasy as a way to escape or experiment. The nurse can encourage the teen to use fantasy constructively to develop creative plans to deal with a stressful situation.

MOTOR ACTIVITY

Engaging in sports, dancing, running, or other physical activity can be an effective tension-releasing strategy, and can also provide an instant peer group. The nurse can encourage physical activity and offer information about protective gear and injury prevention.

Depression is suspected when the adolescent uses words such as down, sad, low, blue, hopeless, worried, bored, or discouraged and exhibits several of the following symptoms:

- Change in weight or appetite
- Insomnia or hypersomnia
- Decreased energy or fatigue
- Loss of interest and pleasure in usual activities
- Out-of-proportion feelings of self-reproach or guilt
- Difficulty concentrating; declining school performance
- Preoccupation with death or suicidal ideation

The nurse needs to refer the adolescent with depression to a mental health specialist.

Suicide

Adolescence is a period of considerable stress, and when coping mechanisms and social supports are inadequate, suicide may emerge as an outcome. Suicide is the third leading cause of death in adolescence to between 15 and 19 years of age (Ball & Bindler, 2008, pg. 1132). In recent years, teen suicide has nearly tripled (Shaw et al., 2005).

Box **21-5** Warning Signs of Suicide Risk in Adolescents

BEHAVIORAL CHANGES
- Increased risk taking
- Increased incidence of accidents
- Substance use and abuse
- Physical violence to self, others, or animals
- Decreased appetite
- Alienation from family or peer group
- Giving away personal items
- Writing letters or notes, essays, and poems with suicidal content

COGNITIVE AND MOOD CHANGES
- Expression of hopelessness
- Increasing rage or anger
- Dramatic swings in affect
- Sleep disorders
- Preoccupation with death
- Difficulty concentrating
- Hearing voices, seeing things or people
- Newfound interest in religion or cult

These figures may not even reflect the full scope of the problem, because many suicides are classified as accidental deaths. Suicide attempts are not included in these statistics, although estimates show that 50 to 200 attempts occur for every successfully completed suicide. Attempts are 3 to 9 times more common in females, but males are 4 times as successful (Evans et al., 2005). Many researchers are convinced that suicide during adolescence is not an impulsive or spontaneous act: it is selected carefully only after other problem-solving methods have failed and suicide is viewed as the only option.

Adolescent suicide can be prevented. Distressed adolescents tend to give clues, both verbally and nonverbally. Any single clue may mean nothing, but when several clues are noted, they should be recognized as important warning signs. Box 21-5 outlines warning signs for parents, teachers, health care providers, and peers to be alert to in preventing adolescent suicide.

When the nurse suspects that an adolescent is suicidal, immediate referral is made to a mental health specialist. A suicide threat should never be ignored, and the adolescent who is in immediate danger of committing suicide should never be left alone (American Academy of Pediatrics, 2006; Shaw et al., 2005).

Values-Beliefs Pattern

Values and beliefs are learned phenomena that serve as guides for decision-making and actions. With the development of abstract thought, adolescents begin to expand their understanding of good and bad or right and wrong, to include autonomous moral principles that have validity apart from the authority of parent or society and instead are based on the individual's beliefs. Their newly discovered maturity in moral reasoning is situational and relational and often is superceded by psychosocial developmental needs and influences. Adolescents may think or feel something is wrong or bad yet may act contrary to that belief because of peer pressure or the need to declare their independence.

Adolescents often align their values and beliefs with a particular religion, philosophical school of thought, social movement or cause, or other formal system, using it to make decisions about what is right or wrong, best or worst, and important or trivial. During adolescence these alignments can change drastically and often, causing strife and concern for parents, yet providing the teen with different ranges of experience from which to base eventual and lasting choices.

According to Kohlberg's theory of moral development (1981), the adolescent begins to make the transition to the postconventional stage, equating what is right with the idea of justice and basing actions on the recognition of the universal principles underlying laws and social agreements. Gilligan, who developed a parallel theory of moral development for females, proposes that the female adolescent sees "good" as involving self-sacrifice and caring for the relationships in her life (Gilligan et al., 1990). As moral reasoning matures, the female adolescent learns to achieve a balance between what is good for her and what is good for others in her network of relationships.

As adolescents struggle with their journey to discover who they are, parents, teachers, and health care providers need to provide positive role modeling, reinforce positive behaviors, and remember how hard their own journeys were. It is often when we like them the least that they need us the most.

ENVIRONMENT
Accidents

Accidents, along with suicide and homicide, continue to be the leading cause of death and injury during adolescence. Newly licensed and inexperienced behind the wheel, it is no surprise that adolescents have a motor vehicle fatality rate 20 times higher than that of any other age group (Dixon & Stein, 2005). Whether drivers, passengers, pedestrians, or cyclists, few adolescents take measures to reduce their risk of injury, with 21% rarely or never using a safety belt and 87% rarely or never using a bicycle helmet (Green & Palfrey, 2002, p. 248).

Nurses encourage teens to wear their safety belts and avoid driving, or riding with someone, under the influence of drugs or alcohol. The tendency to play loud music and change the tune or disc often, as well as the pressure to answer cell phones, can also be distracting, as can a car full of other teens. Recognizing this and that teens have a much higher nighttime crash fatality rate, many states have enacted new driver restrictions and nighttime curfews.

Sports Injuries

Organized sports in and out of school provide adolescents with experiences in competition, teamwork and effort, and conflict resolution. They also provide a valuable means for adolescents to develop self-esteem. However, adolescents are particularly vulnerable to sports injuries. Their coordination skills are developing, their judgment often immature and inadequate, their epiphyses not yet closed, and their extremities poorly protected by stabilizing musculature. They can also become obsessed or driven to perform beyond their capabilities or to the exclusion of all other activities. The use of performance-enhancing substances, such as steroids, which have been unfortunately modeled by many professional athletes, can create another potential extreme scenario that places the adolescent at risk for injury.

The nurse advocates for the proper use of protective gear during all activities and a thorough preparticipation sports examination (see Box 21-2), and also monitors for overuse, overexertion, or overinvestment on the part of the adolescent.

Violence

Adolescents today face an unprecedented risk of injury (American Academy of Pediatrics, 2006) and death from violence in their homes, schools, and communities. Becoming increasingly independent, they test the limits of authority, experiment with a variety of roles, question adult values and authority, and look to peers for affirmation. They may feel pressure to join gangs or feel threatened by them. Many teens report carrying weapons to protect themselves or intimidate others. Adolescents often report a fear of violence

and try to avoid situations where they might be vulnerable to it, including home or even the bathroom at school.

Many studies suggest that witnessing or observing violence, whether in person or projected on the TV, video, or movie screen, results in a higher incidence of violent behaviors. Graphic violence in current music lyrics and videos has also been implicated.

In his documentary, *Bowling for Columbine,* filmmaker Michael Moore made a compelling case that what endangers America most today is not the act of violence or the crime, but our fear of it. Fear is stoked by a media that trumpets every street murder and bank robbery as an imminent threat and elevates shark attacks and escalator mishaps to a national crisis. Children and adolescents with fears that go unresolved have been shown to have an increase in violent behaviors, and fear about others often surfaces as racism. Figure 21-5 outlines the interrelationships of internal and external precipitating factors that increase an adolescent's vulnerability to and for violent behaviors.

Nurses need to engage adolescents, examining and discussing the messages in videos, songs, movies, and television shows. Discussing their developing sense of self, their sense of belonging and where that sense is found, and their fears may help to intercept an adolescent who might otherwise turn to violence. Teens who are valued and nurtured by caring adults have the best chance of emerging from adolescence unscathed.

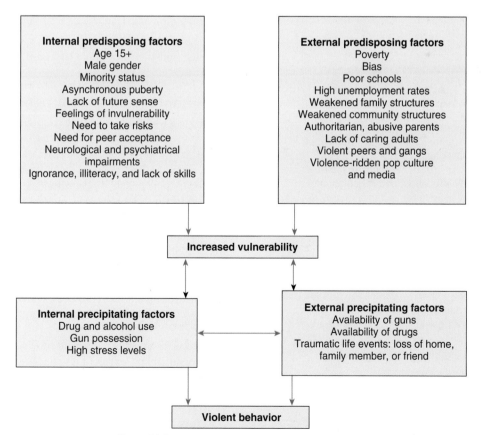

Figure 21-5   Factors contributing to adolescent violence.

Box **21-6** Signs of Substance Abuse

- Accidents
- Agitation
- Appetite loss
- Blackouts
- Bleeding gums
- Chronic cough
- Delusions
- Depression
- Diarrhea
- Dyspnea
- Eye drops
- Headache
- Hoarseness
- Hyperactivity
- Inability to concentrate
- Insomnia
- Lethargy
- Memory loss
- Muscle weakness
- Paranoia
- Rhinorrhea
- Seizures
- Somnolence
- Sore tongue
- Stomach pain
- Taste loss
- Violent outbursts
- Vomiting
- Withdrawal
- Weight loss

From Payne, W. A., & Hahn, D. B. (2002). *Understanding your health* (7th ed.). Boston: McGraw-Hill.

Box **21-7** CRAFFT: Adolescent Substance Abuse Screening Test

A brief screening test for adolescent substance abuse developed by The Center for Adolescent Substance Abuse Research at the Children's Hospital of Boston uses the acronym CRAFFT to guide health care providers when interviewing adolescents about substance abuse:

C—Have you ever ridden in a car driven by someone, including yourself, who was "high" or had been using alcohol or drugs?

R—Do you ever use alcohol or drugs to relax, feel better about yourself, or fit in?

A—Do you ever use alcohol or drugs while you are by yourself, alone?

F—Do your family or friends ever tell you that you should cut down on your drinking or drug use?

F—Do you ever forget things you did while using alcohol or drugs?

T—Have you gotten into trouble while you were using alcohol or drugs?

Two or more affirmative answers suggests a significant problem and warrants referral and follow-up.

From Knight, J. R., Sherritt, L., Shrier, L. A., Harris, S. K., & Chang, G. (2002). Validity of the CRAFFT substance abuse screening test among adolescent clinic patients. *Archives of Pediatrics and Adolescence, 15*(6), 607-614.

Infection

Infectious mononucleosis is a self-limiting viral infection transmitted by direct contact of oropharyngeal secretions. It is prevalent among adolescents and often referred to as the "kissing disease"; however, it can occur in younger children. It is caused by the Epstein-Barr virus. Typically adolescents complain of a sore throat, lymph node enlargement, and lethargy. Both splenomegaly and hepatomegaly can occur, creating a risk for injury.

Rates of meningococcal disease remain highest for infants, but in the past decade rates have increased among adolescents. Reports have identified an increased risk for meningococcal disease among college freshmen who live in dormitories or residence halls. As adolescents prepare for college, nurses need to review their risk and provide them with information on available vaccines.

As adolescents experiment with and explore their sexual development and emerging independence, they often become sexually active, which exposes them to a myriad of sexually transmitted diseases. STDs most commonly include gonorrhea, syphilis, chlamydia, herpes simplex virus, human papilloma virus, trichomonas, hepatitis B, and HIV (see Table 22-3). Considered an epidemic, STDs have the highest rates in adolescents, with minorities, especially African Americans, disproportionately affected (Burns et al., 2008). Inconsistent use of contraceptive and protective devices, increasingly earlier age and frequency of sexual activity, social and peer pressure, and an adolescent's sense of invincibility all contribute to this significant public and adolescent health problem. Although adolescents can be evaluated and treated for STDs, the diseases must be reported and the nurse must be aware of state rules about reporting.

Substance Use and Abuse

Society as a whole is increasingly oriented toward using chemicals such as drugs, alcohol, and tobacco to feel better, look better, act more sociable, stay awake, go to sleep, be sexy or erect, or lose weight. Some of the most famous music, movie, and sports stars openly model substance use and abuse. It is no surprise that adolescents are making the choice to experiment with and use substances at earlier and earlier ages.

Substance use is a precursor to abuse, which emphasizes the need for health care providers to be alert and screen for its presence. Identifying an adolescent with substance use or abuse requires a careful nursing assessment that is conducted in an accepting manner (Boxes 21-6 and 21-7).

Tobacco Use

Most teens begin smoking during adolescence, especially if a close friend, sibling, or parent also smokes (Burns et al., 2008). The highest rate of smoking is among White females, while "smokeless" tobacco, such as snuff and chewing tobacco, is more popular among males. Adolescents begin using tobacco for a variety of reasons, including wanting to appear older, because their friends do, or to imitate adult role models or media images. Advertising by the tobacco industry directed at adolescents has been shown to encourage adolescent smoking.

The nurse's primary prevention focus is on keeping non-smokers from starting and helping smokers to stop. The National Institutes of Health has published guidelines for health care providers to follow, titled The 5 A's for Brief Intervention in Adolescents Who Use Tobacco, which are:

- *Ask* about tobacco use
- *Advise* to quit
- *Assess* willingness to attempt quitting
- *Assist* in quit attempt
- *Arrange* for follow-up

See *www.ahrq.gov/path/tobacco* for more information (Agency for Healthcare Research and Quality, 2008).

Cancer

Adolescents are affected by many of the same cancers as are younger children, such as leukemia, osteogenic sarcoma, lymphomas, and central nervous system tumors. Older adolescents are entering the period of their lives during which cancer of the reproductive and related organs is more common. For females, the focus is on cervical and breast cancer; for males, testicular cancer is of concern.

Peak incidence of breast and cervical cancer is during middle age and is actually rare in the teenage years. Breast self-examination (BSE), which has been highly recommended for more than 30 years, has recently been questioned as a routine practice for most adolescents. The extremely small incidence of breast cancer in teens has caused some health care providers to deemphasize this practice for them. However, most still feel that regular examination of the breasts begins a lifelong habit that should begin as soon as the female adolescent develops (see the Health Teaching box).

Cervical cancer is detected with a Papanicolaou (Pap) smear, obtained from the cervix during a pelvic examination. According to the Center for Young Women's Health at Boston Children's Hospital (*www.youngwomenshealth.org*), factors that increase the risk for cervical cancer include sexual intercourse before age 20, multiple sexual partners or a sexual partner who has had many partners, any history of STDs or exposure to exogenous hormones, and smoking. Sexually active adolescents should have a Pap test performed annually and the American College of Obstetricians and Gynecologists recommends annual pelvic examinations by age 18, even when the young woman is not sexually active. The nurse can explain the purpose and the process involved in conducting a pelvic examination and Pap test.

In June 2006, the Advisory Committee on Immunization Practices (*www.cdc.gov/std/HPV/STDFact-HPV-vaccine.htm*) voted to recommend the first vaccine developed to prevent cervical cancer and other diseases in females caused by certain types of genital human papillomavirus (HPV). The HPV vaccine is recommended for 11- to 12-year-old girls, and can be given to girls as young as 9. The vaccine is also recommended for 13- to 26-year-old girls/women who have not yet received or completed the vaccine series.

Ideally, females should get the vaccine before they are sexually active. This is because the vaccine is most effective in girls/women who have not yet acquired any of the four HPV types covered by the vaccine. Girls/women who have not been infected with any of those four HPV types will get the full benefits of the vaccine.

Females who are sexually active may also benefit from the vaccine, but they may get less benefit since they may have already acquired one or more HPV type(s) covered by the vaccine. Few young women are infected with all four of these HPV types, so they would still get protection from those types they have not acquired. It is not yet known if the vaccine is effective in boys or men. It is possible that vaccinating males will have health benefits for them by preventing genital warts and rare cancers, such as penile and anal cancer. It is also possible that vaccinating boys/men will have indirect health benefits for girls/women. When more information is available, this vaccine may be licensed and recommended for boys/men as well.

Testicular cancer is the number one cancer in adolescent and young adult males. Adolescent males should learn to do a testicular self-examination and continue this practice monthly (see the Health Teaching box). Nurses introduce and teach methods of self-examination to adolescents who naturally are interested in their developing bodies.

SOCIAL PROCESSES
School

Junior high and high school are a new social experience, introducing the adolescent to changing classes, multiple teachers and teaching styles, variable class schedules and homework load, and a variety of peer influences. Adolescents must learn to become accustomed to greater anonymity as they navigate the corridors of larger, more impersonal institutions (Dixon & Stein, 2005). Yet despite these challenges, junior high and high school settings also provide meaningful in-school and after-school learning, peer contact, intellectual stimulation, and activities.

Schools and peers, as opposed to home and parents, become the primary setting through which expectations are shared and standards communicated. Adolescent peer groups serve as sounding boards against which teens test their ideas and gauge their physical, intellectual, psychological, and moral growth (Dixon & Stein, 2005). Nurses ask adolescents about school and their friends, and how they are doing with both. The nurse can also monitor adolescents as they prepare for and make the transition to their next social arena and role whether it is college, vocational training, the military, or another career choice.

Culture and Ethnicity

Cultural and ethnic influences operate throughout childhood and continue into adolescence. The primary difference in adolescence is that teens question, modify, or reject these influences, exchanging them for those of their peers or of the dominant cultural group. First-generation adolescents of immigrant parents have to negotiate two cultures, languages, and sets of expectations. These adolescents live a double life that results in increased stress. Adolescents from minority groups, such as African Americans, Hispanics, Asian Americans, Native Americans, Russian Americans, or Arab Americans, may experience discrimination and rejection as they try to fit in to the dominant adolescent culture. Additional stress may also be experienced when their attempts to fit in to the dominant culture are offensive to the values and beliefs of their own culture.

Young people from minority groups have a particular problem in relation to the culture of adolescence. These teens may desire strongly to fit in to the predominant adolescent culture, which in society is often middle class, White, and Protestant, and they may be able to meet one or two of these criteria but be unable to meet the others because of economics, different appearance, or different education and experiences. Advertising does not emphasize the economically depressed or ethnic-looking model, and the teens' peers are trying every means possible to look and act similar to the dominant culture adolescent. Further pressure comes from their own minority culture when they emulate the majority culture in ways that the family views as offensive to their ideas and beliefs.

Nurses need to recognize and assess for additional stresses experienced by adolescents as they wrestle not only with their own but also with their cultural identities.

Legislation

Many laws and regulations are aimed at adolescents and deal with the minimum age at which they can assume adult responsibilities and decision-making. The rationale for these restrictions is that adolescents, although capable, lack the experience, perspective, and judgment to recognize and avoid choices that might be detrimental to them, so they require protection. A question raised frequently when considering minimum age is whether strict age criteria are appropriate for any adolescent, particularly because development is variable and experiences are diverse.

The restrictions that have recently been questioned most strongly deal with issues related to sexual activity. The U.S. Supreme Court affirmed the right of all individuals to have equal access to contraceptive service, regardless of age or marital status. However, variations occur from state to state and the nurse must be aware of legal age determinants, as well as variations in definitions of **emancipated minors**.

The emancipated minor provision of certain laws recognizes that some adolescents become independent from their families at an early age and assume adult responsibilities. An emancipated minor is an adolescent who has not reached the standard legal age for certain activities, such as consenting to marriage or seeking certain kinds of health or illness care, but who is permitted to accept full responsibility for these decisions because the individual is economically and emotionally separate from the family.

Most often confidentiality is the more important issue for adolescents. The nurse can assure them that information shared will be kept confidential unless the teens pose a risk to themselves or others or state laws mandate that the information be shared (Burns et al., 2008). For example, abuse must be reported, STDs need to be reported, and some states require report of adolescent sexual activity if an age difference of 3 or more years exists between the sexual partners.

Nurses need to familiarize themselves with the legal rights of adolescents in their state and the resources available in their community.

Economics

Identification with peers, the essence of self-image during adolescence, includes dressing alike, having similar possessions, and doing similar things, all of which require economic resources. This can be a major conflict between parents and adolescents. Parents may think that they should have the power to decide how their adolescent spends money. Adolescents may believe, just as strongly, that they know the best ways to allocate resources and determine the amount of money they need.

Ideally, parents and adolescents should negotiate economic questions, with the parents becoming less controlling as the teen gains more experience and expertise in these matters. However, the family with limited economic resources has fewer choices, and adolescents from these families may feel trapped by their circumstance. Poverty is particularly hard on children, and as they become adolescents they often develop a fatalistic view of life (Multicultural Awareness box).

Some adolescents seek employment to earn their own money and have control over it. Others work because their families need the income. It is important for the nurse to assess the economic resources of each adolescent's family and work within them when partnering with the adolescent in health care planning.

Health Care Delivery System

Many health care resources are available to the adolescent. Teens can continue to see their child health care providers in a pediatric center as they did as younger children, but this setting usually is rejected because of the young-child atmosphere.

School-based clinics frequently are available in junior high and high school, and adolescent-focused clinics are available in many communities through both public and private agencies. Each of these clinics serves only adolescents, and the staff is oriented to the needs of this age group. Adolescents frequently have a stronger sense of comfort in these settings than in those in which young children or adults are also served.

Adolescents can also make use of services such as family planning clinics. These settings may designate certain days and hours for teens, whereas other facilities integrate them into the adult-oriented protocols. The pregnant adolescent typically finds prenatal care in an adult-focused setting, although more adolescent-specific programs are being developed. The physical needs of pregnant adolescents may be the same as those of the pregnant adult,

MULTICULTURAL AWARENESS

African American Youths "Choosing" AIDS

Poor, urban African American teens often confront circumstances that the American dream defines as failures, and their disproportionate victimization is manifest in the number of violent crimes that target them. Adolescents in this environment rapidly lose their idealism and learn, instead, to hope for little and expect even less.

In a haunting study, Sylvie Tourigny provided exquisite documentation of a group of impoverished African American teens in inner-city Detroit who deliberately contracted AIDS. Their individual stories of willful seroconversion reveal a world of marginalization, insensitive social policies, and demanding caretaking responsibilities for both themselves and their families.

"I ain't gonna live no 15 years anyway ... you can't be here in the 'hood' and expect to live."

"There is no future to think about anyway."

"There ain't much goin' on for Black girls like me, so this be best ... they'se gonna pay for everything."

"If you got AIDS, you get more."

In an editorial titled "The Complexities of Health Promotion," Morse (2004) asks, "Didn't these teens know that AIDS is terminal?" The answer is yes. However, the attraction of AIDS for these teens was that it would entitle them to much-needed counseling, assistance, and money and yet not cause immediate illness or death. No adolescent should have to choose illness and death for his or her needs to be met.

There is no reason to believe that "choosing" AIDS is only an inner-city problem, confined to African Americans, or even to North America. Nurses need to be the leaders in evaluating health promotion and social services support, assessing whether they are truly available to the poorest and youngest of the poor, prior to contracting disease.

AIDS, Acquired immunodeficiency syndrome.
Based on Morse, J. (2004). The complexities of health promotion. *Qualitative Health Research, 14*(1), 3-4; and Tourigny, S. C. (1998). Some new dying trick: African American youths "choosing" HIV/AIDS. *Qualitative Health Research, 8*(2), 149-167.

but the psychosocial needs are different and should be approached by a professional who has a comprehensive knowledge of their development and responses to stress.

The adolescent is a rapidly changing individual. The nurse who works in an adolescent-focused practice is well prepared in adolescent health-promotion strategies. The nurse should have a thorough understanding of adolescent physical and psychosocial growth and development and recognize each teen as a person.

Adolescents not only tend to be fearful about procedures or possible diagnoses but also need to stay in control of the situation. These conflicting feelings can be difficult to manage simultaneously. By establishing the adolescent as a partner with the health care providers in promoting good health and screening for health risks, the nurse facilitates the adolescent's sense of control (Box 21-8).

The adolescent's questions should be answered thoroughly and honestly. In many instances the adolescent

Box 21-8 HEADSSS Assessment

The HEADSSS Assessment provides a mnemonic that guides health care providers through an adolescent's psychosocial assessment. Responses should be interpreted as those that are indicators of strengths or protection from risk and those that are indicators of risky behavior or situations.
Home and health
Education, employment, eating
Activities, affiliations, aspirations
Drugs
Sexuality
Suicide, depression, self-image
Safety

From Goldenring, J. M., & Rosen, D. (2004). Getting into adolescent heads: An essential update. *Contemporary Pediatrics, 21*(1), 64-90.

is hesitant to voice concerns, so information is offered even when questions are not asked. An effective indirect approach to learning about adolescent concerns, especially about potentially embarrassing or stressful topics, is to say, "Many teenagers ask me about [a topic]. Have you ever thought about this?" or "A lot of young people want to know about [a topic]."

Direct questions are also important, even about sensitive topics: "Have you ever thought about suicide?" "Are you depressed?" "Are you sexually active?" "Do you use birth control and/or protection?" However, asking first about friends and the adolescent's feelings about them may be a good lead-in approach: "Are any of your friends doing drugs?" "How do you feel about it?" Vague or circuitous questions may be interpreted as a sign of discomfort or lack of understanding and may cause the adolescent to be equally vague when responding.

Correct anatomical terms and descriptions of laboratory tests, disease processes, and possible outcomes are essential components in treating adolescents as individuals who are capable of being responsible for their own bodies.

SUMMARY

Adolescence is a period of rapid change, when the integration of family, peer, educational, social, cultural, and community experiences begins to take form in teen's sense of self. Many view adolescence as a construction site in its early stages. Onlookers assume that eventually a recognizable structure will emerge but have no idea what that structure will be. Although many parents, teachers, and health care providers feel that hard hats and steel-reinforced shoes are needed, each is better equipped with an understanding and respect for the adolescent's developmental struggles with physical and cognitive changes, autonomy, body image, peer relations, and identity. The goal, after all, is for the teen to emerge in young adulthood with a healthy body, mind, and spirit.

CASE STUDY

Drug-Facilitated Sexual Assault: Jessica

Sexual assault includes any type of sexual activity that an individual does not agree to. Because of the effects of some drugs, commonly called **date rape** drugs, victims may be physically helpless, unable to refuse or even remember what happened.

Jessica, a 16-year-old high school sophomore, expresses concern to the school nurse that she knows someone who might have had sex "without knowing it." How can the nurse answer these common questions?

Reflective Questions:
1. What are date rape drugs and how can a person be unaware that such a drug has been ingested?
2. What can you do to protect yourself?
3. What do you do if you think you have been sexually assaulted?
4. What can you do when someone you care about has been sexually assaulted?

CARE PLAN

Drug-Facilitated Sexual Assault: Jessica

Nursing Diagnosis: Risk for Powerlessness related to suspected rape/rape trauma syndrome

Definition: At risk for perceived lack of control over a situation and/or one's ability to significantly affect an outcome.

RISK FACTORS (R/T)
• Suspected date rape/rape trauma syndrome
• Acute injury (rape)
• Deficient knowledge
• Disturbed body image
• Situational low self-esteem

EXPECTED OUTCOMES
• Acknowledges personal strength
• Perceived control

• Perceived resources
• Participation in health care decisions
• Increase healthy lifestyle choices
   Goal: Increase individual's sense of power over potential/actual situation for self/others.

SELECTED NURSING INTERVENTIONS
• Active listening
• Risk identification
• Health care information exchange
• Support system enhancement
• Rape-trauma treatment
• Decision-making support
• Health education

Complied from Johnson, M., Bulechek, G. M., Dochterman, J. M., Maas, M. L., Moorhead, S., Swanson, E., & Butcher, H. R. (2006). *NANDA, NOC and NIC Linkages: Nursing Diagnoses, Outcomes & Interventions* (2nd ed.). St. Louis: Mosby; NANDA-International (2009). *Nursing diagnoses: Definitions & classification 2009-2011.* NANDA International. West Sussex, UK: Wiley Blackwell; For further information on developing care plans, see: Carpenito-Moyet, L. J. (2008). *Nursing diagnosis: Application to clinical practice* (12th ed.). Philadelphia: Lippincott, Williams & Wilkins.

REFERENCES

AACAP. (2008). *Teenagers with eating disorders.* Facts for Families (No. 2). Washington, DC: American Academy of Child & Adolescent Psychiatry. Retrieved May 23, 2008, from *www.aacap.org/cs/root/facts_for_families/teenagers_with_eating_disorders.*

Agency for Healthcare Research and Quality. (2008). *AHCRP supported clinical practice guidelines: 18. Treating tobacco use and dependence.* Retrieved January 24, 2009, from *www.ahrg.gov/path/tobacco.*

American Academy of Child and Adolescent Psychiatry. (2004). *When children have children.* Retrieved August 30, 2004, from *www.aacap.org/publications/factsfam/pregnant.htm.*

American Academy of Pediatrics (AAP). (2006). *Teen suicide and guns. Connected Kids: Safe, strong, secure.* Elk Grove, IL: AAP.

American Academy of Pediatrics. (2008). *Bright futures: Guidelines for health supervision of infants, children, and adolescents* (3rd ed.). Elk Grove, IL: American Academy of Pediatrics.

Ball, J. W., & Bindler, R. C. (2008). *Pediatric nursing: Caring for children* (4th ed.). Upper Saddle River, NJ: Pearson Prentice Hall.

Berger, K. S. (2004). *The developing person through the life span* (6th ed.). New York: Worth.

Burns, C. E., Brady, M. A., Dunn, A. M., Starr, N. B., & Blosser, C. (2008). *Pediatric primary care* (4th ed.). New York: W. B. Saunders.

Centers for Disease Control and Prevention (CDC). (2006). Improving the health of adolescents and young adults. Official companion document to *Healthy People 2010: Critical Health Objectives: A Guide for Stats and Communities.* San Francisco: University of California.

Center for Disease Control and Prevention Division of Adolescent and School Health. *Adolescent Health.* Retrieved from *www.cdc.gov/HealthyYouth/ac/index.htm.*

Dixon, S. D., & Stein, M. T. (2005). *Encounters with children* (4th ed.). New York: W. B. Saunders.

Evans, E., Hawton, K., Rodham, K., & Deeks, J. (2005). The prevalence of suicidal phenomena in adolescents: A systematic review of population-based studies. *Suicide and Life Threatening Behaviors, 35,* 239–250.

Gilligan, C., Lyons, N., & Hanmer, T. (1990). *Making connections: The relational worlds of adolescent girls at Emma Willard School.* Cambridge, MA: Harvard University Press.

Green, M., & Palfrey, J. S. (2002). *Bright futures: Guidelines for health supervision of infants, children, and adolescents* (2nd ed., revised). Washington, DC: National Center for Education in Maternal and Child Health Georgetown University.

Greydanus, D. E., Patel, D. R., & Pratt, H. D. (2006). *Essential Adolescent Medicine.* McGraw-Hill.

Gruttmacher Institute. (2006). *U.S. teenager pregnancy statistics—National and state trends and trends by race/ethnicity.* New York: Gruttmacher Institute.

Guyton, A. C., & Hall, J. E. (2006). *Textbook of medical physiology* (10th ed.). Philadelphia, PA: W. B. Saunders.

Hamilton, B. E., Martin, J. A., & Ventura, S. J. (2007). Births: Preliminary Data for 2006. *National Center for Health Statistics.*

Kohlberg, L. (1981). *The philosophy of moral development.* San Francisco, CA: Harper & Row.

National Campaign to Prevent Teen and Unplanned Pregnancy. (2004). *Teen pregnancy—So what?* Retrieved August 30, 2004, from *www.teenpregnancy.org.*

Perrin, K. M., & Dorman, K. A. (2003). Teen parents and academic success. *Journal of School Nursing, 19*(5), 288–293.

Pinyerd, B., & Zipf, W. B. (2005). Puberty-timing is everything. *Journal of Pediatric Nursing, 20*(2), 75–82.

Santelli, J. S., Lindberg, L. D., Finer, L. B., Singh, S., et al. (2007). Recent declines in adolescent pregnancy in the United States: More abstinence or better contraceptive use? *American Journal of Public Health, 97*(6), 969–970.

Seidel, H. M., Ball, J. W., Dains, J. E., & Benedict, G. W. (2006). *Mosby's guide to physical assessment* (6th ed.). St. Louis, MO: Mosby.

Shaw, D., Fernandes, J. R., & Rao, C. (2005). Suicide in children and adolescents: a 10-year retrospective review. *American Journal of Forensic Medicine and Pathology, 26,* 309–315.

Smith Battle, L. (2000). The vulnerabilities of teenage mothers: Challenging prevailing assumptions. *ANS Advances in Nursing Science, 231,* 29–40.

Wood, C. (2005). Reflections on a late start. *Family Medicine, 37*(9), 623–624.

Chapter 22

Elizabeth C. Kudzma

Young Adult

key terms

Achievement-oriented stress
Aerobic exercise
Basal metabolic rate
Binge drinking
Breast self-examination (BSE)
Congenital defects
Congenital rubella syndrome
Coronary artery disease (CAD)
Fetal neural tube defects (FNP)

Genetic impairments
Genital herpes virus
Hepatitis B
Human immunodeficiency virus (HIV)
Human papilloma virus (HPV)
Hypertension
Infertility
Intimacy versus isolation
Maternal mortality rate

Metabolic syndrome
Orchitis
Papanicolaou (Pap) smear
Postconventional level of moral reasoning
Rubella
Stress
Sunscreen protective factor index (SPF)
Testicular self-examination (TSE)

website materials

Assessing Problematic College Drinking Behavior

You are the clinic director and nurse practitioner at a small liberal arts college. Mary, a 19-year-old fresh-man, has generally been a good student, easily mak-ing the adjustment to living away from home during her first 2 months in the dormitory. She comes to you to talk about an episode that occurred the previous weekend and that frightened her. On Saturday night she was at a party at a private residence in a rural, wooded setting away from the campus. She remem-bers consuming five or six alcoholic drinks; however, any memory after midnight is missing. She woke up in a fellow female student's dormitory room without any memory of leaving the party or returning to the dormi-tory. She was able to piece together information from her friends, who told her that she consumed at least nine alcoholic drinks that night and that she left the party with others who were returning to the dormi-tory, but they were not the friends with whom she had been seen with all evening. She is concerned that she may have been drugged or that she may be hav-ing memory lapses. Assessment of her alcohol use in the past reveals that she can recount at least four occasions during which she drank more than seven drinks at a party or family gathering. She describes her family as "social drinkers." Last June, she was involved in a minor car accident that might have been related to her consumption of at least three drinks that afternoon.

1. Do you believe that Mary has a problem with drinking? As what kind of an alcohol user would you classify her? How do you establish appropriate therapeutic communication?
2. What kind of physical symptoms might assist you in making a determination that Mary has a drinking problem?
3. What kinds of monitoring and follow-up mechanisms might assist Mary in keeping her behavior consistent with a treatment plan?

The young adult period encompasses the ages from 18 to 35 years, a time that ranges from the end of adolescence to the beginning of middle adulthood. Formal education, for example, college and graduate school, may delay the onset of this phase of development. The major task of this period is preparing for the assumption of adult responsibilities, rights, and privileges.

AGE AND PHYSICAL CHANGES

The young adult period is a time of many physical and emo-tional changes and is an opportunity for learning by expe-rience and experimentation. All phases of young adult development garner considerable interest. Judging by the increase in books about self-development, more adults are exploring topics in holistic healing and spiritual health and development. Health behaviors, safety practices, diet,

exercise, sexuality, and addictions are widely discussed topics. Preventive health concerns for young adults can be separated into two basic categories: (1) developing behav-iors that promote a healthy lifestyle and (2) decreasing the incidence of accidents, injuries, and acts of violence. *Healthy People 2010 Midcourse Review* reports (and the following *Healthy People 2020*) that injuries are the number one cause of death in children and young adults (U.S. Department of Health and Human Services [USDHHS], 2006).

In 2005, approximately 23.4% of the American popu-lation was composed of adults ages 18 to 35 (U.S. Census Bureau, 2006). The young adult population is projected to be approximately 23.3% of the general population by the year 2010 and 22.9%, in 2015. The percentage of young adults ages 20 to 24 years shows a decline from 9.4% in 1980 to a projected 7.0% in 2010 (U.S. Census Bureau, 2006). A decline in this age group is influenced by birth-rates, and the U.S. Census Bureau (2006) reported that the birthrate per 1000 people for women of all ages in 2003 was 14.1; this rate has been dropping since 1990, when it was more than 16.7 live births per 1000. Health-promotion efforts are particularly important for young adults, because health teaching for this age group has the significant potential to directly influence subsequent generations (*Healthy People 2010* box and the following *Healthy People 2020*).

Young adulthood is generally the healthiest time of life. Physical growth is mostly complete by the age of 20; most concerns related to physiological development are focused on ensuring the optimal functioning of body systems. The young adult's physical abilities are in peak condition, and compensatory mechanisms operate optimally during illness to provide minimal disruption in health patterns. Nursing goals for individuals of this age group are oriented toward prolonging this period of optimal physical energy; devel-oping the mental, emotional, spiritual, and social poten-tial; encouraging proper health habits; anticipating and screening for and, therefore, being able to treat the onset of chronic disease at an early stage; and treating disease when appropriate.

Full adult stature in men is reached at approximately age 21; in women, full growth occurs earlier, typically by age 17. Optimal muscle strength occurs during ages 25 to 30, and then gradually declines by approximately 10% from ages 30 to 60. Manual dexterity peaks in young adulthood and begins to decline in the mid-30s.

Women have greater longevity than do men. Women are considered biologically stronger than men, outlive men, and naturally outnumber men. On the average, in the United States women live 5.2 years longer than do men, an increase of 2.7 years within the past decade (U.S. Census Bureau, 2006). These statistics may be a result in part of female genetic composition or men's greater exposure to environmental and occupational hazards. Men also seek health care services less frequently than do women. The female rate for preventive care is significantly higher than

Healthy People 2010
Selected National Health-Promotion and Disease-Prevention Objectives for the Young Adult

- Increase the proportion of adults who engage regularly 5 or more days a week in moderate physical activity for at least 30 minutes per day. (In 2000, 32% of adults performed the recommended amount of physical activity and 40% of adults engaged in no leisure-time physical activity.)
  - Increase the proportion of adults who perform activities that enhance and maintain muscular strength and endurance. (In 2000, 18% of adults performed those activities and the target is 30%.)
  - Increase the proportion of adults who are at a healthy weight. (42% of adults ages 20 and older were at a healthy weight—target is 60%.)
- Reduce the proportion of adults who are obese. (From 1988 through 1994, 23% of adults age 20 and older were considered obese—target is 15%.)
  - Increase the proportion of worksites that offer nutrition or weight management classes or counseling. (54% of worksites with 50 or more employees offered nutrition or weight management classes/counseling—target is 84%.)
- Reduce cigarette smoking by adults. (In 1998, 24% of adults were current cigarette smokers and the target for 2010 is 12%.)
- Reduce the proportion of adults using any illicit drug during the preceding 30 days. (Illicit drug use in adults age 18 or older in 2002 was 7.9% and the target is 3.2%.)
- Reduce the proportion of adults engaging in binge drinking of alcoholic beverages. (Binge drinking remains fairly stable in adults with the highest current rates of 39% among college-age students.)
- Increase the proportion of sexually active people who use condoms. (In 2002, 23% of sexually active females and 42% of males used condoms and the target is 50% to 54%.)

- Increase the proportion of adults with recognized depression who receive treatment. (In 2002, 58% of adults who were diagnosed with depression received treatment and the target is 64%.)
- Reduce deaths caused by motor vehicle crashes. (In 2002, 15.2 deaths/100,000 vehicle miles traveled occurred and the 2010 target is 8.0.)
  - Increase the number of states that have adopted a graduated driver licensing model law. (In 1999, 23 states had adopted graduate driver licensing and the target is all states.)
- Reduce the number of homicides. (In 1999, 6.0 homicides/100,000 population occurred and the target is 2.8.)
- Increase the proportion of people who have a specific source of ongoing care. (In 1997, 86% of all individuals had health insurance and a usual source of health care; individuals ages 18 to 24 years were the most likely to lack a usual source of primary care.)
  - Increase the proportion of pregnancies that are intended. (In 1995, 51% of pregnancies were intended and the target is 70%.)
- Increase the proportion of women who receive early and adequate prenatal care. (In 1998, 74% received early and adequate prenatal care and the target is 90%.)
  - Reduce the proportion of births occurring within 24 months of a previous birth. (In 1995, 11% of females gave birth within 24 months and the target is 6%.)
  - Increase the proportion of adults 20 years and older who are aware of signs of heart attack and the importance of accessing rapid emergency care. (In 2001, 46% of adults were aware of signs of need for, and access to, emergency care; the target is 50%.)

From U.S. Department of Health and Human Services. (2006). *Healthy people 2010:Midcourse review*. Washington, DC: U.S. Government Printing Office.

the rate for males (67.1 visits per 100 females versus 37.7 visits per 100 males) and reflects the inclusion of multiple prenatal visits in any 1 year (Cherry et al., 2003).

A classic public health indicator of a nation's health resources and services is the **maternal mortality rate**. Since 1980, maternal mortality has been fairly stable in the United States. In 1980 the rate was 9.2 per 100,000 live births; then mortality dropped to 6.6 in 1987, rose to 8.9 in 2002. In 2003 the maternal mortality rate was much higher, 12.1 per 100,000 live births (U.S. Census Bureau, 2006), reflecting inclusion of pregnancy status as a separate item on death certificates in some states. *Healthy People 2010 Midcourse Review* (2006) set a target goal of 4.3 maternal deaths per 100,000 live births, but to

reach this goal there is a need for much more statewide action to identify gaps in research, early prevention, and treatment.

GORDON'S FUNCTIONAL HEALTH PATTERNS
Health Perception–Health Management Pattern

Because excellent physical health frequently is taken for granted, concern about health and well-being is relatively low in individuals in their 20s but begins to increase in individuals in their 30s. Monitoring of specific health parameters is both necessary and appropriate to determine health needs and incipient problems. After the mid-30s, an increased sense of the finiteness of life develops with limitations imposed by work choices, well-being, monetary resources, and the deterioration of physical abilities. For more specific health care management, the young adult age span is split into two age groups (18 to 24 and 25 to 35), according to the preventive services that are required.

The assumption that all adults should have an annual physical examination has been supplanted by increased scientifically based information about health screening measures. Screening services provided in a health-monitoring program need to meet cost-effective criteria. Evidenced-based practice uses best practices information for clinical decisions instead of intuition and unmethodical clinical experience and, as such, forms the current recommended standard of care. Evidence-based approaches ultimately will determine which screening measures are best supported by scientific data (randomized controlled treatment studies), reduce regional variations in use of diagnostic and therapeutic modalities, and close the gap between practice and research (Pravikoff et al., 2003).

Behavioral Health History

A behavioral health history is important for young adults. This type of history focuses on risk factors for unintentional injuries, such as alcohol consumption and seat belt use, which are major causes of death and disability in this age group. The safety focus of nursing health promotion for the younger adult takes different forms, from monitoring seat belt use, to concerns about threats such as bioterrorism and globally spreading infections (USDHHS, 2006). Figure 22-1 lists questions and content that might be included in a health history for young adults focusing on their age-specific behaviors.

Preventive Care

Basic goals of preventive care are to maximize the period of optimal health status and detect incipient health problems at an early stage. At age 18 (approximately the time of graduation from high school), a full health appraisal is recommended. Table 22-1 illustrates preventive care that is important during the young adult period, along with recommended frequency of screening. As a rule, the recommendation for most procedures is a repeat health history and visit at approximately 2-year intervals. Appropriate intervention in the younger age group is directed toward correcting health issues through history assessment and counseling about avoidance of adverse health behaviors. Subsequent counseling sessions focus on rechecking and updating information gathered in earlier meetings.

A physical examination includes measurements of height, weight, BMI, blood pressure, and blood tests, with an emphasis on the need to avoid inactivity and obesity, which are risk factors for many health problems. Clinicians who advise women to perform **breast self-examination (BSE)** to screen for breast cancer should understand that there is currently insufficient evidence to determine if this practice decreases breast cancer mortality, but might likely increase the need for further intervention and biopsy (U.S. Preventive Services Task Force, 2008). Papanicolaou (Pap) smears should be performed within 3 years of the onset of sexual activity or age 21, whichever comes first; the incidence of carcinoma in situ, a precursor of invasive cervical and uterine cancer, is high in this group (1 in 1000 women). **Testicular self-examination (TSE)** is taught to men in this age group, although there is some controversy over whether this practice is effective (U.S. Preventive Services Task Force, 2006) as early testicular cancers often present as benign inflammatory conditions. A rectal examination is not recommended unless symptoms are present.

After age 25 the emphasis is on modifying coronary disease risk factors. Recommendations for screening for young adults are undergoing revision as more information becomes available about the interactive risks of high cholesterol, familial high lipid levels, diabetes mellitus, smoking, and alcohol consumption. Recommended screening intervals for young adults with no known risk factors for coronary heart disease is at least every 5 years starting at age 35 for men and 45 for women (U.S Preventive Services Task Force, 2006). Aging is responsible for some degenerative changes in respiratory and cardiac function, but during the young adult years this decline amounts to less than 1% per year and is largely determined by an individual's fitness level (Huether & McCance, 2007). Because cardiovascular disease (along with cancer and cerebrovascular disease) is a primary cause of death, accounting for more than one half of all deaths (Anderson & Arias, 2003), cardiovascular assessment of the young adult includes determining the presence of hyperlipidemia, hypertension, diabetes, chest pain, or heart disease. A *Healthy People 2010 Midcourse Review* target is to reduce the mean total blood cholesterol levels among adults to 199 mg/dL; the baseline between 1988 and 1994 for adults 20 and older was 206 mg/dL (USDHHS, 2006). In 1999-2002, 17% of persons 20 years of age and older had high total blood cholesterol levels (above 240 mg/dL), down from 21% in 1988–94. Also, in the midcourse review, a secondary goal of increasing the proportion of persons with coronary heart disease who have their LDL-cholesterol treated was adjusted lower to less than 100mg/dL (USDHHS, 2006).This suggests that even more watchfulness regarding prevention is indicated, because the number of adults with lesser risk factors for heart disease and stroke is decreasing at the same time many individuals with risk factors are living with undiagnosed disease (Centers for Disease Control and Prevention, 2004a). Health history questions elicit pertinent information about hypertension and **coronary artery disease (CAD)** in parents and relatives.

Hypertension results from increases in cardiac output, or increases in peripheral resistance, or a combination of both and is the third leading cause of death worldwide. According to the Seventh Joint National Committee Report (JNC VII), the focus of blood pressure assessment is on systolic hypertension, and the risks from systolic

Well Young Adult Behavioral Health History Content

Sociodemographic content and questions:

What organizations (community, church, lodge, social, professional, etc.) are you involved in?_____
_____

How would you describe your community?_____
_____

Hobbies, skills, interests, and recreational activities? _____

Military service? No_____   Yes_____   From _____   to_____

Overseas assignment? No_____   Yes_____

Close friends or immediate family members who have died within the past two years? _____
_____

Names and addresses of relatives or close friends in the area._____
_____
_____

Marital status: S M D W   Length of time _____

Environmental content and questions:

Do you live alone? No_____   Yes_____

When did you last move? _____

Describe your living situation. _____

Number of years of education completed: _____

Elementary?_____   High school?_____   College?_____

Occupation?_____   Employer?_____

How long have you worked for this employer? _____

Are you satisfied with your work situation? No_____   Yes_____

Do you consider your work risky or dangerous? No_____   Yes_____

Is your work stressful? No_____   Yes_____

Over the past two weeks, have you felt depressed or hopeless? No_____   Yes_____

Biophysical content questions:

Have you smoked cigarettes? No_____   Yes_____

How much? Less than ½ pack per day? About one pack per day? More than 1½ packs per day?

Are you smoking now? No_____   Yes_____   Length of time smoking?_____

Have you ever smoked cigars or a pipe? No_____   Yes_____

If yes, how long?_____   Do you smoke cigars or a pipe now? No_____   Yes_____

Do you drink alcohol (wine, beer, or whiskey)? No_____   Yes_____

If you do, how much each day on the average?_____   Each week?_____

Do you consume large amounts occasionally (binge drinking)? No_____   Yes_____

Have you been drunk on work days? No_____   Yes_____

Have you had alcoholic drinks in the morning sometime in the past year? No_____   Yes_____

How much coffee, tea, or cola do you drink? _____

Do you use seat or lap belts? No_____   Yes_____

What type of exercise do you do each week? Describe type and amount. _____
_____

Are you satisfied with your weight? No_____   Yes_____   Body image? No_____   Yes_____

Do you use a bicycle or motorcycle helmet? No_____   Yes_____   Helmet and pads while roller blading? No_____   Yes_____

How much sleep do you usually get each night? _____

Meals: Do you generally eat: three regular meals per day? two meals per day? irregular meals?

Are you sexually active? No_____   Yes_____

If so, are you aware of the risks of sexually transmitted diseases? No_____   Yes_____

For women: Do you perform breast self-examination (BSE) each month? No_____   Yes_____

For men: Do you perform testicular self-examination (TSE) regularly? No_____   Yes_____

Figure 22-1   Common well young adult behavioral health history content. (From U.S. Preventive Services Task Force. [2006]. *Guide to clinical preventive services*. Rockville, MD: Agency for Health Care Research and Quality. Retrieved September 2006, from *www.ahrq.gov/clinic/pocketgd.htm*; Somers, A. R., & Breslow, L. [1979]. Lifetime health monitoring program. *Nurse Practitioner, 4*[40], 50, 54.)

Table **22-1**   Well Young Adult Health Monitoring

| Health Issue | Ages 18 to 24 | | Ages 25 to 35 | |
	Intervention	Frequency (Years)	Intervention	Frequency (Years)
Tobacco use	History and counseling	Each visit	History and counseling	Each visit
Obesity/nutrition/ body mass index (BMI)	History, weight, and counseling	Each visit	History, weight, and counseling	Each visit
Avoid alcohol while driving, swimming, engaging in activities that involve mental and physical alertness	History and counseling	At least once	History and counseling	Every 2
Accidental injury, lap and shoulder belts, bicycle or motorcycle helmets, smoke detectors, safe firearm use	History and counseling	At least once	History and counseling	Every 2
Unintended pregnancy	Counseling	At least once	History and counseling	Every 2
Contraception	Counseling	Individually determined	Counseling	Individually determined
Illegal drug use	History and counseling	At least once	History and counseling	Every 2 to 4
Regular physical activity	History and counseling	At least once	History and counseling	Every 2 to 4
Blood pressure, hypertension	Blood pressure measurement	Every 2	Blood pressure measurement	Every 2 to 4
Breast or testicular cancer	BSE or TSE counseling	Every 1 to 2	BSE or TSE counseling	Every 1 to 2
Vision defects	Examination	Once and refer	Examination	Every 4
Tetanus/diphtheria/ pertussis (Tdap)	Booster	Once if 10 yr since last one	Immunization	Every 10
Hepatitis B	Immunization	If not immunized	Immunization	If not immunized
Diabetes, proteinuria, bacteriuria	Urinalysis	Once	Urinalysis	Every 4
Coronary artery disease	Serum cholesterol level determination, triglyceride level	Once	Serum cholesterol level determination	Every 5
Dental care	Dental examination and cleaning	Every 1 to 2	Dental examination and cleaning	Every 1 to 2
Cervical dysplasia	Gynecological exam; Pap smear	Every 1 to 3	Gynecological exam; Pap smear	Every 1 to 3
STD prevention	Counseling	Individually determined	Counseling	Individually determined
Chlamydia (women)	Chlamydia screen	At gynecological examination, if sexually active	Chlamydia screen	At gynecological examination, if sexually active
Gonorrhea (women)	Vaginal culture	At gynecological examination, if sexually active	Vaginal culture	At gynecological examination

BMI, Body mass index; *BSE,* breast self-examination; *TSE,* testicular self-examination; *Pap,* Papanicolaou; *STD,* sexually transmitted disease.
Modified from U.S. Preventive Services Task Force. (2006). U.S. Preventive Services Task Force. Rockville, MD: Agency for Health Care Research and Quality. Retrieved September 11, 2007, from *www.ahrq.gov/clinic/pocketgd.htm.*

hypertension, which rise beginning with systolic pressures of 115 mm Hg. The risk from diastolic hypertension starts to rise at 75 mm Hg. The focus of attention is on lowering blood pressure toward the new normal goal of 120/80 mm Hg or less (USDHHS, 2006; Chobanian et al., 2003). Each increase in blood pressure over this level exerts a consistent rise in risk for heart attack, stroke, and heart failure. JNC VII also established a new category of "prehypertension" to

better identify individuals at risk for developing treatable hypertension to encourage lifestyle changes before vascular disease is present (USDHHS, 2006).

The Mexican-American population has the lowest percentage of high blood pressure individuals (27%) while the non-Hispanic Black population has the highest (43%) (USDHHS, 2006). More young Black people than young White people die as a result of chronic heart disease or stroke (cerebrovascular accident). Although for the entire population, deaths attributable to coronary heart disease and stroke have declined, the mortality rate remains higher for Blacks (Anderson & Arias, 2003). A wellness target of *Healthy People 2010 Midcourse Review* (2006) is to increase the proportion of young adults 18 years and older with hypertension whose blood pressure is under control from 18% (in 1988 to 1994) to 68% (USDHHS, 2006). A second target of *Healthy People 2010 Midcourse Review* is to reduce the proportion of adults with high blood pressure; from 1988 through 1994, 26% of adults age 20 years and older had high blood pressure. The literature describes a "stroke belt" in the southeastern states, where the incidence of stroke is reported to be above the national average. A target goal of *Healthy People 2010* was to reduce stroke deaths to 48 deaths per 100,000 population and in the *Midcourse Review* (2006) 50% of the target was already attained. Explanations for the change included improved management of blood pressure and atrial fibrillation (USDHHS, 2006).

The **metabolic syndrome** includes a group of cardiovascular risk factors associated with overweight and obesity, particularly abdominal obesity (USDHHS, 2006). This syndrome includes the lethal risks of high lipid levels, insulin resistance, and hypertension. Currently at least one fourth of U.S. adults are estimated to have this cluster of risk factors, placing them at increased risk for CAD. First-step therapy involves lifestyle alterations, including weight management and increase in physical activity (Centers for Disease Control and Prevention, 2004a; USDHHS, 2006).

Diabetes is seventh on the list of leading causes of death in the United States; currently 18.2 million Americans have the disease and nearly one third are unaware that they have it (USDHHS, 2006). Minority populations (Blacks, Native American–Alaska Natives, and Hispanics) are disproportionately affected with Native American populations experiencing twice the rate for new cases recorded in White non-Hispanic populations (USDHHS, 2006). The incidence of diabetes, especially type 2 diabetes (adult onset), and related complications (cardiovascular disease, blindness, and end-stage renal disease) is increasing in the United States (USDHHS, 2006). Of those diagnosed with diabetes, only a few have their blood pressure, glucose levels, and cholesterol levels sufficiently controlled to avoid or delay vascular disease. Because careful control can delay the beginning and progression of long-term complications, early detection and monitoring of diabetes is important.

Decision-Making and Risk Taking

The decision-making of a young adult directly affects health and well-being. Peak physical skills stimulate young adults to be venturesome, daring, enterprising, and aggressive. Young adults have less experience with the death of significant others, and they may take inordinate risks. The leading causes of death in individuals ages 15 to 24 years of age are unintentional injuries, homicide, and suicide (USDHHS,

2006). The prevalence of adverse behaviors associated with sudden death illustrates a developmental lack of fear in young adults. Underuse of seat belts and helmets by motorcyclists and bicyclists is a cause of many accidental injuries and deaths. Some states still do not have laws that require helmets.

Communicable Diseases and Adult Immunization

Communicable (infectious) diseases affect young adults with varying degrees of severity. Although the availability of better drug treatments, vaccines, improved hygiene and food handling, and cleaner water supplies have promoted prevention and control of infectious disease, new disease threats are continually emerging at a rate of approximately one per year. Much of this increase is due to changes in travel, social, sexual, and other behaviors that expose broader populations of individuals to emerging pathogens. Newer threats include drug-resistant tuberculosis, H5N1 bird flu, severe acute respiratory syndrome (SARS), Lyme disease, diarrhea caused by *Escherichia coli* O157:H7, and hantavirus pulmonary disease. Increasingly, new cases of tuberculosis are occurring in foreign-born individuals (USDHHS, 2006), even as the incidence of this disease declined to 6.8 cases per 100,000 of the population. An increase in tuberculosis rates, particularly in some minority groups (Asian American–Pacific Islanders, Blacks, and Hispanics), illustrates that preventive activities must be reinforced and constant vigilance maintained over monitoring and effectiveness for all communicable diseases. The focus of tuberculosis surveillance is moving toward tracking of full completion of the drug protocol. In 2003, SARS, caused by a respiratory virus harbored by the Chinese civet cat, caused a global threat and the monitoring of individuals traveling to and from Asian countries (Fenwick, 2003). Lyme disease climbed from a baseline of 17.4/100,000 population new cases to 32.5 new cases with a goal of 9.7 cases (USDHHS, 2006); the absence of a vaccine for this disease is a significant hindrance to meeting the target (USDHHS, 2006).

Cases of acute **hepatitis B** (HB) infection declined in young adults due to vaccination programs aimed at children, adolescents, and adults in high-risk groups (USDHHS, 2006). A primary way of achieving high levels of vaccination coverage is to identify settings in which unvaccinated young adults can be vaccinated, such as correctional facilities, drug treatment centers, and clinics treating sexually transmitted diseases (STDs) (USDHHS, 2006).

Rubella in young adults is generally a minor disease; however, when the disease is contracted during the first trimester of pregnancy, miscarriage, stillbirth, or **congenital rubella syndrome** (CRS) can result. CRS is associated with loss of hearing, ocular defects, developmental delay and growth retardation, and cardiac malformations. In 2003, seven cases were identified in the U.S. and the target is zero (USDHHS, 2006). New rubella cases appear to be originating in other parts of the world as demonstrated through patterns in viral genotyping (USDHHS, 2006). All women of childbearing age should be screened (titer monitored) for rubella antibodies and those who are not immune should be immunized. Nurses inform women of childbearing age that antibody testing is recommended before pregnancy and that vaccination is available.

Another target of *Healthy People 2010 Midcourse Review* is to reduce the incidence of hepatitis C to 1 case in 100,000 population from the 2.5 new cases per 100,000 population occurring presently (USDHHS, 2006). Chronic hepatitis became a nationally reportable disease in 2003. Individuals most at risk are those who have injected illicit drugs, are on hemodialysis, are seropositive for **human immunodeficiency virus (HIV)**, or have elevated liver function studies.

Although most outbreaks of meningococcal disease are sporadic, young adults living in dormitories may be more susceptible than young adults not living in dormitory settings. Although meningococci are sensitive to the penicillins and many antibiotics, the case fatality rate is high in otherwise healthy adults, and many survivors may have substantial neurological disabilities or loss of hearing. Most at risk are college freshmen living in dormitories, who have a higher case ratio. CDC through the Advisory Committee on Immunization Practices (ACIP) recommends routine vaccination of adolescents, college students, military recruits, and travelers to areas in which the disease is prevalent (Bilukha & Rosenstein, 2005).

Other viral agents, such as genital herpes virus and **human papilloma virus (HPV)**, commonly affect young adults. **Genital herpes virus** infections occur frequently in young adults because of the escalation of sexual activity during this period. HPV is spread through sexual contact, and some forms of the virus in combination with smoking are strongly related to the later development of cervical dysplasia and cancer. The prevalence of HPV infection is 45% among 20 to 24 year olds (Fontenot et al., 2007). The first vaccine to prevent cervical cancer, Gardasil® HPV vaccine, is effective against four types of the virus (HPV types 6, 11, 16, 18); it has become recently available and is recommended for girls and young women ages 9 to 26 years (Fontenot et al., 2007).

Nutritional-Metabolic Pattern

In the *Healthy People 2010 Midcourse Review* (2006), the magnitude of the obesity problem is emphasized in that none of the objectives in the Nutrition and Overweight section met or exceeded their targets. Obesity in the United States is attaining epidemic proportions and is a pressing public health problem. Continue to check *Healthy People 2020* for more updates on obesity.

Many adults value slimness, defined muscle tone, and athletic ability. Regular physical activity increases muscle and bone strength, decreases body fat, aids in weight control, enhances well-being, and reduces depression (USDHHS, 2006). An optimally functioning **basal metabolic rate** in

the young adult permits adequate oxygen intake during normal activity and rest periods. A young male requires approximately 1600 to 1800 calories a day to meet his body's basal metabolic needs, and a young female only 1200 to 1450 calories a day. As growth stops in the late teens, the basal metabolic rate declines.

During the young adult years, caloric intake increases substantially, particularly in men. Increased caloric intake without a corresponding energy expenditure can lead to obesity, which is a precursor to hypertension, coronary disease, and diabetes.

According to information shown in Figure 22-2, 11% of children and adolescents ages 6 to 19 years are overweight or obese and 23% of adults age 20 and older are obese (USDHHS, 2006). During survey periods of 1988 to 1994 and 1999 to 2002, the age-adjusted proportion of adults 20 years and older at a healthy weight decreased from 42% to 33% (goal is 60%); at the same time the proportion of adults who were obese increased from 23% to 30% (goal is 15%) (USDHHS, 2006). Although trends toward increasing weight occurred in all major racial and ethnic groups, the increase was more pronounced for the Black non-Hispanic population (increase from 30% to 39%) (Centers for Disease Control and Prevention, 2005) and the White non-Hispanic population (increase 22% to 30%) rather than for the Mexican American population (29% to 21%) (USDHHS, 2006). In the same survey periods, the prevalence of obesity among males aged 20 years and older increased from 20% to 27% and in females

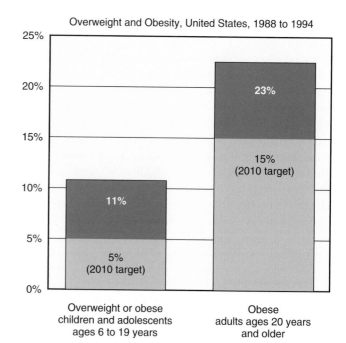

Figure 22-2 Overweight and obesity, 1988 to 1994. (From U.S. Department of Health and Human Services. [2006]. *Healthy people 2010: Midcourse review.* Retrieved September 11, 2007, from *www.healthypeople.gov/data/midcourse/html*)

increased from 25% to 33% (USDHHS, 2006). Reports suggest that intellectually challenged individuals may have 10% more obesity than individuals with normal intelligence (Marshall et al., 2003). To stop or decrease the trend, new behaviors must be learned for nutrition and physical activity.

For many Americans, food sources are abundant, portion sizes have increased, and lifestyles are becoming increasingly sedentary (USDHHS, 2006). More specifically, decreasing fat intake, increasing fruit and vegetable intake, and increasing physical activity must be emphasized. Food-labeling information (now includes trans fats) is now required for processed and packaged foods. Another challenge is the increasing consumption of food prepared and eaten away from home, which is generally higher in fats, cholesterol, and sodium, and lower in fiber and calcium than that prepared at home (USDHHS, 2006). This suggests that the composition of food prepared outside the home promotes weight gain (Frank, 2007). Many states have legislation pending that would require restaurants and fast food outlets to list food composition on menus (Frank, 2007). Collective national action and community involvement are needed to promote healthful diets among all Americans and to reverse the increasing trend to be overweight and obese. With increased obesity and its associated health problems, there will be more access to better pharmaceuticals and increased use of bariatric surgery, although these treatments also must be evaluated for risks and benefits (USDHHS, 2006).

Health professionals are counseled to investigate weight problems by monitoring waist circumference, blood pressure, cholesterol levels, and activity levels rather than solely monitoring weight, to the frustration of many people. Assessments are made of weight and height to calculate body mass index (BMI). Those with a BMI of 25 or less (male waist size of 40 inches or less, women 35 inches or less) should have weight maintenance teaching. Individuals with a BMI of 30 or greater who have tried diets and exercise may be considered for weight-reducing drugs (Manson et al., 2004). A BMI of 40 or more meets the criteria for bariatric surgery in psychologically stable individuals. In persons with comorbidity, bariatric surgery may be suggested with a BMI of 35 or greater (Manson et al., 2004). The focus of professional advice is conservative at first, recommending careful diet appraisal and increase in exercise patterns. Repetitions will probably be necessary, because long-term weight management is a frustrating process.

Proper nutrition is particularly necessary for the young adult female during the childbearing years. Contributing factors to iron deficiency in this age group are regular loss of blood (during menses) and pregnancy. The prevalence of anemia among low-income women in their third trimester of pregnancy increased from 29% in 1996 to 30% in 2003, moving away from a goal of 20% (USDHHS, 2006) (see

Case Study and Care Plan at the end of this chapter). A blood loss of 2 to 4 milliliters per day (1 to 2 mg of iron) can cause iron deficiency anemia; young women who don't eat a healthy diet and have heavy periods or use nonsteroidal anti-inflammatory drugs are specifically at risk for iron deficiency anemia. Iron supplementation is recommended during pregnancy for optimal growth of the fetus and supporting structures (Lowdermilk & Perry, 2007). The CDC recommends that all women of childbearing age consume 0.4 mg of folic acid daily to reduce the risk of **fetal neural tube defects (FNP)**, including spina bifida. Supplementation should include at least the month before pregnancy and the first trimester during pregnancy. The CDC and Food and Drug Administration recommends folic acid fortification of food to prevent neural tube defects (USDHHS, 2006). In addition, the Association of Women's Health, Obstetric and Neonatal Nurses (AWHONN) also recommends fortification of oral contraceptive preparations with folic acid supplementation to provide additional protection to women of childbearing age (Association of Women's Health, Obstetric and Neonatal Nurses [AWHONN], 2004b). Efforts are also being made to reduce health disparities in neural tube defects including the use of better communication modalities with the Hispanic population and other groups that have higher rates of neural tube defects (USDHHS, 2006).

Most adolescents and adult women fail to meet their calcium requirements, placing them at risk for osteoporosis and bone fractures in later life. Low calcium intake is a direct result of low milk consumption related to soft drink ingestion. An increase in calcium-containing foods is therefore recommended, particularly for teens and young women (see Chapter 11).

Elimination Pattern

Patterns of elimination are generally well established by young adulthood. Although eating disorders (anorexia and bulimia) typically begin at an earlier stage of development, they can persist during young adulthood. The fashion industry is widely criticized for using underweight women as young female models, thereby emphasizing excessive thinness as the ideal female standard. Assessment of young adults is directed toward teaching about the common complaints of constipation, hemorrhoids, and occasional diarrhea. While the risk of colon cancer is low in this age group, young adults should be aware that changes in elimination patterns or blood in the stool should be reported to their primary care provider. Young adults should be counseled about drinking adequate amounts of fluid and eating fruits and vegetables, which are sources of fiber, to promote bowel health.

Activity-Exercise Pattern

Inactivity is a predisposing factor to cardiovascular disease and obesity; increasing access to and promoting locations for physical activity is increasingly emphasized. A *Healthy*

People 2010 Midcourse Review goal is to reduce the proportion of adults who engage in no leisure-time physical activity to 20% from approximately 40% in 2002, and to increase the proportion of adults who engage in moderate physical activity for 30 minutes a day to 50% from 32% in 2002 (USDHHS, 2006).

Aerobic exercise, in which oxygen is metabolized to produce energy, develops an optimally functioning cardiorespiratory system. Aerobic conditioning achieves cardiovascular fitness through five periods of moderately intense exercise weekly, for 30 minutes (Physical Activity and Public Health, 2007) or more at a heart rate of approximately 220 minus the age of the person multiplied by 65% to 85%. Young adults are encouraged to engage in fitness activities that increase the heart rate to approximately 150 or more beats per minute. After 5 minutes of activity at this rate, the body is required to make adjustments in cardiovascular capacity by enlarging the lungs and the capillaries in the muscles and the heart. Repeated aerobic exercise, such as swimming, cycling, running, skipping rope, and walking, produces physical fitness and decreases the likelihood of problems caused by inactivity. The major barriers to increasing physical activity seem to be lack of time, access to exercise facilities, and safe environments in which to exercise (USDHHS, 2006).

Radiation and Excessive Sun Exposure

Nurses educate young adults about the risks of sun exposure and tanning, the preventive use of sun-blocking agents, and skin symptoms that might indicate cancer. Sunblocking agents reduce sunburn or other skin damage with the goal of lowering the risk of skin cancer. A number of the agents are rated based on skin type and sensitivity to burning. Many lotions and creams are available with differing radiation protection levels. **Sunscreen protective factor index (SPF)** is a calculation of the effectiveness of various preparations. The agents are rated on a scale by the U.S. FDA. For example, a rating of 30 means the sunscreen provides 30 times the protection of unprotected skin. Active ingredients vary, but the most effective lotions are nonopague combinations of para amino, benzoic acid, ester, and benzophenone (Anderson, 2002). Women's makeup preparations now include sun-blocking agents. Young adults should avoid sunbathing during the 2-hour period before and after noon, because two thirds of the day's ultraviolet light comes through the earth's atmosphere during this time. Ultraviolet light is stronger at different times of the day depending on geographical location. Sunscreens that block both ultraviolet Q and ultraviolet B light are more effective in preventing cancer than those which block only ultraviolet B light (U.S. Preventive Task Force, 2006). Best protection is achieved by applying agents 15 to 30 minutes before exposure, then reapplying every 15 to 30 minutes during exposure to the sun. Further application may be necessary if activities involve swimming, sweating, or rubbing. Sun-protective measures such as sunscreen, sun-protective clothing, and avoidance of ultraviolet light is a part of young adult education.

Sports

Bicycling and motorcycling are encouraged by environmentalists to decrease automobile pollution; this trend is also promoted to relieve traffic congestion, avoid the high costs of fuel and car maintenance, and increase interest in healthy exercise. Cyclists are at risk of being involved in accidents with automobiles. Head injury is responsible for approximately 62% of bicycle-related fatalities. In 1999, only 10 states had mandatory helmet requirements for riders under 15 years of age (USDHHS, 2006). Bicycle helmets are believed to be the single most effective preventive measure available to decrease the incidence of brain and head injury (USDHHS, 2006).

Motorcycles have less occupant protection than do automobiles but are appealing to young adults, primarily because they have high-performance capabilities. Using a motorcycle helmet reduces the chance of dying in an accident by 29% (USDHHS, 2006). A target of *Healthy People 2010 Midcourse Review* is to increase the proportion of motorcyclists using helmets from 67% in 1998 to 79% in 2010 (USDHHS, 2006).

Accidental deaths from drowning are also common in young adults. Swimming, boating, and scuba diving are associated with the high number of water-related fatalities. Hang gliding, parachuting, and flying small aircraft are responsible for a large number of outdoor fatalities. Mountain climbing, hiking in poor weather conditions, downhill ski racing, and bobsledding are other hazardous activities. Most so-called accidents are not random, uncontrollable events, but predictable and preventable if precautions and risks are analyzed (USDHHS, 2006).

Amateur and professional sports activities generally pose few hazards when rules and safety precautions are observed. Relatively few fatalities are associated with the professionally organized contact sports, such as football, hockey, or boxing, but chronic injuries frequently cause discomfort. A study of football hits and accelerations indicates that some of the blows players endure are similar to those experienced in automobile accidents (Bhattacharya, 2004).

A comprehensive history of recreational activities alerts the nurse to specific needs about safety education. Young adults are encouraged to learn and abide by the rules of the sport in which they are engaged. Rules in many sports have evolved from health and safety concerns, enabling the individual to learn the sport well with appropriate instruction.

Sleep-Rest Pattern

Young adults are subject to fatigue induced by work, **stress**, or inactivity. Changes in activity or stressors can help reduce fatigue. Trying out new and challenging tasks can help reduce mental stress. New physical activities, such as learning a new sport or form of exercise, can also provide stimulation.

Cognitive-Perceptual Pattern
Physical and Mental Patterns

Visual acuity is highest at approximately age 20 and begins to decline at approximately age 40, when farsightedness frequently develops. Hearing is also best at age 20; the ability to distinguish high-pitched tones decreases with age. The other senses—taste, smell, touch, and awareness of temperature and pain—remain stable until age 45 to 50.

Further maturation requires young adults to learn skills and behaviors that improve the performance abilities gained as adolescents (Figure 22-3). Factors that an individual young adult may perceive as essential to learn will depend on specific goals, values, attitudes, and practices as influenced by intrinsic (constitutional) and extrinsic (environmental or community) factors. The development of intellectual maturity influences the selection of behaviors and attitudes that affect health and well-being practices.

Piaget's Theory

Jean Piaget's stage of formal operational thought evolves from concrete operational thought in adolescence and extends through the reasoning process of young adults (Piaget, 1972). Achievement of formal operational thinking allows a person to analyze all combinations of possibilities and construct hypotheses that can be tested. Young adult thought becomes more perceptive and insightful; issues can therefore be evaluated realistically and objectively. Young adults are energetic and can therefore contribute substantially to social and occupational decision-making. Although they tend to take greater risks, young adults typically demonstrate the use of appropriate reasoning and analytical approaches.

Intellectual Growth

Organization of information influences memory. Evidence shows that recall performance diminishes with age: at its peak in the twenties, memory starts to diminish during the

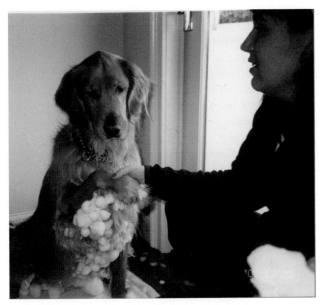

Figure 22-3 Taking care of animal shows adult responsibility.

thirties. Improved strategies for organization of information, however, can enhance recall, and limitation of memory with increasing age is likely a result of retrieval rather than storage mechanisms.

Erikson's Theory

A major goal for young adults is the development of an increased sense of competency and self-esteem (Erikson, 1993). In developing self-esteem, the individual learns to be truly open and capable of trust through the formation of intimate relationships that are characteristic of this period. Erikson (1993) has described this stage of psychosocial development as **intimacy versus isolation** and loneliness.

Erikson's concept of genuine intimacy extends beyond sexual relations to a broader view of mutual psychosocial intimacy with a spouse or lover, parents, children, and friends. Characterized by the reciprocal expression of affection, intimacy requires mutual trust. These interchanges are spontaneous for the young adult; relationships should be free and allow for self-disclosure. Young adults who are unsure of their identity may avoid intimate contact or engage in promiscuous behavior lacking in true intimacy, which can result in isolation and consequent self-absorption. Healthy adults search for continuity, regularity, or unity of meaningful relationships, while avoiding situations of little commitment.

Moral Development

Young adults who have successfully mastered the previous cognitive, social, and moral stages are usually able to recognize or use principled reasoning. Lawrence Kohlberg identifies this ability as the **postconventional level of moral reasoning** (Kohlberg & Lickons, 1986). During this phase, the individual is able to differentiate the self from the rules and expectations of others and to define principles regarding rights in terms of self-chosen principles. The interests of individuals can be weighed against the needs of society and the state, and violations of law can be justified when individual interests are in accord with principles. Gilligan (1982, 2002), who studied the development of moral reasoning in women and girls, asserts that their moral judgments reflect less of a "rights" perspective and more of an emphasis on responsibilities in relationships.

Although development of principled moral reasoning is possible during young adulthood, it may never occur if the cognitive and social factors that stimulate higher reasoning are not present. Acts of personal violence representative of lower moral reasoning should not be present; however, such acts do occur during this period, illustrating the need for addressing moral development concerns at earlier stages of education and socialization.

Self-Perception–Self-Concept Pattern

In non-Western cultures the entrance to adulthood generally is defined and marked by social events such as marriage. In Western societies, maturation is defined through the individual's achievement of financial and residential independence, and is a more drawn-out, gradual process. Two emotional themes regarding the value of work become evident during young adulthood. During their twenties, young adults yearn to explore and experiment, keeping structures temporary and reversible. These individuals may move from job to job and relationship to relationship, remaining in a transient state. At the opposite extreme is the urge to prepare for the future by making firm commitments. During this period, both men and women question their value to society, the merit of their accomplishments, their success as sexual beings, and the probability of attaining their unfulfilled goals.

The U.S. Census Bureau (2006) reports that more than 70% of women ages 25 to 35 were employed in 2005; this percentage is rising and expected to be more than 80% by 2010. As more mothers enter the labor force, the need for child care increases. The gap in earnings, or pay differential, between men and women is also significant. Access to insurance and pension benefits is not always available, especially to high-risk groups such as minorities or people receiving the minimum wage. Even when there is sufficient access to health care, some types of employment expose individuals to occupational risks and hazards.

Many young adults are high achievers and seek opportunities to be challenged. Employment problems can be stressful and traumatic to an individual's self-esteem and self-worth, particularly in the current economic environment. The failure to receive a promotion or a pay raise can accelerate the degree of stress. Employment is more than a source of income; it provides self-esteem and social interaction. Because the adjustment to the job market influences many other aspects of daily living, young adults frequently require assistance in developing coping mechanisms to manage stress. Properly managing the initial stress prevents further complications that can arise if the young adult uses unhealthy stress relievers such as alcohol or drugs.

Young women have many of the same concerns about employment and success as do young men. Many young women postpone childbearing until they have established their careers; many are absent from the job for only a standard maternity leave. Women who return to work when their children are very young frequently risk the emotional strain caused by guilt feelings and role strain. In addition to helping parents cope with the stress of being absent from their children, nurses can help them identify ways to provide high-quality supervision in their absence, either through private baby-sitters, day care programs, or through neighbors, friends, and relatives.

The U.S. workforce is changing dramatically as companies restructure, downsize, "right size," and shift employees around to meet changing market conditions, company mergers, and buyouts. The nature of work is changing with a continued trend toward longer hours, increased use of contracted and temporary workers, and increased telecommuting (USDHHS, 2006). There is increasing concern about "globalization," outsourcing, and jobs, especially in the computer industry, moving overseas. Job stress can lead to increased absenteeism, which is more common in young adults. Nursing interventions in industrial settings are directed toward improving both working conditions and employer-employee relationships. Healthy work sites increase the chance that young adults will have access to comprehensive health-promotion programs.

Roles-Relationships Pattern

Young adult friendships are more enduring than are earlier relationships. The focus of the relationship is the sharing of feelings or confidences as well as common interests. True friendship is characteristic of a person who wants to give rather than receive. Friendships are necessary in a constantly changing society; they provide a source of emotional support and a basis of stability for developing the self-concept.

Establishing interpersonal relationships involves agreeable and purposeful interactions with others. Interpersonal relationships can be created with people of the same or the opposite sex; age is typically a less important factor than it was during adolescence. The formation of intimate relationships develops within or outside a family context and occasionally in the work environment. Cell phone and Internet access facilitates relationships through text messaging, e-mail, and instant messaging. For some the significant other is a person of the same sex, and legislative proposals are active in many states that would legitimize the legal rights of same-sex couples through same-sex marriage or civil union statutes. See the Innovative Practice box about the Gay and Lesbian Wellness Series.

In addition to achieving intimacy, the young adult must accomplish other developmental tasks to achieve true psychosocial maturation. Decision-making about life and career directions is the developmental milestone that heralds the transition from adolescence to adulthood. Decisions usually entail establishing independence from the family of origin. This transition may involve an actual physical move from the parents' home (going away to college, joining the military, or getting an apartment); however, movement away is not the sole indicator of independence. Young adults frequently remain in their parents' home for economic reasons, particularly when life choices involve continued schooling, unemployment, or remaining unmarried. In some cultures, unmarried adults live with their parents until they are married, and newly married young adults share the home of their parents until they begin having their own children.

Individuals in this age group typically choose life partners and begin families; they make decisions about childbearing and the number and education of children. Additional consideration must be given to decisions related to childbearing, such as finances, safety, family support, housing, the relationship with extended family members, and the roles and responsibilities within the nuclear family unit. Young adults who are establishing a family must have open communication about self-development, which includes issues of dual careers, child-rearing practices, and domestic duties.

Family harmony and development are major goals for many young adults. Although family size and structure have undergone dramatic changes in recent decades, concern about each member's health and safety continues to be a primary focus. Family life is influenced by the qualities of individual family members. Typically, economic security, status, place in the community, and healthy patterns of living, such as good nutrition, personal hygiene, and physical fitness, are associated with healthy family adjustment.

Separation and Divorce

About one half of first marriages and 60% of second marriages terminate in divorce (Golden & Hopkins, 2003). About one quarter of all children in the United States are living in single–parent, mother-led families, and one half of the children affected by divorce frequently never see their fathers again. Many stressors contribute to divorce. It is a difficult process, and lingering anger and hostility may remain for years. Socioeconomic factors often place unreasonable stress on marriages. Age at the time of marriage is correlated with duration of marriage, and young adults whose parents have divorced have an increased rate of divorce. Employment has enabled women to leave unhappy marriages that they formerly would have been forced to tolerate. A recent law signed by President Barack Obama assures women equal pay in the workforce.

Although dissatisfaction and unhappiness are frequent precursors to separation and divorce, the decision to dissolve a marriage is not easy. Considerable emotional strain exists for both partners, their children, their families, and close friends. Divorce requires that young adults reevaluate their basic values, individual personality, spiritual beliefs, and ego strength, job potential, and socioeconomic factors to ensure future security for themselves and their children. Divorced young adults frequently suffer severe emotional strain and depression. Some young adults are unable to adjust to role and status changes and to threats to self-concept. For these reasons, support systems in the form of groups, individual counseling, or special social activities are critical. As a result of divorce, many women and their young children are forced to seek emergency shelter in publicly operated homes, including welfare hotels and group shelters.

Many people need support from the nurse to help them work through this difficult period. Nurses help to identify the feelings of guilt, grief, and loss that young adults experience during a separation or divorce. Suggesting that young adults read articles or books on issues related to divorce is helpful, because they provide a reference point for their

---

innovative practice

Gay and Lesbian Wellness Series

The Gay and Lesbian Wellness Series is a multidisciplinary educational program offered through the collaborative efforts of the Be Well! programs of the Tanger Center for Health Management and the Lesbian and Gay Advisory Committee at Beth Israel Deaconess Medical Center in Boston, Massachusetts.

The clinician-teachers encourage clients and employees of the hospital and ambulatory care centers and members of the community, whether gay, straight, or bisexual, to participate in these free educational programs. In 2004, Massachusetts became the first state to implement legislation allowing marriage between individuals of the same sex. The following examples are indicative of educational topics offered at Beth Israel Deaconess Medical Center:

1. *Sexual Orientation and the Workplace: Creating an Open Environment.* Understanding the dynamics of the work environment, whether as a clinician, manager, or support staff, can be challenging when issues of sexual orientation in the workplace are examined. As a gay or lesbian employee, how comfortable do you feel being "out" at work? Alternatively, as a manager of gay and lesbian employees, how successful are you in creating an environment in which staff members feel safe, comfortable, and valued? This class is a discussion of this topic aimed at creating an open environment for all.

2. *A Welcoming Place for All: Improving Access and Quality for Gay and Lesbian Patients.* Underestimating the power of a simple word or gesture in providing care for individuals is easy. Sensitivity to the wording of materials and forms, and the way in which questions are asked, can help gay and lesbian individuals feel safe and comfortable. This class offers the opportunity to learn more about steps you can take to make your department, unit, or practice a welcoming place for all.

3. *Selecting and Communicating with Your Health Care Provider.* Asking the right questions and developing a comfortable and trusting relationship with a primary care provider are challenges for everyone. For gay and lesbian individuals, the task can be especially difficult. Tips are available for enhancing the lines of communication between the client and health care providers.

4. *Supporting and Communicating with Your Gay or Lesbian Child: Understanding Gay and Lesbian Issues in the Family.* Parents of gay and lesbian children frequently have few places to turn for support and information. Struggling with love for one's child and the challenges of accepting the child's sexual orientation can be an overwhelming dilemma.

Contact Information:
Tanger Center for Health Management
Lesbian and Gay Advisory Committee
Beth Israel Deaconess Medical Center
Boston, MA
Telephone: 617-667-4695

---

experiences. The nurse recommends marital counseling by a qualified professional; this may be the most beneficial source of support.

HEALTH TEACHING   Assessment and Education Regarding Firearm Safety

Nurses are taught to perform community and environmental assessments; however, most fail to incorporate assessment of the presence of firearms in the home. Rates of unintentional firearm deaths were highest for individuals aged 15 to 29 years. The potential for suicide in young adults doubles when a firearm is kept in the home. Approximately 25% of families keep at least one firearm in the home, and 74% of these families own more than one firearm. Adults who keep firearms for self-protection are more likely to keep it accessible and loaded, even though there is data that a weapon kept at home is 43 times more likely to be used against a family member or acquaintance. In the past decade, school violence with multiple victims has increased. In 2007, a college student with a history of past mental treatment obtained a gun and shot 32 students and faculty members at Virginia Tech. Five to 13% of high school students reported bringing a firearm to school at least once. Firearm presence in the home is a risk for violence against women. *Healthy People 2010* reports nationwide data that emphasizes the need to reduce firearm deaths, reduce firearm injuries, and reduce the proportion of individuals living in homes with firearms that are unlocked and loaded.

The American Academy of Pediatrics has published a position paper on gun safety and urges all physicians to ask questions about guns when taking client histories. A widely publicized program called ASK requests that parents inquire if guns are present in any home where their child will stay or play: "Is there a gun where my children play?" (Ahmann, 2001). This question should be posed with other questions aimed at ascertaining the adequacy of child supervision in any other site. If there is a gun in the home, the parent can check to see if the gun is stored unloaded in a locked or secure closet, or offer to have the children play in a monitored setting at another location.

The most obvious strategy is to prevent unauthorized access to unlocked and loaded firearms. The best way to accomplish this would be to greatly reduce firearm presence in the general population. Continued technology development may make it more physically difficult for children, adolescents, and unauthorized adults to discharge the firearm. In the meantime, safe storage of firearms and ammunition is important to reducing the number of preventable deaths and injuries caused by firearms.

Complied from FireArm safety: Emergency Room nurses association position statement. *Topics in Emergency Medicine, 27*(3), 233-236; Ahmann, E. (2001). Guns in the home: Nurses' role. *Pediatric Nursing, 27*(6), 587–590, 605; U.S. Department of Health and Human Services. (2006). *Healthy people 2010: Midcourse review.* Retrieved September 11, 2007, from *www.healthypeople.gov/data/midcourse/html.*

Male and Female Risk of Violence

Violence is becoming more prevalent and a global health problem. Although most cite the World Trade Center incident in 2001 and the Iraq War as examples of organized terrorism, worldwide only one fifth of violent acts are related to organized events. Over one half are suicides and another one third are homicides (Centers for Disease Control and Prevention, 2004b). Youth are involved as both the perpetrators and the victims of violence. In the United States their targets tend to be the older adults, children, and women with whom they are familiar (USDHHS, 2006). Homicide (assault) is the second leading cause of death in the 15-year-old to 24-year-old age group and the leading cause of death for Black men in the same age category (U.S. Census Bureau, 2006). Between 1999 and 2002 the homicide rate has remained fairly static at 6.1 deaths/100,000 population; this is a significant decline from the rate seen in the early 1990s and there are ongoing efforts to understand what has contributed to the improvement (USDHHS, 2006). Firearms are involved in approximately two thirds of these deaths, and men have twice the risk of dying as do women. When compared with the general population, mortality statistics are higher for men of poorer populations, in urban areas, and with less formal education. Homicide is closely associated with alcohol and drug abuse and frequently is related to other violent acts, such as robbery. Other risk factors include history of loss of employment, detention or prison experience, access to firearms, abuse in the home, mental illness, social isolation, and homelessness. The presence of firearms in the home

is associated with the increased risk of unintentional and intentional injury to children (Health Teaching box). A target in *Healthy People 2010 Midcourse Review* is to reduce firearm-related deaths from 10.3 per 100,000 population in 2000 to 3.6 per 100,000 population and to reduce the proportion of people living in homes with firearms loaded and unlocked from 19% to 16% (USDHHS, 2006). The firearm-related death rate for young Black men and boys was nearly 5 times the rate for young White men and boys.

Intimate partner violence has serious health consequences for women and men; however, because of social and legal factors, it is probably the most underreported (Hot Topics box). Abuse crosses all socioeconomic, racial, ethnic, religious, and age boundaries. About one in four women and one in seven men during their lifetime reported intimate partner violence or abuse. Women reported higher lifetime and recent-year intimate partner violence than men (Breiding et al., 2008). Nurses and other primary health care providers often fail to assess, detect, or treat violence or abuse in an optimal manner, and more efforts must be made to recognize the scope of the problem and to provide appropriate counseling. Physical assaults by intimate partners decreased in the last decade; this improvement is attributed to increased economic opportunities for women, increasing age at first marriage, and better access to domestic violence services. A target in the *Healthy People 2010 Midcourse Review* is to reduce the rate of physical assault by current or former intimate partners to 3.3 assaults/1000 from 4.4 assaults recorded in 1998 (USDHHS, 2006).

VIOLENCE AGAINST WOMEN

HOTtopics

Assessing the Problem

Epidemiological researchers have attempted to determine the risks for intimate partner violence. Understanding the roots of partner violence has been more difficult than ascertaining determinants of physical disease. Factors associated with intimate partner violence include young age, low income, pregnancy, mental health problems, separation or divorce, and history of abuse (U.S Preventive Services Task Force, 2006). The unequal position of women in a relationship and the manner in which conflict is managed, as well as differences in education and prestige associated with the partners' occupations, are related to risk of violence. Domestic violence is a problem in all age, ethnic, and religious groups; in some cultures attitudes toward women even legitimize the practice. Women who have gained positions of respect and power outside the home through activities in their neighborhood or community are less likely to be abused.

Are Nurses Willing to Take Action?

Some studies indicate that nurses have been reluctant to take action regarding violence against women. Some of the traditional reasons for not taking action are based on paternalistic attitudes, in which the victim is blamed for her part in the social situation that becomes violent. Nursing's strong advocacy stance and emphasis on the communication of nonjudgmental, genuine concern should provide a strong foundation to avoid blaming the victim and to focus on pathological factors that have been identified by much of the health profession's research in this area.

How Can Nurses Recognize Abuse of Women?

Research demonstrates that nurses should be more aware of indicators of partner violence (U.S. Preventive Services Task Force, 2006). These include the presence, as revealed by a health history, of separation or divorce, alcoholism, frequent verbal disagreements, and high levels of conflict. Other warning signs include repeated visits to the emergency room, complaints of headaches or backaches, psychiatric illness, and incidents of bruises, sprains, and lacerations.

What Do You Think?

1. Are nurses less than helpful in their detection and management of violence against women? Why do you think this occurs?
2. Are nurses, because of their education and sensitization to people with mental problems, more or less likely than others to experience violence in their own domestic settings? Explain.

From U.S. Preventive Services Task Force. (2006). *Guide to clinical preventive services*. Rockville, MD: Agency for healthcare Research and Quality. Retrieved September 11, 2007, from *www.ahrq.gov/clinic/pocketgd.html*.

Sexuality-Reproductive Pattern

By young adulthood the menstrual cycle generally is well established in the woman. Cyclical hormonal function is responsible for regularity of the cycle and normal functioning of the ovaries and uterus. The normal duration of menses is 4 to 5 days (range of 2 to 7 days, with a blood loss of 40 mL). Blood loss of over 80 mL per cycle is abnormal and may lead to anemia. Irregularities such as painful menstruation, premenstrual syndrome, and prolonged or heavy bleeding need further assessment. Although these problems are not always abnormal, the symptoms and the individual's reaction to them can signal functional disorders and the need for further investigation and treatment.

Reproductive Problems

Infertility is defined as the lack of conception in the presence of unprotected sexual intercourse for at least 12 months. Approximately 10% to 15% of couples in the United States are believed to be infertile (Lowdermilk & Perry, 2007). Infertility has become more of a public issue since the advance of assistive reproductive technologies, such as in vitro fertilization and gamete intrafallopian transfer, which can enable couples with known reproductive problems to conceive children. These technologies frequently create great stress for the couple and often result in marital conflicts and distress. Generally, infertility is not an issue for those 18 to 25 years old; however, after the age of 25 the diagnosis is more frequent and in vitro becomes more of a choice for some infertile couples. At the other end of this spectrum are those young adult women who choose to be surgically sterilized. In 2002, approximately 2.2% of the 20-year-old to 24-year-old age group were surgically sterile; by the age of 35 this number had jumped to 29.2% (U.S. Census Bureau, 2006).

Common problems of the male reproductive system include **orchitis**, epididymitis, and varicoceles and hydroceles. Mumps in the postpubertal male can cause swelling of the tests, orchitis, and subfertility. External conditions such as fungal infections, contact dermatitis, and eczema; parasites such as scabies and lice; and nonvenereal diseases such as erysipelas, abscesses, and fistulas can occur in the scrotum.

Unintended Pregnancy

According to the CDC, the teen birth rate in the United States has dropped 30% during the past decade; this includes an even steeper decline in pregnancy rates for Black teens ("Michigan teens," 2004). Improved child health and development is associated with healthy planned pregnancies (USDHHS, 2006). Unwanted or unplanned pregnancies can be a considerable source of stress to young adults. Unintended pregnancy is an important public health issue related to increased risk for delayed prenatal care, depression, and other personal and relationship problems (USDHHS, 2006). Despite the advent of modern contraceptives, unintended pregnancy remains a persistent problem. Approximately one half of all pregnancies are intended

(USDHHS, 2006); in 1995 51% of all pregnancies among females aged 15 to 44 years were intended and the target for the U.S. is 70%. Although most young adults consider family planning services as an essential basic health service, health insurance plans historically have tried to limit such services (USDHHS, 2006), but currently abut 86% of employment-based health plans cover contraceptive supplies and equipment (USDHHS, 2006). The current lower pregnancy rates among teens seem to result from more involvement in school activities, contracts between young unmarried couples, effective birth control and pregnancy prevention programs, and expanding job opportunities ("Michigan teens," 2004).

Approximately one half of unintended pregnancies are the result of contraceptive failure (Kaplan, 2007). Both married and unmarried young adults need information about contraceptives (Table 22-2) to decrease the number of unwanted pregnancies and the need for abortions. The nurse's role in contraceptive counseling involves helping individuals to choose the method most appropriate to their needs (Hatcher et al., 2004). New and improved contraceptive agents are continually becoming available, so the nurse continues to learn about current information;

for example, two types of intrauterine devices are now available, the ParaGard T 380A (copper) and the Mirena device (levonorgesterol-releasing), and once inserted they are 99% effective (Kaplan, 2007). Laws and policies in some settings restrict nurses and other health care providers from engaging in certain types of counseling, including abortion counseling. Emergency contraception can reduce the number of unintended pregnancies. In 1999, 80% of family planning agencies offered emergency contraception and the target is 90% for 2010 (USDHHS, 2006). Over-the-counter purchase of emergency contraception, Plan B® is available in several states (10) to women 18 or older (AWHONN, 2004a). Plan B®, which must be started within three days of unprotected sex, works by either altering tubal transport of either sperm or ova, or inhibiting implantation. It will not terminate an existing pregnancy and it does not provide protection against STDs.

Prenatal Care

Access to prenatal care and financing of sufficient care are critical concerns. High-risk and minority women do not receive sufficient prenatal care. Lack of insurance coverage and less-than-adequate referral mechanisms exist. Between

Table 22-2 Summary of Effectiveness, Risks, and Noncontraceptive Benefits of Selected Contraceptive Methods

Contraceptive Method	Risks of Use	Noncontraceptive Health Benefits
OCs (combined and progestin only)	Thromboembolic disorders, CVA, coronary artery disease especially with smoking, hypertension, diabetes, breast cancer	Reduced risk of functional pelvic inflammation, endometriosis, uterine fibroids, endometrial cancer, ovarian cancer, iron deficiency anemia, ectopic pregnancy, irregular cycles
Transdermal (contraceptive patch)	Similar to OCs	Easy verification of presence, weekly application
Implants (Implanon, single rod)	Similar to OCs, data more limited	Similar to OCs, data more limited
Injectable progestin (Depo-Provera)	Prolonged amenorrhea, venous thrombosis, thrombembolism	Bone loss especially in adolescents, unsure of lifetime risk of osteoporosis
Vaginal ring (NuvaRing®)	Similar to OCs, but data more limited	Low-dose hormonal option
Intrauterine contraceptive device (IUD)	Bleeding, anemia, difficult removal, PID, ectopic pregnancy, cramping	Reduced risk of anemia, low cost for long term
Emergency contraception (Plan B®)	Nausea, abdominal pain, delay of menses	Not for routine use
Diaphragm	Toxic shock syndrome, allergy to latex or spermicide, urinary tract infection	Reduced risk of vaginitis, cervicitis
Condom	Allergy to rubber, latex, or spermicide	Reduced risk of STD and HIV transmission
Spermicides*	Sensitivity to agent	Antiviral activity against HPV, decreased activity of other STDs, decreased risk of PID
Sponge	Toxic shock syndrome	Decreased activity of STD organisms
Female sterilization (tubal ligation)	Anesthesia, infection, hemorrhage	One-time procedure
Male sterilization (vasectomy)	Complication rates low, reversal may be difficult	One-time procedure

*Often used in combination with other methods.
OCs, Oral contraceptives; CVA, cerebrovascular accident; HIV, human immunodeficiency virus; STD, sexually transmitted disease; HPV, human papilloma virus; PID, pelvic inflammatory disease.
Modified from Nelson, A, L, Trussell, J, Guest, F., & Kowal, D. (Eds.) (2007). *Contraceptive technology* (18th ed. Revised). New York: Ardent Media.

1990 and 1997 the proportion of mothers receiving care during the first trimester of pregnancy increased from 76% to 83%; the target in *Healthy People 2010 Midcourse Review* is to increase this to 90%. The proportion of mothers receiving early prenatal care needs to increase most in native American, Hispanic/Latino, and Black non-Hispanic mothers (USDHHS, 2006).

Another trend affecting young adults that has moved away (worsened) from the *Healthy People 2010 Midcourse Review* target is birth spacing. In 1995, 11% of females gave birth within 24 months of a previous birth and the target was 6%. Birth intervals of less than 24 months are associated with increased risks of preterm birth, low birth weights (LBW), and babies who are small for gestational age (Conde-Agudelo et al., 2006).

Sexually Transmitted Disease

STDs are a leading cause of infection and almost half of the new infections occurring each year affect persons aged 15 to 24 years. Women ages 15 to 19 and ages 20 to 24 have the highest reported rates of chlamydia and gonorrhea (U.S Preventive Services Task Force, 2006; USDHHS, 2006). The list of STDs (Table 22-3)includes HIV, chlamydia trachomatis infections, genital herpes, HPV, genital mycoplasma infections, cytomegalovirus infections, HB, and bacterial vaginitis, in addition to the more widely known diseases of syphilis and gonorrhea. In particular, chlamydia screening efforts should focus on all sexually active nonpregnant and pregnant women ages 24 or younger in whom the prevalence of chlamydial infection is highest (Meyers et al., 2007). The presence of multiple STDs increases the risk of HIV infection (USDHHS, 2006). STDs cost millions of dollars in screening, treatment, and reporting. In addition to creating a substantial problem for young adults, STDs impose tremendous demands on health care facilities. Many cases are unreported and untreated for lack of screening or failure to recognize symptoms. Many young adults do not understand that STDs can be transmitted from oral and anal sex, not just vaginal intercourse.

Human Immunodeficiency Virus

At the end of 2003, more than 1 million persons were estimated to be living with HIV infection in the United States (USDHHS, 2006). Meeting the treatment or prevention needs of this large group of chronically infected persons, especially HIV-positive low-income Americans, has become a priority. Another challenge is to develop more effective strategies to prevent new infections and improved case finding (USDHHS, 2006). HIV is transmitted by sexual intercourse (oral, vagina, anal), shared needles, and infected blood. Another less common source of transmission is from mother to baby across the placental barrier or through breast milk. The higher level of worry about contracting an STD in young adults is correlated with the implementation of risk-reduction behaviors (Research Highlights box). The incidence of STDs is greatly reduced with proper use

research highlights

Safer Sexual Health Education and Behavior

This descriptive study examined young adults' perceptions of previously taught sexual health information. Young adults were also asked to describe what further information they would like to receive (von Sadovszky et al., 2006). Young adults are at serious risk for contracting sexually transmitted diseases. A convenience sample of 55 young adults were asked questions regarding previously taught sexual health content. Content analysis was used to categorize themes and content.

Most students remembered information taught in middle and high school concerning sexually transmitted infections (STIs). Less than half remembered being taught information about contraception or how to prevent STIs. The majority of students did not feel that the sexual health teachings influenced their current health behaviors. For those who felt the information changed their sexual behavior, the most-cited influencing factor was increased awareness of the risk related to sexual encounters. When asked for a description of an ideal sexual health education program, the majority reported that the instructor must be comfortable with the content, information on STIs should be more detailed, especially about preventing STIs, and more specifics were requested about reproductive system function.

The implications are that young adults have very specific requirements for an effective sexual health education program. It remains to be seen whether additions of the specific content cited by the students would lead to higher rates of learning recall and translate into ability to avoid risky sexual behaviors.

von Sadovszky, V., Kovar, C. K., Brown, C., & Armbruster, M. (2006). The need for sexual health information: perceptions and desires of young adults. *MCN Am J Matern Child Nurs, 31*(6), 373–380.

of condoms. In the *Healthy People 2010 Midcourse Review*, use of condoms in various age groups surpassed targets (USDHHS, 2006), and condom use is considered to be increasing. All sexually active individuals are counseled on the hazards of unprotected sexual activity and on the effective use and limitations of condoms, stressing that they must be used properly and can fail. Condom failures occur at an estimated rate of 10% to 15%; therefore, counseling should stress that condom use is not foolproof. Another success is the decline in perinatal transmission. Rates of HIV perinatal transmission are greatly reduced by drug therapy during pregnancy, changes in obstetric practice, and prohibition of breast feeding in infected mothers. Therefore the U.S. Public Health Service recommends voluntary testing for HIV and counseling as a part of basic prenatal care (U.S. Preventive Services Task force, 2006).

The nurse's role in intervening for STDs includes providing treatment and education, early diagnosis, and treatment. When an individual is suspected of having an STD, the nurse obtains a complete history, including sexual history, sexual contacts, previous treatment and test results, any signs or symptoms of a current infection, recent use of antibiotics, and

Table **22-3** Summary of Selected Sexually Transmitted Diseases

Disease	Causative Agent	Diagnostic Methods	Treatment	Risks or Complications	Nursing Teaching
Viral Diseases:	Treatment doesn't eradicate the underlying infection				
Acquired immunodeficiency syndrome (AIDS)	Human immunodeficiency virus (HIV)	Enzyme immune assay, Western Blot, viral tests	Current recommendations	Opportunistic infections, perinatal transmission	Monitor CD4 T-lymphocyte level and HIV viral load, testing during pregnancy strongly recommended
Hepatitis B	Hepatitis B virus (HBV)	Hepatitis B antibody test	No specific therapy available	Perinatal transmission	Routine vaccination or vaccine prior to pregnancy
Genital herpes	Herpes simplex virus (HSV)	HSV culture, viral test	Acyclovir at first diagnosis or episode	Urethral stricture, lymph node enlargement	Examine partners, abstain from sex while symptomatic
Genital warts	Human papilloma virus (HPV)	Pap, DNA tests, observation of warts, colposcopy, biopsy	Podophyllin, trichloroacetic acid, cryotherapy/laser, valcyclovir, tamiciclovir	Cervical dysplasia, cervical cancer	Offer (Gardisil®) vaccine and counseling, return for treatment as necessary, treat partner
Bacterial/Other STDs:					
Gonorrhea	*Neisseria gonorrhoeae*	Culture	Ceftriaxone, cefixime, fluoroaquinolones no longer recommended	PID, infertility, ectopic pregnancy	Monitor antibiotic treatment, examine partner, repeat culture
Syphilis	*Treponema pallidum*	Fluorescent antibody tests of lesion or exudates, VDRL, RPR	Benzathine penicillin G	Secondary/late syphilis	Monitor treatment, test and monitor partner
Chlamydia	*Chlamydia trachomatis*	Chlamydia monoclonal antibody test, culture	Doxycycline, azithromycin	Infertility, urethral scarring, PID, endocervicitis, neonatal infection	Refer partners for evaluation, condoms to prevent future infection
Bacterial vaginosis (BV)	*Gardnerella vaginalis*	Wet mount: presence of clue cells	Metronidazole (Flagyl)	Asymptomatic infection	Sexual transmission not proven
Trichomoniasis	*Trichomonas vaginalis*	Wet mount: observation of protozoa, Pap	Metronidazole (Flagyl)	Recurrence, excoriation of genital area	Use condoms to prevent new infection
Vulvovaginal candidiasis (VVC)	*Candida albicans, non–C. albicans*	Wet mount: evidence of hyphae and spores	Antifungal medication: miconazole, clotrimazole	Recurrence of disease	Reduce moisture/heat in genital area, recheck in 14 days

Pap, Papanicolaou; *PID*, pelvic inflammatory disease; *RPR*, rapid plasma regain test; *VDRL*, venereal disease research laboratory test.
Based on information from Centers for Disease Control and Prevention. (2006). Sexually transmitted diseases: Treatment guidelines. *Morbidity and Mortally Weekly Report, 55*(36, RR-11), 1–94; Lowdermilk, D. L., & Perry, S. E. (2007). *Maternity & women's care.* St. Louis: Mosby; Nelson, A. L., Trussell, J., Guest, F., & Kowal, D. (Eds.). (2007). *Contraceptive technology* (18th ed.). New York: Ardent Media.

allergic reactions to antibiotics. When treatment is required, the nurse ensures that the person understands the goals of treatment in an attempt to gain cooperation including follow-up care with partners and adherence to the plan of care.

The nurse is an educator not only of the individual, but also of the general public. Appropriate health education for the individual with an STD includes mode of transmission, incubation periods, signs and symptoms, methods of treatment, complications resulting from lack of treatment, and signs of recurrent infections.

Coping–Stress Tolerance Pattern
Assessment of Stress Levels

Stress, the result of forces operating on the individual that disrupt physiological or psychological equilibrium, is an integral part of young adulthood; therefore, a comprehensive health assessment should include questions to determine stress levels. Anxiety, nervousness, depression, or somatic complaints are indicators of stress, as are events such as divorce, loss of employment, failure to be promoted, or financial difficulties. The role of the nurse is to listen, offer support, and demonstrate concern. The nurse also suggests referrals to appropriate health providers and support groups.

Achievement Stress

Achievement-oriented stress differs from the stress of situational crises in that the stress of an overachiever is derived from internal pressures to succeed as measured by self-defined goals. Achievement-oriented stress frequently causes workaholic habits, including loss of sleep and omission of meals. When this behavior becomes extreme, serious physical and emotional consequences can occur, such as nutrition problems or burnout which, in turn, leads to severe emotional and physical exhaustion. Workaholic behaviors may not be perceived by the individual and may not be apparent until changes in bodily functions or behavior occur. Young adults are generally health conscious and willing to alter personal lifestyles and behavior patterns to reduce stress and become healthier. Many people have responded to campaigns for physical fitness, exercise, and nutritional adjustment, which increase their well-being and life expectancy.

Suicide and Depression

Suicide is a leading cause of death in the young adult age group. Suicide occurs because many young adults are unable to cope with the pressures of adulthood. For some people, pressure arises when dealing with interpersonal conflicts such as marital problems, family discord, or the loss of a close relationship; for others, the precipitating event is a lack of personal resources, unemployment, or dissatisfaction with work or school. Many young adults try to solve their problems before the fatal incident but see no positive solutions; in many cases, a prior suicide attempt was a signal for help.

Suicide rates are higher for men than for women; approximately 4 to 5 times as many men as women (18.0 versus 4.2 deaths per 100,000 population in 2003) take their own lives (U.S. Census Bureau, 2006). However, more women are known to suffer from depressive disorders and to unsuccessfully attempt suicide. Young adults are more likely as a group to attempt suicide than are older individuals, and professionals are more likely to attempt suicide than are nonprofessionals. Suicide is more common among single, widowed, and divorced individuals. Chronically ill young adult males may also be more at risk for depression than young adult females because social support systems are more robust within female relationship networks (Kiviruusu et al., 2007).

A quick method of screening young adults who may be depressed requires the nurse to ask two questions. First the nurse asks whether in the last month, the young adult has been bothered by (1) little interest or pleasure in doing things and (2) feeling down, depressed, or hopeless (U.S. Preventive Services Task Force, 2006). A "no" answer to both questions indicates a negative screening result. In 2003, approximately 12.7% of all deaths between the ages of 24 to 35 were classified as suicides (U.S. Census Bureau, 2006). When the health care provider is concerned that the young adult may be at risk for suicide, the following two questions should be asked: (1) "Have these symptoms or feelings that you have been talking about led you to think that you might be better off dead?" and (2) "What thoughts have you had about hurting yourself or even killing yourself?" To question further the nurse can ask, "Have you actually done anything to hurt yourself?" (Depression Management Tool Kit, 2001; U.S. Preventive Services Task Force, 2006). Suicide continues to be a major health problem for young adults; annual rates, especially for men, remain high.

Nursing interventions are directed toward identifying behaviors in individuals who may be contemplating suicide. Physical clues include self-neglect, depression, slowed gait, slumped shoulders, and droopy faces. Presuicidal individuals also tend to exhibit impaired reality testing; feelings of hopelessness, helplessness, and rejection; impaired judgment and decision-making; anxiety; weight loss; insomnia; or a radically changed affect. In addition to identifying presuicidal behaviors, the nurse also investigates relationship patterns to determine behaviors that are complicated by feelings of worthlessness and defeat. When the nurse identifies a young adult at risk for a suicide attempt, referrals to other professionals are indicated.

Values-Beliefs Pattern

Young adults enter their twenties with habits, values, and beliefs acquired during childhood and adolescence. Many acquired habits foster continuance of practices that are hazardous to health and well-being in later life. Prevention is directed toward altering value and belief patterns that encourage poor health practices, reorienting them toward those that support optimal health behaviors. Nursing interventions are more effective when the nurse can describe, discriminate, identify, and align value and belief patterns consistent with practices known to maximize health.

Values Involved in Parenting

Parenthood is envisioned an important developmental stage by most young adults; therefore, health-promotion and health protection activities to ensure healthy offspring are crucial (see Case Study and Care Plan at the end of this chapter). **Genetic impairments**, or **congenital defects** caused by abnormal chromosomes, are responsible for 4% to 6% of perinatal deaths (Lowdermilk & Perry, 2007). Tests are available for about 200 genetic diseases (Lowdermilk & Perry, 2007). Most of the offered genetic testing is for single-gene impairment to mothers and fathers who have a family history of genetic disease. Young adults with a genetic disease must make many important decisions; predicting the transmission of the disease to potential offspring is key.

Values Regarding Prenatal Diagnosis and Genetic Impairment

Prenatal diagnostic procedures have been available since the mid-1960s. This capability has enabled the identification of high-risk pregnancies and requires the cooperation and education of childbearing women and their partners, both of whom must provide accurate family health and obstetrical histories and comply with suggested screening and follow-up measures. Decisions about the advisability of reproduction are based on current information on genetics and known deleterious genetic factors.

The finding of a malformed or genetically impaired fetus may result in a parental decision to terminate the pregnancy. Theological and political debates in addition to legislative mandates have greatly influenced family control over many of these decisions. Genetic counseling is an important nursing intervention for young adults. A genetic specialist gives technical explanations of genetic disorders; however, nurses have a supportive role in helping young adults decide whether to have children or to carry through a pregnancy that is at risk.

ENVIRONMENTAL PROCESSES
Physical
Ethnicity, Race, and Culture

The young adult whose ethnic background is different from that of the dominant culture may encounter prejudice and discrimination, which can occur because of differences in race, creed, language, attitudes, values, preferences, or behaviors. The young adult is susceptible to these prejudices at work, at school, in health care delivery systems, and in the community. Young adults must meet not only personal needs, but also the needs of children or older adults; therefore, nurses continue to consider the values that are common to specific cultures and ethnic backgrounds.

Race and ethnicity are important influencers of health for young adults. Longevity for nonwhite men and women has increased, the result of a decrease in birth-related fatalities and in deaths caused by systemic disabilities. Blacks remain at risk

for specific health problems, and the life expectancy of the average Black person is shorter than that of the average White person.

Race and ethnicity are closely connected to educational and work-related decisions, which subsequently affect choice of residence. Many minority families live in substandard housing or crowded living spaces. A lifestyle of this type, when combined with insufficient economic resources, frequently affects health. Compared with the general population, divorce rates in 2005 were proportionately higher among White women than Hispanic and Black women (U.S Census Bureau, 2006). Poverty is more common among Black families, which often leads to unmet basic needs of food, clothing, and housing and, in turn, leads to decreased regard for health needs.

Accidents

Injuries are the highest cause of death in young adults (USDHHS, 2006). Motor vehicle accidents cause more fatalities than all other causes of death combined. Reducing speed limits contributes to lower fatality rates. Approximately 48 states have seat belt laws, and all states have seat belt requirements for children. All individuals in the car need to use seat belts, because an unrestrained occupant can cause harm to another passenger in a crash (Cummings & Rivara, 2004). The continued high incidence of vehicle accidents in the young adult age group is related to accessibility of cars to young adults and peer pressure on driving behavior; reckless driving and driving under the influence of alcohol and drugs is now viewed as closely connected to violent and abusive behavior (USDHHS, 2006).

Accident-prevention education, long considered appropriate for young children, is an important part of young adult instruction. Most young licensed drivers have participated in driver education courses, and a number of states have adopted progressive licensing programs. "Graduated driver licensing" (GDL) programs have the potential to reduce younger drivers crash rates by 20% to 40% (Shope, 2007). The young adult must understand the potentially fatal consequences of aggressive tendencies or thoughtless risk taking. When young adults are encouraged to reflect on the consequences of their actions, they tend to be more willing to control and change unsafe driving behaviors.

Pollution
Noise

Young adults are exposed to high levels of noise in occupational and recreational settings. Long-term exposure to loud noise is directly related to impaired hearing and can increase irritability and stress. Young adults can be exposed to noises in the work setting from industrial machinery and equipment. Although industrial exposure can be difficult to mitigate, many young adults worsen the situation through recreational exposure, by listening to music or videos at excessively high decibel levels. Ear protection is necessary in some situations to prevent hearing disability. Recognition of hazards and corresponding appropriate preventive education are early nursing strategies for decreasing excessive noise exposure.

Air

Motor vehicles are the largest source of air pollution; vehicles release more than 90 million tons of particles and noxious gases each year, most of which is either carbon monoxide or hydrocarbons. Carbon monoxide in high concentrations is deadly; in lower concentrations it causes headaches, dizziness, and heart palpitations. In sunlight and low-lying areas, automobile exhaust becomes photochemical smog that contains ozone, which irritates the eyes and the respiratory tract. Although air pollution is not a problem only for young adults, they frequently work in dirty, entry-level jobs in industrial settings and may be among the age group that is most affected.

Occupational Hazards and Stressors

Occupational hazards pose a threat of illness, injury, or death in all age groups, and occupational safety standards have contributed greatly to the reduction of work-related accidents. Legislation in 1970, including the Occupational Safety and Health Act (OSHA), has resulted in the improvement of work conditions, along with the provision of health care facilities, in many companies.

Young adults should not be allowed to work in certain industrial settings without vocational training to reduce hazards. Young adults frequently want a challenge and high wages; therefore, they work at hazardous jobs—for example, on offshore drilling rigs, on high bridges, or in nuclear plants. Because of their age, physical stamina, and agility, young adults are suitable candidates for positions that require extreme physical abilities. Occupational training should include education about personal exposure risks, identification of work-related hazards, and identification of situations in which the severity of accidents is connected to personal behaviors or habits. For example, drivers of heavy construction machinery should be particularly observant, avoid reckless behaviors, and avoid fast driving. Working women who are pregnant can expose their fetuses to industrial substances. Proper evaluation and temporary reassignment may be necessary.

Occupational preventive intervention requires that known work hazards and risks be identified early. Health histories should include questions about the place of work, type of work, and young adults' understanding of the risks associated with their occupations. Occupational risk and health are closely related; stress associated with work, the use of alcohol or drugs, and a negative attitude toward work are predictive of occupational injuries. Job counseling aimed at changing the nature of employment can be an appropriate referral for some people with health conditions. Employees in industrial settings should visit a health care provider on a periodic basis for health assessment, update of the health history, and counseling.

Chemical Agents
Drug Use

Misuse of drugs, a major risk for young adults, is associated with injury, disability, violence, homicide, and suicide and is related to social problems (criminal behaviors and maladjustment to accepted norms). Drug abuse may be closely related to an inability to cope appropriately with adult responsibilities. Physical health problems associated with drug misuse account for more than 50% of the major acute and chronic problems of young adults. Heroin users have increased mortality rates because of overdosage or chronic disability associated with hepatitis infections. Drug use is an independent risk factor involved in HIV infections (USDHHS, 2006).

Use of drugs, such as anabolic steroids, to improve athletic performance is increasing. The risks of using steroids are enormous, and preventive education should focus on healthier sports and exercise values. Nursing activities include preventive strategies to curb the problem of drug misuse. Distribution of information on drugs, early treatment of complications, and drug treatment centers are only part of the answer. Nursing efforts aimed at increasing individual awareness and altering drug-taking attitudes and behaviors are of critical importance (Multicultural Awareness box).

Alcohol Use

Alcohol-related accidents among individuals ages 15 to 24 continue to be a leading cause of preventable morbidity, disability, and death. Heavy alcohol use, that is, consuming five or more drinks on at least one occasion within a month, is more common in 18 to 25 year olds than it is

---

MULTICULTURAL AWARENESS

Genetic Variation in Drug Response

Various studies, although limited, indicate genetic differences may be important factors to consider when prescribing certain drugs. Different genetic types tend to metabolize drugs differently, have different binding receptors, or have different environmental influences that change the utilization and uptake. This field of study is called pharmacogenetics. Early clues to variation in drug response were seen when comparing populations from different racial and ethnic backgrounds.

Gene selection favored chances of survival; for example, sickle cell trait developed through selection factors that favored resistance to malaria. Similarly, gene selection factors also favored the prevalence of glucose-6-phosphate dehydrogenase deficiency, which also provides resistance to malaria but causes drug-related red blood cell hemolysis. In a related study of warfarin response, ethnic differences were shown to affect bioavailability and distribution, which were controlled through careful clinical management and dosage regulation (El Rouby et al., 2004).

Continued

MULTICULTURAL AWARENESS

Genetic Variation in Drug Response—cont'd

In studies of people with hypertension, Black individuals responded with a greater decrease in systolic pressure in response to thiazide diuretics (hydrochlorothiazide) and calcium channel blockers. Black individuals have a blunted response to α-blockers, which can be improved by adding a diuretic.

The situation in Asian persons appears to be the exact opposite. In a study of the effectiveness of propranolol in Chinese and White men, the Chinese men had at least twice as much sensitivity as did the White men to propranolol administered at several dosage levels. Studies indicate that Asians are more sensitive to alcohol and its drug effects than are Whites. The most outstanding difference is in the amount of facial flushing, which was experienced by a substantial percentage of Asians compared with the White sample. The alcohol dehydrogenase enzyme is reported to be absent in about one half of Asians.

These examples suggest that nurses should be aware of potential genetic variations that may affect drug metabolism and effectiveness. In individuals who do not respond to certain drugs as expected, the nurse may consider whether this might be related to constitutional factors within the person's genetic makeup. In December 2004, the Food and Drug Administration approved a DNA blood test that analyzes genes in blood known to be related to slow or rapid drug metabolism. Pharmacogenetic research also invites rethinking of managed care practices that restrict diversity of drug use with prescribed drug formulary listings.

This topic is discussed in more detail in Howland, R. H. (2006). Psychopharmacology: A source of clinically concise information about psychopharmacology. Personalized drug therapy with pharmacogenics. Part I: Pharmokinetics. *Journal of Psychosocial Nursing. 44*(1), 13–16; Lea, D. H. (2005). Tailoring drug therapy with pharmacogenetics. *Nursing, 35*(4), 22–23; Kudzma, E. (2001). Cultural competence: Cardiovascular medications. *Progress in Cardiovascular Nursing, 16*(4), 152–160, 169; and El Rouby, S., Mestres, C. A., LaDuca, F. M., & Zucker, M. L. (2004). Racial and ethnic differences in warfarin response. *Journal of Heart Valve Disease, 13*(1), 15–21.

for younger or older adults (USDHHS, 2006). Raising the legal drinking age to 21 reduces not only deaths and injuries connected to motor vehicle accidents, but also homicides and other violent death. A nationwide legal standard of .08% blood alcohol concentration maximum levels for driving while intoxicated (DWI) enforcement and prosecution was achieved (USDHHS, 2006). Alcohol abuse is directly related to chronic conditions such as cirrhosis of the liver. Modifying alcohol consumption in young adults can decrease the frequency of chronic and disabling conditions in later life.

Alcohol consumption is increasing in the young adult population. Twenty-four percent of young adults ages 18 and older report that they have engaged in **binge drinking** in the last 30 days (USDHHS, 2006). Although young adults may drink less frequently than older adults, they tend to consume larger amounts of alcohol at one time; the tendency is toward binge drinking, which causes increased loss of control and is related to an additional risk of automobile accidents. Teens with work schedules of more than 10 hours per week are more often involved in heavy or binge drinking or both. Working more time increases the money available to purchase alcohol and exposes the teen to older adults who drink (Paschall et al., 2004).

Tobacco Use

Smoking is a leading cause of preventable death in the United States; therefore, smoking cessation is the single most important counseling topic for all people because of its potential to lower the risk of contracting many preventable diseases. Smoking was most prevalent among adults aged 18 to 24 years (28.3%) and 25 to 44 years (28.0%) and declined with age (Schoenborn et al., 2003). More than one third of current smokers aged 18 to 24 years started smoking before the age of 16. Cigarette smoking rates among persons 18 and older continued to decline from the 1998 baseline of 24% to a 2003 level of 21% (USDHHS, 2006).

Individuals employed in high-risk occupations are informed of the synergistic relationship between smoking and other environmental exposures including asbestos, coal dust, and radiation. Fear tactics, nagging, preaching, and threats are generally ineffective in convincing people to stop smoking. Major barriers to smoking cessation are the presence of other smokers, particularly in situations where alcohol is also being used.

State enforcement of no smoking policies is important, as Jemal et al. (2003) have reported. Lung cancer death rates declined in states with strong tobacco control enforcement and increased in states where tobacco control was weak. Measures of tobacco control are strongly correlated with smoking cessation rates of young adults ages 30 to 39. Nurses are familiar with the antismoking resources in their communities, enabling them to make the appropriate referrals.

Carcinogens

Young adults can be exposed to environmental carcinogens in their work settings or through unhealthy practices such as having multiple sexual partners. In the work setting, environmental regulations have limited exposure to some hazardous chemicals, but long-term effects on health of exposure to many industrial chemicals remains unknown. In health care, latex, long considered inert and safe, has now been shown to cause long-term immune system disease in some nurses exposed to the agent (or the chemicals that bind it) in surgical gloves.

The risk for developing cervical cancer is related to environmental exposures such as smoking and HPV infection. Cervical cancer has decreased steadily over the years, likely because of the effective use of screening methods, such as **Papanicolaou (Pap) smear** testing. Rates for cervical dysplasia and cancer peak in both White and

Black women between ages 20 and 30. The rate for Black women increases faster than it does for White women over the age of 25. Known risk factors for environmental exposure include smoking, early age of first intercourse, multiple sexual partners, and infection with HPV (USDHHS, 2006).

SOCIAL PROCESSES
Community and Work
Neighborhood Resources

The environment of the community strongly influences the well-being of the young adult and sets the standard for the health of people and families living within a neighborhood. Neighbors can be an excellent source of support, which can be especially important to a young mother who does not have immediate family nearby. Nurses working in the community facilitate the contact of individuals with common interests through community and religious activities and support groups. Community resources for exercise and recreation can make important contributions to the young adult's physical and emotional health (Figure 22-4). When these resources are available, the young adult can have the opportunity to exercise and release stress in a positive fashion.

Health Service Availability

Availability of health services is important. Economic realities, however, influence the effectiveness of resources, particularly for the young adult who lives in an economically depressed area. In some communities, health services are lacking or, when available, are not culturally sensitive or

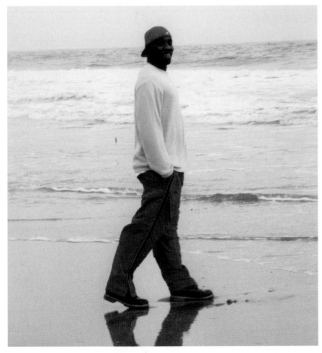

Figure 22-4 Young adults' need for recreation can make important contributions to their physical and emotional health.

adapted to the customs and beliefs of the people who are served. In other communities, access to public transportation can be a critical problem, affecting the ability of the young adult to keep appointments. Young adults ages 18 to 24 years are the least likely of any age group to have a usual source of care; thus, a target of *Healthy People 2010 Midcourse Review* is to increase the proportion of young adults with a usual primary care provider (USDHHS, 2006). Gaps in health care coverage that occur between the end of schooling and achieving full employment with health insurance coverage reduce the access of young adults to primary care.

Culture and Ethnicity

Health delivery methods in the United States are based primarily on Western belief systems, which tend to be rigid in their applications. For example, women seeking birth control information and prescriptions are expected to use health clinics and keep to their schedule of return visits. Because health care provider systems have removed many traditional barriers once assumed to be responsible for poor utilization of services by low-income or minority groups (location and scheduling), nonattendance at scheduled clinic visits frequently is interpreted as noncompliance. Among Native Americans, for example, contraceptive education has gained little acceptance, and fertility rates remain high, primarily because conception control may be viewed as both culturally and religiously objectionable.

Appropriate health strategies and interventions require that nurses identify cultural beliefs and health care practices that are harmful to people. Many cultural practices may be allowed because they do not affect appropriate health care. For example, food cravings are common among many pregnant women. In moderation, following dietary patterns directed by these cravings is not harmful. However, when the craving leads to an unbalanced diet or to pica (eating nonfood substances), the pregnancy can be affected (e.g., the incidence of anemia is higher in women with pica) (Lowdermilk & Perry, 2007).

Legislation

Young adults are one of the major political constituencies in the United States, as seen in the 2008 presidential election; they support many causes and have the time and energy to publicize issues related to the common good. Some of these issues involve the environment, nuclear energy, war, and pollution. Relative to health, predominant issues have involved housing and health care in neighborhoods and rural areas and health, agricultural, and sanitation concerns in foreign countries. Through these efforts, young adults can influence and improve living conditions for future generations.

Economics

One of the young adult's age-related tasks is to choose and develop a lifelong career. This choice is directly related to economic factors; young adults want satisfying occupations that also yield adequate economic returns. To manage financially and maintain a lifestyle in which personal needs can be met, young adults may elect to have fewer children. Caring for aging parents can also cause physical, psychosocial, spiritual, and economic stress.

Although goals vary greatly among young adult couples, they generally are concerned with acquiring material comforts; the desire for housing, transportation, clothing, or recreation generally necessitate that both partners work to meet financial obligations. This desire necessitates the changing of roles and the sharing of responsibilities, and open communication becomes a crucial component. For single parents these challenges can appear insurmountable.

New career opportunities and the economic expansion in the United States during the 1990s have allowed young adults more career choices. During the 1990s and through the first years of the new century, college graduates have had the best choice of employment opportunities in decades. The booming technology industry has provided employment in a wide variety of occupations and start-up companies. Work styles within these companies tend to be different from that in the traditional workplace, including an expectation of longer and more fluid workdays. Internet-based companies provide young adults with jobs that have the potential to give them rapid financial rewards at the cost of long-term job stability. As of the economic downturn in 2008, young adults have been discouraged to the vision that employment will be less available in the immediate future. Due to the high cost of housing many young adults have multiple roommates, creating additional demands and health risks. Some young adults are interested in giving back to society by taking employment at lower salaries in nonprofit agencies involved in education and social issues, such as Habitat for Humanity and going abroad in the Peace Corps or to promote human rights in countries where such rights are nonexistent.

Homelessness

Homeless people in the U.S. were, at one time, primarily single men; today entire families account for approximately one third of the homeless population. More families are seeking subsidized housing, although homelessness is not only a housing issue but results from poor education, lack of employment skills, substandard health care, domestic violence and abuse, and inadequate child and foster care. Poverty is a key factor; welfare benefits are too low to cover rents, and long waits for public housing are common. Housing may be located away from transportation and health care facilities, hindering access to health care (Nunez & Caruso, 2003).

Homeless single men tend to use shelters only for night residence, but families tend to use shelter settings longer, an average of 2 to 11 months, before locating housing. Today's shelters are very different from the temporary places of the past; many provide on-site services and programs to eradicate the causes of homelessness. About 26% of those living in shelters are employed, and many shelters provide child care, after-school programs, and job preparedness training (Nunez & Caruso, 2003). Minorities are significantly and disproportionately represented among the homeless in larger cities, reflecting the large number who live below or near the poverty level.

Dual Careers

For many young adult couples, the increase in unemployment for one of both, different careers, friends, and varying maturity levels place additional strains on their relationship. These circumstances can provide a basis for domestic difficulty. Domestic quarreling tends to precede family disruption, leading to marital separation or divorce. In addition to the emotional strain placed on family members, domestic arguments can result in aggressive acts of abuse and personal injury. Young adults can also be faced with decisions about day care facilities; the couple or mother may need support to resolve guilt feelings related to the separation from the child. Some young adults may also bear responsibilities for caring for aging parents or relatives.

Lifestyles may also include living arrangements with individuals of the same gender or the opposite gender. Although these lifestyles are becoming more acceptable in today's society, attitudes toward varied lifestyles contribute pressures that lead to further stress and uncertainty. Same-sex marriage legislation is a heavily politicized issue. In the U.S. in 2007 only Massachusetts allowed same-sex marriage; however New Jersey, New Hampshire, Connecticut, and Vermont allow civil unions that grant gay couples the same legal rights as in heterosexual marriages.

SUMMARY

Nurses promote health care measures and behaviors at all places where young adults come into contact with the health care delivery system. In community colleges and university settings, efforts can be directed toward health education curricula with emphasis on positive health behaviors, establishment of peer counseling groups, and better utilization of sports and exercise facilities. Workshops on alcoholism, drug abuse, sports or exercise, mental health and self-expression, relationships, and various aspects of sexual care are effective in college populations. At the work site, programs of employee counseling, blood pressure monitoring and treatment, exercise, smoking reduction, cafeteria nutrition management, and stress reduction have also been effective. Employee insurance programs are undergoing continual review to determine an appropriate level of integrated care and coverage. Preventive care, mental health, dental health, and maternity benefits are being analyzed and increased when necessary. Young adults are generally healthy, which challenges the nurse to be even more sensitive, insightful, and creative in implementing care for individuals within this age group.

CASE STUDY

Preparing for Childbearing: Kirsten

Kirsten is a healthy 22-year-old whose favorite sport is running. Since this spring, Kirsten believes that her breathing capacity is diminishing and her levels of energy are decreasing. During her period these symptoms appear to worsen. Last week, while running up a rather steep course, Kirsten became much more weak, dizzy, and fatigued than usual, and her best friend and running partner recommended that she make a doctor's appointment for a physical examination. Kirsten's running partner also noted that she has appeared pale lately.

In the physician's office, Kirsten is noted to have a normal temperature, an elevated heart and respiratory rate, and a blood pressure of 90/60. Kirsten's description of her period is that it tends to be heavy and has been this way for 5 years. For muscle aches and pains caused by running, she usually takes two aspirin tablets every 3 to 4 hours for as long as 7 days. When her running increases during the summer, she takes aspirin continually for 2 to 3 months. Diagnostic testing indicates that her hemoglobin is 7 g/dL, and her red blood cells are pale and small. Kirsten has been in a long-term relationship for several years, her wedding is in several months, and there has been discussion of preconceptual health planning and future children.

Reflective Questions:

1. What common health alteration in young adult women is most likely for Kirsten?
2. What contributing factors place Kirsten at risk?
3. What lifestyle modifications can Kirsten implement to decrease her risk?

CARE PLAN

Preparation for Childbearing: Kirsten

Nursing Diagnosis: Health-Seeking Behaviors Related to Preconceptual Assessment and Preparation for Childbearing

DEFINING CHARACTERISTICS

- Expressed desire to improve overall health to prepare for childbearing
- Expressed thoughts about planning for pregnancy in the near future
- Desire to improve nutritional status before childbearing
- Desire to improve nutritional intake of essential vitamins and minerals (iron and calcium)
- Plan to take multivitamin each day
- Plan to limit foods high in sodium and fat
- Plan to limit alcohol consumption
- Plan for exercise program to increase stamina and flexibility
- Seeks physical examination to rule out problems that might negatively affect pregnancy
- Seeks information on pregnancy risk factors (biophysical, psychosocial, sociodemographic, and environmental)

RELATED FACTORS

- Expressed desire to improve the quality of relationship with husband or partner
- Desire to attend education classes to improve knowledge of childbearing and positive health practices
- Plan for room or housing to accommodate children
- Plan for employment arrangements that accommodate child care

EXPECTED OUTCOMES

- Increase in indices of well-being in person
- Healthy pregnancy and future child
- Increase in self-confidence and awareness preparation for childbearing
- Management of pregnancy risk factors before becoming pregnant
- Making the person aware of resources available for pregnancy and child care

INTERVENTIONS

- Assess current level of wellness regarding preparation for childbearing.
- Identify community resources that provide information regarding preconceptual planning and preparation.
- Identify primary health provider, midwife, or obstetrician, and hospitals with delivery services.
- Assess biophysical risk factors (genetic disorders, nutrition problems, and current medical problems).
- Assess for history of pregnancy loss.
- Test for blood type and Rh factor.
- Screen for sexually transmitted disease, tuberculosis, rubella titer, sickle cell trait.
- Review immunization history, including hepatitis B.
- Assess need to augment diet, particularly to increase intake of calcium and iron.
- Take a multivitamin daily.
- Assess for psychosocial risk factors (mental problems, use of drugs, alcohol, caffeine, and smoking).
- Counsel to avoid alcohol consumption.
- Assess for possible sociodemographic risk factors (poverty, first pregnancy risks of dystocia or PIH, residence [rural or urban], and ethnicity).
- Assess for environmental risks (exposures to chemicals, drugs, pesticides, pollution, smoke, stress, and radiation).
- Assess current employment situation.
- Identify child care arrangements.

PIH, Pregnancy-induced hypertension.
For further information on developing care plans, see: Carpenito-Moyet, L. J. (2008). *Nursing diagnosis: Application to clinical practice* (12th ed.). Philadelphia: Lippincott, Williams & Wilkins.

REFERENCES

Anderson, D. M. (2002). *Mosby's Medical Nursing and Allied Health Dictionary.* St. Louis: Mosby.

Anderson, R. N., & Arias, E. (2003). The effect of revised populations on mortality statistics for the United States, 2000. In *National vital statistics reports* (Vol. 51, No. 9). Hyattsville, MD: National Center for Health Statistics.

Association of Women's Health, Obstetric and Neonatal Nurses. (2004a). AWHONN urges approval of OTC emergency contraception. *AWHONN Lifelines, 8*(1), 65–66.

Association of Women's Health, Obstetric and Neonatal Nurses. (2004b). Fortifying oral contraceptives with folic acid. *AWHONN Lifelines, 8*(1), 12–13.

Bhattacharya, S. (2004). American footballers endure "car crash" blows. *New Scientist.* Retrieved October 22, 2007, from *www.newscientist.com/article.ns?id=dn4534*

Bilukha, O., & Rosenstein, N. (2005). Prevention and control of meningococcal disease. Recommendations of the advisory committee on immunization practices (ACIP). *MMWR, 54*(RR-7), 1–21.

Breiding, M., Black, M., & Ryan, G. (2008). Prevalence and risk factors of intimate partner violence in eighteen U.S. states/territories, 2005. *American Journal of Preventive Medicine, 34*(2), 112–118.

Centers for Disease Control and Prevention. (2004a). Declining prevalence of no known major risk factors for heart disease and stroke among adults—United States, 1991–2001. *MMWR Morbidity and Mortality Weekly Report, 53*(1), 4–7.

Centers for Disease Control and Prevention. (2004b). Violence a growing public health problem in the Americas. *Medical letter on the CDC and FDA, 47,* 1532–1648.

Centers for Disease Control and Prevention. (2005). *Overweight and obesity: Economic consequences.* Retrieved October 22, 2007, from *www.cdc.gov/nccdphp/dnpa/obesity/ economic_consequences.htm.*

Cherry, D. K., Burt, C. W., & Woodwell, D. A. (2003). *National ambulatory medical care survey: 2001 Summary. Advance data from vital and health statistics* (No. 331). Hyattsville, MD: National Center for Health Statistics.

Chobanian, A. V., Bakris, G. L., Black, H. R., Cushmen, W. C., Green, L. A., et al. (2003). The Seventh Report of the Joint National Committee on Prevention, Detection, Evaluation, and Treatment of High Blood Pressure: The JNC 7 report. *Journal of the American Medical Association, 289*(19), 2560–2572.

Conde-Agudelo, A., Rosas-Bermudez, B., & Kafury-Goeta, A. C. (2006). Birth spacing and risk of adverse perinatal outcomes: A meta-analysis. *Journal of the American Medical Association, 295*(15), 1809–1823.

Cummings, P., & Rivara, F. P. (2004). Car occupant death according to the restraint use of other occupants: A matched cohort study. *Journal of the American Medical Association, 291*(3), 342–349.

Depression Management Tool Kit. (2001). *MacArthur initiative on depression and primary care.* Retrieved October 22, 2007, from *www.depression-primarycare.org.*

Erikson, E. H. (1993). *Childhood and society.* New York: W. W. Norton.

Fenwick, A. (2003). On the front line of SARS. *American Journal of Nursing, 103*(9), 118–119.

Fontenot, H., Fantasia, H., & Allen, J. (2007). HPV in adolescents: Making the wake-up call. *ADVANCE for Nurse Practitioners, 15*(10), 73–76.

Frank, G. (2007). Good nutrition on the go. *Advance for Nurse Practitioners, 15*(11), 55–57.

Gilligan, C. (1982). New maps of development: New visions of maturity. *American Journal of Orthopsychiatry, 52*(2), 199–212.

Gilligan, C. (2002). *The birth of pleasure.* New York: Alfred A. Knopf.

Golden, W. E., & Hopkins, R. H. (2003). Divorce. *Internal Medicine News, 36*(17), 22.

Hatcher, R. A., Trussell, J., & Stewart, F. H. (2004). *Contraceptive technology* (18th ed.). New York: Ardent Media.

Huether, S. E., & McCance, K. L. (2007). *Understanding pathophysiology* (4th ed.). St. Louis, MO: Mosby.

Jemal, A., Cokkinides, V., Shafey, O., & Thun, M. (2003). Lung cancer trends in young adults: An early indicator of progress in tobacco control (United States). *Cancer Causes and Control, 14,* 579–585.

Kaplan, C. (2007). Intrauterine contraception. *Advance for Nurse Practitioners, 15*(11), 47–52.

Kiviruusu, O., Huurre, T., & Aro, H. (2007). Psychosocial resources and depression among chronically ill young adults: Are males more vulnerable? *Social Science Medicine, 65*(2), 173–186.

Kohlberg, L., & Lickons, T. (1986). *The stages of ethical development: From childhood through old age.* San Francisco, CA: Harper.

Lowdermilk, D. L., & Perry, S. E. (2007). *Maternity & women's health care* (9th ed.). St. Louis, MO: Mosby.

Manson, J. E., Skerrett, P. J., Greenland, P., & VanItallie, T. B. (2004). The escalating pandemics of obesity and sedentary lifestyle. A call to action for clinicians. *Archives of Internal Medicine, 164,* 249–258.

Marshall, D., McConkey, R., & Moore, G. (2003). Obesity in people with intellectual disabilities: The impact of nurse-led health screenings and health promotion activities. *Journal of Advanced Nursing, 41*(2), 147–153.

Meyers, D., Halvorson, H., & Luckhaupt, S. (2007). Screening for chlamydial infection: an evidence update for the U.S. Preventive Services Task Force. *Annals of Internal Medicine, 147*(2), 134–141.

Michigan teens still having sex, but pregnancy rates are falling. *Women's Health Weekly, 12.* Retrieved October 22, 2007, from *www.obgyn.net/newsheadlines/womens_health-Adolescent_Health-20040205-4.asp.*

Nunez, R., & Caruso, L. (2003, Jan.). Are shelters the answer to family homelessness? *USA Today, 131,* 46.

Paschall, M. J., Flewelling, R. L., & Russell, T. (2004). Why is work intensity associated with heavy alcohol use among adolescents? *Journal of Adolescent Health, 34*(1), 79–87.

Physical Activity and Public Health. (2007). Updated recommendations for adults from the American College of Sports Medicine and the American Heart Association. *Circulation, 116,* 1081–1093. Retrieved April 8, 2008, from *http://circ.ahajournals.org/cgi/ reprint/CIRCULATIONAHA.107.185649.*

Piaget, J. (1972). Intellectual evolution from adolescence to adulthood. *Human Development, 15,* 1–12.

Pravikoff, D. S., Pierce, S., & Tanner, A. (2003). Are nurses ready for evidence-based practice? *American Journal of Nursing, 103*(5), 95–96.

Schoenborn, C. A., Vickerie, J. L., & Barnes, P. M. (2003). *Cigarette smoking behavior of adults: United States, 1997–98. Advance data from vital and health statistics* (No. 331). Hyattsville, MD: National Center for Health Statistics.

Shope, J. T. (2007). Graduated driver licensing: Review of evaluation results since 2002. *Journal of Safety Research, 38*(2), 165–175.

U.S. Census Bureau. (2006). *Statistical abstracts of the United States: 2007* (126th ed.). Washington, DC: U.S. Government Printing Office.

U.S. Department of Health and Human Services. (2006). *Healthy People 2010: Midcourse review.* Retrieved September 11, 2007, from *www.healthypeople.gov/data/ midcourse/html.*

U.S. Preventive Services Task Force. (2008). *Guide to clinical preventive services.* Rockville, MD: Agency for healthcare Research and Quality. Retrieved September 11, 2007, from *www.ahrq.gov/ clinic/pocketgd.htm.*

Chapter 23

Middle-Age Adult

Helene Dixon

- Name three psychosocial and spiritual changes that frequently occur during middle age.
- Explain the normal biological changes that occur as a result of the aging process.
- Identify the major causes of mortality in the middle-age adult.
- Describe frequently occurring health patterns of middle-age adults.
- Discuss the unique health problems related to the occupations of the adult between ages 35 and 65.
- Analyze the influence of psychosocial stressors on the middle-age adult and the ways the individual's culture and occupation can affect these stressors.

key terms

Advance directive	Generativity versus stagnation	Obesity
Body mass index (BMI)	Gingivitis	Osteoarthritis
Calcium	Glaucoma	Osteopenia
Cardiac output	Health care agent	Osteoporosis
Cataracts	Kyphosis	Overweight
Constipation	Living will	Perimenopause
Degenerative joint disease	Macular degeneration	Periodontitis
Durable power of attorney	Menopause	Presbycusis
Functional aerobic capacity	"Midlife crisis"	Presbyopia
		Vitamin D

website materials

evolve These materials are located on the book's website at *http://evolve.elsevier.com/Edelman/*.

- WebLinks
- Study Questions
- Glossary
- Website Resources

  23A: Screening Requirements for Middle-Age Adults
  23B: Community Resources for Health Promotion During Middle Adulthood

Terminal Illness

Charlie Shelton is dying of lung cancer. His wife, Sarah, finds that she must manage a household and provide for their two children (ages 15 and 18) on her own. The elder child plans to enter college next fall, but the Sheltons wonder whether they will be able to afford this. Although Charlie and Sarah worked hard and saved money all their lives, Charlie's long illness continues to deplete their savings. Their parents are helping as best they can, but they live on limited incomes themselves. The hospital bills continue to come, and the Sheltons are overwhelmed.

1. What can health providers do to help the Sheltons during this stressful time?
2. What health-promotion strategies might be suggested and implemented to help them?
3. What community organizations might the health care provider recommend to meet the needs of this family?
4. What responsibilities do health providers and policy makers have to provide health promotion to middle-age adults?

Middle adulthood is defined as the period between 35 and 65. During this dynamic time the adult experiences significant biological, physiological, social, psychological, and spiritual changes. The middle years represent a stage of development set within major economic productivity and family and community responsibilities. This age group makes up nearly 40% of the population of the United States (Boston Women's Health Book Collective & Norsigian, 2005; U.S. Department of Health and Human Services [USDHHS], 2007).

AGE AND PHYSICAL CHANGES

Although their onset is insidious, biological changes come to the forefront during the middle years, affecting most bodily systems. The hair of the adult begins to thin and turn gray. The skin's moisture and turgor decreases, and with the loss of subcutaneous fat, wrinkling occurs. Excessive sun exposure through the years makes some changes more pronounced, especially coursing of facial features.

Fat deposition increases during these years, with increases in weight. The body contour changes as "love handles" and "saddlebags" appear. Sedentary lifestyles and unchanged dietary habits contribute a great deal to these changes. The inactive lifestyle is further compromised by a decrease in energy; "I'm not as young as I used to be" is a common remark. This proclamation is legitimate, because the capacity for physical work actually decreases. The **functional aerobic capacity** decreases, with a resulting decrease in **cardiac output**.

In the musculoskeletal system, bone density and mass progressively decrease. When 55-year-old adults say that they were an inch taller when they were 18, the observation is likely to be true. A 1-inch to 4-inch (2.5-cm to 10-cm) loss in height occurs as a person ages; thinning of the intervertebral disks accounts for approximately 1 inch. However, dramatic losses in height (more than 4 inches) can occur with thoracic **kyphosis**, an angulation of the posterior spine (commonly known as "*hunchback*"). The wear and tear on joints predispose the adult to **degenerative joint disease**, deterioration of the joint(s), with more frequent painful backaches. The general decrease in muscle tone is categorized by many as "*flab*", which reduces physical agility. Degenerative joint disease, specifically **osteoarthritis**, has its peak onset in middle age and can greatly impact activity, including employment. Most frequently the knees and hands, followed by hips, spine, shoulders, and ankles, are involved. In the *Midcourse Review*, six objectives about arthritis moved toward their targets: activity limitations due to arthritis, counseling of adults for weight reduction and exercise, effects of arthritis on paid work, hospitalization for vertebral fracture, and activity limitations due to chronic back pain (USDHHS, 2005). Continue to follow the progress toward these targets in *Healthy People 2020*.

Osteopenia is a condition of subnormally mineralized bone, usually as a result of a rate of bone lysis that exceeds the rate of bone matrix synthesis. **Osteoporosis** is a disorder characterized by abnormal loss of bone density and deterioration of bone tissue, with an increased fracture risk. It occurs most frequently in postmenopausal women who have fair complexions and are small, sedentary individuals, and people on long-term steroid use. It increases with age.

The functional capacity of all organ systems generally decreases. For example, in the gastrointestinal tract, the following chain of events occurs: decreased metabolism leads to less enzyme production, resulting in lower hydrochloric acid levels, which decreases tone in the large intestine. As a result, the middle-age adult may complain of acid indigestion with increased belching.

When the adult leads a sedentary lifestyle as well, the effects of the diminished motility through the gastrointestinal tract can be more pronounced. That Americans eat more refined foods (foods that are low in bulk) than residents of third-world nations is well known. A low-bulk diet can contribute to the problem of **constipation**, a change in bowel habits characterized by decreased frequency or passage of hard, drier stools and difficult defecation, and is believed to be a primary contributor to the increased incidence of colon cancer in the United States. Between ages 25 and 85, a 35% loss of nephron units occurs. The remaining nephrons increase in size and undergo degenerative changes. The entire weight of the kidneys decreases. Because blood supply is also diminished, the glomerular filtration rate is decreased by nearly one half.

Significant changes occur in the cardiovascular system as the blood vessels lose elasticity and become thicker. This process predisposes middle-age adults to coronary artery disease, hypertension, myocardial infarctions, and strokes. Heart disease is the second leading cause of death in middle-age adults (Heron, 2007).

When a previously menstruating woman does not have a period for 1 year, she has reached **menopause**. The median age for menopause is 51 to 52 years. Women now expect to live one third of their lives after menopause. A great deal more must be learned about what causes many of the symptoms that occur in menopause (Mendelsohn & Karas, 2007). Sheehy (1993) conducted interviews of 100 women from their mid-40s to 60s and also interviewed 75 physicians and other experts. Her analysis showed that many of these people felt there was a renewed sexual vitality and surge of mental energy for menopausal women. She characterized menopause as a gateway to a second adulthood. Northrup (2008) and Sheehy (1993) reiterate the importance of taking time to rethink and reprioritize one's life once menopause is in process (Boston Women's Health Book Collective et al., 2006).

During this time, production of ovarian estrogen and progesterone ceases; the remaining estrogen is produced by the adrenal glands. As a result of the diminished estrogen level, a woman's secondary sex characteristics regress, such as loss of pubic hair and decrease in breast size. The female reproductive organs shrink, and vaginal secretions decrease, requiring additional lubrication.

Men experience changes in their sexual response cycle as testosterone levels plateau, then decrease, as they approach the end of the middle years. The testes undergo degenerative changes, the viable spermatozoa diminish, and the volume and viscosity of semen decrease. In men, sexual energy gradually declines; achieving an erection takes longer, but it is sustained longer. Stress, however, can significantly diminish function (Rice, 2000).

Mortality Rates

The leading causes of death during middle adulthood are cancer and heart disease (Miniño et al., 2007; USDHHS, 2007) (Box 23-1). Reducing disabilities and deaths from these chronic conditions are national health-promotion and disease-prevention objectives (Lubkin & Larsen, 2006; USDHHS, 2000, 2005) (*Healthy People 2010* box). Ongoing data of these conditions will be noted in *Healthy People 2020*.

Box 23-1	Leading Causes of Death in Middle-Age Adults

AGES 35 TO 44 YEARS
- Unintentional injuries: 16,471
- Cancer: 14,723

AGES 45 TO 54 YEARS
- Cancer: 49,520
- Heart disease: 37,556

AGES 55 TO 64 YEARS
- Cancer: 96,956
- Heart disease: 63,613

From Centers for Disease Control and Prevention, National Center for Health Statistics, National Vital Statistics Systems. (2007). Washington, DC: U.S. Government Printing Office.

Healthy People 2010

Selected National Health-Promotion and Disease Prevention Objectives for the Middle-Age Adult

Overall Goals

1. Increase the quality of life and years of healthy life.
2. Eliminate health disparities.

Objectives

1. Improve access to high-quality health services.
   - Increase the proportion of people with health insurance to 100% (baseline* is 86% of adults).
   - Increase the proportion of adults who have a specific source of ongoing care (baseline is 84% of adults).
2. Reduce the overall cancer death rate to 158.7 per 100,000 population (baseline is 201.4 per 100,000 population).
3. Reduce new cases of diabetes to 2.5 per 1000 people (baseline is 2.1 new cases per 1000 people).
4. Increase the proportion of adults with disabilities reporting satisfaction with life to 96% (baseline is 87%).
5. Increase the quality, availability, and effectiveness of educational and community-based programs designed to prevent disease and improve health and quality of life.

6. Promote health for all through a healthy environment.
7. Increase the proportion of pregnancies that are intended to 70% (baseline is 51% of pregnancies were unintended).
8. Reduce increases in food-borne illness.
9. Use communication strategically to improve health.
10. Reduce coronary heart deaths to 166 per 100,000 population (baseline is 208 deaths per 100,000 population).
11. Reduce new cases of AIDS among adolescents and adults to 1 per 100,000 population (baseline is 19.5 new cases per 100,000 population).
12. Reduce indigenous cases of vaccine-preventable diseases.
13. Reduce injuries, disabilities, and deaths from accidents and violence.
14. Improve the health and well-being of women, infants, children, and families.
15. Improve mental health and ensure access to appropriate, quality mental health care.

Continued

Healthy People 2010
Selected National Health-Promotion and Disease Prevention Objectives for the Middle-Age Adult—*cont'd*

16. Increase the proportion of adults who are at a healthy weight to 60% (baseline is 42% of all adults).
17. Reduce work-related injuries for full-time workers to 4.6 per 100 (baseline is 6.6 injuries per 100 workers) and deaths to 3.2 per 100,000 workers (baseline is 4.5 deaths per 100,000 workers).
18. Increase the proportion of adults who engage regularly, preferably daily, in moderate physical activity for at least 30 minutes per day to 30% (baseline is 15%).

19. Reduce asthma deaths of adults ages 35 to 64 years to 9 per 1 million (baseline is 17 asthma deaths per 1 million).
20. Promote responsible sexual behaviors, including preventing sexually transmitted diseases.
21. Reduce substance abuse to protect the health, safety, and quality of life for all people.
22. Reduce tobacco use by adults to 12% (baseline is 24% of adults).
23. Increase the proportion of people who have a dilated eye examination at appropriate intervals.

*Baseline year for all objectives is 2000.
AIDS, Acquired immunodeficiency syndrome.
Note: Target and baseline data identified when available.
From U.S. Department of Health and Human Services. (2000). *Healthy People 2010* and (2005) *Healthy People 2010* Midcourse Review. Washington, DC: U.S. Government Printing Office.

Many of these diseases are preventable, entirely or in part, through behavior changes (U.S. Preventive Services Task Force, 2007). Middle adults can influence their own health and that of their children through healthier lifestyles and health promoting care (Buttaro et al., 2003).

Cancer is the leading cause of death in middle adulthood. Death rates from all cancers combined, and the four leading causes of cancer deaths (lung, colorectal, female breast, and prostate), declined by the *Healthy People 2010 Midcourse Review* (USDHHS, 2005). Although there has been a decline in cancer deaths, problems like access to health care still remain (14.8% of the U.S. population does not have health insurance [USDHHS, 2007]). For example, in 2009, the Obama administration will be focusing on health care system changes. Overall, and especially for rural residents, Pap test use within the recommended 3-year interval, primary care provider counseling for exercise, and the proportion of adults practicing skin care prevention remained unchanged from the baseline year, 2000. Use of the fecal occult blood test home kit for colorectal cancer screening decreased (USDHHS, 2005).

Gender and Marital Status

In the middle years, the death rate for men is higher. They are more likely than women to die from heart disease even though adult women under the age of 45 years have a higher rate of heart disease than men of the same age (USDHHS, Women's Health USA, 2007). Although death rates for cardiovascular disease are declining for both sexes, heart disease remains the number one cause of death overall. Risk factors for heart disease include obesity, lack of physical activity, smoking, high cholesterol, hypertension, and old age. Among U.S. adults 61% are overweight (ACS, 2005). (See Chapter 11 for discussion of overweight and obesity.)

Life expectancies for American men and women are now at record highs, 80.4 years for women, and 75.2 years for

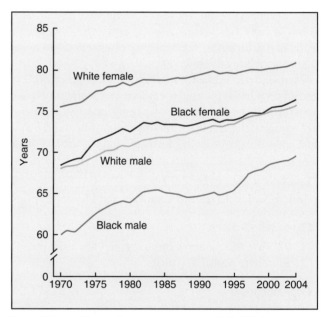

Figure 23-1 Life expectancy by race and sex: United States, 1970-2004. (From Miniño, A., Heron, M., & Murphy, S. [2007]. Deaths: Final data for 2004, *National Vital Results, 55*[19], 7.)

men. Between 2003 and 2004, the largest gain in life expectancy was for Black males. Current trends in life expectancy are noted (Figure 23-1) (Miniño et al., 2007).

Nearly 60% of adults in the United States are married. Married adults report better health than divorced, widowed, or never-married adults. Marriage rates for White adults (61%) are higher than for Hispanic adults (58%) or Black adults (38%). Married adults report they are less likely to smoke, drink heavily, or be physically inactive (NCVS, 2007; U.S. Census Bureau, 2006).

Race, Gender, and Ethnicity

Black Americans are the largest minority race and the second largest ethnic group in the United States. They comprise 13% of the U.S. population. There are 40 million Black Americans. Death rates for all major causes of death are higher for Black Americans than for Whites. Life expectancy is lower for Black men (68.6 years versus 75) and Black women (75.5 years versus 80.2) compared to Whites (U.S. Department of Health and Human Services, 2007).

Cancer is the leading cause of death for Black men and Black women in middle age. Although the incidence and mortality rates from cancer have declined substantially for Black adults since 1993, for all cancer sites and at all stages of diagnosis, Black adults are less likely to survive 5 years after diagnosis than White adults. Researchers believe that this disparity is largely related to factors associated with poverty. Black Americans, while 13% of the population, comprise 24% of the nation's poor (ACS, 2005). Black households have the lowest median income ($31,969), compared to non-Hispanic Whites ($52,423), Hispanics ($37,781), and Asians ($64,238) (DeNavas-Walt et al., 2007).

People who are poor have less access to medical care and are more likely not to have health insurance. Blacks are more likely to be uninsured than non-Hispanic Whites. In an analysis done by the American Cancer Society, those without health insurance were less likely to have had a recent mammogram or to have been screened for colorectal cancer, two of the most common cancers in the United States. In addition, those without insurance who were diagnosed with cancer were more likely to have been diagnosed at an advanced stage, when cancer is more difficult to treat (ACS, 2007). Although poverty and lack of health insurance are important reasons for ethnic and racial disparities in cancer outcomes, there are other reasons as well, including differences in tumor biology and a higher prevalence of coexisting conditions (ACS, 2005). More research is needed on ways to address the racial and ethnic disparities in cancer outcomes.

The second leading cause of death for Black Americans is heart disease. Compared to the general population, they are less likely to be diagnosed with heart disease, but they are 30% more likely to die from it. Hypertension and overweight/obesity are risk factors for heart disease and stroke. Black adults are 50% more likely to have hypertension. 77% of Black women are overweight, compared to 57% of White women. Black adults are 50% more likely to suffer a stroke, compared to White adults. They are 60% more likely to die from it (USDHHS, Office of Minority Health, 2007).

Black Americans share a disproportionate burden of HIV/AIDS. Black men are eight times more likely than non-Hispanic White men to have HIV/AIDS. Black women are 23 times more likely to have HIV/AIDS than non-Hispanic White women. Blacks account for 47% of all persons living with HIV/AIDS in the United States (USDHHS, 2007).

Latino/Hispanic Americans are the largest ethnic minority group in the United States. They comprise 14% of the population. There are 44 million Hispanic Americans. Most Hispanics (60%), are born in the United States. A disproportionate number of Hispanics are poor and lack health insurance.

Compared to 12.4% for the total population, 22% of all Hispanics are poor. Hispanic Americans have the highest uninsured rate of any racial or ethnic group in the United States. Twice as many Hispanic men under the age of 64 (32.7%), report no regular source of health care compared to non-Hispanic White men (14.9%) (ACS, 2006). Results of a major population survey showed that approximately one-third of Hispanics were uninsured at the time they were interviewed or had been uninsured for at least part of the past year. More than one-fourth of Hispanics surveyed had been without health insurance for more than one year (Cohen & Martinez, 2007).

Cancer is the second leading cause of death for Hispanics. Breast cancer is the most common type of cancer in Hispanic women. Hispanic women with breast cancer are less likely to be diagnosed when the disease is at a local stage, and are approximately 20% more likely to die than non-Hispanic White women even when they are diagnosed at a similar age and stage of disease. Overall, the incidence rate of breast cancer is about 40% lower for Hispanic women than for non-Hispanic White women, and the death rate from breast cancer has decreased for both populations. For all cancers combined, the incidence and death rates for Hispanics is lower compared to non-Hispanic Whites. Specific cancers which occur more often in Hispanics are stomach, liver, cervix, acute lymphocytic leukemia, and gallbladder.

Heart disease is the number one cause of death in Hispanic Americans. Hispanic adults are less likely to smoke than non-Hispanic White adults, but almost 80% of Mexican-Americans are overweight. 42.3% of all Mexican-American women are obese (Figure 23-2). Mexican-Americans comprise approximately 60% of the Hispanic population in the United States. Obesity increases the risk of diabetes, hypertension, heart disease, and premature death. Obesity is also associated with increased risk of breast, prostate, colon, and uterine cancer (ACS, 2006).

Genetics

The middle-age adult is at greater risk than is the young adult for diseases known to be associated with genetics (familial characteristics), including diabetes, hypertension, Huntington chorea, arteriosclerosis, gout, obesity, heart disease, and alcoholism.

Some malignancies tend to be hereditary; for example, women with a personal or family history of breast cancer have an increased risk. Additionally, individuals with a family history of colorectal cancer, rectal or colon polyps, or ulcerative colitis are at high risk for colorectal cancer.

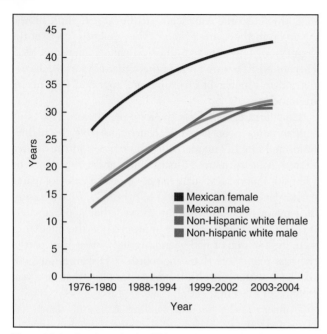

Figure 23-2   Trends in obesity (BMI >30) by gender for Mexican Americans and Non-Hispanic White adults, ages 20 and older, U.S. (From American Cancer Society [2006]. *Cancer Facts & Figures for Hispanics/Latinos 2006–2008,* Atlanta, Georgia.)

GORDON'S FUNCTIONAL HEALTH PATTERNS
Health Perception–Health Management Pattern

To promote health in the middle-age adult, the nurse performs a health assessment that includes the person's values and beliefs, lifestyle patterns, general perceptions of health, and health practices (see the health promotion model by Pender et al., 2005).

Habits

The self-destructive habits of the middle-age adult that have been practiced for years (cigarette smoking, excessive alcohol use, and overeating) begin to have visible consequences. As pressures increase, adults are tempted to turn to substances such as these as a crutch for coping with stress. Prevention is extremely important, primarily because withdrawal from any of these substances is a difficult process.

Risk Factors

The major risk factors for adults in the middle years are environmental and behavioral; they can be changed through teaching, counseling, and other nursing interventions (USDHHS, 2000, 2007). Helping adults to take care of themselves and to change, when indicated, can be accomplished on an individual or group basis.

Some of the health-promotion needs of the middle-age adult include acceptance of aging, the need to exercise, and weight control. Decreasing or stopping cigarette smoking and alcohol consumption can also be identified needs. Preventive health screening is vital. The adult needs input into and control of as many of these behaviors as possible.

Total health risks of middle-age adults are composed of group risks (age, gender, race) and personal risks. Precritical secondary prevention includes periodic selective screening for the detection of disease before it becomes clinically apparent, such as performing a breast self-examination. A suggested screening examination appears in Box 23-2.

Chronic conditions are defined as those that last for more than 3 months. Approximately 20% of the population age 45 to 64 reports limitations caused by chronic conditions (Lubkin & Larsen, 2006). A significant increase is seen between the ages of 45 and 64. Chronic conditions found in the middle-age adult include heart conditions, arthritis, impairments of the back and spine, chronic obstructive lung disease, diabetes, mental and nervous system conditions, and dental disease (Lubkin & Larsen, 2006). Diseases and behaviors for which screening is recommended in the middle-age adult are listed in **Website Resource 23A**.

Nutritional-Metabolic Pattern

Dietary factors are correlated with 5 of the 10 leading causes of death in the United States: coronary heart disease, some cancers, stroke, non–insulin-dependent diabetes mellitus, and atherosclerosis (Centers for Disease Control and Prevention, 2002; USDHHS, 2000, 2007).

Physical activities and nutritional patterns frequently are correlated. The middle-age adult typically leads a more sedentary lifestyle than does the young adult, primarily because of increased responsibilities at work and home and the many convenience devices that infiltrate homes and workplaces. Obesity tends to occur in women (30% to 40%) more than in men (20% to 30%) (Dunphy, 2004). Unfortunately, the less active adult usually fails to alter any dietary habits to compensate, so one of the major health problems of the middle years is obesity.

Obesity

Obesity is defined as a **body mass index (BMI)** of 30 kg/m² or more, and being **overweight** is a BMI over 27.8 kg/m² for adult males and 27.3 kg/m² for adult females. During the survey period 1988–1994 to 1999–2002, the proportion of adults at a healthy weight decreased from 42% to 33% and the proportion of adults who were obese increased from 23% to 30%. (The targets for the year 2010 are 60% and 15% respectively [USDHHS, 2000, 2007].)

"Overweight and obesity substantially raise the risk of illness from high blood pressure, high cholesterol, type 2 (non–insulin-dependent) diabetes, heart disease and stroke, gallbladder disease, arthritis, sleep disturbances and problems breathing, and endometrial, breast, prostate and colon cancers. Obese individuals may also suffer from social stigmatization, discrimination, and lowered self-esteem" (USDHHS, 2005, p. 29). A study including approximately 7000 middle-age people (conducted 26 years ago) revealed that those who had a BMI between 18 and 25 felt better and had a better quality of life than people who were overweight (Daviglus et al., 2003).

Box 23-2 Screening Examination: Ages 35 to 65

DATABASE
- Health history: initial update with nurse or PE
- Health hazard appraisal: initial screening
- Psychological inventories as needed

PHYSICAL EXAMINATION (EVERY 3 TO 5 YEARS UNTIL AGE 40, THEN ANNUALLY) EMPHASIZING
- Weight and height
- Blood pressure, pulse
- Breasts
- Pelvis
- Prostate
- Testicles
- Eyes
- Mouth
- Skin

LABORATORY PROCEDURES
- Pap smear
- Hemoccult: three stools for Hemoccult with PE after age 50
- Colonoscopy or sigmoidoscopy every 3 to 5 years after age 50 as indicated
- Mammography screening at age 35 every 2 years, then yearly after age 50
- Urinalysis: examined at the time of PE
- Lipid profile (men ages 35 to 65; women ages 45 to 65)

- Chest radiograph with PE if heavy smoker
- Tetanus and diphtheria booster every 10 years
- Influenza vaccine: follow current recommendations
- Counseling and testing for HIV as indicated
- Rubella serology (women of childbearing age)

SELF-CARE EDUCATION AND COUNSELING
- With physical examination; individualized according to individual's risk factors
- Injury prevention: seat-belts, helmets, firearms, smoke detectors
- Stress reduction
- Exercise
- Diet: cholesterol, fat, sodium, fiber, multivitamins with folic acid (women of childbearing age)
- Calcium
- Breast self-examination
- Testicular self-examination
- Dental care
- Mouth care
- Sexually transmitted diseases
- Contraception
- Skin protection from ultraviolet light
- Alcohol and other substance abuse
- Smoking cessation
- Possible hormone prophylaxis (perimenopausal and postmenopausal women)

PE, Physician examination; *Pap,* Papanicolaou; *HIV,* human immunodeficiency virus.
Data from American Cancer Society (Massachusetts Division); U.S. Department of Health and Human Services. (2000). *Healthy people 2010.* Washington, DC: U.S. Government Printing Office.

Women with less education and low incomes and Black and Hispanic women are at an increased risk for being overweight. In addition to gender, race, and socioeconomic status, genetics may be a contributing factor. The most significant variables, however, are health behaviors, particularly food intake and exercise and activity patterns. Although an abundance of health information is available, these challenges persist.

As much as 40% of a typical American family's food budget is spent on food in restaurants or for take-out foods, both of which are usually higher in fat (including saturated and trans) and salt content than foods prepared at home (USDHHS, 2000, 2007). Losing and maintaining weight may require an individual to change eating and activity behaviors, but the social, food preparation and consumption behaviors of the family must change as well.

Prevention of obesity is the goal of weight management during the middle years. When the adult is obese, a clear-cut history of the onset is imperative. A lifelong history of obesity is significantly more arduous to alter than that of adult-onset obesity. A decrease in calories should be accompanied by at least 30 minutes of exercise 5 times a week. When calories are reduced and exercise is increased, weight loss is achieved and maintained.

Weight-management resources available to the adult are plentiful. Weight-management programs using behavior modification can be found in varied settings, such as universities and work sites, Weight Watchers, Overeaters Anonymous, and Take Off Pounds Sensibly. If the nurse identifies a need for weight management and no program is available, a self-help group can be initiated. A suggested list of topics generated by the group are assembled. A discussion of basic nutrition with appropriate handouts is a good place to start. Having adults write down their individual goals and keep a 1-week diet log is nonthreatening and helpful for future planning and also gives them some responsibility in the program. Intake food journals assist the individuals in maintaining weight loss outcomes.

High Saturated Fat Diet

Lipid levels and ratios have a significant influence on cardiovascular and cerebrovascular morbidity and mortality rates. The National Heart, Lung, and Blood Institute regards a blood cholesterol level below 200 mg/dL as desirable. For the first time in more than 40 years, the average total cholesterol level for adults in the United States is now 199 (Japsen, 2007). Much of this success is attributed to the use of statin drugs that lower the level of low density lipoproteins (LDL) in the blood. The reference *Coronary Primary Prevention Trial* demonstrates that men at high risk are able to reduce coronary heart disease by approximately 2% for every 1% lower blood cholesterol level. Before initiating medication to reduce cholesterol, persons with high cholesterol are advised to reduce their intake of saturated fat, total fat, and dietary cholesterol, normalize their weight, and increase physical activity. If lifestyle changes are not successful, medication is often advised. Some studies demonstrate the benefits of estrogen on heart health (Parker-Pope, 2007). One pharmaceutical company is currently seeking FDA approval to sell its cholesterol-lowering drug over the counter (Japsen, 2007; USDHHS, 2000).

Calcium

Adequate **calcium** intake is essential for developing and maintaining bone mass. Additionally, calcium is needed for other physiological processes, including muscle contraction and blood pressure regulation. Men and women need a minimal daily intake of 1000 mg of calcium. Pregnant and nursing women need 1200 mg, and postmenopausal women need either 1000 mg (when taking estrogen) or 1500 mg (when not taking estrogen). **Vitamin D** enhances the absorption of calcium (Karch, 2003). When daily intake of calcium is less than adequate, serum calcium level will be maintained by leaching calcium from bone, resulting in osteoporosis. Exercise also contributes to bone mass by increasing mechanical stress on the bones.

Caffeine

Caffeine is a popular stimulant found in coffee, tea, and some soft drinks, such as colas. Caffeine prolongs the amount of time that physical work can be performed and appears to decrease boredom and increase attention span. On the negative side, coffee has come under significant scrutiny from the media recently, with reports of a link between cancer of the pancreas and coffee consumption. There is controversy as to whether daily moderate intake of caffeine has any detrimental effects.

Like alcohol and nicotine, caffeine is readily available and has become an accepted part of daily living. Because caffeine is a strong stimulant with effects that typically are taken for granted, its importance as an addictive substance must be emphasized. Ingestion of 0.5 grams of caffeine (3 to 4 cups of coffee) can increase the basal metabolic rate an average of 10%, and possibly as much as 25% for some people.

Long-term stimulation of the central nervous system results in restlessness, sleep disturbances, cardiac stimulation, and withdrawal effects. Nurses' assessment should screen for stimulating and addicting substances that may be producing these symptoms.

High-Sodium Diet

High-sodium diets play a significant role in hypertension, especially when consumed over many years. The result may be an increase in total body fluids, which increases peripheral vascular resistance. Salt contains approximately 40% sodium and is a contributing factor for hypertension in the 10% to 20% of Americans who are at risk. On average, Americans consume 4 to 5 grams of sodium per day. A major contributor of dietary sodium is the salt found in processed foods.

Over the past 3 decades, many clinical studies have demonstrated the effectiveness of lowering blood pressure by lowering dietary sodium. Other studies have described the relationships between urinary and sodium excretion and the change of blood pressure with age (Joint National Committee, 2003).

Alcohol Abuse

Substance abuse can be a devastating habit. Many adults abuse prescription and illicit drugs and, especially, alcohol. Twenty-three million Americans struggle with a drug or alcohol problem but 85% do not feel they need treatment (USDHHS, 2005).

Initially alcohol appears to be a stimulant, but actually it is a central nervous system depressant and anesthetic. Chronic alcohol use produces tolerance, thereby necessitating a gradual increase in dose to achieve the same effect. Alcohol contributes to problems with safety because of decreased reaction time and depression of the central nervous system.

Alcohol is frequently treated as a nondrug, but alcohol addiction is second only to nicotine addiction. Alcohol is readily available, reasonably inexpensive, and considered a part of social exchange; its long-range physiological and psychological effects are well documented. In the United States, two thirds of adults consume alcohol, and 18 million are problem drinkers. Presently, men outnumber women as alcohol abusers by approximately 5:1, but this ratio is decreasing as more women are exceeding low-risk drinking guidelines (USDHHS, 2005).

The Dietary Guidelines for Americans, issued jointly by the U.S. Department of Agriculture and the U.S. Department of Health and Human Services (*www.nutrition.gov*), defines moderate drinking as no more than one drink a day for women and no more than two drinks a day for men. Women are more vulnerable than men to the effects of alcohol because, pound for pound, women have less water in their bodies and they tend to weigh less than men. This means that a woman's brain and other organs are exposed to more alcohol and to the toxic byproducts of alcohol as it is metabolized. The death rate for female alcoholics is 50% to 100% higher than for male alcoholics. A woman is more likely to drink excessively if her parents, siblings, or other blood relatives have problems with alcohol, if her partner drinks heavily, if she was abused physically or sexually as a child, if she has a history or depression, or if she is able to "hold her liquor" more than others (USDHHS, NIH, 2005).

Alcohol abuse is associated with motor vehicle accidents, homicides, suicides, drowning, heart disease, cancer, liver disease, pancreatitis, and fetal alcohol syndrome. It is a major cause of mental retardation in children (USDHHS, 2000). The alcoholic person is at greater risk for cancer of the larynx, oral cavity, and liver.

The alcoholic may complain of symptoms such as heartburn and gas, stomach distention, poor eating habits, nausea and vomiting, gastric pain, irritation of the mouth, throat, and esophagus, and right upper quadrant pain. Two additional subtle findings are spider angiomata and palmar erythema.

Primary prevention for substance and alcohol abuse is complex, especially because adults consume these agents for many reasons, including peer pressure, loneliness, alienation, frustration, anxiety, and low self-esteem. Heavy drinkers may also be following the example established by influential people in their lives. Merely telling people about the potential physical, emotional, and legal hazards appears to have little effect as a preventive measure. Promoting more realistic portrayals of substance abuse through the media is difficult to implement. Although techniques such as assertiveness training and teaching adults to resist persuasion are helpful, more useful approaches might include helping them learn to manage anxiety and increase their self-esteem. Less anxious and more confident people have greater skills in resisting peer influences to participate in substance abuse; they also are more likely to have fewer episodes of isolation and loneliness.

Early detection and intervention can decrease ongoing and future physical and psychosocial problems resulting from alcohol abuse. Nurses use a variety of screening strategies to identify individuals' perceptions and consequences of drinking. The CAGE questionnaire is the most popular screening tool used in primary care (Dunphy, 2004). The Michigan alcohol screening test (*http://counselingresource. com/quizzes/alcohol-mast/index.html*) and alcohol use disorders identification test (*http://pubs.niaaa.nih.gov/publications/ Assessing%20Alcohol/InstrumentPDFs/14_AUDIT.pdf*) are examples of other screening instruments.

Abnormal laboratory test results, including elevations in aspartate aminotransferase, erythrocyte mean corpuscular volume, and serum glutamyltransferase, are not adequately sensitive and specific and may be a result of other causes including trauma, disease, and medications.

A variety of treatments are known to be effective, but no single "best" intervention has been identified. Effective treatments may be to address other problems using interventions such as pharmacological agents, stress management, acupuncture, individual and family therapy, and supportive environments.

Oral Health

Gingivitis Gingivitis is common among adults who fail to brush their teeth and use dental floss regularly. Redness and swelling develop around the teeth. Bleeding of the gums while brushing the teeth is an early sign of gingivitis. The gums may or may not be tender. When inflammation is not adequately treated and controlled, **periodontitis** involving bone destruction can develop, in addition to tooth loss.

Dental Hygiene and Decay In addition to consuming less carbohydrates (especially sugars), regular oral hygiene and care are major factors in maintaining oral health. However,

44% of Americans aged 40 and older receive annual health care by a dentist, which remained constant from 2000 (USDHHS, 2007). Middle-age adults have responsibility not only for their own care, but also for the care of their children and older parents. Fluoridation of water (vs. bottled) and sealants are additional health choices. Low income is a risk factor. In addition to the overall drop in the number of dentists since the late 1980s (from 57 to 48 per 100,000 people), many dentists do not accept Medicaid nor do they locate their practices in rural or low income areas (USDHHS, 2000, 2007). Untreated dental decay and tooth loss are twice the rate of White non-Hispanics in persons aged 35 to 44 with high school and less than high school education and higher in Black non-Hispanics (USDHHS, 2000, 2007). Regularly scheduled dental care with a dentist and dental hygienist is highly recommended not only for dental hygiene and treatment of dental decay and periodontal diseases such as gingivitis, but also for screening of oral-pharyngeal cancer, which has moved away from the *Healthy People 2010* target.

Elimination Pattern

Aging brings a gradual decrease of tone in the large intestine. As mentioned, this change, accompanied by a sedentary lifestyle and lack of bulk in the diet, predisposes the adult to constipation. Mass media advertising strongly encourage the population to rely on external controls rather than on exercise and dietary means to solve this problem. Consequently, many adults are dependent on taking fiber products as well as laxatives for regular bowel movements.

As discussed, degenerative changes in the nephron units occur during the middle-age years. Usually, however, the middle-age adult does not have any appreciable kidney malfunction. When a woman has had multiple births and little exercise, she may begin experiencing stress incontinence during this time, which can be socially embarrassing (Newman & Giovannini, 2002).

Activity-Exercise Pattern

Regular physical activity increases life expectancy and quality of life. It can help prevent and manage coronary heart disease, hypertension (American Obesity Association, 2004), diabetes, osteoporosis, and depression. Physical exercise has been correlated with lower rates of osteoporosis (National Osteoporosis Foundation, 1998), back injury, stroke, and colon cancer. Effective weight loss programs that incorporate physical activities also make significant contributions to increased life expectancy and quality of life (Kriketos et al., 2000; USDHHS, 2000, 2007).

Despite these benefits, few American adults engage in regular moderate physical activity for at least 30 minutes, 5 or more days a week, as recommended. Only a fraction of adults perform the recommended level, and slightly more report no leisure-time physical activities. By age 75, one in three men and one in two women engage in none. Sedentary behavior increases with age (USDHHS, 2005). Continuous, rhythmic exercise maintained for a sufficient period to stress the cardiac system is desirable. Some suggested activities include brisk walking, jogging, swimming, bicycling, and skipping rope as well as walking for transportation. Activities that focus on skill and coordination should be attempted by the adult over age 40 rather than activities necessitating speed and strength. Moderation is the key, along with increased caution as the adult approaches age 65. Overexertion, evidenced by symptoms of dizziness, tightness in the chest, and unresolving breathlessness, should be avoided.

The nurse initiates an exercise program with the middle-age adult by asking what activities have been enjoyed in the past. When these activities are realistic today, the nurse encourages the individual to rediscover them; when they appear unrealistic, new options should be explored. Additionally, activities are selected with consideration of potential for injury. Anyone at risk for heart disease (heavy smoking, high blood pressure, family history, diabetes, or prolonged lack of exercise) should have a complete history and physical examination before developing a rigorous activity program. For some of these individuals, an exercise test is recommended. Proper equipment, including supportive shoes and thermally appropriate clothing, is also important.

To be health promoting, physical exercise should involve as many muscles as is possible and be performed on a regular basis. Adults should do 30 minutes or more of moderate-intensity (brisk) physical activity on most (or all) days of the week, for a total of 3 to 4 hours. The appropriate level of performance for aerobic exercise is determined by achieving a pulse rate that is established for each individual: taking the number 220, subtracting the person's age, and then computing 75% of that number. A 50-year-old person, for example, should not exceed a pulse rate of 128 ([220–50] × 0.75 = 128).

Despite all these considerations, the kind of activity and style should be an individual choice and approached as something done for oneself and for fun, not as another chore or responsibility of middle age.

Sleep-Rest Pattern

Rest is a frequently omitted consideration for middle-age adults, who spend less time in deep sleep and need less sleep overall than do young adults. This change may be interpreted as insomnia; therefore, middle-age adults may need reassurance that this is common. Regularly scheduled, high-quality sleep and occasional napping when fatigued are healthful guidelines. Cognitive-behavioral therapy has also been demonstrated as effective in treating problems with sleeping (Jacobs, 1998; Jacobs et al., 2004). For further information, see the National Sleep Foundation at *www. sleepfoundation.org*.

Cognitive-Perceptual Pattern

The notion that at age 21 adults reach their peak and that "it is all downhill after that" is a myth. Continued learning is found throughout adulthood in such areas as reasoning, vocabulary, and spatial perception. Decreases can be observed, however, in reaction time and cognitive flexibility.

Intellectual Ability

"Learning" intelligence accumulates through education and life experiences and continues to increase throughout life, as evidenced by the many scholars and artists who are more productive in their middle years than they were as young adults.

The theories of Piaget, Bloom, and Havighurst and Orr are relevant to the middle-age adult. These theorists conclude that the prime time to be in the learner role is when the developmental task for that role is to be accomplished. The adult in the middle years as the learner-performer is a case in point. For example, to balance the responsibilities of caring for children and parents and working, the adult may explore new career options or creative endeavors.

Havighurst defines developmental tasks as the basic tasks of living that must be achieved if the adult is to live successfully. These tasks are dictated by the expectations of society, the physiological changes of the body throughout life, and the individual's own value system and goals. Although initially described in the 1950s, Havighurst and Orr's developmental tasks of middle age remain timely (Havighurst & Orr, 1956) (Box 23-3).

If career goals have been previously identified, then reaching them can be highly rewarding, both psychologically and financially. In addition to career activities, the mature adult has an increased social awareness and assumes more civic responsibility.

In Piaget's theory of cognitive development, formal operations is the final period. This stage begins at approximately age 12 and continues throughout life. Piaget describes the thoughts of adults as being both flexible and effective. The adult can deal efficiently with complex problems of reasoning, including hypothesis testing (Piaget, 1970).

Bloom (1984) developed a hierarchy of cognitive levels in the adult learner. Knowledge is the simplest cognitive level; the adult learner understands and can recall specifics. For example, the individual defines high blood pressure in lay terms.

Box 23-3 Developmental Tasks of Middle Age

1. Helping children become responsible, happy adults
2. Rediscovering or developing new satisfaction in the relationship with one's spouse (for the single adult, this can occur in a relationship with a sibling or significant other)
3. Developing an affectionate, but independent, relationship with aging parents
4. Reaching the peak in one's career
5. Achieving mature social and civic responsibility
6. Accepting and adapting to biological changes
7. Maintaining or developing friendships
8. Developing leisure-time activities

Comprehension is the second level, as indicated by the learner grasping the meaning of the communicated message and relating it to other material. For example, the individual can state one way that obesity influences high blood pressure.

The third level is application. At this level the learner applies knowledge in the form of abstractions and ideas to concrete situations. For example, the hypertensive person begins a weight reduction and exercise program.

In analysis, the fourth level, the adult breaks down material into its constituent parts while noting their relationships. For example, the individual identifies values and life goals in determining actions to be taken for meeting health care needs.

The final levels, synthesis and evaluation, are at times difficult to achieve. The person is able to combine various elements to form a plan and then judge the extent to which the ideas, materials, and so on satisfy the established criteria. For example, people may develop plans to improve their health care and increase their self-care responsibilities. In turn, they may validate their ongoing health care programs in relation to the expected outcomes that they formulated. Genetic, environmental, and personality factors in early and middle adulthood account for the large difference in the ways in which individuals maintain mental abilities. Schaie and Willis (2005) has identified seven of these factors that maintain cognitive function in later life:

1. Absence of chronic diseases
2. Living with favorable socioeconomic factors, including maximal occupational complexity, a low degree of routine, and an intact family
3. Involvement in complex social activities
4. Flexible personality style
5. Marriage to a spouse with high cognitive function
6. Maintaining high levels of performance speed
7. Personal satisfaction with accomplishments in midlife and early old age (see Research Highlights box)

Perceptual Changes

Presbyopia (farsightedness) is common in middle-age adults, even in individuals who have had no previous vision problems. This condition is corrected easily with lenses, which may be needed only for reading or close work. Other visual conditions that may not allow for ready correction include decreased peripheral vision and decreased visual sensitivity in the dark. Both conditions are a result of the cornea becoming less transparent, and both are slow and subtle in development. Because all of these conditions are not readily detected by the individual, middle-age adults should undergo a routine professional eye examination every year. **Glaucoma** is a result of increased intraocular pressure, which can damage the optic nerve. Damage to the optic nerve is irreversible, but vision loss can be prevented if damage is identified early. Peripheral vision is affected. **Cataracts,** opacity of the lens, can develop and cloud the vision in later years of middle age, especially in people who have diabetes.

---

research highlights

Well Being Drops in Middle Age Span the Globe

A large database is developing on the determinants of happiness and well-being, including for example, the relationships with age. In this survey, economists explored the responses of approximately 2 million adults in 80 countries to the following questions:

1. Taken all together, how would you say things are these days? Would you say that you are happy, pretty happy, or not happy?
2. On the whole, are you very satisfied, fairly satisfied, not very satisfied, or not at all satisfied with the life you lead?

Results of the study showed that throughout the world the majority of people in midlife reported lower levels of happiness/satisfaction with life compared with younger and older adults.

Specifically, for example, 41,193 Americans and almost 300,000 Europeans were surveyed throughout 1972 to 2006. In the U.S., unhappiness peaked at 38.6 years for women and at age 52.9 years for men. In contrast, for Europeans the lowest levels of happiness/satisfaction were reported at age 46.5 years for both men and women.

The investigators summarized the lower age person in the modern world, the dip in mental health and happiness comes in slowly, no suddenly in a single year. Only in their 50's do most people emerge from the low period. But encouragingly, by the time you are 70, if you are physically fit, then on average you are as happy and mentally healthy as a 20 year old.

Exploring many variables, the authors concluded that the causes of their findings are unknown, but they propose that one reason why older adults may express more happiness and satisfaction with life than midlife adults is perhaps because "cheerful people live systematically longer," or, as one participant said, "I have seen my school friends die and come eventually to value my blessings during my remaining years" (Oswald & Blanchflower, 2008, pg. 1749).

Oswald A. & Blanchflower D. (2008). Is Well Being 'U'-shaped over the Life Cycle? *Social Science and Medicine;* 66(6), 1733–1749.

Diabetic retinopathy gradually causes rupture of vessels in the retina, which leak into the eye, causing lack of color differentiation and central vision changes.

Other common perceptual changes in middle age are **presbycusis** (impaired auditory acuity) and **macular degeneration**. The first sounds to be lost are higher frequencies, such as a woman's voice. This is important in the work environment and social interaction. Because this process is subtle, middle age is a time for auditory evaluations as a part of routine examinations.

Beginning in the middle years, the sense of taste also diminishes. A progressive loss of taste buds occurs, first affecting those located more anteriorly, which detect sweet and salt, and then the posterior taste buds, which detect bitter and sour. Consequently this change can alter a person's food preferences and present problems for people who insist on adding salt to make up for the deficit. Nurses can suggest using various herbs and spices to enhance flavor.

Self-Perception–Self-Concept Pattern

Levinson's Theory

In Levinson's research on men (1986a, 1986b) and women (1996), a theory on "individual life structures" is posed. Levinson describes age-associated seasons or eras. The midlife transition, beginning at ages 38 to 40 years, appears to include reappraising one's life, integrating the polarities, and modifying one's life structure toward being who one wants to be. Middle-age adults struggle with meaning, value, and direction of their lives.

Erikson's Theory

In Erikson's eight stages of the life cycle (Erikson & Erikson, 1998), the last three stages are related to adulthood. Stage 7, **generativity versus stagnation** or self-absorption, most frequently is associated with the middle-age years.

Erikson identifies generativity as the primary task during this stage. Generativity includes a sense of productivity and creativity, as evidenced by reaching previously established goals (Hornstein, 1986; Reifman et al., 1991; Thomas, 1995). Generativity also encompasses a desire to care for others and is the opposite of stagnation, which is the result of a lack of accomplishment during middle-age's developmental tasks, and self-absorption, the tendency to direct most of one's interest and attention to oneself, thereby excluding others.

Middle age is a time of critical self-review, and some people are sad and disappointed in themselves and their accomplishments. Both women and men question their value to society, the merit of their accomplishments, their success as sexual beings, and the probability of attaining unfilled life goals. Women generally make this life assessment between ages 35 and 50, whereas men do not usually begin until approximately age 40. Because the male life assessment tends to come later, there is a potential problem for couples of approximately the same age. Women begin looking at changes they may want to make in their lives (Apter, 1995), whereas men remain content with the status quo. This type of self-evaluation and lack of effective communication of personal needs to the spouse is a threat to marriage stability (Erikson & Erikson, 1998; Vaillant & Vaillant, 1990).

Physiological Changes

The effect of physiological changes on mental health is nearly as critical during middle age as it is during adolescence. Some of the most obvious changes that influence self-esteem are graying hair, wrinkles, decreased visual and auditory acuity, and changes in body shape (Hot Topics box). The extent to which these changes are tolerated depends largely on the person's level of self-satisfaction

HOT topics

SKIN HEALTH CARE FOR MIDDLE-AGE ADULTS

Wrinkling, xerosis (dry skin), and lentigines (sun spots, liver spots, age spots) begin to be more evident during the forties and fifties, sometimes being manifested even earlier depending on individual amounts of sun exposure, skin irritation, and genetics. Sloughing of the stratum corneum with aging has been projected to happen about twice as quickly as one reaches middle age. There also are changes occurring in the fat and dermis layers that begin around age 40. This causes sagging as the layers separate from each other.

Some middle-age individuals have one or more benign lesions called *seborrheic keratoses,* which are brown or black wartlike papules. Precancerous lesions such as actinic keratoses begin to manifest during the forties, and skin malignancies are more common with aging. There are about 400,000 new cases of basal cell carcinoma each year. These lesions typically occur on sun-exposed areas and have a 99% cure rate with treatment. There are 100,000 new cases of squamous cell carcinoma diagnosed every year. These lesions also have a high cure rate if treated.

Many people use over-the-counter antiaging creams, lotions, sprays, and pills to moisturize and revitalize their skin. For these products to be effective, they must contain at least 5% to 10% α-hydroxy acids (Kucera, 2004). Eye cream should not contain oil but must have antioxidants such as coenzyme Q10 and an anti-inflammatory agent such as vitamin C (Kucera, 2004). Creams containing collagen are not effective, because collagen cannot penetrate the skin. People need to be educated on these over-the-counter products.

Botox (botulism toxin A), a neurotoxin, is effective in managing wrinkles for 4 to 6 months. Another prescriptive treatment is tretinoin (Retin-A), which will decrease pigmented areas such as age spots and hyperkeratosis.

From Kucera, K. (2004). Managing common skin problems in the elderly. *The Clinical Advisor, 7*(6), 23–30.

and acceptance. Some people try to "hold on" to youth by dressing as more youthful counterparts dress, whereas others adapt their attire to their age and position in life.

Prior to 2002, hormone therapy (estrogen alone or estrogen and progesterone) was given to millions of postmenopausal women. Estrogen is still the only therapy approved by the FDA for the treatment of hot flashes associated with menopause. Millions of women took hormone therapy not only to relieve hot flashes, but with the hope that it might prevent heart disease, the number one cause of death in postmenopausal women. All of that changed in 2002, however, when data from the Women's Health Initiative (WHI) showed that postmenopausal women who took estrogen and progesterone actually had higher rates of heart attack and other health problems including stroke, blood clots, and breast cancer. The mean age of women in the WHI study was 63 years. Almost overnight, millions of women stopped using hormone therapy (AACE, 2006; Rossouw et al., 2007).

Follow-up analysis of the WHI data showed that the effects of hormone therapy vary based on a woman's age and the length of time since menopause. In younger postmenopausal women, between the ages of 50 and 59 years, hormone use did not increase the risk of cardiac events, as it did for older women. There is new evidence that hormone therapy may actually turn out to be beneficial for younger postmenopausal women, but for now, hormone therapy is not recommended for the prevention of heart disease (Mendelsohn & Karas, 2007).

Health benefits of hormone therapy include decreased risk for osteoporosis and decreased rates of colorectal cancer (Seaman, 2003). Research is ongoing regarding the risks and benefits of hormone therapy. Currently, the only approved indication for postmenopausal hormone therapy is for the relief of moderate to severe vasomotor symptoms (hot flashes). Only short-term use is advised (1 to 3 years) (Lowdermilk & Perry, 2007).

Increasing numbers of women are now looking for non-hormonal ways to treat hot flashes and other symptoms associated with menopause. Between 1998 and 2000, menopausal women in the United States had more than 100 new natural health products to choose from (Légaré et al., 2007). A law passed to regulate dietary supplements in 1994 does provide some oversight for natural health products but it does not require manufacturers to prove that dietary supplements are either safe or effective (AACE, 2006).

Because there is little scientific data, many midlife women find it difficult to make decisions about using alternative products. Black cohosh, soy, and vitamin E are just a few of the products marketed to women. Even if these products work, women must be cautious about drug interactions that may occur. The use of prescription medication increases with age. The benefits of using alternative therapy may outweigh the risks but more research is needed on the safety profile of natural remedies (AACE, 2006).

It is difficult to separate menopause from the physical and psychological changes that women experience as they age. Stressors common to women in their forties and fifties include raising a family, helping parents as they age, coping with divorce or death of a spouse, retirement, and financial insecurity. Menopause happens in the midst of this. All the events in a woman's life influence her experience of menopause and the **perimenopause**, a period of time that precedes menopause and lasts approximately 4 years. Symptoms such as mood swings, nervousness, agitation, fatigue, and depression are often ascribed to the decline in estrogen levels that occurs during this time. The physiological changes are important, but a woman's experience in menopause is profoundly affected by all the events in her life (Lowdermilk & Perry, 2007).

Men also experience physical and psychological reactions to middle age. The hormonal changes in men are gradual, typically beginning between ages 40 and 55. The symptoms are similar to those experienced by women, with the emotional effects related to other life events, past coping patterns, and general feelings of self-esteem.

Roles-Relationships Pattern

Middle age is frequently a time of reassessment, turmoil, and change. This time has been called **"midlife crisis"**. The turning point occurs for several reasons. Middle-age adults recognize that their physical agility is decreasing; the inevitability of one's own death is recognized, perhaps for the first time. Lifestyle choices have been made and are less flexible than are those made at age 25. The adult identifies mistakes made in the past.

Family

Duvall and Miller (1985) delineate 8 stages of the family life cycle, with stages 5, 6, and 7 in the middle years (see Chapter 7):

Stage 5: families with children, with the oldest child age 13 to 20; lasts approximately 7 years

Stage 6: families launching young adults, from the first leaving until the last; lasts approximately 8 years

Stage 7: families from empty nest to retirement; lasts approximately 15 years

The developmental tasks identified for the families in stages 6 and 7 are similar to those of Havighurst; they focus on changes from a nuclear family to a marital couple with other responsibilities. For example, in stage 6, the parents who are helping their children become independent may also be caring for their aging parents. Additionally, middle-age adults fulfill multiple complex responsibilities within a variety of career, social, and civic positions.

These transitions can be even more challenging for the family headed by a single parent (most typically the mother), which is true of over 10 million American households (out of a total of 35 million). The single most significant health risk in families headed by a single mother is poverty. Nearly one half of all of these families live in poverty, and the median family income for families with two parents is 3 times that of a family headed by a single mother. These inadequate resources make it extremely difficult for middle-age mothers, who are frequently raising grandchildren as well, to fulfill their responsibilities.

Families with young adolescent or young adult children have been described in research studies as both *postparental* and *launching families*. In contrast, criticism of this emphasis on the separation of children (regardless of age) from their families is increasing. Gilligan (1982) criticizes the work of many human development theorists who identify human development in terms of separation from the family. Apter (1990) also challenges the conventional view that adolescent girls must reject their mothers as part of a healthy development. Middle-age parents are encouraged to continue to care for and nurture their adolescent and adult children while recognizing the increasing interdependence of their relationships.

Although many adolescent and young adult children move out of their homes of origin to complete educational or career training, create their own living arrangement, or pursue a career, almost 16 million families had at least one child older than 18 years living at home in 2003, an increase of 7% since 1995 and of 14% since 1985 (USA Today, 2005). Many children of families in these age groups remain dependent on parental help for many more years.

By supporting their children's efforts, parents can increase the self-esteem of their children while being effective role models. The parent assumes less of a parent-child relationship, interacting more on an adult-to-adult level. As the children are "launched," the parents may have uninterrupted time alone and time to share activities. Parents who remove too much care too quickly place their children at risk for depression, substance abuse, violence, and suicide (Silverstein & Rashbaum, 1995).

Family life may also be threatened by older children living at home, opposition to a child's partner, or the inability to establish satisfactory relationships with potential or actual partners or sons-in-law and daughters-in-law. For many parents, the idea of their children leaving home is anticipated with relief that the heavy care responsibilities of parenting are over or with dread over having to fill the void of time and inactivity. The empty nest syndrome may be exacerbated if the husband and wife have never learned to communicate effectively and to enjoy each other's company without the children.

At the other end of the family spectrum, aging parents can place demands on the adult child, primarily because older adults frequently are beset with health problems. A caring relationship is in order, in which the aging parent's need for independence is recognized.

Because of the society's emphasis on youth, the adult must associate feelings of self-worth with personal integrity rather than with bodily appearance or physical prowess. Friends of both genders can provide invaluable support systems. With the newly found free time after children have left home, the middle-age adult can share favorite activities and learn new ones. Middle-age adults should remind themselves how much and how well they are doing, especially considering the complexity of the demands placed on them. Never before in history have families pursued such varied and individual-oriented goals as they do today.

Although for many Americans the concept of family remains of major importance, the perceptions are different from those held by previous generations. Parents and children in most families are involved in numerous activities, as evidenced by a "let's-hurry-or-we'll-be-late" orientation. Even younger children frequently have schedules that must be met if they are to get to their dance, drama, play, or enrichment classes. None of these activities necessarily has a negative effect, but the cumulative influence places heavy demands on all family members. Additionally, many activities in which both children and adults are involved have a certain degree of competitiveness. For example, parents frequently get emotionally involved in the athletic activities of their children to the extent that the failure of a 6 year old to play a winning softball game causes a great deal of parental anguish. One only has to listen to the cheering of parents at a Little League baseball game to note whose self-esteem is at stake. Shouts of "Kill her," "Grab the third baseman," and so on do not tend to engender feelings of team spirit or a notion of playing for the sake of having a good time (Erikson, 1998).

Work

Perhaps the most common role that middle-age adults share is that of a worker. Much of their pride and sense of satisfaction is derived from their work. Work is equated with being "grown up"; one can easily recall the "What do you want to be when you grow up?" questioning of youth. Success and achievement are evaluated in terms of careers and family life. The work ethic still persists, especially with individuals born during the Great Depression and many of their offspring. Much of their conversation evolves from what they do, such as, "My name is Leslie Smith. I am a real estate agent." To be mature is to be a responsible, hard-working individual (Erikson & Erikson, 1998). Research has shown that older adults are more satisfied with their jobs than are younger adults.

Middle-age adults make up most of the work force of 110 million people. Vocations play a major role in their levels of wellness. Approximately 10 million work-related injuries occur every year; 3 million of these are severe, including 3400 to 11,000 deaths and 1.8 million totally disabling injuries (USDHHS, 2000, 2007).

More than 22% of fatal occupational injuries involve motor vehicles; other injuries include falls, nonvehicular injuries, blows, and electrocutions. In decreasing order, workers in mining, agriculture, forestry, fishing, construction, and transportation are at an increased risk of dying from a work-related injury. Although the number of fatal injuries appears to be decreasing, work-related illness and injuries appear to be increasing. The highest nonfatal injuries occur in construction and manufacturing, with high rates also in health services. Thirty percent of nonfatal injuries and illnesses with days away from work continue to be due to overexertion and repetitive motion (USDHHS, 2005). Poor housekeeping and poor design predispose workers to falls and other accidents, expose them to noises and toxic chemicals, and make them susceptible to other illnesses (USDHHS, 2000, 2007).

Many injuries that contribute significantly to the morbidity and mortality of adults can be prevented. Fixing faulty steps, repairing faulty electrical wires, and securing carpets are only a few of the many preventive measures.

Accidents are twice as high among smokers than among nonsmokers. Possible explanations include the loss of attention, the use of one hand for smoking, and irritation of the eyes. Other work-related problems include exposure to harmful substances resulting in lung diseases, cancers, and workplace violence (Health Teaching box).

HEALTH TEACHING   Lifetime Prevention of Cardiovascular Disease in Women

- Smoking cessation and avoiding environmental exposure to tobacco smoke
- At least 30 minutes of moderate-intensity exercise on most, preferably all, days of the week. For women trying to lose weight or sustain weight loss, 60 to 90 minutes of exercise each day is best.
- Eat a variety of fruits and vegetables and whole grain, high-fiber foods. In addition, consume oily fish twice a week, limit alcohol to one drink per day, and consume less than 2.3 grams of sodium each day.
- Weight management
- Daily aspirin, 75 to 325 mg, for women at high risk for cardiovascular disease unless contraindicated. For low-risk women whose blood pressure is controlled, consider daily aspirin, 81 mg, or aspirin every other day, 100 mg, if the benefits are likely to outweigh the risks of gastrointestinal bleeding and hemorrhagic stroke.
- Folic acid should not be used for primary or secondary prevention of cardiovascular disease, although folic acid should be used during childbearing years to prevent neural tube defects in children.
- Neither postmenopausal hormone therapy, nor selective estrogen receptor modulators should be used to prevent cardiovascular disease.

From Sherman, C. (2008). Reducing the risk of heart disease in women. *Clinical Advisor, 11,* 49–53.

The effect of life events on mental health depends on the personal strength of the individual, availability of supports, and the nature and number of events and their significance for the person. Three common examples of life events with potential disruptive effects are divorce, two or more jobs, and caring for aging parents. Their negative effects may be alleviated if assistance is provided early in the process of a change.

Two-or-More-Job Family: Family and Work Responsibilities

More and more women are in the workforce for their own financial well-being or that of their family, especially with the increased cost of living, health care insurance, college expenses, and decreased availability of employer-sponsored pension. Other women, who are postmenopausal and have launched their last child, have a newfound freedom and begin to rediscover themselves, sometimes through a new career. The husband may be a support person in this venture or he may feel threatened by his wife's new pursuits. These role changes can be stressors to the family.

The relationship between marital status, with or without children at home, caring for older parents, and employment status can determine the psychological well-being of the woman in her middle years.

Historically women worked with their husbands within the family farm or business. Only in the few decades immediately after World War II did many middle-class White women stay at home while their husbands went to work. Currently women make up a significant portion of the workforce. Additionally, many women are able to become highly educated and motivated to pursue careers. Both men and women are increasingly taking jobs that do not end at 5:00 PM. The problems and challenges of the workplace are experienced at home as adults bring projects and problems home with them.

Job-related travel has also increased during the last few years for both men and women. Travel by either partner means additional responsibilities for the one who remains at home. Additionally, if one spouse travels far more than the other travels, feelings of resentment may develop, or the common ground for discussion of work events may be altered. The one who stays at home may feel "put upon" when the spouse is perceived as having fun. In contrast, travel is tiring and is not usually as exciting as it appears to observers. The traveling spouse can come home tired and irritable and desire peace and quiet, which may conflict with the expectations of other family members.

Men may feel threatened by highly successful and visible women. For some families, the post-World War II prototype was for the husband to support the family financially and gain status through achievements of work outside the home. As women gain recognition and acclaim for their career accomplishments, even the most "enlightened" man may experience twinges of envy and discomfort. Men have few role models in learning the ways to be a participant in a successful two-career family. Men may need as much, if not more, support than do women in adapting to contemporary family styles. Opportunities to discuss what it means to be a man in today's society can be helpful, such as in support groups with volunteers or professionals who provide services to various agencies and community resources.

In addition to the changes in women and the effect on families of each adult working at one more jobs, the nature of the parental work environment is critical to family coping ability. Work that is emotionally draining, particularly when it is filled with conflict, poses special threats to family stability. When parents come home tired, angry, or frustrated from their experiences at work, they likely have limited emotional support to share with other family members.

When people gain self-esteem from their jobs and generally enjoy going to work, they tend to experience less frustration and dissatisfaction with themselves and their positions, enabling them to give more of themselves to other members of the family (Reifman et al., 1991).

Middle age is important when looking at the career clock. Issues that need to be considered include midcareer changes and preretirement planning. Retirement is a major turning point; to many people, it is the transition from middle age to old age and the period of work to the period of leisure or different work.

Adults are working up to and beyond the age of retirement, and many are entering new careers later in life because they are living longer and are in need of more financial resources to successfully enter the older adult years. As adults progress through the middle years, they become increasingly aware of the time remaining until retirement: "Can I readjust my goals?" "Is there disparity between where I am in my career and where I would like to be?" An example might be the 60-year-old veteran nightclub singer whose goal to cut a solo album remains to be achieved. The heightened awareness of age and the decreased likelihood of finding another suitable job can precipitate increased anxiety or depression in this singer.

Comprehensive health-promotion programs at the work-site contain these elements: "(1) health education that focuses on skill development and lifestyle behavior change in addition to information dissemination and awareness building, preferably tailored to employees' interests and needs; (2) supportive social and physical work environments, including established norms for healthy behavior and policies that promote health and reduce the risk of disease, such as work site smoking policies, healthy nutrition alternatives in the cafeteria and vending services, and opportunities for obtaining regular physical activity; (3) integration of the work site program into the organization's administrative structure; (4) related programs, such as employee assistance programs; and (5) screening programs, preferably linked to health care service delivery to ensure follow-up and appropriate treatment as necessary and to encourage adherence. Optimally, these efforts should be part of a comprehensive occupational health and safety program" (USDHHS, 2000, 2007, pp. 7–28). The efficacy of these programs is beginning to be documented.

Caring for Aging Parents

The needs of aging parents and of the adult's own children can create additional demands during the middle years. The middle-age adult can feel caught between one's children and one's parents. Both children and older parents can present unrealistic, excessive demands and be difficult to please.

Middle-age adults may be faced with having frail and ill parents live within their own family unit or placing them in a nursing home. These dilemmas are complicated by the reality that their parents are growing older and may not have long to live. The recognition of the parents' impending death heightens middle-age adults' awareness of their own aging and mortality.

Difficulties in caring for older parents can be somewhat lessened when potential situations are discussed before a crisis arises. This is particularly true when all members of the middle-adult family are working, space in their home is limited, and the community has few resources for the well or ill older adults. Although institutionalization is undesirable to many families, the care of ill, older parents may eventually require it. By anticipating these needs and preparing for them, middle-age children and their older parents can develop further meaningful relationships with one another.

Divorce

Divorce is a major disruption to the marriage and family and to each individual's short-term and long-term health. As the divorce rate has risen in recent years, individuals and families have been faced with new and multiple problems. When a divorce occurs, each family member must confront the necessity to examine and, in many cases, modify an accustomed style of living and adapting .

In the early 1970s, Wallerstein and her colleagues began a longitudinal study of 131 children of divorce through extensive interviews with the children and their parents. The children are now adults with families of their own and Wallerstein is still following their development through life. The most significant findings of this ongoing study are the long-lasting cumulative and demonstrative effects of divorce, which continue for decades. Although Wallerstein found healing in adults is more or less complete 3 years after divorce; this is not so for the children, who experience the divorce differently from their parents. Even as adults, the children have undercurrents of fears about their abilities to commit to relationships (Wallerstein et al., 2000).

Some of the limitations of Wallerstein's research are: (1) anecdotal methodologies, versus double-blind interviews; (2) the children are primarily White, educated, upper middle class; and (3) the findings are not differentiated from those of high-conflict families, nor are distinctions made between the influences of conflict that caused the divorce and the actual divorce itself. There are many other studies that continue to illuminate these initial findings on the long-term effects of divorce (Fabricius & Luecken, 2007). Continuing research is being done on ways to prevent long-term health problems in the children of divorced parents (Fabricius & Luecken, 2007).

Death

Similar to divorce, death of a spouse can result in grieving for the loss of companionship and the lost planned-for future, free from the responsibilities of work and children. The surviving spouse may be unprepared to be single again, to be the only parent, or to live alone. The loneliness may be exacerbated by ill or dying peers or parents. Middle-age adults become increasingly aware of the finite nature of life, thinking not only of the number of years since birth, but also of the number of years left to live. The midlife review is a common outcome of this recognition.

Sexuality-Reproductive Pattern

Men and women can continue to have a satisfactory pattern of sexual functioning throughout the middle and older adult years. As they would in any other developmental phase, middle-age adults may need counseling to make health-promoting decisions about their sexual and reproductive behaviors and health (Lowdermilk & Perry, 2007).

Unintended pregnancies are high in all ages of American women, but are the highest (77% of all pregnancies) in middle-age women. In contrast, women planning to have children during the fourth and fifth decades of life should know that fertility rates decrease and infant mortality rates increase, especially when mothers are age 44 years and older (USDHHS, 2000). Mothers aged 35 years and older, and those who are Black, had the highest rates of labor and delivery complications (USDHHS, 2005). Additionally, the maternal death rate in women 35 years and older is higher (16.1 per 100,000 live births) than for younger women (USDHHS, 2000). Achieving the *Healthy People 2010* target goal of reducing maternal deaths will require that national, state, and local policies address women's needs before and during pregnancy, and that gaps in research and prevention programs be identified through improved monitoring (USDHHS, 2005).

Median red blood cell folate levels for nonpregnant females aged 15 to 44 years exceeded its target of 220 ng/mL. In addition to food fortification, the "Folic Acid Education Campaign" has contributed to this progress (USDHHS, 2005).

Changes in the reproductive systems of men and women result in changes in sexual function throughout adulthood. During middle adulthood, sexual arousal is slower, orgasms are less intense, and a return to prearousal levels is more rapid, with men having longer refractory periods between erection and ejaculation. When a person continues to be sexually active, these functional changes occur over decades and are minimally noticeable until later in adulthood, unless external factors are present, such as the negative effects of some antihypertensive and antidepressant agents.

After menopause, many women enjoy sex more, especially because no risk of pregnancy exists. Conversely, menopause can bring many challenges to a woman. American culture values women largely for their youth, beauty, and childbearing ability. Middle-age women may confront their own aging for the first time and may be perplexed as to the symptomatic factors and possibly changing roles. Women can experience vaginal dryness, difficulty finding a partner, less interest in initiating sex, and longer times to reach orgasm. No data exist that report decreases in postmenopausal women's interest in and physical capacity for sex (Nelson et al., 2006; Northrup, 2008).

Although men and women frequently enjoy satisfactory sexual relationships throughout the middle adult years, men in their middle age are more vulnerable to sexual dysfunction than are women. Frequently, men first experience problems with premature ejaculation, impotence, and retrograde ejaculation between ages 40 and 50 (Dunphy, 2004).

Abnormal genital bleeding and secondary amenorrhea are common gynecological complaints that indicate serious physical problems. Abnormal genital bleeding is the most common reason for gynecological office visits by adult women. Although pregnancy and menopause are the most common causes of secondary amenorrhea, other conditions related to abnormal pregnancy, functional disorders, physiological changes, and pathological factors must be considered (Buttaro et al., 2003).

As for adolescents and young adults, in the middle-age adult sexually transmitted diseases continue to be a major public health problem. Women and children bear an inordinate share of the burden: sterility, ectopic pregnancy, fetal and infant deaths, birth defects, and mental retardation. Human papillomavirus (HPV), a sexually transmitted disease, causes 90% of all cervical cancers (Lowdermilk & Perry, 2007). As with many other health behaviors and diseases, the full effect on the life of an individual and family may not be realized until middle age.

Adults in middle age represent 71% of all new cases of HIV/AIDS. Nearly three fourths of all people currently living with HIV/AIDS in the United States are men (CDC, 2007). Since the early 1980s, the demographics of HIV/AIDS have changed. An increased proportion of those infected are women, persons under the age of 20, heterosexuals, persons of racial or ethnic minorities, and people who live outside major metropolitan areas (Leone, 2007).

Considered by some to be a "hidden" HIV risk group, adults over the age of 50 now comprise 19% of all people living with HIV/AIDs in the United States. They represent 13% of all new cases (Lindau et al., 2007). The actual numbers may be higher because HIV/AIDS is misdiagnosed, underreported, and undertested in this population. Studies show that older Americans know less about HIV/AIDS than younger people. They are also less likely to discuss sexual behavior with their health care providers. Many health care providers believe it is offensive to ask an older person about her or his sexual activity (amFAR, 2002). Homosexual/bisexual contact (36%) is the most common mode of HIV/AIDS transmission in adults over the age of 50, followed by injection drug use (19%) and heterosexual contact (15%). The CDC now recommends that all persons aged 13 to 64 years, in all health care settings, receive routine testing for HIV (Leone, 2007).

Coping-Stress Tolerance Pattern

Kobasa (1979) studied the concept of stress hardiness, which she identified as including control, commitment, and challenge. Her studies have strong clinical relevance because they strive to answer the question, "Why do some people's illness progress while others improve despite both groups having similar level of stress?" (Harig, 2007).

In a 45-year longitudinal study of 173 men, Vaillant and his colleagues (1990, 2003), found that the extent of tranquilizer use before age 50 was the most powerful negative predictor of both mental and physical health outcomes at age 65. Another important predictor for health outcomes was the maturity of defenses against stress (sublimation, anticipation, altruism, and humor).

Stress and Heart Disease

As reiterated throughout this chapter, heart disease is the second leading cause of death in the middle-age adult. In landmark studies, Haynes et al. (1978) describe the relationship of psychosocial factors to coronary heart disease using the Framingham study (Haynes et al., 1978; Haynes et al., 1980). In the study, 24 measures of psychosocial stress were used. In men, aging worries correlated significantly with systolic and diastolic blood pressure values. Marital disagreement and personal worries correlated significantly with diastolic blood pressure. Both diastolic and systolic pressures correlated significantly with work changes and anxiety in employed women between 45 and 64 years of age. Anger suppressed, anger discussed, tension, and anger symptoms correlated significantly with diastolic blood pressure in this age group.

Among white collar men in this age group, the Framingham type A and ambitiousness scales also correlated significantly with elevated diastolic blood pressure. The correlation of anger symptoms and anger discussed with diastolic pressures was significant for white collar women between ages 45 and 64. The initial findings by Haynes and her colleagues have been supported by many other studies, including those of Spielberger et al. (1983), Kawachi et al. (1996), and Williams et al. (2000).

The death of a parent enhances awareness of one's vulnerability to illness and death. The more opportunities and time people have to prepare for these stressful events, the more likely they will be to feel in control and less likely to feel anxious and helpless. When individuals take on more responsibility for their life, decisions lead to concrete behaviors, such as drafting a will, developing an advance directive (which includes **living will, health care agent**, and appointing a durable power of attorney), and making funeral prearrangements. An **advance directive** is a legal document prepared when an individual is alive, competent, and able to make decisions to provide guidelines for health care providers in the future, when the individual is not able to make decisions because of physical disability (being unconscious) or mental incompetence. By appointing a **durable power of attorney**, the individual designates another person (spouse, son, daughter, or friend) to make health care decisions (especially about how aggressive treatment should be in forestalling death) when an individual becomes unable to make such decisions. The nurse helps middle-age adults anticipate stressors so that they are better prepared to cope and to prevent additional physical, psychosocial, and spiritual stressors, thereby optimizing their health.

Values-Beliefs Pattern

When adults make decisions affecting their lives, it is usually the result of a personal, complex pattern of values and beliefs (McFadden & Gerl, 1990). Much of what people value or believe to be true is formed early in life and can be the most difficult to alter (Rippe, 1996). Normally people do not spend a great deal of conscious thought on abstract explanations of the meaning of life and why certain things are valued. During times of illness or crisis, however, they frequently take time to review their value systems and seek meaning about what is important (Spector, 2003; Stuart et al., 1989) (Innovative Practice box).

A crisis at any age can be a turning point during which both increased vulnerability and increased potential are present. When the crisis is managed successfully, a virtue or strength will evolve. Erikson names *caring* as a middle-age adult virtue that can be developed.

Committed responsibilities for the care and welfare of others promotes moral development. When middle age is lived with generativity, many opportunities are afforded to live life by one's higher principles. The middle adult can differentiate among personal wants and needs, duties demanded by society, and principles by which to live. Kohlberg's work on moral development delineated these phases as conventional and postconventional. His studies of men described stage 3 as an interpersonal definition of morality, whereas stage 4 is a societal definition based on law and order. Kohlberg concludes that most American adults are in these phases of moral development. In contrast, stage 5 is the concern and willingness to sacrifice for the well-being of others (Kohlberg & Lickona, 1986). Subsequent studies by Gilligan on moral development in women and men demonstrate gender differences in describing high morality. Women discussed issues of selfishness versus responsibility, of exercising care with decision-making and avoiding hurting others. Men described terms of *justice, fairness,* and *rights of individuals.* Gilligan (1982, 1990) concludes that women possess a process of moral development different from that of men.

Valuing others, having relationships, and being responsible to others enables middle-age adults to make the transitions of moral development. This process is accomplished through raising children, developing more junior employees, and serving the community. As people fulfill these commitments, they increasingly treat others as equals and gradually develop a sensitivity and desire to change barriers to human worth and equality, such as racial prejudice, homelessness, inadequate access to health care, and weapons stockpiles.

ENVIRONMENTAL FACTORS

Environmental factors are significant variables in health promotion. Placing the emphasis on sanitation and preventing pollution must continue. The complex interactions between physical, biological, and chemical agents threaten health.

innovative practice

Benson/Henry Mind Body Institute of Massachusetts General Hospital Harvard Medical School

MIND/BODY MEDICAL SYMPTOM REDUCTION PROGRAMS

Research demonstrates that 60% to 90% of health care visits are for symptoms such as headaches, insomnia, weakness or fatigue, and gastrointestinal symptoms, all of which are frequently stress related. The Mind/Body Medical Symptom Reduction Programs are designed to help individuals who have chronic illnesses (including life-threatening illnesses) or stress-related symptoms to better manage their health problems and optimize their quality of life. The interventions combine conventional medical care with knowledge about the effects of behaviors and attitudes on health.

The biopsychosocial-spiritual approach of the assessment and treatment plans with clients includes:

- Eliciting the relaxation response, a state of deep rest that changes responses to stress (decreases vital signs, and muscle tenseness, increased mindfulness)
- Enhancing coping skills through cognitive behavioral strategies
- Encouraging exercise or physical activity
- Providing nutritional counseling
- Monitoring and adjusting medication, when necessary, in consultation with the physician

Insurance claims for these outpatient visits are submitted directly to clients' insurance carriers. Because health insurance policies differ, coverage and reimbursement vary. A client advocate helps clients research their specific health insurance coverage and billing requirements.

Research demonstrates that after these interventions:

- Clients with pain reduced their physician visits by 36%.
- Visits to an HMO were reduced by approximately 50% after a relaxation response–based intervention, resulting in significant cost savings.
- Blood pressure was lowered and use of medications decreased in 80% of hypertensive clients; 16% were able to discontinue all of their medications.
- Sleep patterns were improved for 100% of clients with insomnia; 90% reduced or eliminated the use of sleep medication.
- Infertile women reported decreased levels of depression, anxiety, and anger, and a 35% conception rate.
- Women with severe premenstrual syndrome experienced a 57% reduction in physical and psychological symptoms.
- Health-promoting behaviors, such as nutrition, social supports, self-esteem, health responsibility, and exercise, increased after the program and were maintained until a 6-month follow-up.
- Six months after the program, 80% of clients continued to experience improvement of their physical symptoms.
- Anxiety and depression normalized for most participants and were maintained 6 months following the program.
- Women with menopause reported fewer hot flashes, lower blood pressure, improved sleep, and decreased depression, anxiety, and anger.

Contact Information:
Benson Henry Mind Body Institute
Massachusetts General Hospital
Harvard Medical School
824 Boylston Street
Chestnut Hill, MA 02467
Telephone: 617-732-9130

Because there are approximately 100 million workers in the United States, occupational hazards are a serious threat to national health. Exposures to toxic chemicals, asbestos, coal dust, cotton fiber, ionizing radiation, physical hazards, excessive noise, and stress can precipitate numerous health problems. For the middle-age worker, these problems include cancers, lung and heart diseases, decreased hearing, bodily injuries, and mental health problems (USDHHS, 2000, 2007).

Physical Agents

Ionizing radiation is a physical agent that can cause cancer. One example of this is cancer caused by medical procedures that include the use of diagnostic radiography and therapeutic radiation.

Water pollution has become another major concern. Many industrial and agricultural wastes, such as benzene and chlordane, have been recovered in rivers and lakes from which drinking water is obtained. These substances can lead to potential carcinomas and other health problems.

Air pollution from auto emissions, burning fuels, and industrial incineration have warranted smog alerts and air pollution indexes. This issue is especially important to the individual with chronic respiratory or cardiovascular disease (USDHHS, 2007).

Noise pollution in industry is a potential problem for the middle-age adult worker. Hearing loss is the most common occupational disease, but it can be prevented if federal guidelines are followed with regard to noise exposure levels and hearing conservation programs, especially prevention activities aimed at miners and construction workers for whom hearing loss is a major problem (USDHHS, 2005).

Exposure to excessive noise, radiation, sunlight, and vibration can produce problems such as chronic obstructive lung disease, cancer, and degenerative diseases.

Biological Agents

As noted throughout this text, health and disease are influenced by the interactions among the agent, host, and environment. Agent factors can be biological, physical, chemical, or psychological. The biological causes of diseases include bacteria, viruses, rickettsiae, fungi, parasites, and food poisoning. Because these causes are often limited to identifiable occupations, they can be readily diagnosed, treated, and prevented. Many of these agents are transmitted through the air or by contact with certain media, such as water, food, blood, or feces.

Hepatitis A is caused by viral infection, with transmission occurring primarily through the fecal-oral route. This host-agent interaction typically occurs in the middle-age adult living in an environment with poor sanitation and having close contact with an infected person. The person may also be exposed through contaminated food and water. Hepatitis B is transmitted primarily in the blood or plasma of the infected individuals, which is particularly significant for the adult who is employed in a health care setting.

Among medical and dental personnel (with surgeons, oral surgeons, and pathologists at the highest risk), the risk of contracting Hepatitis B is 6 times higher than that of the general population.

There are two other infections that are of particular concern for middle age adults: pneumoniae and varicella/herpes zoster ("shingles"). Both can be prevented through vaccinations, which adults aged 60 years and older are advised to receive (Harpaz et al., 2008; Targonski & Poland, 2007).

Chemical Agents

Chemicals include a wide variety of substances that increase the risk of morbidity and mortality in the middle-age adult. When a home is located near an industry, there is the risk of exposure to toxic chemicals that pollute the air. Contaminants can also be carried home on the clothing from the workplace.

Workers at increased risk include coal miners, wood handlers, and those who work with asbestos and coke. Pneumoconiosis is found in approximately 15% of coal miners, with "black lung disease" implicated in 2178 deaths in 2002 (the *Healthy People 2010* target is 1900). Wood handlers have increased risk of certain cancers. The asbestos worker has an increased risk of mesothelioma and asbestosis. Approximately 2 million workers each year have been exposed to benzene and vinyl chloride, which may be carcinogens (USDHHS, 2000, 2007).

Among American industrial workers, nine out of 10 may be inadequately protected from exposure to at least 10 of the 163 most common hazardous chemicals. More than 2000 of the 50,000 chemicals found in the workplace are suspected human carcinogens (USDHHS, 2000, 2007).

Tobacco

Currently, 23% of men and 18% of women in the United States smoke (USDHHS, 2007). Many 50-year-old adults have a 30-plus-year history of cigarette smoking. Cigarette smokers have nearly twice the heart disease death rates of nonsmokers, with the risk being proportional to the amount of smoke inhaled directly and passively and the number of cigarettes smoked (Brownson et al., 1992). Smoke recipients are at increased risks for heart disease, as well as colds; chronic bronchitis; emphysema; and cancers of the mouth, lungs, esophagus, pancreas, and bladder.

Few smokers realize that cigarettes contain 2000 known chemicals, including tar, nicotine, hydrogen cyanide, formaldehyde, and ammonia. Cigarette smoking is, for most smokers, an addiction to nicotine, which is absorbed into the bloodstream. Nicotine acts on the two divisions of the nervous system: central (brain and the spinal cord) and peripheral (autonomic nervous system and motor and sensory fibers to the arms and legs). Effects of nicotine stimulation can be observed in both electroencephalographic changes and in hand tremors. Nicotine also stimulates the heart, leading to an increased pulse and elevated blood pressure. Although smokers frequently believe that cigarettes have a calming effect, this notion is misleading. Nicotine stimulates the body, whereas carbon monoxide causes lethargy. Smokers may feel calm, although they are actually having their sensations dulled by carbon monoxide. Additive effects such as those from chlorine, cotton dust, and γ-radiation can lower midexpiratory flow values. Profound effects can also be observed with asbestos interaction.

SOCIAL PROCESSES
Culture and Ethnicity

Spector (2008) describes culture as the "sum of beliefs, practices, habits, likes, dislikes, norms, customs, rituals…we have learned from our families during the years of socialization" (p. 1). Spector further relates the ways in which one's cultural background is a component of one's ethnic background. The major ethnic groups of the United States are Asians, Blacks, Native Americans, and Hispanics.

Nurses understand the potential influences their own ethnic cultures have on those of others. The middle-age adult may not interpret dizziness as a possible symptom of hypertension, for example; it may be described simply as a spell. The Black adult's definition of health may be completely different from that of the White health care provider or the Asian person (Perez & Luguis, 2008). The obese adult who has received positive reinforcement throughout life for being pleasingly plump is less motivated to lose weight than is the adult who defines health as being svelte.

The health problems of middle-age adults, even within major ethnic groups, are varied. Recent immigrants who live in crowded urban areas have higher mortality rates than do earlier immigrants of the same cultural group who live in healthier environments. Immigrants' working conditions continue to be poor, with long hours and minimal wages. Modern preventive health care is difficult, if not impossible, to obtain.

Poverty is reported in approximately one third of Native Americans. The middle-age adult Native American is faced with a high rate of tuberculosis, alcohol abuse, inadequate immunization, mental health problems such as depression, and dental problems (Spector, 2008; USDHHS, 2005).

For many women in society, the cessation of menses is associated with aging; the role of the middle-age woman may be shaped by her culture. Nurses who have attained cultural competency can ensure that appropriate health promotion is provided, especially for vulnerable populations and those individuals, families, and communities who have special health care needs.

Economics

Adults in the middle years are frequently at the peak of their careers. Although their net income may be greater than it was during early adulthood, they frequently have significant additional financial obligations. Children may be in college and need financial support, and preretirement planning can stress the budget. The care of an aging parent can be an additional financial burden and can be costly in terms of present lifestyle. When the adult or family members have ongoing health problems, the economic status of the family can be compromised further (Multicultural Awareness box).

The individual's economic status plays a role in the incidence of mental illness. Mental illness is increased in adults at the lower socioeconomic level, with higher rates of anxiety, depression, and phobias.

Health Care Delivery System

The nurse can contact numerous agencies that are geared to middle adulthood. These can be categorized as official, voluntary, and service agencies. Councils of community services frequently publish a directory. Official agencies include those that are state and federally funded, such as public health departments and drug treatment centers. Voluntary agencies include the American Cancer Society, the American Lung Association, and Alcoholics Anonymous. Many educational and self-help programs are sponsored by these organizations. The American Lung Association sponsors a "Stop Smoking" program, which can be conducted on a group basis in a work or community setting. Service agencies include professional organizations, such state nurses' associations, the American Medical Association (sponsor of the Tel-Med program), bar associations, Young Men's Christian Association (YMCA), hospice programs, and the Women's Occupational Health Resource Center. **Website Resource 23B** presents a detailed list of these agencies.

NURSING INTERVENTIONS

By listening, conferring with other individuals in the same environment, and reviewing health and safety data the nurse gains an understanding of the hazards to which an individual is exposed.

As a health educator, the nurse then initiates programs that emphasize helping adults to accept more responsibility for their own health. This effort can be provided on a one-to-one basis or in a seminar fashion. For example, with the goal of early detection of high blood pressure, the nurse in the community or industry might increase consumers' knowledge of hypertension, screen people who have sought health care for any reason, set up mechanisms to screen people outside the health care system, and refer and follow up on all people with elevated blood pressure.

The target groups identified by the nurse frequently have common needs, such as individuals exposed to a particular chemical, smokers, substance abusers, women entering the workplace for the first time, or men nearing retirement. In a work environment, the occupational health nurse can assess absenteeism rates for trends. In gathering data, the nurse can initiate research projects with multidisciplinary input.

The preemployment physical examination not only provides the employer with information about proper placement, but also provides a baseline health assessment. Frequently this examination is the only assessment that the individual has had in years.

The Occupational Safety and Health Administration (OSHA) mandates that the employee have a healthy and safe work environment. Therefore a complete health history is essential. Is there a history of hypertension, arthritis, cancer, or hernia? Is there significant family history? Is the person a smoker? How many packs per day? Does the person take medications? Medical limitations must be addressed; for example, decreased visual acuity means no driving, and dermatitis means no oils, chemicals, or solvents. Removing a worker from a particular job may be indicated if the worker might endanger co-workers, has a disease condition that might be aggravated by the job, or if the worker is taking prescribed medications with potentially harmful side effects.

The nurse in the community and in industry should reiterate some key safety issues to the adult, such as wearing seat belts and observing speed limits. With a decrease in visual acuity, driving at night can be hazardous. The middle-age

MULTICULTURAL AWARENESS

Health Care for Middle-Age Gypsies

Culturally competent and effective health care is imperative for all, especially people with several comorbid conditions who do not have a consistent primary care provider or clinic. Middle-age gypsies, or Roma, are in need of consistent health care but, because they tend to travel from one place to another and do not put down roots, health providers need to understand their beliefs so the episodic interactions will be most productive. It is important to realize the Roma prefer to involve their family when it comes to their health. Hence a family member should be allowed to participate in each interaction with a health provider. This involvement with family will increase the client's compliance with the health regimen. Vivian and Dundes (2004) found that health care providers should be aware that the following variables may affect the Roma's health care: pollution, cleanliness, ideal weight, views on death, and medical procedures.

From Vivian, C., & Dundes, L. (2004). The crossroads of culture and health among the Roma (gypsies). *Image: The Journal of Nursing Scholarship, 36*(1), 86–91.

adult's reaction time is also decreasing, which reinforces the need for periodic driving testing as recommended by the National Highway Traffic Safety Administration.

With an increase in leisure time, the middle-age adult is at greater risk for recreational accidents. As noted, moderation should be stressed. Alcohol is a depressant and should be avoided in activities that require attentiveness.

Protection from burns is essential; 56% of fatal residential fires are cigarette related, such as from smoking in bed. Falls can occur at any age, and safety measures should be considered for the entire family, with preparatory planning for aging parents. A few suggestions to the adult might be to avoid highly waxed floors, poor lighting, high beds, and bathtubs without nonslip bottoms.

Handgun availability is controversial at best; however, approximately 20% of American households have them. When the person believes strongly that it is necessary to have a firearm, safety measures to avoid accidental injury should be discussed, such as security locks and proper storage.

The Occupational Safety and Health Act (1970) was designed to ensure that workers are employed under safe and healthy working conditions. The act is applicable to every employer who is engaged in a business that affects commerce. The employer must ascertain that the workplace is free from recognized hazards and must comply with the act. OSHA has offices in most major cities and can provide recommended standards for occupational agents.

Nurses can participate actively in the safety committee of the industry in which they are employed. When no such committee exists, many protection measures will fall on the nurse. Suggestions include:

1. Tour the facilities on a regular basis. Be familiar with resource books, laws, and codes.
2. Develop a toxicology chart with symptoms of overexposure and recommended treatment. Update this chart frequently.
3. Be a role model in safety issues; wear safety glasses, protective footwear, and gloves, and do not smoke.
4. Discuss the preemployment physical with the employee, with an emphasis on risk factors. Monitor health problems and exposure levels in the work setting.

The worker must be aware of the protective clothing that should be worn, sanitation measures for the work environment, general hygiene measures, and proper immunization. The food handler, for instance, should have an annual tuberculosis skin test, wear clean clothing and appropriate hair protection, and use good hand-washing techniques. The nurse should not assume that workers know how to protect themselves and others.

Since 1996, the National Occupational Research Agenda (NORA) has become the research framework for the National Institute for Occupational Safety and Health (NIOSH) and the nation. Partners work together to identify, research, and address the most critical issues in workplace safety (*http://cdc.gov/niosh/about.html*).

A major challenge for the nurse is to encourage workers to assume responsibility for protecting their own health. Increasingly, organizations are interested in promoting the health of their employees for many reasons, including enhancing their recruiting efforts and minimizing lateness, absenteeism, turnover, physical and emotional inability to work, disability costs, and health and life insurance costs. Health-promotion programs are increasingly recognized for their vital contributions to the financial viability of organizations. It has been validated that providing health care to middle-age adults in homeless centers, showing health-promotion videos during meals, and giving incentives for participating in wellness programs improve health outcomes (Clark, 2002).

Health-promotion programs within an organizational setting can be categorized in one of three levels: (1) awareness, (2) lifestyle change, and (3) supportive environment. The goal of a health program at the level of awareness is to increase the individual's knowledge or interest in a particular health issue, such as smoking cessation. Examples of awareness programs include special events, flyers, lunch seminars, meetings, and newsletters. Changing health behaviors or status are not the goals of awareness programs, but are goals of lifestyle change programs.

Lifestyle change programs last at least 8 to 12 weeks and include assessment, education, and evaluation components to help individuals implement long-term changes in health behavior and status. To maintain these long-term changes and to develop a healthy lifestyle, a supportive organizational environment is needed. This type of environment includes health-promoting physical settings, corporate policies and culture, ongoing programs, and employee ownership of programs (USDHHS, 2000, 2007).

Five models of nurse-managed primary health care delivery at the work site have been proposed as part of the American Nurses Association's program for reform of this nation's health care system, known as Nursing's Agenda for Health Care Reform. Each model is developed to enable employers to fulfill the goal of providing accessible, high-quality, affordable care at locations that are familiar and convenient for employees. These designs help employers introduce or expand health care services at the work site, control health care costs, and meet the health care needs of their employees (*Nursing facts: Nursing's agenda for health care reform*, 2005).

SUMMARY

Nurses help middle-age adults improve their quality of life, both for the present and for the future, through the identification of risk factors, health promotion, and other nursing interventions. Nurses work in a variety of health care settings available to middle-age adults: outpatient clinics, occupational health clinics, and private practice.

Health promotion and disease prevention are aimed at the personal habits and lifestyles of adults to improve their biological, spiritual, and psychosocial development.

Strategies to help an adult achieve a higher level of health include individual and group counseling based on identified risk factors, providing self-help information that is most relevant to the middle-age adult, and describing available resources.

Using these strategies, the nurse can motivate middle-age adults to prioritize their own health and quality of life for the individual middle-age adult, including it as a prerequisite for their own present and future health and particularly preceding the responsibilities in promoting the health and quality of life of younger and older generations. After years of poor health practices, adults can make changes that reduce their risk of disability from chronic disease and promote functioning and quality of life.

CASE STUDY

Caregiver Role Strain: Graham A

Graham A., a 47-year-old divorced woman, was diagnosed with stage 3 ovarian cancer 4 years ago, for which she had a total hysterectomy, bilateral salpingo-oophorectomy, omentectomy, lymphadenectomy, and tumor debulking followed by chemotherapy, consisting of cisplatin (Platinol), paclitaxel (Taxol), and doxorubicin (Adriamycin). She did well for 2 years and then moved back to her hometown near family and underwent three more rounds of second-line chemotherapy. She took on a less-taxing job, bought a house, renewed old friendships, and became more involved with her two sisters and their families.

She developed several complications, including metastasis to the lungs. Then she could no longer work, drive, or care for herself. She had been told by her oncologist that there was nothing else that could be done and that she should consider entering a hospice. She met with her attorney and drew up an advance directive and completed her will. She decided to have hospice care at home and, with the help of her family, set up her first floor as a living and sleeping area. She was cared for by family members around the clock for about 3 days. Graham A. observed that she was tiring everyone out so much that they could not really enjoy each other's company. At this time she contacted the VNA to seek assistance. Her plan was to try to enjoy her family and friend's visits. After assessment the VNA nurse prioritized her problems to include fatigue and caregiver role strain. Other potential problem areas that may need to be incorporated into the care plan include anticipatory grieving and impaired comfort.

Reflective Questions:
1. What are some of the stresses on her middle-age sisters and their families?
2. What resources are available to manage these stresses and support the sisters in caring for their dying sister?
3. Describe Graham A.'s feelings about dependency and loss of autonomy because she is unable to do her own activities of daily living any longer.

CARE PLAN

Caregiver Role Strain: Graham A.

Nursing Diagnosis: Risk for Caregiver Role Strain Related to Sister's Terminal Cancer

DEFINING CHARACTERISTICS
- Ms. A. and sisters are tired of doing all of the daily care for Ms. A.
- Ms. A. and family are at a point where they are accepting Ms. A.'s terminal status.
- Ms. A. and family want to prepare for a death at home.

RELATED FACTORS
- Sisters are missing work and neglecting their own families.
- Sisters need assistance with Ms. A.

EXPECTED OUTCOMES
- Ms. A. and sisters will contact the VNA to assist in planning daily hospice care at home.

- VNA and family will plan realistic care.
- Ms. A. will have enjoyable time with sisters and friends.
- Sisters will have quality time to spend with Ms. A.
- Sisters will be able to voice their grief and anger about their sister's upcoming death.

INTERVENTIONS
- Home health aides are scheduled for 24 hours a day.
- Psychiatric nurse practitioner will meet with Ms. A. and family to schedule therapy time for anticipatory grieving.
- The sisters will meet with a support group for families involved in hospice care at home.
- A schedule will be made to allow each sister time at home, time with Ms. A., and rest.

For further information on developing care plans, see: Carpenito-Moyet, L. J. (2008). Nursing diagnosis: Application to clinical practice (12th ed.). Philadelphia: Lippincott, Williams & Wilkins.

REFERENCES

AACE Menopause Guidelines Revision Task Force. (2006). American Association of Clinical Endocrinologists Medical Guidelines for Clinical Practice for the Diagnosis and Treatment of Menopause. *Endocrine Practice, 12*(3), 315–337.

American Cancer Society. (2005). *Cancer facts & figures for African Americans 2005–2006.* Atlanta, GA: American Cancer Society.

American Cancer Society. (2006). *Cancer facts & figures for Hispanics/Latinos 2006–2008.* Atlanta, GA: American Cancer Society.

American Cancer Society. (2007). *Report Links Health Insurance Status With Cancer Care.* Retrieved December 20, 2007, from *www. cancer.org/docroot/NWS.*

American Obesity Association. (2004). Retrieved June 21, 2004, from *www.obesity. org/subs/fastfacts/aoafactsheets.shtml.*

amFAR Aids Research. (2002). *Seniors Hidden HIV Risk Group.* Atlanta, GA: American Cancer Society. Retrieved December 29, 2007, from *www.amfar.org.*

Apter, T. (1990). *Altered loves: Mothers and daughters during adolescence.* New York: Ballantine Books.

Apter, T. (1995). *Secret paths: Women in the new midlife.* New York: Norton.

Bloom, B. S. (1984). *Taxonomy of educational objectives: Handbook 1, cognitive domain.* New York: Longman.

Boston Women's Health Book Collective & Norsigian, J. (2005). *Our bodies, ourselves: A new edition for a new era.* New York: Simon & Schuster.

Boston Women's Health Book Collective, Norsigian, J., & Pinn, V. (2006). *Our bodies, ourselves: Menopause.* New York: Simon & Schuster.

Brownson, R. C., Alavanja, M. C., Hock, E. T., & Loy, T. S. (1992). Passive smoking and lung cancer in nonsmoking women. *American Journal of Public Health, 82*(11), 1525–1530.

Buttaro, T. M., Trybulski, J., Bailey, P. P., & Sandburg-Cook, J. S. (2003). *Primary care: A collaborative practice.* St. Louis, MO: Mosby.

Centers for Disease Control and Prevention. (2007). *HIV/AIDS surveillance report, 2005* (Vol. 17, Rev. ed.). Atlanta, GA: U.S. Department of Health and Human Services, Centers for Disease Control and Prevention.

Centers for Disease Control and Prevention. National Center for Health Statistics. (2002). *National health and nutrition examination survey, health, United States, 2002.* Retrieved July 31, 2005, from *www.cdc.gov/nchs/nhanes.htm.*

Clark, C. (2002). *Health promotion in communities: Holistic and wellness approaches.* New York: Springer.

Cohen, R., & Martinez, M. (2007). *Health insurance coverage: Early release of estimates from the National Health Interview Survey, January-June 2007.* Washington, DC: Centers for Disease Control.

Daviglus, M., Liu, K., Pirzada, A., Yan, L., Garside, D., Feinglass, J., et al. (2003). Favorable cardiovascular risk profile in middle age and health-related quality of life in older age. *Archives of Internal Medicine, 163*(20), 2460–2468.

DeNavas-Walt, C., Proctor, B., & Smith, J. (2007). *U.S. Census Bureau, Current Population Reports, P60-233, Income, poverty, and health insurance coverage in the United States: 2006.* Washington, DC: U.S. Government Printing Office.

Dunphy, L. (2004). *Management guidelines for nurse practitioners working with adults* (2nd ed.). Philadelphia, PA: F. A. Davis.

Duvall, E. M., & Miller, B. (1985). *Marriage and family development* (6th ed.). New York: Harper Collins.

Erikson, E. H., & Erikson, G. M. (1998). *Life cycle completed.* New York: W. W. Norton.

Fabricius, W., & Luecken, L. (2007). Postdivorce living arrangements, parent conflict, and long-term physical health correlates for children of divorce. *Journal of Family Psychology, 21*(2), 195–205.

Gilligan, C. (1982). *In a different voice: Psychological theory and women's development.* Cambridge, MA: Harvard University Press.

Gilligan, C. (1990). *Mapping the moral domain.* Cambridge, MA: Harvard University Press.

Harig, P. T. (2007). Stress management: a guide for senior leaders. Stress hardiness: beyond jogging. In *Executive wellness: A guide for senior leaders.* Carlisle Barracks, PA: US Army Physical Fitness Research Institute.

Harpaz, R., Ortega-Sanchez, I. R., & Seward, J. F. (2008). Prevention of herpes zoster: Recommendations of the Advisory Committee on Immunization Practices (ACIP). *MMWR Recommendation, 57*(RR-5), 1–30.

Havighurst, R. I., & Orr, B. (1956). *Adult education and adult needs.* Chicago, IL: Center for Study of Liberal Education for Adults.

Haynes, S. G., Feinleib, M., & Kannel, W. B. (1980). The relationship of psychosocial factors to coronary heart disease in the Framingham Study. III. Eight-year incidence of coronary heart disease. *American Journal of Epidemiology, 111*(1), 37–58.

Haynes, S. G., Levine, S., Scotch, N., Feinleib, M., & Kannel, W. B. (1978). The relationship of psychosocial factors to coronary heart disease in the Framingham Study. I. Methods and risk factors. *American Journal of Epidemiology, 107*(5), 362–383.

Heron, M. (2007). Deaths: Leading Causes for 2004. *National Vital Statistics Reports, 56*(5), 1–95.

Hornstein, G. (1986). The structuring of identity among midlife women as a function of their degree of involvement in employment. *Journal of Personality, 54,* 551–575.

Jacobs, G. D. (1998). *Say goodnight to insomnia.* New York: Henry Holt.

Jacobs, G. D., Pace-Schott, E. F., Stickgold, R., & Otto, M. W. (2004). Cognitive behavioral therapy and pharmacotherapy for insomnia: A randomized controlled trial and direct comparison. *Archives of Internal Medicine, 164*(17), 1888–1896.

Japsen, B. (2007). Cholesterol Levels Attain Milestone. *Chicagotribune.com.* Retrieved January 4, 2008, from *www.chicagotribune. com/business/chi-thu.*

Joint National Committee. (2003). The seventh report of the Joint National Committee on detection, evaluation and treatment of high blood pressure. The 7th Joint National Committee on Prevention, Detection, Evaluation, and Treatment of High Blood Pressure. *Journal of American Medical Association, 289,* Retrieved April 21, 2005, from *http://jama.ama-assn.org/cgi/content/full/289,19.2560V/.*

Karch, A. (2003). *Focus on nursing pharmacology* (2nd ed.). Philadelphia, PA: Lippincott.

Kawachi, I., Sparrow, D., Spiro, A., Vokonas, P., & Weiss, S. T. (1996). A prospective study of anger and coronary heart disease: The Normative Aging Study. *Circulation, 94,* 2090–2095.

Kobasa, S. (1979). Stressful life events, personality and health: An inquiry into hardiness. *Journal of Personality and Social Psychology, 37,* 1–11.

Kohlberg, L., & Lickona, T. (1986). *The stages of ethical development: From childhood through old age.* New York: Harper Collins.

Kriketos, A. D., Sharp, T. A., Seagle, H. M., Peters, J. C., & Hill, J. O. (2000). Effects of aerobic fitness on fat oxidation and body fatness. *Medicine and Science in Sports & Exercise, 32*(4), 805–811.

Kucera, K. (2004). Managing common skin problems in the elderly. *The Clinical Advisor, 7*(6), 23–30.

Légaré, F., Stacey, D., Dodin, S., O'Connor, A., Richer, M., Griffiths, F., et al. (2007). Women's decision making about the use of natural health products at menopause: A needs assessment and patient decision aid. *Journal of Alternative and Complementary Medicine, 13*(7), 741–749.

Leone, P. (2007). *Expanded HIV Testing: Practical Screening Cases to Meet New CDC Recommendations.* Retrieved December 27, 2007, from *www.medscape.com.*

Levinson, D. (1986a). A conception of adult development. *American Psychologist, 41,* 3–13.

Levinson, D. (1986b). *The seasons of a man's life.* New York: Ballantine.

Levinson, D. (1996). *The seasons of a woman's life.* New York: Knopf.

Lindau, S., Laumann, E., & Levinson, W. (2007). Sexuality and health among older adults in the United States. *New England Journal of Medicine, 357*(26), 2732–2733.

Lowdermilk, D., & Perry, S. (2007). *Reproductive system concerns. Maternity and women's health care* (9th ed., pp. 145–173). St. Louis, MO: Mosby.

Lubkin, I. M., & Larsen, P. D. (2006). *Chronic illness: Impact and interventions* (6th ed.). Boston, MA: Jones and Bartlett.

McFadden, S., & Gerl, R. (1990). Approaches to understanding spirituality in the second half of life. *Generations, 14,* 35–38.

Mendelsohn, M., & Karas, R. (2007). HRT and the Young at Heart. *New England Journal of Medicine, 356*(25), 2639–2641.

Miniño, A., Heron, M., & Murphy, S. (2007). Deaths: Final data for 2004. *National Vital Statistics Reports, 55*(19), 1–119.

National Center for Health Statistics. (2004). *Married Adults are Healthiest, New CDC Report Shows.* Retrieved September 4, 2007 from *www.cdc.gov/nchs/pressroom/04facts/marriedadults.htm.*

National Osteoporosis Foundation. (1998). *Boning up on osteoporosis: A guide to prevention and treatment.* Washington, DC: The Foundation.

Nelson, H., Vesco, K., Haney, E., Fu, R., Nedrow, A., Miller, J., et al. (2006). Nonhormonal therapies for menopausal hot flashes. *Journal of the American Medical Association, 295*(17), 2057–2071.

Newman, D. K., & Giovannini, D. (2002). The overactive bladder: A nursing perspective. *American Journal of Nursing, 102*(6), 36–46.

Northrup, C. (2008). *The secret pleasures of menopause.* New York: Hay House.

Nursing facts: Nursing's agenda for health care reform. (2005). Washington, DC: American Nurses Publishing. Retrieved July 31, 2005, from *www.nursingworld.org/readroom/rnagenda.htm.*

Parker-Pope, T. (2007). Estrogen Shows Benefit for Heart Health. *Wall Street Journal Online.* Retrieved August 12, 2007, from *www.wsj.com.*

Pender, N. et al. (2005). *Health promotion in nursing practice.* Stamford, CT: Appleton & Lange.

Perez, M. A., & Luguis, R. R. (2008). *Cultural competence in health education and health promotion.* San Francisco: Jossey-Bass.

Piaget, J. (1970). *Structuralism.* New York: Basic Books.

Reifman, A., Biernat, M., & Lang, E. (1991). Stress, social support, and health in married professional women with small children. *Psychology of Women Quarterly, 15,* 431–445.

Rice, V. (2000). *Handbook of stress, coping, and health: Implications for nursing research, theory, and practice.* London: Sage.

Rippe, J. M. (1996). *Fit over forty: A revolutionary plan to achieve lifelong physical and spiritual health and well-being.* New York: William Morrow.

Rossouw, J., Prentice, R., Manson, J., Wu, L., Barad, D., Barnabei, V., et al. (2007). Postmenopausal hormone therapy and risk of cardiovascular disease by age and years since menopause. *Journal of the American Medical Association, 297*(13), 1465–1477.

Schaie, K. W., & Willis, S. L. (2005). *Intellectual functioning in adulthood: Growth, maintenance, decline, and modifiability.* Philadelphia, PA: American Society on Aging.

Seaman, B. (2003). *The greatest experiment ever performed on women: Exploding the estrogen myth.* New York: Hyperion.

Sheehy, G. (1993). *Menopause: The silent passage.* New York: Random House.

Silverstein, O., & Rashbaum, B. (1995). *The courage to raise good men.* New York: Penguin.

Spector, R. E. (2008). *Cultural diversity in health and illness* (6th ed.). East Norwalk, CT: Appleton & Lange.

Spector, R. E. (2003). *Culture care: guide to heritage assessment and health traditions.* East Norwalk, CT: Appleton & Lange.

Spielberger, C. D., Jacobs, G., Russell, S., & Crane, R. S. (1983). Assessment of anger: The state-trait anger scale. In J. N. Butcher & C. D. Spielberger (Eds.), *Advances in personality assessment* (Vol. 2). Hillsdale, NJ: Lawrence Erlbaum Associates.

Stuart, E., Deckro, J., & Mandle, C. L. (1989). Spirituality in health and healing: A clinical program. *Holistic Nursing Practice, 3,* 35–46.

Targonski, P. V., & Poland, E. A. (2007). Pneumococcal vaccination in adults: Recommendations, trends, and prospects. *Cleveland Clinics Journal of Medicine, 74*(6), 408–410, 413–414.

Thomas, S. P. (1995). Psychosocial correlates of women's health in middle adulthood. *Issues in Mental Health Nursing, 16,* 285–314.

U.S. Census Bureau. (2006). *Statistical abstracts of the United States: 2007* (126th ed.). Washington, DC: U.S. Government Printing Office.

U.S. Department of Health and Human Services, Centers for Disease Control and Prevention, National Center for Health Statistics. (2007). *Health, United States.* Hyattsville, MD: The Author.

U.S. Department of Health and Human Services. (2007). *Every American insured.* HHS.gov, Retrieved December 26, 2007, from *www.hhs.gov/everyamericaninsured/.*

U.S. Department of Health and Human Services, Health Resources and Services Administration. (2007). *Women's health USA 2007.* Rockville, MD: U.S. Department of Health and Human Services.

U.S. Department of Health and Human Services. (2007). *The Office of Minority Health.* Retrieved December 26, 2007 from *www.omhrc.gov/templates/browse.*

U.S. Department of Health and Human Services. National Institutes of Health (NIH). National Institute on Alcohol Abuse and Alcoholism. (2005). *Alcohol: A woman's health issue.* Retrieved June 16, 2008, from *http://pubs.niaaa.nih.gov/publications/brochurewomen/women.htm.*

U.S. Department of Health and Human Services. (2007). *Healthy people 2010: Midcourse review.* Retrieved January 29, 2008, from *www.healthypeople.gov/data/midcourse/html.*

U.S. Department of Health and Human Services. (2000). *Healthy people 2010.* Washington, DC: U.S. Government Printing Office.

U.S. Preventive Services Task Force. (2007). *Guide to clinical preventive services.* Rockville, MD: Agency for Healthcare Research and Quality. Retrieved January 29, 2008, from *www.ahrq.gov/clinic/pocketgd07/index.html.*

USA Today. (2005, January 11). *Why grown kids come home.* Retrieved from *www.usatoday.com/educate/college/careers/news4.htm.*

Vaillant, G. (2003). *Aging well: Surprising guideposts to a happier life from the Landmark Harvard Study of Adult Development.* New York: Little Brown.

Vaillant, G., & Vaillant, C. (1990). Natural history of male psychological health, XII: A 45-year study of predictors of successful aging at age 65. *American Journal of Psychiatry, 147*(1), 31–37.

Vivian, C., & Dundes, L. (2004). The crossroads of culture and health among the Roma (gypsies). *Image: The Journal of Nursing Scholarship, 36*(1), 86–91.

Wallerstein, J. S., Lewis, J., & Blakeslee, S. (2000). *The unexpected legacy of divorce: A 25 year landmark study.* New York: Hyperion.

Williams, J., Paton, C., Siegler, I. C., Eigenbrodt, M. L., Nieto, F. J., & Tyroler, H. A. (2000). Anger proneness predicts coronary heart disease risk: Prospective analysis from the Atherosclerosis Risk in Communities (ARIC) Study. *Circulation, 101*(17), 2034–2039.

Chapter 24

Meredith Wallace*

Older Adult

objectives

After completing this chapter, the reader will be able to:

- Describe normal aging changes in the older adult.
- Evaluate morbidity data according to age, gender, and race.
- Discuss nutritional factors that affect the health promotion of the older adult.
- Analyze environmental factors that have an effect on older adults.
- Recognize risk factors that could lead to health problems in older adulthood.
- Enumerate the five most prevalent health conditions and the five leading causes of mortality among older people.
- Discuss environmental, biological, physical, and mechanical agents that contribute to disability, morbidity, and mortality in later adulthood.
- Analyze political and social issues that influence the well-being of the older adult.
- List the leading causes of injury among older adults and suggest preventive measures.
- Identify major resources that are available for older adults.

key terms

Activities of daily living
Alzheimer's disease
Atrophy
Body transcendence versus body preoccupation
Cataracts
Cognition
Constipation
Decubitus ulcer
Delirium
Dementia
Depression
Ego differentiation versus work role preoccupation

Ego integrity versus despair
Ego transcendence versus ego preoccupation
Euthanasia
Glaucoma
Impaction
Impotence
Instrumental activities of daily living
Kegel exercises
Life review
Mild cognitive impairment (MCI)

Mini-Mental State Examination (MMSE)
Multi-infarct dementia
Osteoporosis
Overflow incontinence
Pessaries
Physician-assisted suicide
Polyuria
Reminiscence
Sclerosis
Stress incontinence
Urge incontinence
Urinary incontinence

*The author would like to acknowledge Noah Hendler, Michelle R. Levine, and Dana Zavory for their contributions to this chapter.

website materials

evolve These materials are located on the book's website at *http://evolve.elsevier.com/Edelman/*.

- WebLinks
- Study Questions
- Glossary
- Website Resources

  24A: Yesavage Geriatric Depression Scale: Short Form

  24B: Recommended Adult Immunization Schedule, United States, 2004-2005

THINK About It

Older Adult Smokers

You are the director of a senior center in which 10 of your 40 members smoke. Several of the smoking individuals currently experience health problems. One older woman has chronic obstructive pulmonary disease and avoids using her oxygen because she is not supposed to smoke while the oxygen tank is in the room. One older gentleman has high blood pressure; another one of the smokers has been diagnosed with lung cancer. As director of the center, you would like to help these older adults to stop smoking. You have referred them to their physicians to obtain assistance with smoking cessation. However, all of the participants are Medicare recipients and Medicare does not provide coverage for smoking-cessation programs and/or nicotine-replacement therapy. All involved are on limited incomes and cannot afford to pay the charge of either a behavior management class or nicotine-replacement therapy.

1. What types of resources are available to help you obtain the necessary assistance for these smokers?

2. What policy changes might be instituted within the senior center to prevent secondhand smoke from harming the residents in the center's care?

As a result of health promotion and technological advances, health care professionals now enjoy the gift of caring for an older population. To be caring for a group of human beings that was virtually nonexistent 100 years ago is truly extraordinary. The current standard of living, nutrition, prevention and treatment of infectious diseases, and progress in medical care have increased sharply the survival rate for people living in the United States. Once these individuals reach adulthood, they are likely to survive to old age. In 2003 the number of Americans age 65 and older was approximately 36 million, or 12% of the population. By the year 2050 the percentage is projected to increase to more than 20% of the population (Federal Interagency Forum on Aging-Related Statistics, 2004). The fastest-growing age group in the country is that of adults age 75 and older.

The fastest-growing group within the older adult population is 85 years and older. According to *Healthy People 2010*, individuals age 65 years can be expected to live an average of 18 more years, for a total of 83 years. Individuals age 75 years can be expected to live an average of 11 more years, for a total of 86 years (U.S. Department of Health and Human Services [USDHHS], 2001). (See the development of *Healthy People 2020*.)

The percentages of Whites in the population of adults 65 and older is expected to decrease over the next 30 years, while the percentage of African American, Hispanic, and Asian older adults will continue to rise. Considering this shift in population characteristics, it is imperative that health care providers develop an awareness of the cultural diversity of the population and identify the cultural beliefs that influence health care decisions of older adults (Multicultural Awareness box).

During the past few decades, older adults use the most health care dollars in the last 7 years of their lives. Health care providers waited until they became sick before providing health care. Insurance reimbursement and introduction into the health care system has come late for many, resulting in a high prevalence of illness and limited health-promotion interventions. The misconceptions surrounding health promotion for older adults impede the ability of nurses to provide the best possible care. It is time to overcome these misconceptions and begin to promote the health of older adults rather than wait until they are ill to provide them with health services. Health promotion is as important in later adulthood as it is in childhood. Older adults can derive the same benefits from health-promotion activity as do their younger counterparts; they are not "too old" to stop smoking, start exercising, change their diet, or relinquish other bad health habits. The potential for improvement is great, and nurses have a key role in changing common societal misconceptions and in creating new fields of knowledge surrounding health promotion and older adults.

The many physical, economical, spiritual, and role changes of aging that will be discussed in this chapter are compromised by the great diversity of cultural backgrounds in this country. Older adults who have immigrated to the

United States have brought with them different languages, spiritual patterns, eating habits, views toward modern medicine, and other customs foreign to U.S. culture. Furthermore, in other cultures older adults are more frequently respected than they are in the United States. Throughout this chapter, cultural norms and behaviors will be discussed within each functional health pattern.

AGE AND PHYSICAL CHANGES

Although the need to promote the health of the older population is great, numerous challenges are presented in fulfilling this need. As stated, one of the great challenges to health promotion among older adults lies in the misconceptions about its benefits. Another challenge concerns separating the normal changes of aging from pathological processes and illness. Normal age-related changes frequently are regarded as inevitable and irreversible. However, an extraordinary amount of variability exists in the age-related changes that occur in each individual. Exposure to environmental injury, illness, genetics, stress, cultural influences, and many other factors combine to influence the aging process. Most researchers agree that biological changes show that growth and development peak during the thirties, with subsequent linear decline until death. These normal changes must be distinguished from pathological changes to focus health-promotion interventions on behaviors that can and should be changed. For example, older adults experience a decline in their respiratory vital capacity. Therefore when recommending exercise programs, these people must start gradually, allowing them to experience the exercise free from respiratory distress. These changes will be discussed specifically under each section of the physiological and psychological processes.

Another challenge to promoting the health of older adults lies in the prevalence of chronic illness. Although chronic illness is not a normal change of aging, years of environmental assault, poor health behaviors, and stress have placed older adults at a high risk for developing these illnesses. Generally health deteriorates with aging through an accumulation of chronic disorders and disabilities. According to the Centers for Disease Control and Prevention (CDC), chronic conditions significantly limit daily activity for 39% of people over 65 years of age. Although older Americans make up 12% of the population, they account for nearly three to five times more health care costs than their younger counterparts, reflecting an increase of 25% in health care expenditures of this population (Centers for Disease Control and Prevention and the Merck Company Foundation, [2007]). Table 24-1 lists the percentage of older adults with chronic conditions. Illness impairs the individual's capacity and motivation to learn new health-promoting behaviors. This prevalence of illness clearly indicates that this population has a great need for health promotion, although it is one of the most difficult in which to effect change.

MULTICULTURAL AWARENESS

How Different Cultures Care for Older Adults

How fortunate is today's society to enjoy the variety of many cultures? Individuals and families who immigrated to the United States in the early 1900s are now spending their later years as citizens of this country. Although many older adults have lived in the United States for many years, remembering the countries they came from is of great importance. An understanding of the individual cultural backgrounds of older adults allows nurses to provide care that is respectful of the whole individual.

Schmall (1996) indicates that five major cultural groups in the United States display differing attitudes toward older adults. Most White Anglo-Saxon Protestants show less respect for older adults and their role in the family than do other cultures, in which older men and women tend to share in the family structure more equally. Parents are expected to live away from and not be overly dependent on their adult children. Although this view represents the mainstream American culture, other distinct and important cultures within the United States should be recognized and respected.

The Black culture generally has a greater respect for older adults and their family role than do White cultures. Black people also place a value on kinship and the extended family that is no longer present in White cultures. East Asians have an especially high level of respect for older adults: the older an individual is, the more respect that individual is given. Additionally, the oldest son in East Asian cultures assumes responsibility for the care of the aging parents. Hispanic cultures give more overt respect to older adults than do White cultures. In many families, aging parents live in households that consist of numerous extended family members. Finally, Native American cultures have a high level of respect for older adults because of their years of accumulated wisdom and knowledge, and they are frequently sought out for advice.

Knowledge of the different cultures in the United States provides the nurse with a broader understanding of the psychosocial mechanics underlying an individual's illness. Understanding the older adult's role within the family gives the nurse the information that is needed to develop an appropriate plan of care. Many of them will be well cared for by family members, and others do not expect or value care from their families. Additionally, the role that older adults are expected to fulfill within their culture, such as grandparent, primary caregiver, or family decision maker, must be considered when nurses are attempting to understand the value of health and illness to the older adult. Although nurses generally believe that the health of the individual should come first, an understanding of the culture can help in planning; for example, an aging Hispanic grandfather prefers to be home when his grandchildren return from school rather than at the clinic receiving dialysis treatments in the afternoon. Enhanced cultural competency among nurses has great potential for improving health care and quality of life for older adults.

Data from Schmall, V. L. (1996). Family influences. In A. G. Lueckenotte (Ed.), *Gerontologic nursing*. St. Louis: Mosby, pp. 136–166.

Table **24-1**	Average Percentage of People Age 65 and Older Who Have Chronic Health Conditions	
Chronic Condition	**Women**	**Men**
Hypertension	54	52
Arthritis	54	43
Heart disease	26	37
Cancer	19	24
Diabetes	17	19
Asthma	12	10
Chronic bronchitis or emphysema	10	11
Stroke	8	10

From Centers for Disease Control and Prevention, National Center for Health Statistics, *National Health Interview Survey* (2008).

It is important to note that health-promotion practices among older adults vary by cultural background. In a study of 13 older Korean immigrants in the United States, older Korean immigrants did not practice healthy lifestyles, but were shown to have improved health outcomes with structured programming (Sin et al., 2005). In order to improve the health-promotion practices of immigrants to the United States and other cultural groups, cultural norms and behaviors must be taken into consideration. In a study of Chinese Americans, older adults began to shift dependence for health needs from traditional family caregivers to friends and neighbors (Pang et al., 2003).

Goals of Health Promotion

The U.S. Department of Health and Human Services (2007) has developed *Healthy People 2010: National Health-Promotion and Disease Prevention Objectives* (see further developing *Healthy People 2020*) for health-promotion programs for the older population (*Healthy People 2010* box). These goals focus on increasing health-promotion programs and decreasing morbidity and mortality related to various disease states. In 2005, half way through the *Healthy People 2010* project period, a midcourse review of the status of the national objectives was conducted. Data were collected to measure the progress of the goals and to revise and reword the goals to make sure they were accurate and scientifically relevant. Through this process it was determined that many goals focusing on older adults are being met. Importantly, the life expectancy continues to improve throughout the nation. Years in good or better health and years free of activity limitations and chronic illness have also increased slightly.

As the population of older adults continues to rise, the number of cultural backgrounds within this population will increase and diversify. Cultural background and race have an effect on the prevalence of disease in the United States. The CDC and Merck Company Foundation (2007) report that the five major cultural groups share eight leading causes of death. Heart disease and cancer are the first and second leading causes, respectively, with stroke, respiratory diseases, flu, pneumonia, Alzheimer's disease, diabetes, and other causes following with varying disease rates depending on cultural background.

THEORIES OF AGING

The study of how and why people age has continued over many years and has been the source of a great deal of debate. Until fairly recently the cause of death on many older adults' death certificates was listed simply as "old age." As the study of gerontology has progressed, researchers have begun to question the physiological, social, and psychological reasons why people die. At the 55th annual meeting of the Gerontological Society of America, Butler and Olshansky (2002) explored these questions in a presentation entitled, "Has Anyone Ever Died of Old Age?"

Despite this attention, the debates among those studying biogerontological, psychogerontological, and sociogerontological theories of aging continue. There is no formula to predict how a person will age or how long that individual will live. Many theories continue to be tested today. Included in the most prevalent research are the roles of both genetics and diet in aging. Genetic markers to predict the development of disease will play a large role in determining how a person will age and longevity. In addition, researchers report that calorie-restricted diets have shown an increase in longevity in animals (Heilbronn et al., 2006). The role of antioxidants in binding free radicals is also being researched as an important influence on increasing longevity (Tse & Benzie, 2004). Although no consensus has yet been reached that describes the entire aging process, theories continue to be forthcoming and are very exciting. Explanations of each of these theories is extremely interesting but beyond the scope of this book. Some of the theories used to explain aging are listed in Box 24-1.

Box **24-1**	Theories of Aging

- Growth hormone secretion theory
- Waste product theory
- Cross-linkage theory
- Rate of living theory
- Wear and tear theory
- Social theories of aging
- Gene regulation theory
- Somatic mutation theory
- DNA damage theory
- Free radical theory
- Error theory
- Programmed cell loss theory
- Neuroendocrine theory
- Immunological theory
- Autoimmune theory

DNA, Deoxyribonucleic acid.

GORDON'S FUNCTIONAL HEALTH PATTERNS
Health Perception–Health Management Pattern

The most important factor in maintaining health is the older adult's motivation. Nurses who care for older adults know that all the best nursing in the world cannot make an individual do something believed to be unnecessary. A primary factor in the older adult's motivation to promote personal health is the perception of health and its subsequent management.

The *Harvard Women's Health Watch* (Forestalling frailty, 2003) reports five major activities older adults should engage in to promote health and prevent frailty. These include: (1) maintaining healthy weight and diet, (2) staying active, (3) practicing fall prevention, (4) maintaining relationships, and (5) keeping regular medical appointments. Helping an

---

Healthy People 2010
Selected National Health-Promotion and Disease Prevention Objectives for the Older Adult

- 1-9. Reduce hospitalization rates for three ambulatory care–sensitive conditions (pediatric asthma, uncontrolled diabetes, and immunization-preventable pneumonia and influenza in older adults).
- 2-9. Reduce the overall number of cases of osteoporosis.
- 6-3. Reduce the proportion of adults with disabilities who report feelings such as sadness, unhappiness, or depression that prevent them from being active.
- 6-4. Increase the proportion of adults with disabilities who participate in social activities.
- 6-5. Increase the proportion of adults with disabilities reporting sufficient emotional support.
- 6-6. Increase the proportion of adults with disabilities who report satisfaction with life.
- 6-7. Reduce the number of people with disabilities in congregate care facilities, consistent with permanency planning principles.
- 6-8. Eliminate disparities in employment rates between working-age adults with and without disabilities.
- 7-12. Increase the proportion of older adults who have participated during the preceding year in at least one organized health-promotion activity.
- 8-22. Increase the proportion of people living in pre-1950s housing that have tested for the presence of lead-based paint.
- 10-1. Reduce infections caused by key food-borne pathogens.
- 12-6. Reduce hospitalizations of older adults with heart failure as the principal diagnosis.
- 14-5. Reduce invasive pneumococcal infections.
- 14-28. Increase hepatitis B vaccine coverage in high-risk groups.
- 14-29. Increase the proportion of adults who are vaccinated annually against influenza and were ever vaccinated against pneumococcal disease.
- 15-1. Reduce hospitalization for nonfatal head injuries.
- 15-15. Reduce deaths caused by motor vehicle crashes.

- 15-27. Reduce deaths from falls.
- 15-28. Reduce hip fractures among older adults.
- 17-3. Increase the proportion of primary care providers, pharmacists, and other health care professionals who routinely review with their clients aged 65 years and older and those with chronic illnesses or disabilities all newly prescribed and over-the-counter medicines.
- 19-1. Increase the proportion of adults who are at a healthy weight.
- 19-2. Reduce the proportion of adults who are obese.
- 19-17. Increase the proportion of physician office visits made by clients with a diagnosis of cardiovascular disease, diabetes, or hyperlipidemia that includes counseling or education related to diet and nutrition.
- 19-18. Increase food security among U.S. households and, in so doing, reduce hunger.
- 21-4. Reduce the proportion of older adults who have had all their natural teeth extracted.
- 22-1. Reduce the proportion of adults who engage in no leisure-time physical activity.
- 22-2. Increase the proportion of adults who engage regularly, preferably daily, in moderate physical activity for at least 30 minutes per day.
- 22-3. Increase the proportion of adults who engage in vigorous physical activity that promotes the development and maintenance of cardiorespiratory fitness 3 or more days per week for 20 or more minutes per occasion.
- 22-4. Increase the proportion of adults who perform physical activities that enhance and maintain muscular strength and endurance.
- 24-9. Reduce the proportion of adults whose activity is limited because of chronic lung and breathing problems.
- 24-10. Reduce deaths from chronic obstructive pulmonary disease among adults.
- 27-10. Reduce the proportion of nonsmokers exposed to environmental tobacco smoke.

Modified from U.S. Department of Health and Human Services. (2007). *Healthy people 2010: National health promotion and disease prevention objectives.* Washington, DC: U.S. Government Printing Office. Retrieved April 12, 2007, from *www.health.gov/healthypeople.*

older adult to understand the importance of these factors for maintaining health is an essential nursing role needed to form positive health perceptions and effective health management patterns.

Health maintenance behaviors include exercise, good nutrition, sexual safety, and appropriate sleep-rest patterns. Health maintenance practices also includes regular health care checkups, which will provide early detection and management of disease. Although these behaviors are important for all older adults, the perception of these activities and the ability to practice good health behaviors varies by cultural groups. It is essential that nurses are culturally competent and understand the cultural values that guide behavior. In so doing, the nurse will be most effective in helping the older adult to form a positive health perception and practice good health behaviors.

Nutritional-Metabolic Pattern

Brownie (2006) reports that between 5% and 10% of older adults living independently are malnourished with that rate increasing to almost 85% among institutionalized

older adults. These statistics underscore the problems of maintaining good nutrition. Problems with access to food are compounded by the effect of normal changes of aging. Declines in gastrointestinal organ function can lead to changes in digestive metabolism and the absorption and elimination of nutrients. Additionally, a deterioration of the smell, vision, and taste senses and the high frequency of dental problems makes maintaining adequate daily nutrition even more difficult. Cultural food preferences and lifelong eating habits, such as diets high in fat and cholesterol, are other obstacles to maintaining optimal nutrition.

The living environment further affects nutritional status. Community-dwelling seniors are at high risk for nutritional disorders, because access to food may be limited. Institutionalized older adults do not have a problem with availability of food, but the meals served in institutions frequently contain excessive fat, cholesterol, or salt and a lack of fiber. Additionally, fresh fruit and vegetables are less available, and the nutritional value of produce is reduced significantly when the food is canned or cooked.

---

innovative practice

Geriatric Assessment

The health care system, with its emphasis on acute care, busy office schedules, and fragmented delivery systems, often frustrates older people and their families. The very old or frail person's health problems frequently are overlooked, ignored, or only partially treated. Many communities have a health care service that uses a team approach to meet the special needs of older adults. This service is known as *geriatric assessment*.

GOALS OF GERIATRIC ASSESSMENT

- Maintain health and health maintenance practices
- Minimize hospitalizations
- Establish complete diagnoses that are frequently overlooked, including hearing impairment, vision deficits, early dementia, depression, poor nutrition, and falls
- Decrease overprescription of medications

Geriatric assessment uses an interdisciplinary team consisting of a geriatric nurse practitioner, physical therapist, and a social worker. Each member of the team evaluates the person from a health care, functional, cognitive, or psychosocial point of view. Additional members of the team might include a geriatric psychiatrist, geriatrician, nutritionist, pharmacist, dentist, or podiatrist. The program team evaluates the home environment, advance directives, falls, incontinence, vision and hearing impairments, memory loss, depression and anxiety, functional decline, deconditioning, caregiver stress, economic resources, and quality-of-life issues. The team is coordinated by the geriatric nurse practitioner.

Geriatric assessment is not meant for all older people. The people who benefit are the frail ones. A typical person who might benefit from geriatric assessment would be:

- Over age 80
- Falls frequently
- Is losing weight because of poor nutrition
- Is depressed because of loss of spouse and friends
- Has mild memory loss
- Has been hospitalized 3 times in 2 months
- Takes more than five medications regularly and frequently gets them confused
- Has no close family in the community
- Is in need of health teaching

Geriatric assessment usually identifies the strengths and weaknesses of these people. Following the assessment, the geriatric nurse practitioner begins developing a plan of care to address usable strengths and assist with weaknesses.

The primary care physician, family physician, or internist is a key link between the geriatric assessment team and the individual, primarily because this provider carries out the team's recommendation and monitors the person's progress. In most cases the nurse practitioner coordinates between the team and the person's primary physician and family.

Geriatric assessment clinics are available in many larger cities. As the U.S. health care system changes from its costly system of treating acute health problems with frequent office and hospital visits to a more cost-controlled, coordinated, comprehensive health management system, geriatric assessment will play a key role in identifying individual strengths, correcting problems, and maintaining the health and quality of life of older citizens.

Courtesy Carole Lium Edelman.

Finally, institutional food tends to be unappealing, and most institutions are not able to adapt their meals to the cultural diversity of their residents.

Anorexia, or lack of appetite, can accompany disease. Medications or a lack of dentures can also cause older people to eat less than is optimal. Those in acute care hospitals or long-term care facilities may experience a lack of appetite as a result of illness. The hospital stay is a time during which good nutrition is most important to heal wounds and to restore energy; however, a lack of interest in or energy for eating during these stays places the older adult at a high risk of developing nutritional disorders.

Rank and Hirschl (2005) report that slightly more than half of all Americans use food stamps to acquire and maintain nutrition at some point in time in their lives, including older adulthood. Good nutrition helps prevent cancer, obesity, and gastrointestinal disorders and provides older adults with the energy required to function in all **activities of daily living**. Good nutrition can be measured by ascertaining whether the individual is meeting the recommended daily allowance (RDA) for caloric intake established by the National Academy of Sciences and the National Research Council. The RDA is 2000 to 2800 calories for men ages 51 to 75 years and 1650 to 2450 for men 76 years and older. The range for women 51 to 75 years of age is between 1400 and 2200 calories; for women 76 years and older, 1200 to 2000 calories are recommended (Wolf, 2006).

The nurse assists the older adult in maintaining the highest possible nutritional level. Teaching about the food needed to maintain optimal nutritional status is of utmost importance. In addition to food stamps, there are several other federally supported nutrition assistance programs available to the older adult, including commodity supplemental food program, child and adult food program, older adult nutrition program (Meals on Wheels), and the emergency food assistance program. However, Wellman and Kamp (2004) report that only 6% to 7% of the people who really need these programs use them. The nurse may assist the older adult in acquiring transportation to obtain food and applying for these programs. Nurses who work in institutional settings are charged with the difficult task of encouraging good nutrition on the resident and administrative level. Residents who frequently do not want to eat institutional food should be encouraged to eat the types of food that they enjoy. Encouraging family members to bring in food that the resident enjoys is helpful. A pleasant setting with socialization can also enhance the desire to eat. The reader may refer to Chapter 11: Nutrition Counseling for more information to help older adults achieve improved levels of nutrition.

Elimination Pattern

Bowel and bladder functions in the older adult are altered by the normal changes of age. The bladder retains its tonus, but its capacity decreases. Large bowel motility also decreases as people age. In addition to some of the normal changes of aging, diet plays a significant role in problems with intestinal motility and constipation. Increased incidence of nutritional disorders, particularly decreased intake of fluids and fiber, contributes in large part to elimination problems. Many medications frequently taken by older adults cause elimination concerns. Lack of physical activity and changes in environment that decrease privacy also contribute. To maintain healthy bowel hygiene, the nurse encourages the older adult to have adequate fluids, roughage, and exercise.

Constipation is a major problem for older adults and has far-reaching effects on their quality of life. Researchers report that constipation requires excessive nurse staffing costs (Lagman, 2006). By encouraging older adults to exercise and change their fluid and dietary intake, nurses can help reduce their incidence of constipation. Exercise has a rapid and favorable effect on constipation. Dietary modifications, such as the increase of fiber and fluid, can stimulate the colon and resolve constipation.

Urinary incontinence affects approximately 30% of community-dwelling older adults and half of nursing home clients (Mauk, 2005) and is associated with considerable expense and reduction in quality of life (DuBeau et al., 2006). The causes of urinary incontinence are summarized in Box 24-2. The three major types of incontinence among older adults include **stress incontinence**, which is most common and occurs during exercise, laughing, coughing, or sneezing; **urge incontinence**, or the inability to delay voiding after the bladder is full; and **overflow incontinence** caused by an obstruction in the elimination system, such as an enlarged prostate gland or urethral stricture.

Incontinence results in threats to both psychological and physical health, including depression, urinary tract infections, pressure ulcers, and falls (Wyman, 2003). Despite the high prevalence of the problem, older adults frequently fail to report incontinence to their health care providers because of its embarrassing nature (Vinsnes et al., 2001). Accepting incontinence as a manageable problem and seeking appropriate treatment is important for continued health and self-esteem.

Incontinent older adults in all cultural groups tend to avoid physical and social activities because of this problem.

Wyman (2003) describes several treatment categories. The first method includes lifestyle modifications and health-promotion behaviors to decrease incontinence, such as weight loss, exercise, and diet. Voiding schedules are most effective when the person can select specific times during the day for urination. After developing a schedule, the individual is instructed to use the toilet 30 minutes before this time each day. This technique may prevent incontinence.

Prompted voiding is another method to decrease incontinent episodes. The individual is reminded or asked about voiding. A structured bladder training program allows older individuals to develop a voiding schedule that is progressive by increasing the time between voids and ensuring that adequate fluids are taken from 7:00 AM to 7:00 PM. Postponing

Box **24-2** | **Causes of Urinary Incontinence Among Older Adults**

DELIRIUM

- New onset of UI may be associated with delirium from acute underlying conditions requiring diagnosis and treatment.

RESTRICTED MOBILITY

- Acute conditions causing immobility may precipitate UI; environmental manipulation and scheduled toileting are appropriate while rehabilitative efforts are undertaken.

INFECTION

- Acute cystitis may precipitate urge UI. Asymptomatic bacteriuria, with or without pyuria, should not be treated in the absence of symptoms of acute UTI.

INFLAMMATION

- Atrophic vaginitis and urethritis can cause irritative voiding symptoms, including UI.

IMPACTION

- Fecal **impaction** may be associated with UI and fecal incontinence.

POLYURIA

- Poorly controlled diabetes with glucosuria can contribute to urinary frequency and UI.
- Excess intake of caffeinated beverages may exacerbate symptoms.
- Edema from congestive heart failure or venous insufficiency can cause nocturia and exacerbate nocturnal UI.

PHARMACEUTICALS

- Rapid-acting diuretics (urge UI)
- Psychotropic drugs (sedation, immobility)
- Anticholinergic agents, α-antagonists, calcium channel blockers, narcotics (urinary retention)
- α-Antagonists (stress UI)
- Alcohol (sedation, immobility, **polyuria**)

UI, Urinary incontinence; UTI, urinary tract infection.
Modified from Ouslander, J. G. (June, 2000). Incontinence management in LTC. *Annals of Long-Term Care, 8*(6), 35–41.

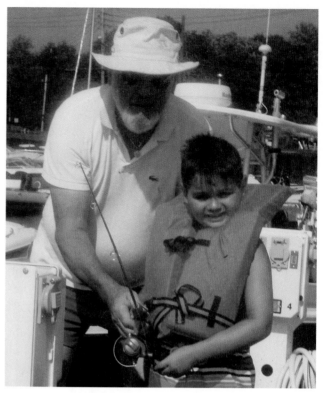

Figure 24-1   A grandparent teaches his grandson how to fish.

voids by using relaxation, imagery, or distraction is essential to the success of this management strategy. This type of training is difficult, however, and relies on a good working relationship between the individual and the nurse.

Anti-incontinence devices, such as **pessaries**, are often helpful. In addition, pelvic floor or **Kegel exercises** may be taught to improve the musculature of the urinary system. To perform Kegel or pelvic floor exercises, the first step is to locate the muscle that requires strengthening. The individual is instructed to squeeze around the finger for 10 seconds. Repetitions of 10 cycles of 10 seconds each 6 times a day will result in fewer accidents in a period of approximately 2 weeks. Supportive interventions such as disposable pads may be used to avoid embarrassment as well.

Activity-Exercise Pattern

The benefits of regular exercise in promoting health and preventing disease are widely accepted. The overwhelming evidence of the positive effects of exercise has led the U.S. Department of Health and Human Services to develop within its program *Healthy People 2010* (see the developing *Healthy People 2020*) national objectives for increasing the numbers of adults who exercise regularly. Exercise becomes increasingly more important among older adults as it has the capacity to reduce, stop, or reverse physical decline (Melov et al., 2007). Despite the many benefits of exercise, Friis et al. (2003) report that older adults do not often participate in exercise programs. Although exercise is not popular among this age group, no physiological or psychological explanation has been found to explain this decline. Normal changes of aging, pathological conditions, and environmental deterrents do not prevent the older adult from exercising (Figure 24-1).

Teaching the many benefits of exercise is the first lesson in motivating older adults to participate. With respect to the role that culture plays on the value of exercise, individual counseling is needed to identify exercises that can be enjoyed and continued (Figure 24-2). The nurse assists in designing an appropriate exercise program that will maintain strength, flexibility, and balance. Walking is broadly reported as the most widely accepted form of exercise among older adults. Friis et al. (2003) found that 38% of

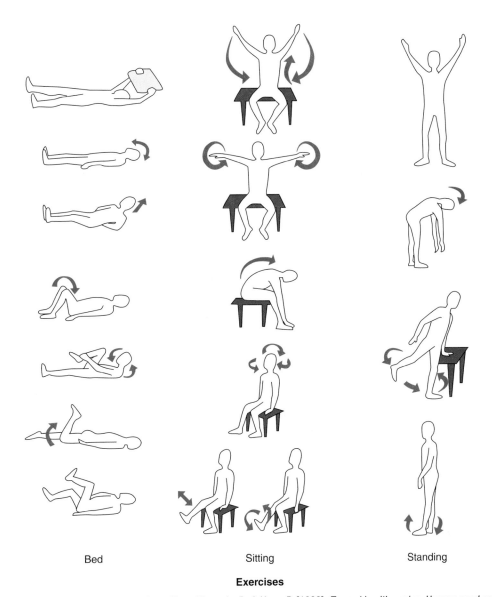

Bed   Sitting   Standing

Exercises

Figure 24-2   Bed-lying, sitting, and standing exercises. (From Ebersole, P., & Hess, P. [1998]. *Toward healthy aging: Human need and nursing response* [3rd ed.]. St. Louis: Mosby).

men and 26% of women in their study walked for exercise. Walking is an exercise that can be done in both community settings and health care facilities.

Other popular activities for older adults include weight-bearing and aquatic exercises. Weight-bearing and muscle-building exercises help to maintain functional mobility, promote independence, and prevent falls. Weight-bearing exercises are shown to be highly effective in reducing bone wasting common to osteoporosis. Recent research shows that regular exercise promotes bone mineral density among older adults (Melov et al., 2007). Older individuals who suffer from arthritis find aquatic exercise a pain-free way to promote their health and increase their functional ability. Exercising in the water is also an effective and enjoyable activity for those without arthritis. The effects of exercise on the older adult are extensive.

Box **24-3**   **Benefits of Exercise in the Older Adult**

- Better sleep
- Reduced constipation
- Lower cholesterol level
- Lower blood pressure
- Better digestion
- Weight loss
- Socializing opportunities

Box 24-3 lists many benefits that can be derived from participating in an exercise program.

Before beginning any exercise program, an older person who has not been exercising should consult a physician or nurse practitioner. After the program begins, activity levels should be increased gradually. Adherence to exercise is a major problem for all populations. The best tools available to encourage continued exercise among older adults are to communicate the role of exercise in maintaining their quality of life, to help them choose an exercise that they enjoy with others, and to choose one that is easily accessible (Binder et al., 2002).

Sleep-Rest Pattern

Inability to sleep well is one of the most frequent complaints of older adults (Westley, 2004). The high prevalence of sleep disorders in this population indicates that they experience a great need for assistance in getting to sleep and staying asleep. Quan and Zee (2004) state that 45% of the sample in their research study reported difficulty falling asleep and remaining asleep, 33% reported snoring, and 27% reported daytime sleepiness. Sleep complaints result from several normal aging changes that occur among older adults of all cultural backgrounds. The changes result in a decrease in the total hours of sleep that are required, an increase in nocturnal awakenings, shorter periods of sleep, and a decrease in slow-wave activity.

The benefits of a good night's sleep are numerous. Overall increases in energy, motivation to continue a high quality of life, and improved immune function are only a few. Nurses assist older adults in achieving a good night's sleep through assessment that might reveal possible causes of sleep disturbances. Teaching about the normal changes can reassure older adults that their sleep patterns have changed but are not necessarily harmful. Having this information may decrease anxiety. Increasing physical activity can also help them fall asleep more readily in the evening or night hours. Increased pain medication or alternative pain-relief methods can help those who suffer from painful conditions obtain better rest at night.

Residents of nursing facilities or people in acute care facilities may have difficulty adjusting to the environment at night. Adjustments in noise and lighting can help these individuals sleep better. Emotional disorders frequently can be identified, and therapy and medication can be administered during the day to help them sleep peacefully at night. Finally, daytime napping has been viewed as inhibiting a good night's sleep in this population.

Sleep medications may be helpful for short-term use. However, Frighetto et al. (2004) report that benzodiazepines should be used cautiously because of the possibility of rebound and morning insomnia, as well as hangover effect and daytime sedation.

Cognitive-Perceptual Pattern
Cognition

Thinking processes (**cognition**) in old age have been the subject of intensive study over the past few decades. Brain weight decreases with aging, and a shift occurs in the proportion of gray matter to white matter. The ways in which these changes are manifested in individuals varies because of culture, heredity, lifestyle, environmental exposures, and many other factors. No consensus has been reached as to the ways in which these changes translate into human behavior.

There is a common belief that most older adults will eventually develop dementia; however, cognitive problems are not a normal change of aging. **Mild cognitive impairment (MCI)** is a pathological collection of symptoms that results in memory loss, language difficulties, and impairments in judgment and reasoning. A review of **instrumental activities of daily living** will help the nurse identify changes in higher executive functions, such as paying bills, taking medications as ordered, using the phone, and driving safely. It is estimated that 10% of older adults over the age of 65 will develop Alzheimer's disease with this number increasing to 50% in the 90 and over age group (Beatty, 2006).

Dementia is an illness of the cognitive system and is not accepted as a normal change of aging. Dementia is defined by the World Health Organization (2007) as "A syndrome due to disease of the brain, usually of a chronic or progressive nature, in which there is a disturbance of multiple cortical function, calculation, learning capacity, language, and judgment. Consciousness is not clouded. Impairments of cognitive function are commonly accompanied and occasionally preceded by deterioration in emotional control, social behavior or motivation" (p. 1). Cognitive alterations are key symptoms indicating changes in physiological function among the aged. Preliminary reports from a recent Mayo Clinic (2006) study suggest that about 12% of those over the age of 70 have mild cognitive impairment. People with MCI are three to four times more likely to develop Alzheimer's than those without such impairment.

Two main types of dementia exist. The first type is **multi-infarct dementia**, which is caused by the death of brain tissue and diagnosed through brain imaging. Tissue death may be caused by of a lack of blood flow to the brain from a cerebral vascular accident (CVA) or from another cause. The other main type of dementia is **Alzheimer's disease**, the most common type, which makes up about 50% of all dementia diagnoses. The Alzheimer's Association estimates that approximately 5 million U.S. adults have Alzheimer's disease. Other dementias include Parkinson-related dementia, Huntington disease, Creutzfeldt-Jakob disease, Pick disease, and Lewy body dementia. Each one involves cognitive processes as defined above, although cognitive symptoms may vary depending on the area(s) of the brain affected by the disease (Alzheimer's Association, 2007).

The symptoms of dementia include forgetfulness, inattentiveness, disorganized thinking, altered levels of consciousness, perceptual disturbances, sleep-wake disorders, psychomotor disturbances, and disorientation. All older adults should be assessed for dementia and again if these symptoms arise. One tool that has been used successfully to screen for cognitive impairments among older adults is the **Mini-Mental State Examination (MMSE)** (Folstein et al., 1975) (Figure 24-3). This instrument was developed to assess the baseline mental status of older adults and to evaluate change or decline in mental functioning.

Mini Mental Status Examination Sample Items

Orientation to Time

"What is the date?"

Registration

"Listen carefully,

I am going to say three words.

You say them back after I stop.

Ready? Here they are...

HOUSE (pause), CAR (pause), LAKE (pause).

Now repeat those words back to me."

[Repeat up to 5 times, but score only the first trial.]

Naming

"What is this?"

[Point to a pencil or pen.]

Reading

"Please read this and do what it says."

[Show examinee the words on the stimulus form.]

CLOSE YOUR EYES

Figure 24-3   Mini Mental State Examination sample items. (Reproduced by special permission of the Publisher, Psychological Assessment Resources, Inc., 16204 North Florida Avenue, Lutz, Florida 33549, from the Mini Mental State Examination, by Marshal Folstein and Susan Folstein, Copyright 1975, 1998 by Mini Mental LLC, Inc. Published 2001 by Psychological Assessment Resources, Inc. Further reproduction is prohibited without permission of PAR, Inc. The MMSE can be purchased from PAR, Inc., by calling 800-331-8378 or 813-968-3003.)

The MMSE is based on a 30-point scale that measures level of awareness and orientation, appearance and behavior, speech and communication, mood and affect, disturbances in thinking, problems with perception, and abstract thinking and judgment. The higher the older adult scores on the examination, the more intact the mental status is presumed to be. When the scale is 23 or lower, the individual is determined to have a problem with cognition. It is important to note that this instrument has been criticized for its cultural insensitivity, and it is difficult to use among individuals who speak languages other than English and among those with visual impairments and low literacy.

The MMSE is relatively easy to perform after a little practice and has been used for initial and subsequent evaluation of older adults in a variety of settings. The most effective way to perform the assessment is to make the person comfortable and establish a rapport. Eliminating noise and promoting attention and concentration will allow individuals to answer questions to the best of their ability. After the examination, the score can be computed and used as a basis for care planning.

Nonpharmacological techniques for managing the problems associated with dementia include developing and keeping routines; working in a calm, gentle, and unhurried manner; encouraging self-care activity; and reducing sensory overload. Interventions to keep the older adult safe include curtailing wandering behavior and preventing falls, cuts, and bruises. Medications to treat Alzheimer's disease are known as cholinesterase inhibitors. These medications are most effective during the early stages of the disease and act by increasing the levels of acetylcholine in the brain to prevent further loss and improve cognitive status.

Researchers are testing the effectiveness of an Alzheimer's vaccine. Brain swelling in the study participants, however, has slowed testing on this vaccine. In 2002, researchers halted a clinical trial of the first Alzheimer's vaccine after about 6% of the 375 volunteers with Alzheimer's developed brain inflammation. The vaccine, a synthetic form of beta-amyloid protein, was designed to trigger the body's immune system to create antibodies against beta-amyloid. Researchers tracked the health of 159 of the subjects for four and a half years, and found that the 25 persons who had built up an antibody response did better on memory tests and were less dependent on their caregivers. Several laboratories are now in the process of testing another vaccine they believe is safer and just as effective (Shute, 2007).

Another medication that has shown some promise in treating Alzheimer's disease is Namenda, or memantine. The action of memantine differs from that of cholinesterase inhibitors but works well in combination with this class of drugs and appears to be well tolerated. Lithium is also being suggested as a possible medication to suppress the development of α-amyloid plaque formation among people who already have the disease. However, the cardiovascular and central nervous system side effects of this medication make it difficult for the older adult to tolerate.

Stereotypes suggest that older people are less capable of learning and lose their intellectual capacity, but research has not supported this notion. Consistent with the two previous studies, expectations for intellect increased from adolescence to young adulthood; however, these expectations did not then decline from middle age to old age, instead appearing to increase nearly linearly across all age groups. Also, as expected, the expected mean-level differences across age groups appeared smaller in this study than the previous studies following the separation of target age and role information. Nonetheless, the majority of the findings again showed strong agreement between the pattern of personality expectations for age and the actual pattern of personality changes exhibited over the life span (Wood & Roberts, 2006).

Nurses encourage older individuals to take classes, read, engage in stimulating conversation and entertainment, keep their minds active, and continue learning throughout their lives. They are encouraged to continue with self-care activities rather than to relinquish them to caregivers. Because some memory impairment may be present in cognitively healthy older adults, memory aids and familiar environments are to be encouraged (Research Highlights box).

---

research highlights

Assisted Living Facilities for Older Adults

The number of assisted living facilities has increased greatly over the past decade because older adults have been attracted by the facilities' philosophical emphasis on maintaining independence and privacy. A study by Hawes et al. (2003) examined the extent to which these facilities are meeting the philosophical ideals of older adults that they aim to serve. The data revealed that only 11% of the 11,459 facilities offered a high level of services and privacy. Aging in place, or the ability of the older adult to live in the facility when health conditions decreased functional ability, was limited by the policies in these facilities. The authors concluded that the practice of assisted living facilities does not always live up to their philosophy.

Data from Hawes, C., Phillips, C. D., Rose, M., Holan, S., & Sherman, M. (2003). A national survey of assisted living facilities. *The Gerontologist*, *43*, 875–882.

Sensory Factors

Older adults experience several age-related changes in the five senses. Because of the normal and pathological changes associated with their senses, individuals of all cultural backgrounds and in all settings can benefit from nursing interventions. A variety of structural changes cause visual acuity to decrease, color discrimination to become less acute, pupil size and constriction ability to decrease, and peripheral vision to diminish. The lens of the eyes become yellow and predisposes them to **cataracts**. The older adult is at increased risk for **glaucoma**, a group of eye disorders characterized by increased intraocular pressure. Because of the normal changes in the aging eye and the high risk for disease, a baseline eye assessment should be done early in this stage of life. Based on the normal changes and any disease processes assessed, follow-up eye appointments should be scheduled at least annually. Safety, particularly while driving, is a concern for older adults and society. Nurses should encourage them to take driving classes that will help them deal with the diminishment of certain senses and learn how to become safer drivers as these changes occur.

Hearing deficits are common in old age, resulting from inner ear **atrophy** or **sclerosis** of the tympanic membrane. The inner ear can also undergo a number of changes, including those that are cell degenerative and nerve related. Sound threshold changes, with an associated difficulty in understanding what others are saying. Similar to the changes of the eye, changes in hearing and high risk for pathology indicate that older adults should begin regular ear and hearing screening early in this stage of life. On the recommendation of the audiologist, audiological testing should be conducted at least annually. Hearing aids can assist those with hearing loss to communicate more effectively. Wallhagen and Strawbridge (2003) report that there is a relationship between hearing impairment and cognitive impairment in this population. Several studies also point to a significant correlation between hearing loss and loss of cognitive functions. Most of these studies show such a correlation without being able to show whether the hearing loss caused the reduction in cognitive performance or if both the hearing loss and the cognitive decline are parts of a common, general age-related degeneration (Arlinger, 2003).

The nurse assesses, on an ongoing basis, for the buildup of wax to ensure optimal hearing (see the Case Study and Care Plan at the end of this chapter).

Taste changes with aging because of a loss of taste buds. The flavors of sweet, sour, salty, and bitter become blurred with this loss. The sensations brought about by touch may also diminish with sensory nerve losses, especially in the presence of debilitating diseases such as diabetes, stroke, or Parkinson's disease. The ability to smell and the acuity of the olfactory nerve also decrease with age. Because of the loss of smell and taste sensations, older adults have the tendency to use large, perhaps unsafe, amounts of salt and sugar in their food. Teaching about safe cooking and seasoning of food may be appropriate. Additionally, cognition related to common danger signals such as smoke or rotten food is impaired. Older adults should be taught to check the dates on their food packages frequently and be attentive when cooking and preparing meals. The United States Dietary Association (USDA, 2005) recommends that infants and young children, pregnant women, older adults, and those who are immuno-compromised should not eat or drink raw (unpasteurized) milk or any products made from unpasteurized milk, raw or partially cooked eggs or foods containing raw eggs, raw or undercooked meat and poultry, raw or undercooked fish or shellfish, unpasteurized juices, and raw sprouts.

The loss of taste and smell sensations, combined with the many other problems of obtaining appropriate nutrition, makes dental care of vital importance to this population. Lack of fluoridated water and preventive dentistry during the developmental years have caused tooth and gum problems to prevail in the older population. Tooth loss among adults is a common contributor to decreased taste sensation. In fact, *Healthy People 2010* has established goal 21-4, to decrease the number of older adults who have had all of their natural teeth extracted (USDHHS, 2007). The inability to chew and swallow food in a comfortable manner works synergistically with decreased smell and taste sensations and other problems to inhibit proper nutrition. The American Dental Association recommends that adults be seen for oral hygiene and counseling at least twice a year. During the initial evaluation, follow-up visits should be scheduled to ensure that teeth and gums remain in good condition or that appropriate dental devices are being used.

Skin changes, becoming thinner, wrinkled, and more fragile. Although sweating decreases and injuries take longer to heal, the skin remains capable of sensing and carrying out its protective role. However, chronic disease can place an individual at risk for decreased sensation throughout the body. Cerebral vascular accidents (CVAs) (strokes) or neuropathies resulting from diabetes are two examples of diseases that disrupt the ability to feel pain and pressure through the skin. This lack of sensation can threaten safety. When older adults are homebound, information about cooking on a hot stove and bathing and showering is provided to prevent burns. The nurse should perform frequent skin assessments to detect alterations in skin integrity at an early stage.

The potential for skin impairment is common for those who suffer sensory deprivation from physical disease or dementia. A pressure sore (**decubitus ulcer**) is a localized area of tissue necrosis that develops when soft tissue is compressed between two bony prominences or between a bony prominence and an external surface for a prolonged period. In addition to prolonged pressure on the skin, friction, moisture, shearing, and lack of nutrition place the older adult at risk of developing a decubitus ulcer, which is difficult to treat. Preventing the ulcer is the best method for maintaining intact skin. People at risk for decubitus ulcers should shift their position at least every 2 hours to distribute pressure appropriately throughout all areas of

the skin. Elevating the lower extremities and maintaining proper body alignment are imperative to prevent decubitus ulcers. Specialty beds are readily available in most care settings to decrease pressure and assist in positioning individuals who are at risk. Positioning pillows and other orthopedic devices provide ways to help maintain the proper support of body parts and body alignment. Proper nutrition, including zinc and vitamins C and E, will help prevent this skin problem.

Self-Perception–Self-Concept Pattern

The variability of self-concept in the older adult is similar to the variability that is seen in the general population. As in all aspects of health, culture, environment, family, lifestyle factors, and heredity combine to form self-concept. Self-concept includes an individual's attitudes, perception of abilities (cognitive, affective, or physical), body image, identity, general sense of worth, and general emotional pattern. Personality traits tend to remain constant throughout life.

Erikson's Theory

The prevailing belief holds that adults no longer grow either emotionally or physically in their later years. Although the rate of physical decline exceeds the rate of physical growth, no evidence was found that emotional growth declines in any way. One needs only to view the classic film *Driving Miss Daisy* to understand that older adults go through many developmental changes in the 30 to 40 years that often make up older adulthood. Erikson's theory of development (1982) asserts that older adults must pass through developmental stages as do infants, children, and younger adults. As in all stages of psychosocial development, unsuccessful passage through a stage yields psychological illness, and successful passage through the stage promotes health (Erikson, 1982).

Ego integrity versus despair is the developmental stage of older adults (Erikson, 1982). The quality associated with successful passage of this stage is integrity, defined as an honest acceptance of the life that has passed and the stage of life that is currently being lived. Individuals who have reached this stage are said to be at peace with themselves. The inability to reach this stage leads to fear of death and despair that life has been lived in vain. Based on the expanding life span, this stage of development was expanded into three additional stages: (1) **ego differentiation versus work role preoccupation**, which involves achieving identity apart from work; (2) **body transcendence versus body preoccupation**; which focuses on adjusting to normal and aging changes, and (3) **ego transcendence versus ego preoccupation**, which involves accepting death (Erikson, 1997).

Nurses working in all settings are charged with helping older adults successfully pass through Erikson's psychosocial stages, enabling them to reach ego integrity. Two successful methods of assistance for older adults at all cognitive levels are *reminiscence* and *life review*. Haight (2005) defines these as, "**Reminiscence** is a multifaceted, multipurpose, naturally occurring mental phenomenon manifested across the life span in a variety of forms and contexts. **Life review** is one of those forms of reminiscence but it differs in that it is more intense and has more depth." Haight et al. (2000) found a positive effect of reminiscence on reducing depression. The typical reminiscence session takes the form of a semistructured, 45-minute to 1-hour meeting focusing on positive memories and the process, rather than product.

Roles-Relationships Pattern

Although the general framework of self-perception remains constant throughout the life span, the source of an individual's self-perception often changes with older adulthood. The formation of the self that has focused on a person's role in the family changes when the children become independent or a spouse passes away. Roles such as daughter, son, sister, brother, wife, or husband may be lost because of death or illness. The loss of these roles can bring a great deal of sadness and possibly depression to the older adult. On the other hand, with the loss of these roles, a new role, such as grandparenting, frequently evolves (Figure 24-4). In the United States, 5.8 million, or 3.6%, of grandparents are raising grandchildren (Simmons & Dye, 2003). The role of grandparent frequently brings great joy and happiness at a time when the older adult feels loss; however, grandparents who rear grandchildren encounter several issues. A study by Ross and Aday (2006) investigated the degree of stress in 50 African American grandparents (M = 63.12 years) who are raising their grandchildren and identified the importance of caregiver characteristics, the caregiving situation, and specific coping strategies that influence stress. Data were collected via interview at senior centers and

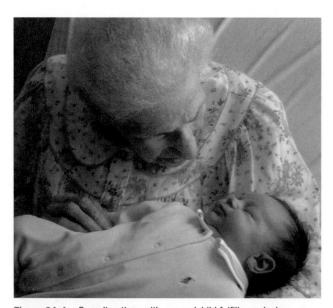

Figure 24-4 Spending time with a grandchild fulfills a relaxing pleasure for the older adult.

churches in Harris County, Texas. The instruments used to measure stress and coping were the Parenting Stress Index and the Ways of Coping Questionnaire. Of grandparents, 94% reported a clinically significant level of stress. Use of professional counseling, special school programs, and length of caregiving longer than 5 years were associated with less stress. Coping strategies significantly correlated with less stress included accepting responsibility, confrontive coping, self-control, positive reappraisal, planned problem solving, and distancing. This study adds to the limited information about custodial grandparents and suggests counseling, support groups, and education to help them manage stress associated with their caregiving situation more effectively.

Encouraging and supporting older adults in this role is necessary to help them fill the void left by the loss of their job or spousal roles, and to prevent the stress and strain of this caregiver role.

With the average life span increasing, older adults can spend many more years in retirement than did previous generations. There were approximately 49 million social security beneficiaries at the end of 2006 (Social Security Administration, 2007) up from an estimated 27.2 million retirees reported in December 1997. In a large government study regarding retirement influences (USDHHS, 2007), respondents who said they were completely retired in 2002 were asked about four possible influences on their decisions to stop working: poor health, wanting to do other things, not liking their work, and wanting to spend more time with family. More than one third of those who retired between 2000 and 2002 said that spending more time with their families was a very important reason for retirement, and roughly one fourth also cited "wanting to do other things." Poor health was a very important factor for 35% of retirees in the 55 to 59 age category, but the importance of poor health as a motivating factor for retirement dropped consistently with increasing age. In keeping with findings noted earlier in this chapter about enjoyment of work, fewer than 10% of respondents were motivated to retire by a strong dislike of their work.

Another researcher used 2000 HRS data to gauge people's overall retirement satisfaction (Panis, 2003). When retirees were asked how satisfying their retirement has turned out to be, a majority (61%) said "very satisfying." One third of respondents reported moderate satisfaction, and only 7% indicated that their retirement was not at all satisfying.

Further assaults on the individual's self-concept may include a lowered income, loss of friends, disease, and disability. Volunteering can be an effective method for older adults to continue to feel engaged in the working environment as a productive, contributing member of society. Older adults who volunteer have an external incentive for getting dressed in the morning; they take a great amount of pride in their work. Filling a volunteer position can remedy negative feelings about retirement and other role changes.

Federal and state funding has created a number of subsidized work programs for older adults. With the assistance of this funding through private agencies and local Area Agencies on Aging, they are given the opportunity to work for pay. Although the pay may not be comparable with that earned before retirement, the earnings can be a necessary supplement, after the age of 70, to Social Security benefits. These programs allow older adults to work with children in day care centers, with disabled and ill older adults at home, and in administrative positions. Nurses should provide interested individuals with information about these programs.

Leaving home, widowhood, retirement, and relocation can elicit profound feelings of loss. Older adults who remain engaged in a variety of activities and relationships are happier and healthier. Personality, and its expression over time, is considered as a major determinant of how engaged or active a person will be late in life. Other variables such as culture, health, bereavement, and habit affect activity as well.

Health-promotion activities center on an understanding of the individual's usual behavior and any unexpected or unexplained deviation in that behavior. Nurses help older adults identify the meaning of their lost roles and the results of those losses, and to work through reactions to the loss. In more traumatic cases, support groups, such as bereavement groups, can be helpful. The nurse supports those going through role changes by eliciting reactions and facilitating communication about these reactions. Significant others, such as children, neighbors, and friends, can provide important ongoing support. The nurse is integral in helping older adults develop and explore their new role as grandparents.

Sexuality-Reproductive Pattern

Within the World Health Organization's (2004) definition of sexuality, it states that "physical, emotional, mental and social well-being of an older adult is related to sexuality." A great deal of debate has taken place over the presence or absence of sexual desire among older adults. Society generally believes that older adults do not participate in sexual relationships. The myths regarding sexual activity among older adults include the following:

- Older adults are no longer interested in sex.
- Medical illnesses common to older adults prevent them from having sex.
- **Impotence** is a normal aging change (Wallace, 2000).

The most accurate predictor of sexual interest in older adulthood is the enjoyment and frequency of sex at a younger age. No data were found to show that men or women lose interest in sexual activity as they age. Older adults also fulfill the human need to touch and be touched. Touch is an overt expression of closeness and an integral part of sexuality. Although the need to express sexuality continues, older adults are susceptible to many disabling medical conditions, such as cardiac problems, arthritis, and normal aging changes, and these can make the expression of sexuality difficult. In both genders, reduced availability of sex hormones results in less rapid and less extreme vascular responses to sexual arousal. The lack of circulating hormones in both men and women results in changes in four areas of the sexual system: arousal, orgasm, postorgasm, and extragenital changes. Management of a medical condition can hinder sexual response.

Nurses are in an ideal position to help older adults fulfill their sexual desires by helping them to compensate for normal aging changes and disabling medical conditions and medications. Knowledge is essential to the successful fulfillment of sexuality. In a study of 68 older adults living in the community, Walker and Ephross (1999) found that the group was able to answer only 67% of sexual knowledge questions correctly.

After making a sexual assessment, nurses can intervene at an early point to prevent or correct problems, but they frequently choose not to consider sexuality when planning care. One of the reasons for this refusal is that nurses believe the societal myths about older adults' sexuality. Without proper training and experience, they are not sufficiently confident to venture into this delicate area.

One method in which they may gain knowledge is through a game aimed at educating nursing staff about sexual dysfunction in older adults. This may be accomplished through staff development in-services in which nursing staff are asked to role play older adults in the situation and discuss feelings associated with lack of ability to fulfill relationships. The expression of sexuality among older adults results in a higher quality of life achieved through fulfilling a natural desire. In long-term care facilities, the need to address sexual needs of the residents is great because of their many disabilities. In the community setting nurses have access to the entire family unit in their natural surroundings. The information that is necessary to make a sexual assessment is readily accessible.

Many nurses believe that acquired immunodeficiency syndrome (AIDS) and other sexually transmitted diseases are not problems for older adults. However, the number of older adults who have contracted the human immunodeficiency virus (HIV) has risen sharply over the past decade. Of all AIDS cases 11% to 15% are among people aged 50 and older and this number is projected to increase with the rising lifespan (*www.HIVoverfifty.org*). Older adults should use proper precautions, such as a barrier method, to prevent the spread of disease. Nurses use universal precautions to protect themselves from HIV and other blood-borne pathogens. Older adults should follow the safer sex guidelines recommended by the CDC.

Coping-Stress Tolerance Pattern

An individual's ability to cope with the common stresses of older adulthood is a key factor in maintaining self-concept and subsequent integrity. As people age, they tend to encounter many losses, such as the loss of a home, physical functioning, spouses, friends, and siblings. The nurse who cares for the older adult can be extremely helpful in the coping process. In a sample of 99 older adults, it was found that continually thinking about a loss or bad event was not as effective as trying to find the positive and developmental benefits of losses. In a study aimed at exploring the relationships between cognitive–emotion regulation strategies and depressive symptoms, significant relationships between depressive symptoms and the cognitive emotion regulation strategies of Rumination, Catastrophizing, and Positive Reappraisal were found. Whereas Rumination and Catastrophizing were positively related (the more the strategy was used, the more symptomatology), Positive Reappraisal was negatively related. In addition, Self-blame showed significant positive effects in all samples but the older adults. None of the samples showed significant relationships between depressive symptoms and other-blame. (Garnefski & Kraaij, 2006). Cultural background has a profound effect on the manner in which coping with stresses occurs. After assessing the most appropriate way in which the individual desires to cope with a situation, the nurse may help create an appropriate environment for coping. The spirituality of older adults is also an important consideration for the care of older adults. Spirituality is very individualistic and may be exercised privately or through a religious framework. However, the impact of spirituality on quality of life has been well documented among older adults and often has a strong relationship with older adults' ability to cope and manage stress related to illness and life changes.

Depression

Among older adults, **depression** mainly affects those with chronic medical illnesses and cognitive impairment, causes suffering, family disruption, and disability, worsens the outcomes of many medical illnesses, and increases mortality (Alexopoulos, 2005). Aging-related and disease-related processes, including arteriosclerosis and inflammatory, endocrine, and immune changes, compromise the integrity of frontostriatal pathways, the amygdala, and the hippocampus, and increase vulnerability to depression. Heredity factors might also play a part. Psychosocial adversity—economic impoverishment, disability, isolation, relocation, caregiving, and bereavement—contributes to physiological changes, further increasing susceptibility to depression or triggering depression in already vulnerable older individuals (Alexopoulos, 2005).

According to *Healthy People 2010* (USDHHS, 2007) (see *Healthy People 2020*), adults and older adults have the highest rates of depression. Rates are especially high among those with coexisting medical conditions. Research further reports that 12% of older people hospitalized for problems such as hip fracture or heart disease are diagnosed with depression. Rates of depression in nursing home residents range from 15% to 25%. The cause of this increase is not completely understood. The numerous losses experienced by older people may be partly to blame. Depression is also caused by physiological changes in the aging body. As a manifestation of an individual's self-concept, this disease has been

the subject of detailed study. Although it appears to affect older adults in much the same way that it affects younger individuals, certain patterns of symptoms and older adults' overall susceptibility are different from those of younger counterparts.

Nurses are integral in helping to diagnose and manage depression in older adults. Depression can be found in all care environments. Some common behaviors include sullen affect, lack of appetite and weight loss, sleeplessness, fatigue, decreased ability to think or concentrate, psychomotor agitation, decreased participation in daily living activities and social activities, and suicidal ideation. Many instruments are available to assist nurses in assessing for this commonly occurring disorder. The Geriatric Depression Scale (Yesavage et al., 1983) is available in several formats, with 30, 15, 5, and 1 question, and is easily administered. This scale is presented in **Website Resource 24A**. Positive results on the screening examinations require referral to social services for a diagnostic workup. After depression is diagnosed, successful management may include antidepressant medications and psychosocial therapy.

Suicide

According to the CDC and unpublished mortality data from the National Center for Health Statistics, suicide rates increase with age and are highest among Americans age 65 years and older (CDCP, 2007). Men accounted for 83% of suicides among people age 65 years and older in 1997. From 1980 to 1997, the largest relative increases in suicide rates occurred among people 80 to 84 years of age. The rate for men in this age group increased 8% (from 43.5 to 47.0 per 100,000). Firearms (71%), overdose (liquids, pills, or gas) (11%), and suffocation (11%) were the three most common methods of suicide used by persons aged 65+ years (National Strategy for Suicide Prevention, 2007).

The reason for the high number of suicides in the older adult population continues to be explored. The elevated rate of depression helps the medical community understand the motive of many older adults. Many older adults have serious medical illnesses that provide an explanation for wanting to die. Risk factors for suicide include social isolation, alcohol abuse, psychosis, bereavement, and serious medical illness. Waern et al. (2003) found that family conflict, serious physical illness, loneliness, and both major and minor depressions were associated with suicide in the 75+ group. Economic problems predicted suicide in the younger but not in the older adults. Older adult suicide victims with depression (major or minor) were less likely to have received depression treatment than their younger counterparts.

The importance of different aspects of life also varies by culture. Some older adults may visit a health care provider with a somatic complaint before the suicide attempt as, perhaps, a final call for help. Nurses working with the older population are aware of their high rate of suicide and are alert for the risk factors. Suicide threats are taken seriously and interventions are implemented to keep the older adult safe.

Lourde, K. (2008). Community needs dictate move to home care. *Provider, 34*(1), 18–21.

HOT Topics

COMMUNITY NEEDS DICTATE MOVE: HOME CARE UTILIZATION BY OLDER ADULTS

About 90% of home health users are age 75 and older, and more than half are women. About 43% have limitations in one or more ADLs, compared with 9% of beneficiaries in general. The numbers of Medicare beneficiaries using home health care in 2006 was 2.9 million, a 6.1 % increase over 2005 utilization. With the increase in the population of older adults over the age of 85, as well as the approaching baby boomer generation moving into older adulthood, a continued increase in home care is expected, because most older adults want to be in their own homes surrounded by their loved ones, in addition to being on their own schedule.

The chronic illness that frequently accompanies old age raises a concern for ethical care. Many members of society believe that with the increased life span, individuals can be subjected to more suffering. A solution to ending the suffering of those with chronic illness has been **euthanasia**, or **physician-assisted suicide**. In many states, people are lobbying to legalize physician-assisted suicide. The American Nurses Association maintained in their 1994 position statement that nurses should refuse to participate in assisted suicide. Nurses help society to understand the many benefits of older adulthood and celebrating the extended life span rather than deeming it wasteful. Nurses caring for chronically ill older adults have the added burden of determining which ones are at risk for wanting physician-assisted suicide and helping them to live free of pain and discomfort. Nurses are instrumental in ensuring that the older person experiences a pain-free death by advocating for an appropriate pain-management program and working with other health care professionals toward this end (Hot Topics box).

Values-Beliefs Pattern

Every older adult for whom nurses have the opportunity to care will have a different sense of spirituality, which will have a profound influence on the person's motivation and ability to live a healthy lifestyle. Using a large sample of American adults, analyses demonstrate that subjective spirituality and tradition-oriented religiousness are empirically highly independent and have distinctly different correlates in the personality domain, suggesting that individuals with different dispositions tend toward different styles of religious/spiritual beliefs (Saucier & Skrzypinska, 2006). Although no universal sense of spirituality exists among older adults, many researchers report that spiritual resources are related to mental health.

Nurses may find themselves in a difficult position in attempting to promote the spiritual health of individuals.

One reason for this perceived difficulty may be the nurse's discomfort with the person's belief system. Spirituality can play a significant role in meaning-making in relation to attitudes and beliefs about the world, self, and others. A spiritual process of meaning-making (or seeking significance in an event) can touch on all aspects of life, including work, interpersonal relationships, general philosophy of living, attitudes, and/or whatever that person's "God" may be (Gall et al., 2005).

There may be as many different spiritual values and beliefs as there are individuals. Varying spiritual values make helping older adults actualize their spirituality, and thus acquire a high quality of life, difficult for nurses. Because of the highly personal quality of spirituality, an unobtrusive and sensitive presence by the nurse is needed to allow the person in any setting to achieve spiritual health. Additionally, spiritual assessment tools are available to guide nurses with the right questions to help get to the root of the person's spirituality. Open-ended questions, such as, "What is your perception of a higher being and spirituality?" can encourage discussions about the person's innermost spirituality.

ENVIRONMENTAL PROCESSES
Accidents

Falls are a leading cause of morbidity and mortality among older adults. In 2003, more than 1.8 million older adults were treated in emergency departments for fall-related injuries and 421,000 were hospitalized. Moreover, more than 13,700 older adults died of fall-related injuries. The annual direct cost of falls is currently approximately $19 billion, but is expected to exceed $43.8 billion by 2020 (CDC, 2007). The CDC reports that White men have the highest fall fatality rates, followed by White women, Black men, and Black women (CDC, 2006a).

Some of the causes of falls in older adults are neuromuscular dysfunction, osteoporosis, stroke, and sensory impairment. Although a fall in a younger individual may not be problematic, a fall in an older adult can have devastating consequences. Because of the higher risk of osteoporosis in the older population, a fall can result in a fracture. **Osteoporosis** is a disease of bone loss common to women age 70 and older and men age 80 and older. The disease occurs 6 times more frequently in women than it does in men. The rapid decline in estrogen secretion at the onset of menopause signals the calcium in the bones to move into the bloodstream, which allows the bones to become weak and brittle. Because of this weakness, falls in older adults with osteoporosis frequently result in fractures, which places these individuals in a spiral of iatrogenic risk, beginning with weeks of immobilization and possibly resulting in decubitus ulcers, psychological trauma, pneumonia, and even death.

Risk factors for osteoporosis include a small, thin frame; White or Asian ancestry; family history; excessive thyroid medication or high doses of cortisone-like drugs for asthma, arthritis, or cancer; a diet low in dairy products and other sources of calcium; physical inactivity; smoking cigarettes;

and drinking alcohol. Osteoporosis typically is diagnosed after an older adult sustains a fracture. However, bone density testing is readily available to diagnose individuals at risk before a fracture occurs. Sufficient calcium intake remains vitally important and will continue to reduce the normal bone loss of aging. Most women need 1000 mg a day before menopause and 1500 mg a day after menopause. Consuming this amount of calcium from today's average diet is nearly impossible; therefore, a calcium supplement is essential. For the prevention of osteoporosis and the optimal health maintenance of both psychological and physical well-being in the older adult, physical activity is necessary.

A program to prevent falls is essential in the care of older adults. Because many factors contribute to falls, risk assessment is essential. Recommendations for prevention are abundant in the literature. Close (2005) recommends that all older adults should be screened for falls using valid and reliable fall assessment instruments. Moreover, if a prior fall was sustained, the older adult remains at very high risk for falling again and fall prevention strategies should be implemented. By identifying the risks and assessing an older adult's vision, hearing, medication usage, blood pressure, mobility, and other factors, falls can be predicted and prevented (CDCP, 2007).

Several fall risk assessments have been developed. These instruments are easy to use and can be employed in acute or long-term care or in home settings. After completing the assessment, scores can assist in preventive care planning. Nurses in all settings will then be prepared to implement environmental, physiological, and psychological interventions.

Table 24-2 lists frequent causes of accidents that occur in the home and nursing interventions to prevent them. Home care nurses are in an ideal position to prevent injuries. During the initial and subsequent assessments, the nurse can evaluate individuals' homes for common factors leading to poisoning, fires, and falls, such as frayed wires on electrical appliances that can produce sparks and start fires or improperly labeled cleaning products that can be accidentally ingested. Health teaching should incorporate the concept of accident prevention for all older adults living not only in the community, but also in acute care and long-term care facilities.

The older adult's ability to feel changes in heat and cold may be impaired due to normal and pathological changes of aging. This process can cause older adults to die from the effects of heat waves or cold spells. During periods of heat and humidity, older people should increase fluid and salt intake; they should stay in cool quarters, remain quiet, have more rest periods, and refrain from going outdoors when the temperature goes above 90° F. Sweating, which tends to be delayed and reduced in older adults, can be facilitated by wearing light-colored, lightweight cotton clothing. If sweating ceases or is inadequate, the older person can be at risk for heat stroke. Heat stroke can contribute to sepsis, myocardial infarction, and CVAs, particularly in people with diabetes. Reduced body heat can also present problems in the older

Table **24-2**	Safety Risk Areas and Related Interventions
Area of Attention	**Intervention**
Stairways	Secure handrails
	Stairways illuminated with light switches at both top and bottom
	Nonskid treads for steps
Bedroom	Night lights
	Tacked-down carpet
	Discourage use of throw rugs
	Furniture securely placed that will not obstruct clear pathways
	Extension cords and telephone wires secured and not in walking areas
Bathroom	Handrails used near tub and toilet
	Nonskid mats in tub area
	Bath thermometer for tub hot water
Kitchen	Nonflammable, lightweight clothing when cooking
	Dishes and cooking devices at reasonable heights
	Use stepstools according to specifications and only when not alone
	Keep off wet floor and refrain from using slippery wax
	Never climb on chairs
	Keep emergency numbers near the telephone
	Locks should to be easy to open in times of emergency
	Cook at front of the stove rather than at the back
Living Room	Furniture that is easy to get in and out of
	Fire detectors installed at appropriate places
Outdoors	Stairs free of breaks and cracks, clear of snow and ice
	Safe handrails
	Good lighting for stairs and walkways

adult. Symptoms of and interventions for hypothermia are listed in Box 24-4.

Preventing Injury

Many causes of death by injury exist for older adults. Some of these causes are motor vehicle accidents, falls, suffocation, fires, and poisoning. Because of normal age-related changes and the increased incidence of illness, older adults can experience a decrease in muscle strength and reaction time and may subsequently become more vulnerable to environmental hazards. Decreased sensory acuity and impaired balance further diminish their ability to interpret the environment (CDCP, 2006a).

As the percentage of older adults living in the United States increases, the number of older drivers also increases. Between the years 1994 and 2004, there was a 17% increase in the number of older licensed drivers, making up 15% of all licensed drivers and 15% of all traffic fatalities. Older individuals are at a high risk for hospitalization and death

Box 24-4 Nursing Interventions for Hypothermia

SYMPTOMS
- Cold to touch
- Slow respirations
- Bradycardia
- Low blood pressure
- Slurred speech
- Drowsiness
- Temperature 95° F rectally

INTERVENTIONS
- Warm hands and feet
- Cover with blanket
- Set room temperature to 70° F
- Wear cap to bed at night
- Wear several layers of clothing
- Increase activity
- Decrease alcohol intake

from motor vehicle injuries because of the many changes in their neuromuscular and sensory abilities, which slow response time in emergency situations. The National Center for Statistics and Analysis (2005) reports that most older adult traffic fatalities occur during the daytime and involve other vehicles. Interestingly, in two-vehicle fatal crashes involving both older and younger drivers, the older driver's vehicle was more than twice as likely to be struck than the younger person's indicating a decline in defensive driving as opposed to an increase in aggressive driving among older adults. Older drivers involved in fatal automobile accidents had the lowest blood alcohol level. A survey of 2046 older adults showed that older adults limited or stopped driving because of medical problems or problems with eyesight (Ragland et al., 2004). Some were concerned about getting in an accident or stopped driving because they didn't have anywhere to go.

Older adults are encouraged to relearn how to drive so as to adapt to their neuromuscular and sensory changes. Nurses working in the community may encourage older drivers to contact AARP for driving classes designed to meet their needs. Attending these classes frequently allows savings on car insurance.

Biological Agents

A large emphasis is placed on immunizing young children against disease. However, older adults can require commonly available vaccines that have been shown to lower both morbidity and mortality. In many cases, older adults have not received primary immunization against diphtheria and tetanus. Lack of immunity leaves them vulnerable to illness and death from these two diseases. **Website Resource 24B** lists immunization schedules for older adults.

Influenza

Influenza is a major cause of morbidity and mortality in older adults. The 80 and older population experiences an estimated 200,000 hospitalizations and 36,000 deaths per year due to flu (CDC, 2006b). Despite the increase in immunization rates and recent Medicare reimbursement for the vaccine, influenza immunization rates among older adults in senior housing is approximately only 30% to 60% while the number of older adults receiving the vaccine has improved greatly. The CDC (2006b) reports that influenza vaccination levels increased from 33% in 1989 to 66% in 1999 among older adults, surpassing the *Healthy People 2000* objective of 60%. The vaccine, composed of inactivated whole virus or virus subunits grown in chick embryo cells, is given annually to older adults, especially those with chronic conditions such as pulmonary or cardiac problems and those in long-term care facilities. Vaccination is contraindicated in people who have experienced a reaction to it, and caution should be exercised in administering it to people who have allergies to eggs. A *Healthy People 2010* goal (14-29 a-b) is to increase the number of older adults who are vaccinated annually against influenza and ever vaccinated against pneumococcal disease (USDHHS, 2007). (See developing *Healthy People 2020*.)

Pneumococcal Infections

Estimates indicate that pneumococcal infections were responsible for approximately 90,000 deaths in 1999 (National Institute of Allergy and Infectious Diseases, 2004). Nevertheless, many older adults remain unvaccinated. The CDC recommends that older adults should receive the pneumococcal vaccination. Boosters are recommended among older adults who received the vaccine before the age of 65, if more than five years have passed and among older adults who have received a transplant, have chronic kidney disease, or a compromised immune status. However, many barriers, such as the prevailing myth that receiving the vaccination will result in the disease, prevent older adults from receiving immunization.

Tuberculosis

Commonly referred to as *consumption*, tuberculosis (TB) was the leading killer among infectious diseases from the 19th century into the mid-20th century. The TB organism usually is inhaled and deposited in the lung, where it replicates and causes morbidity and mortality in all populations, especially older adults. The TB epidemic was virtually wiped out with the introduction and appropriate use of various medications. In 1984, however, TB rates began to rise again. The increase in poverty, homelessness, drug and alcohol abuse, and AIDS has produced multiple strains of drug-resistant TB. The CDC estimates that there were 14,097 active cases of TB the United States in 2005 (CDCP, 2007).

The chances of acquiring TB in public areas with adequate ventilation are not significant. Ultraviolet rays from the sun kill the virus. The major risk comes from close contact with individuals who are carrying the TB organism. Nurses who suspect TB infection in older adults should look for these signs and symptoms: cough, fatigue, anorexia, nausea, fever, night sweats, and weight loss. However, atypical symptoms, such as **delirium**, frequently occur in older adults. A tuberculin skin test will indicate exposure to the TB organism, and a chest radiograph can confirm the presence of the disease in the person's lungs.

Therapy for TB includes isoniazid (300 mg a day) and rifampin (600 mg a day) orally for 9 months. Unfortunately, because of the possibility of concomitant altered liver function in older adults, side effects are possible. People must be instructed to take the medications exactly as ordered and not to skip a dose, because undertreatment leads to drug-resistant strains.

Drug Use

Normal changes of aging have a significant influence on drug use in the older adult. The way in which medications are absorbed, distributed, metabolized, and cleared from the body is affected by changes in organ systems and illness. Even when medications are taken as prescribed, age-related changes and disease can increase the risk of undesirable side effects. In addition to problems caused by the processing of drugs, prescription and nonprescription drug use is much higher in the older adult population than it is in the general population. Morley (2003) reports that the use of excessive and often inappropriate medication among older adults remains a significant problem.

One problem in this population is drug-drug interactions. Evidence suggests that as a person ages, the chance of experiencing a drug reaction is increased, and each prescribed or over-the-counter preparation that is taken multiplies the possibility of an adverse reaction. The Beers criteria, developed from the Health Care Financing Administration Guidelines for Potentially Inappropriate Medications in the Elderly, present medications known to place older adults at risk for adverse reactions. Federal government regulations (Omnibus Reconciliation Act) developed in 1987, implemented in 1990, and revised in 1997, have attempted to curtail the large use of unnecessary medications by older adults in long-term care facilities. As a rule, nurses should take a medication history to assess for past drug reactions. Medications should be started at their lowest effective dose and slowly increased as needed.

Many older adults who reside at home take their medications independently. Although self-medication with prescription and over-the-counter medications is an effective method of disease management, little is known about the process of taking medications after the person leaves the health care practice or facility. Although it is often assumed that medications are taken as ordered, sensory disturbances; lack of knowledge; and alternative drug, alcohol, and nutrition practices may present challenges to medication self-administration that interfere with medical management of health problems. Amoako et al. (2003) conducted a study of 39 older adults who lived independently to determine their over-the-counter self-medication practices. The researchers concluded that people may not be aware of risks associated with interactions between medications, as well as concomitant alcohol and caffeine use. Moreover, the Food and Drug Administration (FDA) estimates that between 4% and 18% of adverse drug reactions occur because of misuse or overdosing of over-the-counter medications with an annual cost of $784 million.

One of the major barriers to drug adherence in the older adult is affordability. Prescription drug costs continue to rise annually and Medicare does not usually pay for medications. Recently the Medicare Prescription Drug Improvement and Modernization act of 2003 approved prescription discount drug cards for Medicare recipients. These cards are available to more than 7 million of Medicare's 41 million participants. To be eligible for the discount cards, older adults must apply and, depending on their income, a fee of $30 may be charged. The cards provide discounts on some drugs, but not all. The *American Journal of Nursing* (AJN) (2004) reports that older adults with higher incomes may save more by using other prescription drug plans or by shopping around.

The use of illegal drugs among older adults is a problem that has been around since the beginning of time, but it remains widely unrecognized by health care professionals. Because of this lack of acknowledgment, drug abuse frequently is overlooked. In fact, some of the problems of older adults, such as accidents, neglected personal hygiene, malnutrition, noncompliance, and memory loss, may actually be signs of substance abuse. New tools designed to detect the problems of substance abuse are being developed that will help nurses assess this problem and make referrals to treatment programs.

Alcohol Use

Alcohol problems among older adults have been underestimated and hidden. The National Institute on Alcohol and Alcoholism reports that for women of all ages and for men over 65, more than seven drinks per week or more than three drinks per occasion is considered a risk. It is estimated that the number of adults over age 50 who abuse or are dependent on alcohol will increase 2.5 fold over the next 20 years (Gfroerer et al., 2003).

A report from Brown University (2005) indicates that older adults with alcohol problems were often undiagnosed, but those who received treatment specific to their needs could achieve positive health outcomes. However, a major barrier to treatment is lack of detection. Alcohol abuse in seniors frequently goes unnoticed, because the symptoms can be similar to those of other common problems of aging, and the affected individuals are no longer in the work force where they could be observed. The longer the problem remains undetected, the greater it becomes.

Older adults are more vulnerable to the effects of alcohol, because their systems do not detoxify and excrete as efficiently as do those of younger people. Alcoholism predisposes them to accidents, nutritional deficiencies, disease, and decreased function. Interestingly, when older adults seek treatment for their alcoholism, their prognosis is many times better than it is for their younger counterparts. When alcohol abuse is suspected, referral to a treatment program will help the person conquer the problem and return to a higher level of functioning.

Tobacco Use

Cigarette smoking causes cardiovascular disease, several kinds of cancer (lung, larynx, esophagus, pharynx, mouth, and bladder), and chronic lung disease. Cigarette smoking also contributes to cancer of the pancreas, kidney, and cervix (CDC, 2006c). Aging men of today are perhaps the first generation to smoke practically throughout their adult lives. The results of smoking occur slowly over time, and problems usually are not experienced until lung damage has occurred. Research demonstrates that because smoking can initiate and promote disease processes, it is one of the most important negative predictors of longevity. Other diseases common to smokers are chronic obstructive pulmonary diseases, including bronchitis, asthma, emphysema, and bronchiectasis. Smoking is a particular problem for older adults because of the large number of medications they take and the potential for drug interactions. Nicotine-drug interactions can cause many problems.

Older adults can experience the benefits of smoking cessation even after the age of 65. These people may be more motivated to quit smoking than when they were younger, because they are likely to see some of the damage that smoking has caused and anticipate that smoking cessation will restore their health. Nurses in acute care settings are in an ideal position to assist them in making the commitment to quit smoking while recovering from an acute illness. Nurses in long-term care and community settings also have the opportunity and access to resources to help motivate individuals to quit. Behavioral management classes are available to community-dwelling older adults, who may also be candidates for other nonmedical interventions and nicotine-replacement therapy.

Cancer

Cancer rates for older adults are disproportionately high in the United States. Although only 12% of the population is considered as older adults, more than 50% of all diagnosed cancers are found in this population. The reason for the large proportion of cancer in this country is unknown. Theories include longer exposure to carcinogens, increased susceptibility to cancer in the older body, decreased cellular healing ability, loss of tumor-suppressing genes, and decreased immune function. Although the exact cause cannot be determined, cancer is a significant problem for older adults in the United States.

The types of cancer common to older adults are listed by gender in Table 24-3. Prostate cancer is the leading cancer among men of all races and ages and is clearly the most common male cancer and the second leading cause of death from cancer in men in the United States. Estimates are that 8% of all men in the United States will be diagnosed with

Table **24-3** 2008 Estimated U.S. Cancer Deaths	
Men	**Women**
294,120	**271,530**
Lung and bronchus 31%	Lung and bronchus 26%
Prostate 10%	Breast 15%
Colon and rectum 8%	Colon and rectum 9%
Pancreas 6%	Pancreas 6%
Leukemia 4%	Ovary 6%
Liver and intrahepatic bile duct 4%	Leukemia 3%
Esophagus 4%	Non-Hodgkin lymphoma 3%
Urinary bladder 3%	Uterine corpus 3%
Non-Hodgkin lymphoma 3%	Brain and other nervous system 2%
Kidney and renal pelvis 3%	Liver and intrahepatic bile duct 2%
Other 24%	Other 25%

From Cancer Statistics. (2008). A Presentation from the American Cancer Society (2008). Retrieved July 11, 2007, from *www.cancer.org/docroot/PRO/content/PRO_1_1_Cancer_Statistics_2008_Presentation.asp.* Text reprinted by the permission of the American Cancer Society, Inc. from *www.cancer.org.* All rights reserved.

prostate cancer during their lifetime. Early detection of prostate cancer allows treatment while it is still localized in the prostate gland and highly curable. Evidence suggests that by using a combination of screening techniques, more cases of prostate cancer can be detected earlier. There are three key components of an appropriate prostate screen: (1) symptomatology, (2) prostate-specific antigen, and (3) a digital rectal examination. The four major treatment options for prostate cancer are surgery, radiation therapy, watchful waiting, and hormone therapy.

Breast cancer is the most common cancer in older women of all ages and races in the United States. It is surpassed only by lung cancer as the cause of mortality in women. Reports suggest that one in nine women will develop breast cancer in her lifetime. Three quarters of all breast cancers occur in women over 50. The risk is increased in women whose close female relatives (mothers or sisters) have had the disease. Women who have never had children or had their first child after age 30 appear to have an increased risk. The causes of breast cancer remain unclear. The best protection is early detection and prompt treatment. The American Cancer Society recommends that women have annual mammograms and breast examinations beginning at age 40 and practice monthly breast self-examination.

Nurses help older adults change the habits that place them at high risk for developing cancer. Following nutritional guidelines (as suggested earlier in this chapter), reducing stress, adopting a program of regular exercise, and smoking cessation are a few of the approaches that nurses can advise to promote individual wellness. Periodic monitoring and screening in the form of regular visits with a primary health care provider or community screening can alert older adults to early signs and symptoms of cancers that occur during the later years.

SOCIAL PROCESSES
Environments of Care

The incidence of chronic and acute illnesses, the subsequent decline in functional status, changes in economic status, and changes in family structure frequently place older adults in situations for which they are admitted to acute care facilities or must make a temporary or permanent move into another housing situation or a long-term care facility. When providing health-promotion services to older adults, nurses must take into account that they might live in a number of different settings.

When older adults leave their homes, they enter a continuum of care extending from the acute care facility to the long-term care or community setting (Figure 24-5). Nurses who work in each of the settings on the continuum can promote health to this population in many ways. From the acute care setting through each stage of the continuum until

they return home, opportunities are available for nurses to introduce older adults and their families to community resources (Table 24-4). The acute care nurse has the opportunity to present health-promotion strategies at a time during which individuals perceive the greatest need to change their lifestyle to return to a healthy status. In most cases an acute care admission is a perfect opportunity to introduce health-promotion teaching. However, the acute care nurse may feel frustrated by the inability to see the results of this teaching and may therefore give it a low priority in the plan of care.

Some older adults will rapidly grasp material that they believe will prevent future hospital admissions and restore their health. Visiting nurse appointments, transportation, homemaking and chore services, adult day care, and assistance with grocery shopping or home-delivered meals will help them return to the home care environment better prepared to recover from the illness. Helping older adults to locate adult day care programs, smoking-cessation programs, stress-management workshops, or weight-loss and exercise programs before leaving the hospital will encourage them to enter these programs immediately after discharge, while they are motivated.

Long-term care nurses are able to locate and plan community resources during the resident's stay. Some of the community services discussed will allow a return home to an environment in which health promotion can continue. Community resources that may help older adults who are discharged from long-term care facilities include adult day care programs, support groups and medical resources, telephone information, and referral services. In addition to their role in individual care planning, long-term care nurses can be more involved in institutional policy changes. Recommendations about smoking policies and healthy diets may prompt interdisciplinary changes that will result in improved health for the entire institution.

The geriatric care manager who sees people in their original residences or in housing complexes may be charged with individual health-promotion planning. Home care nurses provide health care information and services to both individuals and their families. The resources available to community health nurses frequently are rich and enable the nurses to draw on a variety of sources to assist them in promoting the health of community-dwelling older adults. Transportation, home-delivered meals, assistance with housekeeping, socialization, exercise programs, and self-help groups are only a few of the health-promotion resources available within the community. Nurses in all settings may take the opportunity to call the town or city older adult services office for information on the many resources available.

Despite the vast growth in geriatric care services across environments of care, there remains a substantial deficiency in the quality of palliative care and an underutilization of Hospice services at the end of life. In fact, 90% of American people indicated that they would prefer to die in their own home, yet only 20% to 25% can expect to die at home or at

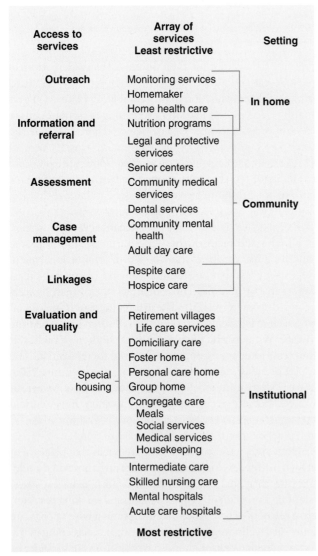

Figure 24-5   Continuum of care for older adults. (From Wetle, T. [1982]. *Handbook of geriatric care.* East Hanover, NJ: Sandoz.)

HEALTH TEACHING   Sleep and the Older Adult

When you believe that you suffer from poor sleep, ask your health care provider about what is considered normal for adults your age. Follow these suggestions to improve your sleep:
- Plan a regular bedtime and wake-up schedule.
- Pursue activities and hobbies.
- Avoid daytime napping; consider any nap you take as part of your sleep total for the day.
- Exercise will help you fall asleep easily, but avoid exercise immediately before bedtime.
- Avoid caffeine after 10:00 AM.
- Avoid drinking too much alcohol.
- Avoid some over-the-counter medications, such as cough syrup and allergy medicine.
- Avoid sleeping medications.
- Avoid tobacco products.

To further your getting a good night's sleep, your bedroom should include the following:
- Quiet surroundings
- Darkness
- Coolness and comfort
- A firm and comfortable mattress

Contact your health care provider if you are experiencing any of the following:

- Sleepiness while driving
- Depression, anxiety, or severe personal stress
- Trouble doing your usual daily activities

How will my health care provider find the cause of my sleep problem?

To find the cause of your sleep problem, your health care provider may:
- Ask you many questions about your health and your family's health
- Ask your sleep companion questions about your sleeping habits
- Ask you to complete a sleep log; in the sleep log, you record whether you were tired during the day, when you fell asleep, how well you slept, and when you woke up
- Perform tests, which may include a blood test or having you fall asleep in a laboratory so that your sleep can be observed
- Refer you to a sleep specialist

What usually causes sleep problems in older adults?

Sleep problems can be caused by many things, including medications; medical conditions such as angina, asthma, or anxiety; poor sleeping habits; and sleep disorders.

Modified from Grand Jean, C. K., & Gibbons, S. W. (2000). Assessing ambulatory geriatric sleep complaints. *Nurse Practitioner, 25*(9), 29–32, 35–36.

a loved one's home (Benoliel, 2001). In the United States a substantial impediment to dying at home is access to home care and knowledge about services that would facilitate a "good death." Hospice care at the end of life is an extremely valuable, yet underused, resource. Hospices cared for only one of every two persons dying from cancer in America in 1995 and the majority of hospice clients were 65 years of age or older (Hoffman, 2005).

There are approximately 3200 hospice programs in the United States. Although inpatient programs are available, hospice originated within a home care model focused on the value of life and the belief that dying is a natural extension of the living process. Consequently, hospice clients are empowered to live with dignity, alert and free of pain. The goal of hospice care is to facilitate a "good death" for individuals. Families and loved ones are consistently engaged in caregiving for the dying and helping them maintain the highest possible quality of life. The environment aims to promote multidimensional aspects of quality of life within the context of differing cultural and spiritual values and beliefs. Nurses in all settings may identify and refer individuals for hospice and facilitate usage of these services to enhance palliative care in all care settings.

The AARP provides many services to people over age 50, including excellent educational materials and community program packages. The topics reflect a broad range of concerns and generally are presented in a self-help manner. Among the topics covered are smoking, exercise, nutrition, and wellness. Each program serves as a guide to negotiate a system or learn more about a health problem. These topics are written in lay terms, are easily understandable, and are printed in large letters to accommodate vision changes. This self-help method is especially important for those who feel uncomfortable addressing questions on finances or sexuality to nurses and physicians.

Two additional environments of care have emerged over the last half of the 20th century in the United States: (1) continuing care retirement communities (CCRCs) and (2) assisted living facilities (ALFs). CCRCs are full-service communities offering long-term contracts that provide older adults with a continuum of care, extending from retirement services through assisted living to skilled nursing, all in one location. The mission behind CCRCs is "aging in place." CCRCs are very expensive and require an entrance fee ranging from $60,000 to $700,000, and a monthly payment ranging from $2500 to $4000. Residence in a CCRC requires commitment to a long-term contract that specifies the housing, services, and nursing care provided. ALFs are defined as homelike settings that promote resident autonomy, privacy, independence, dignity, and respect while providing necessary support. Wallace (2003) reports that the lower cost of ALFs in comparison with that of skilled nursing facilities and the greater emphasis on functional autonomy makes these facilities appealing to older consumers and their families. Although ALF residents have many long-term health care needs, it is important to realize that the role and availability of nurses in these facilities varies greatly by state guidelines.

Table 24-4 Long-Term Care Housing and Assessment Continuum

	Independent Living	Retirement Community	Assisted Living	Nursing Facility
Description	Provides a living arrangement that integrates shelter and services for older people who are functionally and socially independent	Provides a living arrangement that integrates shelter and services for older people who do not need 24-hour protective oversight	Provides a living arrangement that integrates shelter and services for frail older people who are functionally and socially impaired and require 24-hour protective oversight	Provides a living arrangement that integrates shelter with medical, nursing, psychosocial, and rehabilitation services for older people who require 24-hour nursing supervision
Primary services	-A- Environmental security Possibly coordination of resident services (transportation, activities, housekeeping) Or no services are available	-B- "A" plus: Meals (1 to 3 per day) Transportation Activities Housekeeping assistance Assistance with coordination of community-based services	-C- "A & B" plus Assistance with activities of daily living Medication monitoring 24-hour protective oversight	-D- "A, B, & C plus" Medication administration 24-hour nursing supervision
Mobility	Capable of moving about independently OR ambulatory with cane or walker Independent with wheelchair, but needs help in an emergency	Capable of moving about independently Able to seek and follow directions Able to evacuate independently in emergency OR ambulatory with cane or walker Independent with wheelchair, but needs help in an emergency	Mobile, but may require escort or assistance resulting from confusion, poor vision, weakness, or poor motivation OR requires occasional assistance to move about, but is usually independent	May require assistance with transfers from bed, chair, toilet OR requires transfer and transport assistance Requires turning and positioning in bed and wheelchair
Nutrition	Able to prepare own meals; eats without assistance	Able to prepare own meals; eats without assistance. Generally a minimum of one meal a day is available	All meals and snacks are provided. May require assistance getting to dining room or requires minimal assistance (opening cartons or other packages, cutting food, or preparing trays)	May be unable or unwilling to go to dining room. May be dependent on staff for eating or feeding needs OR fully dependent on staff for nourishment (includes reminders to eat or feeding)
Hygiene	Independent in all care, including bathing	Independent in all care, including bathing and personal laundry	May require assistance with bathing or hygiene OR may require assistance, initiation, structure, or reminders. Resident may be able to complete tasks	May be dependent on staff for all personal hygiene
Housekeeping	Independent in performing housekeeping functions (includes making bed, vacuuming, cleaning, and laundry)	Independent in performing housekeeping functions (includes making bed, vacuuming, cleaning, and laundry) OR may need assistance with heavy housekeeping, vacuuming, laundry, and linens	Housekeeping and laundry services provided	Housekeeping and laundry services provided

Dressing	Independent and dresses appropriately	Independent and dresses appropriately	May require occasional assistance with shoelaces, zippers, or medical appliances or garments OR may require reminders, initiation, or motivation	May be dependent on staff for dressing
Toileting	Independent and continent	Independent and completely continent OR may have incontinence, colostomy, or catheter, but independent in caring for self through proper use of supplies	Same as "retirement community" OR may have occasional problem with incontinence, colostomy, or catheter and may require assistance in caring for self through proper use of supplies	May have problem with incontinence, colostomy, or catheter and requires assistance OR may be dependent and unable to communicate needs
Medications	Responsible for self-administration of all medications	Responsible for self-administration of all medications OR may arrange for family or home health agency to establish a medication administration system	Able to self-administer medications OR facility staff may remind or monitor the actual process OR facility staffed by RN or LPN who administers medications	Medications administered by staff personnel or self if assessed as capable
Mental status	Oriented to person, place, and time. Memory intact, but has occasional forgetfulness AND able to reason, plan, and organize daily events. Mentally capable of identifying needs and meeting them	Oriented to person, place, and time AND memory is intact, but has occasional forgetfulness without consistent pattern of memory loss AND able to reason, plan, and organize daily events. Mentally capable of identifying environment needs and meeting them	May require occasional direction or guidance in getting from place to place OR may have difficulty with occasional confusion that may result in anxiety, social withdrawal, or depression OR orientation to time or place or person may be impaired	Judgment can be poor and may attempt tasks that are not within capabilities OR may require strong orientation and reminder program. May need guidance in getting from place to place OR disoriented to time, place, and person OR memory is severely impaired
Behavioral status	Deals appropriately with emotions and uses available resources to cope with inner stress	Deals appropriately with emotions and uses available resources to cope with inner stress AND deals appropriately with other residents and staff OR may require periodic intervention from staff to resolve conflicts with others to cope with situational stress	May require periodic intervention from staff to facilitate expression of feelings to cope with inner stress OR may require periodic intervention from staff to resolve conflicts with others to cope with situational stress	May require regular intervention from staff to facilitate expression of feelings and to deal with periodic outbursts of anxiety or agitation OR maximal staff intervention is required to manage behavior

RN, Registered nurse; LPN, licensed practical nurse.
Modified from Steven Bender (geriatric social worker), Colorado Springs, CO.

Cultural Diversity

The percentage of White older adults is expected to decrease from 1990 to 2030, while the percentage of Black, Asian, and Hispanic members of the population is expected to rise. These changes in cultural background bring unprecedented challenges to the Western health care delivery system. Challenges continue to present in the way that each culture perceives disease origin and management, and the traditional manner in which health is maintained or improved will be changed.

Nurses must be aware of the cultural diversity of older adults for whom they care and the cultural beliefs that influence health care decisions of older adults. Cultural competence refers to the ability of nurses to understand and accept the cultural backgrounds of individuals and provide care that best meets the persons' needs—not the nurses' needs. In order to develop cultural competence the first step is to examine personal beliefs and the effect of these beliefs on professional behavior. This may best be accomplished by conducting personal cultural assessments. After identifying personal cultural biases that influence care, nurses must bracket these beliefs to make sure they do not affect delivery of care. After this step is accomplished, it is important to increase understanding about population-specific health-related cultural values, beliefs, and behaviors. It is important to remember that although an older person may be part of a cultural group, the individual may have become acculturated while living in the United States. A cultural history is therefore an essential first step in determining the person's health care beliefs and practices. When conducting cultural assessments, it is necessary to remember that some of the standardized assessment tools, such as the Geriatric Depression Scale and the MMSE, are available in languages other than English. Caution should be taken in interpreting a tool that has not been formally translated, because the meanings of many words change with cultural background.

The final stage in attaining cultural competence is to develop skills for working with culturally diverse populations. This entails the development of knowledge in working with culturally diverse populations and consistently using those skills with older adults. Conducting cultural assessments, using translation services, and providing culturally competent care are integral components to developing culturally competent institutions and improving care.

Health Care Delivery System

This chapter has brought the need for health-promotion services for older adults into the limelight. Few health care plans pay for health-promotion services. Medicare (the primary health insurance coverage for older adults) offers little coverage for preventive services. Although these people require a wide range of services that ideally exist on a continuum, not all services on this continuum are available regardless of care setting.

Medicare and other federal expenditures for older adults (direct or indirect) constitute a large part of the federal budget. Most goes to old age and retirement programs, disability, and Medicaid. Because of the large percentage of the federal budget consumed by Medicare, this insurance program is undergoing much scrutiny. Legislation to cut the Medicare budget is under review. Lawmakers anticipate that approximately $49 billion in savings could come from more effective use of health maintenance organizations and prospective payment systems instituted in the home. Regardless of the nature of funding cuts, illness prevention contributes to financial stability of the older adult. Nurses will play a key role during the years of Medicare reform in promoting health not only to prevent illness, but also to prevent older adults from losing all their savings and becoming impoverished.

Medigap policies have been promoted to pay for the health care coverage not afforded by Medicare, including prescription drugs (see Drug Use section for discussion of Medicare prescription discount cards). There are approximately nine Medigap policies. Each one provides varying levels of coverage. Choices about whether to purchase coverage for durable health care supplies, prescription medications, and other medical charges must be made to select the most appropriate policy. The charge for the policy varies according to the level of coverage selected. Federal legislation is being explored to improve coverage for prescription medications by Medicare.

Unfortunately, many people are not financially prepared for older adulthood. Although some individuals receive supplemental income from pensions or individual retirement accounts, this situation is rare. Most live on limited incomes. Several resources are available to help those with limited finances live quality lives. Medicaid, authorized by Title 19 of the Social Security Act, is designed to help older adults who are receiving public assistance to pay for medical expenses. Both federal and state governments fund the Medicaid program. To qualify for Medicaid, an individual must have limited income and assets. The coverage afforded by Medicaid is more extensive than that of Medicare. For example, Medicaid covers stays in long-term care facilities, transportation, and prescription drug services. Medicare covers these services only in limited and medically acute situations. Frequently older adults and their caretakers desire the more extensive coverage provided by Medicaid. These individuals are required to "spend down" their assets to be eligible.

Other resources are available to help older adults live this last stage of life in a high-quality manner. Food stamps are available to those who meet certain economic criteria. Food stamps can help them obtain nutritious food at participating markets without depleting their limited budgets. Supplemental medication payment programs assist some in purchasing their prescription medications. When income criteria are met, older adults may be entitled to purchase medications by paying only small co-payments rather than paying the large amount of money that frequently is charged.

Careful financial planning before the onset of illness is ideal to avoid the need to spend down assets and to help the older adult live at a desirable income level. This task can be accomplished through meeting with lawyers and financial planners as early in life as 30 years of age. Completing advance directives, including naming a conservator in advance of illness, assists caregivers, physicians, clergy, and the family in making difficult decisions at the end of life, when the affected person is no longer able to make them. The better prepared the older adult is, the easier it is to receive appropriate care and treatment during times of illness. Reverse annuity mortgages are one option for increased income during the later years. A reverse annuity mortgage is obtained when a bank or private business purchases the home of an older adult. The bank pays the person a set amount of money each month until the house is paid for in its entirety. The senior continues to live in the home. This approach provides the person with necessary funds and negates the need to move and sell the house if an illness arises.

Long-term care insurance is a newer option for those planning for the possibility of long-term care. As with other insurance programs, younger adults can purchase a policy, now widely available from reputable insurance agents. A premium is paid each month that entitles the beneficiary to receive long-term care benefits at home, in assisted living, in day care, or in a long-term care facility. Older individuals are cautioned to explore the many options available for this type of insurance. The benefits and coverage vary, and exclusions frequently are written into the contract to prevent care in certain situations. An important feature of these policies is the option to hire a personal caregiver if the need should arise.

Because population shifts have created a large number of older adults in the United States, political movements toward protecting older adults' rights are abundant and strong. Nowhere is there more political activity than among the groups responsible for social policy and aging. However, this large number has created problems of consistency, equity, and authority. Several large programs, including those directed by the Social Security Administration, the Health Care Financing Administration, and the Department of Veterans Affairs, have coordination problems because of their size and the large number of cases they handle.

The nurse who specializes in the care of older adults can do a great deal to promote their health and well-being through education, research, and practice. Educational curricula should be evaluated continually to ensure that content is appropriate and accurate with respect to aging. The quality of care depends on the clinician's knowledge base. Education for the older person is equally important and begins with an assessment of the individual's level of understanding of health-promotion activities.

Health-promotion research for this population is only beginning. A great deal more remains to be done in exploring the concepts of health promotion, relating these concepts,

and developing and testing hypotheses. Research may best begin with an attempt to debunk commonly held beliefs. Defining some of the concepts of health promotion, such as quality of life and functional ability, will yield immeasurable amounts of information that can be tested. Eventually, with the commitment of qualified nurses, health promotion will be respected for the integral role it plays in the quality of life of these people.

SUMMARY

Life expectancy is now beyond 75 years for both men and women, with the fastest-growing age group being those older than 85. This phenomenon is indeed wonderful. However, aging causes physiological changes in many bodily functions. Although some of these changes are benign, older adults have a higher frequency of illness than the younger population. The many physical, emotional, and role changes of aging are complicated by the great diversity in cultural backgrounds. Older adults who have immigrated to the United States have brought with them different languages, spiritual patterns, eating habits, views toward modern medicine, and other customs foreign to U.S. culture. Culturally competent health-promotion services are integral to helping them lead high-quality lives throughout their extended life spans.

Many problems of old age are related to lifestyle. Changes in nutritional needs, sleep patterns, and activity level are required to adapt to normal and pathological processes. Psychological health depends on reassessing spirituality, self-concept, and role functions. Change and adaptation are possible. With the assistance of nurses and other health care professionals, older adults can be empowered to live their final years with integrity.

Some of the dysfunctional aspects of aging have extrinsic causes, such as environmental pollution. Older adults are as susceptible as any age group is to society's problems, such as homelessness, mistreatment, and drug and alcohol abuse. In conjunction with physiological and pathological changes, cancer, TB, and other disorders can result. Internal and public policy changes will continue to help older adults live in a world in which old age can be the most rewarding stage of life.

CASE STUDY

Unsafe Driving: Larry Johnson

Larry Johnson, a healthy 75-year-old man, lives in his own apartment and is completely independent in ADLs and IADLs. Last Friday morning, Larry left his apartment complex at 8:09 AM to go to the store. While backing out of his driveway, he failed see a school bus passing on the intersecting street, and his car struck the bus. Although no one was injured, this incident indicated the need for a sensory and neurological assessment. The assessment revealed both hearing and visual deficits.

ADLs, Activities of daily living; *IADL*, instrumental activities of daily living.

CARE PLAN

Unsafe Driving: Larry Johnson

Nursing Diagnosis: Risk for Injury Related to Unsafe Driving

DEFINING CHARACTERISTICS

- Altered response time
- Change in vision or hearing

RELATED FACTORS

- Past accident
- Stressful life events
- Receipt of traffic tickets
- Witnessed poor driving

EXPECTED OUTCOMES

- Client will have realistic expectations of ability to drive.
- Client and nurse will set appropriate limitations on driving.

- Client will take a driver refresher course.
- Client will have no further accidents.

INTERVENTIONS

- Assist Larry in registering for a renewal driving program.
- Assist Larry in finding alternative modes of transportation until visual and hearing alterations are corrected and instead of driving in the evening.
- Schedule hearing and vision appointments for Larry and assist in transportation to appointments.

For further information on developing care plans, see: Carpenito-Moyet, L. J. (2008). *Nursing diagnosis: Application to clinical practice* (12th ed.). Philadelphia: Lippincott, Williams & Wilkins.

REFERENCES

American Journal of Nursing. (2004). Pick a card—Any card? *American Journal of Nursing, 104,* 24–26.

Alexopoulos, G. S. (2005). Depression in the elderly. *The Lancet, 365,* 1961–1970.

Alzheimer's Association. (2007). *What is Alzheimer's Diseases?* Retrieved July 11, 2007, from *www.alz.org/Resources/Glossary.asp.*

Amoako, E. P., Richardson-Campbell, L., & Kennedy-Malone, L. (2003). Self-medication with over-the-counter drugs among elderly adults. *Journal of Gerontological Nursing, 29*(8), 10–15.

Arlinger, S. (2003). Negative consequences of uncorrected hearing loss—a review. *International Journal of Audiology, 42,* S17–S20.

Beatty, G. (2006). Shedding light on Alzheimer's. *Nurse Practitioner, 31*(9), 32-45.

Benoliel, J. Q. (2001). Illness, crisis, & loss. *Journal of Thanatology and Human Rights, 9*(1), 8–14.

Binder, E. F., Schechtman, K. B., Ehsani, A. A., Steger-May, K., Brown, M., Sinacore, D. R., et al. (2002). Effects of exercise training on frailty in community-dwelling older adults: Results of a randomized, controlled trial. *Journal of the American Geriatrics Society, 50,* 1921–1928.

Brownie, S. (2006, April). Why are elderly individuals at risk of nutritional deficiency? *International Journal of Nursing Practice, 12* (2), 110–118.

Brown University. (2005). Update: late-life alcohol abuse: Finding solutions to a hidden medical problem. *Geriatric Psychopharmaology, 9*(1), 1, 5–6.

Butler, R., & Olshansky, S. J. (2002). Has anybody ever died of old age? *The Gerontologist, 42* (Special Issue 1), 285–286.

Centers for Disease Control and Prevention. (2007). *Preventing falls among older adults.* Retrieved July 19, 2007, from *www.cdc.gov/ncipc/duip/preventadultfalls.htm.*

Centers for Disease Control and Prevention. (2006a). *National Center for Injury Prevention and Control.* Web-based Injury Statistics Query & Reporting System (WISQARS) [online]. Retrieved July 19, 2007, from *www.cdc.gov/ncipc/wisqars.*

Centers for Disease Control and Prevention. (2006b). *Key Facts About Influenza and Influenza Vaccine.* Retrieved July 19, 2007, from *www.cdc.gov/flu.*

Centers for Disease Control and Prevention. (2006c). *Smoking & Tobacco Use Fact Sheet.* Retrieved July 19, 2007, from *www.cdc.gov/tobacco/datastatistics/factsheets/healtheffects.htm.*

Centers for Disease Control and Prevention. (2007). *Falls among older adults.* Retrieved July 19, 2007, from *www.cdc.gov/ncipc/pubres/unintentional_activity/2004/04_FallOAdults.htm.*

Centers for Disease Control and Prevention. (2007). *Suicide: Facts at a glance.* Retrieved July 19, 2007, from *www.cdc.gov/ncipc/factsheets/suifacts.htm.*

Centers for Disease Control and Prevention. (2007). *TB Elimination: Trends in Tuberculosis, 2005.* Retrieved July 19, 2007, from *www.cdc.gov/tb.*

Centers for Disease Control and Prevention and The Merck Company Foundation. (2007). *The state of aging and health in America 2007.* Retrieved from *www.cdc.gov/aging.*

Centers for Disease Control and Prevention, National Center for Health Statistics, National Health Interview Survey (2008).

Close, J. C. (2005). Prevention of falls in older people. *Disability and Rehabilitation, 27,* 1061–1071.

DuBeau, C., Simon, S., & Morris, J. (2006, September). The effect of urinary incontinence on quality of life in older nursing home residents. *Journal of the American Geriatrics Society, 54*(9), 1325–1333.

Erikson, E. H. (1982). *Life cycle completed: A review.* New York: W. W. Norton.

Erikson, E. H. (1997). *The life cycle completed.* New York: W. W. Norton.

Federal Interagency Forum on Aging-Related Statistics. *Older Americans 2004: Key Indicators of Well-Being. Federal Interagency Forum on Aging-Related Statistics.* Washington, DC: U.S. Government Printing Office. November 2004.

Folstein, M. F., Folstein, S. E., & McHugh, P. (1975). "Mini-mental state." A practical method for grading the cognitive state of patients for the clinician. *Journal of Psychiatric Research, 12,* 189–198.

Friis, R. H., Nomura, W. L., Ma, C. X., & Swan, J. H. (2003). Socioepidemiologic and health-related correlates of walking for exercise among the elderly: Results from the longitudinal study of aging. *Journal of Aging & Physical Activity, 11,* 27–31.

Frighetto, L., Marra, C., Bandali, S., Wilbur, K., Naumann, T., & Jewesson, P. (2004). An assessment of quality of sleep and the use of drugs with sedating properties in hospitalized adult patients. *Health and Quality of Life Outcomes, 2*(17), 1–10.

Gall, T. L., Charbonneau, C., Clarke, N. H., Grant, K., Joseph, A., & Shouldice, L. (2005). Understanding the nature and role of spirituality in relation to coping and health: A conceptual framework. *Canadian Psychology, 46,* 88–104.

Garnefski, N., & Kraaij, V. (2006). Relationships between cognitive emotion regulation strategies and depressive symptoms: A comparative study of five specific samples. *Personality and Individual Differences, 40,* 1659–1669.

Gfroerer, J., Penne, M., Pemberton, M., & Folsom, R. (2003). Substance abuse treatment need among older adults in 2020: The impact of the aging baby-boom cohort. *Drug & Alcohol Dependence, 69,* 127–135.

Haight, B. K., Michel, Y., & Hendrix, S. (2000). The extended effects of the life review in nursing home residents. *International Journal of Aging & Human Development, 50*(2), 151–168.

Haight, B. K. (2005). Reminiscence. In J. Fitzpatrick, & M. Wallace (Eds.), *Encyclopedia of nursing research.* New York: Springer.

Harvard Medical School. (2003). Forestalling frailty. *Harvard Women's Health Watch,* 27.

Heilbronn, L., de Jonge, L., Frisard, M., DeLany, J., Larson-Meyer, D., Rood, J., et al. (2006). Effect of 6-month calorie restriction on biomarkers of longevity, metabolic adaptation, and oxidative stress in overweight individuals: A randomized controlled trial. *Journal of the American Medical Association, 295*(13), 1539–1548. Retrieved July 11, 2007, from CINAHL database.

Hoffman, R. L. (2005). The Evolution of Hospice in America: Nursing's Role in the Movement. *Journal of Gerontological Nursing, 31*(7), 26–34.

Lagman, R. L. (2006). Constipation—Not a Mundane Symptom. *Journal of Supportive Oncology, 4*(5), 223–224.

Mauk, K. (2005, August). Health matters: Promoting health and wellness. Conservative therapy for urinary incontinence can help older adults. *Nursing, 35*(8), 20–21. Retrieved July 11, 2007, from CINAHL database.

Mayo Clinic. (2006). *Mild cognitive impairment.* Retrieved July 19, 2007, from *www.mayoclinic.com/health/mild-cognitive-impairment/DS00553.*

Melov, S., Tarnopolsky, M. A., Beckman, K., Felkey, K., & Hubbard, A. (2007). Resistance exercise reverses aging human skeletal muscle. *PLoS One, 5,* 1–9.

Morley, J. (2003). Hot topics in geriatrics (Editorial). *Journal of Gerontology Medical Sciences, 58A,* 30–36.

National Center for Statistics and Analysis. (2005). *Traffic Safety Facts: Older population.* Retrieved July 19, 2007, from *www.nrd.nhtsa.dot.gov/pubs/810622.pdf.*

National Institute of Allergy and Infectious Diseases. (2004). *Pneumococcal pneumonia.* Retrieved May 10, 2005, from *www.niaid.nih.gov/factsheets/pneumonia.htm.*

National Strategy for Suicide Prevention. (2007). *At a glance—suicide among the elderly.* Retrieved July 19, 2007, from *http://mentalhealth.samhsa.gov/suicideprevention/elderly.asp.*

Pang, E. C., Jordan-Marsh, M., Silverstein, M., & Cody, M. (2003). Health-seeking behaviors of elderly Chinese Americans: Shift in expectations. *The Gerontologist, 43,* 864–874.

Panis, C. W. A. (2003). Retrieved at *www.rand.org/pubs/drafts/2008/DRU3021.pdf.*

Quan, S., & Zee, P. (2004). Evaluating the effects of medical disorders on sleep in the older patient. *Geriatrics, 59*(3), 37-47. Retrieved July 11, 2007, from CINAHL database.

Ragland, D. R., Satariano, W. A., & MacLeod, K. E. (2004). Reasons given by older people for limitation or avoidance of driving. *The Gerontologist, 44,* 237–244.

Rank, M., & Hirschl, T. (2005, May). Likelihood of using food stamps during the adulthood years. *Journal of Nutrition Education & Behavior, 37*(3), 137–146. Retrieved July 11, 2007, from CINAHL database.

Ross, M. E., & Aday, L. A. (2006). Stress and coping in African American grandparents who are raising their grandchildren. *Journal of Family Issues, 27,* 912–932.

Saucier, G., & Skrzypinska, K. (2006). Spiritual but not religious? Evidence for two independent dispositions. *Journal of Personality, 74*(5), 1257–1292.

Shute, N. (2007). New Alzheimer's drugs on the horizon. *U.S. News & World Report,* June 12, 2007. Retrieved July 18, 2007, from *http://health.usnews.com/usnews/health/articles/070612/12alzheimersdrugs.htm.*

Simmons, T., & Dye, J. L. (2003). *Grandparents living with grandchildren: 2000.* Retrieved May 6, 2005, from *www.census.gov/population/www/cen2000/briefs.html.*

Sin, M., Belza, B., Logerfo, J., & Cunningham, S. (2005, September). Evaluation of a community-based exercise program for elderly Korean immigrants. *Public Health Nursing, 22*(5), 407–413.

Social Security Administration. (2007). *Social Security Beneficiary Statistics.* Retrieved August 20, 2007, from www.ssa.gov/OACT/STATS/OASDIbenies.html.

Tse, M., & Benzie, I. (2004, December). Diet and health: Nursing perspective for the health of our aging population. *Nursing & Health Sciences, 6*(4), 309–314.

U.S. Department of Health and Human Services (USDHHS). (2001). *Healthy people 2010.* Washington, DC: U.S. Government Printing Office.

U.S. Department of Health and Human Services. (2007). *Healthy people 2010: National health promotion and disease prevention objectives.* Washington, DC: U.S. Government Printing Office. Retrieved April 12, 2007, from *www.health.gov/healthypeople.*

U.S. Department of Health and Human Services (USDHHS). (2007). *Health & Retirement Study.* Retrieved July 17, 2007 from *www.nia.nih.gov/NR/rdonlyres/D164FE6C-C6E0-4E78-B27F-7E8D8C0FFEE5/0/HRS_Text_WEB.pdf.*

United States Dietary Association (USDA). (2005). *Dietary guidelines for Americans, 2005.* Retrieved July19, 2007, from *www.health.gov/dietaryguidelines/dga2005/document/html/chapter10.htm.*

Vinsnes, A. G., Harkless, G. E., Haltbakk, J., Bohm, J., & Hunskaar, S. (2001). Healthcare personnel's attitudes towards patients with urinary incontinence. *Journal of Clinical Nursing, 10,* 455–462.

Waern, M., Rubenowitz, E., & Wilhelmson, K. (2003). Predictors of suicide in the old elderly. *Geronotology, 49,* 328–334.

Walker, B. L., & Ephross, P. H. (1999). Knowledge and attitudes toward sexuality of a group of elderly. *Journal of Gerontological Social Work, 31,* 85–107.

Wallace, M. (2000). Sexuality and intimacy. In A. G. Lueckenotte (Ed.), *Gerontologic nursing* (pp. 244–256). St. Louis: Mosby.

Wallace, M. (2003). Is there a nurse in the house? The role of nurses in assisted living: Past, present, and future. *Geriatric Nursing, 24*(4), 218–221, 235.

Wallhagen, M., & Strawbridge, S. S. (2003). Hearing impairment and cognitive frailty: A five year longitudinal study. *The Gerontologist, 43*(Special Issue 1), 20–21.

Wellman, N., & Kamp, B. (2004, Fall). Federal food and nutrition assistance programs for older people. *Generations, 28*(3), 78–85.

Westley, C. (2004). Sleep: Geriatric self-learning module. *MEDSURG Nursing, 13*(5), 291–295.

Wolf, G. (2006). Calorie restriction increases life span: A molecular mechanism. *Nutrition Reviews, 64*(2 Part 1), 89–92.

Wood, D., & Roberts, B. W. (2006). The effect of age and role information on expectations for big five personality traits. *Personality social psychology Bulletin, 32*(11), 1482–1496.

World Health Organization. (2004). Sexual health—A new focus for WHO. *Progress in Reproductive Health Research, 67,* 1–8.

World Health Organization. (2007). *Definition of dementia.* Retrieved August 20, 2007, from *www.neuroland.com.*

Wyman, J. F. (2003, Mar.). Treatment of urinary incontinence in men and older women. *American Journal of Nursing, 114* (Suppl.), 26–35.

Yesavage, J., Brink, T., Rose, T., Lum, O., Huang, V., Adey, M., et al. (1983). Development and validation of a geriatric depression screening scale: A preliminary report. *Journal of Psychiatric Research, 17,* 37–49.

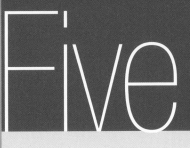

Unit Five

Challenges in the Twenty-First Century

Health Promotion in the Twenty-First Century: Throughout the Life Span and Throughout the World

objectives

After completing this chapter, the reader will be able to:

- Identify global trends and directions for health promotion and disease prevention.
- Discuss problems and implications related to emerging diseases (Community-Associated Methicillin-Resistant *Staphylococcus Aureus*; Multidrug-resistant tuberculosis; and severe acute respiratory syndrome).
- Describe problems and implications related to human immunodeficiency virus/acquired immunodeficiency syndrome.
- Discuss problems and implications related to violence.
- Discuss problems and implications related to bioterrorism.

key terms

Anthrax (*bacillus anthracis*)
Bioterrorism
Botulism
Centers for Disease Control and Prevention
Community-Associated Methicillin-Resistant *Staphylococcus Aureus* (CA-MRSA)

Human immunodeficiency virus/acquired immunodeficiency syndrome (HIV/AIDS)
Malnutrition
Multidrug-resistant tuberculosis (MDR-TB)
Plague
Severe acute respiratory syndrome (SARS)

Smallpox (*variola major*)
Tularemia
Violence
Viral hemorrhagic fevers
World Health Organization
United Nations Millennium Development Goals (MDGs)

website materials

evolve These materials are located on the book's website at *http://evolve.elsevier.com/Edelman/*.
- WebLinks
- Study Questions
- Glossary

Health Challenges in a Developing Country

Rosa lives in Mombasa, Kenya, with her three children, ages 14, 11, and 4 years. She has been a widow for 10 years and has no family members to help her support her family. Her husband's brothers all succumbed to AIDS several years ago, and Rosa has no way to return to what family she has left in the interior of Kenya. Rosa and her children share a room in the harbor with Huwayda, another widow with no children and no family. There are no cooking facilities or running water in the room, so Rosa, Huwayda, and the children must cook on a charcoal fire outside in the street. Water must be hauled from a public well four blocks away. Everyone sleeps on mats on the floor, and it is the oldest child's responsibility each morning to sweep the floor. Rosa can earn a little money by sweeping out local shops before they open in the morning. Huwayda works at the fish market and brings home what leftovers she can from the fish, fruit, and vegetable stalls. None of the children attends school and none has ever been to a clinic or doctor for immunizations or preventive care. Local missionaries provide what food they can to Rosa and Huwayda.

1. What kind of developmental problems would you anticipate that the children might encounter?

2. Visit the World Health Organization Website (*www. who.org*) to identify the incidence and prevalence of HIV and AIDS in Kenya.

3. Who in this family is most at risk for contact with an HIV carrier?

4. What other kinds of health problems do you see not only for the children but for Rosa and Huwayda as well?

Scenario courtesy Doug and Laura Kreftig, Maryknoll Missionaries in Mombasa, Kenya. July, 2004. *AIDS,* Acquired immunodeficiency syndrome; *HIV,* human immunodeficiency virus.

In the new millennium the gap in life expectancies between people in developed and developing cultures has been widening. In many developed nations, such as Japan, France, and the United States, people have a life expectancy at birth ranging from 78 to 82 years (Central Intelligence Agency [CIA], 2007), whereas residents of some countries in Africa, such as Botswana and Swaziland, can have a life expectancy as low as 32 years, due primarily to high rates of HIV infections (CIA, 2007).

In 2002, there were 57 million deaths worldwide: Over 10 million deaths were among children younger than 5 years, and around 98% of these deaths happened in developing countries (World Health Organization [WHO], 2003). The leading causes are related to pregnancy, labor, and postpartum conditions, lower respiratory tract infections, diarrhea, and malaria (Hageman et al., 2006). Malnutrition contributes to all of these causes (WHO, 2003). Researchers in East Timor reported that almost 32% of 880 hospitalized children younger than 12 years old experienced undernutrition (Bucens & Maclennan, 2006). Of these malnutrition cases, 61% were severe and the mortality rate was approximately 13%. In rural Honduras, results showed that 42.4% of boys and girls (*n* = 798) aged 7 to 12 years had stunted growth (a long-term condition of illness and/or inadequate food intake) related to malnutrition (Gray et al., 2006) (Figure 25-1).

International statistics also illustrate a shift in developed countries from infectious diseases to chronic diseases as a primary influence on people's life expectancy. This shift is related to cultural components such as exercise, diet, and smoking (Health Teaching box), among other factors. However, urgent interventions are needed in many developing countries to combat and prevent infectious diseases such as HIV infection.

Emerging infections (i.e., methicillin-resistant *Staphylococcus aureus* and tuberculosis), varied forms of intercultural

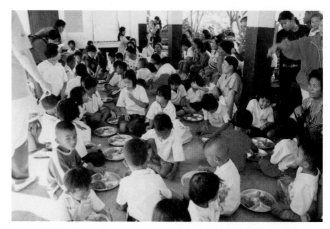

Figure 25-1   Lunchtime for school children in a remote area of Thailand. The food was made possible through donations from health care providers.

and interpersonal violence, and **bioterrorism** also pose great worries and risks to develop and developing countries (Huttlinger, 2004). This chapter presents information on malnutrition, emerging infections, HIV infection, bioterrorism, and violence and discusses their important implications for the future.

MALNUTRITION

The **World Health Organization** (WHO, 2000) defines **malnutrition** as "bad nourishment" that can be associated with "either too much or too little food intake and [is] not limited to the wrong types of food." Malnutrition is characterized by "inadequate or excess intake of protein, energy, and micronutrients such as vitamins." In general, malnutrition can be classified into three categories: protein-energy malnutrition, micronutrients deficiencies, and obesity (WHO, 2000). This chapter will address only protein-energy malnutrition because it is the most serious among the three types (WHO, 2000).

HEALTH TEACHING   Smoking Cessation

Tobacco use is a risk factor for more than 25 diseases, including lung cancer, which is one of the leading causes of cancer-related mortality throughout the world. Negative health effects from smoking account for 438,000 deaths (almost 20% of all deaths) each year in the United States (CDC, 2006b). Tobacco use causes more deaths than other causes of deaths combined (AIDS, illegal drug and alcohol use, motor vehicle injuries, suicides, and murders [CDC]). In Australia, more than 18,000 people annually die prematurely due to smoking (The Non Smokers' Movement of Australia, 2006). Smoking in Australia also causes more deaths than all other death causes combined (alcohol and drug use, violence, motor vehicle injuries, poisoning, drowning, fires, falls, lightning, electrocution, snakes, spiders, and sharks).

According to WHO (2004c), worldwide one third of male adults and one fifth of teenagers aged 13 to 15 years old smoke. Although smoking is on the decline in developed countries, rates in developing countries are rising alarmingly, especially among youths.

- In Cambodia, in the male population, 67% in urban areas and 86% in rural areas smoke. Most smokers are older (50 to 70 years) and monks.
- In China, among the whole population, 67% of men and 4% of women smoke. Among teenagers, smoking rates are 30% for males and 8% for females. One third of cigarettes worldwide are smoked by Chinese, and about 3000 people die daily in China from smoking-related illness.
- In Japan, 51% of the male population smoke. The number of female smokers has increased dramatically during the past 10 years to about 10%. There are very few smoke-free public areas in Japan due to weak laws against tobacco consumption.
- In Malaysia about 50% of the men smoke. There are approximately 50 teenage (younger than 18) new smokers each day. Among teenage boys (12 to 18 years), 30% smoke. Smoking among teenage girls is rapidly rising, from 4.8% to 8% between 1996 and 1999.
- In the Philippines, approximately 60% of the men smoke, and 40% of teenage boys are smokers. There are no laws in the Philippines to prevent children from buying cigarettes.
- In South Korea, 67% of the men smoke. The smoking rate among female adults rose nearly twofold from 3.9% in 1989 to 6.7% in 1997. Throughout the world, South Korea is the eighth largest tobacco market.

School-based interventions and personal contact with teenage groups by nurses can help prevent this harmful activity. A thorough assessment of tobacco use is a necessary part of the health intake.

Compiled from Centers for Disease Control and Prevention. (2004b). *Factsheet: Actual causes of death in the United States, 2000*. Retrieved March 11, 2004, from *www.cdc.gov/nccdphd/factsheets/death_causes2000.htm*; World Health Organization. (2004c). *Smoking statistics: Factsheet*. Retrieved March 11, 2004, from *www.cdc.dov/tobacco/research_data/adults_prev/mmwr5253_highlights.htm*.

Protein-Energy Malnutrition

Protein-energy malnutrition is widespread, especially in resource-poor countries, and can be fatal (WHO, 2000). It can be severely harmful to the mental and physical development of individuals, especially young children under the age of 5 (WHO, 2008). Children born to undernourished mothers have been reported to be at high risk for low birth weight, birth defects, low immunity levels and infection susceptibility, growth retardation, learning disabilities, mental retardation, blindness and, most severely—premature deaths (WHO, 2000, 2004a, 2008). Worldwide, one out of two deaths among children younger than 5 years old stems from protein-energy malnutrition (WHO, 2008). One out of four children are underweight and one out of three are stunted (WHO, 2000).

Severe Malnutrition

Protein-energy malnutrition can be lethal. WHO (2004a) defines severe protein-energy malnutrition as the presence of serious wasting and/or edema. Severe wasting is defined as the weight of a child being less than 70% (or <3 standard deviations) of the median weight-for-height (WHO, 2004a). Severe wasting is caused by loss of subcutaneous and skeletal muscle and is highly noticeable as underdeveloped buttocks, thighs, and upper arms. It is also characterized by sunken eyes, visible ribs, and protruding shoulder blades (WHO, 2004a). Children with severe wasting usually have a distended abdomen and an overall appearance similar in a sense to an older adult. In general, these children are irritable, anxious, and cry easily; yet they will often have an absence of tears while crying due to lachrymal gland atrophy (WHO, 2004a).

Edema in children with under-nutrition is caused by the leaking of potassium from cells, leading to an electrolyte imbalance and fluid retention in the feet, lower legs, arms, and face. The skin of children with edema is abnormally dark with peeling patches and is sensitive to the touch.

WHO (2004a) classifies severe malnutrition into three types: *marasmus, marasmic-kwashiorkor,* and *kwashiorkor.* Children with *marasmus* usually experience severe wasting without any sign of edema; those with *marasmic-kwashiorkor* typically demonstrate both severe wasting and edema; while those with *kwashiorkor* generally have only edema (WHO, 2004a).

When treating children with severe malnutrition who have a co-existing infection of diarrhea or pneumonia, both malnutrition and the co-existing infection need to be addressed simultaneously. A common mistake in clinical practice is that health care providers often try to treat the infection before addressing malnutrition problems. Such a mistake can cause fatal outcomes (WHO, 2004a). According to the WHO's guidelines for management of severe malnutrition among children, necessary treatments should be included to address problems related to: hypoglycemia, hypothermia, dehydration, electrolyte imbalance, infections, micronutrient deficiencies, feeding, physical growth, and mental and behavioral development (WHO, 2004a). A follow-up should be set up before the child leaves a hospital for long-term care and treatment in the community. Parents must be educated about appropriate food, psychosocial stimulation, and regular follow-ups to ensure recovery and appropriate immunizations (WHO, 2004a).

WHO Proposed Model

Generally, poverty causes food insecurity, which, in turn, leads to severe protein-energy malnutrition (WHO, 2000a). A model (Figures 25-2 and 25-3) proposed by WHO illustrates how "Turning the Tide" of malnutrition can replace the "Downward Spiral" of malnutrition and ensure better health and the well-being of children across the globe.

WHO (2000) has worked collaboratively with various organizations and institutions at the global level to create several initiatives to address the malnutrition issue. These include the "Baby Friendly Hospital Initiative" programs to manage nutrition needs during emergencies, global nutrition data banks, and a global network of collaborating centers in nutrition (WHO, 2000).

The "Baby Friendly Hospital Initiative," launched in 1992 by WHO and the United Nations Children's Fund (UNICEF), has as its goal to promote exclusive breastfeeding during the first four months of life when it is most required by the infant (WHO, 2000). The program involves at least 170 countries and over 16,000 hospitals (WHO, 2000). Through

the initiative, a mother starts breastfeeding as soon as her child is born and continues to breastfeed her child exclusively, unless medically otherwise indicated or until the child is 4 months old. This results in avoiding supplemental food and drink until the older child is ready for such intake (WHO, 2000).

The management of nutrition needs during emergencies was established by WHO in collaboration with many organizations, such as international humanitarian aid agencies, UNICEF, the Office of the United Nations High Commissioner for Refugees, and the World Food Programme (WHO, 2000). The goal is to assist people who are experiencing tragedies from wars, political and social turbulences, natural disasters, food shortages, and other complex crises (WHO, 2000). In response to such emergencies, these organizations work closely to rapidly assess needs and to provide for their fulfillment (WHO, 2000). The most recent example of this type of crisis management was the distribution of food and services to people in Sichuan province of China after the 8.0 earth quake that struck May 12, 2008. To learn more about this event as reported by the United Nations (UN, 2008), please follow the link: *www.reliefweb.int/rw/RWB.NSF/db900SID/EGUA-7F4P4B?OpenDocument.*

The global nutrition data banks developed by WHO help in the practical and valuable exchange of information related to malnutrition and include several different databases (as listed below). Please follow the links associated with the database names to learn more about them:

- Global Database on Child Growth and Malnutrition: *www.who.int/nutgrowthdb/en/*
- Global Database on Iodine Deficiency Disorders (IDD): *www.who.int/vmnis/iodine/en/*
- The Micronutrient Deficiency Information System (MDIS): *www.who.int/nutrition/databases/micronutrients/en/index.html*

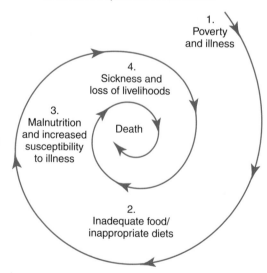

Downward Spiral

Malnutrition is the single most important risk factor for disease. When poverty is added to the picture, it produces a downward spiral that may end in death. At the personal level:

- Poor people may eat and absorb too little nutritious food, making them more disease-prone.

- Inadequate or inappropriate food leads to stunted development and/or premature death.

- Nutrient-deficient diets provoke health problems; malnutrition increases susceptibility to disease.

- Disease decreases people's ability to cultivate or purchase nutritious foods.

- The downward spiral of poverty and illness can end in death.

A downward spiral that ends in death

1. Poverty and illness
4. Sickness and loss of livelihoods
3. Malnutrition and increased susceptibility to illness
Death
2. Inadequate food/inappropriate diets

Figure 25-2   Downward spiral of malnutrition. (Reproduced with the permission from the World Health Organization.)

- Global Database on Vitamin A Deficiency (VAD): *www.who.int/vmnis/vitamina/en/*
- Global Database on Anaemia: *www.who.int/vmnis/anaemia/en/*
- Global Database on Breastfeeding: *www.who.int/research/iycf/bfcf/*
- Global Database on Obesity & Adult Body Mass Index (BMI): *www.who.int/bmi/index.jsp*
- Global Database on National Nutrition Policies & Programmes: *www.who.int/nutrition/databases/policies/en/index.html*

Note: A very useful and comprehensive link created by WHO (2006) about nutrition publications and documents can be found at: *www.who.int/hac/crises/international/middle_east/Nutrition_guidinglist%20_2_.pdf.*

The global network of collaborating centers in nutrition led by WHO (2000a) includes 24 institutions around the world (Figure 25-4). This global network carries out specialized nutrition activities. Examples are:

- Research, development, and technology application for nutrition;
- Training, including research training, in nutrition

Turning the Tide of Malnutrition

This need not be so. Better nutrition is a prime entry point to ending the malnutrition maelstrom. Better health means stronger immune systems, which means less illnesses. Healthy people feel stronger, can work better, and may have more earning opportunities to gradually lift them out of both poverty and malnutrition. Healthier, more productive societies are a potential outcome.

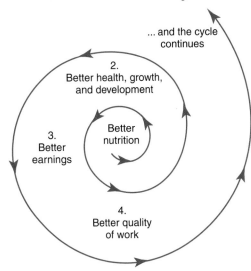

Figure 25-3 Turning the tide of malnutrition. (Reproduced with the permission from the World Health Organization.)

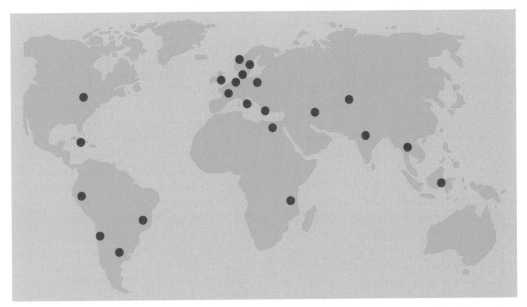

As of February 2000, there were WHO collaborating centres in: Argentina, Brazil, Chile, Cuba, Denmark, Egypt, France, Greece, India, Indonisia, Islamic Republic of Iran, Italy, Kazakhstan, Netherlands, Norway, Peru, Poland, Sweden, Thailand, United Kingdom of Great Britain and Northern Ireland, United Republic of Tanzania, and USA.

Figure 25-4 WHO nutrition collaborating centers. (Reproduced with the permission from the World Health Organization.)

- Collaborative nutrition research with, or under, WHO supervision
- Coordination of nutrition-oriented activities carried out by multiple institutions (WHO, 2000a, p. 19)

EMERGING INFECTIONS

Community-Associated Methicillin-Resistant *Staphylococcus Aureus* (CA-MRSA)

The most common cause of skin/soft-tissue infections in the United States is *Staphylococcus aureus* (Fridkin et al., 2005). When the infections become invasive and resistant to antibiotics, infected persons require hospitalization with a mortality rate of 20% to 25%, despite highly active antibiotic treatments (Centers for Disease Control and Prevention [CDC], 2003a; CDC, 2003b; Fridkin et al., 2005). Since it was first identified in 1961, Methicillin-Resistant *Staphylococcus aureus* (MRSA) infection was found to be limited in health care settings until the past two decades (Bradley, 2005; Brown & Ngeno, 2007). It is now recognized that **Community-Associated Methicillin-Resistant *Staphylococcus aureus* (CA-MRSA)**, a Staph bacterium resistant to many antibiotics and found in community settings both in the rural and urban areas, poses new risks in the United States and other countries (Brown & Ngeno, 2007; CDC, 2006a; Groom et al., 2001).

CA-MRSA spreads more easily, has higher recurrence rates, and causes more skin problems and serious damage than the traditional healthcare-associated MRSA (HA-MRSA) found in hospital settings (Siegel et al., 2006; Fekete, 2007a). The infection's most severe systemic complications may include pneumonia and death among infected individuals due to its voluminous toxin genes (Fekete, 2007a), especially Panton-Valentine leukocidin, which has significant potential for further spread (Bradley, 2005). More than three different *S. aureus* strains are found to cause CA-MRSA infections. However, in the United States, the most common strains are USA-300 and USA-400 and these strains are different from USA-100 and USA-200, strains of HA-MRSA found in health care settings (Siegel et al., 2006; Fekete, 2007a).

CA-MRSA cases have been reported by emergency departments, schools, correctional facilities, dormitories, and military stations (CDC, 2003a,b; Fleming et al., 2006; Kazakova et al., 2005) with 94,000 infected individuals reported in the United States in the year 2005 (Zeller et al., 2007). Persons who are generally healthy can contact the bacteria through close skin-to-skin contact, cuts or abrasions in the skin (Cooper, 2007; Long et al., 2006), crowded conditions, and poor hygiene (i.e., sharing clothing items and towels) (CDC, 2005a). Also, those who have been on or have previously taken antibiotic therapy have a greater risk of infections than those who do not have a history of previous antibiotic intake (Fekete, 2007a).

Most CA-MRSA cases are mild, which include skin or soft tissue infection (i.e., a boil or abscess). Usually, the infected area resembles a red, swollen, and painful "spider bite" (CDC, 2005a). Pus or other drainage may be present. If the infection is limited to skin, it could be difficult to distinguish CA-MRSA from HA-MRSA (Fekete, 2007a). Among severely CA-MRSA–infected people, complications may include serious necrotizing infection, septicemia, pneumonia, and death (CDC, 2005a). To diagnose CA-MRSA infections, a culture is taken by obtaining a specimen from the infection site (i.e., a small biopsy of skin or drainage and/or a sample of sputum, blood, or urine).

CA-MRSA skin infections, such as boils or abscesses, may be treated by incision and drainage. Antibiotic regimens guided by sensitivity test results should be administered to the infected individuals (Fekete, 2007a). Intravenous antibiotic treatment should be considered among hospitalized clients who show signs of oral therapy nonadherence (Fekete, 2007a). Oral antibiotics may include sulfamethoxazole/trimethoprim, clindamycin, doxycycline, minocycline, and linezolid (Fekete, 2007a). Phage therapy, the use of a bacterial virus that targets specific bacteria, has been seriously considered by some scientists and pharmaceutical companies as a possible route for treating MRSA, despite concerns about increased regulations regarding protection of human rights by the Food and Drug Administration (Thacker, 2003). To prevent MRSA cross-infection, meticulous hand washing has been found to be a helpful and cost-effective everyday practice (Fekete, 2007a).

In the United States, MRSA outbreaks are reportable in many states. Examples of reportable states include Connecticut (the first state to require such reports), Indiana, Kentucky, New Jersey, New York, Ohio, Vermont, and others. Announcing its position on the issue, the New York Department of Health (2007) stated, "Our goal is to reduce the prevalence of these antibiotic-resistant bacteria in the community and to quickly identify and properly treat the infections. The medical community should be on the alert to even minor infections that could be caused by MRSA and treat them properly." The Indiana State Department of Health (2007) said, "MRSA is not a new disease, nor is it specific to Indiana or to school settings. Because MRSA is so common, it is not reportable in Indiana. However, outbreaks of MRSA (or any disease) are reportable."

Whether or not CA-MRSA infection is reportable in a given area, having knowledge of this disease is essential to enable health care professionals to provide appropriate infection control initiations. Standard Precautions, a combination and expansion of Universal Precautions and Body Substance Isolation, are required among health care professionals to prevent cross contamination (Siegel et al., 2006).

Severe Acute Respiratory Syndrome (SARS)

Severe Acute Respiratory Syndrome (SARS) is a viral respiratory illness caused by SARS-associated coronavirus (SARS-CoV) (CDC, 2005b). It is an infectious, flu-like disease that emerged in south Guangdong, China, in

November 2002 and infected people globally by the spring of 2003. WHO alerted the world regarding international travel warnings when a number of SARS cases were reported from China, Hong Kong, Taiwan, Vietnam, Singapore, and Canada (CDC, 2005b; Lingappa et al., 2004; Weingartl et al., 2004). In 2003, 8098 people were infected and 774 died from this outbreak (CDC, 2005b). In the same year in the United States, eight people had a positive test result for the virus; the disease has not spread more widely in the U.S. community.

Based on the sequence analysis of SARS-CoV, it is suggested that the virus is different from any other coronavirus and might have evolved and lived in a domesticated animal host. However, a research study that inoculated pigs and chickens intravenously, intranasally, ocularly, and orally with SARS-CoV failed to show that these animals are amplifying hosts for the virus (Weingartl et al., 2004). The origins of SARS-CoV remain unclear (Lingappa et al., 2004). Nevertheless, animal traders carry antibodies to SARS-CoV and indigenous animals in Guangdong province are hosts for a SARS-like coronavirus (CDC, 2005b).

SARS is spread by close person-to-person contact, especially by respiratory droplets. "Close contact means having cared for or lived with someone with SARS or having direct contact with respiratory secretions or body fluids of people with SARS. Examples of close contact include kissing or hugging, sharing eating or drinking utensils, talking to someone within 3 feet, and touching someone directly. Close contact does not include activities like walking by a person or briefly sitting across a waiting room or office" (CDC, 2004a, p. 1). The virus can be deposited on the mucous membranes of the mouth, nose, or eyes of a person who is within 3 feet when an infected person coughs or sneezes. Also, a person who touches infectious droplets on a surface of an object and then touches the mouth, nose, or eye(s) can become infected (CDC, 2004a).

SARS Symptoms

Normally when a person is infected by the SARS virus, early symptoms include a fever of more than 100.4° F (38.0° C), headache, malaise and body aches, diarrhea (10% to 20% of SARS clients), and mild respiratory symptoms (for some people). Dry cough develops 2 to 7 days later. Most people end up experiencing pneumonia (CDC, 2004a). The **Centers for Disease Control and Prevention** (CDC) responded to the 2003 SARS outbreak by working closely with WHO and other international sectors to:

- Provide 24-hour coordination and response
- Deploy health professionals to help with on-site investigations around the world
- Provide help and support for health departments locally and nationally in identifying and investigating possible SARS cases and causes
- Initiate a new system to alert travelers who may have been exposed to SARS (CDC, 2004a)

In 2003, WHO announced that the last chain of human transmission of SARS-CoV was broken on July 5, 2003. However, all countries should be vigilant for its reemergence, as there have been reports of SARS-CoV cases due to (1) laboratory accidents in Taiwan, China, and Singapore and (2) contacts with animal hosts and environmental contamination in China. Every country in the world should be prepared for episodes of recurrence and be able to detect promptly and respond to the reemergence of SARS-CoV transmissions in humans (WHO, 2004a).

HIV/AIDS

Throughout the world, almost 40 million people are living with **Human immunodeficiency virus/acquired immunodeficiency syndrome (HIV/AIDS)**, with 24.7 million in sub-Saharan Africa, 7.8 million in South/Southeast Asia, 1.7 million in Latin America, 1.7 million in Eastern Europe and Central Asia, 1.4 million in North America, 750,000 in East Asia, 740,000 in Western/Central Europe, 460,000 in Middle East/North Africa, 250,000 in the Caribbean, and 81,000 in Oceania (islands in the pacific and vicinity) (Joint United Nations Programme on HIV/AIDS, 2008). In sub-Saharan Africa, life expectancy has been reduced by more than 20 years because of HIV/AIDS. Botswana, Lesotho, Swaziland, and Zimbabwe are being hit particularly hard by the disease, despite the fact that antiretroviral medicines have been used to decrease mother-to-child transmission in these areas (Joint United Nations Programme on HIV/AIDS, 2008).

In developed countries, HIV prevalence rates in the adult population are much lower than those in developing countries. For instance, the rate is approximately at 0.6% in the United States and less than 0.1% in Japan. In Lesotho, the 2007 rate was 23.2% (CIA, 2009a) and 26.1% in Swaziland (CIA, 2006b).

People in sub-Saharan countries are trying to reduce HIV transmission rates (Research Highlights box). Yet this effort is complicated by the existence of certain unique cultural practices. Traditional sexual cleansing, a cultural practice performed among particular tribes in sub-Saharan African countries, is usually undertaken after the spouse of a survivor has died. In this ritual, the widow or widower is required to have penetrative sex with a *cleanser* to avoid misfortune and to chase away the spirit of the dead from the self and the community (Ayikukwei et al., 2007; Malungo, 2001). The cleanser could be anyone, ranging from an in-law to a stranger, or commercial performer (Ayikukwei et al., 2007; Malungo, 2001). However, in Zambia, a study showed that 69% of widowers and widows are choosing to use combined alternative practices (i.e., sliding over a half-naked person, body-brushing, cow jumping, hair cutting, mud throwing at the widow/widower) instead of traditional sexual cleansing (Malungo, 2001). Such alternative practices are helpful in that they do not pose any HIV infection risks for the survivors as does sexual cleansing.

The Kenya Ministry of Health reported that 99% of adult Kenyans are aware of HIV transmission modes,

research highlights

Prevention of Mother-to-Baby (Vertical) Transmission Through the Use of Nevirapine

A randomized trial study was conducted from November 1997 to April 1999 to compare vertical transmission rates among 645 mother-baby pairs in Uganda. One group of 313 HIV-infected pregnant women was randomly assigned regimen A, a single dose of 200 mg NVP, an inexpensive antiretroviral drug, at the onset of labor. Their babies also received NVP (2 mg/kg) within 72 hours after birth. For regimen B, another 313 pregnant women received ZDV 600 mg orally at the onset of labor and 300 mg every 3 hours until delivery. Their babies received ZDV 4 mg/kg orally twice a day for 7 days. Nineteen mother-baby pairs received placebo. Most babies (99%) in the total sample were breastfed for a median of 9 months' duration. HIV testing for infants was performed 5 times. The first testing was done at birth, and subsequently at 6 to 8 weeks, 14 to 16 weeks, 12 months, and 18 months after birth.

Results revealed that single-dose NVP prophylaxis for the mothers and their babies significantly decreased vertical transmission at 14 to 16 weeks compared with those who received ZDV. At 18 months, the infants who received NVP maintained a significantly lower rate of transmission than those given ZDV (15.7% versus 25.8%). However, infant mortality rates between the two groups were about the same at 18 months of age (12%). The results of this study have shed new light for developing countries in terms of using affordable short-course NVP prophylaxis to prevent mother-to-baby transmission. It is projected that this regimen could prevent 246,000 infants (out of 800,000) a year from getting the virus from their mothers.

Data from Jackson, J. B., Musoke, P., Fleming, T., Guay, L. A., Bagenda, D., Allen, M., et al. (2003). Intrapartum and neonatal single-dose nevirapine compared with zidovudine for prevention of mother-to-child transmission of HIV-1 in Kampala, Uganda: 18-month follow-up of the HIVNET 012 randomized trial. *The Lancet, 362*(9387), 859–867.

including awareness of the context of sexual cleansing (Ministry of Public Health, 2005); in contrast to Zambia, however, the ritual of sexual cleansing persists widely in Kenya. Luo (a tribe in Kenya) members believe that this ritual will help the widow and her community avoid misfortune (Ayikukwei et al., 2007). The female widow needs to be cleansed by having sex after the period of mourning over her husband's death is over. The mourning period can last from 1 to 12 months (Ayikukwei et al., 2007). Although, there have been some movements to modify the cleansing procedures (e.g., dress code, mourning period), having sex with a cleanser is still a requirement for Luo members (Ayikukwei et al., 2007).

The ritual of sexual cleansing can clearly contribute to the spread of HIV. Other cultural practices in areas of Africa that can also cause HIV transmission, and are performed widely, include promiscuity among heterosexual individuals (Seckinelgin, 2003), group circumcision, and genital tattooing (Patel & Cobbs, 2004).

In terms of gender, women with HIV in African countries are more vulnerable to progression to AIDS than their male counterparts, due to their unequal socioeconomic status. African females in general are the caretakers for the sick in their families and they can lose their property when they become widows. In Kenya, a widow in Luo clans is ostracized by her community members and not allowed to join any social functions immediately upon her husband's death (Ayikukwei et al., 2007). To be accepted back to the community, the Kenyan widow needs to undergo traditional sexual cleansing.

Despite the importance of culture in relation to HIV transmission in Africa, Gausset (2001) argued that cultural beliefs and practices should not take central blame for the spread of HIV:

> In the context of AIDS, some of the beliefs and practices of specific African cultures have been seen as accelerating the spread of the virus, or at least as barriers to understanding and preventing the epidemics. I will argue that the major problems relating to AIDS prevention involve the negotiation of safe sex, rather than these "cultural barriers," and that the problems linked to this negotiation are comparable to those found in the West.
>
> (Gausset, 2001, p. 510)

However, addressing HIV/AIDS problems without taking people's cultural beliefs and practices into account is dangerous and superficial. As discussed earlier, studies conducted by Ayikukwei et al. (2007) and Malungo (2001) demonstrated the significant role that the culture (especially as it promotes sexual cleansing) plays in spreading the virus.

Helping HIV-positive individuals to live in their culture with a high quality of life is also important. An interpretive phenomenology study among seven HIV-positive postpartum women in Thailand found that focusing on religious practices (e.g., meditation, reading religious stories) and beliefs (e.g., Karma and the Five Precepts) helped the Buddhist participants to live more peacefully with their HIV infection (Ross, Sawatphanit, & Suwansujarid, 2007). Thus, taking religious beliefs and practices into account can enable health care providers to better assist clients in their cultural setting.

The challenge of HIV/AIDS is complex and its solution requires multidisciplinary and multidimensional approaches. Ordinary people, community leaders, health care professionals, and organizations at all levels must work collaboratively. Together, we can consider gender/social inequalities and cultural/religious beliefs and practices as we work to identify barriers to understanding and facilitate the reduction of HIV infections. Support from all parties will enable us to set priorities and fight HIV/AIDS more effectively.

Tuberculosis and Multidrug-Resistant Tuberculosis (TB)

HIV/AIDS is a major cause of increased TB rates in sub-Saharan Africa, where at least 60% of TB clients are identified as being infected with HIV (Williams & Dye,

2003). Although TB rates have declined in the United States since 1992 (Blumberg et al., 2005), TB remains a persistent problem for many other nations, especially in Asia, Eastern Europe, and Latin America, due to its comorbidity with HIV (DeAngelis & Flanagin, 2005; Dye et al., 2005).

In general, the starting treatment of TB consists of four drugs (isoniazid, rifampin, pyrazinamide, and ethambutol) and lasts six to nine months. Recently, latent TB infection has begun to be treated in the United States to prevent its progression to TB. It is recommended that testing for latent TB infection be performed with persons: (1) who contact individuals with TB; (2) who have HIV; and (3) who recently immigrated to the United States from countries with high rates of TB (Blumberg et al., 2005). If tested positive for latent TB, isoniazid is to be given for nine months (Blumberg et al., 2005).

TB has been a predisposing factor for **multidrug-resistant tuberculosis (MDR-TB)**, an increasing problem throughout the world. In general, countries with high MDR-TB prevalence rates poorly control TB (WHO, 2007b). There are approximately 500,000 MDR-TB worldwide cases per year, with half of the cases in China and India (WHO, 2007b). Costs related to MDR-TB are found to be much higher than costs related to TB due to the high expenses of second-line drug use, prolonged treatment duration, and productivity loss (Kang et al., 2006; Ormerod, 2005). MDR-TB causes high social and financial burdens, particularly among resource-poor countries. A study in South Korea found that the total cost of MRD-TB treatment is approximately $1680 to $7637 per drug-susceptible TB clients, which is 7 to 22 times higher than that of normal TB (Kang et al., 2006).

Causes of MDR-TB are believed to be related to both the physician and the client (Ormerod, 2005). Inappropriate treatment of drug-susceptible TB by the physician combined with the person's noncompliance during such treatment can lead to MDR-TB, demonstrating resistance to at least two basic anti-TB drugs: isoniazid and rifampicin (Di Perri & Bonora, 2004; Ormerod, 2005).

The MDR-TB strain in former Soviet Union countries is severe, as evidenced by the fact that half of MDR-TB (Beijing-family strains) cases in these countries are resistant to all four first-line drugs (isoniazid, rifampin, pyrazinamide, and ethambutol), compared to only 12% in other world regions (Drobniewski et al., 2005; WHO, 2007b).

A strong suspicion of MDR-TB should be held when a person has a history of TB treatment failure. In developed countries, TB can be confirmed by a specific testing method called "whole-blood interferon Υ (IFN-Υ) assay," which is more expensive and more accurate than tuberculin skin testing (TST), normally used in developing countries (Kang et al., 2005). MDR-TB drug use in developed countries also includes an appropriate combination of ethambutol, pyrazinamide, and streptomycin, plus second-line drugs (i.e., Fluoroquinolones), based on individualized susceptibility patterns (Di Pierri & Bonora, 2004). However, in developing countries where susceptibility testing is not affordable, a WHO regimen is normally recommended

(Ormerod, 2005). Despite all of these endeavors in developing countries to treat MDR-TB, client outcomes are usually much worse than those in developed countries with individualized treatment (Ormerod, 2005). In fact, successful management of MDR-TB requires considerable expertise (Di Perri & Bonora, 2004). At the international level, the **United Nations Millennium Development Goals (MDGs)** recommends "Directly Observed Therapies (DOTS)," an approach initiated by WHO to control TB. In this program, the client is observed by the giver of medications to ensure that the client really swallows the anti-TB drugs. At present, the United Nations MDGs programs are directed toward more careful evaluations of the effects of DOTS. (More detailed information about DOTS can be found at: *www.who.int/tb/dots/en/* and *www.stoptb.org/wg/dots_expansion/default.asp?AM=DEWG.*) Also, the Stop TB Department is working for the Global Fund (the most significant source of external funding internationally supported by WHO to combat TB) in collaboration with its partners in order to:

- Support and monitor maximal use of funding granted by Global Fund among developing countries.
- Promote countries' National TB Strategic Plans and finance their related activities.
- Simplify access to and implementation of funding granted by Global Fund.
- Reinforce the capacity of National TB Programmes (NTPs), other TB implementers, and technical assistants to implement policies and procedures provided by Global Fund (WHO, 2007c).

At the international level, the Stop TB Working Group on DOTS-Plus for MDR-TB was created in 2002 to combat MDR-TB. Also, prices of some second-line drugs have been reduced by 95%, with the first DOTS-Plus pilot projects launched in many countries. The pilot projects of DOTS-Plus in developing countries were found to be successful and cost-effective, with 70% of 1047 MDR-TB clients treated (WHO, 2007b). Despite the success of the DOTS-Plus project, the expansion of surveillance and monitor trends of global anti-TB drug resistance is a real challenge due to a severe lack of qualified personnel. The Stop TB Working Group on DOTS-Plus for MDR-TB has the goal of enabling all health care providers to diagnose and treat TB clients and manage MDR-TB as a routine in collaboration with DOTS expansion. As a result, 56% of MDR-TB-positive clients will be treated (instead of <2% at present) by the year 2015. Of these, it is expected that at least 75% will have successful treatment and the number of MDR-TB cases will be reduced from an estimated 533,000 in 2005 to 193,000 in 2015 (WHO, 2007b).

VIOLENCE

Violence can happen to individuals anywhere, regardless of gender, age, or nationality, and is a major leading cause worldwide of physical, sexual, reproductive, and mental health problems. Thus, violence costs nations immeasurable amounts of money each year in terms of health care, law enforcement, and productivity loss (WHO, 2007d). Worldwide, it is estimated that about 1.6 million people at all ages lose their lives to violence annually (WHO, 2007d). Approximately 875,000 children under the age of 18 died in 2002 as a result of an injury (e.g., burns) or violence (WHO, 2007e). In 2004, 5292 youths in the United States aged 10 to 24 were murdered—an average rate of 15 victims per day (CDC, 2007a).

A study examining intimate partner violence among 24,097 women in 10 different countries reported that lifetime numbers of incidences of physical abuse ranged from 13 (Japan) to 61 (Peru), with the incidences of sexual violence ranging from six (Japan, Serbia, and Montenegro) to 59 (Ethiopia) (Garcia-Moreno et al., 2006). The differences between these prevalence rates in different countries were not explained by age, partnership status, or education. Participants reported that physical violence was often accompanied by sexual violence. In some countries, however, such as Bangladesh, Ethiopia, and Thailand, many women only reported sexual violence. Results of the study confirm that intimate partner violence is a common problem worldwide. Yet, violence rates in developed countries are lower than those in developing countries.

Definition of Violence

Violence is defined differently in different parts of the world, depending on people's beliefs and cultures. The definition proposed by WHO is used in this chapter. According to WHO (2007a), violence is defined as:

> intentional use of physical force or power, threatened or actual, against oneself, another person, or against a group or community, that either results in or has a high likelihood of resulting in injury, death, psychological harm, maldevelopment or deprivation. The definition encompasses interpersonal violence as well as suicidal behaviour and armed conflict. It also covers a wide range of acts, going beyond physical acts to include threats and intimidation. Besides death and injury, the definition also includes the myriad and often less obvious consequences of violent behaviour such as psychological harm, deprivation and maldevelopment that compromise the well-being of individuals, families and communities.
>
> (WHO, 2007a)

In response to violence, WHO has proposed a four-step public health approach, which includes: (1) defining the problem; (2) identifying risk and protective factors; (3) devising and testing means of dealing with violence; and (4) applying successful means at a large scale (CDC, 2007b; WHO, 2007d). Successful response prevention of violence should be based on rigorous research and collaboration among health care professionals and other experts in areas such as epidemiology, criminology, education, and economics (Figure 25-5).

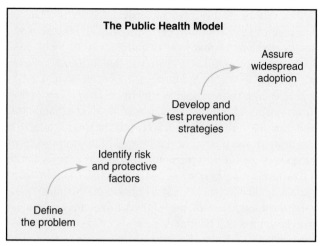

Figure 25-5 The Public Health Approach to Violence Prevention. (Reproduced with the permission from the National Center for Injury Prevention and Control, Division of Violence Prevention.)

The CDC is an example of an organization in the United States that is applying the above four-step public health model. Activities, projects, and funding support by the CDC are outlined below as an exemplar:

Step 1: Defining the Problem

In order to understand the magnitude of violence in the United States, different data sources are needed. Such sources may include police reports, medical examiner files, vital records, client charts, population-based surveys, and research results. Extrapolations of the data from these sources can help us learn about violence frequencies, places, trends, and perpetrators. The CDC has provided funding to studies deemed to be helpful in defining violence problems. The National Violent Death Reporting System (NVDRS) is an example of a project funded by the CDC to ensure that timely, complete, and accurate data are collected about violent deaths for different states in the United States. It is hoped that the data will enable each state to have a clearer picture of violence in order to respond to the violence effectively (CDC, 2007b).

Step 2: Identifying Risk and Protective Factors

A "Risk Factor" is defined as "a characteristic that increases the likelihood of a person becoming a victim or perpetrator of violence," and a "Protective Factor" as "a characteristic that decreases the likelihood of a person becoming a victim or perpetrator of violence" (CDC, 2007c). Knowing risk and protective factors can help responsible organizations and personnel to estimate violence magnitudes and devise appropriate measures to prevent it. It is important to note that identified risk factors should not be used to blame victims of violence, but as part of a focus for interventions. To support step 2 endeavors, the CDC is funding a study examining the association between exposure to violent media (e.g., from videogames and news related items to serious violent behavior in the media) and identifying risk and protective factors, particularly among youth, about the effects of violent media.

Step 3: Devising and Testing Means for Dealing with Violence

In this step, data on violence from all available sources are extrapolated and assessed. Based on the evidence, programs and interventions are planned. Such programs and interventions are then implemented, tested, and rigorously evaluated to determine their effectiveness. An example of step 3 activities is the *Choose Respect* project, a communication initiative for 6th- to 8th-grade students to guide adolescents in forming healthy relationships in order to prevent dating violence.

Step 4: Applying Successful Means at a Large Scale

After a program has been tested successfully for its effectiveness, large-scale dissemination should be provided. At this stage, communities are encouraged to adopt a program tailored to their own problems and needs. An evaluation of the program should be performed in each community. Training, networking, technical assistance, and process evaluations are to be supported by all involved parties. An example of step 4 activities initiated by the CDC is the National Youth Violence Prevention Resource Center with its goal to prevent youth violence and suicide. In this project, a website, toll-free hotline, and fax-on-demand service were created as helpful resources for youth. Any interested community can request more information from the CDC.

Forms and Context of Violence

WHO classifies violence into three major categories: interpersonal, suicide/self-harm, and collective.

Interpersonal Violence

Interpersonal violence is a violence committed by an individual or a small group of people in a wide range of acts and behaviors (emotional, physical, sexual, and psychological). The violence could happen to people of any age (adolescents, children, and older adults). It could also happen anywhere, including the home, workplace, neighborhood, and unfamiliar places.

Whereas violence in the community (e.g., youth violence or crimes) is highly visible, violence in the home is usually hidden. The impact of such hidden violence is complicated by the fact that authorities or health personnel are less willing or prepared to deal with it (WHO, 2007d).

Risk factors for interpersonal violence may include a victim's low self-esteem, low self-control, and personality/conduct disorders. Other risk factors are reported to be lack of social support, dysfunctional family structure, family history of violence, and drug and alcohol abuse (WHO, 2007d). For example, a study among 447 students in grades 6 through 12 reported that male students who experienced

violence at home were more inclined to use violence and guns at school than those who did not (Slovak et al., 2007). Arriaga and Foshee (2004) examined dating violence among 1965 8th and 9th graders in 14 middle schools and found that 14% (n = 284) of these adolescents were perpetrators of dating violence themselves. Another 26% (n = 503) experienced dating violence as victims at some point in their lives. Also, results showed that dating violence among friends had a stronger impact than parental violence on the participants' dating violence. Thus, those with friends who are perpetrators or victims of dating violence tend to become perpetrators or victims themselves (Arriaga & Foshee, 2004). Interestingly, girls were more likely to be perpetrators than boys in this study. However, their violence behaviors were less severe than those of boys.

Culture and gender inequality are also significant factors of interpersonal violence. For instance, research results in rural south India showed that wife beating is not only acceptable in some communities, but also a hallmark of manhood (Krishnan, 2005). Chinese immigrant men (living in the New York Metropolitan area and New Jersey) who believe that wife beating is legitimate are likely to beat their wife more than those who do not believe so (Jin et al., 2007).

Mothers who are victims of violence and their children are at risk for physical, emotional, psychological, and developmental damage. Pregnant victims of physical violence have increased risk of complications, such as hemorrhage, preterm births, and fetal loss (Peedicayil et al., 2004). Abused mothers can also become emotionally and/or physically abusive to their own children as a way to project their anger (Hornor, 2005; Lutenbacher et al., 2004).

It is important for health care providers to understand the seriously negative impact that interpersonal violence can have on individuals. They should be able to identify such violence and be aware of helpful resources for their abused clients and children. Local domestic violence crisis contact information (i.e., numbers and counseling services) should be readily provided to their clients. Children of the victims who witness domestic violence might also need to see a counselor for therapeutic interventions (Hornor, 2005).

Suicide and Self-Harm

It is estimated that 815,000 people committed suicide in 2000. Eastern European countries have the highest suicide rates in the world. The lowest rates are found in Latin America and some Asian countries. In general, the older that a person is, the higher is his/her possibility of committing suicide. For instance, the global rates among people aged 75 years or older are three times higher than those among people aged 15 to 24 (WHO, 2007f). However, it is found that people at a younger age are the most vulnerable group to commit suicide in Turkey, where older adults are taken care of by younger family members and usually enjoy their lives with their family and grandchildren (Oner et al., 2007).

Other factors contributing to suicide include low socio-economic status and stressful life events (e.g., unemployment, social crisis, loss of loved ones, problematic relationships with a family member, friend, or significant other). Although such factors are generally common in people's lives, only people with particular vulnerability and self-harm tendencies tend to kill themselves due to such problems. Vulnerability and self-harm tendencies are often found among individuals who use alcohol or drugs, have a history of being abused as a child, and are experiencing depression or schizophrenia (WHO, 2007f). Other medical factors include severe pain and/or physical illnesses. People who have a history of attempted suicide in the past six months are at a higher risk for later suicidal attempts.

Gender is also found to be a significant factor of suicide. A study in China showed that females have higher suicide rates than males (Ji et al., 2001). Conversely, research in Turkey among 17,327 people who committed suicide showed that 61.1% were men and 38.9% women. Hanging (48.2%) and firearms (19.2%) were the two most frequently used methods for suicide. However, women in the study used chemicals (drugs, etc.) more than men. Reasons for suicide included illness (33.8%; found more among men) and unsatisfactory relationships (33.0%; found more among women) (Oner et al., 2007). Coinciding with this study, Ziherl and Zalar (2006) found that among 16,522 people who committed suicides and 15,057 who attempted suicides in the Republic of Slovenia, hanging was the most prevalent means for completing suicide. People with a history of suicide attempts are 773 times more likely to attempt another suicide, as compared to those without such a history (Ziherl & Zalar, 2006).

Bipolar disorders have been found to be another predictor of suicides, with rates 20 times higher than those of the general population (Simon et al., 2007). Results of a study in California among 32,360 individuals with a diagnosis of BD revealed that a comorbidity of anxiety disorders was significantly related to more frequent suicide attempts and suicide deaths (Simon et al., 2007). In this study, men had lower rates of suicidal attempts, but higher rates of suicidal deaths than their women counterparts. It is crucial for health care professionals to be vigilantly alert for risk factors related to suicidal attempts, and to find appropriate ways to successfully prevent such attempts.

Collective Violence

Collective violence is defined as the instrumental use of violence by a particular group of people for specific political, economic, or social objectives. Such violence may include armed conflicts within or between states or nations, genocide, terrorism, repression, and other abuses of human rights (WHO, 2007a).

In the 20th century, it is estimated that 191 million people lost their lives due to armed conflict. More than half of these people were civilians. In the year 2000, more than 300,000 people died because of collective violence. The majority of victims lived in the poorer regions of the world.

Besides death, the aftermath of collective violence includes physical and psychological disabilities that exert burdens on families, communities, and nations. Young children and refugees are among the most vulnerable to the aftermaths of disease and post-traumatic stress disorders related to violence. A study among 3415 Palestinian students in the 10th and 11th grades revealed collective violence to be associated with the students' depressive symptoms, and that such violence had a stronger effect on female students than their male counterparts. This may be due to their culture's allowance of more freedoms to boys, such as being able to move around outside the domestic or school areas (Giacaman et al., 2007). Also, those students who lived in refugee camps were more negatively affected than those who lived in the city because of the poor living conditions found in the camps (Giacaman et al., 2007).

WHO (2007f) is committed to working with its partners at the regional, national, and international levels to prevent violence. Its goal is to identify and implement preventive strategies. Data collection systems are used to support and evaluate the success of their strategies. In this effort, political commitment and momentum are required from a wide variety of concerned parties to strengthen and increase violence prevention endeavors in the next five years (WHO, 2007f).

BIOTERRORISM

Whether it was the juxtaposition of the anthrax poisonings with the US terrorist attacks of September 2001 or just an outgrowth of fear of biological weapons, the public has heard more about bioterrorism in the past 6 years than at any previous time. Fear of bioterrorism persists because of new reports of biological warfare, including the most recent attack that involved a Russian spy who was poisoned with ionizing radiation (polonium-210). The fear also stems from the knowledge that biological weapons are inexpensive to produce and relatively easy to disseminate.

(Fekete, 2007b, p. 1149)

The above remark reflects what many people in different nations feel about bioterrorism. As health care professionals, we are required to be knowledgeable about possible diseases/agents that could be used for bioterrorism and how we should respond to such action.

Bioterrorism is classified by the CDC (2007c) into three different categories: A, B, and C. These categories are based on: (1) how easy the disease or agent might be spread; (2) the potential negative impact it could have on public health; (3) the extent to which it could cause public panic or social disruption; and (4) the degree to which it would require the public to prepare for an attack.

Category A Diseases/Agents

Category A diseases/agents include various biological agents and pathogens that are not usually seen in the United States and pose the highest risks and priority. They include

Anthrax, **Botulism**, **Plague**, **Smallpox**, **Tularemia**, and **Viral hemorrhagic fevers.**

Anthrax *(Bacillus Anthracis)*

Since the anthrax mailing attacks to a few recipients in the United States in 2001, no other attacks have been reported (Fekete, 2007b). These unfortunate mail recipients contacted the bacillus either cutaneously or inhalationally (Fekete, 2007b). Cutaneous anthrax contactors developed erythema (red inflamed area similar to cellulitis) on exposed areas of the hands, arms, or face that later transformed into painful vesicles and then necrotic painless, depressed, black eschar. Inhalation contactors had fever, dyspnea, cough, and chest discomfort (CDC, 2007c). Usually, a respiratory failure and hemodynamic collapse will follow. Other symptoms may include lymphangitis and painful lymphadenopathy. It is recommended that persons received a complete treatment of doxycycline or ciprofloxacin for 60 days (Fekete, 2007b).

Smallpox *(Variola Major)*

It is believed that smallpox was eradicated in 1977. However, there are fears that a strain kept in a laboratory could be used as a bioweapon (Fekete, 2007b). Smallpox symptoms usually resemble influenza symptoms, which include fever and myalgias, followed by a rash. Rashes in smallpox can be differentiated from those of chickenpox (varicella). A rash from smallpox is most prominent on the face and extremities with the same stage of lesion development. A rash of chickenpox is more prominent on the trunk, with different stages of lesion development and resolution.

Smallpox vaccination was given to those (military and civil health care personnel) considered to be at the highest risk of infection in 2003. Cardiac toxicity (especially myopericarditis), was reported as a side effect of the vaccine. Although such a side effect is rarely fatal, careful case selection for general vaccination is needed (Fekete, 2007b). At this point, it is unknown whether the vaccination of older people (who received their vaccination long ago when smallpox was widespread) can prevent them from being infected today (Fekete, 2007b).

Category B Diseases/Agents

Category B diseases/agents are those that pose the second highest risks for world and national security. They include Brucellosis; Food safety threats (e.g., *Salmonella* sp., *Escherichia coli* O157:H7, *Shigella*); Glanders; Melioidosis; Psittacosis; Q fever; Ricin toxin; Staphylococcal enterotoxin B; Typhus fever; Viral encephalitis; and Water safety threats (e.g., *Vibrio cholerae, Cryptosporidium parvum*).

Category C Diseases/Agents

Category C diseases/agents are emerging pathogens that could be reproduced for mass dissemination. They include emerging infectious diseases such as Nipah virus and hantavirus.

Epidemic and Pandemic Alert and Response (EPR)

At the national level, health care providers should be alerted to any unusual symptoms indicative of infectious outbreak related to bioterrorism. In turn, if a bioterrorist action is suspected, health care providers should report it to their local or state health department. According to the CDC (2007c), indications of bioterrorism include "(1) an unusual temporal or geographic clustering of illness (e.g., persons who attended the same public event or gathering) or patients presenting with clinical signs and symptoms that suggest an infectious disease outbreak (e.g., >2 patients presenting with an unexplained febrile illness associated with sepsis, pneumonia, respiratory failure, or rash or a botulism-like syndrome with flaccid muscle paralysis, especially if occurring in otherwise healthy persons); (2) an unusual age distribution for common diseases (e.g., an increase in what appears to be a chickenpox-like illness among adult patients, but which might be smallpox); and (3) a large number of cases of acute flaccid paralysis with prominent bulbar palsies, suggestive of a release of *botulinum* toxin." To learn more about clinical diagnosis, management, and responses to bioterrorism, refer to the CDC website available at *www.bt.cdc.gov and www.cdc.gov/mmwr/preview/mmwrhtml/mm5041a2.htm.*

At the international level, responses to bioterrorism also have been prepared. WHO is a core organization responding to needs for such preparation at this level. WHO works collaboratively with agencies in many countries to gather reports of suspected outbreaks and rumors regarding bioterrorism through advanced technologies from all sources available, both formally and informally.

The Global Public Health Intelligence Network (GPHIN), a significant source of informal information related to outbreaks, was also collaboratively established by Health Canada and WHO. Its multilingual capabilities are Internet-based, constantly searching data worldwide to identify information regarding disease outbreaks that can put international public health sectors at risk (WHO, 2007g).

The 2005 International Health Regulations (IHR)—legally-binding regulations across countries led by WHO—are embraced by most nations throughout the world. IHR's mission is to provide legal frameworks to ensure health security among nations without unnecessary international traffic and trade interference (WHO, 2007g). An example of the 2005 IHR function is a notification about emerging infections (SARS, or a new human influenza virus) or threats (e.g., chemical spills, nuclear melt-downs) that can have a negative impact on populations across borders (WHO, 2007g). To learn more about International Health Regulations, go to: *www.who.int/ features/qa/39/en/index.html.*

IMPLICATIONS

The health-promotion and disease-prevention priorities that have been outlined in this chapter present challenges for all health care professionals. This is an opportune context for health care providers, as individuals and as a collective profession, to play a key role in emerging systems that must emphasize health promotion and disease prevention to bring their clients greater longevity and quality of life. The principles of primary prevention, cultural diversity, and multidisciplinary teamwork in health-promotion policy development are critical to an era bringing dramatic changes in health care and life styles (McCullagh, 2004). Through a perspective on the development of community-based, health-promotion programs, health care professionals can bring a balance to decisions that will be made about the appropriate use of traditional and newer health care resources.

With rapidly advancing health technology, developing an international declaration on health, human rights, human genetics, and public health policy is of great significance (WHO, 2007b) (Multicultural Awareness box). The preventive services delivered by health care providers, including efforts such as health assessment, screening, and counseling, are necessary tools to empower individuals to

promote and maintain optimal health and well-being. It is important to help individuals, families, and communities become active participants in defining their health needs, in making informed decisions to meet these needs, and ultimately, in bringing about improvements in health status and quality of life. Appropriate models must be generated (see Figures 25-3 and 25-5).

The demand for primary health care providers will continue to spur the need for more advanced practice nurses, including nurses with PhDs. This demand can be met if undergraduate students are introduced early to concepts of health promotion and disease prevention (McCullagh, 2004) with an emphasis on cultural diversity and with a global perspective. In this way, health promotion, quality of life, and socioeconomic justice might become increasingly valued in cultures throughout the world.

Although some baccalaureate nursing programs in America focus on cultural diversity and international health, nursing programs in other countries, such as Australia, Japan, South Korea, and Thailand, do not (Lambert et al., 2004). Curricula with cultural diversity global frameworks that develop concepts and experiences directed toward malnutrition, emergent diseases, HIV/AIDS, bioterrorism, violence, and the like to maximize quality of life will enable nurses to fulfill innovative roles in reformed health care systems around the world. Faculty and students will increasingly work together in interdisciplinary teams with and in communities, using an expanding variety of health-promotion services. The team will be guided by national and international standards.

Nursing faculty will bring the strength of tested nursing theories to their teaching, practice, and research (McCullagh, 2004). Curricula that provide experiences directed toward evidence-based practice and international nursing will enable health care providers to fulfill innovative roles in a reformed health care system. Given the increasing focus on cultural diversity and self-care in disease prevention and health promotion, nurses can respond directly to the health needs of individuals, families, communities, and groups by focusing on health promotion and disease prevention tailored to particular cultures and spiritual beliefs and by supporting new ways to work and live.

In the area of research, understanding health care practices and the impact of culture on people from different nations will enable health care professionals to create appropriate health-promotion and disease-prevention interventions. Thus, international collaborative research is important (Chiang-Hanisko et al., 2006).

A heightened need exists to test individual, family, community, and group interventions that optimize the health and well-being of both healthy and ill populations in cultures.

A successful action research program conducted in Thailand promoted self-reliance and self-esteem among HIV-positive pregnant women. With a combination of counseling, advocacy, education, and services that the researchers provided to participants at both the hospital and home,

MULTICULTURAL AWARENESS

Health and Health Promotion in a Native American Tribe: The Navajo

The Navajo people of the *Dine' Bike'yah* live on a vast land on which the four states of Arizona, Utah, New Mexico, and Colorado intersect. The *Dine'* hold this land as sacred and as an integral part of their lives. The Navajo believe that health is a part of the *Hozho'*, which is a personal sense of well-being and rightness with the world and is all inclusive. For the Navajo, health is not separate from the overall state of balance among the body, mind, spirit, and the surrounding environment. When one of these is out of balance, *Hozho'* is not achieved. *Hozho'* is everything that a Navajo thinks of as being good, in terms of good and evil or favorable and unfavorable. The Navajo strive to maintain *Hozho'* and to live in harmony with all things that surround them. The goal of Navajo life in this world is to live to attain maturity with *Hozho'* and to die of old age, the result of which incorporates beauty, harmony, and happiness or *sa'ah naagh"ii bik'eh hozho'*. When the body, spirit, or mind fall out of *Hozho'*, a traditional healer or medicine man is sought. In many instances, the medicine man recommends that the individual seek both Western medicine and the traditional ways to cure the problem.

Since 1955, trends in Navajo health have demonstrated a progressive improvement, particularly in the areas of maternal and infant mortality. However, on the increase are lifestyle-related diseases and premature deaths for which health-promotion activities can have an effect. Among these lifestyle-related diseases are adult-onset diabetes, AIDS, and alcohol and substance abuse. Health care providers who work with the Navajo must address all health-promotion and disease-prevention activities in terms of an appreciation for the cultural and economic realities and the needs of this community.

Compiled from Anonymous. (n.d.). *Navajo Land.* Retrieved June 4, 2008, from *www.discovernavajo.com/culture.html*; The Official Navajo Nation Visitor Guide. (2002). *Navajo cultural history and legends.*

most women from the study felt that they could move on with their lives with higher self-esteem than before participating in the project (Sawatphanit et al., 2004). A support group inspired them to have hope and let go of tension related to their infection. Education provided by the nurses encouraged them to use condoms with their partners to prevent them from getting more HIV viruses. Additionally, counseling enabled the women to solve other problems in their lives more effectively (Sawatphanit et al., 2004). Understanding HIV-positive women's life stories is important in promoting nurse-client relationship and the clients' quality of life (Ross, Sawatphanit Draucker, & Suwansujarid, 2007; Ross, Sawatphanit Suwansujarid, & Draucker, 2007).

To be advocates for newly emerging priorities for disease prevention and health promotion, nurses in the 21st century need to:

1. Participate in policy development for health promotion as the health care of individuals in acute settings shifts from hospitals to home and community settings. Attention to health-promoting environments and behaviors in home and community settings provides an entry point to the development of community-based models of primary care that emphasize health promotion and disease prevention.
2. Influence public expectations about health promotion. Presentations and other forms of public dialogue and education will help raise awareness of the value of individual and community health promotion. Nurses have the collective capacity to change the philosophy of the system from selling health care in the marketplace to creating a milieu for changing health behaviors. Encouraging meaningful community participation in addressing health issues provides a significant opportunity to narrow the gap between what is possible in terms of health promotion in each country and what is reality. As mentioned earlier, violence and emerging diseases are among the challenges today that require heightened public awareness.
3. Promote equitable access to preventive health care. Given the higher rates of preventable conditions among populations in resource-poor countries, a need to promote the justified distribution and utilization of preventive health services is apparent. Internationally, community-based efforts that combine public and private resources should be targeted to those most in need of health care. Delivery models that focus on integrating preventive and primary care should be expanded.

Preventive health care delivery should be based on broad research agendas that encompass multiple health and social science perspectives. Health care providers should participate in areas of research that will cost-effectively influence both personal and community health. Service delivery can also benefit from expanded health service research agendas that foster collaboration among disciplines and countries. Most important, preventive health care should be adapted to the health and social problems of specific groups and cultures.

Alternate approaches to health-promotion and preventive service delivery should be used where most effective to meet new international health challenges, including mobile vans, school and worksite clinics, and other community-based, collaborative actions (Innovative Practice box).

innovative practice

Haitian Health Foundation: A Charitable Outreach to Neighbors in Need

A volunteer effort of health professionals initiated in Haiti in 1982 by Dr. Jeremiah Lowney and his wife, Virginia, has grown into an outpatient health care facility supported by a nondenominational foundation called the Haitian Health Foundation, Inc. (HHF). In 1985, after working for 4 years in Port au Prince, HHF moved its outreach to Jeremie, Haiti, at the suggestion of Mother Teresa of Calcutta, to bring health care, hope, and opportunity to this especially poor and remote area. The clinic at Jeremie employs 105 people, including two full-time physicians, one full-time dentist, 10 registered nurses, two licensed professional nurses, a medical technician, a dental assistant, and 70 to 80 auxiliary personnel (all Haitians). The clinic provides health care to 350 to 400 Haitians daily.

The Haitian Agents de Sante program currently employs villagers in 936 villages surrounding Jeremie. This program was initiated by a nurse who enlisted an individual who had a seventh-grade education in each village. After being educated in health promotion, the person became the Health Agent of that village. These Health Agents are trained by HHF to provide preventive and basic health care and education. Many villages have also begun mothers' groups, by which women can share experiences and knowledge relating to nutrition, health care, and other topics that have an effect on their quality of life. Breast-feeding classes and immunization programs are available.

Another program was begun by building a food distribution pavilion. This building will be used to store and distribute food to more than 1000 children and pregnant women 3 times a week. The pavilion will also be used to educate participants in nutrition and preventive health care. Much of the education in these programs is accomplished through song, primarily because this approach appears to enable the Haitians to remember what is being taught.

For more than 8 years, another education program has provided access to schools for poor children in a country in which education is neither free nor mandatory. As of 2004, 1250 students were attending school through this program. Tuition, uniforms, books, and shoes are provided by HHF funds or through the Save-a-Family Program.

The HHF relies heavily on the generosity of donors and the many volunteers who donate their time and talents to supplement the staff in Haiti. Volunteers travel to Jeremie at their own expense from America, Canada, and Europe to share their skills and resources with the poor. These volunteers include health care providers, electricians, plumbers, teachers, clergy, and students.

These programs are only a few examples of the health-promotion programs sponsored by the HHF. These efforts show how dedicated professionals can make a difference, even in third world countries in which health care resources are rare.

Courtesy Jeremiah Lowney, MD, MPH.

SUMMARY

This chapter has presented priority issues and future directions for health professions in the areas of health promotion and disease prevention from a world perspective. Current emerging challenges and health care reform efforts pose significant opportunities for health care providers, educators, and researchers. With an enduring emphasis on (1) individuals, families, communities, and the environments in which people live, work, and play and (2) health promotion and disease prevention, health care professionals today are critical links for promoting national and international health. Nurses in the new millennium are required to have sufficient vision, expertise, and to truly make a difference in the health of their clients. Through leadership, creativity, and determination, health care providers can establish a healthier future for all people around the globe.

CASE STUDY

Nutrition: Don

Don is a 4-year-old boy who is brought to a rural health department clinic by his grandmother. Don and his family are recent immigrants from Laos and have lived in this area for less than a year. This is Don's first visit to the clinic. Don looks weak with sunken eyes and dry mouth. His weight is less than 70% (or <3 standard deviations) of the median weight-for-height with underdeveloped buttocks, thighs, and upper arms. Through a translator, Don's grandmother tells the community health nurse that Don has had diarrhea for more than two days and that the family hardly makes ends meet. Don's parents are seasonal farm workers and are at work today. Don's grandmother is his caretaker during the day.

CARE PLAN

Nutrition: Don

Nursing Diagnosis: Altered nutrition—Less than body requirement related to inadequate food intake and diarrhea as evidenced by the weight of less than 70% (or <3 standard deviations) of the median weight-for-height, underdeveloped buttocks, thighs, and upper arms, and sunken eyes and dry mouth

DEFINING CHARACTERISTICS

- A weight of less than 70% (or <3 standard deviations) of the median weight-for-height
- Underdeveloped buttocks, thighs, and upper arms
- Sunken eyes, dry mouth, and a history of diarrhea

RELATED FACTORS

- Poverty, lack of knowledge about available resources

SHORT-TERM EXPECTED OUTCOMES

Grandmother will:
- Increase health-promotion and health-maintenance knowledge regarding Don's nutrition
- Increase health-promotion and health-maintenance practices regarding Don's nutrition

- Gain access to available resources, such as Food Stamps and the Women, Infants and Children Program

NURSING INTERVENTIONS

- Give Don fluids/food per protocol.
- Observe Don's fluids/food intake and monitor his signs and symptoms.
- If necessary, refer Don to an appropriate health setting.
- Assess grandmother's knowledge and practices about Don's nutrition.
- Educate grandmother about negative effects of malnutrition on Don's growth and development.
- Educate grandmother about appropriate food choices for Don.
- Assist family to access and connect with available nutrition community resources.
- Assist Don's parents to access community career center.
- Provide for follow-ups to monitor Don's physical progress (body weight for age and height) and family's access to available resources.

LONG-TERM EXPECTED OUTCOME

- Don will show no sign of malnutrition.

REFERENCES

Arriaga, X. B., & Foshee, V. A. (2004). Adolescent dating violence: Do adolescents follow in their friends', or their parents' footsteps? *Journal of Interpersonal Violence, 19,* 162–184.

Ayikukwei, R. M., Ngare, D., Sidle, J. E., Ayuku, D. O., Baliddawa, J., & Greene, J. Y. (2007). Social and Cultural Significance of the Sexual Cleansing Ritual and its Impact on HIV Prevention Strategies in Western Kenya. *Sexuality & Culture, 11*(3), 23–50.

Blumberg, H. M., Leonard, M. K., Jr., & Jasmer, R. M. (2005). Update on the treatment of tuberculosis and latent tuberculosis infection. *JAMA, 293*(22), 2776–2784.

Bradley, S. F. (2005). Staphylococcus aureus pneumonia: Emergence of MRSA in the community. *Seminars in Respiratory and Critical Care Medicine, 26*(6), 643–649.

Brown, P. D., & Ngeno, C. (2007). Antimicrobial resistance in clinical isolates of *Staphylococcus aureus* from hospital and community sources in southern Jamaica.

International Journal of Infectious Diseases, 11(3), 220–225.

Bucens, I. K., & Maclennan, C. (2006). Survey of childhood malnutrition at Dili National Hospital, East Timor. *Journal of Paediatrics and Child Health, 42*(1-2), 28–32.

Centers for Disease Control and Prevention. (2003a). Methicillin-resistant *Staphylococcus aureus* infections among competitive sports participants—Colorado, Indiana, Pennsylvania, and Los Angeles County, 2000-2003. *MMWR, 52,* 793–795.

Centers for Disease Control and Prevention. (2003b). Methicillin-resistant *Staphylococcus aureus* infections in correctional facilities—Georgia, California, and Texas, 2001-2003. *MMWR, 52,* 992–996.

Centers for Disease Control and Prevention. (2004a). *Fact sheet: Basic information about SARS.* Retrieved from *www.cdc.gov/ncidod/SARS/factsheet.htm.*

Centers for Disease Control and Prevention. (2004b). *Factsheet: Actual causes of death in the United States, 2000.* Retrieved March 11, 2004, from *www.cdc.gov/nccdphd/factsheets/death_causes2000.htm.*

Centers for Disease Control and Prevention. (2005a). *Community-Associated MRSA Information for Clinicians.* Retrieved December 24, 2007, from *www.cdc.gov/ncidod/dhqp/ar_mrsa_ca_clinicians.html#4.*

Centers for Disease Control and Prevention. (2005b). *Severe acute respiration syndrome (SARs).* Retrieved December 24, 2007, from *www.cdc.gov/ncidod/sars/faq.htm.*

Centers for Disease Control and Prevention. (2006a). *Understanding intimate partner violence.* Retrieved December 27, 2007, from *www.cdc.gov/ncipc/dvp/ipv_factsheet.pdf.*

Centers for Disease Control and Prevention. (2006b). *Health effects of cigarette smoking.* Retrieved December 29, 2007, from *www.cdc.gov/tobacco/data_statistics/Factsheets/health_effects.htm.*

Centers for Disease Control and Prevention. (2007a). *Web-based Injury Statistics Query and Reporting System (WISQARS).* Retrieved December 27, 2007, from *www.cdc.gov/ncipc/wisqars/default.htm.*

Centers for Disease Control and Prevention. (2007b). *Violence prevention: The public health approach to violence prevention.* Retrieved December 26, 2007, from *www.cdc.gov/ncipc/dvp/PublicHealthApproachTo_ViolencePrevention.htm.*

Centers for Disease Control and Prevention. (2007c). *Recognition of illness associated with the intentional release of a biologic agent.* Retrieved December 22, 2007, from *www.cdc.gov/mmwr/preview/mmwrhtml/mm5041a2.htm.*

Central Intelligence Agency. (2007). *The world factbook.* Retrieved December 22, 2007, from *www.cia.gov/library/publications/the-world-factbook/rankorder/2102rank.html.*

Chiang-Hanisko, L., Ross, R., Ludwick, R., & Martsolf, D. (2006). International collaborations in nursing research: Priorities, challenges and rewards. *Journal of Research in Nursing, 11*(4), 307–322.

CIA. (2009a). *The world factbook: Lesotho.* Retrieved July 31, 2009, from *www.cia.gov/library/publications/the-world-factbook/geos/lt.html.*

CIA. (2009b). *The world factbook: Swaziland.* Retrieved July 31, 2009, from *www.cia.gov/library/publications/the-world-factbook/geos/wz.html.*

Cooper, C. (2007). *Governor Rell Directs Health Department to Hold Symposiums on MRSA in Schools and Other Community Settings.* Retrieved December 21, 2007 from *www.ochd.org/MRSA/MRSA%20school%20fact%20sheet_OCHD.pdf.*

DeAngelis, C. D., & Flanagin, A. (2005). Tuberculosis. *JAMA, 293*(22), 2693.

Di Perri, G., & Bonora, S. (2004). Which agents should we use for the treatment of multidrug-resistant Mycobacterium tuberculosis? *Journal of Antimicrobial Chemotherapy, 54*(3), 593–602.

Drobniewski, F., Balabanova, Y., Nikolayevsky, V., Ruddy, M., Kuznetzov, S., Zakharova, S., et al. (2005). Drug-resistant tuberculosis, clinical virulence, and the dominance of the Beijing strain family in Russia. *JAMA, 293,* 2726–2731.

Dye, C., Watt, C. J., Bleed, D. M., Hosseini, S. M., & Raviglione, M. C. (2005). Evolution of tuberculosis control and prospects for reducing tuberculosis incidence, prevalence, and deaths globally. *JAMA, 293,* 2767–2775.

Fekete, T. (2007a). Emerging infections: What you need to know, Part 1. *Consultant, 47*(12), 1013–1016.

Fekete, T. (2007b). Emerging infections: What you need to know, Part 2. *Consultant, 47*(13), 1149–1156.

Fleming, S. W., Brown, L., & Tice, S. E. (2006). Community-acquired methicillin-resistant *Staphylococcus aureus* skin infections: Report of a local outbreak and implications for emergency department care. *Journal of the American Academy of Nurse Practitioner, 18,* 297–300.

Fridkin, S. K., Hageman, J. C., Morrison, M., Sanza, L. T., Como-Sabetti, K., Jernigan, J. A., et al. (2005). Methicillin-resistant *Staphylococcus aureus* disease in three communities. *New England Journal of Medicine, 352,* 1436–1444.

Garcia-Moreno, C., Jansen, H., Ellsberg, M., Heise, L., & Watts, C. H. (2006). Prevalence of intimate partner violence: Findings from the WHO multi-country study on women's health and domestic violence. *Lancet, 368,* 1260–1269.

Gausset, Q. (2001). AIDS and cultural practices in Africa: The case of the Tonga (Zambia). *Social Science and Medicine, 52,* 509–518.

Giacaman, R., Shannon, H. S., Saab, H., Arya, N., & Boyce, W. (2007). Individual and collective exposure to political violence: Palestinian adolescents coping with conflict. *European Journal of Public Health, 17,* 361–368.

Gray, V. B., Cossman, J. S., & Powers, E. L. (2006). Stunted growth is associated with physical indicators of malnutrition but not food insecurity among rural school children in Honduras. *Nutrition Research, 26,* 549–555.

Groom, A. V., Wolsey, D. H., Naimi, T. S., Smith, K., Johnson, S., Boxrud, D., et al. (2001). Community-acquired methicillin-resistant *Staphylococcus aureus* in a rural American Indian community. *JAMA, 286,* 1201–1205.

Hageman, J. C., Uyeki, T. M., Francis, J. S., et al. (2006). Severe community-acquired pneumonia due to *Staphylococcus aureus,* 2003-04 influenza season. *Emerging Infectious Diseases Journal, 12,* 894–899.

Hornor, G. (2005). Domestic violence and children: Effects of domestic violence on children. *Journal of Pediatric Health Care, 19*(4), 206–212.

Huttlinger, K. (2004). Perspectives on international health. In M. Stanhope, & J. Lancaster (Eds.), *Community and public health nursing* (5th ed.). St. Louis: Mosby.

Indiana State Department of Health. (2007). *Information and talking points for MRSA.* Retrieved February 26, 2007, from *www.lakeland.k12.in.us/documents/MRSA_Talking_Points.pdf.*

Ji, J., Kleinman, A., & Becker, A. E. (2001). Suicide in contemporary China: A review of China's distinctive suicide demographics in their sociocultural context. *Harvard Review of Psychiatry, 9,* 1–12.

Jin, X., Eagle, M., & Yoshioka, M. (2007). Early exposure to violence in the family of origin and positive attitudes towards marital violence: Chinese immigrant male batterers vs. controls. *Journal of Family Violence, 22,* 211–222.

Joint United Nations Programme on HIV/AIDS. (2008). *2008 report on the global AIDS epidemic.* Geneva: Author.

Kang, Y. A., Choi, Y-J., Cho, Y-J., Lee, S. M., Yoo, C-G., KIM, Y. W., et al. (2006). Cost of treatment for multidrug-resistant tuberculosis in South Korea. *Respirology, 11*(6), 793–798.

Kang, Y. A., Lee, H. W., Yoon, H. I., Cho, B., Han, S. K., Shim, Y-S., et al. (2005). Discrepancy between the tuberculin skin test and the whole-blood interferon gamma assay for the diagnosis of latent tuberculosis infection in an intermediate tuberculosis-burden country. *JAMA, 293,* 2756–2761.

Kazakova, S. V., Hageman, J. C., Matava, M., Srinivasan, A., Phelan, L., Garfinkel, B., et al. (2005). A clone of methicillin-resistant *Staphylococcus aureus* among professional football players. *New England Journal of Medicine, 352,* 468–475.

Krishnan, S. (2005). Do structural inequalities contribute to marital violence? Ethnographic evidence from rural South India. *Violence against Women, 11,* 759–775.

Lambert, V. A., Lambert, C. E., Daly, J., Davidson, P. M., Kunaviktikul, W., & Shin, K. R. (2004). Nursing education on women's health care in Australia, Japan, South Korea, and Thailand. *Journal of Transcultural Nursing, 15,* 44–53.

Lingappa, J. R., McDonald, L. C., Simone, P., & Parashar, U. D. (2004). Wrestling SARS from uncertainty. *Emerging Infectious Disease, 10*(2), 167–170.

Long, T., Coleman, D., Dietsch, P., McGrath, P., Brady, D., Thomas, D. et al. (2006). Methicillin-Resistant *Staphylococcus aureus* Skin Infections among Tattoo Recipients— Ohio, Kentucky, and Vermont, 2004-2005. *JAMA, 296,* 385–386.

Lutenbacher, M., Cohen, A., & Conner, N. M. (2004). Breaking the cycle of family violence: Understanding the perceptions of battered women. *Journal of Pediatric Health Care, 18*(5), 236–243.

Malungo, J. R. S. (2001). Sexual cleansing (Kusalazya) and levirate marriage (Kunjilila mung'anda) in the era of AIDS: Changes in perceptions and practices in Zambia. *Social Science & Medicine, 53*(3), 371–382.

McCullagh, M. C. (2004). Health promotion. In S. J. Peterson, & T. S. Bredow (Eds.). *Middle range theories: Application to nursing research* (pp. 290–301). Philadelphia: Lippincott Williams & Wilkins.

Ministry of Public Health. (2005). *Thailand health profile 2001–2004.* Bangkok, Thailand: Printing Press, Express Transportation Organization.

New York Department of Health. (2007). *State Health and Education Departments Issue Guidance to Schools on MRSA.* Retrieved on December 17, 2007 from *www.health.state.ny.us/press/releases/2007/2007-10-25_mrsa_school_guidance.htm.*

Oner, S., Yenilmez, C., Ayranci, U., Gunay, Y., & Ozdamar, K. (2007). Sexual differences in the completed suicides in Turkey. *European Psychiatry, 22*(4), 223–228.

Ormerod, L. P. (2005). Multidrug-resistant tuberculosis (MDR-TB): Epidemiology, prevention and treatment. *British Medical Bulletin, 73,* 17–24.

Patel, M. & Cobbs, C. G. (2004). Infections from body piercing and tattoos. In O. Schlossberg (Ed.). *Infections of Leisures.* Washington DC: ASM Press.

Peedicayil, A., Sadowski, L. S., Jeyaseelan, L., Shankar, V., Jain, D., Suresh, S. et al. (2004). Spousal physical violence against women during pregnancy. *BJOG, 111,* 682–687.

Ross, R., Sawatphanit, W., Draucker, C., & Suwansujarid, T. (2007). The lived experiences of HIV-positive, pregnant women in Thailand. *Health Care for Women International, 28*(8), 731–744.

Ross, R., Sawatphanit, W., & Suwansujarid, T. (2007). Finding peace (*Kwam Sa-ngob Jai*): A Buddhist way to live with HIV. *Journal of Holistic Nursing, 25*(4), 228–235.

Ross, R., Sawatphanit, W., Suwansujarid, T., & Draucker, C. B. (2007). Life story and depression of an HIV-positive, pregnant Thai woman who was a former sex worker: Case study. *Archives of Psychiatric Nursing, 21*(6), 32–39.

Sawatphanit, W., Ross, R., & Suwansujarid, T. (2004). Development of self-esteem among HIV-positive pregnant Thai women: Action research. *Journal of Science, Technologies, and Humanities, 2*(2), 55–69.

Seckinelgin, H. (2003). *HIV/AIDS, global civil society and people's politics: An update.* London: Oxford University Press.

Siegel, J. D., Rhinehart, E., Jackson, M., & Chairello, L. (2006). *Management of multidrug-resistant organisms in health care settings.* Retrieved December 31, 2007, from *www.cdc.gov/NCIDOD/DHQP/pdf/ar/mdroGuideline2006.pdf.*

Simon, G. E., Hunkeler, E., Fireman, B., Lee, J. Y., & Savarino, J. (2007). Risk of suicide attempt and suicide death in patients treated for bipolar disorder. *Bipolar Disorders, 9*(5), 526–530.

Slovak, K., Carlson, K., & Helm, L. (2007). The influence of family violence on youth attitudes. *Child and Adolescent Social Work Journal, 24,* 77–99.

Stratton, R. J. (2007). Malnutrition: Another health inequality? *Proceedings of the Nutrition Society, 66,* 522–529.

Thacker, P. D. (2003). Set a microbe to kill a microbe: Drug resistance renews interest in phage therapy. *JAMA, 290*(24), 3183–3185.

The Non Smokers' Movement of Australia. (2006). *Fact Sheet: Statistics on smoking.* Retrieved on December 29, 2007 from *www.nsma.org.au/facts/figures.htm.*

The Official Navajo Nation Visitor Guide. (2002). *Navajo cultural history and legends.* Retrieved June 4, 2008, from *http://ashtloguild.org/natani/navajovalues.htm.*

United Nations. (2008). *United Nations stands ready to support quake reconstruction over long-term.* Retrieved from June 5, 2008, from *www.reliefweb.int/rw/RWB.NSF/db900SID/EGUA-7F4P4B?OpenDocument.*

Weingartl, H. M., Copps, J., Drebot, M. A., Marszal, P., Smith, G., Gren, J. et al. (2004). Susceptibility of pigs and chickens to SARS coronavirus. *Emerging Infectious Diseases, 10,* 179–184.

Williams, B. G., & Dye, C. (2003). Antiretroviral drugs for tuberculosis control in the era of HIV/AIDS. *Science, 12,* 1535.

World Health Organization. (2000). *Turning the tide of malnutrition: Responding to the challenge of the 21st century.* Geneva: WHO, 2000 (WHO/NHD/00.7).

World Health Organization. (2003). *The World Health report 2002: Reducing risks, promoting healthy life.* Geneva: Author.

World Health Organization. (2004a). *Serious childhood problems in countries with limited resources: Background book on management of the child with a serious infection or severe malnutrition.* Geneva: Author.

World Health Organization. (2004b). *WHO SARS international reference and verification laboratory network: Policy and procedures in the inter-epidemic period.* Retrieved April 13, 2005, from *www.who.int/csr/resources/publications/en/SARSReferenceLab.pdf.*

World Health Organization. (2004c). *Smoking statistics: Factsheet.* Retrieved March 11, 2004, from *www.cdc.gov/tobacco/research_data/adults_prev/mmwr5253_highlights.htm.*

World Health Organization. (2006). *WHO publications and documents, and documentation to which WHO has contributed.* Retrieved June 5, 2008, from *www.who.int/hac/crises/international/middle_east/Nutrition_guidinglist%20_2_.pdf.*

World Health Organization. (2007a). *Cumulative Number of Confirmed Human Cases of Avian Influenza A/(H5N1) Reported to WHO.* Retrieved December 17, 2007, from *www.who.int/csr/disease/avian_influenza/country/cases_table_2007_12_14/en/index.html.*

World Health Organization. (2007b). *Global fund grant support and guidance.* Retrieved December 23, 2007, from *www.who.int/tb/dots/planningframeworks/gf_proposals/en/index.html.*

World Health Organization. (2007c). *Stop TB Working Group on DOTS-Plus for MDR-TB Strategic Plan 2006-2015.* Retrieved December 23, 2007, from *www.stoptb.org/wg/dots_plus/assets/documents/Stop%20TB%20Working%20Group%20on%20DOTS%20Final.pdf.*

World Health Organization. (2007d). *World report on violence and health.* Retrieved December 23, 2007, from *www.who.int/violence_injury_prevention/violence/world_report/en/abstract_en.pdf.*

World Health Organization. (2007e). *Child injuries and violence.* Retrieved December 24, 2007, from *www.who.int/violence_injury_prevention/child/en/.*

World Health Organization. (2007f). *Third Milestones of a Global Campaign for Violence Prevention Report 2007.* Retrieved December 27, 2007, from *www.who.int/violence_injury_prevention/publications/violence/milestones_2007/en/index.html.*

World Health Organization. (2007g). *What are the International Health Regulations?* Retrieved December 27, 2007, from *www.who.int/features/qa/39/en/index.html.*

World Health Organization. (2008). *Challenges.* Retrieved March 10, 2008, from *www.who.int/nutrition/en/print.html.*

Zeller, J. L., Burke, A. E., & Glass, R. M. (2007). MRSA infections. *JAMA, 298,* 1826.

Ziherl, S., & Zalar, B. (2006). Risk of suicide after attempted suicide in the population of Slovenia from 1970 to 1996. *European Psychiatry, 21*(6), 396–400.

Zinderman, C. E., Conner, B., Malakooti, M. A., LaMar, J. E., Armstrong, A., Bohnker, B. K. (2004). Community-acquired methicillin-resistant *Staphylococcus aureus* among military recruits. *Emerging Infectious Diseases Journal, 10,* 941–944.

Index